Fourth Edition

Schaechter's Mechanisms of Microbial Disease

15/8/08

Fourth Edition

Schaechter's Mechanisms of Microbial Disease

N. CARY ENGLEBERG

Division of Infectious Diseases
Departments of Internal Medicine and
Microbiology and Immunology
University of Michigan Medical School
Ann Arbor, Michigan

VICTOR DiRITA

Unit for Laboratory Animal Medicine and
Department of Microbiology and Immunology
University of Michigan Medical School
Ann Arbor, Michigan

TERENCE S. DERMODY

Elizabeth B. Lamb Center for Pediatric Research
Departments of Pediatrics and Microbiology and Immunology
Vanderbilt University School of Medicine
Nashville, Tennessee

Lippincott Williams & Wilkins
a Wolters Kluwer business
Philadelphia · Baltimore · New York · London
Buenos Aires · Hong Kong · Sydney · Tokyo

Acquisitions editor: *Betty Sun*
Developmental editor: *Kathleen H. Scogna*
Marketing manager: *Jennifer Kuklinski*
Production editor: *Jennifer P. Ajello*
Art Director: *Doug Smock*
Compositor: *Maryland Composition, Inc.*
Printer: *RR Donnelley & Sons-Willard*

351 West Camden Street
Baltimore, MD 21201

530 Walnut Street
Philadelphia, PA 19106

Third Edition, 1999

Library of Congress Cataloging-in-Publication Data

Schaechter's mechanisms of microbial disease / [edited by] Cary Engleberg, Victor DiRita,
Terence Dermody. — 4th ed.
   p. ; cm.
   Rev. ed. of: Mechanisms of microbial disease / edited by Moselio Schaechter. 3rd ed. c 1998.
   Includes bibliographical references and index.
   ISBN-13: 978-0-7817-5342-5
   1. Medical microbiology. 2. Communicable diseases—Pathogenesis. I. Schaecter, Moselio. II.
Engleberg, Cary. III. DiRita, Victor J. IV. Dermody, Terence. V. Mechanisms of microbial
disease. VI. Title: Mechanisms of microbial disease.
   [DNLM: 1. Communicable Diseases—microbiology. 2. Bacteria—pathogenicity. 3.
Communicable Diseases—physiopathology. 4. Fungi—pathogenicity. 5. Viruses—pathogenicity.
QW 700 S293 2007]
QR46.M463 2007
616.9′041--dc22

          2005034409

To purchase additional copies of this book, call our customer service department at **(800) 638-3030** or fax orders to **(301) 223-2320**. International customers should call **(301) 223-2300**.

Visit Lippincott Williams & Wilkins on the Internet: http://www.LWW.com. Lippincott
Williams & Wilkins customer service representatives are available from 8:30 am to 6:00 pm, EST.

06 07 08 09 10
1 2 3 4 5 6 7 8 9 10

Preface

The previous editions of this book were designed by its original editor-in-chief, Moselio Schaechter, to present major concepts in microbiology and infectious diseases in a pathobiological framework and within the context of clinical cases. This format lends itself to an active form of studying and is easily adaptable to problem-based learning. It is particularly appropriate for use in revised medical curricula that feature a synthesis of basic microbiology and clinical infectious diseases, or those that follow an "organ system" approach to the basic sciences.

KEY FEATURES AND APPROACH

The use of the text in these variously structured courses is facilitated by the presentation of the material in three distinct sections. Part I presents basic concepts of microbiology as well as immunology and pharmacology as these disciplines relate to infections. Part II describes the major infectious agents and the diseases they cause, and Part III illustrates how the major systems of the body are affected by infection.

This textbook is intended to be used in courses on medical microbiology or infectious diseases for medical students, allied health professionals, graduate students, or advanced undergraduates. Because the purpose of this book is to develop a conceptual framework for understanding infection, it highlights certain agents and diseases of special biological or clinical importance and does not attempt to describe the microbial world in an exhaustive fashion.

One of the most distinctive features of the previous edition has been retained: in many of the chapters on individual infectious agents, the reader will find boxed sections labeled "Paradigm." Those sections present discussions of certain general principles that are best illustrated by the agents described in that chapter but also can be applied to other organisms.

NEW TO THIS EDITION

This new edition retains the basic conceptual framework of past editions credited to Dr. Schaechter in its new title, but it has been revised to reflect many of the recent changes that have taken place in the field as well as new features to facilitate learning. Several new chapters have been added or revised by new authors. The updated text is as current as possible, realizing that new information in the field is accumulating at such dazzling speed that it risks becoming outdated before the ink dries. Because this edition is printed in full color, virtually all the illustrations are either new or recolored.

For the first time the book is accompanied by electronic material, including additional color images, answers to the questions posed in the printed text, and more than 300 multiple-choice test items composed in the format of the U.S. Medical Licensing Examination with explanations of the correct answers. Although the printed text contains all the important core information, the electronic supplement allows for further enrichment and consolidation of the material for students who choose to access it.

Cary Engleberg

Victor DiRita

Terence S. Dermody

Acknowledgments

Many colleagues and friends have helped us in the past in preparing this book. Their names appear in the previous editions. For this revision we received invaluable advice from Moselio Schaechter, the originator of the text and editor of the first three editions. We were also helped by Jim Chappell, David Friedman, and Powel Kazanjian. Our heartfelt thanks go to them for their kind and thoughtful suggestions. We are particularly grateful to our senior developmental editor, Kathleen Scogna, who provided thoughtful direction on format and style as well as the patience and discipline to bring the various elements of the project together in a coherent manner. We thank Betty Sun, acquisitions editor, for helping to formulate the framework of the fourth edition and for her support through the course of the project. We thank Jennifer Ajello, who was instrumental in bringing the book to completion in the most efficient possible manner. We offer special thanks to Matthew Chansky for creating a style for the color artwork that is both coherent and visually pleasing. We are grateful to Dru Lundeng for expert editorial assistance, to Carolyn Campbell and Carrie Lapham for secretarial support, and to Suzy and Alexander Engleberg for management of the text and image files. Finally, our appreciation and love go to Margot, Michael, David, Kathleen, Victor, Amalia, Suzy, Roderick, and Alexander for their support and indulgence through the arduous task of making this book a reality.

Contributors

David Acheson, MD
Director of Food Safety and Security
Center for Food Safety and Applied Nutrition
U. S. Food and Drug Administration
College Park, MD
Chapter 60 (with James Nataro): Digestive System
Infections

C. Alan Anderson, MD
Assistant Professor
Department of Neurology
University of Colorado Health Sciences Center and
School of Medicine
Denver, CO
Chapter 56 (with Kenneth L. Tyler): Prion Diseases

Elliot J. Androphy, MD
Professor
Department of Medicine
University of Massachusetts Medical School
Worcester, MA
Chapter 40: Human Papillomaviruses and Warts

Robert L. Atmar, MD
Associate Professor
Departments of Medicine and Molecular Virology and
Microbiology
Baylor College of Medicine
Houston, TX
Chapter 37 (with Mary K. Estes): Rotaviruses,
Noroviruses, and Other Viral Agents of Gastroenteritis

Joseph T. Barbieri, PhD
Professor
Departments of Microbiology and Molecular Genetics
Medical College of Wisconsin
Milwaukee, WI
Chapter 9: Damage by Microbial Toxins

Joel B. Baseman, PhD
Professor and Chair
Department of Microbiology and Immunology
University of Texas Health Science Center
San Antonio, TX
Chapter 29 (with Joseph G. Tully): *Mycoplasma*:
Curiosity and Pathogen

Jeffrey M. Bergelson, MD
Associate Professor
Departments of Pediatrics and Microbiology
University of Pennsylvania School of Medicine
Philadelphia, PA
Chapter 31 (with Terence S. Dermody): Biology of
Viruses

Suzanne F. Bradley, MD
Associate Professor
Department of Internal Medicine
Divisions of Infectious Diseases and Geriatrics
University of Michigan Medical School
Ann Arbor, MI
Chapter 66: Sepsis
Chapter 74: Fever: A Clinical Sign of Infection

William J. Britt, MD
Professor
Department of Pediatrics
Division of Pediatric Infectious Diseases
University of Alabama
Birmingham, AL
Chapter 42: Betaherpesviruses and
Gammaherpesviruses: Cytomegalovirus and
Epstein-Barr Virus

Sandro K. Cinti, MD
Assistant Professor
Division of Infectious Diseases
University of Michigan Medical School
Ann Arbor, MI
Chapter 57 (with Philip C. Hanna): Biological Agents
of Warfare and Terrorism

Jenifer Coburn, PhD
Assistant Professor
Departments of Geographic Medicine and Infectious
Diseases
Tufts University School of Medicine
Boston, MA
Chapter 25 (with John Leong): *Borrelia burgdorferi*
and Lyme Disease

Laurie Comstock, PhD
Assistant Professor
Channing Laboratory
Harvard Medical School
Boston, MA
Chapter 15: *Bacteroides* and Abscesses

Peggy A. Cotter, PhD
Assistant Professor
Department of Molecular, Cellular, and Developmental Biology
University of Santa Barbara
Santa Barbara, CA
Chapter 4: Genetic Approaches to Studying Bacterial Pathogenesis

James E. Crowe, Jr., MD
Professor
Department of Pediatrics
Vanderbilt University School of Medicine
Nashville, TN
Chapter 34: Paramyxoviruses: Measles, Mumps, and Respiratory Syncytial Virus

Richard T. D'Aquila, MD
Professor
Departments of Medicine and Microbiology and Immunology
Vanderbilt University School of Medicine
Nashville, TN
Chapter 44: Antiviral Treatment Strategies

Roberta L. DeBiasi, MD
Associate Professor
Departments of Pediatrics and Neurology
University of Colorado Health Sciences Center
Denver, CO
Chapter 61 (with Kenneth L. Tyler): Infections of the Central Nervous System

Mark Denison, MD
Professor
Department of Pediatrics
Vanderbilt University School of Medicine
Nashville, TN
Chapter 32 (with Vincent Racaniello): Picornaviruses and Coronaviruses

Peter Dull, MD
National Center for Infectious Diseases
Division of Bacterial and Mycotic Disease
Meningitis and Special Pathogens Branch
Centers for Disease Control and Prevention
Atlanta, GA
Chapter 14 (with David Stephens): Neisseriae: Gonococcus and Meningococcus

Roman Dziarski, PhD
Professor
Department of Microbiology and Immunology
Northwest Center for Medical Education
Indiana University School of Medicine
Gary, IN
Chapter 6: Innate Immunity

John R. Ebright, MD
Associate Professor
Department of Internal Medicine
Wayne State University School of Medicine
Detroit, MI
Chapter 24 (with Jack Sobel, MD): Syphilis: A Disease with a History
Chapter 69 (with Jack Sobel, MD): Sexually Transmitted Diseases

Kathryn M. Edwards, MD
Professor
Department of Pediatrics
Vanderbilt University School of Medicine
Nashville, TN
Chapter 45 (with Natasha B. Halasa): Vaccines and Antisera for the Prevention and Treatment of Infectious Diseases

Barry I. Eisenstein, MD
Executive Vice President
Research and Development
Cubist Pharmaceuticals
Lexington, MA
Chapter 2 (with Moselio Schaechter): Normal Microbial Flora

Mary K. Estes, PhD
Professor
Departments of Medicine, Molecular Virology and Microbiology and Medicine
Baylor College of Medicine
Houston, TX
Chapter 37 (with Robert L. Atmar): Rotaviruses, Noroviruses, and Other Viral Agents of Gastroenteritis

George Fogg, MD, PhD
Lecturer
Department of Pediatrics and Communicable Diseases
Division of Infectious Diseases
University of Michigan School of Medicine
Ann Arbor, MI
Chapter 12: Streptococci and Enterococci: Sore Throats and Beyond

Donald E. Ganem, MD
Professor
Department of Microbiology and Immunology
University of California, San Francisco
San Francisco, CA
Chapter 43: Viral Hepatitis

Joanna B. Goldberg, PhD
Professor
Department of Microbiology
University of Virginia
Charlottesville, VA
Chapter 18: *Pseudomonas aeruginosa*: A Ubiquitous
Pathogen

Diane E. Griffin, MD, PhD
Professor and Chair
W. Harry Feinstone Department of Molecular Biology
and Immunology
Johns Hopkins Bloomberg School of Public Health
Baltimore, MD
Chapter 33: Arthropodborne Viruses

Richard K. Groger, MD, PhD
Instructor of Medicine
Department of Medicine, Division of Infectious
Diseases
Washington University School of Medicine
St. Louis, MO
Chapter 71 (with William G. Powderly): Acquired
Immunodeficiency Syndrome

David Haas, MD
Associate Professor
Departments of Medicine and Microbiology and
Immunology
Vanderbilt University Medical School
Nashville, TN
Chapter 23: Mycobacteria: Tuberculosis and Leprosy

Natasha B. Halasa, MD
Assistant Professor
Department of Pediatrics
Vanderbilt University School of Medicine
Nashville, TN
Chapter 45 (with Kathryn M. Edwards): Vaccines and
Antisera for the Prevention and Treatment of
Infectious Diseases

MeiLan King Han, MD
Assistant Professor
University of Michigan Health Center
Division of Pulmonary and Critical Care
Ann Arbor, MI
Chapter 62 (with Fernando Martinez): Respiratory
System Infections

Philip C. Hanna, PhD
Associate Professor
Department of Microbiology and Immunology
University of Michigan Medical School
Ann Arbor, MI
Chapter 57 (with Sandro K. Cinti): Biological Agents of
Warfare and Terrorism

Adolf W. Karchmer, MD
Professor
Harvard Medical School
Chief
Division of Infectious Diseases
Beth Israel Deaconess Medical Center
Boston, MA
Chapter 67: Intravascular Infection

Carol A. Kauffman, MD
Professor
Department of Internal Medicine
University of Michigan Medical School
Chief, Infectious Diseases
Department of Internal Medicine
Veterans Affairs Ann Arbor Health Care System
Ann Arbor, MI
Chapter 46: Introduction to the Fungi and Mycoses
Chapter 47: Endemic Mycoses
Chapter 48: Systemic Mycoses Caused by
Opportunistic Fungi
Chapter 49: Subcutaneous, Cutaneous, and
Superficial Mycoses
Chapter 50: Antifungal Agents

Gary Ketner, PhD
Professor
Department of Molecular Microbiology and
Immunology
Johns Hopkins Bloomberg School of Public Health
Baltimore, MD
Chapter 39: Adenoviruses

John Leong, MD, PhD
Associate Professor
Departments of Molecular Genetics and Microbiology
University of Massachusetts Medical School
Worcester, MA
Chapter 25 (with Jenifer Coburn): *Borrelia burgdorferi*
and Lyme Disease

Preeti N. Malani, MD
Assistant Professor
Department of Internal Medicine
Divisions of Geriatrics and Infectious Diseases
University of Michigan Medical School
Ann Arbor, MI
Chapter 68 (with Mark A. Zacharek): Head and
Neck Infections

Fernando Martinez, MD
Professor
Division of Pulmonary and Critical Care
Department of Internal Medicine
University of Michigan Medical School
Ann Arbor, MI
Chapter 62 (with MeiLan King Han): Respiratory
System Infections

Stephen Melville, PhD
Associate Professor
Department of Biology
Virginia Polytechnic Institute and State University
Blacksburg, VA
Chapter 20: Clostridia: Diarrheal Disease, Tissue
Infection, Food Poisoning, Botulism, and Tetanus

Roger Melvold, PhD
Professor and Chair
Department of Microbiology and Immunology
University of North Dakota School of Medicine and
Health Sciences
Grand Forks, ND
Chapter 7 (with Carl Waltenbaugh): Adaptive
Immunity

Joseph J. Nania, MD
Assistant Professor
Department of Pediatrics
Vanderbilt University School of Medicine
Nashville, TN
Chapter 65 (with Jeffrey Parsonnet): Infections of the
Bones, Joints, and Muscles

James Nataro, MD
Professor
Department of Pediatrics
Chief
Section of Molecular Diagnostics
Center for Vaccine Development
Division of Infectious Diseases and Tropical
Pediatrics
University of Maryland Medical School
Baltimore, MD
Chapter 60 (with David Acheson): Digestive System
Infections

Lindsay E. Nicolle, MD, FRCPC
Professor
Departments of Internal Medicine, Medical
Microbiology
University of Manitoba
Winnipeg, Manitoba, Canada
Chapter 63: Urinary Tract Infections

E. Turner Overton, MD
Instructor
Division of Infectious Disease
Department of Internal Medicine
Washington University School of Medicine
St. Louis, MO
Chapter 70 (with William G. Powderly): Infections of
the Immunocompromised Patient

Peter Palese, PhD
Professor and Chair
Department of Microbiology
Mount Sinai School of Medicine
New York, NY
Chapter 36: Influenza and Its Viruses

Timothy G. Palzkill, PhD
Associate Professor
Department of Molecular Virology and Microbiology
Baylor College of Medicine
Houston, TX
Chapter 5 (with Cary Engleberg): Biological Basis for
Antibacterial Action

Jeffrey Parsonnet, MD
Associate Professor
Department of Microbiology and Immunology
Director, Infectious Diseases Training Program
Dartmouth-Hitchcock Medical Center
Lebanon, NH
Chapter 65 (with Joseph J. Nania): Infections of the
Bones, Joints, and Muscles

Richard M. Peek Jr, MD
Associate Professor
Department of Medicine and Cancer Biology
Vanderbilt University School of Medicine
Nashville, TN
Chapter 22: *Helicobacter pylori*: Pathogenesis of a
"Slow" Bacterial Infection

Marnie L. Peterson, PhD, PharmD
Assistant Professor
Experimental and Clinical Pharmacology
University of Minnesota
Minneapolis, MN
Chapter 11 (with Patrick M. Schlievert): Staphylococci:
Abscesses and Toxin-Mediated Diseases

William G. Powderly, MD
Professor
Department of Infectious Diseases
Washington University School of Medicine
St. Louis, MO
Chapter 70 (with E. Turner Overton): Infections of the
Immunocompromised Patient
Chapter 71 (with Richard K. Groger): Acquired
Immunodeficiency Syndrome

Charles G. Prober, MD
Professor
Departments of Pediatrics and Microbiology and
Immunology
Stanford University School of Medicine
Stanford, CA
Chapter 72: Congenital and Perinatal Infections

Vincent Racaniello, PhD
Higgins Professor
Department of Microbiology
Columbia University College of Physicians and
Surgeons
New York, NY
Chapter 32 (with Mark Denison): Picornaviruses and
Coronaviruses

Jane E. Raulston, PhD
Associate Professor
Departments of Pathology and Microbiology
James H. Quillen College of Medicine
Johnson City, TN
Chapter 27 (with Priscilla B. Wyrick): Chlamydiae:
Genital, Ocular, and Respiratory Pathogens

Charles E. Rupprecht, VMD, PhD
National Center for Infectious Diseases
Division of Viral and Rickettsial Diseases
Viral and Rickettsial Zoonoses Branch, Rabies Section
Centers for Disease Control and Prevention
Atlanta, GA
Chapter 35: Rabies

Moselio Schaechter, PhD
Professor Emeritus
Department of Molecular Biology and Microbiology
Tufts University School of Medicine
Boston, MA
Chapter 2 (with Barry I. Eisenstein): Normal
Microbial Flora
Chapter 3: Biology of Infectious Agents

Patrick M. Schlievert, PhD
Professor
Department of Microbiology
University of Minnesota
Minneapolis, MN
Chapter 11 (with Marnie L. Peterson): Staphylococci:
Abscesses and Toxin-Mediated Diseases

Robert T. Schooley, MD
Professor and Head of the Division of Infectious
Diseases
University of California, San Diego
San Diego, CA
Chapter 38: Human Retroviruses: AIDS and Other
Diseases

Daniel S. Shapiro, MD
Department of Laboratory Medicine
Lahey Clinic
Burlington, MA
Chapter 73: Zoonoses

David R. Snydman, MD
Professor
Department of Medicine
Tufts University School of Medicine
Boston, MA
Chapter 59: Principles of Epidemiology
Chapter 75: Health Care–Associated Infections
Chapter 76: Foodborne Diseases

Jack D. Sobel, MD
Professor
Department of Internal Medicine
Wayne State University School of Medicine
Chief
Detroit Medical Center
Division of Infectious Diseases
Detroit, MI
Chapter 24 (with John Richard Ebright): *Treponema
pallidum* and Syphilis: A Disease with a History
Chapter 69 (with John Richard Ebright): Sexually
Transmitted Diseases

Patricia G. Spear, PhD
Professor
Department of Microbiology and Immunology
Northwestern University
Chicago, IL
Chapter 41: Alphaherpesviruses: Herpes Simplex Virus
and Varicella-Zoster Virus

David Stephens, MD
Professor and Executive Vice Chair
Department of Infectious Diseases
Emory University School of Medicine
Atlanta, GA
Chapter 14 (with Peter Dull): Neisseriae: Gonococcus
and Meningococcus

Dennis L. Stevens, MD, PhD
Professor
Department of Medicine
University of Washington School of Medicine
Seattle, WA
Chief, Infectious Disease Section
Veterans Affairs Medical Center
Boise, ID
Chapter 64: Infections of the Skin and Soft Tissue

Michele Swanson, MD
Associate Professor
Department of Microbiology and Immunology
University of Michigan Medical School
Ann Arbor, MI
Chapter 21 (with Cary Engleberg): *Legionella*: Parasite
of Amebas and Macrophages

Joseph G. Tully, PhD
Department of Microbiology
Division of Special Operations
Walter Reed Army Institute of Research
Washington, DC
Chapter 29 (with Joel B. Baseman): *Mycoplasma*:
Curiosity and Pathogen

Kenneth L. Tyler, MD
Revler-Lewin Family Professor of Neurology
University of Colorado Health Sciences Center
Chief
Neurology Service
Denver Veterans Affairs Medical Center
Denver, CO
Chapter 56 (with C. Alan Anderson): Prion Diseases
Chapter 61 (with Roberta L. DeBiasi): Infections of the
Central Nervous System

David H. Walker, MD
Professor and Chair
Department of Pathology
University of Texas Medical Branch
Chair
Department of Pathology
John Sealy Hospital
Galveston, TX
Chapter 26: Cat Scratch Disease, Bacillary
Angiomatosis, and Other Bartonelloses
Chapter 28: Rocky Mountain Spotted Fever and Other
Rickettsioses

Carl Waltenbaugh, PhD
Professor
Department of Microbiology and Immunology
Feinberg School of Medicine
Northwestern University
Chicago, IL
Chapter 7 (with Roger Melvold): Adaptive Immunity

Jeffrey Weiser, MD
Associate Professor
Departments of Microbiology and Pediatrics
University of Pennsylvania School of Medicine
Philadelphia, PA
Chapter 13: Pneumococcus and Bacterial Pneumonia

Priscilla B. Wyrick, PhD
Professor and Chair
Department of Microbiology
James H. Quillen College of Medicine
Johnson City, TN
Chapter 27 (with Jane E. Raulston): Chlamydiae:
Genital, Ocular, and Respiratory Pathogens

Mark A. Zacharek, MD
Senior Staff Otolaryngologist
Henry Ford Health System
Detroit, MI
Chapter 68 (with Preeti N. Malani): Head and Neck
Infections

PAST CONTRIBUTORS

We acknowledge several individuals who contributed to previous editions of this book and whose work formed a basis for many of the updated chapters in this edition:

David W.K. Acheson

George M. Baer

Neil Barg

Michael Barza

John M. Coffin

Roger G. Faix

Bernard N. Fields

Janet Gilsdorf

Sherwood L. Gorbach

Penelope J. Hitchcock

George S. Kobayashi

Donald Krogstad

Gerald T. Keusch

David W. Lazinski

Zell A. McGee

Gerald Medoff

Cody Meissner

Edward N. Robinson, Jr.

David Schlessinger

Arnold L. Smith

John Spitznagel

Gregory A. Storch

Stephen E. Straus

Francis P. Tally

Debbie S. Toder

Ellen Whitnak

Victor L. Yu

Figure Credits

CHAPTER 3

Figure 3-2. Adapted from DiRienzo JM et al. The outer membrane proteins of the Gram-negative bacteria: biosynthesis, assembly, and function. Ann Rev Biochem 1978;47:481.

Figure 3-8. Adapted from Blumberg P, Strominger JL. Interaction of the penicillin with the bacteria cell wall: penicillin-binding proteins and penicillin-sensitive enzymes. Bacteriol Rev 1974;38:291–335.

Figure 3-9. Adapted from Kaback HR. Ion gradient coupled transport. In: Andreoli TE, Hoffman JS, Sanastil DD, et al. Physiology of Membrane Disorders. New York: Plenum Publications, 1986:287–407.

Figure 3-12. Courtesy of Drs. C. C. Brinton and J. Carnham.

Figure 3-14. Adapted from Boyd RF, Hoerl BG. Basic Medical Microbiology. Boston: Little, Brown, 1986.

CHAPTER 4

Figure 4-5. Adapted from Neidhardt et al. Physiology of the Bacterial Cell. Sunderland, MA: Sinauer Associates, Inc., 1990.

Figure 4-6. Adapted from Neidhardt et al. Physiology of the Bacterial Cell. Sunderland, MA: Sinauer Associates, Inc., 1990.

CHAPTER 5

Figure 5-1. Adapted from Strehler BL. Implications of aging research for society. Fed Proc 1975;34:6.

Figure 5-2. Adapted from Gale EF et al. The Molecular Basis of Antibiotic Action, 2nd Ed. New York: John Wiley & Sons, 1981.

CHAPTER 6

Figure 6-4. From Knobel HR, Villinger W, Isliker H. Chemical analysis and electron microscopy studies of human C1q prepared by different methods. Eur J Immunol 1975;5:78–82.

Figure 6-5. From Bhakdi S, Tranum-Jensen J. Mechanism of complement cytolysis and the concept of channel-forming proteins. Phil Trans Roy Soc London, series B 1984;306:311.

Figure 6-6. Adapted and colorized from Rubin E, Farber JL. Pathology, 3rd Ed. Baltimore: Lippincott Williams & Wilkins, 1999:fig 2-30.

CHAPTER 7

Table 7-1. Adapted from Vivier E, Malissen B. Innate and adaptive immunity: specificities and signaling hierarchies revisited. Nature Immunology 2005;6:17–21.

Figures 7-1 through 7-14. Adapted from Doan TT, Melvold R, and Waltenbaugh C. Concise Medical Immunology. Baltimore: Lippincott Williams & Wilkins, 2005.

CHAPTER 9

Figure 9-3. From Bell CE, Eisenberg D. Crystal structure of nucleotide-free diphtheria toxin. Biochemistry 1997;36:481.

CHAPTER 11

Figure 11-1. From Koneman EW et al. Diagnostic Microbiology, 5th Ed. Baltimore: Lippincott Williams & Wilkins, 1997:color plate 11-1C.

CHAPTER 13

Figure 13-1. Courtesy of Dr. Stuart S. Sagel.

Figure 13-2. From Marler LM, Siders JA, Allen SD. Direct Smear Atlas: A Monograph of Gram-Stained Smear Preparations of Clinical Specimens. Baltimore: Lippincott Williams & Wilkins, 2001.

Figure 13-4. From Wood WB Jr. Studies on the cellular immunology of acute bacterial infections. Harvey Lectures 1951–1952;47:72–98.

Figure 13-5. From Marler LM, Siders JA, Allen SD. Direct Smear Atlas: A Monograph of Gram-Stained Smear Preparations of Clinical Specimens. Baltimore: Lippincott Williams & Wilkins, 2001.

CHAPTER 14

Figure 14-1. From McClatchey KD, Alkan S, Hackel E, et al. Clinical Laboratory Medicine, 2nd Ed. Philadelphia: Lippincott Williams & Wilkins, 2001.

Figure 14-6. From McGee Z et al. Pathogenic mechanisms of *Neisseria gonorrhoeae*: observation on damage to human fallopian tubes in organ culture by gonococci of colony type I or type 4. J Infect Dis 1981;143:413–422.

CHAPTER 15

Figure 15-1. Courtesy of Coy Laboratories, Ann Arbor, MI.

Figure 15-2. Courtesy of A. Tzianabos.

CHAPTER 17

Figure 17-1. Adapted from Taussig MJ. Processes in pathology and microbiology, 2nd Ed. Oxford, UK: Blackwell Scientific Publications, 1984.

Figure 17-2. From Rubin E, Farber JL. Pathology, 3rd Ed. Baltimore: Lippincott Williams & Wilkins, 1999:fig 9-21.

Figure 17-3. Courtesy of Dr. Stanley Falkow. Panel B reproduced with permission from Jones BD, Ghori N, Falkow SJ. J Exp Med 1994;180:15–23.

CHAPTER 18

Figure 18-2. From McClatchey KD, Alkan S, Hackel E, et al. Clinical Laboratory Medicine, 2nd Ed. Philadelphia: Lippincott Williams & Wilkins, 2001.

CHAPTER 19

Figure 19-1. From Muse KE et al. Scanning electron microscopy study of hamster tracheal organ cultures infected with *Bordetella pertussis*. J Infect Dis 1977;136:771–777.

Figure 19-3. Adapted from a figure provided courtesy of Dr. W. E. Goldman.

CHAPTER 20

Figure 20-1. From Koneman EW et al. Diagnostic Microbiology, 5th Ed. Baltimore: Lippincott Williams & Wilkins, 1997:color plate 14-3D.

Figure 20-2. From Schering Slide Library, Schering Corp., Kenilworth, NJ, copyright owner. All rights reserved.

CHAPTER 22

Figure 22-2. From Blaser MJ, Parsonnet J. Parasitism by the "slow" bacterium *Helicobacter pylori* leads to altered gastric homeostasis and neoplasia. J Clin Invest 1994;94:4–8.

Figure 22-3. Adapted from Blaser MJ, Parsonnet J. Parasitism by the "slow" bacterium *Helicobacter pylori* leads to altered gastric homeostasis and neoplasia. J Clin Invest 1994;94:4–8.

Figure 22-4. Rubin E, Farber JL. Pathology, 3rd Ed. Baltimore: Lippincott Williams & Wilkins, 1999:fig 13-14. Originally from Mitros FA: Atlas of Gastrointestinal Pathology. New York: Gower Medical Publishing, 1988.

CHAPTER 23

Figure 23-2. Adapted from Centers for Disease Control and Prevention. Tuberculosis morbidity—United States, 1997. MMWR Morb Mortal Wkly Rep 1998;47:253–257; Centers for Disease Control and Prevention. Tuberculosis morbidity among U.S.-born and foreign-born populations—United States, 2000. MMWR Morb Mortal Wkly Rep 2002;51:101–104.

Figure 23-3. Adapted from Myers JA. The natural history of tuberculosis in the human body. JAMA 1965;194:1086.

CHAPTER 24

Figure 24-1. Courtesy of Dr. E. M. Walker, Department of Microbiology and Immunology, UCLA School of Medicine, Los Angeles, CA.

Figure 24-2. Adapted from Taussig MJ. Processes in Pathology and Microbiology, 2nd Ed. Oxford, UK: Blackwell Scientific, 1984.

Figure 24-3. From Goodheart HP. A Photoguide of Common Skin Disorders: Diagnosis and Management. Baltimore: Lippincott Williams & Wilkins, 1999.

CHAPTER 25

Figure 25-2. Courtesy of Dr. Roberta O'Connor.

Figure 25-3. Courtesy of the American Lyme Disease Foundation.

Figure 25-4. Adapted with permission from the American Lyme Disease Foundation.

Figure 25-5. Adapted from the Centers for Disease Control and Prevention, Atlanta, GA, http://www.bt.cdc.gov.

Figure 25-6. Courtesy of the American Lyme Disease Foundation.

CHAPTER 26

Figure 26-2. From Goodheart HP. Goodheart's Photoguide of Common Skin Disorders, 2nd Ed. Philadelphia: Lippincott Williams & Wilkins, 2003.

CHAPTER 28

Figure 28-4. From McClatchey KD, Alkan S, Hackel E, et al. Clinical Laboratory Medicine, 2nd Ed. Philadelphia: Lippincott Williams & Wilkins, 2001.

CHAPTER 29

Figure 29-1. Courtesy of Dr. Gary Shackleford.

Figure 29-2. From Koneman EW et al. Diagnostic Microbiology, 5th Ed. Baltimore: Lippincott Williams & Wilkins, 1997:color plate 16-1A&B.

Figure 29-3. From Hu PC et al. Surface parasitism by *Mycoplasma pneumoniae* of respiratory epithelium. J Exp Med 1977;145:1328.

CHAPTER 30

Figure 30-1. Courtesy of Dr. D. J. Krogstad.

CHAPTER 31

Figure 31-1. Paramyxovirus: © Science Photo Library. Smallpox virus: Courtesy of Frederick A. Murphy, DVM, PhD, University of California-Davis, Davis, California. Influenza virus: Courtesy of Pete Palese, PhD, Mount Sinai School of Medicine, New York, New York. All other images from T. S. Baker, N. H. Olson, and S. D. Fuller. Adding the Third Dimension to Virus Life Cycles: Three-Dimensional Reconstruction of Icosahedral Viruses from Cryo-Electron Micrographs. Microbiol. Mol. Biol. Rev. 63:862-922, 1999.

Figure 31-2. Redrawn from Dermody TS, Tyler KL. Introduction to viruses and viral diseases. In: Mandell GL, Bennett JE, Dolin R, eds. Mandell, Douglas, and Bennett's Principles and Practice of Infectious Diseases, 5th Ed. New York: Churchill Livingstone, 2000:1536–1552.

Figure 31-3. Redrawn from Taussig MJ. Processes in Pathology and Microbiology, 2nd Ed. Oxford, UK: Blackwell Scientific Publications, 1984.

Figure 31-4. Redrawn from Taussig MJ. Processes in Pathology and Microbiology, 2nd Ed. Oxford, UK: Blackwell Scientific Publications, 1984.

CHAPTER 32

Figure 32-2. Adapted from Flint SJ, Enquist LW, Racaniello VR, Skalka AM. Principles of Virology, 2nd Ed. Washington, DC: ASM Press, 2004.

Figure 32-3. Adapted from Flint SJ, Enquist LW, Racaniello VR, Skalka AM. Principles of Virology, 2nd Ed. Washington, DC: ASM Press, 2004.

Figure 32-5. Adapted from Ogra PL, Karzon DT. Formation and function of poliovirus antibody in different tissues. Prog Med Virol 1971;13:156–193.

CHAPTER 34

Figure 34-1. Adapted from Knipe DM, Howley PM, eds. Field's Virology, 4th Ed. Philadelphia: Lippincott Williams & Wilkins, 2001:ch 41, fig 2.

Figure 34-3. From Rubin E, Farber JL. Pathology, 3rd Ed. Baltimore: Lippincott Williams & Wilkins, 1999:fig 12-32.

CHAPTER 35

Figure 35-1. Courtesy of Dr. Makonnen Fedaku, Centers for Disease Control and Prevention, Atlanta, GA.

Figure 35-2. From Rubin E, Farber JL. Pathology, 3rd Ed. Philadelphia: Lippincott Williams & Wilkins, 1999:fig. 28-9.

CHAPTER 37

Figure 37-1. Courtesy of A. Kapikian.

Figure 37-2. Adapted from Field BN et al. Virology. New York: Raven Press, 1990.

CHAPTER 38

Figure 38-1. World Health Organization. The world health report 2004–changing history. Available at: http://www.who.int/whr/2004/en/report04_en.pdf. Accessed October 28, 2005.

Figure 38-5. Courtesy of Dr. M. Gonda.

CHAPTER 39

Figure 39-1A. From Stewart PL, Burnett RM, Cyrklaff M, Fuller SD. Image reconstruction reveals the complex molecular organization of adenovirus. Cell 1991;67:145–154.

Figure 39-1B. Redrawn from Philipson L, Pettersson U. Advances in tumor virus research. In: Advances in Virus Research, vol 18. New York: Academic Press, 1971.

Figure 39-3A. From Kelly TJ Jr. Adenovirus DNA replication. In: Ginsburg HS, ed. The Adenoviruses. New York: Plenum Publishing, 1984:278, 298.

Figure 39-3B&C. Redrawn from Kelly TJ Jr. Adenovirus DNA replication. In: Ginsburg HS, ed. The Adenoviruses. New York: Plenum Publishing, 1984:278, 298.

CHAPTER 40

Figure 40-1. Courtesy of Dr. K. V. Shah.

Figure 40-2. From Goodheart HP. Goodheart's Photoguide of Common Skin Disorders, 2nd Ed. Philadelphia: Lippincott Williams & Wilkins, 2003.

Figure 40-3. Courtesy of Dr. Benjamin Barankin.

Figure 40-4. From Rubin E, Farber JL. Pathology, 3rd Ed. Baltimore: Lippincott Williams & Wilkins, 1999:fig 17-19A.

CHAPTER 41

Figure 41-3B. From Rubin E, Farber JL. Pathology, 3rd Ed. Baltimore: Lippincott Williams & Wilkins, 1999:fig 9-7A.

Figure 41-4A & B. From Rubin E, Farber JL. Pathology, 3rd Ed. Baltimore: Lippincott Williams & Wilkins, 1999:figs 9-5, 9-7B.

Figure 41-5. From Hsiung GD, Mayo DR, Lucia HL, Landry MI. Genital herpes: pathogenesis and chemotherapy in a guinea pig model. Rev Infect Dis 1984;6:33–50.

CHAPTER 42

Figure 42-1. Modified from figure provided by Dr. Jay Nelson and Andrew Townsend, Oregon Health Sciences University, Portland, OR.

Figure 42-3. Photographs provided by Dr. D. Kelly, Dept. of Pathology, Children's Hospital of Alabama, Birmingham.

CHAPTER 43

Figure 43-1. Adapted from Ganem D, Schneider RJ. Hepadnaviruses. In: Knipe DM, Howley PM, eds. Field's Virology, 4th Ed. Philadelphia: Lippincott Williams & Wilkins, 2001:ch 86, fig 2.

Figure 43-2. Courtesy of Dr. John Jerin.

Figure 43-3. Adapted from Ganem D, Schneider RJ. Hepadnaviruses. In: Knipe DM, Howley PM, eds. Field's Virology, 4th Ed. Lippincott Williams & Wilkins, 2001:ch 86, fig 7.

CHAPTER 44

Figure 44-2. Adapted from Freed EO, Martin MA. HIVs and their replication. In: Knipe DM, Howley PM, eds. Field's Virology, 4th Ed. Philadelphia: Lippincott Williams & Wilkins, 2001:ch 59, fig 30.

Figure 44-4. Adapted from Crumpacker C. Antiviral therapy. In: Knipe DM, Howley PM, eds. Field's Virology, 4th Ed. Philadelphia: Lippincott Williams & Wilkins, 2001:ch 15, fig 12.

Figure 44-6. Modified from Corey L et al. Intravenous acyclovir for the treatment of primary genital herpes. Ann Intern Med 1983;98:914–921.

Figure 44-7. Redrawn from Straus S et al. Suppression of recurrent genital herpes with oral acyclovir. Trans Assoc Am Phys 1984;97:278–283.

CHAPTER 46

Figure 46-2. From Koneman EW et al. Diagnostic Microbiology, 5th Ed. Baltimore: Lippincott Williams & Wilkins, 1997:color plate 19-6E.

Figure 46-4. From Koneman EW et al. Diagnostic Microbiology, 5th Ed. Baltimore: Lippincott Williams & Wilkins, 1997:color plate 19-1C.

Figure 46-5. Adapted from Koneman EW et al. Diagnostic Microbiology, 5th Ed.

Baltimore: Lippincott Williams & Wilkins, 1997:fig 19-5.

CHAPTER 47

Figure 47-3. From Kauffman CA. Fungal infections in older adults. Clin Infect Dis 2001;33:550–555.

Figure 47-4B. From Rubin E, Farber JL. Pathology, 3rd Ed. Baltimore: Lippincott Williams & Wilkins, 1999:fig 9-59B.

Figure 47-6. From Rubin E, Farber JL. Pathology, 3rd Ed. Baltimore: Lippincott Williams & Wilkins, 1999:fig 9-62.

Figure 47-8B. From Rubin E, Farber JL. Pathology, 3rd Ed. Baltimore: Lippincott Williams & Wilkins, 1999:fig 9-60.

Figure 47-9. From Rubin E, Farber JL. Pathology, 3rd Ed. Baltimore: Lippincott Williams & Wilkins, 1999:fig 9-61.

CHAPTER 48

Figure 48-2. From Rubin E, Farber JL. Pathology, 3rd Ed. Baltimore: Lippincott Williams & Wilkins, 1999:fig 9-54A.

Figure 48-4. Courtesy of Dr. Leonor Haley, Centers for Disease Control and Prevention, Atlanta, GA.

Figure 48-6. From Koneman EW et al. Diagnostic Microbiology, 5th Ed. Baltimore: Lippincott Williams & Wilkins, 1997:color plate 19-1C.

Figure 48-10. From Grossman ME, Roth J. Cutaneous Manifestations of Infection in the Immunocompromised Host. Philadelphia: Lippincott Williams & Wilkins, 1995: fig 1-51.

Figure 48-11. From Rubin E, Farber JL. Pathology, 3rd Ed. Baltimore: Lippincott Williams & Wilkins, 1999:fig 9-72A.

Figure 48-13. From Rubin E, Farber JL. Pathology, 3rd Ed. Baltimore: Lippincott Williams & Wilkins, 1999:fig 9-72B.

CHAPTER 49

Figure 49-1. Watanakunakorn C. Photo quiz. Clin Infect Dis 1996;22:765.

CHAPTER 52

Figure 52-2. Redrawn from Friedman MJ. Erythrocytic mechanism of sickle cell resistance to malaria. Proc Natl Acad Sci USA 1978;75:1994.

Figure 52-7. Courtesy of Drs. M. S. Bartlett and J. W. Smith, Indiana University School of Medicine.

Figure 52-10. Redrawn from Ross R, Thompson D. Proc Roy Soc London, series B 1910;82:411–415.

CHAPTER 53

Figure 53-3. Courtesy of Dr. Stanley L. Erlandsen, Washington University School of Medicine, St. Louis, MO.

CHAPTER 55

Figure 55-8A. From Kean BH, Sun T, Ellsworth RM. Ophthalmic parasitology. New York: Igaku-Shoin, 1991:212.

Figure 55-8B. Courtesy of Dr. H. Zaiman, Charlottesville, VA. From a pictorial presentation of parasites. In: Sun T. Parasitic Disorders: Pathology, Diagnosis, and Management, 2nd Ed. Baltimore: Lippincott Williams & Wilkins, 1999.

CHAPTER 56

Figure 56-2A. From the National Creutzfeldt-Jakob Disease Surveillance Unit, Western General Hospital, Crewe Road, Edinburgh, UK.

Figure 56-2B. From Rabinstein, AA. Abnormal diffusion-weighted magnetic resonance imaging in Creutzfeldt-Jakob disease following corneal transplantations. Arch Neurol 2002;59:637.

Figure 56-3. From Rubin E, Farber JL. Pathology, 3rd Ed. Baltimore: Lippincott Williams & Wilkins, 1999:fig 28-109.

Figure 56-4. Adapted from Beisel CE, Morens DM. Variant Creutzfeldt-Jakob disease and the acquired and transmissible spongiform encephalopathies. Clin Infect Dis 2004;38:697–704.

Figure 56-5. From Collie DA. Diagnosing variant Creutzfeldt-Jakob disease with the pulvinar sign: MR imaging findings in 86 neuropathologically confirmed cases. AJNR 2003;24:1560.

CHAPTER 57

Figure 57-1. Bush LM, Abrams BH, Beal A, Johnson CC. Brief report: Index case of fatal inhalational anthrax due to bioterrorism. N Engl J Med 2001;345:1607–1610. Copyright © 2001 Massachusetts Medical Society.

Figure 57-2. Jernigan JA et al. Bioterrorism-related Inhalation Anthrax: The First 10 Cases Reported in the United States. Emerg Infect Dis 2001;7(6):933–944.

Figure 57-3. Public Health Image Library, Centers for Disease Control and Prevention, Atlanta, GA, http://www.bt.cdc.gov.

Figure 57-4. Public Health Image Library, Centers for Disease Control and Prevention, Atlanta, GA, http://www.bt.cdc.gov.

Figure 57-5. From Knipe DM, Howley PM, eds. Field's Virology, 4th Ed. Philadelphia: Lippincott Williams & Wilkins, 2001:ch 85, fig 3.

Figure 57-6. From Knipe DM, Howley PM, eds. Field's Virology, 4th Ed. Philadelphia: Lippincott Williams & Wilkins, 2001:ch 85, fig 1A.

CHAPTER 60

Figure 60-3. Modified from Cawley JR. Infectious diarrhea. Am J Med 1985;78(suppl 6B):65–71.

CHAPTER 61

Figure 61-2. Redrawn from Menkes JH. Viral neurological infections in children. Hosp Pract 1977;12:100–109.

Figure 61-4. Courtesy of Dr. E. J. Bottone, Mount Sinai Hospital, New York, NY.

CHAPTER 63

Figure 63-1. Redrawn from Fass RJ et al. Urinary tract infection: Practical aspects of diagnosis and treatment. JAMA 1973;225:1509–1513.

Figure 63-3. Redrawn from Fass RJ et al. Urinary tract infection: Practical aspects of diagnosis and treatment. JAMA 1973;225:1509–1513.

CHAPTER 64

Figure 64-1. Fleisher GR, Ludwig W, Baskin MN. Atlas of Pediatric Emergency Medicine. Philadelphia: Lippincott Williams & Wilkins, 2003:fig 11-37.

Figure 64-2. From Goodheart HP. Goodheart's Photoguide of Common Skin Disorders: Diagnosis and Management. 2nd Ed. Philadelphia: Lippincott Williams & Wilkins, 2003:fig 5-2.

Figure 64-3. From Barankin B. The Barankin Dermatology Collection. Baltimore: Lippincott Williams & Wilkins, 2003.

Figure 64-4. From Rubin E, Farber JL. Pathology, 3rd Ed. Baltimore: Lippincott Williams & Wilkins, 1999:fig 9-11.

Figure 64-5. From Smeltzer SC, Bare BG. Brunner and Suddarth's Textbook of Medical-Surgical Nursing, 9th Ed. Philadelphia: Lippincott Williams & Wilkins, 2000:fig 51-01.

Figure 64-7. From Sweet RL, Gibbs RS. Atlas of Infectious Diseases of the Female Genital Tract. Philadelphia: Lippincott Williams & Wilkins, 2005:fig 9-2.

CHAPTER 67

Figure 67-1. Adapted from Rodbard S. Blood velocity and endocarditis. Circulation 1963;27:18–28.

Figure 67-2. From Rubin E, Farber JL. Pathology, 3rd Ed. Baltimore: Lippincott Williams & Wilkins, 1999:fig 11-34.

Figure 67-3A. From Rubin E, Farber JL. Pathology, 3rd Ed. Baltimore: Lippincott Williams & Wilkins, 1999:fig 11-34.

CHAPTER 73

Figure 73-3. Data from the Centers for Disease Control and Prevention, Atlanta, GA.

Table of Contents

Part I: Principles   *1*

Part II: Infectious Agents   *139*

SECTION 1   **BACTERIA**

Part III: Pathophysiology of Infectious Diseases *553*

Principles

Establishment of Infectious Diseases

Barry I. Eisenstein and Moselio Schaechter

B oth students and physicians confront a large number of facts about infectious agents and the diseases they cause. What is the best way to manage this large amount of material? Given the magnitude of the task, memorizing bits of information would be difficult and unproductive. The better approach is to develop a conceptual framework on which to hang a multitude of facts. This framework consists of two generalizations based on the features that characterize all forms of parasitism:

1. In all infectious diseases, the following events take place:
   Encounter: the agent meets the host.
   Entry: the agent enters the host.
   Spread: the agent spreads from the site of entry.
   Multiplication: the agent multiplies in the host.
   Damage: the agent, the host response, or both cause tissue damage.
   Outcome: the agent or the host wins out, or they learn to coexist.
2. Each of these events requires the breach of host defenses. The manner in which a parasite combats host defenses distinguishes it from other parasites.

ENCOUNTER

Most of us first encounter microorganisms at birth. Microbiologically speaking, we lead a sterile existence while in our mother's womb. First, the fetal membranes shield the fetus well from the microorganisms in the uterine environment. Second, the mother is not a likely source of microorganisms for the fetus. The mother's blood carries infectious agents only sporadically and in small numbers. In addition, the placenta is a formidable barrier to the transmission of microorganisms to the fetus. Such transmission is possible, however, and some diseases are transmitted to the fetus through the placenta. Examples of these so-called congenital infections are **rubella** (German measles) and **syphilis** or those caused by **HIV** or **cytomegalovirus (CMV).**

The first encounter with environmental microorganisms usually takes place at birth. During parturition the newborn comes in contact with microorganisms present in the mother's vaginal canal and on her skin. Thus, the newborn faces the challenge of living in the intimate company of a bewildering number of microorganisms. The mother, however, does not send the newborn into the world totally unprotected. Through her circulation she endows the fetus with a vast repertoire of specific antibodies. Some immunological protection is also provided by the mother's milk

3

(colostrum), which also contains maternal antibodies. However, these acquired defenses soon wane and the child must cope on its own. The microbial challenge is renewed time and again as we come in contact with new organisms throughout our lives. Most organisms rapidly disappear from our bodies, but some are adroit colonizers and become part of the normal flora. A few cause disease.

Endogenous Versus Exogenous Encounters

Microbial diseases are contracted in two general ways, exogenously and endogenously.

Exogenously Acquired Diseases

Exogenously acquired diseases result from encounters with agents in the environment. Thus, we "catch" a cold from others, or we get typhoid fever from eating or drinking contaminated food or water. There are various ways in which disease-causing agents can be acquired from the environment: food, water, air, objects, insect bites, or humans or animals with whom we share our environment. Many agents are readily transmitted among humans through the exchange of bodily fluids—for instance, by sneezing, touching, or sexual intercourse. The way we encounter a disease agent often suggests a mode of prevention (Table 1-1); for example, infection by an agent spread through the fecal-oral route can be dramatically reduced by ensuring that wastewater and drinking water are maintained separately. Prevention has been successful for many serious epidemics, at least in the developed countries of the world. With the exception of vaccination, most preventive measures involve improving sanitation and the standard of living, rather than employing medical procedures.

Endogenously Acquired Diseases

Endogenously acquired diseases are caused by agents present in or on the body. Members of the microbial flora that are normally found on our skin or mucous membranes may cause disease, usually when they penetrate into deeper tissues. Thus, a cut can lead to the production of pus caused by the staphylococci that inhabit healthy skin. The encounter with the agent took place long before the disease—namely, at the time the skin was colonized by the staphylococci. A distinction must be made between **colonization** and **infectious disease.** Colonization simply denotes the presence of microorganisms in a site of the body that may or may not lead to tissue damage and signs and symptoms of disease. It does suggest, however, that the microorganisms have invaded that site of the body and can multiply there.

Normal Flora

The difference between endogenous and exogenous infections is sometimes quite sharp. However, in many other instances the demarcation is less clear because it is difficult to define precisely which organisms constitute the **normal flora** (see Chapter 2). For example, some people harbor certain strains of virulent streptococci in their throat for a considerable period but only rarely come down with strep throat. Are these streptococci members of the normal flora? The answer is yes, if *normal flora* refers to organisms in or on the body that are not in the process of causing disease. The answer is no if this kind of streptococcus is considered not found in the throats of approximately 95% of all healthy people. No easy way exists out of this ambiguity, and the terms *exogenous infection* and *endogenous infection* must be used tentatively. Obviously, if we cannot define precisely the composition of normal flora, we cannot always distinguish between endogenous and exogenous infections.

table **1-1**	**Examples of Encounters and Disease Prevention**				
TYPE OF CONTACT	**EXAMPLE**	**TYPE OF AGENT**	**SOURCE**	**STRATEGY FOR PREVENTION**	**PREVENTIVE AIM**
Inhalation	Common cold	Virus	Aerosol from infected persons	None	
	Coccidioidomycosis	Fungus	Soil	None	
Ingestion	Typhoid fever	Bacterium	Water, food	Sanitation	Lower infecting dose
Sexual contact	Gonorrhea	Bacterium	Person	Social behavior	Avoid contact
Wound	Surgical infections	Bacteria	Normal flora surroundings	Aseptic techniques	Avoid contact
Insect bite	Malaria	Protozoan	Mosquito	Insect control	Eliminate vector

Another consideration that must also be kept in mind is that even for highly virulent microbes, exposure does not always lead to disease. For example, even at the height of deadly bubonic plague and typhus epidemics, most people were likely to have encountered the disease agent, but only about half the population became sick.

Thus, human encounters with microbes are quite varied, and disease is not inevitable in every case. Humans display an idiosyncratic pattern of response to infectious agents; even within one individual, the pattern can change with age, nutritional state, and many other factors.

ENTRY

Most of the tissues we normally think of as being inside the body are topologically connected with the outside (Fig. 1-1). For instance, the surface of the lumen of the intestine, the alveoli of the lung, the bile canaliculi, and the tubules of the kidney are in direct contact with the exterior environment. In fact, this is true of almost all the organs contained within the thorax and abdomen. In principle, an insect could crawl from the mouth to the anus without penetrating any mucous membranes, although it would have to go through several valves and sphincters. In reality, these "external" sites of the body employ powerful mechanisms to keep out invading microorganisms. With the exception of much of the digestive tract and the lower reaches of the genitourinary system, these sites are normally sterile.

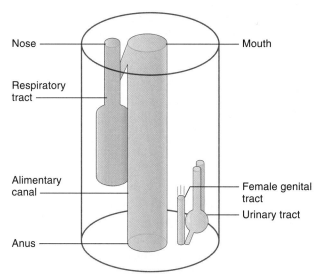

FIGURE 1-1 ▪ **A schematic diagram showing the regions of the body in direct contact with the exterior.** These include the outer aspects of the digestive, respiratory, and urogenital systems. These systems account for most of the organs of the thorax and abdomen. The main systems that do not have such direct connections are the musculoskeletal, nervous, circulatory, and endocrine systems. In women the genital tract is connected to the peritoneal cavity via the fallopian tubes.

The term *entry* then can be used in two senses: it means either the **ingress** of microorganisms into body cavities that are contiguous with the outside environment or the **penetration** of microorganisms into deeper tissue after crossing an epithelial barrier. Both aspects of entry are discussed in detail here.

Ingress: Entry Without Crossing Epithelial Barriers

Obviously microorganisms enter the intestine by being swallowed and enter the lung by being inhaled. External microorganisms can also enter the urinary tract or the genital system. To cause disease, microorganisms do not have to enter deep into tissues but can stay only on mucosal surfaces. Examples of serious infectious diseases that occur without bacterial penetration through epithelial surfaces are **cholera, whooping cough,** and infections of the urinary bladder.

Inhalation

To enter the respiratory system, microorganisms face a series of aerodynamic and hydrodynamic obstacles. Microorganisms are inhaled in **aerosol droplets** or **dust particles** contained in the air we breathe. They take a circuitous path through the respiratory tract because they must navigate through complex anatomic structures such as nasal turbinates, the oropharynx, and the larynx. Accordingly, the surgical removal of the larynx (with its nooks and crannies) predisposes an individual to diseases of the lower respiratory tract. Microorganisms that arrive in the lower reaches of the respiratory tree face the powerful upward-sweeping action of the ciliary epithelium. As expected, persons in whom this ciliary elevator is impaired (e.g., heavy smokers) are more likely to get sick with pneumonia. Colonization of these sites requires that the microorganisms be able to stick to the epithelial surface.

Ingestion

When contaminated food or water is ingested, microorganisms face a powerful host defense, the acid in the stomach. The stomach is a chemical disinfection chamber where many microorganisms are destroyed. Its effectiveness in killing microbes, however, is determined by the length of time the microorganisms spend in the stomach, which in turn depends on the kind and amount of the food eaten. Even after great destruction, some bacteria and yeasts escape the stomach alive, although their original number may have been reduced a millionfold or more. In addition, the way that bacteria are ingested can influence their level of acid sensitivity because certain foods can protect the microbes from acid killing. Finally, some species have inherently greater resistance to acid and are therefore infectious at lower doses.

Bacteria, fungi, parasites, and viruses that escape the stomach's acid barrier enter the duodenum. There they meet the enzymes of the pancreatic juice, the bile salts, and the strong sweeping force of **peristalsis.** Not unexpectedly, very few microbes can colonize the duodenum or anywhere else in the upper reaches of the small intestine. Toward the ileum, the environment is more favorable to bacterial life, but even there the few organisms that gain a foothold must avoid being washed away. Indeed, bacteria found in this region have special mechanisms that allow them to adhere to the epithelial cells of the intestinal mucosa. As will be discussed in Chapter 2, several surface components of these bacteria serve as **adhesins.** The main adhesins are the hairlike pili (fimbriae) and the surface polysaccharides. As mentioned previously, bacteria at this site may cause disease without penetrating the mucosal epithelium. Cholera and its milder relative **travelers' diarrhea** are the manifestations of the local production of powerful toxins in the intestine that affect the epithelial cells. The bacteria that produce these toxins need not enter the host cells to cause disease.

Penetration: Entry Into Tissues After Crossing Epithelial Barriers

Penetration into tissues takes many forms. Some microorganisms pass directly through epithelia, especially mucous membranes that consist of a single cell layer. To penetrate the skin, which is tough and multilayered, most infecting agents must be carried across by insect bites or await breaks in the skin surface. On the other hand, certain worms can burrow unaided through the skin and invade the host. An example is the hookworm, which can be acquired by walking barefoot on contaminated soil.

To penetrate mucosal epithelial cells, many agents first interact with specific **receptors** on the surface of the host cell. This phenomenon has been studied intensively in viruses, some of which have a complex mechanism for attachment and internalization. For instance, influenza viruses have **surface components** that bind to receptors on the surface of sensitive host cells. Binding is soon followed by the uptake of the virus particles by the cells. These two functions, **attachment** and **internalization,** are also the subjects of intensive study in relation to bacteria, many of which are able to induce their own uptake into host cells after attachment. Unlike viruses, however, not all bacteria must enter host cells to replicate; some can replicate to high levels on the mucosal epithelium.

Microorganisms can also be actively carried into tissues by white cells or macrophages that lie outside the body. For instance, macrophages that reside in the alveoli of the lungs, known as **dust cells,** can pick up infectious agents by phagocytosis. Most of the time, microorganism-containing macrophages are carried upward on the ciliary epithelium, but occasionally infected macrophages can reenter the body and carry their load of microorganisms into deeper locations. This mechanism of **cell-mediated entry** can function in other mucous membranes as well. For example, it is thought that HIV, the virus that causes AIDS, may be sexually transmitted by the penetration of virus-laden macrophages from semen.

Insect Bites

Insect bites can lead to the penetration of viruses (viral encephalitis, yellow fever), bacteria (plague, typhus), protozoa (malaria, sleeping sickness), or worms (river blindness, elephantiasis). In the case of protozoa and worms, residence in the insect is part of their complex life cycles. The **life stage** of the parasite in the insect is often quite different from that found in the human host. Insects also spread diseases by carrying microorganisms on their surfaces and by contaminating foodstuffs or a person's skin. A particularly unsavory example of insect transmission is that of the so-called reduviid bugs, which defecate at the same time they bite. Parasites contained in the insect's feces are then introduced by scratching the bite area. A serious protozoal infection, **Chagas disease,** is transmitted in this manner.

Cuts and Wounds

Penetration from cuts and wounds is a common occurrence that often goes unnoticed because it does not usually lead to symptoms of disease. For example, brushing one's teeth or even defecating can cause minute abrasions of epithelial membranes. A small number of bacteria can then enter in the bloodstream, but they are rapidly removed by the filtering mechanisms of the lymphoreticular system. However, if internal tissues are damaged or the defense mechanisms disrupted, circulating bacteria may gain a foothold and cause serious diseases. An example is **subacute bacterial endocarditis,** a devastating disease in the preantibiotic era. The infection was usually caused by oral streptococci that invaded the heart valves damaged by a previous disease, usually rheumatic fever.

Organ Transplants and Blood Transfusions

Yet another way for organisms to penetrate into deeper tissue is through organ transplants or blood transfusions. For instance, cornea transplants have been known to result in the infection of recipients with a virus that causes a slow degenerative disease of the central nervous system, **Creutzfeldt-Jakob disease.** Kidney transplants sometimes result in infections by CMV, perhaps because of virus residing in the transplanted kidney. However, the transplanted organ is not always the source of infection. Because the immune response of transplant recipients must be suppressed to avoid graft rejection, an **endogenous virus** may take advantage of these weakened host defenses and begin to multiply.

Of the infectious agents that can be acquired through blood transfusions, none causes greater concern than HIV. However, many others, such as **hepatitis B virus (HBV)** can also be transmitted in this manner. Screening of blood in blood banks is imperative.

Inoculum Size

The likelihood that organisms from the flora of the skin or mucous membranes will cause disease depends on many factors. Among them is the size of the **inoculum,** the number of invading organisms. An encounter with a small number of organisms is unlikely to result in an infection; it usually takes many infecting agents to overcome the local defenses. An example that illustrates the importance of inoculum size is infection acquired from a contaminated hot tub. At times the water can become a veritable culture broth with as many as 100 million bacteria (*Pseudomonas*) per milliliter. In such numbers, bacteria that are normally harmless can overcome the normal defenses of the skin and cause skin infection all over the body. Medical professionals are also aware of the importance of inoculum size in infection. For example, before making an incision in the skin, a surgeon prepares the area to reduce the number of bacteria that could invade a surgical wound. Infections are almost inevitable if large numbers of microorganisms are deposited in deeper tissues, either from dirty skin or from contamination by soil or other microbial-rich material. Treatment of patients with open wounds thus requires careful attention to sterile techniques, even in the modern era of powerful antimicrobial drugs.

SPREAD

The term *spread* has two shades of meaning. It suggests direct, **lateral propagation** of organisms from the original site of entry to contiguous tissues, but it can also refer to **dissemination** to distant sites. Either way, microorganisms spread and multiply only if they overcome host defenses. It should be kept in mind that spread can precede or follow microbial multiplication in the body. For instance, the parasite that causes **malaria** enters the body through a mosquito bite and is distributed throughout the bloodstream before it has a chance to reproduce. On the other hand, staphylococci that infect a cut must multiply locally before spreading to distant sites.

The role of **host defenses** in impeding the spread of microorganisms requires a fair understanding of the immune response and of the innate defense mechanisms. Host defenses are discussed in detail in Chapters 6 and 7 and are a central theme of this book. For now, it is important to keep in mind the dynamic nature of host–parasite interactions: For every host defense mechanism, microbes have developed a strategy to overcome

it. The host, in turn, adapts to these new challenges, eliciting yet different responses from the agents. This intricate counterpoint is played out, sometimes over extended periods, and one of three things can happen: the host wins out, the parasite overcomes the host, or host and parasite learn to live with one another in an uneasy truce.

Anatomical Factors

Because the pattern of spread of microorganisms from a given site is often dictated by **anatomical factors,** a knowledge of human anatomy often helps us understand infectious diseases. Consider the example of a localized infection, a bacterial abscess of the lung. The abscess could burst and allow the organisms to escape into the bronchial tree or, if the abscess is pointed outwards, to the pleural cavity. Spread in one or the other direction has different consequences: in the first case it could lead to a generalized pneumonia; in the second, to pleurisy. Another example is an infection of the middle ear, a condition more common in children than in adults. The age difference is explained in part by developmental changes that take place in the eustachian tubes with growth. These conduits are nearly horizontal in children and become more steeply inclined with age. For this and other reasons, the eustachian tubes of children do not drain as well as those of adults.

Spread of microorganisms is greatly influenced by **fluid dynamics.** Infected fluids in the interior of the body tend to flow along fascial planes. For example, infection of one site of the meninges will usually result in generalized meningitis, because there are no barriers to impede the spread of the infected cerebrospinal fluid. The same is true for the pleura, the pericardium, and the synovial cavities. Of course, the most extensive liquid system of the body, the blood, is replete with defense mechanisms. All the liquids of the body (blood, lymph, cerebrospinal fluid, synovial fluid, urine, tears, etc.) contain unique antimicrobial defense factors. If these are overcome, disease results.

Active Participation by Microbes

Infectious agents are not always passive participants in the process of spread; some contribute to it by actively moving. Thus, worms wiggle, ameba crawl, some bacteria swim. Although some of these movements appear random, others are probably in response to chemotactic signals. Spread can also be facilitated by chemical rather than mechanical action. For instance, streptococci manufacture a variety of extracellular hydrolases that allow them to break out of the walled defenses erected by the inflammatory response. These organisms make a protease that breaks up fibrin, a hyaluronidase that hydrolyzes the hyaluronic acid of connective tissue and may allow the organism to spread, and a deoxyribonuclease that reduces the viscosity of pus caused by release of DNA from lysed white cells. Some bacteria make elastases, collagenases, or other powerful proteases. Such organisms can break through natural surface barriers or spread through thick viscous pus that would otherwise impede their expansion. At a more superficial site, fungi that cause athlete's foot make keratin-hydrolyzing enzymes that help them spread through the horny layers of the skin. These factors confer clear selective advantages on the microorganisms that produce them.

MULTIPLICATION

Rarely do infectious agents cause disease without first multiplying within the body. As previously stated, the number of microorganisms we inhale or ingest (the size of the inoculum) or the number that survives initial host barriers is usually too small to produce symptoms directly. Infectious agents must reproduce before their presence is noted by symptoms (Fig. 1-2). One exception to the rule are agents that cause disease through the production of a toxin, such as *Clostridium botulinum*, which produces the botulinum toxin that leads to botulism. This condition is an **intoxication,** not an infection.

In most infections, symptoms manifest some time after the organisms enter the host. This **incubation period** reflects the time needed for the infectious agents to overcome early defenses and grow to a certain population size. The subject of how hosts defend themselves

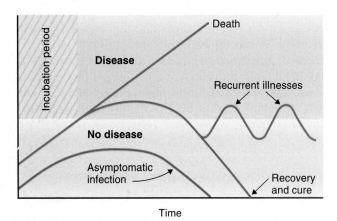

FIGURE 1-2 ▪ **Microbial multiplication and clinical manifestations of disease.** The number of microorganisms present in a patient must exceed a given threshold to cause disease. If the number is below that threshold, no signs and symptoms of disease will be apparent. In some cases the numbers oscillate above and below the threshold, resulting in recurrent bouts of disease. Note that this drawing is idealized; in reality the threshold of overt disease is not fixed but varies with the physiological state of the host.

against microbial multiplication is a lengthy and varied one. A later section in this chapter discusses how defense mechanisms sometimes go overboard and actually contribute to tissue damage in infections.

Environmental Factors That Influence Multiplication

The physical environment of the body selects for microbes that grow within certain ranges of temperature, osmotic pressure, and pH. Those that are almost always found associated with a host tend to have a narrow **temperature optimum.** On the other hand, microbes that are also found in the environment, such as *Pseudomonas*, can grow at lower temperatures as well. Replication of some viruses, such as poliovirus, is limited to within a few degrees over normal human body temperature. Fever then may be a defense mechanism that helps restrict the disease. Fungi that cause athlete's foot do not grow well at temperatures above around 30°C and are thus found only on the cooler body surfaces. It follows that in most circumstances these fungi cannot cause internal diseases. As with nutritional requirements, the optimal temperature range for growth is often dictated by the habits of the organism.

Subversion of Host Defenses

When a microbe causes an infection, it creates a hostile environment for itself because it impels the host to mobilize defenses that impair its growth. In most cases the host prevails, but the existence of infectious diseases demonstrates that this is not always true and that microorganisms can thwart or evade the host defenses. Microbial countermeasures do not contribute directly to tissue damage, yet they can be thought of as virulence factors because they are essential for the microbe to be pathogenic. Generally, each species of infectious agents develops a unique spectrum of survival strategies. For every successful infection by a microbe, the question is, how does it survive in its particular location of the body? Part of the answer is known, but by no means all of it.

Host defenses do not operate in isolation but are interrelated. The strategies that microbes use to subvert them are correspondingly complex. Two types of strategies exist: **complement and phagocytosis,** which make up constitutive defenses, and **humoral and cellular immunity,** which make up induced defenses. A microbe invading a host that has not previously encountered it will meet these defenses in that order. Many microbial countermeasures are known from in vitro experimental situations, and it is not always possible to determine if they also operate in human disease. This is the subject of intensive research that has clear therapeutic and prophylactic implications.

One type of microbial defensive strategy is making, or appropriating from the host, a protective covering. For example, some microbes produce extracellular capsules that block recognition and binding by both complement and antibodies and prevent phagocytosis by leukocytes. This is the strategy of such important mucosal pathogens as the pneumococcus or the meningococcus. Notwithstanding their protective properties, these capsules are themselves immunogenic and antigenic and thus have become the basis of vaccines used to prevent pneumonia and meningitis. Another way that bacteria avoid immune recognition is by altering their surface antigens in a genetically programmed way. Certain pathogens, such as the gonococci or the salmonellae, can modify surface structures that are recognized by the immune system.

Many microbes survive in the body because they do not cause too much damage to the host. The best adapted of them cause no disease at all, elicit no inflammatory response, and actually are a help to the host by providing nutrients in the gastrointestinal tract (e.g., vitamin B_{12}) or crowding out potential pathogens (on the skin and mucosal surfaces). They may even stimulate the immune system to raise useful cross-protective antibodies (e.g., protection against meningococci may be the result of the colonization by related but nonpathogenic commensal species). Among the most successful pathogens are those that cause sexually transmitted diseases. In some cases these bacteria cause minimal disease (e.g., chlamydial infection, gonorrhea), whereas in other cases disease comes on slowly or as part of a chronic process (e.g., syphilis). When nonpathogenic strains cause trouble, it is a result of their getting into places they do not belong, such as when the mixed flora of the bowel gets into the peritoneal cavity with the rupture of an appendix.

In contrast, the occasional highly pathogenic invaders with their well-developed set of toxins cause significant acute damage and disease but may end up killing the host (thus biting the hand that feeds them). For example, dead-end processes like lethal meningitis do not, by themselves, promote bacterial survival.

DAMAGE

There are nearly as many kinds of damage as there are infectious diseases. The type and intensity of the damage depend on the tissues and organs affected, which makes it difficult to make generalizations. An important, if not intuitively obvious, point is that damage is not always caused by activities of the invading agent alone but is often the consequence of a vehement host response. What causes damage in an infection such as pneumonia caused by pneumococci? These organisms make no known toxins, and their invasion of the lung alveoli is manifested chiefly by the extensive production of pus in the affected sites. Pus is the result of acute inflammation, the outpouring of white blood cells and liquid from the circulation. As in many other infections, the symptoms of pneumonia are due mainly to a forceful host response. In chronic infections, such as tuberculosis, the symptoms of disease can almost invariably be ascribed to the host response, with the microbe being relatively passive but able to stimulate a host response that causes the symptoms of the disease.

Mechanisms of Direct Damage

Although damage from microbial infection is often the result of the immune response, microbes are not always just innocent bystanders. Some bacteria produce extracellular toxins that are directly responsible for tissue damage. Some of these toxins, such as those of botulism and tetanus, are among the strongest poisons known. Toxins cause damage in various ways: some just help bacteria spread in tissues, others lyse host cells, yet others stop cell growth, and still others exaggerate normal physiological mechanisms. By depressing or augmenting particular functions, a toxin can kill a person without directly damaging any cells. No abnormal lesions result; rather, the toxin acts by causing hyperactivity of a normal process.

One of the most dramatic manifestations of infection is cell death. This comes about in a variety of ways: direct action of cytolytic toxins, activation of cell-killing white blood cells, or induction of programmed cell death. The damage caused by the death of tissue cells is most serious when it occurs in essential organs, such as the brain or the heart. It should be noted that in some serious and even life-threatening infectious diseases, cell death is not a distinctive feature even though the agents multiply intracellularly. In the prime example, tuberculosis, the infected cells survive, yet the infection results in far-reaching and pervasive damage. However, cell death is often a prominent feature, especially of acute infections.

With many of the common Gram-negative bacteria (see Chapter 3), the host response is elicited by a major component of their surface, a lipopolysaccharide known as **endotoxin.** In small amounts endotoxin elicits fever and mobilizes certain defense mechanisms. In large amounts it results in shock and intravascular coagulation. Thus, the host response to the presence of these bacteria depends on the **amount** of endotoxin present.

Immune Response

The immune response is complex and has multiple functions. Because of its complexity, the immune response can go awry in many ways and cause damage. **Innate immunity** refers to immune mechanisms that are always present and available for action. These responses tend to be less specific than acquired, adaptive immunity, but since they require no prior exposure to a pathogen to be active, they represent the first line against microbial invasion. Alternatively, **adaptive immune responses** are usually classified as humoral when they lead to the production of circulating antibodies or as cellular when special immune system cells seek out and destroy infected cells. Both responses can cause damage.

Humoral Immunity

Infecting agents elicit the formation of specific antibodies. In the circulation and tissues, antibodies combine with the infecting agents or with some of their soluble products. These antigen–antibody complexes evoke an inflammatory response by facilitating the activation of a complex set of serum proteins, the **complement system**. In the presence of antigen–antibody complexes, these proteins are activated by a series of proteolytic reactions, called the **classical pathway** of activation. The complement system can also be activated by the presence of microorganisms alone, through a process called the **alternative pathway.** The products of these proteolytic cleavages are pharmacologically active compounds. Some work on platelets and white cells to produce substances that increase vascular permeability and vasodilation. The result is edema, the outpouring of fluids into tissues. Other complement factors act on white blood cells, some as chemotaxins, others to make bacteria more easily phagocytized. These activities result in the mobilization of powerful defenses against invading microorganisms and inflammation.

Antigen–antibody complexes are sometimes deposited on the membrane of the glomeruli of the kidneys, resulting in impairment of kidney function, a condition called **glomerulonephritis**. This condition is seen in the aftermath of certain streptococcal and viral infections. Similar effects also take place in blood vessels, leading to visible skin rashes.

Cellular Immunity

A different type of response is expressed via special cells of the immune system and is called **cell-mediated immunity (CMI)**. This complex phenomenon leads to the activation and mobilization of macrophages, the powerful phagocytic cells that participate in the later stages of inflammation to clean up debris and remaining microorganisms.

CMI is associated with chronic inflammation, the histological changes that limit the spread of infections but also cause lesions in tissues. These damaging activities are characteristic of chronic infections, often caused by intracellular microorganisms and viruses. An example is chronic tuberculosis, in which the main damage to tissue is caused by CMI. The immune response is elicited by the tubercle bacilli, which are able to persist in cells for a long time. Pathological changes associated with CMI lead to the production of **tubercles** or **granulomas** and eventually to destruction of tissue cells.

It is worth repeating that although the immune responses can cause tissue damage, in most instances the price is well worth it. This point is illustrated in people who have genetic or acquired defects in their immune systems. Unfortunately, such people are no longer a medical rarity. The advent and spread of AIDS has placed hundreds of thousands of persons in this category. Immunocompromised patients are ravaged and later killed by microorganisms that cause little or no disease in healthy persons. In the immunocompetent person, for example, active tuberculosis causes much damage, but death only occurs after many years. In the immunocompromised patient, the disease can become rampant in a much shorter period.

OUTCOME

No infectious disease, be it mild or life threatening, is simple. Various properties of the invading agent and the host lead to an intricate and ever-changing interplay. It is not always possible to discern the relative roles of the known properties, let alone those that still await discovery. To complicate matters, humans are beset by a huge number of possible invaders. New ones emerge apparently under our very eyes, to be added to the long list.

Conclusion

The student of medical microbiology faces a demanding challenge. The fascination of the topic may not suffice to overcome its inherent problem of tremendous detail. The conceptual framework used in this chapter, which is based on the fact that all host–parasite interactions have steps in common, may be useful in mastering many of the details of microbiology. If these steps are kept in mind, the myriad facts will fall logically into place. As indicated at the beginning of this chapter, parasite and host must encounter one another, and the parasite must enter the host, spread, multiply, and eventually cause damage. All these steps require the breaching of host defenses. When studying the pathogenesis of infectious diseases, it is essential to remember that the outcome of microbial infection is usually the net result of offensive measures taken by the microbe and counteroffensive measures taken by the host.

Normal Microbial Flora

Barry I. Eisenstein and Moselio Schaechter

The human body normally contains thousands of species of bacteria and a smaller number of viruses, fungi, and protozoa. Most are commensal organisms, meaning they coexist with humans without causing harm. The members of the normal flora change with time, but their number at any instant is still formidable. Each person possesses an individualized spectrum of species and strains. In the words of the Romans, *suum quique*, to each his own.

What Is the Normal Flora?

Members of the normal flora are defined as microorganisms frequently found on or in the body of healthy persons (Fig. 2-1). Some of these organisms are found only in the bodies of humans or animals; others can also live freely in the environment.

A precise roll call of the organisms that constitute the normal flora is usually not possible, as discussed in Chapter 1. Consider, for instance, the meningococcus or the pneumococcus, both true pathogens capable of causing meningitis, pneumonia, or septicemia. Because both pathogens are found in the throats of about 10% of healthy people, they can be counted as members of the normal flora in these individuals but not in 90% of the population. Coming and going as sporadic denizens of a person's throat, such organisms could be called **transient** members of the normal flora of that individual. Obviously, these pathogens do not usually cause trouble in most colonized individuals. Not as obvious is that disease caused by either of the two organisms does not occur without prior **colonization.** Thus, colonization is necessary, but insufficient, for meningococcal or pneumococcal disease. Long-term colonization is not a universal prerequisite for all infections, many of which develop soon after entry of the infectious agent into the body. An example is the common cold.

The problem with many of the definitions in this field is that they are not absolute. The same problems that arise in precisely identifying the normal microbial flora pertain to terms such as **pathogenicity** and **virulence.** (These two terms are not identical, but the distinction between them is subtle.) As subsequent chapters will show, definitions of such terms depend not only on the properties of the infectious agent but also on the state of the defenses of the host. In addition, disease seldom results from the activities of the agent alone but often reflects the **responses of the host** as well. In many cases the signs and symptoms of infection are actually caused by the host's inflammatory response to the infection. A good analogy: firefighters occasionally add to the property destruction resulting from a fire by producing water damage as they try to contain the flames.

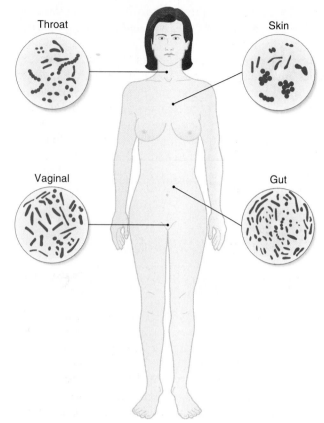

FIGURE 2-1 ▪ **The normal bacterial flora in a healthy person.** The typical bacteria seen in the microbe-laden sites of the body are shown in schematic fashion. Gram-positive bacteria are shown in purple, Gram-negative bacteria in red.

The objective of all living organisms, microbes included, is to grow and reproduce. In the human body the most successful microbe is the one that can rapidly and efficiently become two microbes. In describing the nature of success among organisms, pathogenicity or virulence is not considered. In fact, the most virulent pathogens, those that kill their hosts, may be poorly adapted for survival and represent recent biological associations. After all, why would guests paying no rent want to set fire to the house in which they live? Before exploring the world of pathogens (the "misfits"), it is instructive to consider first the body's normal guests who behave well—keeping in mind, though, that even the most domesticated among them can cause trouble if given the opportunity.

What Parts of the Body Are Typical Sites?

Among the parts of the body colonized by the normal flora, the following usually contain large amounts of microorganisms:

Skin: moist areas especially, such as the groin and between the toes

Respiratory tract: nose and oropharynx
Digestive tract: mouth and large intestine
Urinary tract: anterior parts of the urethra
Genital system: vagina

Bacteria, and to a lesser extent fungi and protozoa, reside and actively proliferate at these sites. Other parts of the body contain small numbers of microorganisms, most of which are in transit and do not usually colonize. Examples include the rest of the respiratory and digestive tracts, the **urinary bladder,** and the **uterus.** Finding pathogenic microorganisms at these sites is highly suggestive of disease but not proof. At the other extreme are certain tissues and organs that are usually sterile. The presence of microorganisms at these sites is usually diagnostically significant. These sites include **blood, cerebrospinal fluid, synovial fluid,** and **deep tissues** in general.

The number of bacteria in sites that contain thriving microbial communities varies widely. In some areas bacteria are almost as densely packed as is physically possible. For instance, the gingival pockets around teeth contain wall-to-wall bacteria. Normal feces are about one-third bacteria by weight. If the average bacterium were about $1\ \mu m^3$ in volume, the densest possible packing would result in a mass of 1×10^{12} per milliliter. Numbers like that are actually approached in certain parts of the body. In contrast, sites that are not quite as hospitable, such as the skin, mouth, and vagina, may harbor populations on the order of 1 million to 10 million bacteria per milliliter of fluid or per gram of scrapings.

How Do Microorganisms Persist in the Body?

To colonize the human body, invading microorganisms must be able to resist host mechanisms that could dislodge or kill them, as well as compete successfully with other microbial species. Picture a bacterial cell entering the mouth and the problems it faces trying to remain there. Strong liquid currents will wash the organism away unless it adheres to the surface of the teeth or the mucous membranes. In addition, saliva contains antibacterial compounds, such as enzymes and antibodies, although these substances are not equally damaging toward all bacterial species. At sites of the mouth not exposed to the flushing action of saliva, such as the crevasses of the gums, the bacterial cell will find a large resident flora already occupying the likely adherence sites. These resident organisms also produce antimicrobial substances, such as acids derived from their metabolism of sugars that may be hostile to the invader.

Although certain body sites are normally extensively colonized, trouble from the microbes only occasionally occurs at these sites. One example is the pneumonia caused by respiratory defenses lowered by, say, a poor cough reflex following a stroke or by smoking-induced paralysis of the ciliary clearance mechanisms. Under these conditions "aspiration pneumonia" is likely to occur. The bacteriologic etiology of such a pneumonia is highly dependent on the kinds of organisms that colonize the mouth or throat at the time of the aspiration. If the person is unlucky enough to be colonized with a virulent strain of pneumococcus, a small amount of material aspirated from the mouth or pharynx into the lungs is sufficient to cause severe pneumonia. In fact, most cases of pneumococcal pneumonia are not associated with obvious aspiration at all but rather with imperceptible microaspirations. If the oropharynx is not colonized with virulent bacteria, a significantly larger amount of aspirated material (i.e., a larger inoculum) must reach the lungs to cause disease.

Colonization involves both microbial and host factors. For example, an adhesive protein called **fibronectin** coats the mucosal surfaces of epithelial cells and has a strong predilection for Gram-positive organisms (see Chapter 3). Fibronectin is probably important in determining the nature of the bacterial flora in the mouth and pharynx, as suggested by the following findings. The oropharynx of individuals in poor general health, including many hospitalized patients, becomes deficient in fibronectin. With low levels of this protein, Gram-negative organisms tend to displace Gram-positives. The high incidence of Gram-negative pneumonia in hospitalized patients can be explained in part by adherence specificity.

The example of the mouth can be extended to the large intestine, vagina, perineum, skin, and other sites normally laden with microbes. It follows that colonization by new organisms is an unlikely event and that the successful colonizer must be unusually adept at resisting both host and microbial defenses. On the other hand, colonization of sites that are normally sterile or carry a sparse load of microorganisms (e.g., deep tissues and the small intestine) is not affected by microbial competition. Not surprisingly, host defenses are typically more intensive at such susceptible sites. Obviously, throughout our long history of coexistence and coevolution

with the microbial world, our bodies have designated territories that are safe to share—preferably, only with well-behaved guests—and others that are off limits. Foreign devices, such as plastic catheters stuck into arteries and veins, are notorious for upsetting the delicate ecological balance between microbes and host tissues.

The attributes that permit microbes to colonize the body make a long list and, to a large extent, determine what makes each pathogenic organism distinct. Such attributes will be discussed in detail in the chapters on individual organisms. Table 2-1 lists the classes of microbial properties that allow successful colonization.

Site Preferences of Some Infectious Agents

At first glance it may seem that microorganisms usually cause disease only in specific organs. To some extent, that statement is true: hepatitis viruses affect the liver; encephalitis and rabies viruses, the brain; the common cold viruses, the nasal epithelium. Some bacteria, like the cholera bacillus, have strong predilections (the small intestine, in this case), whereas others, like the staphylococcus, may infect almost any site of the body. Such preferences are known as **tissue tropism.** In some cases tissue tropism can be attributed to tissue-specific cellular properties, such as the presence of specific receptors on the surfaces of certain cells (e.g., fibronectin, with its affinity for Gram-positive bacteria). In other instances physical properties—the temperature of the organ, for instance—determine the tropism.

The complexities of tissue tropism can be illustrated using the gonococcus as an example. This bacterium most often causes infection of the urethra, but it can also affect the throat, rectum, or eyes. Where the lesion occurs in this disease depends on the **site of entry** of the organism. Pharyngeal and rectal gonorrhea are the result of nonvaginal intercourse, whereas ophthalmia (eye infection) is caused by the infection of the eyes of a neonate as it passes through the birth canal of the infected mother. Thus, the gonococcus has no absolute predilection for the mucous membrane of a given organ. What

table **2-1**	Issues in Bacterial Colonization
ANTICOLONIZING PROPERTY OF THE HOST	**HOW BACTERIA OVERCOME THE PROPERTY**
Sweep microbes away by liquid currents	Adhere to epithelial cells (e.g., gonococci stick to the mucous membrane of the urethra)
Kill microbes with host phagocytes	Avoid being taken up (e.g., the pneumococcus is surrounded by a slimy capsule that impairs uptake by neutrophils) Kill the phagocyte (e.g., certain streptococci produce a toxin that punches holes in the neutrophil membrane)
Starve microbes for lack of needed nutrients	Derive needed nutrients from host cells (e.g., certain staphylococci lyse red blood cells and use their hemoglobin as a source of iron)

about tissue other than mucosal epithelia? Some strains of gonococci survive in circulation and show a marked predilection for certain organs, such as the joints. Gonococcal arthritis is one of the most common complications of gonorrhea. Therefore, it is clear that gonococci have strong tropism for certain deep tissues, not only for epithelial membranes.

Affinity for host cell receptors is seen clearly in viruses and may explain why, in general, these agents are often tissue and organ specific. Influenza virus, for example, relies for its attachment on special glycoproteins found on the surface of respiratory epithelial cells. HIV, the virus that causes AIDS, attaches to protein receptors found selectively on certain lymphocytes and macrophages. Many research efforts, particularly in novel forms of antiviral therapy, are aimed at discovering ways to neutralize the action of receptors, thereby precluding infection by the agents that recognize them.

The temperature of an organ sometimes determines the location of the infectious agent. For example, the viruses of the common cold thrive in the nasal epithelium and not in internal organs, where high temperatures inhibit the viruses' growth. Likewise, the spirochete of syphilis is sensitive to higher-than-normal body temperatures, which induced certain physicians of the preantibiotic era to try to cure syphilis by injecting patients with the agent of malaria. Another example is the fungus that causes athlete's foot, which is confined to the skin because it does not grow at body temperature (athlete's foot of the liver is impossible).

Role of the Normal Flora

The most easily perceived manifestation of normal flora activity is the production of the various odors associated with epithelial surfaces of the human body. A germ-free human would not need deodorant. Beyond that, however, the normal flora plays a critical role in health and disease, as illustrated by the following examples.

Common Source of Infection

The normal flora is the source of many opportunistic infections. When commensal organisms find themselves in unaccustomed sites of the body, they may cause disease. For example, anaerobic bacteria, usually of the genus *Bacteroides*, are carried harmlessly in the intestines of normal persons but produce abscesses if they penetrate into deeper tissues via traumatic or surgical wounds. When *Bacteroides*-carrying fecal contents are spilled in the peritoneal cavity, as in the case of a burst appendix, the consequences can be dire. Staphylococci

from the skin and nose, or streptococci and Gram-negative cocci from the throat and mouth, are also responsible for this class of infections. In fact, *Staphylococcus epidermidis*, a prevalent species on the skin, has a strong propensity to attach to plastic prosthetic surfaces and can thus cause severe bloodstream infections in patients with intravenous catheters. Likewise, *Escherichia coli,* a normal inhabitant of the gastrointestinal tract, is the most common cause of urinary tract infection. In fact, physicians see more patients with diseases resulting from the normal flora than from agents acquired outside the body.

These facts point out that the definition of virulence is elusive and that no microorganism is intrinsically either benign or pathogenic. Under the right circumstances any microorganism that can grow in the body can cause disease. However, members of the normal flora do not all have the same pathogenic potential. Some cause disease more readily than others because they are endowed with special virulence properties. For example, when peritonitis is caused by the release of intestinal bacteria through a break in the gut wall, the resulting infection is usually caused by only a few bacterial species.

Virulence is not intrinsic to the microorganisms but depends also on the degree of immune competence of the host. Members of the normal flora often invade organs and tissues in immunocompromised patients. Thus, the yeast *Candida*, a harmless commensal found in about one third of all healthy people, is a common cause of bloodstream infection in patients undergoing vigorous cancer chemotherapy. *Pneumocystis carinii*, a common inhabitant of the lungs of healthy persons, can cause a specific kind of pneumonia and is one of the principal causes of death in patients with AIDS.

Immune Stimulation

Our repertoire of antibodies (immunoglobulins) partly reflects antigenic stimulation by the normal flora. In general, we do not have high antibody titers to the bacteria, viruses, and fungi that inhabit our body. Nonetheless, even in low concentrations, our antibodies serve as a defense mechanism, a clear benefit from our normal flora. Among the antibodies produced in response to bacterial stimulation are those of the IgA class, which are secreted through mucous membranes. Although the role of these immunoglobulins is not well understood, they likely are an important first line of defense and interfere, possibly on a daily basis, with the colonization of commensal organisms in deeper tissues.

Antibodies elicited by the antigenic challenge of the normal flora sometimes cross-react with normal tissue components. Relevant examples are antibodies against ABO blood group antigens. People that belong to the A group have anti-B antibodies, and conversely, B-group individuals have anti-A antibodies. People in the O group make both anti-A and anti-B antibodies. None of these antibodies is found in the newborn. What is the source of antigenic stimulation for these antibodies? On reflection the source is not obvious. Why should one make antibodies against a blood group different from one's own? Few of us come in contact with red blood cells of a different type, through transfusions of the wrong type of blood. The answer to this puzzle is that bacteria from the intestinal flora contain antigens that cross-react with both A and B blood antigens. These constituents are the source of antigenic stimulation. We make antibodies against foreign blood group antigens but not against those of our own group, because we are immunologically tolerant to the "self" antigens but not to the "foreign" ones.

This type of **cross-reactivity** does not usually cause disease. In fact, some evidence demonstrates that cross-reactivity between bacterial antigens can be protective. For example, antibodies against various bacteria that normally reside in the bowel have been shown to cross-react with the polysaccharide capsule of meningitis-producing strains of meningococci; the presence of the antibodies is protective against this form of bacterial meningitis. By contrast, it is possible for antibodies cross-reactive to microbial antigens to play an insidiously harmful role in health. For instance, the serious disease systemic lupus erythematosus is associated with the production of antibodies against the body's DNA. Some evidence suggests that the antigens setting off the production of these antibodies are not nucleic acids but may be cross-reacting bacterial lipopolysaccharides.

The importance of just a single molecule from the normal flora was demonstrated by experiments with germ-free mice. Animals colonized by the commensal organism *Bacteroides fragilis* expressing a wild type polysaccharide structure developed a healthy immune system. However, animals colonized with a polysaccharide mutant of *B. fragilis* had decreased numbers of splenic T-cells, atypical thymus development and aberrant Th1 cytokine responses.

Keeping Out Invaders

In some sites of the body, the normal flora helps keep out pathogens. Commensal bacteria have the physical advantage of **previous occupancy,** especially on epithelial surfaces. Some commensal bacteria produce substances that inhibit newcomers, such as antibiotics or lethal proteins called bacteriocins. It is not surprising, therefore, that colonization by a new species or a new strain is not a frequent event.

When most of the normal flora is wiped out with antibiotics, both exogenous and endogenous microorganisms are given the opportunity to cause disease. For example, after mice are given certain antibiotics, the infecting oral dose of a *Salmonella* strain decreases almost

a millionfold. Patients treated with antibiotics that are particularly effective in the gut may suffer from diarrhea caused by toxins produced from the overgrowth of a particular organism, *Clostridium difficile*. Severe infections with this bacterium result in a serious disease called pseudomembranous colitis (see Chapter 20). This organism is a minor member of the normal flora but can grow to a large population density when its neighbors are suppressed.

Role in Human Nutrition and Metabolism?

The normal flora of the intestine plays a role in human nutrition and metabolism, but little is known about the extent of its influence. Why has it proved difficult to investigate this role? Obviously, humans cannot be made "germ free" at will. Most of the information comes from work with animals, and its relevance to human nutrition is uncertain. Nonetheless, it is likely that a biomass as huge and metabolically active as that residing in the large intestine plays a role in the nutritional balance of the host. It is known, for instance, that several intestinal bacteria, such as *E. coli* and *Bacteroides*, synthesize vitamin K and thus may be important sources of that vitamin for human beings and animals.

The metabolism of several key compounds involves their excretion from the liver into the large intestine and their return from there to the liver. This enterohepatic circulatory loop is particularly important for sex steroid hormones and bile salts. The compounds are excreted through the bile in conjugated form as glucuronides or sulfate but cannot be reabsorbed in that form. Members of the intestinal bacterial flora make glucuronidases and sulfatases that deconjugate the compounds. The extent to which these activities are physiologically important is not yet known, but they have prompted some to call the large intestine a "second liver."

Source of Carcinogens?

The flora of the large intestine may produce **carcinogens.** The compounds we ingest are chemically transformed by the varied metabolic activities of the gut flora. Many potential carcinogens are active only after being modified. Some of the known modifications are carried out by enzymes of intestinal bacteria. For example, the artificial sweetener cyclamate (cyclohexamine sulfate) is converted to the active bladder carcinogen cyclohexamine by bacterial sulfatases. Evidence does implicate the normal flora as a risk factor for some cancers, but the importance is difficult to assess; consequently, this is a subject of considerable scrutiny (Box 2-1).

How Do We Study the Normal Flora?

Much of what we know about the role of the normal flora in nutrition and prevention of disease comes from studying animals reared under sterile conditions—the so-called germ-free animals. Rats and mice resemble humans in many physiological properties but differ in important details. Nonetheless, germ-free-animal research has produced interesting information.

A small mammal can be reared in the germ-free condition if it is placed in a sterile chamber after a cesarean birth. Chickens can be hatched from eggs whose shell surfaces have been sterilized. The germ-free chamber is equipped with gloves and ports to allow manipulation and the exchange of food and other material without breaking the sterile barrier. Many species of animals breed under these conditions, and large colonies can be established. It is even possible to obtain germ-free rats and mice from commercial suppliers.

In general, rodents thrive under germ-free conditions as long as their diets are supplemented with vitamins. They even gain weight faster than do conventional animals. As expected, a germ-free rodent's concentration of immunoglobulins is reduced, especially if its diet is chemically defined and does not contain antigenic compounds. One of the more interesting characteristics of germ-free animals is that the histology of their intestines is quite different from the usual. The most visible difference is in the lamina propria, which has only a few lymphocytes, plasma cells, and macrophages. By contrast, in conventional animals, the same tissue is heavily infiltrated with these cells. This finding suggests that the "normal" intestine is in a constant state of chronic inflammation.

Members of the Normal Flora

What types of microorganisms constitute the normal flora? Most are bacteria. We also carry viruses, fungi, protozoa, and occasionally worms, but in the healthy person these microorganisms are present in smaller numbers than are the bacteria. In the early days of microbiology, it was thought that most bacteria of the body were aerobes or facultative anaerobes. For a long time *E. coli* was believed to be one of the principal members of the fecal flora. This erroneous conclusion was based on the observation that most members of the normal bacteria flora are strict anaerobes and do not grow on media incubated in the ordinary manner in air. Only by using special techniques of anaerobic cultivation has it been realized that in the gingival pocket or in feces, strict anaerobes outnumber the others by 100 to 1 or more. Bacteria do not have to be located far from the air to find anaerobic conditions, because oxygen is not very soluble in water. Furthermore, the small amount of oxygen that diffuses into deeper tissue layers can readily be used by host cells or by actively metabolizing aerobes and facultative anaerobes. Thus, anaerobic conditions can be found a fraction of a millimeter below the surface.

Table 2-2 shows the distribution and occurrence of the most prominent bacteria in selected parts of the human body. It should be understood that the organisms listed, although the most frequently encountered, repre-

table **2-2**	**Frequent Types of Normal Bacterial Flora**					
	GRAM-POSITIVE			**GRAM-NEGATIVE**		
SITE	**COCCI**	**RODS**	**COCCI**	**RODS**	**OTHER**	
Skin	Staphylococcus	Corynebacterium, Propionibacterium acnes		Enteric bacilli (on some sites)		
Oropharynx	α-Hemolytic streptococci, Micrococcus	Corynebacterium	Neisseria	Haemophilus	Spirochetes	
Large intestine	Streptococcus (enterococci)	Lactobacillus Clostridium		Bacteroides Enteric bacilli		
Vagina	Streptococcus	Lactobacillus		Bacteroides	Mycoplasma	

sent only a minute fraction of the number of genera and species represented. The total number of taxonomic groups is probably well in the thousands. For example, in a particularly detailed study, the intestinal flora of just one person yielded about 400 distinct species of bacteria.

Newborn babies become colonized very rapidly by a varied microbial flora, especially in their intestines. In animals and probably in humans, organisms appear according to a specific time sequence. The earliest colonizers are *E. coli*, streptococci, and some clostridia. Within 24 hours or so, lactobacilli appear, followed within a few days by the major anaerobes that characterize the normal intestinal flora.

Little is known about why species vary in their colonizing capacity and in their ability to compete with others. It seems likely that specific properties of bacteria, such as their pili, allow them to attach and survive in various microenvironments within the intestine. Thus, the microbial flora is different at the base of the intestinal crypts, in the mucus that covers the villi, and in the lumen of the gut. Normally, the intestinal flora of one individual is remarkably constant. This stability suggests that each successful colonizer is equipped with powerful devices to withstand the challenge from newly ingested microorganisms.

Conclusion

Our knowledge about the role of the normal flora in health and disease is derived largely from a few circumstances, including studies with germ-free animals and observation of patients on antibiotics. We are left with the realization that from an immunological and microbiological point of view, the normal flora contributes to the maintenance of health mainly by excluding potential invaders and possibly by long-term immunological stimulation. Nutritionally, the microbial biomass within us plays a role in recycling certain important compounds and probably in supplying vitamin K. However, members of the normal flora are opportunistic pathogens and may cause disease when present in tissues and organs not typically colonized. We do not have the choice of living in a germ-free environment. In our microbe-laden world, it is reasonable to conclude that the normal microbial flora is adapted to do more good than harm.

Biology of Infectious Agents

Moselio Schaechter

What do future health practitioners want to know about microbes? Mainly, how pathogenic microbes harm the host and what can be done about it. Knowing this requires more than understanding how microbes cause disease. For example, features of bacterial anatomy and metabolism have suggested targets for the successful development of powerful antibiotics. Similarly, unraveling the details of viral structures and metabolism has led to the production of protective vaccines and to antiviral therapy.

Prokaryotic and Eukaryotic Pathogens

The world of pathogenic microbiology spans the largest cleft in the living world—the one between the prokaryotes and the eukaryotes. Bacteria belong to the prokaryotes, whereas fungi, protozoa, and worms are eukaryotes. There is another group of prokaryotes, the archaea, but none have yet been found to be of medical importance. Prokaryotes lack nuclei and other internal membrane-bound organelles. They do not carry out endocytosis and are incapable of ingesting particles or liquid droplets. Prokaryotes differ from eukaryotes in important biochemical details, such as the composition of their ribosomes and lipids (Fig. 3-1). Prokaryotes are usually haploid, with a single chromosome and extrachromosomal plasmids; most eukaryotes have a diploid phase and many chromosomes.

Differences in organization between prokaryotes and eukaryotes have important consequences for the way they synthesize certain macromolecules. For instance, the lack of a nuclear membrane allows prokaryotes to simultaneously synthesize proteins and messenger RNA molecules. In other words, **translation** (protein synthesis) can be coupled to **transcription** and therefore begin rapidly on new messenger RNA (mRNA) chains. In eukaryotes the two processes cannot be directly linked. Transcripts of heterogeneous nuclear RNA must first be processed in the nucleus before they are transported across the nuclear membrane to the ribosomes in the cytoplasm. Only then can eukaryotic protein synthesis take place.

Table 3-1 compares the regulation of gene expression between *Escherichia coli*, a bacterium, and the best known of the unicellular eukaryotes, a yeast. A review of basic biochemistry and molecular biology may be appropriate to understand this material.

Bacteria's Complex Envelopes and Appendages

Going from the outside inward, bacteria are surrounded by a complex set of surface layers and appendages that differ in composition from species to species. Some of these structures are useful only in certain environments, such as the human body, and may be dispensable under laboratory conditions. These surface components often determine whether an organism can survive in a particular environment and cause disease.

Like all cells, bacteria have an essential structure, the **cytoplasmic membrane**. Most bacteria also possess structures outside the membrane—namely, a **cell wall**—and some have an **outer membrane, flagella, pili,** and a **capsule.** These outer structures can amount to 10 to 20% of the dry weight of the cell (as in other organisms, the wet weight of bacteria is about two-thirds water). The reason for the extra layers outside the cell membrane becomes clear if one considers the stresses that bacteria must face in natural surroundings. For example, intestinal bacteria such as *E. coli* are exposed to bile salts that would dissolve an unprotected cell membrane.

Bacteria use envelope layers and appendages to adhere to surfaces and for protection from phagocytes and other threats.

During colonization by microbes, the immune system of the host first senses the surface components of the invading microbes. Consequently, many of the properties of the surface constituents are relevant both to the establishment of infection and to the response of the host to the organisms. The strongest antibody response to bacterial antigens is usually directed to surface antigens.

Protection of the Cytoplasmic Membrane

Bacteria use three principal means to protect their cytoplasmic membrane from environmental stresses, such as low osmotic pressure or the presence of detergents. These solutions are represented by the **Gram-positive, Gram-negative,** and **acid-fast** bacteria. Figure 3-2 illustrates the first two.

Gram staining (named after Dr. H. C. J. Gram, the Danish microbiologist who devised the method in

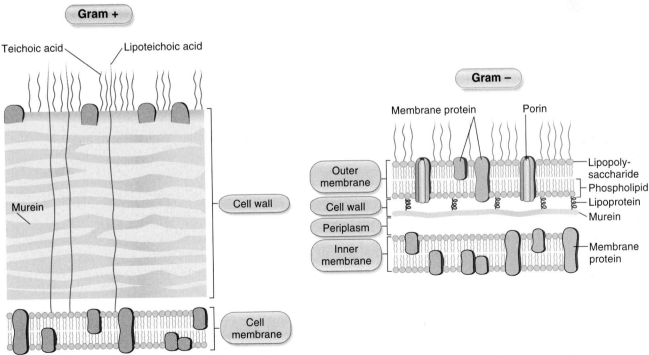

FIGURE 3-2 ▪ **The envelope structure of Gram-positive (left) and Gram-negative (right) bacteria.** Capsules and appendages are not shown, nor are surface proteins like the M protein of streptococci. Note the 20-fold greater amount of peptidoglycan, or murein, in the Gram-positive. The outer membrane of the Gram-negative envelope has a covering of lipopolysaccharide molecules. The Gram-negative's outer membrane also has pores made of trimers of porin, which permit the entry of small hydrophilic molecules.

table **3-2**	**Gram Stain and Acid-Fast Procedures**
GRAM STAIN	**ACID–FAST STAIN**
1. Stain with crystal violet (purple)	1. Stain with hot carbol–fuchsin (red)
2. Modify with potassium iodide	2. Decolorize with acid alcohol; only acid-fast remain red
3. Decolorize with alcohol; only Gram-positives remain purple	3. Counterstain with methylene blue: acid-fast remain red; others become blue
4. Counterstain with safranin: Gram-negatives become pink; Gram-positives remain purple	

1884) divides most bacteria into two groups, nearly equal in number and importance. The staining procedure is central in microbiology and, in due course, should be learned by every medical student. In brief, Gram staining depends on the ability of certain bacteria (the Gram-positives) to retain a complex of a purple dye and iodine when challenged with a brief alcohol wash (Table 3-2). Gram-negatives do not retain the dye and can later be counterstained with a red dye, safranin. This distinction turns out to be correlated with fundamental differences in the cell envelopes of the two classes of bacteria.

Gram-Positive Solution

A gram-positive bacterium protects its cytoplasmic membrane with a thick **cell wall.** The major constituent of the wall is a complex polymer **unique to bacteria,** composed of sugars and amino acids called **murein,** or **peptidoglycan** (Fig. 3-3). Murein is the critical component in maintaining

the shape and rigidity of both Gram-positives and Gram-negatives but plays a larger role in protecting the cell membranes of Gram-positives.

How does murein contribute to the defense of cell integrity? Murein is composed of glycan (sugar) chains that are cross-linked to one another via peptides. The overall structure of murein is similar in all cases, but some variation in chemical details occurs (Fig. 3-4). This polymeric fabric is wrapped around the length and width of the bacterium to form a sac of the size and shape of the organism. Depending on the shape of the murein sac, bacteria may be shaped like rods (**bacilli**), spheres (**cocci**), or helices (**spirilla**). The rigid murein corset allows bacteria to survive in media of lesser osmotic pressure than that of their cytoplasm. In the absence of a rigid structure to push against, the membrane bursts and the cells lyse. This can be demonstrated experimentally by removing the murein with **lysozyme,** a murein-hydrolytic enzyme present in many human and animal tissues. Treatment with lysozyme causes bacteria to lyse in a low-osmotic-pressure environment. If lysozyme-treated bacteria are kept in an isoosmotic medium, they

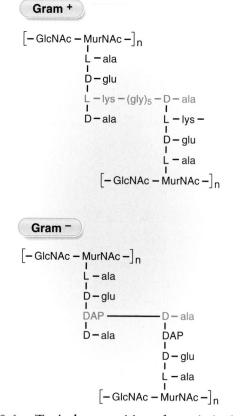

FIGURE 3-4 ▪ **Typical composition of murein in Gram-positive and Gram-negative bacteria.** In Gram-positives, peptide chains are cross-linked through a peptide (a pentaglycine in *Staphylococcus aureus*) between the free amino group of lysine and the terminal carboxyl group of a D-alanine residue. In the Gram-negatives, the cross-link is between diaminopimelic acid and D-alanine.

FIGURE 3-3 ▪ **Structure of murein.** The polysaccharide (glycan) strands consist of alternating units of N-acetylglucosamine and N-acetylmuramic acid connected to a peptide. Some of the peptides of one strand are cross-linked to those of another. Because of cross-linking, murein has a two-dimensional structure resembling a chain-linked fence.

FIGURE 3-5 ▪ **Teichoic acid structure.** The repeating units of ribitol and glycerol teichoic acids are shown. The chains in Gram-positive organisms vary in length and amounts.

do not lyse but become spherical. Such structures are called **spheroplasts.**

The cell wall of a Gram-positive is composed of many layers of the saclike murein. The layers are so thick that they impede the passage of hydrophobic compounds. The reason for this is that the sugars and charged amino acids of murein make the highly polar structure surrounding these cells a dense hydrophilic layer. Thus, many Gram-positives can withstand certain noxious hydrophobic compounds, including bile salts in the intestine. (The feature that makes bacteria Gram-positive—the ability to retain the dye–iodine complex—also seems to depend on the characteristic murein structure of the Gram-positive wall.)

Gram-positive walls contain other unique polymers, such as **teichoic acids,** which are chains of ribitol or glycerol linked by phosphodiester bonds (Fig. 3-5). Teichoic acids will be discussed in connection with individual groups of bacteria, because some of these acids appear to play a role in pathogenesis.

Gram-Negative Solution

Gram-negatives have adopted a radically different solution to the problem of protection of the cytoplasmic membrane. These bacteria build a completely different structure, an **outer membrane,** outside the murein cell wall (see Fig. 3-2). The outer membrane is chemically distinct from the usual biological membranes and is able to resist damaging chemicals. It is a bilayered structure, but its outer leaflet contains a unique component in addition to phospholipids. This component is a bacterial **lipopolysaccharide (LPS),** a complex molecule not found elsewhere in nature and one that deserves further attention.

LPS has three components (Fig. 3-6):

- **Lipid A:** This lipid anchors LPS in the outer leaflet of the membrane. Lipid A is an unusual glycolipid composed of disaccharides to which are attached short-chain fatty acids and phosphate groups.
- **Core:** This component consists of a short series of sugars that are nearly the same in most Gram-negative bacteria and includes two characteristic sugars, **keto-deoxyoctanoic acid** and a **heptose.**
- **O antigen:** This is a long carbohydrate chain of up to 40 sugars in length. The hydrophilic carbohydrate chains of the O antigen cover the bacterial surface and exclude hydrophobic compounds. The importance of the O-antigen chains is shown with mutants deficient in their biosynthesis. Mutants that make either no O antigen or merely shortened chains become sensitive to hydrophobic compounds such as bile salts and antibiotics to which the wild type is resistant.

Thus, exclusion of hydrophobic compounds in Gram-negative bacteria, as in Gram-positive bacteria, relies on surrounding the cells with hydrophilic polysaccharides,

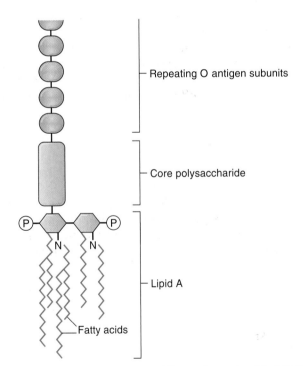

FIGURE 3-6 ▪ **The structure of lipopolysaccharide (LPS).** LPS consist of three portions. Lipid A is a phosphorylated disaccharide to which fatty acids are attached. The fatty acids vary with the organism but are always responsible for the hydrophobicity of the molecule. In a typical *Salmonella*, region I shows a characteristic series of sugars in the polysaccharide: the core polysaccharide, which consists of a variable and an invariant portion, and the O antigen, made up of repeating sugar subunits. Highly variable, the O antigen is the main reason for the different antigenic specificities among Gram-negative bacteria.

although these polysaccharides differ in structure and organization in the two groups. Because of its lipid nature, the outer membrane of Gram-negatives could be expected to exclude hydrophilic compounds as well. If so, nothing could cross the membrane. However, by dealing with the problem of protecting the cytoplasmic membrane, the Gram-negative bacteria appear to have created a new one. How do they transport their nutrients? One possible solution would be to use the same active transport devices of the cytoplasmic membrane copied in the outer membrane. However, this not only would be wasteful but probably would be incompatible with the protective role assigned to the outer membrane. Once again, bacteria have found an interesting solution. The outer membrane has special **channels** that permit the passive diffusion of hydrophilic compounds like sugars, amino acids, and certain ions. These channels consist of protein molecules with holes, aptly called **porins.** Porin channels are narrow—just the right size to permit the entry of compounds of up to 600 to 700 daltons (see Fig. 3-2). The channels are small enough that hydrophobic compounds come in contact with the polar "wall" of the channel and are thereby excluded.

Certain **hydrophilic** compounds that are sometimes necessary for survival are larger than the exclusion limit of porins. These larger molecules include vitamin B_{12}, sugars larger than trisaccharides, and iron in the form of chelates. Each hydrophilic compound crosses the outer membrane by a unique permeation mechanism that uses proteins especially designed to translocate that compound. Thus, the outer membrane allows the passage of small hydrophilic compounds; excludes hydrophobic compounds, large or small; and allows the entry of some larger hydrophilic molecules by specially dedicated mechanisms.

The dual-membrane system of Gram-negative bacteria creates a compartment called the **periplasmic space,** or **periplasm,** on the outside of the cytoplasmic or inner membrane. This compartment contains the murein layer and a gel-like solution of components that facilitate nutrition. Among these components are degradative enzymes (phosphatases, nucleases, proteases, etc.) that break down large and impermeable molecules to "digestible" size. In addition, the periplasm contains so-called **binding proteins** that help soak up sugars and amino acids from the medium. It also contains enzymes that inactivate antibiotics such as penicillins and cephalosporins, the β-lactamases. Gram-positive bacteria do not have a defined periplasmic compartment and secrete similar enzymes into the medium.

The outer membrane barrier constitutes both an advantage and a disadvantage for Gram-negative bacteria. For example, some bacteriophages use outer membrane proteins as attachment sites for infecting their host bacteria. On the other hand, the outer membrane confers considerable resistance to many antibiotics. Broadly speaking, Gram-negative bacteria are more resistant to antibiotics, especially penicillin. In general, this complex architecture must work very well because in nature (but not necessarily in the human body) Gram-negatives outnumber Gram-positives. The peculiarly Gram-negative solution to the problem of protecting the cytoplasmic membrane has unexpected biological consequences. The lipopolysaccharide of the outer membrane is highly reactive in the host. The lipid A component has a large number of biological activities. It elicits fever and activates a series of immunological and biochemical events that lead to the mobilization of host defense mechanisms. In large doses this compound, also known as **endotoxin,** can cause shock and even death (see Chapter 9). The O-antigen portion, as the name denotes, is highly antigenic. O antigens come in many varieties, each defining a species or a subspecies of Gram-negative bacteria.

Acid-Fast Solution

A few bacterial types, notably the tubercle bacillus, have developed yet another way to confront environmental challenges to the cytoplasmic membrane. Their cell walls contain large amounts of **waxes,** which are complex long-chain hydrocarbons with sugars and other modifying groups. Having such a protective cover, these organisms are relatively impervious to many harsh chemicals, including acids. If a dye is introduced into these cells—for instance, by brief heating—it cannot be removed by dilute hydrochloric acid, as would be the case in all other bacteria. These organisms are therefore called acid fast or acid resistant (see Table 3-2).

The waxy coat is interlaced with murein, polysaccharides, and lipids. This covering enables the organisms not only to resist the action of many noxious chemicals but also to avoid being killed by white blood cells. The cost of this protection, however, is that these organisms grow very slowly, possibly because the rate of uptake of nutrients is limited by the waxy covering. Some, like the human tubercle bacillus, divide once every 24 hours.

Murein and Antibiotics That Inhibit Its Synthesis

The uniqueness of the bacterial murein makes it a natural target for antibiotics. Drugs that block its formation lead to lysis and death of susceptible bacteria. It is not surprising, therefore, that some of the most clinically effective antibiotics—the **penicillins, cephalosporins,** and **carbapenems** (collectively, the β-lactams)—act by inhibiting murein synthesis. They are among the antibiotics that are most unequivocally bactericidal and least

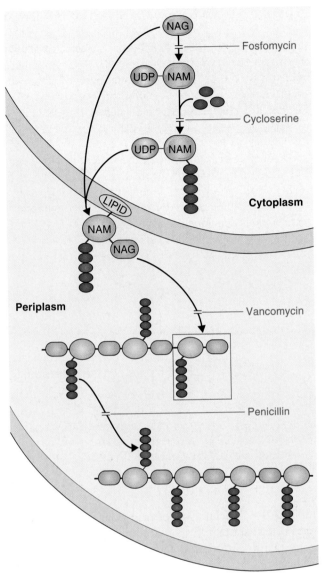

FIGURE 3-7 ▪ **Biosynthesis of murein, indicating the site of action of a number of antibiotics.** The successive steps occurring in the cytoplasm, at the cytoplasmic membrane, and outside the membrane (in the periplasm of Gram-negatives; in the murein layer of Gram-positives) are indicated, along with the points of attack of cycloserine, bacitracin, vancomycin, and penicillin.

toxic to humans. The critical steps in their mode of action are presented in Figure 3-7.

Murein, like many other polysaccharides, is synthesized from nucleotide-bound building blocks. These monomeric precursors consist of uridine diphosphate plus either N-acetylglucosamine (GlcNAc) or N-acetylmuramic acid (an unusual sugar, the 3-O-D lactic acid derivative of GlcNAc). The latter has a peptide chain attached to it (see Fig. 3-3). The monomeric units are made in the cytoplasm and transferred from uridine diphosphate to a **lipid carrier** in the membrane (see Fig. 3-7). Disaccharides are then linked to a growing chain of

murein. This step is inhibited by the antibiotic **vancomycin.** Regeneration of the lipid carrier is inhibited by another antibiotic, **bacitracin.**

The final reaction in murein synthesis is transpeptidation. The long chains of disaccharides are cross-linked to make a two-dimensional network (see Fig. 3-3). Cross-linking requires the formation of a peptide bond between D-alanine on one chain and the free N terminus of a lysine or a diaminopimelic acid on the other chain. The link is formed with the **subterminal** D-alanine, the **terminal** D-alanine being cleaved away in the process. Thus, the reaction is the exchange of one peptide bond (that between the two D-alanines) with another—a true transpeptidation. The amino acids that make up the peptides vary in different organisms, but the D-alanine cross-bridge to either lysine or diaminopimelic acid is universal. Penicillins and cephalosporins inhibit this reaction.

The reason why penicillin inhibits transpeptidation may lie in its stereochemical similarity with the D-alanine–D-alanine dimer (Fig. 3-8). In the presence of the drug, the transpeptidase becomes confused: instead of synthesizing an intermediate D-alanine–enzyme complex, it makes a lethal penicilloyl–enzyme complex.

Antibiotics that inhibit murein synthesis almost invariably kill bacteria by lysing them. In contrast with lysozyme, these drugs do not affect the murein itself, only its synthesis. How then do they cause lysis? When treated with these drugs, the cells continue to synthesize their cytoplasmic components and increase in mass. Because the enlarged cytoplasm is not restrained by a properly cross-linked murein sac, the cell contents extrude and the cells lyse. Cells that are not growing are not lysed by penicillin because they are not increasing in mass. Would it therefore be advisable to administer an antibiotic that inhibits cell growth at the same time that the patient is receiving penicillin?

Penicillin   **D-ala–D-ala**

FIGURE 3-8 ▪ **The resemblance of part of the penicillin structure to the backbone of the D-alanine–D-alanine dimer.** The arrows indicate the bonds broken during covalent attachment to the enzyme involved.

The simple concept that cells lyse by outgrowing their coats encounters some difficulties. First, cultures treated with penicillin usually include a small number of "persisters," bacteria that stop growing but do not lyse. Second, for some types of bacteria, penicillin is bacteriostatic, not bactericidal. These bacteria are called "tolerant." What is the explanation for persisters or tolerant bacteria? It appears that tolerant organisms are deficient in an **autolysin,** a bacterial enzyme that cleaves murein. Bacteria use such an enzyme to break open some bonds of murein at the septum, which permits the separation of daughter cells during cell division. Normally, the activity of autolysin is tightly controlled. Treatment with penicillin may arouse it to more-unrestrained action. The role of autolysin in penicillin-induced lysis is well illustrated by pneumococci, which are extraordinarily susceptible to lysis. Autolysin-defective mutants are found among penicillin-resistant derivatives; even strong detergents do not lyse these mutants. Thus, rather than a spontaneous explosion, lysis involves active steps of self-destruction.

There are exceptions to the universal use of murein to maintain bacterial cell integrity. The mycoplasmas are a group of bacteria that have no murein and consequently are not rigid and have almost no defined shape. As expected, they are resistant to penicillin. Some, like an agent of pneumonia, *Mycoplasma pneumoniae,* contain sterols in their membranes, an unusual feature among prokaryotes. It is puzzling how mycoplasmas cope well without rigid cell walls. Although these organisms are quite delicate in culture, they are common in the human body and in the environment. Other exceptions to the ubiquity of mureins exist, especially among a separate group of prokaryotes, the archaea. In addition, some bacteria, such as the anthrax bacillus, have an outside covering made up of especially tough proteins, called the S layer. Thus, bacteria safeguard their integrity with a variety of strategies.

Cytoplasmic Membrane

The cytoplasmic membrane of bacteria is a busy place. It assumes functions that in eukaryotic cells are divided up among the plasma membrane and intracellular organelles. Most critical is its role in the uptake of substrates from the medium. Bacteria take up mainly small-molecular-weight compounds and only rarely macromolecules and phosphate esters. Such compounds are usually hydrolyzed by enzymes in the periplasm or the surrounding medium, and the resulting breakdown products—peptides, oligosaccharides, nucleosides, and phosphate, among others—can then be transported across the cytoplasmic membrane.

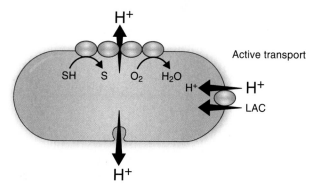

FIGURE 3-9 ▪ **Mechanisms of transport.** The three types of transport in *E. coli* are facilitated diffusion, group translocation, and active transport with the *lac* permease.

The cytoplasmic membrane contains specific carrier proteins, called **permeases,** that facilitate the entry of most metabolites. In some cases the carrier facilitates the equilibration of a compound inside and outside the cell (Fig. 3-9). However, carrier-mediated transport usually requires the expenditure of energy. This permits the internal concentration of certain substances to be as much as 10^5 times higher than that in the medium surrounding the cell.

Transport Across the Cytoplasmic Membrane

The three main versions of transport are illustrated in Figure 3-9.

1. **Facilitated diffusion:** A substance, such as glycerol, is carried across the membrane down a concentration gradient. This mechanism does not concentrate compounds in the inside of the cells relative to the outside

environment. Uptake is driven by intracellular use of the compound. For instance, the concentration of free glycerol inside cells is lowered by its phosphorylation to glycerol-3-phosphate. More glycerol is then taken up to equilibrate with the outside concentration.

2. **Group translocation:** Also known as phosphorylation-linked transport, this energy-dependent mechanism is used to transport certain sugars. Substances transported in this manner are chemically altered in the process. The example of glucose is shown in Figure 3-9. The sugar binds to a specific carrier in the membrane (e.g., the enzyme E_2 shown in the figure). Subsequent enzymatic steps yield glucose-6-phosphate, which can then be further metabolized.

3. **Active transport:** Energy is used to drive the accumulation of substrate. A substrate—for instance, the sugar lactose—is concentrated unchanged inside the cell, which makes the transport of additional molecules energetically unfavorable. To drive the transport of lactose, the cells use energy stored in an electrochemical gradient of protons, the **proton motive force.** This gradient is generated by the extrusion of protons from the cell, resulting from the oxidation of metabolic intermediates like reduced nicotinamide adenine dinucleotide (NADH) or by hydrolysis of adenosine triphosphate (ATP). Lactose is accumulated intracellularly by coupling its **energetically unfavorable** transport with the **energetically favorable** reentry of protons into the relatively alkaline cytoplasm of the cell. Thus, transport of this type takes place via a **symport,** which requires the simultaneous uptake of positive hydrogen and sugar molecules.

Each type of transport system involves specific protein molecules. Some proteins aid the process by modifying or concentrating substrates in the periplasmic space of Gram-negatives. These **binding proteins** are specific for sugars, nucleotides, and so on. The periplasmic space also contains nucleosidases, nucleases, peptidases, proteases, and other hydrolytic enzymes. The actual transport process is carried out by membrane-bound carriers, or **permeases,** which are involved in all three types of transport. We do not have a physical picture of how permeases respond to the proton gradient, but we know that they assume different configurations inside and outside the cytoplasmic membrane. Thus, permeases have a high affinity for substrate on the outside and low affinity on the inside. However they work, they are essential for transport. For example, in the much-studied lactose system, cells that lack a functional permease remain impervious to the sugar, even when soaked in concentrations approaching syrup.

The three mechanisms of transport are used to different extents by different bacteria. In general, few substrates equilibrate across membranes without the expenditure of energy. Among the energy-requiring mechanisms, group translocations are used to a different extent. *E. coli,* for instance, transports a wide variety of

sugars in this way, whereas strictly aerobic bacteria use it little. All in all, active transport dominates the repertoire of transport mechanisms in bacteria, especially when nutrients must be concentrated from the medium to support cell growth.

Uptake of Iron

The uptake of iron deserves special mention. Free iron is extremely scarce in the blood and many tissues because it is bound by proteins like transferrin or ceruloplasmin. It is essential for the growth of bacteria, and many species that inhabit the human body have developed ingenious mechanisms to obtain the amounts of this element they need for growth. They excrete chelating compounds, known as **siderophores,** that bind iron with great avidity. Each organism can take up its own particular form of complexed iron; individual complexes are unique enough to be less digestible for other organisms. However, in response to the competition for iron, many bacteria have multiple siderophores and uptake systems, thus trying to gain an edge on the other organisms in the same environment; some can efficiently extract iron from transferrin, an advantage at our expense.

Other Functions of the Bacterial Membrane

The cytoplasmic membrane of bacteria is also where **cytochromes** are located and **oxidative metabolism** is carried out. It thus performs the role of the mitochondria of eukaryotic cells. The membrane is also the location of nascent proteins destined either for secretion or incorporation in the membrane itself. Some bacteria secrete as much as 10% of all the proteins they make, including toxins and other virulence factors. The nascent peptide chains that a hydrophobic "signal sequences" at the N termini are translocated from ribosomes across the cytoplasmic membrane by an energy-requiring mechanism. Note that Gram-negative bacteria have the added problem of transporting proteins to the outer membrane. It is not known exactly how that takes place.

Some bacteria have also an exceptional ability to take up enormously long DNA molecules. The phenomenon was first demonstrated by genetic transformation of pneumococci and occurs among other bacteria. Little is known about bacteria's mechanism of uptake of DNA, but like active transport, it depends on the proton motive force.

In spite of its versatility and range of activities, the cytoplasmic membrane of bacteria is rarely the site of useful antibiotic action (see Chapter 5). Could one possible reason for this be that the membrane's overall structure is similar to that of the eukaryotic cell membrane?

DNA and Chromosome Mechanics

The genome of most bacteria consists of a **single circular chromosome** of double-stranded DNA. However, some species have a linear chromosome, and others have more than one. The chromosome of *E. coli* has about **5 million base pairs.** This codes for about 2,000 to 3,000 genes, over half of which have been identified. The total DNA sequence of hundreds of bacterial genomes is at hand, and many more are forthcoming.

Bacteria must solve a demanding topological problem in organizing their DNA because it is a long, thin molecule. If stretched out, DNA would be about 1,000 times the length of the cell. If a bacterium were to be magnified to the size of a human being, its DNA would be about a mile long. The DNA is coiled in a central irregular structure called the **nucleoid.** Its physical state is unknown and somewhat mysterious, because in the test tube a solution 100 times more dilute is a gel. Roughly all that is known about the physical state of the DNA is that it is twisted into **supercoils** (analogous to twisted telephone coils) and that this condition is indispensable for its organization, its replication, and the transcription of a number of genes. Supercoiling depends on balancing the actions of two topoisomerases. One of these, **DNA gyrase,** introduces supercoils into circular DNA, an action counteracted by a second enzyme, **topoisomerase I,** which relaxes the supercoils by making single-strand nicks.

Like all macromolecular synthesis, DNA replication has three stages: initiation, elongation, and termination. Replication takes place bidirectionally; that is, DNA synthesis starts at a precise place on the chromosome, the **replicative origin,** and proceeds away from it in both directions. The two moving polymerase complexes meet halfway around the chromosome. To replicate, the DNA helix in *E. coli* must unwind and rotate at some 6,000 rpm. One wonders how this can take place without entanglement of the tightly coiled nucleoid.

The **timing of chromosome replication** is a highly regulated process and is coupled to growth and cell division. At a given temperature the **rate of DNA polymerase movement is nearly independent of the growth rate** of the cells. In *E. coli*, DNA replication takes 40 minutes, whether the cells are growing slowly or quickly. In slow-growing cells (e.g., those dividing once every 100 minutes) one round of synthesis occurs in each division cycle, and no DNA is synthesized during the remaining 60 minutes. In fast-growing cells (e.g., those dividing every 20 minutes), initiation of rounds of replication is adapted to produce new chromosomes as often as the cell divides (Fig. 3-10). Since each chromosome requires 40 minutes to be synthesized, replication will initiate

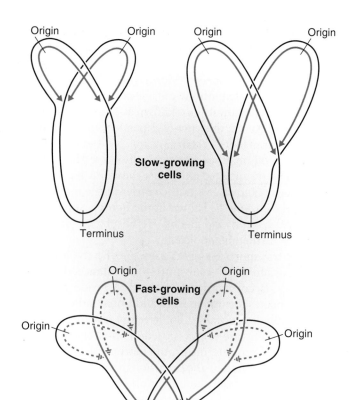

FIGURE 3-10 ▪ **Replication of DNA in slow-growing and fast-growing *E. coli*.** Replication begins at a specific site, the origin, and proceeds in both directions toward a terminus. The process takes about 40 minutes at 37°C. In a culture doubling every 20 minutes, the process must initiate every 20 minutes—that is, before the previous round of replication has terminated. In such cultures the DNA is undergoing multifork replication.

again on a strand long before its own replication has completed. Thus, chromosome replication in bacteria is regulated by how often the process gets started—that is, by the frequency of initiation of DNA synthesis.

How do antibiotics inhibit DNA metabolism? Most inhibitors of DNA replication bind to DNA and are too toxic for clinical use. An interesting exception is **metronidazole,** a drug that is inert but can be selectively modified to an active form by some bacteria. This compound contains a nitro group that must be **partially** reduced to render the molecule active. Full reduction to the amino state makes the molecule inactive again. Partial reduction is achieved by anaerobic bacteria but only rarely by the cells of the human body or by aerobic bacteria.

Partially reduced metronidazole is incorporated into the DNA of the bacteria. This is an example of **lethal synthesis** because the metronidazole-containing DNA molecules are unstable. It follows that metronidazole and related drugs are particularly useful against anaerobic bacteria and against amebas, which also grow anaerobically. These drugs, however, are not ideal. To a small extent, the partial reduction to active agents occurs in normal tissue, leading to possible mutagenesis and perhaps carcinogenesis.

Other DNA inhibitors act selectively by binding to specific enzymes involved in DNA supercoiling. **Nalidixic acid,** for example, inhibits DNA gyrase and is bactericidal. The more-stable fluorinated derivatives of nalidixic acid, the **fluoroquinolones,** interfere with DNA gyrase or topoisomerase and cause double-stranded DNA breaks.

Gene Expression: Uniqueness of Prokaryotic RNA Polymerase and Ribosomes

The bacterial cytoplasm is composed largely of proteins (about 40% of the dry weight, with about 1 million molecules per cell) and RNA (up to 35% of the dry weight in rapidly growing cells). Bacterial **ribosomes** have smaller subunits and smaller RNA molecules than do their eukaryotic counterparts. Bacterial ribosomal RNAs make up the small and large ribosomal subunits with 21 and 35 different proteins, respectively. These subunits join in the complete ribosomes, which move along messenger RNA molecules to synthesize proteins.

The large requirement for proteins makes **protein synthesis** the **principal biosynthetic activity** of rapidly growing bacteria. A large proportion of a bacterium's energy and metabolic building blocks is devoted to the assembly of the protein-synthesizing machinery, including ribosomes and RNA polymerase. Over a considerable range of growth rates, **RNA is made at a rate proportional to the number of RNA polymerase molecules** engaged in the process of transcription. Likewise, the rate of protein synthesis is proportional to the cellular concentration of ribosomes. This suggests that, as with DNA replication, the rate of polymerization of single chains of RNA or protein remains constant whether cells are growing rapidly or slowly. Thus, the synthesis of the principal macromolecules of bacteria is **regulated mainly by the frequency with which each chain is initiated** and **not** so much by altering their rate of manufacture of each molecule (i.e., the speed of **chain elongation**).

Antibiotics act selectively at **initiation** or **elongation** of macromolecular synthesis. For example, **rifampin,** a powerful inhibitor of bacterial transcription, acts at the initiation step. How does it recognize this step? The drug binds strongly to molecules of RNA polymerase that are floating freely in the cytoplasm but much less strongly to polymerase molecules that are bound to DNA. As a result, a polymerase that is bound to DNA and has initiated RNA synthesis will not be inactivated by rifampin until it completes its round of RNA synthesis and is released from the DNA. Rifampin is clinically useful, particularly in the treatment of tuberculosis and leprosy, in part because it is relatively nontoxic. The reason is that mammalian RNA polymerases do not bind rifampin.

Apart from the murein-inhibiting β-lactams and DNA inhibitors, the largest class of **clinically useful antibiotics** consists of those that **inhibit protein synthesis.** Some of these antibiotics work by binding to ribosomes, either to the large or the small subunit (Table 3-3). The reason that bacteria are selectively targeted is that the ribosome of prokaryotes is different from that of eukaryotes. Among the ribosomally active antibiotics are **chloramphenicol** and **macrolides** (such as **erythromycin**), which **block the formation of peptide bonds** by binding at or near the aminoacyl transfer RNA (tRNA) binding site on the large ribosomal subunit. After some time, the previously synthesized peptidyl tRNA is released and hydrolyzed. The ribosomal subunits are then released from the mRNA and are free to rejoin other mRNA molecules to start another abortive cycle. This leads to a truncated version of the ribosome cycle (Fig. 3-11). As a result, when ribosomally active antibiotics are withdrawn, many free ribosomes are present and ready to resume normal protein synthesis. This explains why the **action of these drugs is reversible** and why they are **bacteriostatic** and not **bactericidal.** It should be pointed out that this does not necessarily diminish their usefulness. When bacteria are kept in check by bacteriostatic drugs, they are usually cleared from tissues by the host defense mechanisms.

One important group of protein synthesis inhibitors, the **aminoglycosides,** is **bactericidal.** How they kill bacteria has not yet been satisfactorily explained, but some hints exist. Aminoglycosides, like **streptomycin, gentamicin,** and **neomycin,** are taken up by bacteria and bind to the smaller 30S ribosomal subunit. This is their critical site of action, as demonstrated by the finding that a single amino acid change in a mutated 30S ribosomal protein leads to resistance to these drugs. Binding of aminoglycosides has many effects on ribosome function; for instance, it enhances the interaction of the 30S and 50S subunits and inhibits the elongation of peptide chains. Typical of the action of this group of antibiotics is the accumulation of free ribosomes as aberrant 70S particles and not as 30S and 50S subunits. This coincides with cell death. Accumulating 70S ribosomes results in abortive attempts to initiate protein synthesis. However, these atypical ribosomes bind to mRNA and therefore block the function of normal ribosomes still unaffected by the drug. The inhibition of protein synthesis by aminoglycosides is apparently irreversible, because once the drug is taken up it cannot be removed from the cell. Thus, cells treated with these drugs

table **3-3**	Antibiotics: Mechanisms of Action of Commonly Used Antimicrobial Agents
ANTIBIOTIC	**ACTION**
Cell wall inhibitors	
β-lactams: Penicillins, cephalosporins, carbapenems, monobactams	Interfere with cell wall cross-linking through interaction with penicillin-binding proteins (transpeptidases); autolysis
Glycopeptides: vancomycin	Interfere with incorporation of new subunits into growing murein chains
Imidazoles: fluconazole, itraconazole, voriconazole, posaconazole	Blocks synthesis of ergosterol required for fungal cell wall integrity
Echinocandins: caspofungin, mycofungin	Blocks β-glucan synthesis, a major constituent of fungal cell walls
Inhibitors of membrane function	
Lipopeptide antibiotics: daptomycin	Forms channels in cell membranes of Gram-positive bacteria resulting in K+ leakage and metabolic death
Polyene: amphotericin B	Bind to sterols in eukaryotic cell membranes, leading to membrane leakiness and, at high levels, lysis
Folate antagonists	
Sulfonamides: sulfamethoxazole, sulfadiazine	Competitive inhibitor of dihydropteroate synthesis; blocks synthesis of tetrahydrofolate and cell-linked metabolic pathways
Trimethoprim	Inhibition of bacterial dihydrofolate reductase
Protein synthesis inhibitors	
Aminoglycosides: gentamicin, tobramycin, streptomycin, amikacin, neomycin	Bind to 30S subunit of bacterial ribosome; cause translational misreading and inhibit elongation of protein chain; kill by blocking initiation of protein synthesis
Macrolides: erythromycin, azithromycin, clarithromycin, clindamycin	Bind to ribosome 50S subunit; inhibit protein synthesis at chain elongation step
Ketolides: telithromycin	
Streptogramins: dalfopristin, quinupristin	
Chloramphenicol	
RNA synthesis inhibitors	
Rifampin	Binds to bacterial RNA polymerase and blocks transcription (synthesis of RNA) at initiation step
DNA synthesis inhibitors	
Metronidazole, nitrofurans	Partially reduced nitro groups give addition products on DNA that lead to cidal strand breakage
Fluoroquinolones: ciprofloxacin, levofloxacin, gatifloxacin, moxifloxacin, gemifloxacin	Interfere with DNA replication by inhibiting the action of DNA gyrase or topoisomerase
Nalidixic acid	

cannot recover, which is one reason why the aminoglycosides are bactericidal.

Capsules, Flagella, and Pili: How Bacteria Cope in Various Environments

The morphological variety of bacteria is not limited to walls and membranes. Some bacteria, but by no means all, have other exterior structures such as **capsules, flagella,** and **pili.** These components are dispensable; that is, they are important for survival under certain circumstances but not others. The **capsule** is a slimy outer coating made by certain bacteria. Under laboratory conditions the capsule is not needed, and the organisms may grow well without it. Capsules usually consist of high-molecular-weight polysaccharides that make the bacteria slippery and difficult for white blood cells to phagocytize. As you will see, pneumococci, meningococci, and other bacteria that are likely to encounter phagocytes during their infective cycle are indeed encapsulated. In the laboratory, colonies of encapsulated bacteria on agar plates are viscous and shiny. Colonies of nonencapsulated organisms are usually smaller and appear dull.

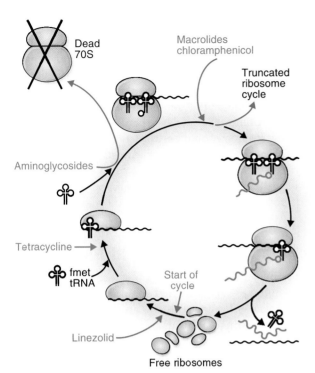

FIGURE 3-11 ▪ **Antibiotic blockage of the ribosome cycle.** The normal cycle of 30S and 50S subunits in and out of polysomes is recalled, with the assembly of a 70S initiation complex, elongation of the polypeptide chain as the ribosome moves across the messenger RNA, and release of all components on completion of the polypeptide. Points of blockage by antibiotics are shown. Linezolid blocks the assembly of the initiation complex; tetracycline inhibits aminoacyl transfer RNA binding; aminoglycosides provoke formation of "dead" aberrant initiation complexes; and chloramphenicol and macrolides block elongation, leading to premature dissociation of the active complex.

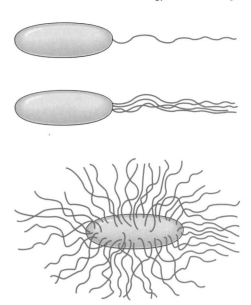

FIGURE 3-13 ▪ **Arrangement of flagella in some types of bacteria.**

Protruding through the surface layers of many bacteria are two kinds of filaments, **flagella** and **pili** (Fig. 3-12). Flagella are long, helical filaments that endow bacteria with motility. Many successful pathogens are motile, which probably aids their spread in the environment and possibly in the body of the host. Depending on the species, a single bacterial cell may have one flagellum or many flagella (Fig. 3-13). In some, the flagella are located at the ends of the cells (polar) and in others at random points around the periphery (peritrichous, or "hairy all over"). This distinction is useful in taxonomy and in diagnostic microbiology. Pili (also

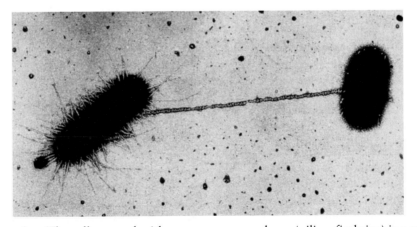

FIGURE 3-12 ▪ **E. coli mating.** The cell covered with numerous appendages (pili or fimbriae) is a genetic donor connected to a recipient cell (without appendages) by the so-called F pilus. The F pilus is a specialized structure (sex pilus) controlled by genes on the fertility, or F plasmid. The F pilus has been labeled by special virus particles that infect donor cells via the F pilus. The other pili surrounding the cell have no role in conjugation but are required by E. coli for colonization and pathogenicity in the intestinal and urinary tracts of humans and animals.

called **fimbriae**) are involved in the attachment of bacteria to cells and other surfaces, as discussed later in the chapter.

Bacterial Chemotaxis

The movement caused by flagella is used by bacteria for **chemotaxis**—that is, movement toward substances that attract and away from those that repel. Considerable research has shown that bacterial chemotaxis is based on the following sophisticated mechanism: Flagella spin around from their point of attachment at the cell surface. Each flagellum has a **counterclockwise helical pitch,** and when there are several on one bacterium, they array themselves into coherent **bundles** as long as they all rotate counterclockwise. When the flagella are arranged in these bundles, they beat together, and the bacteria **swim in a straight line** (Fig. 3-14). However, when flagella

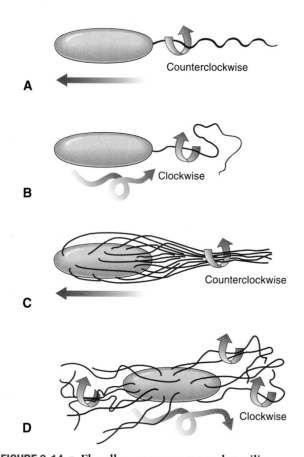

FIGURE 3-14 ▪ Flagellar arrangement and motility.
A. A bacterium moving smoothly right to left when its single polar flagellum rotates counterclockwise; this is the same direction as the thread of the helix formed by the flagellin molecules in the flagellum. **B.** The same bacterium tumbles generally left to right when the flagellum rotates clockwise. **C.** With a peritrichous bacterium, counterclockwise rotation produces a coherent bundle of flagella and smooth movement. **D.** Tumbling produced by clockwise rotation is extreme.

rotate clockwise, they get in each other's way and cannot form bundles. As a result, the bacteria **tumble** in random fashion. The two types of motion, swimming and tumbling, account for bacterial chemotaxis. In the absence of **attractants** or **repellants,** bacteria alternate indifferently between swimming and tumbling. When an attractant is sensed, swimming lasts longer than tumbling, whereas swimming stops more quickly when a repellant is present. The net result is movement toward attractants and away from repellants. Chemotaxis has a role in pathogenesis, probably in guiding bacteria toward cellular targets or possibly away from white blood cells.

Bacterial Adhesion and Pili

Whether by active chemotaxis or by more-passive mechanisms, microbes are attracted to specific tissues. Such **tissue tropism** often involves the **attachment** of surface components of the organisms to **specific receptors** present on the cells of certain tissues. The bacterial structures most often involved in attachment are the **pili,** or fimbriae. These are protein filaments shorter than flagella and distributed, often in large numbers, over the surface of some bacteria. Bacteria that can conjugate have, in addition, specialized **sex pili.** These structures are rather different from the "common pili." They are much longer and link the donor (male) and recipient (female) cells during transfer of DNA by conjugation (see Chapter 4). Attachment to cells or other bacteria via pili involves the attachment at the tip of the pili followed by their retraction into the cell (a process that resembles the use of grappling hooks).

How Bacteria Change their Surface Components

Pili are also highly changeable and permit some organisms to put on a succession of disguises that enables them to outflank the immune system. This has been studied in detail in the gonococcus. Gonococci have a large number of genes that code for variants of the protein **pilin,** which polymerizes to form pili. Each version of pilin is antigenically distinct and elicits the formation of different antibodies. In the presence of antibodies to one type of pilin, there is rapid selection for variants of gonococci that have switched to the synthesis of another antigenic type of pilin. Thus, they keep one step ahead in this quick-change scenario. Only one (or a few) of the large repertoire of pilin genes is active at any time. The molecular basis for the shift from one pilin to another is that pilin genes contain two types of sequences: one codes for a constant portion of the pilin protein that is not very antigenic, and the other (of which there are many varieties in one genome) codes for a variable region that is highly antigenic. At intervals, a constant region will recombine with a variable region to form a gene that codes for a complete pilin protein. The result is that many varieties of pilin genes can arise and be expressed, allowing the organisms to survive for long periods in the face of the host immune response. It is easy to see why attempts to immunize against gonococci using a particular pilin vaccine have failed so far.

Such specific rearrangements of portions of genes are not unique. A comparable shuffling of constant and variable portions of genes gives rise to the magnificent variety of antibodies made by the body. In microbes, analogous mechanisms have been found in yeast, in the bacteria that cause relapsing fever (*Borrelia*), and in the protozoa that cause sleeping sickness (trypanosomes). By a related mechanism, organisms that cause food poisoning and other illnesses, the *Salmonella*, undergo rapid changes between expression and nonexpression of genes that code for the protein of flagella. This change in flagellar synthesis is called **phase variation** and is based on the control of a gene for flagellar protein. The gene can be inverted on the chromosome but can be expressed in only one of the two orientations.

Nutrition and Energy Metabolism

Bacteria survive and grow in a large variety of habitats. Whatever the habitat, all bacteria must synthesize cellular constituents in a coordinated manner to grow. The required building blocks must either be provided at suitable levels in the medium or be synthesized in proper amounts by the organisms themselves. Based on their nutritional requirements, bacteria can be divided into two large groups: In one are the **photosynthetic** or **chemosynthetic** bacteria that subsist on carbon dioxide and minerals, using either light or chemical energy. The other includes all the **organisms that need preformed organic compounds.** All pathogenic microbes fall in the second group, but within it they have many gradations of nutritional needs. Some, like *E. coli*, are satisfied with glucose and some inorganic material (Table 3-4). Other pathogenic bacteria, like their human host, are unable to make one or more essential metabolites—vitamins, amino acids, purines, pyrimidines, and so on—which must be supplied as growth factors.

Bacteria also have a wide range of responses to oxygen. At the extremes are the **strict aerobes,** which must have oxygen to grow. An example is the tubercle bacillus, which thrives in the portions of the body that are well oxygenated, such as the lungs. At the other extreme are the **strict** or **obligate anaerobes,** bacteria that cannot grow in the presence of oxygen, such as the organisms that cause botulism and tetanus. The largest number of bacteria that are medically important can grow whether or not oxygen is present. They are called

table **3-4**		**Glucose-Minimal Medium**
COMPOUND	**GRAMS PER LITER**	**MAIN SOURCE OF**
Na_2HPO_4	6.0	Phosphorus, buffering power, osmotic strength
KH_2PO_4	3.0	Phosphorus, buffering power, osmotic strength
NH_4Cl	1.0	Nitrogen
$MgSO_4$	0.012	Magnesium, Sulfur
$CaCl_2$	0.011	Calcium
Glucose	2.0	Energy, carbon-building blocks

Note: pH adjusted to 7.0.

facultative anaerobes and include *E. coli* and other intestinal bacteria.

Their various responses to oxygen mirror the ways bacteria oxidize substrates to obtain energy. Strict aerobes perform **respiration** only; in a series of coupled oxidation–reductions, the **final electron acceptor** is **molecular oxygen.** Strict anaerobes usually carry out **fermentation,** where the final electron acceptor is an **organic molecule.** Examples of organic electron acceptors are pyruvate, which is reduced to lactate in the lactic acid fermentation, and acetyl coenzyme A, which is reduced to alcohol in ethanol fermentation. Facultative anaerobes are capable of either form of metabolism, depending on whether oxygen is present or absent. Thus, they will respire in the presence of oxygen and ferment in its absence. (To make matters more complex, some anaerobes, called anaerobic respirers, carry out respiration using compounds such as nitrate or sulfate instead of oxygen as final electron acceptors.)

Per molecule of substrate oxidized, respiration yields more energy than fermentation. Therefore, fermentative organisms must turn over more substrate to obtain the same amount of energy. The industrial microbiologist takes advantage of this for the purpose of maximizing either the yield of cell mass or the amount of metabolic products formed. Under what conditions of oxygenation would you grow yeast in a fermentation tank if the intended product were yeast cake or alcohol?

We have mentioned that *E. coli* can use glucose as its sole organic source. It can also use other compounds, such as lactose, fructose, or one of several amino acids. The list includes more than 30 known substances, but this is not particularly impressive compared with species of *Pseudomonas*, which can grow on any of several hundred organic compounds. No wonder such nearly omnivorous *Pseudomonas* have been used by genetic engineers to construct strains for use in the degradation of environmental pollutants. And no wonder *Pseudomonas* species are omnipresent in the water supply and the soil, where they can take advantage of a great variety of substrates.

Although *E. coli* and *Pseudomonas* can manage on meager solutions of glucose and a few salts, they do not disdain richer fare. When *E. coli* is given a mixture of amino acids, sugars, vitamins, and other compounds, it will use what is provided rather than making the compounds endogenously. The result is sparing of energy and biosynthetic potential, and faster growth. In the laboratory it is possible to culture bacteria in media that are truly spartan, the so-called **minimal media,** which are water solutions of glucose, ammonia, phosphate, sulfate, and other minerals (see Table 3-4). Conversely, the bacteria can be grown in a rich medium, a **nutrient broth** that contains meat extract and soluble partial hydrolysates of complex proteins. Add **agar** to these solutions and you have the corresponding **solid media.**

Some bacteria can grow only in complex media and have nutritional requirements that rival or exceed those of humans. Called **nutritionally fastidious,** these organisms include highly parasitic species found only in the rich environment of the human body. For example, staphylococci or streptococci can grow only if provided with a long list of compounds. As expected, bacteria that can get by with only a few nutrients, like *E. coli* or *Pseudomonas,* can also exist in less-rich habitats, such as bodies of water. The ecology of an organism then usually gives good hints of its nutritional requirements.

Certain bacteria have never been cultured in artificial media and only replicate inside host cells. These bacteria, like *Chlamydia,* are known as **obligate intracellular parasites.** Other bacteria, such as *Treponema pallidum* (the causative agent of syphilis) or *Mycobacterium leprae* (which causes leprosy) should, in principle, be able to grow in laboratory media because they replicate extracellularly in the host. However, microbiologists have not figured out how to get them to do it.

Growing and Resting States

When bacteria find themselves in a suitable environment, they grow and eventually divide. The time it takes for a bacterium to become two is called the **generation time** or **doubling time.** For example, *E. coli* requires about 20 minutes to double in a rich nutrient broth and 1 hour in a glucose-minimal medium at 37°C. For a time, the bacteria grow in an unhindered manner and are physiologically all alike. Such a steady state does not exist for long in nature, however, because the environment usually undergoes rapid changes. Growth will stop once the population reaches a certain cell density and the nutrients in the environment become exhausted or toxic metabolites accumulate.

Bacterial Growth Measurement and a Few Definitions

How is bacterial growth measured? The most direct way is to take samples at various times and count the number of bacteria under a microscope using a hemocytometer chamber. This tedious procedure has been superseded by electronic particle analyzers that detect bacteria as tiny semiconductors in an electric field. Either procedure measures the number of bacteria as physical particles. In other words, they give the body count, with no discrimination between living and dead bacteria. This is known as the **total count.** The total count can also be conveniently estimated by measuring a property proportional to the number of bacteria present—for instance, the turbidity of a liquid culture.

Often it is important to determine the number of **living** or **viable** bacteria. This number is determined by a **colony count,** which is carried out by placing an appropriate dilution on solid growth medium. Since colonies arise from living bacteria, the number of colonies multiplied by the dilution factor is the number of **colony-forming units (CFUs)** originally present. Note that if bacteria grow in clumps, like staphylococci, or in chains, like streptococci, the number of CFUs is an underestimate of the total number of living bacteria present.

Law of Growth

Balanced growth can be described mathematically as follows. Let N be the number of bacteria and t the time, then

$$dN/dt = Nk$$

where k is the **growth rate constant.** By integration we obtain the **law of growth:**

$$N_t = N_0 e^{kt}$$

where N_t is the number of bacteria at time t and N_0 is the initial number of bacteria at $t = 0$. The law of growth describes a **geometric progression,** which holds for many situations. In some circumstances leading to cell death (for instance, sterilizing heat or antiseptic chemicals), the decrease in viable bacteria may be described by the same equation but with a negative constant. The same equation also describes the decay with time of a radioactive isotope or the kinetics of degradation of unstable messenger RNA molecules in cells (or the law of compound interest, which Benjamin Franklin called "the eighth wonder of the world").

Growth in the Real World

If balanced growth went unchecked, a single bacterium dividing twice an hour would produce a mass as large as that of Earth in just 2 days. Instead, when bacteria grow to a certain density, they either exhaust required

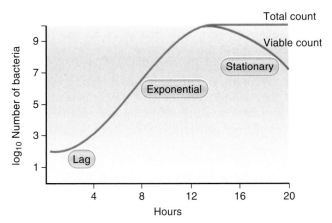

FIGURE 3-15 ▪ The growth of a bacterial culture. Bacteria in the inoculum sometimes resume growth slowly (lag phase, hours 0 to 5). They then enter the exponential phase of growth (hours 5 to 10). When foodstuff is exhausted or toxic material accumulates, they enter the stationary phase (hours 10 onward). During the stationary phase bacterial cultures may lose their viability, as reflected in the viable count, often without losing cell integrity (maintaining a constant total count).

nutrients or they accumulate toxic levels of metabolites (Fig. 3-15). They may run out of the carbon source, a required inorganic compound, or essential amino acids or vitamins. For aerobic bacteria, crowding leads to the exhaustion of oxygen, which is poorly soluble in water. Toxic metabolites may be hydrogen peroxide, which is the case for some anaerobes that lack catalase, or acids formed by fermentation, which results in a pH too low to be compatible with growth. Which of these factors actually slows down growth first depends on the strain of bacteria and on the composition of the culture medium. For example, in a well-buffered medium, *E. coli* may exhaust nutrients before the pH drops, while the converse may be true in poorly buffered media. The stage of the culture where growth stops is known as the **stationary phase.**

The explosiveness of exponential growth means that even a small number of bacteria can rapidly initiate an infection. An example of unhampered growth that leads to dangerous illness is acute bacterial meningitis in a child. Bacteria that cause this disease, such as the meningococci, grow so rapidly in the patient that the physician must intervene with great speed to avoid a fatal outcome. However, not all pathogens are fast growing. For example, tubercle bacilli divide every 24 hours or so even under optimal conditions. The disease they cause is chronic and takes considerable time to be manifested.

In the tissues of the body (as well as in the environment), bacteria are often **stressed** by nutritional limitations or by the damaging action of the defense mechanisms. Consequently, bacterial populations in the

body are rarely fully viable. To permit them to adapt to such conditions, bacteria do not cease all metabolic activities when they stop growing. Instead, although they cease net growth, they continue some synthetic activities that permit them to make specific constituents needed for adaptation. To use a laboratory example, when *E. coli* cultures exhaust glucose, they continue to carry out a low level of protein synthesis, sufficient to adapt to the use of other nutrients, such as other sugars that may be present. Energy and building blocks are supplied by turnover of cell material not needed in the stationary phase. Major sources of amino acids are the ribosomes and preexisting proteins not greatly used under these conditions. Their breakdown products can also be utilized to supply energy. This process of feeding on itself gives bacteria adaptability and postpones death, which might otherwise occur by random degradative events in the absence of synthetic activities.

Bacteria are exposed to countless **injuries** and have developed special adaptive mechanisms to cope with many of them. For example, damage to the DNA of *E. coli* by ultraviolet light activates a set of genes that code for proteins capable of repairing the damage. This is known as the **SOS response.** Other protective responses are turned on when bacteria are starved for the source of carbon, nitrogen, or phosphorus; when the temperature is raised abruptly; or when anaerobic cultures are suddenly exposed to oxygen. In each case the rapid rate at which the bacteria implement their coping mechanism is a tribute to the powers of bacterial adaptation.

Even when they are **not growing**, bacteria can still **cause damage** to their host. First, nongrowing bacteria are still immunogenic and can elicit immune responses with both beneficial and detrimental results. Second, production of toxins often starts or accelerates when bacteria enter the stationary phase. In some cases we can fathom the reason for this timing, because toxin production provides certain bacteria with nutrients. For example, some streptococci make enzymes that lyse red blood cells and proteases that degrade hemoglobin. The organisms are thus supplied with amino acids plus a source of iron. Why do these organisms make their hemolysins mainly in the stationary phase? Clearly, as long as they are growing, they must already be supplied with the necessary iron and amino acids. Why should they then expend energy to make hemolysins?

Cessation of growth of some bacterial species initiates **sporulation.** This results in the production of metabolically inert **spores** extraordinarily resistant to chemical and physical insults. During sporulation the "mother cell" eventually lyses. The cytoplasmic contents that are released sometimes contain large amounts of toxins. This happens in tetanus, gas gangrene, and other diseases caused by sporulating bacteria.

The relationship between microbial growth and pathogenesis is far from simple but should be kept in mind when attempting to understand the etiology and course of infections.

Mechanisms of Adaptation

Both over short periods and throughout evolutionary times, bacteria are selected for their efficient and economical ways of coping with the environment. **Inefficient strains are rapidly lost** in competition with others that use their resources more effectively. Metabolic efficiency is characterized by metabolic **parsimony;** that is, bacteria tend not to make constituents they cannot use at the time. There are important exceptions to this statement, but generally it illustrates the economy and efficiency of the bacterial way of life.

We know a great deal about the mechanisms bacteria use to adapt to changing environmental conditions. As more information is gathered, it becomes evident that a large number of mechanisms operate a certain way under specific circumstances. One example is a culture of *E. coli* growing in a minimal medium to which is added to it an excess of the amino acid leucine. Within seconds the endogenous synthesis of leucine will be stopped, and the cells will use the exogenously supplied leucine exclusively. From the point of view of the economy of the bacteria, this is desirable because it saves the metabolic energy expended for biosynthesis of leucine. The same phenomenon would occur if other amino acids, purines, pyrimidines, or other metabolites were added.

Regulation of Enzyme Activity

How did the bacteria switch off the synthesis of leucine? When the enzymes of the metabolic pathway dedicated to the synthesis of leucine were studied, it was found that the first enzyme in the pathway is inhibited by leucine and will not function in its presence. This inhibition is the result of the **allosteric** properties of the enzyme—that is, its ability to change conformation by the binding of an effector, in this case leucine. Why was the first enzyme and not the others in the pathway affected? The reason is economic: stopping the flow of substrates at the very beginning of the pathway eliminates waste of unusable metabolites. This effect is known as **feedback** or **end-product inhibition.**

Regulation of Enzyme Synthesis

Feedback inhibition suffices to stop the synthesis of leucine in the leucine-fed culture. If this were all, the organisms would still synthesize the biosynthetic enzymes for leucine, at a cost of considerable energy. This is wasteful and might place the organisms at a selective disadvantage vis-à-vis more-efficient ones. To avoid such an unnecessary expenditure, the cells rapidly turn off the synthesis of the enzymes of the leucine biosynthetic pathway. How is this done? It is a characteristic of prokaryotic cells that genes for the enzymes involved in a metabolic pathway are often strung together in a multigenic segment of DNA called an **operon. Transcription** of all the genes of an operon into mRNA can be turned on or off together by throwing a single regulatory switch. At one end of the operon where transcription starts is a series of regulatory sequences that do not code for amino acids but are recognized by the regulatory mechanisms. One of these sequences is the **promoter** site, where RNA polymerase binds to initiate the synthesis of mRNA. Two such mechanisms of **regulation of gene expression** used to switch operons on and off are discussed here.

The operons involved in the biosynthesis of amino acids, such as leucine, are sometimes regulated by a mechanism called **attenuation.** This is how it works, still taking leucine as an example: A small stretch of mRNA is synthesized from the beginning of the coding sequence of the leucine operon, regardless of the presence or absence of leucine. The RNA polymerase now encounters a region called the **attenuator,** where in the presence of leucine, **transcription is terminated.** This achieves the desired effect of not making the unneeded biosynthetic enzymes. In the absence of leucine, when the biosynthetic enzymes become essential, the secondary structure of the nascent mRNA at the attenuator region is altered in such a way that transcription, and therefore translation, can proceed. Details of how this works are shown in Figure 3-16.

Another mechanism for turning on or off the synthesis of enzymes is found in the case of many enzymes involved in the utilization of sugars. Taking the utilization of lactose as an example, if this sugar is the sole carbon source, the bacteria must make the enzyme β-galactosidase, which is necessary to convert lactose into glucose and galactose. In the absence of lactose, as in the case of a culture growing solely on glucose, the synthesis of β-galactosidase is unnecessary and wasteful. The synthesis of the enzyme is regulated (Fig. 3-17). At the beginning of the operon, just past the promoter, there is a regulatory sequence known as the **operator,** where a protein called the **repressor** binds. When the repressor binds to the operator, transcription cannot begin. In the presence of lactose, however, the repressor undergoes a conformational change to render it incapable of binding to the operator. Note that the lactose repressor is an allosteric protein, capable of undergoing conformational changes under the influence of an effector. The result is that when lactose is added to a culture, the repressor becomes inactive and cannot bind to the operator, thus allowing the synthesis of β-galactosidase, to proceed. β-galactosidase is an example of an **inducible enzyme,** which is made on demand, compared with a **constitutive enzyme,** which must be made at all times, such as RNA polymerase. In the case of β-galactosidase, lactose (or more precisely, one of its metabolites) is known as the **inducer.**

FIGURE 3-16 ▪ **Regulation of enzyme synthesis by attenuation.** Transcription stops when a termination stem and loop structure involving sequences C and D is formed. The middle of the drawing shows how the absence of leucine causes ribosomes to stop at sequence A and to prevent the formation of the CD stem-and-loop structure. This allows RNA polymerase to continue transcription past this region. On the bottom, when abundant leucine is present, ribosomes continue to sequence B, allowing the formation of the CD termination stem-and-loop structure. In this case RNA polymerase cannot proceed and transcription stops.

Overview of Regulation

Regulation of gene expression by attenuation, repression, or other mechanisms results in the relatively rapid switching on and off of gene expression. The reason is that mRNA molecules in bacteria are relatively short lived and undergo rapid turnover. Thus, after the synthesis of an enzyme is stopped, the amount of residual enzyme produced will be very small. In addition, what enzyme is left may be subject to feedback inhibition, and little of its product will be made. Note that all forms of regulation come at energy cost. Thus, feedback inhibition requires that the protein be more complex than just what is needed for catalytic activity. Regulation of enzyme synthesis by attenuation depends on the synthesis of a stretch of mRNA that will not be used if the enzymes of the operon are not made. Using a repressor to regulate an operon likewise requires the constitutive synthesis of protein repressor molecules. The energy cost of making regulatory devices is weighted against the greater disadvantage that cells would have in not being able to switch major biosynthetic pathways on and off. Thus, free-living cells like bacteria must balance their powers of efficiency and adaptability.

The theme of efficiency and adaptability to environmental changes recurs throughout this book, especially in discussing how microbes cope with the changes they encounter when entering the body and certain body tissues and organs.

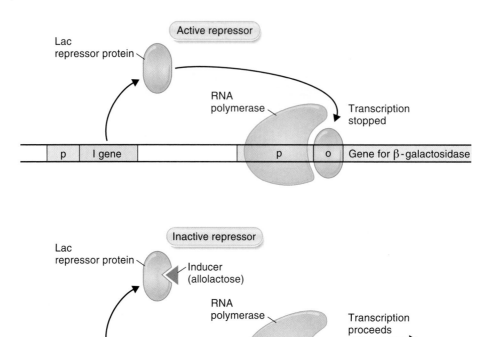

FIGURE 3-17 ■ **The operon model: regulation of β-galactosidase synthesis by repression.** The repressor protein for the genes encoding enzymes for lactose utilization exists in two states: active, when the sugar inducer is absent, and inactive, when the inducer is present. The top of the figure shows that when the inducer (allolactose, a derivative of lactose) is absent, the repressor is in the active form and binds to the operator, thus preventing transcription from taking place. In the bottom of the figure, the repressor is inactivated by the inducer and cannot bind to the operator. Transcription can then proceed, and the enzyme β-galactosidase is formed.

Conclusion

Bacteria share many biochemical attributes with eukaryotic cells, including the use of the same building blocks (amino acids, nucleotides, etc.) and analogous energy metabolism and polymerizing machinery. They differ, however, in their body plan, being smaller and more compactly constructed than their eukaryotic counterparts. In addition, bacteria face the challenges of living freely in highly changing environments. They possess specialized structures that help them cope when facing scarcity of food or toxic compounds, and they are remarkably efficient in how they regulate the expression of their genes under various circumstances. They do not all use the same strategies but have a wide-ranging repertoire of ways to adapt to the environment, including the human body.

Genetic Approaches to Studying Bacterial Pathogenesis

Peggy A. Cotter

Traits that render bacteria pathogenic are called **virulence factors.** Originally, this term referred to substances that are produced by a microorganism and can, by themselves, harm the host. Classic examples of virulence factors are bacterial toxins such as those discussed in Chapter 9. With the increased understanding of molecular mechanisms in bacterial pathogenesis that has occurred over the last few decades, the term has been redefined to include any component of a microbe that is required for or potentiates its ability to cause disease. This chapter focuses on the techniques that have been used to discover virulence factors and to study pathogenic mechanisms. Some basic genetic concepts are also introduced.

The number and nature of virulence factors expressed by bacterial pathogens vary as widely as the strategies the pathogens employ to establish infection and cause disease. At one end of the spectrum are organisms like *Clostridium botulinum* (see Chapter 20), a Gram-positive anaerobic bacterium with a propensity to grow in improperly prepared canned foods. A single protein toxin expressed by *C. botulinum* (botulism toxin) can cause lethal food poisoning in humans when ingested, even in the absence of the bacteria themselves. At the other end of the spectrum are bacteria like *Salmonella enterica*, serovar Typhi (see Chapter 17), which are able to adhere to, invade, and/or induce cytotoxicity in a variety of human cell types as they travel through the gastrointestinal tract, across the gut mucosa, and into deeper tissues to eventually cause a lethal systemic infection. Progress in understanding mechanisms of bacterial pathogenesis has revealed that although each organism expresses its own repertoire of virulence factors and virulence-related functions, many microbes use similar approaches to solve common biological problems.

How are these bacterial virulence factors identified and studied in the laboratory? Researchers have traditionally used biochemical approaches, and these types of investigations continue to reveal structure–function relationships telling us much about how toxins and other virulence factors work. Epidemiological approaches that correlate the virulence of naturally isolated strains with their clinical properties have also been extremely useful. The most commonly used approaches for identifying virulence factors and studying bacterial pathogenesis today, however, are genetic in nature. Driven by advances in molecular biotechnology, the development of broadly applicable genetic tools, and increasingly creative screening and selection strategies, these approaches have led to dramatic advances in our understanding of the molecular interactions that occur between bacterial pathogens and their mammalian hosts.

Complementation Approaches

Genetic complementation refers to the ability of a gene to produce a functional product that overcomes a mutant phenotype, typically caused by a mutation in the same gene. Thus, when an extrachromosomal copy of gene X is expressed in a bacterium that has a mutation in the chromosomal gene X, the function normally supplied by the gene X product is expressed and the cells are wild type. A variation of complementation has been used to identify virulence genes in a variety of pathogenic bacteria. In these cases, rather than restoring a wild-type phenotype to a mutant, the gene products expressed extrachromosomally confer one or more pathogenic traits on a nonpathogenic bacterium.

An example of such an approach was first used in the mid-1980s. Isberg and colleagues investigated the mechanism by which *Yersinia pseudotuberculosis* (a relative of *Yersinia pestis*, the plague bacillus) penetrates cells lining the small intestine, an early and important step in the disease caused by this organism. The researchers hypothesized that *Y. pseudotuberculosis* possesses at least one gene that encodes proteins mediating penetration (or invasion) of animal cells. They hypothesized further that expression of that gene in *Escherichia coli* would confer on that nonpathogenic, noninvasive bacterium the ability to penetrate mammalian cells. In other words, they believed it was possible for *E. coli* to gain a function—host cell invasion—by acquiring a single gene from *Y. pseudotuberculosis*.

Their hypotheses proved to be correct and led to the identification of a gene they named *inv*, which encodes a protein, named invasin, that allows *E. coli* (and even latex beads) to invade eukaryotic cells in culture. Other researchers soon used this approach to identify many important virulence factors in a variety of human pathogens. To illustrate the power of the approach, the following paragraphs describe the steps Isberg and colleagues took and highlight the genetic and molecular biological processes involved. The basic steps are illustrated in Figure 4-1.

Constructing Plasmid Libraries

Isberg and colleagues hypothesized that a single *Y. pseudotuberculosis* gene (or perhaps a cluster of linked genes) would allow *E. coli* to invade mammalian epithelial cells in culture. To test this hypothesis, they needed a collection of *E. coli* bacteria—a library composed of bacteria, each containing a unique, relatively small fragment of the *Y. pseudotuberculosis* genome (enough to contain, on average, about five genes).

The first step in constructing the genomic library was to isolate DNA from the organism of interest (*Y. pseudotuberculosis* in this case) and cut it into a large number of fragments using **restriction endonucleases**—

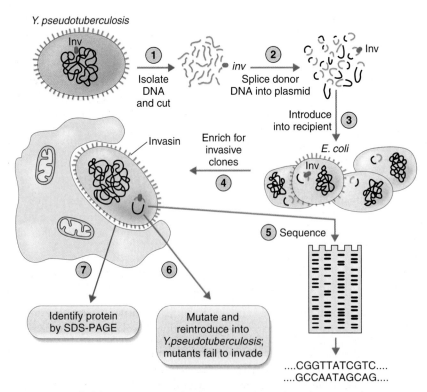

FIGURE 4-1 ▪ General scheme used to identify invasin.

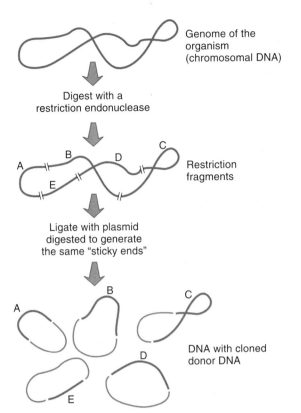

FIGURE 4-2 ▪ Creating a genomic library. The DNA of an organism is cut into restriction fragments (here labeled **A** through **E**), which are ligated with plasmid DNA that was cut with a restriction endonuclease that generates the same "sticky ends." After ligation these recombinant plasmids are transformed into *E. coli*.

Labels in figure:
Genome of the organism (chromosomal DNA)
Digest with a restriction endonuclease
Restriction fragments
Ligate with plasmid digested to generate the same "sticky ends"
DNA with cloned donor DNA

enzymes that work like molecular scissors, cutting both strands of the DNA at specific sequences (Fig. 4-2). Several hundred restriction endonucleases with different specificities are available commercially. These enzymes typically recognize specific short sequences in the double-stranded DNA (four to six bases in most examples) that read the same on the top strand from 5′ to 3′ as they do on the bottom strand. The enzyme cuts the DNA asymmetrically such that fragments with overhangs ("sticky ends") are generated.

Next, the large fragments of *Y. pseudotuberculosis* DNA generated by restriction endonuclease digestion were cloned into a **plasmid** so they could be introduced into *E. coli* and stably maintained. (Plasmids are small, extrachromosomal, usually circular DNA molecules capable of replicating independently within bacterial cells.) Cloning was accomplished by allowing the fragments to anneal (via their complementary sticky ends) with plasmid DNA that had been cut with a restriction endonuclease that generates the same 5′ overhangs as the one that generated the fragments in the library. Then the loosely joined molecules were covalently linked using the enzyme DNA ligase. The resulting circular plasmid molecules containing fragments of *Y.*

pseudotuberculosis DNA were then introduced into *E. coli* by the mechanism of **transformation.** This process enabled bacteria to take up naked DNA from their surroundings. Strains with this ability are said to be "competent." Some bacteria are naturally competent, while others, like *E. coli*, are not but can be coaxed to take up extracellular DNA by treating them in a way that changes their surface properties before adding plasmid DNA.

The plasmid used by Isberg and colleagues contained a gene-encoding ampicillin resistance; therefore, the bacteria that had taken up the plasmid (transformants) could be selected by plating on agar containing ampicillin. Each colony that arose represented a single transformant that contained a plasmid with, potentially, a separate piece of the *Y. pseudotuberculosis* genome.

Positive Selection for a Virulence Trait

The next step in the process was to determine if any of the bacteria in the *E. coli* library contained plasmids with a *Y. pseudotuberculosis* gene capable of giving *E. coli* the ability to invade mammalian cells. One way to find such bacteria would be to test each member of the library (at least 1,000 different bacteria) individually for their invasion ability. Although not an impossible task, it is very labor intensive. Isberg and colleagues used a clever scheme to decrease the workload. They used the invasion phenotype itself to enrich the culture for the bacteria containing the desired plasmid.

The procedure was as follows (Fig. 4-3). Pooled bacteria from the *E. coli* library were grown in liquid culture. Then aliquots were added to mammalian epithelial cells using plates with multiple wells to allow for large-scale screening. The bacteria and mammalian cells were coincubated for 1 hour, after which the bacteria were washed out of the wells and discarded. Fresh medium containing gentamicin was then added. Gentamicin is a powerful bactericidal antibiotic that cannot get into mammalian cells, which means that bacteria that remain extracellular will be killed but those that have penetrated the tissue culture cells will live. After another hour of incubation, the gentamicin-containing medium was washed away, the mammalian cells were gently lysed, and the surviving bacteria were plated on agar containing ampicillin. Theoretically, only bacteria that penetrate the mammalian cells can be recovered in this type of genetic approach called a **positive selection.** In practice, however, the procedure is rarely completely effective. The bacteria that Isberg and colleagues recovered were therefore tested individually for their ability to invade mammalian cells. Most did enter mammalian cells at a rate significantly greater than *E. coli* containing the plasmid with no *Y. pseudotuberculosis* DNA (the negative control), demonstrating the usefulness of this enrichment strategy. Those clones were characterized further.

FIGURE 4-3 ▪ **Enrichment for *E. coli* containing a *Y. pseudotuberculosis* gene conferring invasion ability.** The steps in the enrichment protocol are shown.

Molecular and Genetic Analysis of Cloned DNA

The next step was to determine the gene(s) responsible for conferring the invasive phenotype to *E. coli*. The researchers isolated plasmid DNA from the *E. coli* that were able to invade mammalian cells and characterized the *Y. pseudotuberculosis* DNA present on the plasmid. This was done by a time-consuming approach in which fragments of the cloned *Y. pseudotuberculosis* DNA were subcloned onto additional plasmids to identify smaller fragments that conferred the phenotype. The nucleotide sequence of the smallest fragment that could confer invasion was then determined.

DNA sequencing is now routine, and the complete genomes of many pathogens have been determined. If a study such as this were performed today, the nucleotide sequence of just a small piece of *Y. pseudotuberculosis* DNA from the plasmid would be determined. Then the sequence corresponding to the rest of the gene(s) would be identified by computer and downloaded from a sequence database. At the time that Isberg and colleagues performed their study, however, DNA sequencing was quite labor intensive. It was therefore prudent and customary to first identify the minimal DNA fragment conferring the desired phenotype before beginning a sequencing project. Inspection of the nucleotide sequence revealed an open reading frame (ORF), which the researchers named *inv*, with the potential to encode a protein of about 103 kDa, which they named invasin. Further biochemical analysis proved that the *inv* gene does in fact encode such a protein and that the protein is in the outer membrane.

Recombinant Methods for Generating Chromosomal Mutations

Although compelling, the experiments described in the previous section did not prove that *inv* and its product were responsible for allowing *Y. pseudotuberculosis* to invade host cells. For the definitive proof, at least by the standards of genetics, Isberg and colleagues had to construct a strain of *Y. pseudotuberculosis* containing a **loss-of-function mutation** at the *inv* locus. Such a mutation would lead to complete abrogation of the *inv* function. Many varieties of these types of mutants can be created. Substitution of a single nucleotide in a gene for a different one can result in an amino acid substitution in the protein that completely abrogates its function, decreases its functionality, or even confers on the protein a new function. If a stop codon is introduced, the truncated protein produced can similarly have little, no, or different activity. Deletion mutations, in which most or all of the gene is removed from the chromosome, are nearly always loss-of-function mutations.

Isberg and colleagues used the following approach to create a *Y. pseudotuberculosis* strain with a loss-of-function mutation in the *inv* gene. The first step was to mutate the *inv* gene present on the plasmid on which it was identified. Using restriction endonucleases that cut the *inv* gene at locations near the 5′ and 3′ ends of the gene, the researchers replaced the majority of the ORF with a different gene, one encoding a protein that confers resistance to kanamycin, an antibiotic that kills both *E. coli* and *Y. pseudotuberculosis* (Fig. 4-4). A DNA fragment containing the mutated *inv* gene (comprising the kanamycin resistance gene plus about 500 base pairs of flanking DNA both 5′ and 3′ to *inv*) was then cloned into a plasmid with two important features: (1) it could be introduced into *Y. pseudotuberculosis* by **conjugation,** and (2) it was a **suicide plasmid** for *Y. pseudotuberculosis*, meaning that it could not replicate in *Y. pseudotuberculosis*.

Conjugation is a mechanism by which genetic material is transferred one way from a donor cell to a recipi-

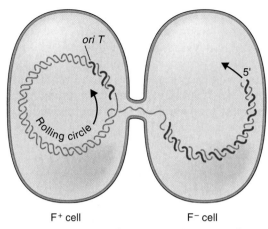

F⁺ cell   F⁻ cell

FIGURE 4-5 ▪ **Transfer of F plasmid from an F⁺ to an F⁻ cell.** A single DNA strand generated by replication is transferred from the donor to the recipient cell. The complementary strand is then synthesized in the recipient to reconstitute the complete F plasmid.

ent cell in a process that requires cell-to-cell contact (Fig. 4-5). The donor cell contains a conjugative plasmid (e.g., the F plasmid of *E. coli*) with genes encoding a conjugation (or sex) pilus that forms a bridge between the donor and recipient cells. The conjugative plasmid also contains an origin of transfer and additional genes that encode proteins mediating the transfer of a single strand of DNA, beginning at the origin of transfer, from the donor cell into the recipient cell. The complementary strand is synthesized inside the recipient cell to reconstitute the complete plasmid. Conjugation is typically several orders of magnitude more efficient than transformation; therefore, by cloning the mutated *inv* gene on a conjugative plasmid, the researchers greatly increased the probability of introducing the plasmid containing the mutated *inv* gene into *Y. pseudotuberculosis*.

The reason for using a suicide plasmid was that the researchers wanted to replace the wild-type *inv* gene on the chromosome with the mutated allele they had constructed on the plasmid. After using conjugation to introduce the plasmid into *Y. pseudotuberculosis*, the bacteria were plated on medium containing kanamycin (as well as an antibiotic that would kill the conjugation donor strain but not *Y. pseudotuberculosis*). Because the plasmid could not replicate in *Y. pseudotuberculosis*, **exconjugates** (cells that had received the conjugative plasmid) would be resistant to kanamycin only if the plasmid, or at least the part of the plasmid containing the kanamycin resistance gene, had integrated into the *Y. pseudotuberculosis* chromosome. In that case the event most frequently leading to kanamycin-resistant colonies would be homologous recombination between sequences on the plasmid and sequences on the chromosome (i.e., the 5′ and 3′ ends of the *inv* gene). A single recombination event would lead to integration of the entire plasmid into the chromosome and the creation of a merodiploid strain containing one wild-type copy of *inv*

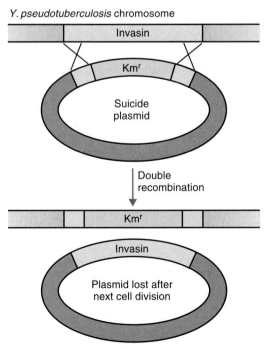

FIGURE 4-4 ▪ **Replacing the wild-type *inv* gene with a kanamycin resistance gene.** A majority of the *inv* gene contained on a suicide plasmid is replaced with a gene conferring kanamycin resistance (Km^r). After mobilization of the plasmid into *Y. pseudotuberculosis*, kanamycin-resistant exconjugants, which have undergone a double recombination event, are selected.

and one mutant copy of *inv*. However, if two recombination events occurred, one within the 5′ region of homology and one within the 3′ region, the wild-type *inv* gene would be replaced with the mutated *inv* gene. Although not the case for most bacteria, it turns out that in *Y. pseudotuberculosis*, exconjugates resulting from double recombination events are obtained from this type of experiment much more frequently than those resulting from single recombination events.

The mutant *Y. pseudotuberculosis* strain the researchers constructed was greatly impaired for cell invasion, doing so at a frequency that was only 0.1% of that of its wild-type parental strain. To rule out any effects of inserting the antibiotic on downstream genes (called **polar effects**), a wild-type copy of *inv* was introduced into the *inv* mutant on a plasmid that could replicate in *Y. pseudotuberculosis*. This **complemented** strain was able to invade mammalian cells at a rate indistinguishable from wild-type *Y. pseudotuberculosis*. Because this complementing plasmid contained only the *inv* gene and no downstream genes, the invasion defect displayed by the strain containing the insertion mutation in *inv* had to be caused by the lack of expression of a functional invasin protein.

Transposon-Based Methods for Virulence Gene Discovery

Transposons, first discovered in maize by Barbara McClintock in 1940, are found in all major branches of life. Achieving a mechanistic understanding of how transposons function led to the development of incredibly powerful genetic tools that have been used by plant, animal, and bacterial biologists.

Transposable Elements

Transposable elements ("hopping genes") are DNA segments that can insert themselves into and excise themselves from DNA molecules. These elements can therefore "hop" from one chromosomal location to another, from a chromosome to a plasmid, or vice versa. The two steps, integration and excision, are carried out by different mechanisms. There are two varieties of transposable elements: the **insertion sequence (IS)**, which has the minimal genetic information for transposition, and **transposon (Tn)**, which carries extra genes in addition to those required for transposition.

An IS element is a relatively small DNA sequence, about 1 to 2 kilobase pairs long, with two characteristic properties: First, it contains specific sequences located at its ends that are inverted repeats of one another and are required for the integration and excision processes (Fig. 4-6). Second, an IS element encodes within its core region an enzyme (called **transposase**) that recognizes the inverted repeat sequences and catalyzes the integration and excision of the IS element into and out of a DNA molecule. The integration process often results in duplication of a short stretch of DNA at the insertion site; therefore, an IS element is usually flanked by a small direct repeat sequence.

A transposon is more complex. It is composed of two IS elements flanking a core region that often contains genes encoding antibiotic resistance. Usually, the transposase of only one of the IS elements is functional, and the sequences of the "inner" inverted repeats have changed such that the entire Tn translocates from place to place via a reaction that is catalyzed by the functional transposase and involving the outermost inverted repeat sequences.

When a Tn inserts into an ORF, it almost always disrupts the function of the ORF, usually creating a loss-of-function mutation. If the Tn contains an antibiotic-resistant gene (as most do), it also marks its location in the chromosome by conferring antibiotic resistance.

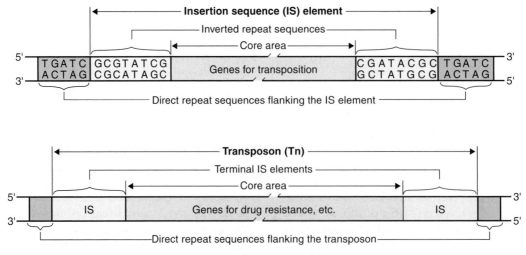

FIGURE 4-6 ▪ Insertion sequences and transposons.

Thus, a Tn can be mapped easily, transduced (along with flanking DNA) into another bacterium, and cloned (along with flanking DNA) onto a plasmid. These features make transposons extremely useful tools, and geneticists have used and modified them extensively over the years.

Transposable Reporter Genes to Identify Commonly Regulated Traits

Tn5 is a transposon that has undergone considerable "evolution" in the laboratory. It contains a gene encoding kanamycin resistance (Km^r). Originally, researchers performed transposon mutagenesis with Tn5 by introducing it into a bacterium on a suicide plasmid and then selecting for Km^r colonies that formed as a result of the Tn5 hopping from the plasmid to the chromosome. Next, pools of mutants were screened for a particular mutant phenotype (a different colony morphology or failure to grow under certain conditions, for example), and then the disrupted gene was mapped, cloned, and characterized by virtue of the Km^r gene. However, because Tn5 encodes a functional transposase, it is capable of translocating repeatedly; therefore, the mutations it creates are not stable. To circumvent this problem, geneticists moved the transposase gene from within Tn5 to another location on the suicide plasmid. The resulting "mini-Tn5," which lacks a functional transposase, cannot translocate again after the suicide plasmid containing the functional transposase gene is diluted out of the recipient bacterial cell. Mini-Tn5 thus creates stable mutations, facilitating mapping, cloning, and characterization experiments.

In the 1980s Tn5 was modified further to enable it to "report" information regarding the expression pattern of the gene into which it had inserted. With this new Tn5, researchers can identify genes whose expressing is influenced by specific factors that might be predicted to be important during infection, like temperature or the availability of iron. Of these reporter genes, the *E. coli lacZ* gene, encoding β-galactosidase, is perhaps the most commonly used. Chromogenic substrates are available that allow bacteria expressing *lacZ* (Lac$^+$ colonies) and those not expressing *lacZ* (Lac$^-$ colonies) to be distinguished easily on plates, allowing for efficient screening strategies, and sensitive quantitative enzymatic assays can be performed on cells grown in liquid culture. Specific antibodies for detecting the β-galactosidase protein are also available.

Mini-Tn5–*lacZ* contains a promoterless *lacZ* gene (the entire ORF from start codon to stop codon as well as enough sequence 5′ to the ATG to include the native ribosome binding site) located just inside the IS element. If mini-Tn5–*lacZ* inserts into a gene "downstream" from its promoter (i.e., such that the gene into which it has inserted is transcribed in the same direction as the promoterless *lacZ* gene), then *lacZ* transcription will be under the control of the promoter of the disrupted gene. Thus, levels of β-galactosidase activity will reflect (report) the transcription pattern of the disrupted gene. Mini-Tn5–*lacZ* can be used to identify genes that are regulated in response to specific environmental conditions. For example, to find genes that are expressed at 37°C but not 25°C, Km^r mini-Tn5–*lacZ* insertion mutants can be plated on a medium containing X-gal (a chromogenic substrate for β-galactosidase that produces a blue product when cleaved) and incubated at 37°C. Blue colonies can then be restreaked or replica plated onto the same medium and incubated at 25°C. Those that form white colonies at 25°C would have the desired expression pattern. Many additional easily screened or selectable reporter genes have been incorporated into mini-Tn5, including *gusA* (encoding β-glucuronidase), *luxAB* (encoding luciferase), and genes encoding resistance to antibiotics such as chloramphenicol, tetracycline, and streptomycin.

Mini-Tn5 took another evolutionary step with the development of Tn-*phoA*. The *E. coli phoA* gene encodes alkaline phosphatase, an enzyme that is active only after transportation to the periplasm. A chromogenic substrate for alkaline phosphatase analogous to X-gal, called X-P, is available. PhoA$^+$ bacteria will form blue colonies when plated on agar containing X-P, and PhoA$^-$ bacteria will form white colonies. The truncated *phoA* gene present on Tn-*phoA* lacks a promoter, a ribosome-binding site, ATG, and the nucleotides encoding the signal sequence (the first roughly 40 amino acids of the PhoA protein) used by the cellular secretion machinery to direct the alkaline phosphatase enzyme across the cytoplasmic membrane and into the periplasm. Therefore, Tn-*phoA* mutants will form blue colonies only if Tn-*phoA* has inserted into a gene such that an in-frame fusion is created and the N terminus of the fusion protein (encoded by the nucleotides at the 5′ end of the disrupted gene) contains a signal sequence for secretion across the cytoplasmic membrane. Tn-*phoA* mutagenesis is used therefore to identify genes that encode proteins secreted across the cytoplasmic membrane (and possibly also across the outer membrane of Gram-negative bacteria). Tn-*phoA* has been particularly useful in the identification of virulence factors because usually, perhaps always, they are proteins that are either surface associated or secreted. A schematic showing how Tn-*phoA* mutagenesis was used to identify virulence genes in *Vibrio cholerae* is shown in Figure 4-7. In this experiment the investigators already knew that some virulence genes in *V. cholerae* are maximally expressed at ph 6.5 in high osmolarity. So they tested PhoA$^+$ fusions for a similar pattern of expression before testing the strains in a mouse model.

Negative Selection for Identifying Essential Genes

Transposon mutagenesis is most useful when the desired phenotype can be easily screened—as with the reporter transposons incorporating *lacZ* or *phoA*—or better yet, selected. In a **screen,** the entire population is examined, and the desired mutants are identified based on an observable

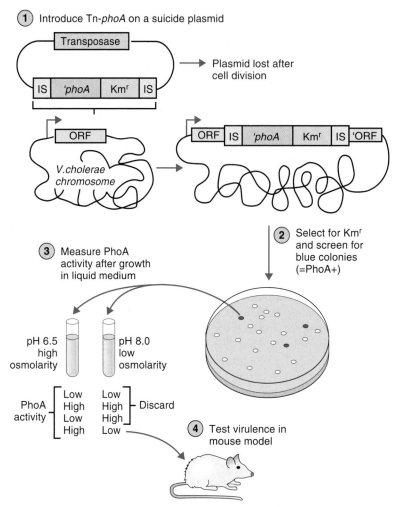

FIGURE 4-7 ■ General Tn-*phoA* mutagenesis scheme used to identify virulence genes in *V. cholerae*.

altered phenotype, such as a difference in colony color or morphology on a specific medium, lack of production of a specific protein as determined by Western blot analysis, or an inability to adhere to mammalian cells in culture. In a **selection,** only mutants with the desired phenotype (such as resistance to a specific antibiotic) survive; therefore, a mutant that is present in a population at a frequency of 1 per 10^6 or less can be identified easily. Selection schemes are clearly much more powerful than those involving screens because they allow for the detection of very rare events with little effort. Unfortunately, it is not always possible to design a selection-based mutagenesis scheme, particularly if survival of the desired mutant is decreased. The desired selection is a **negative selection,** used to find mutants unable to grow under particular conditions.

Hensel and colleagues designed a clever strategy to solve this problem. They were studying the mechanisms by which *Salmonella typhimurium* causes systemic infection in mice, a well-established model for typhoid fever in humans that is caused by *Salmonella typhi* (see Chapter 17). Although many *Salmonella* virulence genes had been identified, the researchers hypothesized that many more existed, some of which may not be identifiable using any of the in

vitro–based schemes developed up to that time. Their desire was to determine the contribution to virulence of every gene in the *S. typhimurium* chromosome. Specifically, they were after genes that were essential for the bacterium to survive during growth within the host but not within laboratory media. Although, as previously described, it is relatively simple to perform transposon mutagenesis and collect enough mutants to be certain that every nonessential gene in the genome has been mutated (within the population), it would be extremely labor intensive and prohibitively expensive to test each mutant individually to determine whether it had lost the ability to cause a lethal, systemic infection in mice. Hensel and colleagues wanted to infect mice with pools composed of hundreds of different mutants and determine which mutants were attenuated. The problem was, how do you identify the mutants that do not survive?

"Signature-Tagged" Transposons

Hensel and colleagues wanted to be able to create a population of random mutants, each marked to make it relatively easy to distinguish from the rest of the population. Although it is simple and straightforward to produce large numbers of random mutants using transposon mutagenesis, the individual mutants cannot be easily identified because the transposons are identical and the mutants differ only in the chromosomal location of the Tn. To overcome this problem, the researchers created a pool of transposons that were each "tagged" with a unique 40–base pair stretch of DNA (a molecular signature). The tags were synthesized in vitro as oligonucleotides with 40–base pair random sequences in the center, flanked by recognition sequences for the restriction endonuclease *Hin*dIII and invariable "arms" that served as primer binding sites for amplification using the **polymerase chain reaction (PCR)**. The population of random tags was amplified using PCR and cloned into mini-Tn*5* present on a suicide plasmid, creating a source of tagged mini-Tn*5*s (Fig. 4-8).

Creating Transposon Pools

The tagged mini-Tn*5*s were introduced into *S. typhimurium* on a suicide plasmid by conjugation, and mu-

tants on whose chromosomes the tagged mini-Tn*5*s had hopped were selected on plates containing kanamycin. Each mutant was stored in a well of a 96 well microtiter dish and a total of 1,510 individual mutants was isolated and stored.

Screening for Mutants in Animal Models of Infection

To identify mutants with this approach, Hensel and colleagues used the following procedure (see Fig. 4-8). Bacteria from each well of a microtiter dish were replica-plated onto two identical membranes, the bacteria were lysed, and the DNA was denatured to separate the two strands and attached to the membranes by cross-linking. These membranes were saved for use later in the procedure. Bacteria from each well were also grown together in liquid medium in vitro, forming the "input pool." An aliquot of this culture was used to infect mice by intraperitoneal injection.

FIGURE 4-8 ■ **Signature-tagged mutagenesis to identify virulence genes in *S. typhimurium*.**

Three days later, bacteria recovered from the spleens of the infected mice were plated on standard laboratory medium, and about 10,000 colonies were combined, forming the "recovered pool." Chromosomal DNA was isolated from the two pools of bacteria (the input pool and the recovered pool), and PCR was used to amplify the sequence tags. Radioactive nucleotides were used in the amplification to label the products. Because recognition sequences for the restriction endonuclease *Hind*III were incorporated into the sequence tags, the unique 40–base pair portions of the tags could be liberated by digesting with this enzyme. The labeled, unique sequence tags generated from the input pool were incubated with one of the membranes containing DNA from each of the mutant bacteria, and the tags generated from the recovered pool were incubated with the other membrane. The incubations were carried out under conditions in which the tags could anneal with the complementary sequences present in the chromosomal DNA.

After extensive washing, the membranes were exposed to x-ray film, and the patterns obtained for the two blots were compared. The membrane incubated with labeled tags amplified from the input pool caused black spots on the film corresponding to every well of the microtiter dish. This was expected because all the mutants, and thus all the sequence tags, should have been represented in the input population. The membrane incubated with labeled tags amplified from the recovered pool caused black spots on the film corresponding to most, but not all, of the wells. A well for which a black spot was not obtained contained mutants that were not present in the recovered pool, potentially because the transposons in these mutants disrupted genes required for survival in the host. Of 12 pools tested (representing 1,152 different mutants), 40 such mutants were identified.

The DNA sequence flanking the transposon insertion in 28 of the 40 mutants was determined. Thirteen of the insertions were in previously identified *S. typhimurium* virulence genes. This result validated the usefulness of the screening approach. Six of the mutations were in genes with sequence similarity to known genes in other pathogenic bacteria but which had not previously been identified as virulence genes in *S. typhimurium*. In this class were genes for a specialized secretion system, called a **type III secretion system** (see Chapters 16 and 17) that has since been demonstrated to be required for macrophage survival of *Salmonella*. When these mutants were tested for virulence individually, they were each found to be greatly attenuated. Nine of the mutants identified in the screen were in genes with no similarity to database entries and therefore represented potentially novel virulence genes.

The power of this approach cannot be overstated. Because pools of 96 mutants could be screened simultaneously, 1,152 mutants were tested using only 24 mice (2% of the number that would have been required to test them individually). This represents a significant savings in effort, time, and mice. In addition, because signature-tagged mutagenesis finds genes essential for survival in the host, it is an exceptional method for potential new antimicrobial targets for therapeutic purposes.

Promoter-Trapping Methods

Several approaches have been developed to identify virulence genes based on their predicted pattern of transcriptional activity during infection. The approach, called **in vivo expression technology (IVET)**, was designed to isolate promoters that are active under specific conditions. Once a promoter is identified, the genes and gene products whose expression it drives can be identified and characterized.

IVET differs significantly from most of the genetic approaches used to identify and characterize virulence genes, which require that the gene be expressed either within the pathogen itself or in a surrogate such as *E. coli* grown in or on laboratory medium. For example, the discovery of *inv* by Isberg and colleagues required its expression in *E. coli* growing in Luria Bertani (LB) broth. These approaches are dependent on, and limited by, the ability to mimic in the laboratory the environmental conditions that the bacteria are exposed to in the host during infection. Mahan, Slauch, and Mekalanos hypothesized that specific conditions exist in the host that laboratory conditions cannot (or do not) adequately reflect, and that some virulence genes are expressed *only* under those specific conditions. To test their hypothesis, the researchers devised a genetic strategy designed to identify genes expressed in vivo but *not* in vitro. They employed this strategy to study *S. typhimurium* genes, using murine infection as the in vivo condition and MacConkey lactose agar as the in vitro condition.

Constructing Promoter Libraries

The first goal of the IVET approach was to identify *S. typhimurium* genes expressed in vivo—that is, during murine infection. It had been demonstrated previously that *S. typhimurium purA* mutants are completely avirulent. The *purA* gene encodes an enzyme required for purine biosynthesis. *S. typhimurium* can import purines from its surroundings; therefore, *purA* mutants can grow in the laboratory if purines are supplied in the medium. *PurA* mutants are completely unable to establish murine infection, indicating that purines are not readily available to *S. typhimurium* within the in vivo niches it colonizes in the mouse. Mahan and colleagues exploited this fact to design a **selection** scheme to identify genes expressed in vivo.

First, the researchers constructed an *S. typhimurium* strain containing a deletion mutation in the *purA* gene. It was important to use a deletion mutation, which is non-revertible, rather than a point mutation, which could potentially revert to wild type during infection, eliminating the basis for selection. Next Mahan and colleagues constructed a plasmid (pIVET1) with the following characteristics (Fig. 4-9): (1) It could be introduced into *S. typhimurium* by conjugation. (2) It was a suicide plasmid for *S. typhimurium* but not *E. coli*; that is, it could replicate autonomously in *E. coli* but not *S. typhimurium*. (3) It contained a gene encoding ampicillin resistance (called *bla*, for β-lactamase). (4) It contained a site upstream of the *purA* gene into which foreign DNA fragments could be cloned. (5) It contained a promoterless *lacZ* gene immediately downstream of *purA*, with no transcriptional termination signals between *purA* and *lacZ*. (6) It contained no sequences with homology to the *S. typhimurium* chromosome.

The researchers isolated chromosomal DNA from wild-type *S. typhimurium*, digested it with a restriction endonuclease, and ligated the resulting DNA fragments in the cloning site upstream of *purA*. The resulting plasmids were used to transform *E. coli*, and transformants were selected on agar containing ampicillin. These transformants, representing a chromosomal library of *S. typhimurium*, were pooled.

Plasmid-Based Recombination for Operon Fusion

The pIVET1 derivative plasmids were introduced into the mutated Δ*purA* strain of *S. typhimurium* by conjugation, and exconjugates were selected on agar containing purines and ampicillin. Because pIVET1 is a suicide plasmid for *S. typhimurium* with no homology to the *S. typhimurium* chromosome, ampicillin-resistant

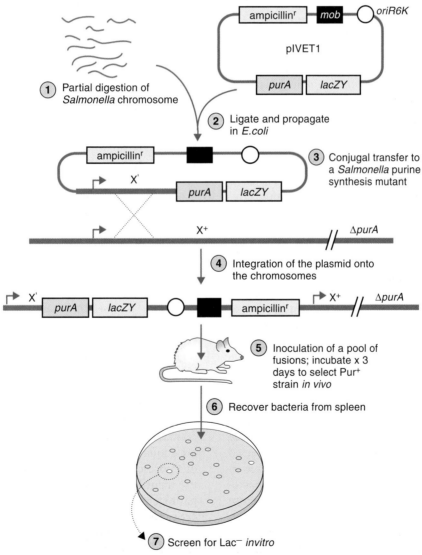

FIGURE 4-9 ▪ **In vivo expression technology (IVET) used to identify virulence genes in *S. typhimurium*.**

exconjugates will take place only if homologous recombination occurs between the *S. typhimurium* sequences cloned into the pIVET1 derivative and the *S. typhimurium* chromosome, resulting in integration of the entire plasmid into the chromosome (see Fig. 4-9). If the *S. typhimurium* sequences on the plasmid happen to contain a transcriptional promoter oriented in the same direction as *purA* and *lacZ*, then on integration of the plasmid, transcription from this promoter will drive transcription of *purA* and *lacZ* when it is active. Note that if the entire promoter region is present within the fragment cloned into pIVET1, transcription of the native gene on the chromosome will not be altered because these sequences will also be present upstream of the native gene. Mahan and colleagues pooled ampicillin-resistant exconjugates.

Selection of Promoters Active During Infection

The pooled exconjugates (containing integrated pIVET1-derivative plasmids) were injected into mice intraperitoneally. Three days later the mice were euthanized and bacteria were recovered from their spleens (see Fig. 4-9). Because *purA* mutants of *S. typhimurium* are avirulent, the only bacteria that could be recovered from a spleen three days postinoculation would be those in which the *purA* gene on the integrated plasmid was expressed in vivo. For such recovery to occur, the *S. typhimurium* chromosomal DNA fragment cloned into the pIVET1 plasmid either must contain a promoter oriented to directing transcription of *purA* (and *lacZ*), or it must contain an internal fragment of a gene or operon oriented so that when the plasmid integrates into the gene, the upstream promoter directs expression of *purA* (and *lacZ*). Note, however, that if the fragment contains only an internal fragment of a gene or operon, the gene or operon will not be transcribed in the exconjugates because it will have been separated from its promoter by integration of the plasmid. If the gene or operon is essential for virulence, then although *purA* transcription will be restored in vivo, the strain will not survive in the mouse. Passage of the exconjugates' pool through the mouse thus provides a selection for strains containing integrated plasmids that contain promoters expressed in vivo.

Because the goal of this approach was to find genes expressed in vivo and not in vitro, the next step in the analysis was to determine if any of the promoters selected on the basis of expression in vivo were not expressed in vitro. To do this, Mahan and colleagues plated the bacteria recovered from the mice onto MacConkey lactose agar. MacConkey lactose agar is a differential medium on which Lac$^+$ bacteria form red colonies and Lac$^-$ bacteria form white colonies. Most of the recovered bacteria formed red colonies. That result was expected because most genes required for *S. typhimurium* to grow in vivo

(such as those encoding ribosomal proteins and RNA, RNA polymerase, cell wall constituents, and other "housekeeping" functions) are also required for growth in vitro. Five percent of the bacteria recovered from the mouse spleens formed white colonies on MacConkey lactose agar, indicating that the integrated plasmids contained promoters expressed in vivo but not in vitro. These were the clones Mahan and colleagues were looking for. They chose 15 strains for further characterization. To confirm that those strains contained plasmids with in vivo–induced promoters, they infected mice with each strain individually and measured β-galactosidase activity in bacteria recovered from the spleens of mice as well as from bacteria grown in a standard laboratory medium. In all cases β-galactosidase activity was greater in bacteria recovered from mouse spleens than in bacteria grown in a laboratory medium.

To identify the in vivo–induced genes, the researchers determined the nucleotide sequences of the *S. typhimurium* DNA fragments containing the in vivo–induced promoters and compared the sequences they obtained with those present in GenBank. Five genetic loci were identified. Two had no significant homology to sequences present in GenBank and therefore represented potentially novel virulence genes. Some of the genes identified with this approach were involved in quite ordinary aspects of bacterial physiology, raising the question of how we define virulence factors. Enzymes involved in amino acid, nucleic acid, or transfer RNA biosynthesis do not fit the classic definition of a virulence factor. However, expression of these enzymes occurs in vivo and is required for virulence yet dispensable for growth in vitro. Thus, these enzymes represent "components that are required for or that potentiate the organism's ability to cause disease" and thus fit an expanded definition of a virulence factor. While a debate regarding whether factors that fall into this category represent true virulence genes will undoubtedly continue for some time, there is no question that learning that these factors are essential for *S. typhimurium* to cause a lethal infection reveals information regarding the types of environments it encounters within the host to do so. Furthermore, given their requirement for growth during infection, the genes identified by IVET also represent attractive therapeutic targets.

A variation of IVET, termed differential fluorescence induction (DFI), was subsequently developed. The basic features of library construction and pooling of strains are similar to IVET, but the key feature of DFI is its use of fluorescence as a reporter. The method was designed to identify promoters specifically upregulated by pathogens that can survive within professional phagocytic cells, which represent a major defense against infection (see Chapter 6). A number of important pathogens, such as *Salmonella typhi* (see Chapter 17), *Legionella pneumophila* (see Chapter 21), and *Mycobacterium tuberculosis* (see Chapter 23), to name just a few, can sur-

FIGURE 4-10 ▪ Differential fluorescence induction (DFI) technique used to identify genes expressed by *S. typhimurium* during intracellular survival in macrophages.

vive within professional phagocytes. A state-of-the-art approach, DFI uses **fluorescence-activated cell sorting (FACS)** of pooled libraries of bacteria in which promoter DNA has been randomly fused to a fluorescent reporter gene, such as *gfp*, which encodes green fluorescent protein (Fig. 4-10). Promoters that are activated by bacteria within the phagocyte cause the phagocyte to become highly fluorescent, which causes it to be sorted from the rest of the nonfluorescent population. The basic elements of DFI are shown in Figure 4-10.

Antibody-Based Approaches

In addition to performing their primary and critically important functions in clearing current infections and preventing new ones, our adaptive immune responses also provide powerful tools for studying bacterial pathogenesis. Antibodies are particularly useful because they are easily obtained from serum, and a plethora of reagents and protocols that take advantage of their specificity and binding characteristics have been developed. Indeed, because pathogen-specific antibodies are induced to very high levels in response to infection, relatively simple yet highly sensitive antibody-based protocols are used routinely in clinical laboratories to diagnose many bacterial and viral infections. Pathogen-specific antibodies have

also been extremely useful for identifying, purifying, and characterizing virulence factors. An antibody-based approach designed to identify virulence genes expressed exclusively in vivo is described here.

In vivo–induced antigen technology (IVIAT), first suggested by Handfield and colleagues in 2000, uses the host antibody response to identify proteins expressed by the bacteria during infection but not during growth in standard laboratory conditions. Although similar to IVET in that its goal is to identify factors expressed *only* in vivo, IVIAT does not rely on the use of animal models. This represents a significant advantage because animal models that reproduce, at least to some extent, the natural course of infection do not exist for many human pathogens. The rationale behind IVIAT is as follows: On exposure to a particular pathogen, production of a large population of pathogen-specific antibodies are induced. Each antibody in the population recognizes a single epitope and therefore, most likely, a single factor expressed by the bacteria during the course of infection. As discussed earlier, most factors expressed during infection are also expressed during growth in vitro. Antibodies that recognize such factors should be present in the population of induced antibodies. However, if, as hypothesized, some bacterial factors are expressed *only* during infection, antibodies that recognize these in vivo–induced antigens should also be present in the population of induced antibodies. The goal of IVIAT is to isolate this population of antibodies and use it to identify the in vivo–induced antigens. Deb and colleagues were the first to publish a study using this approach. They used IVIAT to identify virulence genes in *Mycobacterium tuberculosis,* the causative agent of tuberculosis (TB), which kills about 3 million people annually (see Chapter 23).

Preparing Convalescent Sera

The first objective of the IVIAT approach is to isolate a population of antibodies that recognize bacterial factors expressed only during infection. Deb and colleagues began by collecting and pooling sera from 25 TB patients. The pooled convalescent serum theoretically contained antibodies recognizing all *M. tuberculosis* factors expressed in vivo. To remove the antibodies recognizing factors expressed by *M. tuberculosis* in vitro, a lysate of *M. tuberculosis* grown on Lowenstein-Jensen agar was prepared and immobilized on a nitrocellulose membrane, and the membrane was incubated with the pooled serum. Antibodies that bound to the factors present on the membrane were removed when the membrane was removed from the serum sample (Fig. 4-11). This absorption procedure was repeated multiple times, resulting in depletion of antibodies recognizing in vitro–expressed antigens

from the pooled serum, and leaving behind the antibodies that recognize *M. tuberculosis* factors expressed in vivo but not in vitro. For reasons that will become apparent in the following sections, a lysate of *E. coli* was also prepared, bound to nitrocellulose, and used to deplete the serum of anti–*E. coli* antibodies.

Phage-Based Expression Libraries

The next objective of the IVIAT approach is to use the absorbed serum to identify in vivo–induced factors. Because the genes encoding these factors are, by definition, not expressed during growth in vitro, the researchers needed to activate transcription of these genes artificially. They accomplished this by constructing an **expression library.** The goal of constructing an expression library is to express all or part of every protein that the bacterium is capable of producing in at least one member of the library. A commonly used expression library is **bacteriophage λgt11.**

Bacteriophage, or simply phage, are viruses that infect bacteria. When some phages, called **temperate phages,** infect bacteria, they can take one of two path-

FIGURE 4-11 ▪ **In vivo–induced antigen technology (IVIAT) used to identify in vivo–induced antigens in *M. tuberculosis.***

ways of growth. In one pathway, they incorporate their genomes into that of their host and replicate in a benign, quiescent state in which most of their genes are not expressed or are expressed at low levels. Bacteria in which phage are replicating this way are called **lysogens,** and many pathogenic bacteria are actually lysogens in which important virulence factors are expressed from the phage genome. An example of this is *Corynebacterium diphtheriae,* which produces a potent toxin by virtue of being lysogenic for a toxin-encoding phage (see Chapter 9). Under conditions of DNA damage and possibly other stresses, lysogens can be induced, and the phage **lytic growth** program is activated. During lytic growth, phage take over the host cell transcription and translation machinery to express phage genes and proteins at very high levels, assemble 100 or more phage particles per bacterial cell, and then lyse the bacterial cell and infect neighboring cells. On a lawn of bacteria growing on an agar plate, a single phage can form a **plaque** (a clearing zone resulting from the lysis of infected bacteria) containing 10^8 to 10^9 phage particles in a matter of hours.

The expression phage λgt11 is a modified form of the well-studied temperate phage λ. This modified phage has been engineered to contain a *lacZ* gene with a unique restriction endonuclease cleavage site just downstream of the transcription and translation initiation sites. Moreover, the promoter driving expression of *lacZ* in λgt11 is inducible by isopropyl-β-D-thiogalactopyranoside (IPTG). Deb and colleagues isolated *M. tuberculosis* chromosomal DNA, generated fragments of about 3 kilobase pairs, and inserted them into λgt11 DNA using restriction enzymes and DNA ligase. The recombinant λ chromosomes were packaged into phage particles in vitro and used to infect lawns of *E. coli.* The first several hours of infection were allowed to proceed in the absence of IPTG. Under these conditions, phage genes were expressed, but *lacZ* and any fusion proteins resulting from insertion of *M. tuberculosis* DNA were not expressed. For the last few hours of the infection process, IPTG was added to the medium. The presence of IPTG results in high levels of transcription from the *lacZ* promoter. If inserting *M. tuberculosis* DNA into *lacZ* results in the formation of an in-frame fusion between *lacZ* and an *M. tuberculosis* open-reading frame, a fusion protein is synthesized at high levels, and when λ lyses the bacterial cells to infect neighboring cells, the fusion protein is released.

The λgt11 expression library system has been developed such that every step is very efficient. It is relatively easy to construct a library of expression phages in which every open-reading frame of the bacterial genome is represented as a fusion protein in at least one member of the library. Because the infection process is so efficient and tiny plaques can contain high levels of the fusion proteins, it is also easy to set up conditions such that thousands of plaques can be produced on a single lawn of *E. coli* growing on an agar plate, which can then be screened for expression of the desired protein.

Screening Expression Libraries with Sera

The next step in the process was to identify recombinant λ phage expressing the in vivo–induced *M. tuberculosis* genes. Lawns of *E. coli* were infected with the phage library such that about 1,000 plaques formed on each plate. Then a nitrocellulose membrane saturated with IPTG was placed on top of the lawn. The IPTG induced transcription of the *lacZ* promoter and therefore expression of the LacZ fusion proteins resulting from insertion of *M. tuberculosis* open-reading frames, and proteins that were released from the bacterial cell bound to the nitrocellulose membrane. The membranes with their bound proteins were then incubated with the absorbed serum. Any proteins recognized by antibodies present in the serum would be bound by those antibodies. The membranes were washed to remove unbound antibodies and then incubated with antihuman antibodies to which the enzyme horseradish peroxidase (HRP) was conjugated. After additional washing steps, the membrane was incubated with a substrate for HRP that produces a dark brown product when cleaved. The position of any brown spots on the membrane therefore indicated the position of λ phage expressing fusion proteins recognized by the absorbed serum. Because the serum was depleted of antibodies that recognize *M. tuberculosis* proteins expressed in vitro and *E. coli* proteins, the fusion proteins should have represented *M. tuberculosis* proteins expressed only in vivo. The IVIAT approach is obviously very useful for identifying genes whose products can stimulate an immune response and which therefore might be valuable components in vaccine development.

Genomic Approaches

As previously mentioned, DNA sequencing technology is now so fast and efficient that determining the complete nucleotide sequence of entire genomes has become almost routine. For most bacterial pathogens, the genomic sequence of at least one strain is known and publicly available, and for some organisms the sequences of several strains have been determined, allowing comparative analyses. The availability of genome sequence information has revolutionized all aspects of microbiology: many diagnostic tests are now based on genomic sequence information; epidemiological studies are much more sensitive and sophisticated; and the ability to identify, clone, and mutate genes specifically, accurately, and efficiently has increased the pace of research enormously.

Transcriptome Analysis

With the availability of genomic sequence information and the advent of **microarray** technology, it is now possible to measure the relative transcription level of every gene in a bacterial chromosome at the same time. Moreover, gene expression patterns (or transcriptomes) in bacteria grown under various environmental conditions can be compared simultaneously so that genes that are differentially expressed in response to specific conditions can be identified. Thus, while some of the approaches described in the preceding sections allow the identification of individual genes expressed preferentially or exclusively in vivo, microarray-based approaches have the potential of identifying *all* the genes with that expression pattern. A typical analysis was performed by Merrell and colleagues, who were studying *Vibrio cholerae* pathogenesis.

DNA Microarrays

Merrell and colleagues wanted to identify in vivo–induced genes in *V. cholerae* on a genome-wide scale. Their goal was to identify all the *V. cholerae* genes transcribed at a higher rate when the bacteria were colonizing the human intestine than when growing under standard laboratory conditions. The first step was to construct a microarray of the *V. cholerae* genome. A fragment of every open-reading frame identified from the nucleotide sequence of the *V. cholerae* genome (which happens to be composed of two separate circular chromosomes) was amplified by PCR and placed (or printed), using a special robot, onto a discrete spot on a microscope slide coated with poly-lysine to which the DNA molecules would bind and be immobilized (Fig. 4-12). Using this technique, thousands of individual DNA fragments, each corresponding to a different gene, were spotted onto a single square inch area of the slide such that the identity of the gene present in each location was known.

RNA Isolation

The next step was to isolate total cellular RNA from bacteria grown under the two conditions to be compared. For the in vitro–grown sample, Merrell and colleagues grew *V. cholerae* in a standard laboratory medium to

stationary phase. To obtain bacteria grown in vivo, the researchers obtained stool samples from cholera patients in Bangladesh. As discussed in Chapter 16, *V. cholerae* causes severe diarrhea that is characterized by "rice water" stools. Merrell and colleagues found that not only did these stools contain incredibly high numbers of bacteria (10^8 to 10^9 per milliliter, which is similar to the density obtained after overnight growth in a standard laboratory medium), but also they were nearly all *V. cholerae*. Sufficient in vivo–grown *V. cholerae* bacteria could therefore be obtained rather easily to isolate enough RNA to do several experiments.

Complementary DNA Synthesis and Fluorescent Labeling

Next the researchers synthesized complementary DNA (cDNA) from the RNA samples. For the RNA isolated from in vitro–grown bacteria, the cDNA was synthesized using deoxycytidine triphosphate (dCTP) conjugated to Cy5, a fluorescent dye that emits red light; and for the RNA isolated from in vivo–grown bacteria, the cDNA was synthesized using dCTP conjugated to Cy3, a fluorescent dye that emits green light.

Probing DNA Microarrays

The Cy3- and Cy5-labeled cDNA samples were then mixed together and incubated with the microarray, first under denaturing conditions to separate all the DNA strands and then under renaturing conditions to allow the Cy3- and Cy5-labeled cDNA molecules to hybridize with complementary DNA molecules immobilized on the glass slide. The slide was then washed to remove all unbound cDNA molecules and analyzed using a special microarray fluorescence scanner. For every spot on the microarray, the level of green and red fluorescence was recorded, and the data were reported as a ratio of the two. A high green-to-red ratio resulted when more Cy3-labeled cDNA was present in the sample, indicating a

FIGURE 4-12 ▪ Microarray scheme used to compare the transcriptomes of *V. cholerae* grown in vitro and in vivo.

higher level of expression of that particular gene in the bacteria recovered from the stool samples than in the bacteria grown in vitro. Reciprocally, a low green-to-red ratio indicated a higher level of expression in the in vitro–grown bacteria than in those recovered from the cholera patients. A ratio of one, or very close to one, indicated approximately equal expression in the in vitro– and in vivo–grown bacteria.

Merrell and colleagues' analysis identified 237 differentially regulated genes: 44 that were expressed more highly in the bacteria recovered from the stool samples and 193 that were expressed more highly in the in vitro–grown bacteria. Some of the in vivo–induced genes were the same as those identified using other approaches, including those involved in the ability of *V. cholerae* to mount an acid-tolerance response, and some were previously unidentified *V. cholerae* genes. Genes that were repressed in vivo included many involved in chemotaxis.

Proteome Analysis

All the approaches described in this chapter so far have focused on identifying and characterizing genes involved in pathogenesis. However, it is not the genes that allow pathogenic bacteria to grow in or on host tissues to cause disease; it is their protein products. Although protein levels in bacteria frequently reflect gene transcription levels, biological influences that affect the stability, half-life, posttranscriptional, cotranslational, and degradative modifications of proteins cannot be deduced from transcriptional analyses. Therefore, major goals toward understanding mechanisms of pathogenesis have been to identify and characterize directly the entire protein profile (or **proteome**) expressed by pathogenic bacteria. A comparison of the proteome expressed by bacteria grown in vitro with that of those recovered from an infected host, analogous to the transcriptome comparison described earlier, should be especially informative. Recent advances in two-dimensional polyacrylamide gel electrophoresis (2D-PAGE) technologies, coupled with increased ability to recover proteins and determine their amino acid sequences using highly sophisticated mass

spectrometry and mass peptide finge gies, are beginning to make such analy is expected that approaches that comb and proteomic techniques will represent advance in this field.

Analyzing The Host Response

Just as bacteria alter their gene expression profile sponse to the environments they encounter during course of infection, their mammalian hosts also acti and repress different classes of genes in response to ba terial infection. Using a microarray approach, Relma and colleagues examined gene transcription responses in human peripheral blood mononuclear cells exposed to a variety of bacterial pathogens. They found very similar gene expression responses to killed bacteria and to common bacterial components, such as LPS. Of interest to questions of infection and immunity, however, is that qualitative and quantitative differences in responses to various live bacterial pathogens were observed. Although much characterization remains to be done, Relman and colleagues proposed the intriguing hypothesis that different pathogens may induce distinct "signature" responses in their hosts that could provide a basis for their identification. If true, bacterial infections could be diagnosed in the future by analyzing the gene expression profile in cells obtained from a peripheral blood specimen rather than culturing the organism from the primary site of infection.

Conclusion

The experimental "case studies" described in this chapter demonstrate how a combination of genetic, biochemical, molecular biological, and cell biological approaches can be used to identify and characterize bacterial virulence genes and their products, improving the understanding of the mechanisms of microbial pathogenesis. Such information is crucial to the development of new diagnostic tests, vaccine strategies, and therapeutic agents.

Bacterial Pathogenesis

55

...printing technolo-
...is possible, and it
...ne both genetic
...he next major

...s in re-
...g the
...ate
...c-

...is for
...al Action

...alzkill and Cary Engleberg

Killing microorganisms is relatively simple as long as it is not selective. Among the substances that can kill microorganisms are heat, radiation, and strong acids. Targeting specific microbes while sparing host cells and tissues is much more difficult. According to Paul Ehrlich, a pioneer of modern chemotherapy, what we want is a "specific chemotherapy" to kill the microbes and not ourselves. Paradoxically, we depend on the microbial world to provide us with many of the chemotherapeutic agents that we need to kill bacteria.

How and When Were Antibiotics Discovered?

One way organisms in the environment—soil, water, or areas of the human body—attempt to gain an advantage over other organisms is by secreting specific chemicals. Some secrete antibiotics, and others employ more subtle methods of competition. Chapter 3 described how microorganisms secrete iron-chelating compounds and are capable of reabsorbing their own iron-bearing products. In this manner microbes reduce the iron concentration to levels that do not permit the growth of other organisms unable to scavenge iron more efficiently. Thus, in complex environments competition for nutrients combines with the action of antibiotic substances to produce a balanced microbial ecology.

In the last 30 years we have taken advantage of this natural warfare for our own purposes, borrowing antibiotics from one organism to combat others. The result has been a medical revolution of immense proportions. Figure 5-1 shows the increase in human longevity since the introduction of antibiotic therapy. Now, because we take for granted the use of antibiotics, it is difficult to recapture the early impact of modern chemotherapy. Ask older family members how they feared the loss of a loved one from pneumonia or postoperative infection, or talk to older physicians about how powerless they were when treating children with meningococcal meningitis or subacute bacterial endocarditis.

However, there is a price to pay for our therapeutic progress. The selective pressure exerted by antibiotics on bacteria is so great that within one human generation, many bacteria have responded by becoming resistant, often to several antibiotics.

The first important antimicrobial agents were not true antibiotics but synthetic **antimetabolites.** Ehrlich's seminal work derived from his findings that dyes used in histochemistry became bound to cell-specific receptors. "Why then," he asked,

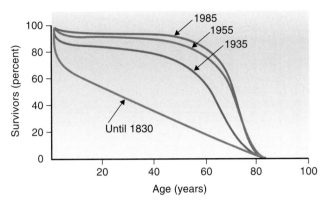

FIGURE 5-1 ▪ **Survival of human populations as a function of age.** Average life expectancy (50% level) remained at 25 until l830. Between 1830 and l935 the impact of sanitation, public health, and immunization extended life expectancy. Antibiotics (along with better nutrition and health education) added an average of another 8 years. Note that more recent medical breakthroughs have not extended average life expectancy very much.

"should not such dyes be made toxic for specific organisms?" As validation of Ehrlich's intuition, workers in the mammoth German chemical industry systematically synthesized thousands of compounds and tested them for biological effects. In 1934 Domagk found that one of those compounds, prontosil, cured a fatal streptococcal infection in mice. It was then shown that prontosil was inactive in pure cultures of bacteria in vitro but was hydrolyzed in vivo to the active drug **sulfanilamide.** Cures with this first sulfa drug, or **sulfonamide,** were soon reported. These findings gave impetus to the efforts to purify penicillin, a true antibiotic produced by the mold *Penicillium* and first detected by Alexander Fleming in 1928. A new era had arrived; the search for new antimetabolites and antibiotics has continued ever since.

What Is the Basis for Selective Antimicrobial Action? The Example of Sulfonamides

Early on researchers discovered that extracts from yeast contain a substance that antagonizes the action of sulfonamides. When purified, the substance was found to be *p*-aminobenzoic acid (PAB; Fig. 5-2), a component of folic acid. The similarity in the structure of PAB and sulfanilamide is obvious. Following this lead, hundreds of thousands of antimetabolites have been tested for possible therapeutic value. In the sulfa class alone, thousands

FIGURE 5-2 ▪ **Inhibition of folic acid synthesis (by sulfa) and function (by other antibacterial drugs).** The addition of sulfanilamide instead of *p*-aminobenzoic acid to dihydropteroic acid inhibits the synthesis of folic acid. In addition, the resulting analog functions as a "lethal product."

of derivatives with small and large modifications have been studied; about 25 are still in use.

The competition between sulfonamide and PAB in bacteria is illustrated in Figure 5-3. When more sulfonamide is added, proportionally more PAB is required to counteract its action. This type of antagonism is called **competitive inhibition.** The mechanism of action was clarified when the function of PAB became better

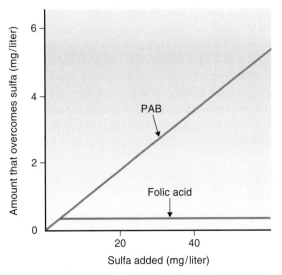

FIGURE 5-3 ▪ **PAB overcomes sulfa addition competitively; folic acid, noncompetitively.**

known. Because PAB is a constituent of folic acid (see Fig. 5-2), it was inferred that sulfa drugs inhibit the synthesis of that vitamin and thus the coenzymes that contain it. The main coenzyme is tetrahydroformyl folic acid (THFA), which functions in reactions that add a carbon unit to synthesize nucleosides and certain amino acids (see Fig. 5-2). Therefore, researchers reasoned that folic acid should suppress the action of sulfa drugs, and further, that if bacteria were given enough folic acid to satisfy their growth requirements, no amount of a folic acid inhibitor synthesis could suppress their growth. In contrast to PAB, antagonism of sulfas by folic acid is **noncompetitive**. This expectation was subsequently confirmed (see Fig. 5-3).

The effectiveness of sulfa drugs against bacteria depends on the different ways body cells and bacteria synthesize and use folic acid. Body cells require **preformed** folic acid, which explains why they are unaffected by sulfonamides. Sulfonamides inhibit the *synthesis* of the compound, not its *utilization*. On the other hand, the folic acid we require must be present in the circulation and tissues. Why then cannot bacteria use this and escape sulfonamide action? The reason seems to be that many bacteria that make folic acid lack a system for the uptake of preformed folic acid and cannot benefit from its presence in the environment. These bacteria must synthesize their own folic acid, which makes them susceptible to sulfa drugs. Folic acid everywhere, and not a molecule to save them!

What Limits the Efficacy of Antimicrobial Drugs?

The mechanism of action of a drug is only one of the properties that determine its potential usefulness. This book describes many others, including pharmacodynamics, cost, and the likelihood of patient compliance. Briefly considered here are three kinds of limitations on the efficacy of antimicrobial drugs that are related directly to their modes of action: the speed with which the drugs work, the sensitivity of the microbial target, and the side effects on the host.

Speed of Action

The practical efficacy of drugs sometimes depends on how fast they stop bacteria in their tracks. The case of sulfanilamide is instructive: when the drug is added to a culture of susceptible bacteria, growth is inhibited after about two to four generations. The reason for the delay is that each bacterium contains enough preformed folic

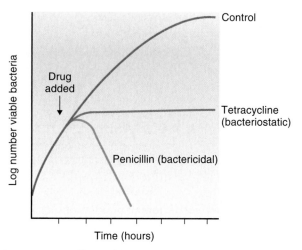

FIGURE 5-4 ■ **Effect of bacteriostatic and bactericidal drugs on the growth of bacteria.** Note that certain bacteriostatic drugs may not inhibit growth for some time. In the case of sulfa drugs, the lag is the result of the time required to use up preformed folic acid in the bacteria.

acid to meet the demands of up to 16 daughter cells. Only after 16 cells are formed does the drug become effective. Inhibition by sulfonamides then is dependent on the continued growth of the bacteria.

Other things being equal, **bactericidal** agents, which kill microorganisms rapidly, are preferable to **bacteriostatic** ones, which inhibit growth reversibly (Fig. 5-4). Organisms that remain alive in the presence of a drug can still harm the host, either by continuing to produce toxins or by becoming resistant to the drug and eventually resuming growth. Bactericidal drugs have been clearly shown to work better when the body's defenses are insufficient to clear the invading agents. Important examples are bacterial endocarditis, bacterial meningitis, and infections in patients with low numbers of circulating neutrophils (agranulocytopenia). Nevertheless, the preference for bactericidal agents depends on the circumstances. For example, an inhibitor of protein synthesis, such as erythromycin, is bacteriostatic but stops the synthesis of protein toxins abruptly. In contrast, penicillin kills bacteria but not immediately: during the lag before the drug exerts its lytic effect, the organisms continue to produce toxins. Therefore, in experimental infections of mice with an agent of gas gangrene, *Clostridium perfringens*, a static drug protected the animals better than a cidal one. Thus, in practical terms, static antibiotics can be more useful in some circumstances. Ultimately, inhibition of bacterial growth gives the defense mechanisms of the body an opportunity to get rid of the organisms.

The distinction of **static versus cidal** should not be taken as absolute. First, a drug may act differently in different organisms. For example, the modified aminoglycoside, spectinomycin, is static for *Escherichia coli* and cidal for gonococci. Second, some drugs show odd kinetics of action that make them difficult to classify. For example, rifampin rapidly kills 99% of *E. coli* cells in vitro but is static for the remaining 1%, perhaps because these bacteria are particularly resistant during a phase of their cell cycle. In other cases a combination of two static drugs may achieve a cidal action. Despite these ambiguities, the criterion of static versus cidal is generally useful in considering the outcome of drug therapy. In the future, drugs may be developed that work in other ways, for example, inhibiting virulence factors (e.g., toxins or adhesins). Because such drugs would not affect the growth of microorganisms in vitro, their action would only be manifested during infection in vivo.

Sensitivity of the Target

The efficacy of antimicrobial drugs depends on the degree of sensitivity of the intended target organisms. Every agent is effective against a defined range or **spectrum** of organisms. Broad-spectrum antibiotics, which are effective against a wide range of bacteria, might be thought to be preferable to drugs with narrow spectra. However, several practical considerations, such as cost, argue against the widespread use of broad-spectrum antibiotics. These drugs should be reserved for appropriate situations, such as when the etiological agent cannot be determined before therapy begins or for immunocompromised patients who may be subject to simultaneous infection by several agents.

The spectrum of microbial susceptibility depends not only on the organisms but also on the conditions of the infection. For example, aminoglycosides are taken up poorly by bacteria under anaerobic conditions. Thus, these drugs are ineffective against anaerobes. Also, the level of a drug achievable at the site of infection limits its usefulness. For example, nitrofurantoin is concentrated in the urine and is effective in many cases of uncomplicated urinary tract infections. However, the rapid excretion of this drug prevents it from achieving effective levels in blood or tissues. Consequently, susceptible organisms outside the urinary tract are not affected by nitrofurantoin.

Side Effects

An important limitation is that antimicrobial drugs may have side effects on the host. In antimicrobial chemotherapy the object is to optimize the **therapeutic index,** the ratio between the effective and the toxic dose. It is important to keep in mind that the degree of selectivity chosen depends on the plight of the patient. Certain inhibitors of folic acid metabolism, like methotrexate, are very toxic in humans but are useful as anticancer agents.

Infectious agents that do not penetrate into deep tissues are special cases in therapy. Topical applications for skin infections are less likely to produce side effects. This lack of side effects permits extensive use of agents that can harm host cell membranes, such as the antibacterial drug polymyxin and the antifungal antibiotic nystatin. Drugs against intestinal worms, which are topologically located outside body tissues (see Fig. 1.1), are also less likely to cause side effects.

Occasionally, an astute clinical observation can turn a side effect to an advantage. Some derivatives of sulfonamides act as a diuretic and cause blood acidosis and alkaline urine. Although these effects are weak, they led to the synthesis of an important group of modern diuretics. Similarly, some sulfa drugs produce hypoglycemia, which led to the development of new drugs for the treatment of diabetes.

How Are Antibiotics Selective?

In the case of sulfa drugs, selectivity is based on the fact that, unlike humans, bacteria must synthesize their own folic acid. Any step in metabolism, whether unique to microorganisms or not, is a potential target for antimicrobial action. All that is needed is selective toxicity. In the same pathway as that affected by sulfonamides, the drug **trimethoprim** blocks the function rather than the synthesis of folic acid (see Fig. 5-2). Trimethoprim inhibits the enzyme dihydrofolate reductase, which catalyzes the reduction of dihydrofolate to tetrahydrofolate. This enzyme is necessary for human cells as well as for bacteria, but the amount needed to cause 50% enzyme inhibition is 0.005 mM for bacteria, 0.07 mM for protozoa, and 250 mM for mammals. Thus the drug can be used against bacteria and protozoa at concentrations that do not harm humans.

This example of efficacy is based on the relative insensitivity of the host compared with bacterial targets. In another example, both host cells and bacteria are sensitive to tetracycline. However, unlike mammalian cells, bacteria concentrate the antibiotic. As a result, tetracycline is effective against even intracellular organisms (e.g., chlamydiae).

The armamentarium of antimicrobials includes drugs that affect the synthesis or function of every class of microbial macromolecules. Extreme selectivity is achieved when the biochemical target is absent in the host cells. The best examples are the β-lactam antibiotics (e.g., penicillin), which affect the biosynthesis of the murein layer of the bacterial cell wall (see Chapter 3). No comparable structure exists in mammalian cells, which are therefore totally insensitive to the action of these antibiotics. Nonetheless, even β-lactams can have undesirable side effects. Some individuals cannot take them because they have a strong allergic reaction. Also, administration of broad-spectrum β-lactams can lead to the destruction of the normal flora. This effect can lead to colitis, overgrowth by fungi, and other complications. Even a nearly perfect antibiotic comes with a price tag.

How Do Microbes Circumvent the Action of Antibiotics?

The destructive power of antibiotics is so pervasive that within a few years of their introduction, resistant organisms can supplant susceptible ones. At what point in the action of antibiotics does resistance come into play? The action of antimicrobial drugs can be broken into a sequence of three steps: First, the drugs must associate with the bacteria and penetrate their envelope. Second, they must be transported to an intracellular site of action. Third, they must bind to their specific biochemical target. Resistance to drugs can occur at each step. Microorganisms, like sophisticated biochemists, have developed a multitude of ways to become resistant. Resistance poses a serious problem when it arises in a pathogenic microbe capable of causing damage to human hosts. Following are the clinically relevant mechanisms of resistance:

- Synthesis of enzymes that break down the drug molecule
- Chemical modification of the drug that interferes with its function
- Prevention of access to the target site by inhibiting uptake

- Prevention of access to the target site by increasing export of the drug from the microbial cell
- Modification of the target site

All these mechanisms have been recognized in clinical pathogens, but the most common is the last one. Some of the examples introduced in Chapter 3 are treated more fully in the following paragraphs. A more extensive list of mechanisms of antibacterial resistance is shown in Table 5-1.

β-lactams and Enzymes that Inactivate Them

Chapter 3 summarized the effects of penicillins and cephalosporins on cell wall formation and their consequences for bacterial survival. This group of drugs is large, and for various reasons, their efficacy varies greatly.

These antibiotics contain a β-lactam ring (Fig. 5-5). Particular side chains located on the β-lactam ring permit the drugs to penetrate the outer membrane of Gram-negative bacteria, thus extending the list of susceptible organisms. In effect, these drugs become "broad-spectrum antibiotics" by virtue of modification of their β-lactam rings. Other modifications may allow these drugs to be more easily absorbed or more resistant to stomach acid, thus making them effective oral chemotherapeutic agents.

An example of drug development is the transformation of cephalosporin. The original drug is more resistant to inactivating enzymes but less potent than is penicillin. The addition of new side chains created a so-called second generation of cephalosporins with greater potency, especially against Gram-negatives. A third generation with a somewhat different spectrum has been synthesized

table **5-1**	Most Common Mechanisms of Resistance to Antibacterial Agents		
AGENT	**PLASMIDBORNE**	**RESISTANCE MECHANISM**	
Penicillins, cephalosporins	Yes	Hydrolysis of β-lactam ring by β-lactamase	
Methicillin	No	Change in penicillin-binding protein (not in β-lactamase)	
Tetracyclines	Yes	Efflux pump pushes drug out of cell	
Aminoglycosides (gentamicin, tobramycin, amikacin, streptomycin, etc.)	Yes	Enzymatic modification of drug by R plasmid encoded enzyme; drug has reduced affinity for ribosome, and transport into cell is reduced	
Sulfonamides	Yes	Sulfanilamide-resistant dihydropteroate synthase	
Trimethoprim	Yes	Trimethoprim-resistant dihydrofolate reductase	
Erythromycin	Yes	Enzymatic modification (methylation of 23S ribosomal RNA)	
Chloramphenicol	Yes	Acetylation of hydroxyl groups of chloramphenicol transacetylase; interference with transport into cell	
Oxazolidinones	No	Mutations in 23S ribosomal RNA	
Quinolones (naladixic acid, ciprofloxacin, etc.)	No	Mutations in genes encoding DNA gyrase and topoisomerase IV	
Vancomycin	Yes	Change in binding site in the peptidoglycan target	

Penicillin

Cephalosporin

FIGURE 5-5 ▪ **Core structure of penicillin and cephalosporin.** The R groups specify the particular antibiotic; arrows indicate the bonds broken during function and during inactivation by β-lactamases, respectively.

with further modifications of the side chains. (see Fig. 5-5). Cephalosporins in this class have two important advantages: First, they extend the spectrum of activity to organisms that were resistant to most of the previous cephalosporins, including *Pseudomonas*, an opportunistic pathogen, and *Haemophilus influenzae*, an important pathogen in pulmonary infections and meningitis. Second, unlike the previous cephalosporins, they penetrate well into the central nervous system. This ability has made them especially useful in the treatment of Gram-negative meningitis.

The bactericidal action of the β-lactam antibiotics requires the following steps:

1. Association with the bacteria.
2. Penetration through the outer membrane and the periplasmic space (only in Gram-negatives).
3. Interaction with penicillin-binding proteins on the cytoplasmic membrane.
4. Activation of an autolysin that degrades the cell wall murein.

The principal mechanism of resistance to the β-lactams is the elaboration of inactivating enzymes, the β-lactamases. So far, more than 300 β-lactamases have been identified, a small number of which account for most of the clinically encountered resistance. They can be divided into two major categories, the penicillinases and the cephalosporinases. A fair degree of cross-over occurs within these categories; that is, a cephalosporinase can also inactivate a penicillin, and vice versa, but with different efficiency.

In general, Gram-positive bacteria such as the staphylococci produce extracellular β-lactamases. Secreted into the medium, these enzymes destroy the antibiotic before it comes in contact with the bacterial surface. Gram-positive bacteria often make β-lactamases

in large amounts after induction by the corresponding antibiotic. Adding more of the drug only induces formation of greater amounts of enzyme, and as a result, resistance usually cannot be overcome even with massive doses. In Gram-negatives, β-lactamases are found in the periplasm or bound to the inner membrane. They are often constitutively produced; that is, they are produced at a constant rate that does not increase with addition of greater amounts of the drugs. Therefore, resistance in these organisms can sometimes be overcome with higher doses of the antibiotic.

β-lactamase–dependent resistance to penicillins and cephalosporins is widespread among pathogenic bacteria. It has become so common in staphylococci, both those acquired in hospitals and in the community, that infecting strains of these organisms must be considered penicillin-resistant unless proven otherwise by antibiotic susceptibility tests.

Development of β-lactam resistance among Gram-negative bacteria differs from that of Gram-positives. With few exceptions, such as the gonococcus, Gram-negative organisms are resistant to the first drug of this group, the original penicillin G. However, when challenged with newer drugs to which they are susceptible, the Gram-negatives have eventually developed resistance. For example, before 1974 *H. influenzae* was universally susceptible to the penicillin derivative ampicillin. This antibiotic was considered the drug of choice in treatment of *H. influenzae* infections. However, in 1975 it became apparent that 10 to 20% of the isolates of *H. influenzae* elaborate an ampicillin-degrading β-lactamase. This enzyme is encoded on a highly promiscuous plasmid, which probably accounts for the rapid spread of ampicillin resistance in this organism.

A similar reversal has occurred with gonococcus. This organism used to be universally susceptible to penicillin, although higher levels of the drug have been gradually required over the last 30 years. In 1976 highly penicillin-resistant strains were isolated in two widely separated areas of the world. The gene coding for the relevant β-lactamase is carried on a **transposon,** which hops to other strains of gonococci and to other aerobic Gram-negatives. Thus, we can no longer rely on penicillin as the universal agent for the treatment of gonorrhea.

These examples illustrate the role of transferable genetic elements in the spread of β-lactamase resistance. The role of plasmids and transposons in the transfer of resistance has increased in importance since the early days of the antibiotic era. The first strains that became antibiotic-resistant harbored chromosomal genes and only later were replaced by strains with plasmidborne resistance. This trend for the genes to become associated with a mobile genetic element has facilitated the development of resistance in previously susceptible organisms. If this trend continues to include other important β-lactam–susceptible pathogens, such as the meningococci and certain streptococci, it would be a serious blow to our ability to treat some important infectious diseases.

Other mechanisms of resistance to β-lactams are also important. In Gram-negative bacteria, β-lactams must be able to pass through outer membrane pores to make contact with the antimicrobial targets, **penicillin-binding proteins (PBPs)**. Resistance can occur in some Gram-negative organisms when spontaneous mutations in the outer membrane **porins** lead to exclusion of β-lactams to the periplasmic space. Alternatively, many Gram-positive organisms have become resistant by altering the PBPs themselves so they fail to bind β-lactams. This type of β-lactam resistance has been most important in the emergence of penicillin-resistant *Streptococcus pneumoniae* and methicillin-resistant *Staphylococcus aureus*. Most strains of *S. aureus* are already resistant to penicillins by virtue of a β-lactamase. However, acquisition of an altered PBP in many strains has resulted in resistance to all penicillins and cephalosporins, including ones that were specifically designed to resist the staphylococcal β-lactamase, like methicillin. For this reason, these strains have the blanket designation of **methicillin-resistant *Staphylococcus aureus* (MRSA)**. They are responsible for some of the worst outbreaks of hospital-acquired infection in recent history. These strains must be treated with antimicrobials from another class, such as the cell wall–inhibiting cyclic glycopeptide, vancomycin, or newer antistaphylococcal drugs, such as linezolid, or daptomycin. Unfortunately, resistance to all these agents has also been reported (as discussed later).

Finally, some strains of pneumococci and staphylococci are inhibited rather than killed by certain levels of β-lactams. This form of partial resistance is called **tolerance.** In the case of tolerant pneumococci, the drugs are bacteriostatic and not bactericidal because these strains lack sufficient levels of the suicidal **autolysin.** Bacterial tolerance might explain some of the relapses that occur following treatment of staphylococcal and streptococcal infections. However, compared with drug inactivation by β-lactamases, tolerance accounts only for a small percentage of clinically important resistance.

Vancomycin: Resistance by Target (Cell Wall) Modification

Vancomycin, a glycopeptide antibiotic in constant clinical use since the 1950s, has been a mainstay of therapy for resistant Gram-positive infections. Since this antibiotic is given intravenously, it is most commonly used in hospitalized patients, many with nosocomial (hospital-acquired) infections. Vancomycin has been particularly valuable against MRSA strains for which it has been, until recently, the only useful drug available.

Since the late 1980s many strains of *Enterococcus* have acquired resistance to vancomycin by acquisition of a set of plasmidborne genes. These genes act in concert to produce an altered peptidoglycan precursor. Instead of the usual D-alanine–D-alanine terminus, these modified precursors have D-alanine-D-lactate. The normal D-alanine–D-alanine is the target for vancomycin, whereas D-alanine-D-lactate is not. Bacteria with this modified terminus are resistant to vancomycin (Fig. 5-6).

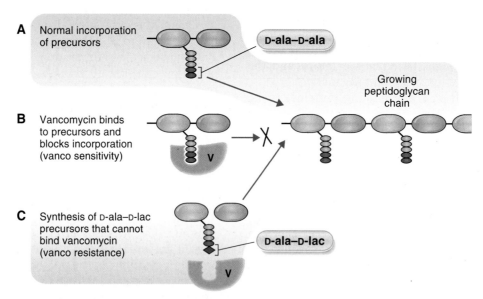

FIGURE 5-6 ▪ **Mechanism of vancomycin resistance. A.** Normally, peptidoglycan precursors composed of two sugars and a five-amino-acid peptide are exported from the bacterial cell and added to a growing peptidoglycan chain as the cell wall enlarges. **B.** Vancomycin inhibits peptidoglycan chain elongation by binding to the D-ala–D-ala terminal peptides on the precursor. **C.** The basis of vancomycin resistance in *Enterococcus* is the production of precursors with D-lactate in the position of the terminal D-ala. This blocks the binding of vancomycin and allows the precursor to be incorporated.

Patients infected with strains of **vancomycin-resistant** *Enterococcus* (VRE) are extremely difficult to treat because these strains are usually also resistant to β-lactams and aminoglycosides. Fortunately, enterococci are not aggressively invasive pathogens. However, since the recognition of VRE, microbiologists have expected that their plasmidborne vancomycin resistance genes would eventually be transferred to the more virulent *Staphylococcus aureus*. This concern was realized in the early part of this century. Strains of **vancomycin-resistant** *S. aureus* (VRSA) have now been identified in patients who were coinfected with MRSA and VRE and on long-term treatment with vancomycin. As of this writing, the VRSA isolates have been contained and do not circulate in the general population. However, it is generally regarded as simply a matter of time before these highly resistant staphylococci take hold and become more prevalent. Eventually, this could result in the evolution of untreatable *S. aureus* strains, a situation akin to that of the preantibiotic era.

Quinolones: Resistance by Target and Efflux Alteration

The quinolone antibiotics act by inhibiting the action of bacterial topoisomerases, including **DNA gyrase** (in Gram-positive bacteria) and **topoisomerase IV** (in Gram-negatives). Quinolones kill bacteria by trapping the topoisomerases in the act of cutting DNA and thus promoting the formation and persistence of double strand breaks in the bacterial chromosome. Nalidixic acid was the first quinolone used clinically and was effective for treating urinary tract infections caused by Gram-negative bacteria. More recently developed **fluoroquinolone** antibiotics are used to treat infections caused by both Gram-negative and Gram-positive bacteria, and these agents are now widely used. Resistance to fluoroquinolone antibiotics is mainly the result of mutations in the genes encoding the target enzymes DNA gyrase and topoisomerase IV, which cause reduced binding of the drugs. Another important source of resistance is the elimination of quinolones from the bacterial cell by **efflux pumps**. A role for efflux in resistance has been demonstrated in both Gram-negative bacteria, such as *Pseudomonas aeruginosa*, and Gram-positive bacteria, such as *Staphylococcus aureus*.

Antiribosomal Antibiotics

The effectiveness of the second-largest class of antibacterial agents, the antiribosomal antibiotics, is based on structural differences between the ribosomes of bacteria and those of eukaryotic cells; in eukaryotic cells, ribosomes have larger RNA molecules and more protein components. Typical drugs of this group, including streptomycin and erythromycin, bind to bacterial but not mammalian ribosomes. The difference is not always absolute and does not completely explain the selective toxicity of all the drugs of this class. First, some antibiotics like tetracycline target mammalian and bacterial ribosomes in vitro. Second, mammalian cells have bacterial-like ribosomes in their mitochondria, and these are sensitive to many of the drugs of this class. Researchers believe that some of these drugs are not toxic because they cannot pass through the plasma membrane. Recent additions to the antiribosomal antibiotics are the **oxazolidinones**, including linezolid. These agents bind to the 50S subunit of bacterial ribosomes to prevent the assembly of the translational complex and the initiation of protein synthesis.

Other toxic side effects of these antibiotics cannot be anticipated from their mechanisms of action. Examples are chelation of magnesium by tetracyclines with attendant bone and tooth malformation in children, or toxicity of aminoglycosides for the renal tubules and inner ear.

Aminoglycosides: Resistance by Transport or Drug Inactivation

Perhaps the most complex mechanism of action of all antiribosomal antibiotics is that of the aminoglycosides. Their action results from the following steps:

1. Penetration of the outer membrane of Gram-negatives.
2. Association with a two-stage active transport system in the cell membrane. (This system is one way and irreversible, unlike that of tetracycline or most metabolites.)
3. Binding to the 30S ribosome subunit to inhibit protein synthesis, primarily at or near the initiation step, and to increase "miscoding" by the ribosomes and the production of "nonsense proteins."

Two major mechanisms of resistance to aminoglycosides have been recognized in Gram-negative bacteria. Obligate anaerobic bacteria may inactivate the transport of aminoglycosides. However, a more common mechanism in clinically important isolates involves **modifying enzymes**. Various aminoglycoside-modifying enzymes may modify these antibiotics by the addition of acetyl, adenyl, or phosphoryl groups to the drug molecules rendering them inactive. Several distinct enzymes have been identified in coliforms, pseudomonads, and staphylococci. Each one can inactivate more than one but usually not all aminoglycosides. Thus, a given strain can become resistant to, say, gentamicin and tobramycin but remain fully susceptible to amikacin. Usually, the aminoglycoside-inactivating enzymes are encoded by genes carried on plasmids or transposons, and more than one enzyme may be carried by one plasmid.

Tetracyclines: Resistance by Drug Excretion

Resistance to antiribosomal antibiotics can take many forms because these drugs must go through many steps to reach their targets. Tetracyclines, for example, must do the following:

1. Bind to the cytoplasmic membrane, which, in the case of Gram-negatives, requires passage through the outer membrane and the periplasmic space.
2. Be transported across the cytoplasmic membrane by an active transport mechanism. This transport mechanism involves two components: an initial rapid uptake and a second phase of slower uptake.

Resistant strains do not accumulate tetracycline within the cell. The reason is not, as might be expected, failure to take up the drug. Rather, the intracellular concentration is kept low by an exit mechanism that actively excretes the drug. Tetracycline resistance has been found in almost all bacteria, including Gram-positives, Gram-negatives, aerobes, and anaerobes.

Macrolides: Resistance by Target (Ribosome) Modification

The macrolide antibiotics and their derivatives are represented in clinical medicine by **erythromycin, clindamycin, azithromycin,** and **clarithromycin.** Like tetracyclines, macrolides can be transported out of the bacterial cell by efflux pumps, creating a low level of resistance. However, a more significant degree of resistance occurs by a particularly interesting mechanism of drug target alteration—methylation of the 23S ribosomal RNA. This modification renders the 50S ribosomal subunits resistant to the drugs. The **methylase** involved is usually made from a plasmid gene under highly regulated conditions: little enzyme is formed during growth in the absence of a macrolide, but it is rapidly induced in the presence of a macrolide. A newer agent in this category, **telithromycin,** has been modified to bind to two separate sites on the 23S ribosomal RNA. It retains its capacity to inhibit the 50S ribosomal subunit even in the presence of the methylase. In addition, it cannot be exported from the cell by most efflux pumps. Consequently, telithromycin may be active against bacteria that are resistant to the other macrolides.

Oxazolidinones: Resistance by Target Modification

Unlike most of the antibiotics previously mentioned, oxazolidinone antibiotics such as **linezolid** are not derived from naturally occurring antimicrobial substances. They are entirely synthetic, much like the sulfonamides described earlier in this chapter. Consequently, preexisting resistance genes such as those that encode β-lactamases, aminoglycoside-modifying enzymes, or ribosomal methylases do not exist. Nevertheless, resistant bacteria have been identified and isolated. In all cases so far, resistance has been the result of point mutations in the 23S RNA of the 50S ribosomal subunit. These mutations presumably block the binding of linezolid to the ribosome.

Selectivity and Limitations of Antifungal Agents

Moving up the phylogenetic tree to the eukaryotic pathogens, the differences between host and parasite begin to narrow. For example, most of the antibiotics that inhibit fungal ribosomes are also active against human ribosomes and are therefore too toxic to use. In general, therapeutic agents against fungi, viruses, and animal parasites are often quite toxic. Nevertheless, antifungal agents with selective toxicity do exist.

Especially interesting examples are the **polyenes** (see Chapter 50), which bind more avidly to ergosterol in the membranes of fungi than to cholesterol in the membranes of higher eukaryotes. The margin of safety is often considerable. For example, yeasts are about 200-fold more sensitive to the polyene antibiotic **amphotericin B** than are cultured human cells. Nevertheless, the efficacy of amphotericin B is limited by toxicity to blood cells and damage to membranes of kidney cells. To some extent, this toxicity has been limited by conjugating the drug to lipid complexes.

The **imidazoles** are another group of agents with greater specificity for a fungal target than for a similar target in the host. The target is cytochrome P450 demethylase, which is involved in sterol synthesis. These antifungal agents can be used topically to treat local infections or systemically to treat invasive disease. Similarly, **echinocandins** are inhibitors of another component of the fungal cell wall, β-glucan, which is not present in human cells.

If One Antibiotic Is Good, Are Two Better?

A potent argument for counteracting drug resistance in microorganisms can be made for the administration of several antibiotics at once. Mutants resistant to some antibiotics occur with frequencies of 10^6 to 10^9 per generation. Thus, because of the rapid growth of bacteria in human infection, outgrowth of resistant mutants can easily take place and become a significant clinical risk. However, two antibiotics given simultaneously can theoretically reduce the chance that a bacterium will completely evade antibiotic destruction. For example, assume that resistance to drug A arises with a frequency of 10^6 per generation. If drug B has a similar frequency of resistant mutants and is given simultaneously, the chance of a single bacterium becoming resistant to both antibiotics is 10^6 times 10^6, or 10^{12}, which is vanishingly small.

An excellent example of this concept currently in practice is combination therapy with sulfamethoxazole and trimethoprim. Although both drugs act on one-carbon metabolism, their sites of action are different, and resistance to one does not influence resistance to the other. Another example is the obligatory combination of drugs used to treat tuberculosis. Treatment of active tuberculosis with a single agent is invariably associated with clinical failure and the emergence of drug-resistant strains. Multidrug therapy for this disease is therefore considered essential.

The use of drugs in combination is not without problems. In fact, three outcomes are possible:

1. **Synergism:** The effectiveness of the drugs together is greater than that of either drug alone. For example, enterococci are naturally tolerant to penicillins and resistant to gentamicin. However, when penicillin is given along with gentamicin, the bacteria become permeable to gentamicin, which exerts a bactericidal effect in the cytoplasm.
2. **Antagonism:** The action of one drug reduces the effectiveness of the other. Thus, when tetracycline is given with penicillin, it blocks protein synthesis, preventing the cell growth required for penicillin to cause lysis. The result is dominance by the weaker bacteriostatic drug.
3. **Indifference:** Each drug works no better and no worse alone or in combination.

Further cautions are warranted with multiple drug administration. Drugs can show **synergism in toxicity** as well as in antimicrobial action (an example is the heightened damage to the kidney by the joint administration of vancomycin and an aminoglycoside). Finally, in a hospital setting the main sources of drug resistance are the members of the resident bacterial flora. Therefore, the decision to administer multiple drugs and which ones to choose should be governed by the spectrum of multidrug resistance of the dominant organisms in that hospital.

Are Supergerms a Threat?

Some of the genes that lead to antibiotic resistance are chromosomal and thus are inherent in the genome of the species. But many resistance genes are plasmidborne and are probably acquired from other bacteria (see Table 5-1).

Resistance genes, both chromosomal and on plasmids, predate the use of antibiotics. Such genes have been found in strains stored before the introduction of the drugs or in isolates from areas where antibiotics have never been deliberately introduced. The selective pressure of the widespread use of antibiotics has resulted in an increasing frequency of resistant bacteria. In broad terms the spread of resistance genes increases with the use of drugs in a particular geographic area or medical center. Multiple resistance genes may accumulate in a given strain by the effective mechanism of gene transposition. This process could lead to the emergence of "supergerms," microorganisms resistant to a large number of antimicrobial agents. Near-supergerm status has been achieved by occasional isolates resistant to 15 or more antibiotics. Particular examples are strains of enterococci resistant to most available antibiotics. In contrast, meningococci, group A streptococci, and the spirochete of syphilis remain nearly as susceptible to penicillin today as they were when the drug was first used. The reasons for this persistent susceptibility are not clear.

Conclusion

The countermeasures taken against resistant organisms include continued development of more effective antibiotics (such as the cephalosporins). Certainly, the war between effective therapy and drug resistance is unlikely to abate, but the battles must continue to be fought and won. The alternative would be to give up what many physicians and historians of science regard as a key difference between modern medicine and the Dark Ages.

Innate Immunity

Roman Dziarski

We have a unique ability to shape our environment. Largely, our sanitary lifestyle determines the extent to which we encounter exogenous microorganisms, including potential pathogens. Our health is influenced by such external factors as cleanliness and nutrition. Thus, defenses against infectious diseases begin with the way we affect our environment and one another. For example, children who live in crowded, inadequately ventilated housing and eat a diet lacking in protein are more likely to contract infectious diseases such as tuberculosis than are other children. The reason is twofold: poor nutrition diminishes the effectiveness of body defenses, and crowding makes the encounter with tubercle bacilli more frequent. The adults in such households may already have tuberculosis and in close quarters become ready sources of contagion. Defenses against such events are clear: good nutrition, adequate housing, and treatment of the ill. While these favorable conditions occur readily in affluent societies, they have to be fostered with care and sacrifice in the developing countries of the world.

Physicians share with others their concern for defense against infectious diseases. Good food in sufficient quantity, uncontaminated water, and protection from insects and rodents—these are the primary business of the sanitary engineer and the social scientist. Other activities are mainly medical, such as immunizations and treatment of human carriers or patients likely to contribute to the spread of disease (see Chapter 56). This chapter focuses on the body's own defense mechanisms.

Functions and Components of the Innate Immune System

Throughout life the body surfaces tolerate a rich and complex flora that is usually harmless but can cause opportunistic infections. In contrast, domains of the body just a few micrometers beneath the epidermis or the mucous membranes are usually free of microorganisms. Host defenses intensify as microorganisms encounter the skin and mucous membranes. This and the next chapter explore how the body maintains this microbial gradient, from microorganism-associated surfaces to aseptic intercellular and intracellular tissue domains. The question is important because a breakdown of the gradient is usually what infection is about.

CHAPTER 6 Innate Immunity **67**

table **6-1**	Components of the Innate Immune System	

COMPONENT	MAIN FUNCTION
Cellular	
Skin and mucous membranes (epithelial cells)	Mechanical and chemical defenses
Phagocytic cells (neutrophils, macrophages)	Ingest and kill bacteria and fungi
Proinflammatory cells (macrophages, mast cells, eosinophils, basophils, platelets)	Induce host defenses and inflammation
Natural killer cells	Kill virus-infected cells and tumor cells
Antigen-presenting cells (dendritic cells, macrophages)	Recognize, process, and present antigens to lymphocytes Initiate adaptive immune responses
Humoral	
Antimicrobial peptides	Kill microorganisms
Complement	Enhances phagocytosis (opsonization) Induces inflammation Kills some microorganisms
Cytokines	Activate innate and adaptive defenses
Chemokines	Attract leukocytes
Kinins	Induce inflammation
Acute phase proteins	Enhance cellular and humoral defenses
Enzymes	Kill and digest microorganisms
Inflammation	
Increased blood supply (erythema)	Brings more antimicrobial cells and proteins to the site of infection
Increased vascular permeability (edema)	Brings more antimicrobial proteins to the site of infection
Chemotaxis (induration)	Infiltration of infection site with white cells

Innate immunity is the body's first line of defense against infections. It is present in all metazoans, and in plants and invertebrate animals it is the only (and very effective) defense against infections. Vertebrates, including humans, have not only innate immunity but also adaptive immunity (also known as acquired immunity), which is the second line of defense (see Chapter 7).

Following are the functions of innate immunity:

■ Recognize microbes that are encountered by the host
■ Prevent infection of the host by either eliminating the microbes or allowing them to exist on body surfaces as normal flora that is not harmful (or beneficial)
■ Initiate adaptive immune responses and influence the nature of those responses based on the type of the invading microorganism
■ Serve, in some cases, as an effector mechanism for adaptive immune response

As shown in Table 6-1, the components of the innate immune system that perform these functions are either **cellular,** consisting of various types of cells, or **humoral,** consisting of various secreted soluble peptides, proteins, and other mediators. The interaction of these components in the body with the invading microbe often, but not always, leads to a constellation of responses called **inflammation.** The purpose of inflammation is to amplify the body's defenses by increasing blood supply to the site of infection and by bringing more antimicrobial proteins and white cells to fight the infection.

This chapter discusses how the innate immune system functions and how it protects us from infections.

Skin and Mucous Membranes

Before microorganisms can enter the normally aseptic regions of the body, they must pass through the barriers of the skin, the conjunctivae of the eyes, or the mucous membrane of the respiratory, alimentary, or urogenital tracts. Each barrier has its own protective mechanisms, which can be broadly classified as mechanical, chemical and molecular, and microbial (Table 6-2).

Mechanical barriers are highly effective, especially in the skin, which is covered with a thick layer of **keratinized epithelium.** The mucous membranes of the mouth, pharynx, esophagus, and lower urinary tract are composed of several layers of epithelial cells, whereas

table 6-2 Defenses on the Skin and Mucous Membranes

COMPONENT	MAIN FUNCTION
Mechanical	
Keratinized epithelium in the skin	Offers protection against microorganisms
Desquamation of stratified epithelium	Removes microorganisms attached to its surface
Epithelial cells joined by tight junctions	Offers protection against microorganisms
Mucus-coated hair in the nose	Trap particles
Mucus-coated ciliated epithelium	Removes particles from the respiratory tract
Coughing and sneezing	Expel particles
Flow of urine	Cleanses the urethra
Chemical and molecular	
Low pH in the stomach	Kills many bacteria, fungi, or parasites, and inactivates many viruses
Antimicrobial peptides (constitutive and induced)[a]	Kill many microorganisms
Defensins (skin, intestine, mucous membranes)	Kill bacteria and fungi
Phospholipases (in intestinal Paneth cells and tears)	Kill bacteria
Dermcidin (in sweat glands)	Kills bacteria and fungi
Ribonucleases (on the skin)	Kill bacteria and fungi
Fatty acids (from sebaceous glands of the skin)	Inhibit bacterial growth
Enzymes	
Lysozyme (in tears, sweat, saliva, and serum)	Hydrolyses bacterial cell wall peptidoglycan
Amidase (in the skin and serum)	Hydrolyses bacterial cell wall peptidoglycan
Microbial antagonism	
Normal flora bacteria and fungi	Compete for nutrients with potential pathogens
	Produce antimicrobial factors (bacteriocins)

[a] See Table 6-3.

those of the lower respiratory, gastrointestinal, and upper urinary tracts are delicate single layers of epithelial cells, often endowed with specialized functions. Membranes of the alveoli and the intestine are thin because they serve as exchangers of gases, fluids, and solutes. Although all epithelia have protective **tight junctions** that do not allow passage of microorganisms, these epithelia are easily traumatized, especially when subjected to high pressure or abrasions. In fact, trauma occurs daily in the colon during defecation and in the mouth during vigorous toothbrushing.

Many mucous membranes are covered by a protective layer of **mucus** that provides a mechanical and chemical barrier, yet permits proper function. Mucus is a giant cross-linked gel-like structure made up of glycoprotein subunits. It entraps particles and prevents them from reaching the mucous membrane. Mucus is hydrophilic and allows diffusion of many substances produced by the body, including antimicrobial peptides and enzymes such as **lysozyme** and **peroxidase.** Its viscous properties enable it to bear substantial weight and yet be readily moved by the motion of the cilia of the underlying cells.

To afford additional protection, skin and mucous membranes are rich in chemical and molecular antimicrobial factors (see Table 6-2). Some of these factors are constitutive (always present), such as low pH in the stomach; fatty acids on the skin; and lysozyme, a bacteriolytic enzyme in tears, sweat, and saliva.

The most potent antimicrobial factors are **antimicrobial peptides** (Table 6-3). One of the most active peptides is **phospholipase A_2 (PLA_2)**, which is an enzyme that destroys bacterial cytoplasmic membrane. **Defensins** are cysteine-rich small peptides (3 to 5 kDa), which are ubiquitous in all vertebrates and invertebrates, and which in humans are subdivided into two families, α-defensins and β-defensins, based on their structure. Six α-defensins and four β-defensins have been well characterized in humans, but recent analysis of the human genome revealed 34 defensin genes, which highlights the significance of this family of antimicrobial peptides. Defensins, like most other antimicrobial peptides, are highly cationic, enabling them to bind to the negatively charged cell walls of bacteria and fungi and to kill them by pore formation and permeabilization of their cell membranes.

table **6-3** **Antimicrobial Peptides**

PEPTIDE	LOCATION	ACTIVE AGAINST
Phospholipases (PLA$_2$ most active)	PMN primary granules Intestinal Paneth cells Tears Serum	Gram-positive bacteria Gram-negative bacteria together with BPI
α-Defensins	PMN primary granules Intestinal Paneth cells	Bacteria, fungi, some parasites and viruses
β-Defensins	Induced in epithelial cells (skin, respiratory tract, genitourinary tract)	Bacteria and fungi
Ribonucleases	Constitutive and induced in epithelial cells (skin, genitourinary tract, intestinal tract) PMNs, monocytes	Bacteria and fungi
Dermcidin	Sweat glands	Bacteria and fungi
BPI	PMN primary granules	Gram-negative bacteria
Cathelicidins (CAP18 in humans)	PMN secondary granules	Bacteria and fungi
Serprocidins (cationic serine proteases: elastase, proteinase 3, cathepsin G)	PMN primary granules	Bacteria and fungi
Lysozyme	Phagocyte granules Tears, saliva Serum Intestinal Paneth cells	Gram-positive bacteria (hydrolyses peptidoglycan)

BPI, bactericidal permeability-increasing protein; CAP, cationic antimicrobial protein; PMN, polymorphonuclear leukocyte.

Many antimicrobial peptides are constitutively present on the skin and mucous membranes, such as PLA$_2$, α-defensins, and ribonucleases (RNases) in the intestinal Paneth cells. Other antimicrobial peptides, such as β-defensins and RNases, are present in low levels on epithelial surfaces of the skin and mucous membranes, and their increased production can be induced by high numbers of bacteria or by proinflammatory cytokines released from macrophages following exposure to bacteria.

The enzyme **lysozyme** is present in large amounts in tears, sweat, saliva, and serum. It hydrolyses **peptidoglycan,** the main structural component of bacterial cell walls. Lysozyme acts mainly on Gram-positive bacteria, although many bacterial species have evolved resistant modifications of their cell wall chemistry. Gram-negative bacteria, however, are resistant because their peptidoglycan substrate is shielded by their outer membranes. In this case, lysozyme can work synergistically with other antimicrobial peptides or complement. Damage to the outer membrane of Gram-negative bacteria can allow lysozyme to access its substrate. **Amidase** is another enzyme in the skin and serum that hydrolyses bacterial cell wall peptidoglycan, although in contrast to lysozyme, it does not have a direct bacteriolytic activity. However, peptidoglycan-lytic enzymes are important not only in killing bacteria but also in removing proinflammatory peptidoglycan from the tissues. Many antimicrobial peptides and bacteriolytic enzymes are also present in the granules of phagocytic cells (which will be discussed later) and can be released from the granules into the surrounding tissues by a process called **exocytosis.**

The innate immune system prevents colonization of the skin and mucous membranes by potential pathogens but allows colonization by limited numbers of the nonpathogenic bacteria and fungi of the normal flora. The **normal flora** is unique for each area of the body (see Chapter 2) and is beneficial to the host because it protects the skin and mucous membranes from colonization by pathogenic microorganisms. Called **microbial antagonism,** this protection is likely accomplished by competition for nutrients with potential pathogens and by production of antimicrobial factors (bacteriocins) by the normal flora. However, in immunocompromised patients, the normal flora can cause opportunistic infections that are quite severe or even life threatening.

The barrier function of skin and mucous membranes is seldom breached except by injuries, such as burns, cuts, or wounds. Once microorganisms have traversed the skin, they encounter powerful defenses in the underlying soft tissues. However, these defenses do not work at full capacity under all conditions. For instance, abrasions or lacerations impair the local vascular and lymphatic circulation and interfere with soluble and cellular defense mechanisms, thus rendering the underlying connective tissue vulnerable. When this occurs, substantially fewer microorganisms are required to cause infection. For example, many chronically debilitated patients suffer from decubitus ulcers (bed sores) that become contaminated and are constantly infected with normally harmless organisms on the skin. When an injury introduces foreign bodies, such as splinters or particles of soil, the impairment of the defensive mechanisms is even more profound. Moreover, pathogenic microorganisms have developed many virulence mechanisms (discussed in subsequent chapters) that allow them to escape the body defenses, either by evasion or by resistance mechanisms.

When a microorganism crosses the protective epidermis of the skin or the epithelia of mucous membranes, it encounters the next line of defense mechanisms: phagocytic cells, proinflammatory cells, natural killer (NK) cells, and antigen-presenting cells. Once in the body, microorganisms are also confronted by humoral defenses, of which complement is the most powerful. We will discuss all these defense mechanisms in this chapter.

Recognition Strategies of the Innate Immune System

One of the central questions in immunology is how the immune system is able to recognize the invading (and potentially dangerous) microbes and discriminate between potentially dangerous microorganisms and nondangerous materials in the host or the environment (clothing, food, etc.). During its long evolution and coexistence with microorganisms, the innate immune system developed three recognition strategies: detection of microbes through pattern recognition receptors, detection of danger signals from damaged tissues, and detection of a missing self (host).

The first and most frequently used strategy is recognition through receptors specific for microbial molecules that are not present in the host. These are called **pattern recognition receptors,** because they recognize characteristic structures present in microbes but not in mammals (Table 6-4). These structures are found in microbial products that are essential for survival of the microbes and thus cannot be easily changed, dispensed with, or substituted. Several pattern recognition receptors are located on the cell membrane of phagocytic cells, lymphocytes, endothelial cells, and epithelial cells (although not all these cells express all pattern recognition receptors).

The largest family of pattern recognition receptors is called **toll-like receptors** (**TLRs**) because of their homology to a fruit fly *Drosophila* receptor called toll. As shown in Table 6-4, TLRs recognize many essential microbial molecules, including essential cell wall components (peptidoglycan, lipoteichoic acids, lipopeptides, lipopolysaccharide), flagella, bacterial DNA (which has unmethylated cytidine phosphate guanosine (CpG) nucleotide motifs not found in mammalian DNA), fungal cell walls, and viral double-stranded or single-stranded RNA. Some of the same molecules are also recognized by another pattern recognition receptor, **CD14** (*CD* stands for "cluster of differentiation" and refers to cell surface molecules characterized by different stages of differentiation for various types of leukocytes). The TLRs and CD14 allow the host cells (especially macrophages and dendritic cells) to recognize most microbes (bacteria, fungi, viruses), alert the host to their presence, start proinflammatory defense response, and start adaptive immune responses. Other pattern recognition receptors, such as the **scavenger receptor, mannose receptor,** and **β-glucan receptor,** present primarily on phagocytic cells, recognize various bacterial or fungal surface molecules, and allow the host cells to phagocytize them.

Some pattern recognition receptors are intracellular. One such receptor, **protein kinase R,** recognizes intracellular viruses and induces synthesis of the antiviral substance interferon. Interferon is released from the virus-infected cell and inhibits the growth of viruses in other host cells. Another family of intracellular pattern recognition receptors includes the proteins with **nucleotide oligomerization domain (NOD),** a common structural feature of these molecules. NOD proteins recognize fragments of peptidoglycan from bacterial cell walls and allow the cells to produce proinflammatory cytokines, which enhance antimicrobial responses. The need for intracellular recognition of bacteria stems from the ability of some bacteria (for example, *Shigella* and *Listeria*) to enter the host cells and escape into the cytoplasm, a strategy that allows these bacteria to avoid recognition and destruction by phagocytic cells and other extracellular antimicrobial mechanisms.

Several of the pattern recognition receptors are **secreted,** or soluble (see Table 6-4). Some of these molecules enable or enhance responses of the host cells to microbial products. For example, soluble CD14 and lipopolysaccharide-binding protein enhance responses to bacterial lipopolysaccharide. Other secreted pattern recognition receptors enhance phagocytosis or activate complement (phagocytosis and activation of complement are discussed later in this chapter).

The clinical significance of these pattern recognition receptors has been only recently realized by identification of patients who suffer from severe recurrent pyogenic bacterial infections resulting from a genetic defect

table **6-4** **Pattern Recognition Receptors**

RECEPTOR	RECOGNITION OF	MAIN EFFECT
Cell membrane		
TLRs	Bacterial, viral, and fungal components (see below)	Activation of macrophages and dendritic cells to secrete proinflammatory mediators, mature, and initiate adaptive immune response
TLR2 (plus TLR1 or TLR6)	Peptidoglycan (all bacteria) Lipoteichoic acid (Gram-positive bacteria) Lipopeptides (many bacteria) Lipoarabinomannan (*Mycobacterium*) Zymosan (fungal cell wall)	
TLR3	Double-strand RNA (viruses)	
TLR4	Lipopolysaccharide (Gram-negative bacteria)	
TLR5	Flagella (many bacteria)	
TLR7 and TLR8	Single-strand RNA (viruses)	
TLR9	Bacterial DNA	
CD14	Lipopolysaccharide (Gram-negative bacteria) Peptidoglycan (all bacteria) Lipoteichoic acid (Gram-positive bacteria)	Activation of macrophages to secrete proinflammatory mediators
Scavenger receptors	Negatively charged polymers (bacteria and fungi)	Phagocytosis by macrophages
Mannose receptor	Mannose-containing polymers (bacteria and fungi)	Phagocytosis by macrophages
β-glucan receptor (dectin-1)	β-glucan (fungi)	Phagocytosis by macrophages
N-formylmethionyl peptide receptor	Bacterial proteins	Chemoattraction of PMNs and macrophages
Intracellular		
Protein kinase R	Double-strand RNA (viruses)	Induces expression of a viral-inhibitory protein, interferon
NOD1 and NOD2	Peptidoglycan (bacteria)	Activation of macrophages and epithelial cells to produce proinflammatory mediators
Secreted		
Soluble CD14	Lipopolysaccharide (Gram-negative bacteria)	Activation of CD-14 negative cells (e.g. endothelial cells) to secrete proinflammatory mediators
Lipopolysaccharide- binding protein	Lipopolysaccharide (Gram-negative bacteria)	Activation of macrophages to secrete proinflammatory mediators
Mannose-binding lectin (collectin)	Mannose-containing polymers (bacteria and fungi)	Activation of complement
Surfactant proteins (collectin)	Bacteria, fungi, viruses	Opsonization (enhancement of phagocytosis)
Serum amyloid P (pentraxin)	Bacteria	Activation of complement Opsonization
C-reactive protein (pentraxin)	Bacterial polysaccharides	Activation of complement Opsonization

CD, cluster of differentiation; NOD, nucleotide oligomerization domain; PMN, polymorphonuclear leukocyte; TLR, toll-like receptor.

in signal transduction pathways activated by **TLRs.** Another genetic defect recently discovered is a mutation in an intracellular recognition protein, **NOD2.** The mutation is present in many patients with **Crohn's disease,** a chronic inflammatory bowel disease associated with the inability to properly control the responsiveness to bowel bacteria.

The second recognition strategy of the innate immune system is to detect danger signals produced by tissue damage, which would usually be found in tissue-damaging infections. For example, uric acid crystals released from damaged cells can induce proinflammatory responses in dendritic cells. However, it is still not clear what receptors recognize such danger signals.

The third recognition strategy of the innate immune system is to detect a missing or changed self. This strategy is used by the specialized NK cells, which can recognize the host's own cells (self) that do not express a normal set of major histocompatibility complex (MHC) class I molecules. The functions of these cells will be discussed later in this chapter.

Consequences of Recognition: Effector Mechanisms

The consequences of recognition by the innate immune system depend on the type of tissue and the recognition system (cells or soluble factor; see Table 6-1). Constitutive innate immunity is an immediate response based on presynthesized antimicrobial factors and effector cells ready to act. Keratinocytes, epithelial cells, and several specialized cells (e.g., Paneth cells present in the crypts in the intestine, or cells in sweat and sebaceous glands) produce many antimicrobial peptides (see Table 6-3). When a microbe comes in contact with the skin or mucous membranes, it is confronted by mechanical barriers and antimicrobial factors. When a microbe escapes these mechanisms and penetrates the skin or mucous membranes, it is phagocytized and killed by phagocytic cells (neutrophils and macrophages) present in blood and tissues. The presence of microbes on the skin or mucous membranes or in tissues also triggers **induced innate immunity,** which amplifies and supplements the initial constitutive response. This response consists of the following:

- **Increased production of antimicrobial peptides** by keratinocytes, epithelial cells, and specialized cells in the tissues; this action enhances the killing of microorganisms.
- **Secretion of numerous mediators of inflammation,** such as cytokines, chemokines, and vasoactive products, by macrophages, mast cells, eosinophils, basophils, and platelets; this action induces inflammation.
- **Activation of complement,** which enhances phagocytosis (opsonization), chemotactic attraction of phagocytic cells, inflammation, and direct killing of some microorganisms.
- **Activation of clotting cascade and generation of bradykinin,** a nonapeptide that has proinflammatory effects; this action increases vascular permeability, vasodilation, hypotension, pain, and smooth muscle contraction.

- **Chemotactic attraction of phagocytic cells and lymphocytes** to the site of infection.
- **Acute phase response,** which involves greatly increased production of many defense proteins and proinflammatory mediators, collectively known as acute phase proteins (which include C-reactive protein lipopolysaccharide binding protein, serum amyloid P, and fibrinogen). Acute phase response is induced in the liver by proinflammatory cytokines, such as interleukin 1 (IL-1) and IL-6 and tumor necrosis factor-α (TNF-α), produced by proinflammatory cells (mainly macrophages) in response to infection.
- **Inflammation** induced by a combined action of the previously mentioned mediators (as discussed later in this chapter).

These responses have various sensitivities to microbial stimulation depending on the local need of a given tissue. The extent of the response is also usually proportional to the need—that is, the location and the extent of the infection. For example, external tissues (skin and mucous membranes) constantly come in contact with microorganisms, which are usually controlled by constitutively produced antimicrobial peptides. Therefore, these tissues respond only to high numbers of microorganisms; responsiveness to low numbers of microorganisms would induce constant unnecessary inflammation. By contrast, the immune cells in tissues that are normally sterile (have no microorganisms), especially macrophages and leukocytes, are highly sensitive to very low amounts of microbial products. The reason for this high responsiveness is the need for detection of low numbers of microorganisms in normally sterile blood and tissues, because any appearance of microorganisms in the tissues indicates that these microorganisms breached the first line of defense (skin and mucous membranes) and need to be immediately eliminated. Epithelial cells from skin and mucous membranes, however, are highly responsive to cytokines produced by macrophages, because cytokine production means that an infection is already being established in the tissues.

Severe clinical manifestations of infection include fever, inflammation, and **septic shock.** They are the price we pay for high responsiveness to microorganisms to fight the infection. Although usually very effective and self-limiting, this high proinflammatory response unfortunately sometimes results in death of the patient because of an irreversible septic shock.

Complement

The complement system has many components (Table 6-5), mediates a large number of biological effects, and interacts with other complex systems, such as blood clotting and adaptive immune responses. Complement derives its name from the original belief that it complements, or completes, the action of antibodies. Only later

table 6-5 — Components of the Complement System[a]

COMPONENT	ROLE IN THE COMPLEMENT CASCADE
Classical pathway	
C1q	Binds to Fc region of Ig in antigen–antibody complexes; this binding leads to the activation of C1r
C1r	C1r is cleaved on activation to generate C1r, a serine protease that cleaves C1s
C1s	C1s is cleaved to produce, a serine protease; which, in turn, cleaves C4 and C2
C4	Is split by C1s into C4a and C4b; C4b binds to the surface membrane and becomes part of the C3 convertase
C2	Binds to C4b and is cleaved by C1s into C2a, which is a serine protease component of the C3/C5 convertase, and C2b that diffuses away
C3 (also part of the lectin and alternative pathways)	Cleaved by C4b2a into the anaphylatoxin C3a, and C3b which is an opsonin and is also part of the C3/C5 convertases
Lectin pathway	
MBL	Binds to mannose-containing carbohydrates on bacterial and fungal cells, analogous to C1q in the classical pathway, associates with MASP-1 and MASP-2
MBL-associated proteases-1 and -2 (MASP-1 and MASP-2)	Serine protease that associates with MBL and activates C4 and C2 by cleaving them, similar to C1s
Alternative pathway	
Factor B (B)	Analogous to C2 in the classical pathway
Factor D (D)	A serine protease that activates factor B by cleaving it
Properdin (P)	Binds to the C3–C5 convertase of the alternative pathway and stabilizes it
Membrane attack complex	
C5	Cleaved by the convertase complex; C5a is an anaphylatoxin, C5b is the anchoring protein for C6
C6	Binds to C5b and this complex becomes the anchor for C7
C7	Binds to the C5bC6 complex, and then C5bC6C7 inserts into the membrane and becomes an anchor for C8
C8	Attaches to C5bC6C7 and produces a stable membrane-associated complex that can bind C9
C9	Polymerizes at the site of the C5–C8 complex; this completes formation of the fully lytic membrane attack complex
Complement receptors	
Complement receptor type 1(CR1, CD35)	Accelerates dissociation of the C3 convertases, enhances phagocytosis of C3b- or C4b-coated microorganisms
Complement receptor type 2 (CR2, CD21)	Activates B cells, cell surface receptor for Epstein-Barr virus
Complement receptor type 3 (CR3, CD11b/CD18)	Adhesion protein (integrin family), important in phagocytosis of iC3b-coated microorganisms
Complement receptor type 4 (CR4, CD11c/CD18)	Member of the integrin family of proteins, important in phagocytosis of iC3b-coated microorganisms
C3a receptor	Release of vasoactive products from mast cells
C5a receptor	Release of vasoactive products from mast cells, chemotactic attraction of phagocytic cells

[a] The proteins that regulate complement activity are listed separately in Table 6-6.
CD, cluster of differentiation; MBL, mannose-binding lectin.

FIGURE 6-1 ■ **Activation of complement through the classical, lectin, and alternative pathways.**

did researchers realize that it plays a crucial role in body defenses even in the absence of antibodies. The complement system is normally barely "on" and must be **activated** to become a significant part of the defense mechanisms (Fig. 6-1). Once activated, it functions to enhance the antimicrobial defenses in several ways:

- Makes invading microorganisms susceptible to phagocytosis (opsonization)
- Lyses some microorganisms directly
- Activates antimicrobial systems of phagocytes
- Produces substances that are chemotactic for white blood cells
- Promotes the inflammatory response

The complement system can be activated in one of three ways. The three activation pathways are known as **classical, lectin,** and **alternative** (see Fig. 6-1). Each pathway starts out separately, but the three eventually converge to make the same products. The classical pathway is usually set in motion by the presence of antigen–antibody complexes. It is the most prominent pathway and was described first, hence its name. The lectin and alternative pathways are elicited independently of antibodies, often by microbial surface components like mannose-containing polysaccharides (lectin pathway) or bacterial lipopolysaccharides (alternative pathway). In either case, activation results from proteolytic cleavage of inert larger proteins. Some important steps in activation by either pathway depend on the function of protein complexes made by binding several of the cleaved fragments.

Nomenclature

The complement system has more than 35 proteins, most of which are present in plasma and a few that are part of cell membranes. Complement proteins constitute 15% of plasma globulins, which amounts to more than 3 g per liter. The nomenclature of complement components is complicated by their sheer numbers and by the chronology of their discovery. The major components of the classical pathway are designated by the letter C followed by a number, for example, **C3** (see Table 6-5). When the component is cleaved in the process of activation, its fragments receive an additional letter, *a* or *b*. Thus, **C3a**

and **C3b** are the products of proteolytic cleavage of C3. The *a* usually designates a small soluble peptide, whereas the *b* denotes a larger peptide that may bind to cell surfaces. Cleavage products often bind to form an active enzyme, for example, C4b2a. Components of the lectin pathway are designated by abbreviations and numbers (such as **MASP-1**), and components of the alternative pathway are designated by letters (such as **B, D, P**), except for C3b, which is used by all three pathways. What an alphabet soup it is!

Role of Complement in Host Defenses: Overview of the Functions of Complement Proteins

Activation of the complement system is involved in several important aspects of host defenses. Two activities of complement are specifically directed toward enhancing phagocytosis, which is probably the most effective of the constitutive defenses against microorganisms. These activities are the recruitment of white cells by **chemotactic proteins**, such as C5a (Fig. 6-2), and the facilitation of phagocytosis by proteins called **opsonins** (Fig. 6-3).

Complement activation also induces acute inflammation by generating **anaphylatoxins** (C3a and C5a), which act by causing release of vasoactive mediators from mast cells. This activity can be considered beneficial, insofar as the inflammatory response helps fight invading microorganisms. However, they can also have negative, possibly quite severe, effects. In persons with hypersensitivity disorders, the inflammatory response damages sensitive tissues, especially by causing leukocytes to secrete their lysosomal enzymes in inappropriate ways (see Chapter 7).

Other components of complement make the so-called **membrane attack complex (MAC)**, which is responsible for the lysis of Gram-negative bacteria, enveloped viruses, and foreign cells. They may even lyse infected tissue cells

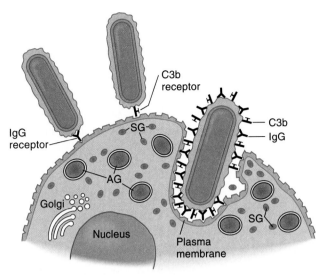

FIGURE 6-3 ▪ **Opsonization enhances phagocytosis.** This schematic representation shows how *Escherichia coli* is opsonized with immunoglobulin (IgG) and complement component C3b. The Fc and C3b ligands on the bacteria attach to the phagocyte through specific receptors. The mechanism of this interaction probably resembles that of a zipper or perhaps Velcro. Thus, sequential binding leads to the ingestion of the bacteria by the phagocytic membrane until the vesicle formed is pinched off as a new organelle inside the phagocyte. Meanwhile, degranulation (the fusion of granules with the phagocytic vesicle) forms a chamber in which bacteria are destroyed. The secondary granules (SG) and the azurophil granules (AG), also known as primary granules, fuse their membranes with that of the nascent phagosome, thus making a phagolysosome. Because phagocytes tend to be "sloppy" eaters, there is some "drooling," and the enzymes and surfactant proteins enter the surrounding fluid, contributing to the tissue changes of inflammation.

that appear alien because they display viral or other foreign proteins in their cell membranes. This activity is particularly important in killing bacteria that resist phagocytosis, such as meningococci and gonococci. Indeed, genetic deficiencies of the proteins involved in the formation of the MAC result in increased susceptibility to infections by these particular organisms.

Crucial Step in Complement Activation: Cleavage of C3

The three pathways of complement activation converge at a key biochemical step, the **cleavage of component C3** (see Fig. 6-1). From that point the remaining steps of all three pathways are the same. The enzymes responsible for this activity, **C3 convertases**, yield fragments C3a and C3b. Both components are pharmacologically active. **C3a**, which diffuses into the surrounding fluid, is an **anaphylatoxin**. **C3b**, which has an active thioester group

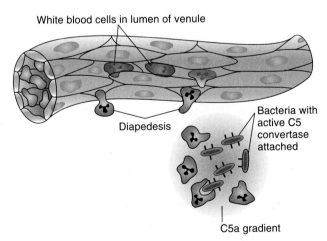

FIGURE 6-2 ▪ **Chemotactic action of C5a diffusing from bacteria toward a postcapillary venule.**

that covalently binds to hydroxyl groups of carbohydrates or proteins on the antigen (e.g., bacterium), is an **opsonin**. C3b binds to **complement receptor type 1 (CR1)** on phagocytic cells and thus greatly enhances binding of the opsonized bacteria to phagocytic cells (see Fig. 6-3). C3b also binds to CR2 on B cells and enhances B-cell activation and production of antibodies in the adaptive immune response. In addition, C3b becomes part of the C3 convertase of the alternative pathway, and a part of C5 convertase (as discussed later in the chapter and shown in Fig. 6-1).

C3 Convertase of the Classical Pathway

Activation of complement by the classical pathway is usually initiated by the presence of antigen–antibody complexes and thus is set off as the result of an adaptive immune response. The immune complexes are recognized by a protein complex called **C1**, composed of three proteins, **C1q, C1r, and C1s**. C1q is made up of six subunits, each shaped like a tulip (Fig. 6-4). The globular "head" of C1q binds to the Fc portion of antibodies in antigen–antibody complexes (the *c* in *Fc* stands for "constant" or "crystallizable"). One IgM molecule is sufficient for C1q binding, but two closely adjacent IgG molecules are needed. For this reason IgM is a very potent C activator, whereas only high concentrations of IgG can activate C. C1q binds only to antibodies bound to

antigens, which prevents C activation by free antibodies always present in the serum, and ensures that only antigen–antibody complexes activate the classical pathway. Following binding to the antigen–antibody complex, C1q converts C1r into a protease that carries out the next step in the pathway, the cleavage of C1s. The activated enzyme C1s in turn cleaves C2 and C4 into fragments **C4b2a**, which bind covalently to the antigen and become the **C3 convertase** of the classical pathway (see Fig. 6-1), and C4a and C2b fragments that are released.

C3 Convertase of the Lectin Pathway

The lectin pathway is activated by binding of the **mannose-binding lectin (MBL)**, which is a C1q analog, to mannose-containing polysaccharides, frequently present in the cell walls of many bacteria and fungi. This results in activation and complexing of MBL with the MBL-associated proteases **MASP-1** and **MASP-2**, which then cleave **C4** and **C2** to generate **C4b2a**, which is the same **C3 convertase** as in the classical pathway (see Fig. 6-1). From that point the activation of the lectin pathway proceeds the same as the classical pathway.

C3 Convertase of the Alternative Pathway

How is the alternative pathway activated? C3 is constantly cleaved at a very low level even without complement activation. Such cleavage generates C3b in plasma, but normally specific inhibitors inactivate most of these fragments. In the presence of microorganisms, some C3b fragments survive by binding covalently to their surfaces. Such **surface-bound C3b** is protected from inactivation and can participate in subsequent complement reactions. This C3b binds **factor B**, a protein homologous to C2, to form **C3bB** complex. **Factor D** then cleaves factor B from the C3bB complex to yield **C3bBb** complex, which is **C3 convertase** of the alternative pathway. Binding of **factor P** (properdin) to **C3bBb** stabilizes this enzyme. **C3bBb** then complexes with another C3b fragment, to yield another enzyme (**C3b3bBb**) that splits C5 (see Fig. 6-1).

Late Steps in Complement Activation: The Membrane Attack Complex

Once C3b is formed by either pathway, the downstream steps in complement activation can take place (see Fig. 6-1). C4b2a3b of the classical and lectin pathways or C3b3bBb of the alternative pathway cleaves C5a to produce two important fragments, C5a and C5b. **C5a**, like C3a, is an **anaphylatoxin**, as well as a powerful **chemoattractant** for phagocytes. The other fragment, **C5b**, is involved in making the final product of the complement cascade, the **membrane attack complex.** This armor-

FIGURE 6-4 ■ **Electron micrograph of complement component C1q x500,000.** In this lateral view of C1q, six terminal subunits are connected to a central subunit by fibrillar strands. Mannose-binding lectin (MBL), which has a similar function to C1q in activation of the lectin pathway, has a similar structure.

FIGURE 6-5 ▪ **Membrane attack complex (MAC) seen under the electron microscope. A.** MACs inserted into complement-lysed red blood cell membranes. On top portion, MACs are shown in their lateral projections. **B.** Isolated MACs in a detergent solution: a MAC on end (e) and MACs on their side (s).

piercing weapon can punch holes in bacteria and, in some cases, in tissue cells (Fig. 6-5). The MAC damages cells and bacteria by inserting donut-shaped multimers of C9 (which are assembled with the help of components C5b, C6, C7, and C8) into their membranes. The resulting hole makes cells permeable to ions and metabolites. Water enters the cells and raises their pressure, which eventually causes the cells to lyse.

Regulation of Complement Activation

The complement system is programmed to destroy. It must therefore be strictly regulated. On one hand, the complement activation pathway can amplify itself: each active enzyme can split and activate many complement

molecules. Fortunately, on the other hand, each activated component has its inhibitor (Table 6-6). The inhibition usually involves one of three mechanisms: (1) a suicide substrate mechanism, in which an inhibitor forms a covalent bond with the active site of the enzyme (e.g., C1 inhibitor binds to C1r and C1s); (2) proteolytic digestion of the active fragments into smaller inactive fragments (e.g., digestion of C4b and C3b by factor I); or (3) inhibition of association of complement components (e.g., inhibition of MAC formation by CD59). Without inhibition, all complement in the body would eventually be activated and massive inflammation would ensue. The adjacent host cells are also protected from the damage by activated complement components by several membrane proteins that inhibit complement activation or inactivate the activated components (see Table 6-6).

table **6-6**	Proteins That Regulate Complement Activity
COMPONENT	**FUNCTION**
Soluble serum proteins	
C1 inhibitor (C1 INH)	Inhibits enzymatic activity of C1r and C1s of the classical pathway and MASPs of the lectin pathway by suicide substrate mechanism
C4 binding protein (C4bp)	Binds to C4b and enhances the decay of C4b2a classical and lectin pathway C3 convertase
Factor H (H)	Binds to C3b and enhances the decay of the alternative pathway C3 convertase
Factor I (I)	Proteolytically inactivates C4b and C3b
Anaphylatoxin inactivator (ANA-IN)	Proteolytically inactivates the anaphylatoxins, C3a and C5a
S-protein (S; vitronectin)	Inhibits insertion of the MAC into the lipid bilayer by binding to the C5b-7 complex
Membrane proteins	
Complement receptor type 1 (CR1, CD35)	Accelerates dissociation of both C3 convertases
Membrane cofactor protein (MCP)	Cofactor for factor I-mediated cleavage of C3b
Decay accelerating factor (DAF, CD55)	Accelerates dissociation of both C3 convertases
Membrane inhibitor of reactive lysis (MIRL, CD59)	Binds to C9 and prevents MAC formation
Homologous restriction factor (HRF)	Blocks MAC insertion into the surface of cells

These plasma and membrane inhibitors ensure that the activation of complement occurs locally and is limited to the microbial surface at the site of infection.

The importance of complement and its appropriate regulation is demonstrated by genetic deficiencies of complement components. Patients lacking complement components that participate in the activation cascade suffer from more frequent and more severe bacterial infections. The impact of MAC deficiencies on susceptibility to infections with *Neisseria* was mentioned earlier in the chapter. Patients with C3 deficiencies suffer from infections with pyogenic bacteria, such as *Streptococcus pneumoniae*, *Staphylococcus aureus*, and *Haemophilus influenzae*. MBL and the lectin activation pathway were discovered by studying a group of children with recurrent pyogenic bacterial infections and failure to thrive. Their serum could not opsonize a yeast, *Saccharomyces cerevisiae* (which has mannose polymers in its cell wall), with C3; the serum was found to be deficient in MBL.

Deficiencies in complement inhibitors often result in overactivation of complement and inflammatory diseases. The genetic deficiency of C1 esterase inhibitor permits activation of the classical and lectin pathways with the uncontrolled production of anaphylatoxins. The result may be **hereditary angioedema,** a potentially fatal condition that causes laryngeal edema and airway obstruction. Another serious hereditary disease, **paroxysmal nocturnal hemoglobinuria,** manifests as bouts of intravascular hemolysis partly caused by complement-induced host cell lysis. This condition results from defective function of the inhibitory proteins CD55 (DAF) and CD59 (MIRL) on the surface of red blood cells. Each red blood cell binds as many as 1,000 molecules of C3b per day. The reason these cells are not normally lysed is that they have inhibitory proteins on their surfaces. In patients with this disease, these inhibitors do not function because they are not properly inserted in red blood cell membranes.

Microbial View of Complement

Complement killing by insertion of the MAC affects not only bacteria but also **enveloped viruses.** Not surprisingly, sensitive microorganisms have evolved countermeasures, some of which are discussed in Chapter 8. An interesting example of microbial defenses against complement is provided by herpes simplex virus. One of the glycoproteins of herpes simplex virus, glycoprotein C, contains a region that has an amino acid sequence similar to that of part of CR1. This amino acid sequence allows glycoprotein C to bind complement component C3b, thereby interfering with the rest of the complement cascade and with complement-mediated killing of the virus.

Several viruses have evolved to take advantage of complement receptors to enter host cells. Epstein-Barr virus uses CR2 to enter B cells and epithelial cells. Some viruses (e.g., HIV) or bacteria (e.g., *Mycobacterium*) not only have developed resistance to the lytic action of complement but also activate complement and use the C3b that deposits on its viral or bacterial surface to enter host cells through C3b receptors.

Leukocyte Chemotaxins: Sounding the Alarm

We have already seen that a product of complement activation, C5a, is an attractant for neutrophils and monocytes. It is not the only one; chemically distinct **chemotaxins** are also made by bacteria and by nucleated blood cells. Prominent among the latter are the leukotrienes, which are lipid products of cell membrane metabolism, and IL-8 and numerous other chemokines (discussed later), products of monocytes and macrophages.

The chemotaxins made by bacteria have an interesting origin. Many bacterial proteins "mature" after their synthesis, when a peptide is clipped off from their N terminus. The first amino acid in the peptide is N-formylmethionine, the initiator amino acid in prokaryotic protein synthesis. Eukaryotic cells do not use this device. The clipped peptide is recognized by the host as a strong chemoattractant for phagocytes. Its activity depends on its amino acid sequence and can be remarkably potent. N-formylmethionyl-leucyl-phenylalanine, for example, is active at concentrations of 10^{-11} molar. That is an extremely sensitive way for the host to detect bacterial proteins.

Chemotaxins enhance and direct the motility of phagocytic cells. As these compounds diffuse from their source, a concentration gradient is formed in the surrounding tissues. If the tissues are inflamed, neutrophils are already poised for action on the vascular endothelia. When neutrophils sense the chemotaxins, they travel along the gradient, cross the endothelial cells, and move tissues toward the microorganisms. This chemical homing mechanism guides the neutrophils precisely and efficiently to their targets.

Opsonization and Opsonins

Phagocytic cells alone can phagocytize bacteria, but without enhancing cofactors this process in inefficient. In the presence of substances called **opsonins,** neutrophils and macrophages will phagocytize many more bacteria. The term *opsonin* is related to the Latin word *opsonium*, which means "relish," an apt term for making bacteria more appetizing to phagocytes.

Several substances normally serve as opsonins, including the **C3b** component of complement and IgG antibodies (see Tables 6-4 and 6-5). C3b binds covalently to the surface of bacteria and forms a ligand that is recognized by receptors on neutrophils, monocytes, and macrophages. Microorganisms coated with C3b become anchored to the surface of phagocytes, which facilitates their uptake (see Fig. 6-3). Three receptors for C3b and its various cleavage products are located on white blood cells: **CR1, CR3,** and **CR4** (see Table 6-5).

Phagocytes

Of all the constitutive antimicrobial defenses of the body, the most potent is the cellular response. It consists of the influx of neutrophils, eosinophils, and monocytes into infected tissues. The properties of these and other white blood cells are listed in Table 6-7.

Neutrophils

Neutrophils are actively motile phagocytic cells produced in the bone marrow (see Table 6-7). They differentiate from stem cells over a period of about 2 weeks. Together with eosinophils and basophils, they are also known as **polymorphonuclear leukocytes (PMNs)** because of their segmented nucleus, or as **granulocytes** because of their granules. They produce four kinds of granules—primary, secondary, tertiary, and secretory vesicles—of which the first two kinds, azurophil (primary) and specific (secondary) are the largest and most easily visible under the microscope. These granules have many antimicrobial factors (see Tables 6-3 and 6-8). When they mature, in numbers of about 10^{10} per day, about 5% enter the peripheral blood and circulate for an average of 6.5 hours. Half these neutrophils enter the capillary bed where they **marginate**—that is, they adhere to the endothelium of venules. In response to distress signals from the tissues (complement components and cytokines such as IL-1 and TNF-α), the endothelium in the involved region expresses a set of adhesion molecules that bind more firmly to the neutrophils. When summoned by chemotaxins, the neutrophils cross the endothelium by **diapedesis** through the cell junctions, traverse the basement membrane, and enter the extravascular tissue spaces (see Fig. 6-2).

Neutrophils and monocytes can be enticed into foci of infection by gradients of many chemoattractants, such as the C5a complement component, formylated bacterial proteins, and chemokines. But what ensures that these phagocytes will arrive precisely where they are needed?

The answer to the question is that neutrophils and monocytes, as well as the endothelial cells to which they must adhere, become sticky (see Fig. 6-2). The molecular explanation is simple: it is the result of sugars on glycosylated surface proteins. These glycoproteins on the endothelial cells are **selectins** (which mediate weak binding) and **integrin ligands** (which mediate strong binding). They bind to **integrins** on the phagocytes. However, stickiness introduces a problem: blood cells that originate in the marrow must enter the bloodstream and be able to circulate there without sticking too firmly. For their part, the endothelial cells lining the blood vessels must avoid becoming too sticky, to allow circulation of the blood cells. At the proper time, however, both leukocytes and endothelial cells must be able to stick to each other. The transition

table **6-7**	**White Blood Cells**	
CELL	**SOURCE**	**FUNCTION**
Neutrophil	Bone marrow stem cells to peripheral blood	Adherence, chemotaxis, diapedesis Phagocytosis Degranulation Antimicrobial action, oxidative and nonoxidative
Eosinophil	Similar to neutrophil	Antiparasitic action, nonoxidative and oxidative
Basophil	Similar to neutrophil	Release of proinflammatory vasoactive mediators
Monocyte	Bone marrow stem cells Promonocyte to peripheral blood	Adherence, chemotaxis Diapedesis Phagocytosis Antimicrobial actions, secretion of cytokines
Macrophage	Monocytes of the peripheral blood	See monocytes Synthesis of many important molecules, including cytokines (TNF-α, IL-1, IL-6, IL-12, IL-15, and others), chemokines (IL-8 and others), complement components, plasminogen activator and other proteases, lysozyme, cell membrane components, including major histocompatibility complex class I and class II molecules Functions in adaptive immunity through antigen recognition, antigen processing, antigen presentation, and regulation of immune responses
T lymphocyte	Bone marrow stem cells via thymus	Helper, effector, and regulatory functions in adaptive immune response
B lymphocyte	Bone marrow stem cells	Antibody production in adaptive immune responses
NK cell	Bone marrow stem cells	Killing of virus-infected cells and tumor cells

IL, interleukin; TNF, tumor necrosis factor.

table **6-8**	**Antimicrobial Substances Associated with the Azurophil and Specific Granules of Neutrophils**		
GRANULE TYPE	**O$_2$-INDEPENDENT**	**O$_2$-DEPENDENT**	**OTHER**
Azurophil (primary)	α-Defensins Phospholipase A$_2$ (PLA$_2$) Azurocidin (CAP37) BPI Elastase Cathepsins G, D, B Lysozyme	Myeloperoxidase[a]	
Specific (secondary)	Lactoferrin Lysozyme Cathelicidin (CAP18)	NADPH oxidase[b] cofactors	Bacterial chemotaxin receptors C5a receptors Collagenase Gelatinase Vitamin B$_{12}$–binding protein

[a] Myeloperoxidase together with Cl and hydrogen peroxide form a potent antimicrobial system.
[b] This enzyme complex forms with fusion of specific granule membranes with the cytoplasmic membrane. The specific granules contribute the cytochrome component of the complex and the flavoprotein, while the neutrophil cytoplasmic membrane contributes an NADPH oxidase to the complex.
BPI, bactericidal permeability-increasing protein; CAP, cationic antimicrobial protein.

from loosely adherent to tightly adherent is critical for the leukocytes when they leave the circulation and move through the tissues. Clearly, leukocytes and endothelial cells are subject to regulatory mechanisms that induce stickiness of these cells at the proper time. Complement components such as C5a and cytokines such as IL-1, TNF-α, and IL-8 play such directive and regulatory roles, attracting leukocytes and stimulating endothelial cells, upregulating their stickiness, and causing them to produce additional cytokines and prostaglandins.

The importance of glycoprotein receptors for endothelial cells that are present on neutrophils is illustrated in people with congenital defects in these proteins. Neutrophils of these patients are unable to pass through the vascular endothelium and fail to orient, bind, and ingest particles. Such defective neutrophils are unable to form pus. Patients with this condition are said to have congenital **leukocyte adhesion deficiency (LAD)** and suffer recurrent, often fatal infections. Neutrophils of LAD patients do not pass through endothelia because their receptors fail to bind to the endothelial cells. The reason for failure to bind and to ingest bacteria is a defect in one of the cellular receptors for C3b (called Mac-1 or CD11b, which is one of the integrins). These molecules are of great interest to the pharmaceutical industry, which is attempting to discover drugs to control leukocyte adhesion functions.

In a healthy person, sticking of leukocytes to endothelial surfaces is most intense in the submucosa of the alimentary tract. The large intestine has an enormous microbial population just one cell layer away from the host's aseptic tissues. This abundant flora generates large amounts of chemotaxins that recruit the bulk of the normally available neutrophils. Thus, the submucosa of the gut is in a constant state of low-level inflammation, which keeps the microbial flora of the lumen in check.

When the bone marrow fails to make neutrophils in reaction to toxic chemicals or radiation or for other reasons, infections emanate from the gut.

Monocytes and Macrophages

Slower to arrive at the sites of microbial invasion are the **monocytes.** These circulating members of the mononuclear family eventually settle in tissues and become known as resident **tissue macrophages.** Although monocytes and macrophages share a common progenitor with neutrophils, their kinetics of maturation and appearance are substantially different. Unlike the neutrophils, monocytes continue to differentiate after they leave the bone marrow. Most importantly, monocytes and macrophages function in both innate and adaptive immune responses, a point that will be elaborated later in this chapter and in Chapter 7.

In general, monocytes and macrophages come into play slowly, often hours after neutrophils have been actively combating invading microorganisms. Neutrophils play a role in recruiting mononuclear cells because they release a granule protein (**azurocidin** or CAP37) that is a potent attractant specific for monocytes. The delay in monocyte activity is seen in patients who become neutropenic from chemicals or radiation. If the neutropenia develops slowly, there is time for monocytes to replace the disappearing neutrophils. The risk of infection is much smaller in these patients than in those with an abrupt onset of neutropenia.

Tissue or resident macrophages exist throughout the body and have different names and functions, depending on the tissue. Thus, they are called **Kupffer cells** in the liver, **alveolar macrophages** in the lungs, **osteoclasts** in the bone, and **microglia** in the brain. All these tissue macrophages phagocytize invading microorganisms. Tissue macrophages contribute greatly to the inflammatory response by releasing IL-1, which enhances sticking of neutrophils to the capillary endothelia, and TNF-α, which activates newly arrived neutrophils. In addition, tissue macrophages release an activator of the acute phase reaction (IL-6) and many chemokines (including IL-8) that attract neutrophils. These macrophages are replenished by the arrival and differentiation of monocytes from the bone marrow. The most active macrophages arise from monocytes delivered to sites of inflammation.

Eosinophils

The eosinophils parallel the neutrophils in lifestyle and function. Although they are not efficient in phagocytosis, they can readily **exocytose** (release to the outside) their granules. Their target is usually animal parasites rather than bacteria. Indeed, the increase of these cells in the circulation, **eosinophilia,** is the hallmark of multicellular parasitic diseases such as schistosomiasis or trichinosis. The reason for this specificity is not known. It has been shown that the cytoplasmic granules of the eosinophils carry large amounts of an enzyme known as **eosinophil peroxidase,** as well as specific cationic proteins. These compounds have the power to kill certain parasites. Thus, eosinophils have an anti-infectious armamentarium similar to that of neutrophils but specifically targeted to certain protozoa and worms, which are too large to be phagocytized by neutrophils.

How Do Phagocytes Kill Microorganisms?

Once near their microbial target, neutrophils and other phagocytes can begin their antimicrobial action (see Figs. 6-3, 6-6, and 6-7). To start the process, they must attach and ingest the microorganisms, either spontaneously or with the aid of **opsonins** (substances that enhance phagocytosis, as described earlier in this chapter). The membranes of neutrophils contain the receptors for chemotaxins and opsonins. After chemotaxins bind to these membranes, the receptor molecules are internalized and replaced with new ones. What makes chemotaxis so effective is that neutrophils are extraordinarily motile. Neutrophils move by recombining their cytoplasmic microfilaments and their microtubules. **Actin** and **myosin** in microfilaments are affected by the protein **gelsolin** (which invites the comparison of neutrophils with muscle cells). The result is a morphological alteration of the cell shape. During chemotaxis, the portion of the cell that faces upstream in the chemotactic gradient forms a structure called a **lamellipodium,** where the cytoplasm is densely packed with microfilaments. The portion of the cell that faces downstream in the gradient forms a knoblike structure, the **uropod.**

FIGURE 6-6 ▪ **Phagocytosis of *Escherichia coli* by a neutrophil visualized by transmission electron microscopy.** Shown here are lobes of the segmented nucleus (N) and two bacteria engulfed and seen within a phagosome (P).

Engulfing of bacteria or other particles of suitable size takes place by formation of a pouchlike structure, the **phagosome,** which invaginates, displacing the nucleus and the granules toward the uropod (see Figs. 6-6 and 6-7). The cytoplasmic granules soon discharge their contents into the phagosome by fusion of their membranes (a process called degranulation), forming a new structure known as the **phagolysosome.** The phagolysosome quickly pinches off from the plasma membrane and becomes a separate cytoplasmic organelle. By the time the pinching off is completed, the fusion of the granules is well under way, and bacteria are already coated with antibacterial proteins. Thus, like poisonous snakes that disable their prey before swallowing them, neutrophils kill bacteria before they completely ingest them.

Bacteria become enfolded into the plasma membrane of the neutrophils by a zipperlike action, with the receptors on the phagocyte surface progressively attaching to the ligands on the bacterial surface (see Figs. 6-3 and 6-7). This binding stimulates two mechanisms that lead to the killing of bacteria. One mechanism is set in motion by a vigorous burst of oxidative metabolism that leads to the production of hydrogen peroxide and other compounds lethal to microorganisms (see Fig. 6-7). This is **oxygen-dependent killing.** The second mechanism also results in the discharge of toxic compounds from the

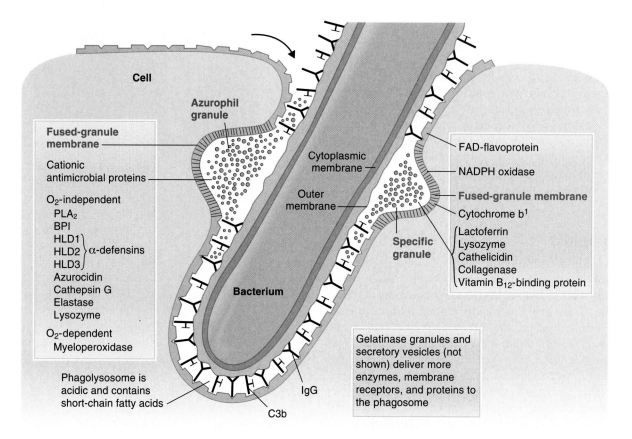

Cell

Azurophil granule

Cytoplasmic membrane

Outer membrane

Fused-granule membrane

Cationic antimicrobial proteins

O_2-independent
PLA$_2$
BPI
HLD1
HLD2 } α-defensins
HLD3
Azurocidin
Cathepsin G
Elastase
Lysozyme

O_2-dependent
Myeloperoxidase

FAD-flavoprotein

NADPH oxidase

Fused-granule membrane

Cytochrome b^1

Lactoferrin
Lysozyme
Cathelicidin
Collagenase
Vitamin B$_{12}$-binding protein

Specific granule

Bacterium

Phagolysosome is acidic and contains short-chain fatty acids

IgG

C3b

Gelatinase granules and secretory vesicles (not shown) deliver more enzymes, membrane receptors, and proteins to the phagosome

FIGURE 6-7 ■ **Fusion of the phagosome and the granules.** Fusion between the membranes of the specific granules and the cytoplasmic membrane, together with proteins from the cytosol, completes the enzyme complex that generates reduced oxygen species, including H_2O_2, which then forms antimicrobial hypochlorite from chloride by the action of myeloperoxidase. Fusion of specific and azurophil granules with the phagosome also activates oxygen-independent mechanisms and delivers many antimicrobial proteins to the phagosome.

granules into the phagosome. This is known as **oxygen-independent killing.** The granules of these cells may be considered enlarged lysosomes, packed with large amounts of powerful hydrolytic enzymes and other active substances. They are contained within unit membranes (see Fig. 6-7). **Azurophil,** or **primary granules,** contain a variety of enzymes and several cationic proteins that are also powerfully antibacterial (see Tables 6-3 and 6-8). **Specific,** or **secondary, granules** contain a cytochrome, the iron-binding protein **lactoferrin,** a collagenase, and other proteins.

Oxygen-Dependent Killing

How does the oxidative process kill microorganisms? The mechanism is complex and involves several radicals and chemical species. A highly active, multicomponent **NADPH oxidase** rapidly reduces molecular oxygen to superoxide, O_2^-, which in turn becomes H_2O_2 in the following reaction:

$$2 O_2^- + H_2O \rightarrow H_2O_2 + O_2$$

The components of the NADPH oxidase include at least four proteins. Two of them, the cytochrome **Phox 91**

(*Phox* stands for "phagocyte oxidase") and **Phox 22** are inserted into the cytosolic membrane by fusion of the specific granules with the phagosome. There they are joined by the cytosolic proteins **Phox 47** and **Phox 67** to form the completed oxidase. Separating NADPH oxidase components into different subcellular compartments ensures that the active enzyme is assembled only inside the phagolysosomes following phagocytosis and prevents generation of toxic oxygen products outside the phagolysosome.

Hydrogen peroxide, while bactericidal, does not work alone in killing microorganisms within phagocytes. Rather, an enzyme called **myeloperoxidase** uses peroxide to convert chloride ions into the highly toxic **hypochlorous ions,** the same chemical found in common bleach (see Fig. 6-7 and Table 6-8). Myeloperoxidase is delivered to the phagolysosome by fusion with the azurophil granules.

The importance of these oxidative processes in neutrophil microbicidal action is illustrated in children with **chronic granulomatous disease,** a congenital defect caused by mutations involving the NADPH oxidase Phox proteins, most often Phox 91. Such defects render the phagocytes incapable of producing the reduced oxygen products. The cells can phagocytize and degranulate, but they fail to kill the ingested bacteria. Interestingly, microorganisms that lack catalase, such as the streptococci, obligingly release H_2O_2 into the phagocytic vacuole when phagocytized, thereby committing suicide. Thus, pneumococci (a species of streptococci) do not cause disease any more frequently in such patients than they do in normal persons. The incidence of chronic granulomatous disease is about 4 per million. Mutations involving Phox 91 make up 70 to 80% of the cases of chronic granulomatous disease and are X chromosome linked. These patients develop subcutaneous abscesses, lung abscesses, hepatic abscesses, lymphadenitis, pneumonias, and osteomyelitis.

Oxygen-Independent Killing

Oxygen-independent killing mechanisms are also triggered by the binding of opsonized bacteria to the plasma membrane of neutrophils (see Fig. 6-7 and Table 6-8). Specific granules seem to fuse to phagosomes first and deliver several bactericidal proteins, such as **cathelicidin** (CAP18), lysozyme (the enzyme that disrupts the cell wall of many bacteria), and lactoferrin (an iron-binding protein that effectively reduces the amount of iron available to the microorganisms). The azurophil granules discharge **antimicrobial cationic proteins** into phagosomes. Each of these substances has a unique antimicrobial spectrum, but they tend to affect Gram-negative bacteria more than Gram-positives. These proteins usually damage microbial membranes through direct insertion into the membranes (e.g., **defensins**) or through enzymatic activity (e.g., **PLA$_2$**). They also act synergistically; for example, sensitivity of Gram-negative bacteria is much greater to a mixture of **bactericidal permeability-increasing protein (BPI)** and phospholipase A$_2$ (PLA$_2$) than to each peptide individually. The activity of these proteins may account for the survival of some children with chronic granulomatous disease. The oxygen-independent mechanisms also account for bacterial killing under the highly anaerobic conditions found in deep abscesses.

Deficiencies in cationic proteins have been described in patients with chronic skin infections and abscesses. A genetic disease known as the **Chediak-Higashi syndrome** is caused by the formation of large granules in neutrophils, which are poorly functional and substantially reduce the killing power of these cells.

How do various kinds of bacteria differ in their sensitivity to the two bactericidal mechanisms of neutrophils? In general, organisms found in the gut, such as Gram-negative rods, are readily killed by the oxygen-independent mechanism. Gram-positive bacteria, like those found on the skin and in the upper respiratory epithelia, tend to be resistant to oxygen-independent killing and are killed chiefly by the oxygen-dependent pathway. Does this reflect the abundance of oxygen in the skin and its absence in the gut?

Killing by Monocytes and Macrophages

Together, monocytes and macrophages serve to mop up what is left at the scene of the battle between microorganisms and neutrophils. They phagocytize the microorganisms and the debris left by neutrophils. Their mechanisms of chemotaxis, phagocytosis, and microbial killing resemble those of the neutrophils. **Nitric oxide,** a simple chemical made by macrophages in some animal species as the result of activation by interferon-γ and TNF-α, has been shown to play an important role in the killing of microorganisms by macrophages in mice. However, human monocytes and macrophages do not make nitric oxide in any significant amounts; thus, the contribution of nitric oxide to microbial killing by these cells is negligible. In humans nitric oxide is made in small amounts by fibroblasts, some neurons, and cells of the vasculature, where nitric oxide may perform some vasoactive and transmitter functions.

An important point is that monocytes and macrophages, unlike the neutrophils, continue to differentiate after they leave the bone marrow and become activated when properly stimulated. In addition, these versatile cells synthesize several complement components and cytokines. Activated macrophages phagocytize more vigorously, take up more oxygen, and secrete a large quantity of hydrolytic enzymes. In general, they are better prepared to kill microorganisms and, appropriately, have been called the "angry" macrophages. Macrophage activation is elicited by substances made in response to the presence of microorganisms, like complement fragment C3b and interferon-γ. They are also activated by a variety of other compounds, such as endotoxin of Gram-negative bacteria. Some bacteria, fungi, and protozoa can grow within unstimulated macrophages, but in general they are killed when these cells become activated. Perhaps the most important property of macrophages is their participation in the recognition of antigens and induction of adaptive immune responses, which is discussed later in this chapter.

Inflammation: Complex Response to Infection and Injury

The combined action of the various defense mechanisms discussed so far in this chapter results in **inflammation**, which further amplifies both innate and adaptive immune defenses. Inflammation is a process that occurs in vascularized tissues in response to injury. Early signs of inflammation are confined locally and include pain, swelling, or both and a sense of heat and throbbing of the injured part. The inflamed site appears red, shiny, hot, and painful to the touch as the result of alterations ocal blood vessels and lymphatics. These rapid anges, which are called **acute inflammation,** are dynamic and undergo predictable and continued evolution. The tissues may return to normal or become scarred. The outcome depends on the extent of damage done by trauma, by the infecting microorganisms, or by the inflammatory response itself. If acute inflammation does not cure the problem, it may change character and become a **chronic inflammation.**

Many **mediators** induced by various mechanisms cause inflammation (Table 6-9). They include **complement-generated split products; histamine** released from mast cells, basophils, and platelets; lipid mediators (**prostaglandins** and **leukotrienes** generated from arachidonic acid, and **platelet-activating factor** generated from phospholipids in the cell membranes of mast cells and other cells); and **kinins** (mainly bradykinin) generated in plasma during activation of the clotting system.

Cytokines (literally, "cell movers") are 10- to 25-kDa polypeptides secreted from microbe-activated proinflammatory cells (primarily macrophages and lymphocytes). They have multiple proinflammatory effects. Produced locally in small amounts, the cytokines **tumor necrosis factor** (TNF-α), **IL-1,** and **IL-6** locally activate other proinflammatory cells and endothelial and epithelial cells, enhance their defensive activity, and induce production of more cytokines and chemokines. When produced in large amounts, these cytokines enter circulation and have endocrine-like effects. They induce fever, increased lipolysis in adipose tissues, mobilization of amino acids from muscles (to be used in synthesizing defense proteins), and synthesis of acute phase proteins in the liver (which enter circulation and enhance body defenses). The cytokines mentioned here also enhance the function of antigen-presenting cells and lymphocytes that participate in adaptive immune responses. Excessive production of cytokines (especially TNF-α) and other mediators of inflammation induce **septic shock,** which can be fatal.

Many microbe- or cytokine-activated host cells, including macrophages and endothelial cells, produce numerous **chemokines,** which are cytokines with chemotactic properties. More than 100 chemokines and chemokine receptors have been identified to date, which is a testimony to the complexity of chemotactic events and their importance for host defenses. Classified into two families based on a structural motif of two cysteines separated by one amino acid (CXC) or two adjacent cysteines (CC), chemokines are named **CXCL** or **CCL** (*L* stands for "ligand") and numbered consecutively. Similarly, chemokine receptors are named CXCR or CCR (*R* stands for "receptor") and numbered. Chemokines are usually chemotactic for many cell types, but in general most of the chemokines of the CXC group (which includes the well-known chemokine IL-8) are chemotactic for neutrophils. Chemokines of the CC group are primarily chemotactic for T lymphocytes, although some are also chemotactic for eosinophils, basophils, and

other cells. High induction of CXC chemokines by various bacteria is responsible for accumulation of large amounts of **pus** (which is primarily composed of PMN exudate and bacteria) at the site of infections.

The combined action of the mediators of inflammation results in the following:

■ **Increased blood supply** (manifested as erythema or redness), which brings more antimicrobial cells and proteins to the site of infection
■ **Increased vascular permeability** (manifested as edema or swelling caused by accumulation of fluid), which brings more antimicrobial proteins to the site of infection
■ **Chemotaxis** (manifested as induration or hardening of the lesion caused by accumulation of cells), which causes infiltration of the site of infection with phagocytic cells and lymphocytes attracted to the site of infection by chemotactic factors

Inflammation is essential for defenses against infections; therefore, patients with infections should generally *not* be treated with anti-inflammatory agents. However, excessive or uncontrolled inflammation, or inflammation induced by noninfectious causes, may cause substantial damage to the tissues and needs to be treated. Such a condition is called hypersensitivity. Because hypersensitivities often result from exaggerated adaptive immune responses, they will be discussed in Chapter 7.

Natural Killer Cells

NK cells are large granular lymphocytes that have cytotoxic activity for other cells. In this aspect they resemble cytotoxic T cells. However, NK cells are neither T cells nor B cells because they do not have the markers characteristic of T or B lymphocytes. They also do not have the T- or B-cell antigen receptors and the associated signal transduction molecules that make B and T cells antigen specific (see Chapter 7). Therefore, they do not recognize antigens through the types of receptors that T and B cells use, and they do not need to be selected and generated in adaptive immune responses directed to specific antigens. The name natural killer thus stems from their readiness to kill other cells without the need for time-consuming antigen-driven selection in adaptive immune response. NK cells constitute 5 to 20% of mononuclear cells in peripheral blood and spleen but are rare in other lymphoid organs.

NK cells kill virus-infected cells before those cells can produce mature infective viral particles. This function is important because viruses can only grow inside the living host cells, using their biochemical machinery to produce more viruses. Once the virus enters the host cell, however, it is not visible and thus not susceptible to extracellular host defenses. Therefore, virus-infected

table **6-9**   Mediators of Inflammation

MEDIATOR	SOURCE	MAIN EFFECT
C3a (peptide)	Complement	Anaphylatoxin, causes histamine release from platelets and mast cells, which increases vascular permeability
C5a (peptide)	Complement	Chemotaxis of PMNs
		Anaphylatoxin, causes histamine release from mast cells and platelets
Histamine (decarboxylated histidine)	Mast cells	Increased vascular permeability
	Basophils	Vasodilation
	Platelets	
Prostaglandins (lipids)	Arachidonic acid from membranes of mast cells and other leukocytes, by cyclooxygenase pathway	PGE_2, PGI_2 (prostacilin): vasodilation, edema
		TXA_2 (thromboxane A_2): vasoconstriction
Leukotrienes (lipids)	Arachidonic acid from membranes of mast cells and other leukocytes, by lipoxygenase pathway	LTB_4: chemotaxis LTC_4, LTD_4, LTE_4: vasoconstriction, increased vascular permeability
Platelet activating factor (lipid)	Mast cells	Release of vasoactive products from platelets
	Basophils	Increased vascular permeability
	PMNs, Macrophages	Adhesion of PMNs to endothelial cells
	Endothelial cells	
Bradykinin (peptide)	Plasma	Increased vascular permeability
		Vasodilation
Cytokines (peptides)		
TNF-α	Macrophages	Endothelial cell and PMN activation
		Inflammation
		Fever
		Shock
		Fat and protein catabolism
		Acute phase protein synthesis in liver
IL-1	Macrophages	Endothelial cell activation
	Endothelial cells	Inflammation
		Fever
		Acute phase protein synthesis in liver
IL-6	Macrophages	Acute phase protein synthesis in liver
	Endothelial cells	Fever
	T cells	B cell growth and differentiation
Chemokines (peptides)		
CXC family[a] (includes IL-8)	Macrophages	Chemotactic attraction of PMNs
	Endothelial cells	
CC family[a]	Macrophages	Chemotactic attraction of T lymphocytes
	Endothelial cells	

[a] More than 50 chemokines are divided into two families based on a structural motif of two cysteines separated by one amino acid (CXC) or two adjacent cysteines (CC).
IL, interleukin; PMN, polymorphonuclear leukocyte; TNF, tumor necrosis factor.

FIGURE 6-8 ▪ **Function of NK cell killing and inhibitory receptors.** Activating receptors (NKRs) on NK cells engage glycoproteins on autologous host cells. Inhibitory receptors (e.g., KIRs) engage major histocompatibility complex (MHC) class I–peptide complexes on autologous host cells. **A.** Engagement of inhibitory receptors is dominant and prevents NK cell activation and killing. **B.** If a virus-infected host cell does not express MHC class I peptide complexes, inhibitory receptors on NK cells are not engaged and binding of activating NKRs to glycoproteins on host cells activates NK cells and induces killing of virus-infected cells.

cells must be destroyed before they can make more infective viruses. Cytotoxic T cells can do this by using T-cell antigen receptors that recognize viral peptides bound to host MHC class I antigens exposed on the surface of infected cells (see Chapter 7). How can NK cells discriminate between virus-infected and uninfected cells? NK cells can also kill some tumor cells. How can they discriminate between malignant or nonmalignant cells?

NK cells use the previously mentioned missing or changed self strategy to detect virus-infected cells or tumor cells. NK cells have on their surface two types of receptors. The first is the **natural killer receptor** (**NKR**). NK cells have several types of NKRs, but in general they are lectins that bind to various glycoproteins present on many cells in the body. Thus, many host cells are potential NK targets. Engagement of NKRs triggers the killing of target cells. However, this would induce the killing of many healthy cells in the body. Therefore, NK cells also

have a second type of receptor, the **killer inhibitory receptors** (**KIRs;** also called killer Ig-like receptors e.g., CD158), which prevent the killing action of the NKRs. KIRs bind to self MHC class I molecules on target cells. Because all healthy cells in the body express MHC class I molecules (see Chapter 7), KIRs inhibit killing of normal healthy cells by NK cells. However, virus-infected cells or some tumor cells often have missing or changed MHC class I molecules and therefore do not engage KIRs but still have glycoproteins that engage NKRs. In the absence of inhibition by KIRs, NKRs trigger the killing of these target cells (Fig. 6-8). What a clever way to dispose of unwanted infected cells or tumor cells.

NK cells are stimulated by the macrophage-derived cytokines IL-15 and IL-12. **IL-15** is a growth factor for NK cells, and **IL-12** induces **interferon-γ** production in NK cells and enhances their cytolytic activity. Interferon-γ in turn activates macrophages and inhibits growth of viruses in host cells. The activity of NK cells is also enhanced by **IL-2**, produced by helper T cells in adaptive immune response (see Chapter 7). NK cells, similarly to T cells, also express **CD2** molecule, which binds to CD58 (also called lymphocyte function-associated antigen-3, or LFA3), which is expressed on many cells in the body. CD2–CD58 binding stabilizes interaction between killer cells and target cells and enhances the effectiveness of killing. NK cells also have **FcγRIIIa receptors** (CD16), which bind the Fc portion of IgG when complexed with the antigen. This allows NK cells to function as killer cells in the so-called **antibody-dependent cell-mediated cytotoxicity (ADCC)**, which is the killing of target cells coated with the antibody IgG. This type of killing is also sensitive to inhibition by KIRs, which ensure that only unhealthy cells are killed.

Although the recognition mechanisms of target cells by NK cells and cytotoxic T cells are different, the **mechanism of killing** by both cell types is the same. NK cells, similar to cytotoxic T cells, have granules filled with **granzymes** and **perforin** (see Chapter 7). On engagement of the target cells, the content of the granules is released onto the surface of the target cell. In the low Ca^{+2} environment of the granules, perforin is a monomeric molecule, but in the presence of high extracellular Ca^{+2}, it aggregates and inserts itself into the membrane of target cells in a manner very similar to the assembly of the membrane attack complex of the complement. This destroys the permeability of the membrane and allows granzymes (also released from the granules) to enter the target cells. **Granzymes** are serine proteases that cleave and activate intracellular caspases in target cells, which triggers target cell death by **apoptosis** (programmed cell death).

Initiation of Adaptive Immune Responses by Innate Immunity

From the examples cited in the previous sections, it is obvious how tightly the functions of the innate and adaptive immune systems are intertwined and how they complement each other and depend on each other for full activity. This section considers another important concept: the innate immune system is required for the initial recognition of antigen and initiation of the adaptive immune response.

The main function of innate immunity is to provide immediate protection against infections and to defend the host and eliminate less severe infections with low-virulence microorganisms. In infections with more pathogenic microorganisms, that can evade or resist the elimination by the innate immune system, the adaptive immunity must

develop to eliminate these infections (adaptiv will be discussed in detail in Chapter 7).

Another important function of the inna system is to recognize, process, and present antigens to lymphocytes, the cells required to initiate adaptive immune responses. This function is performed by **antigen-presenting cells,** such as **dendritic cells** (e.g., **Langerhans cells** in the skin) and **macrophages.** These cells use pattern recognition receptors, like TLRs (see Table 6-4), to recognize the antigen (the antigen could be the entire microorganism or isolated microbial products). This interaction induces uptake of the antigen by dendritic cells or macrophages, stimulates them, and induces their migration into the lymph nodes adjacent to the site of infection (Table 6-10). The dendritic cells or macrophages mature

table **6-10**	**Sequence of Events in Initiation of Adaptive Immunity to Extracellular Antigens by Innate Immunity**

SEQUENCE OF EVENTS
Microbial antigen
↓
Recognition by dendritic cell through pattern recognition receptors (e.g., TLRs)
↓
Uptake of the antigen
↓
Migration of dendritic cells into the lymph nodes and maturation into antigen-presenting cells
↓
Expression of T-cell costimulatory molecules on dendritic cells (B7, also known as CD80/CD86)
↓
Processing of the antigen and loading of antigenic peptides into MHC class II molecules
↓
Presentation of the antigenic peptide–MHC complex to T helper cells
↓
Secretion of T cell–activating cytokines
↓
Activation, proliferation, and differentiation of antigen-specific T cells
↓
Generation of effector cells specific for the antigen
↓
Elimination of the antigen

MHC, major histocompatibility complex.

into functional antigen-presenting cells. This maturation involves expression of T-cell costimulatory molecules on dendritic cells or macrophages (mainly **B7**, also known as **CD80/CD86**), which are absolutely required for the activation of helper T cells (see Chapter 7).

Antigens that are not recognized by dendritic cells or macrophages through the pattern recognition receptors (and do not stimulate these cells) are unable to induce maturation of these cells and expression of this costimulatory molecule. Such antigens, therefore, are not immunogenic or very poorly immunogenic. This mechanism ensures that the adaptive immune response is triggered by potentially dangerous microbial products recognized by pattern recognition receptors. The dendritic cells process the antigen, digesting the antigen into peptides, loading the peptides into MHC class II molecules, and expressing the MHC class II–peptide complexes on the surface of the antigen-presenting cells. The complexes are then presented to helper T cells that have the T-cell antigen receptor specific for a given combination of the antigenic peptide and MHC class II molecules. This interaction induces activation, proliferation, and differentiation of antigen-specific helper T cells, which are required for the initiation of the adaptive immune response to the antigen. (The entire process of the adaptive immune response will be discussed in more detail in Chapter 7.)

The type of antigen and the way the antigen is recognized and processed by dendritic cells dictates the direction of the adaptive immune response. The example given in Table 6-10 describes the response to an extracellular antigen, which typically would be presented to Th1 cells as an MHC class II–bound peptide. This antigen would also be available to B cells, would be processed by B cells, and would activate Th2 cells, which would then induce B-cell antibody response to this antigen (see Chapter 7).

If the antigen comes from an intracellular pathogen present in a macrophage or dendritic cells but is not readily available as an extracellular antigen to B cells, the antigen would be processed only by the macrophages and dendritic cells (but not by B cells) and would primarily induce Th1 cells (but not Th2 cells). Macrophages and dendritic cells, on contact with the antigen, secrete cytokines that direct maturation of the helper T cells either into Th1 or Th2 cells. These two types of T helper cells secrete different cytokines and induce different types of responses: Th1 cells induce cell-mediated responses that primarily activate macrophages through interferon-γ, and Th2 cells help B cells to differentiate into antibody-secreting plasma cells (see Chapter 7).

If the antigen is a virus whose proteins are being synthesized by host cells, peptides derived from these viral proteins are delivered to MHC class I molecules, which triggers generation of cytotoxic T cells. Cytotoxic T cells recognize viral antigenic peptides bound to MHC class I molecules (see Chapter 7).

Thus, the way the antigen-presenting cells respond to the antigen, process the antigen, and present the antigen to T cells determines what type of adaptive immune response is induced: antibody production is induced by extracellular antigens, a cell-mediated T-cell response is induced by intracellular pathogens delivered to MHC class II molecules, and a cytotoxic T-cell response is induced by intracellular viral antigens delivered to MHC class I molecules.

Another way the innate immune system affects the generation of adaptive immunity is through activation of complement. Activation of complement can enhance adaptive immune responses because B cells have CR2 receptors for the C3b complement split product. Thus, coating an antigen with C3b enhances its delivery to the B cells in the spleen and lymph nodes, and enhances B cell–antigen interaction and B cell–antibody response to the antigen.

Innate Immunity as an Effector Mechanism of Adaptive Immunity

Some components of the innate immune system are also used as effector mechanisms of adaptive immunity. Cell-mediated responses generate cytokine-secreting Th1 cells, which secrete large amounts of **interferon-γ** (also known as **macrophage-activating factor**, or MAF), whose primary function is to activate macrophages. Activated macrophages become very efficient in killing pathogens, such as *Mycobacterium tuberculosis*, which can normally survive and grow in nonactivated macrophages. Interferon-γ is produced by Th1 cells generated in the adaptive immune response to *Mycobacteria*. Thus, macrophages function as effector cells for the T-cell responses to *Mycobacteria*. Many other examples of close cooperation between the effector mechanisms of the innate and adaptive immunity have been already given, such as activation of complement by antibodies, which enhances phagocytosis and induces inflammation, or antibody-dependent killing by NK cells. Thus, innate immunity is indispensable not only for early protection against infections but also for the development of adaptive immune responses and for some of the effector functions of adaptive immunity.

Conclusion

It is apparent that innate immunity is *not* a static constitutive defense that has little specificity, handles all microbial invaders in the same way, and is separate from adaptive immunity (as was earlier believed, thus its old name, nonspecific resistance). Innate immunity is a complex and dynamic web of microbial recognition systems that are specific for various microorganisms and swiftly generate various antimicrobial responses precisely tailored to the microbial invader that challenges the host. Moreover, innate immunity is intricately connected with adaptive immunity because it serves as the recognition system for the antigens and is required for efficient initiation of adaptive immune responses. It also often directs which type of adaptive immune response is induced and in some cases serves as the effector mechanism of adaptive immunity.

Adaptive Immunity

Carl Waltenbaugh and Roger Melvold

We live in a world populated by microorganisms with the ever-present potential for microbial attack. Although physical (e.g., skin and membranes) and chemical (e.g., microbicidal molecules secreted by some skin cells) barriers are usually very effective in preventing the entry of microbes into the body, sometimes they are not enough. If these physical and chemical barriers are breached, microbes invade and a "state of war" ensues, the outcome of which determines our very survival or extinction. The immune system becomes actively involved in resisting and eliminating infection. Humans use two immune systems to combat invasion by infectious organisms: the innate immune system, discussed in Chapter 6, and the adaptive immune system (also known as the acquired immune system). This chapter focuses on the constituents and functions of the adaptive immune system.

Innate Versus Adaptive Immune Systems

The innate immune system uses a limited number of genetically encoded receptors (e.g., pattern recognition receptors and toll-like receptors) to detect foreign organisms. In contrast, the adaptive immune system employs subsets of an elite set of leukocytes called **lymphocytes,** which have the capacity to generate a large number of antigen-specific cell surface receptors by random gene rearrangement. Bone marrow–derived lymphocytes (**B lymphocytes,** or **B cells**) generate **B-cell receptors (BCRs),** and thymus-derived lymphocytes (**T lymphocytes,** or **T cells**) generate **T-cell receptors (TCRs).** Further diversity is added by some degree of flexibility in the precision of the cutting and joining of these genes (**junctional diversity**) and, in the case of BCRs, the accumulation of small mutations (**somatic hypermutation**) as the B cells undergo periods of intense proliferation. The number of possible receptors becomes immense, with estimates exceeding 10^{15} possible specificities.

Another key difference between the two systems is the way they respond to attack. Unlike cells of the innate immune system, those of the adaptive immune system, once stimulated to respond, have the ability to recall previous exposures to the same stimulus and to modify their response accordingly, a process called **memory.** Additional features that distinguish innate and adaptive immune responses are summarized in Table 7-1.

table **7-1**	Hallmarks of Innate and Adaptive Immune Responses	
	INNATE IMMUNITY	**ADAPTIVE IMMUNITY**
Receptors	Germline encoded	Generated by somatic genetic recombination, junctional diversity, and somatic mutation
Receptor distribution	Expressed by a variety of cell types	Clonally expressed on lymphocytes
Receptor repertoire	Limited	Vast
Memory	None	Both the magnitude and quality of a response to an epitope is altered by previous exposures to that same epitope

Adapted from Vivier E, Malissen B. Innate and adaptive immunity: specificities and signaling hierarchies revisited. Nat Immunol. 2005;6(1):17–21.

Cells and Molecules of the Adaptive Immune System

Cells of the innate immune system are morphologically distinct. In contrast, lymphocytes of the adaptive immune system generally look alike, although they vary in size from small (4 to 7 μm), to medium (7 to 11 μm), to large (11 to 15 μm). Lymphocytes are broadly categorized according the antigen-specific receptors they generate by gene rearrangement and the organs in which they develop. They may be likened to the soldiers of the adaptive immune system, and like soldiers they often display combinations of additional surface molecules that, in essence, serve as molecular "badges of rank." Some of these badges are useful for identifying a lymphocyte's function and its role in immune defense. Even the most basic appreciation of adaptive immune mechanisms depends on understanding the role that soluble molecules and molecular badges play in immune function. These molecules include **immunoglobulins**, BCRs, TCRs, **cluster of differentiation (CD)** molecules, **human leukocyte antigen (HLA)** molecules, **cytokines**, and **complement**.

Synthesized by B cells, **immunoglobulins** also serve as the BCRs. When activated some B cells differentiate further into **plasma cells** that produce and secrete large quantities of immunoglobulin. **Immunoglobulin** is a generic term for a diverse group of globular molecules found in the blood and tissue fluids. They include immunoreactive molecules of the gamma (γ) globulin group of serum proteins, so named because they migrate slowly in the γ region of an electrophoretic field. An **antibody** is an immunoglobulin that specifically binds to a known **ligand** or epitope. An **epitope** is the smallest molecular structure recognized by a specific receptor. An **antigen,** such as a microbe, may be viewed as a collection of (sometimes) repeating and/or unique epitopes. For purposes of clarity, the term *immunoglobulin* is used in this chapter in reference to the general structural characteristics of these molecules,

and the term *antibody* is used in reference to their functional activities.

T cells also use a set of cell surface receptors, the TCRs, that recognize and bind to antigen but are distinct from antibodies. Other molecules (or "badges") such as **CD3, CD4,** and **CD8** associate with and assist the TCRs in antigen recognition. Many more than 250 cell surface CD molecules serve as useful indicators of the functional capacities of leukocytes and other cells of the body.

HLA molecules are the products of distinct genetic loci within the major histocompatibility complex (MHC), which encodes proteins of three different types called MHC class I, II, or III molecules. Cytokines are protein molecules that act as soluble messengers between cells that affect cell behavior. *Complement* is a collective term for a set of serum proteins involved in both innate and adaptive defense mechanisms. The role of the classical, lectin, and alternative complement pathways in innate immune defenses has already been discussed (Chapter 6).

Immunoglobulins: Structure and Synthesis

The basic structural element for all immunoglobulins is the **immunoglobulin monomer**. It contains four polypeptides: two *identical* light (L) and two *identical* heavy (H) glycoprotein chains linked by disulfide bonds (Fig. 7-1). There are five types of heavy chains, termed α (alpha), δ (delta), ε (epsilon), γ (gamma), and μ (mu) as well as two types of light chains, termed κ (kappa) and λ (lambda). The amino acid sequence of the heavy chain of an immunoglobulin determines the serological **class** or **isotype** of the immunoglobulin molecule. A single immunoglobulin molecule is composed of one or more monomers (Table 7-2).

Heavy and light chains can be further divided into **regions** or **domains,** homologous portions containing approximately 110 amino acids and an intrachain disulfide bond (see Fig. 7-1). Light chains contain two regions, a **variable** (V_L) and a **constant** (C_L) domain. Heavy chains contain a single variable (V_H) and three or four constant (C_H1, C_H2, C_H3, and sometimes C_H4) region domains. Constant regions of the heavy and light

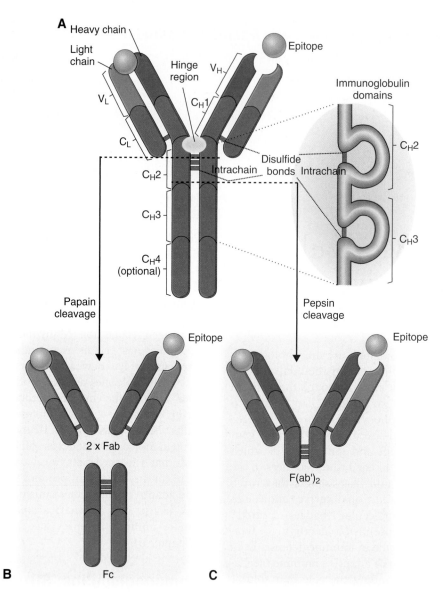

FIGURE 7-1 ▪ **Immunoglobulin landmarks. A.** The immunoglobulin monomer contains two identical heavy and two identical light polypeptide chains. The polypeptides are organized into variable or constant domains, each containing approximately 110 amino acids and an intrachain disulfide bond (see insert). A light chain contains a single variable (V_L) and a single constant (C_L) region domain. Each heavy chain contains a single variable (V_H) and three or four constant region domains (C_H1, C_H2, C_H3, and for some isotypes C_H4). Disulfide bonds link a single light chain to a single heavy chain and link the heavy chains. Some isotypes are built from two or five monomers to form dimers or pentamers (see Table 7-2). Together, V_LV_H form a combinatorial epitope- (or antigen) binding pocket. **B.** Enzymatic cleavage of the immunoglobulin monomer by papain yields three fragments: two Fab fragments and one Fc fragment. Disulfide bonds link peptides within each fragment. Each Fab fragment is monovalent, containing a single epitope-binding site. **C.** Pepsin cleaves the monomer's heavy chains below the disulfide bonds to create two Fab′ fragments (the prime mark ′ indicates extra amino acids) linked by disulfide bonds, $F(ab′)_2$. The $F(ab′)_2$ fragment has valency of two, retaining the two epitope binding sites of the original immunoglobulin monomer.

chains determine immunoglobulin isotype. Variable regions are so named because they exhibit great variation in amino acid sequence in immunoglobulin molecules produced by various B cells. The amino acid sequence determines the conformation structure of an individual V_H or V_L region. Disulfide bonds link a single heavy chain with a single light chain, and the combination of the V_H and V_L regions forms a pocket that constitutes

the epitope-binding region of the immunoglobulin molecule. Disulfide bonds also link the heavy chains to form an immunoglobulin monomer. Following are some landmarks of immunoglobulin monomers (see Fig. 7-1):

▪ Fab (*ab* stands for "antigen-binding") fragment is produced by papain cleavage of the monomer and contains only a single epitope-binding site (V_H,C_H1,V_L,C_L).

table 7-2 Immunoglobulin Isotypes

ISOTYPE	HEAVY CHAINS[a]	HEAVY SUBCLASS	ASSOCIATED CHAINS	FORMULA[a]	NUMBER OF MONOMERS[b]	SUBCLASS	VALENCE	MW	DIAGRAM
IgM	μ			2 Hμ[c] 2L	1		2	180,000	T7-2a
			J chain	5 [2 Hμ 2L] + J	5		10	900,000	T7-2b
IgG	γ			2 Hγ 2L	1		2	150,000	T7-2c
		$γ_1$		2 H$γ_1$ 2L	1	IgG_1	2	150,000	
		$γ_2$		2 H$γ_2$ 2L	1	IgG_2	2	150,000	
		$γ_3$		2 H$γ_3$ 2L	1	IgG_3	2	150,000	
		$γ_4$		2 H$γ_4$ 2L	1	IgG_4	2	150,000	
IgA[d]	α			2 H α 2L	1	IgA	2	170,000	T7-2d
			J chain and SC	2 [2 H$α_1$ 2L] + J + SC	2	sIgA	4	390,000	T7-2e
IgD	δ	δ		2 Hδ 2L	1		2	180,000	T7-2f
IgE	ε	ε		2 Hε 2L	1		2	190,000	T7-2g

[a]Each monomer contains 2 identical heavy (H$_{isotype}$) and 2 identical (κ−κ or λ−λ) light (L) chains.
[b]A single monomer is expressed on the B-cell surface; IgM is secreted as a pentamer by plasma cells.
[c]The carboxyl-terminal portion of the μ chain cytoplasmic tail differs significantly from the μ chain present in the pentameric secreted form of IgM.
MW, molecular weight; SC, secretory component.
[d]IgA is synthesized as a monomer or dimer. Special epithelial cells add SC to the dimer and transfer it to the external surface.

■ **Fc** (*c* stands for "constant" or "crystallizable") fragment is produced by papain cleavage of the monomer to produce a fragment containing C_H2, C_H3, and (sometimes) C_H4 portions of the heavy chains. Epitope engagement by the epitope-binding site of the intact immunoglobulin monomer causes conformational changes in the Fc region that may trigger a number of biologic activities, including activation of the classical pathway of complement and binding to specific cell surface receptors on neutrophil, lymphocytes, macrophages, and dendritic cells.

■ **F(ab′)₂** is produced by **pepsin cleavage** of the immunoglobulin monomer to yield a fragment containing two linked epitope-binding sites.

■ **Hinge region** is a proline-rich region between the C_H1 and C_H2 domains that allows flexibility of the Fab portions of the monomer.

Many other immune and nonimmune-related proteins have been found to share a degree of structural homology with immunoglobulins, including a certain degree of sequence homology and the presence of intrachain disulfide bonds. These proteins are collectively identified as members of the **immunoglobulin supergene family,** or **Ig superfamily.**

Immunologists estimate that a typical adaptive immune system in a single individual has the ability to recognize and respond to more than 10^{15} epitopes. Two major theories have been proposed to account for the genetic basis of immune recognition. The **germline theory** holds that a unique gene encodes each immunoglobulin and TCR. This theory is untenable because the number of unique genes would need to be several thousand times greater than the entire human genome. Alternatively, the **somatic mutation theory** states that a single germline gene undergoes multiple mutations to generate diversity. This scheme would require an unimaginable mutation rate. The adaptive immune system has, in fact, developed an elegant solution, **chromosomal rearrangement** of separate gene segments, which also employs some elements of both the germline and somatic mutation theories.

DNA chromosomal rearrangement is responsible for a significant portion of immunoglobulin diversity. This rearrangement is accomplished by the removal of nucleotides (both at the DNA and RNA levels) to bring together genes that were previously separated. Light- and heavy-chain gene clusters on chromosomes 2 (κ light chains), 22 (λ light chains), and 14 (heavy chains) encode the basic building blocks for this process. For a pre-B cell to generate a light κ or λ chain, one of 35 ($V_L\kappa$) or 30 ($V_L\lambda$) variable (V_L) genes recombine with one of 4 ($J_L\kappa$) or 5 ($J_L\lambda$) light chain–joining (J_L) segments and a single constant ($C_L\kappa$ or $C_L\lambda$) segment (Fig. 7-2). Thus, κ light chains are a union of three genes ($V_L\kappa J_L\kappa C_L\kappa$), as are λ

light chains ($V_L\lambda$-$J_L\lambda$-$C_L\lambda$). Likewise, a pre-B cell must combine one of 65 heavy-chain variable (V_H) segments with one of 27 diversity (D_H) segments and one of 6 joining (J) segments and a single constant region ($C_H\mu$, $C_H\delta$, $C_H\gamma$, $C_H\alpha$, or $C_H\varepsilon$).

A cautionary note on terminology: *variable genes* refer to the DNA level, one of the types of genes that are rearranged to encode *variable regions* that are part of the immunoglobulin polypeptides. Although both maternal and paternal immunoglobulin alleles are inherited, a single B cell can express only one $V_L J_L C_L$ combination and one $V_H D_H J_H$ combination to the exclusion of all others. The restriction of light- and heavy-chain expression to a single member of the chromosome pair encoding them, either maternal or paternal, is termed **allelic exclusion.** Heavy and light chains may be expressed from both paternal chromosomes, from both maternal chromosomes, or from one each.

Now for the math. Because combinations apparently are generated at random, this process can generate 175 κ chain variable regions (35 $V_L\kappa$ × 5 $J_L\kappa$) and 120 λ chain variable regions (30 $V_L\lambda$ × 4 $J_L\lambda$) and amino acid sequences for at least 295 different light-chain variable regions (sum of the κ and λ variable regions). Heavy-chain gene recombination can generate at least 6,210 different heavy-chain variable regions (45 V_H × 23 D_H × 6

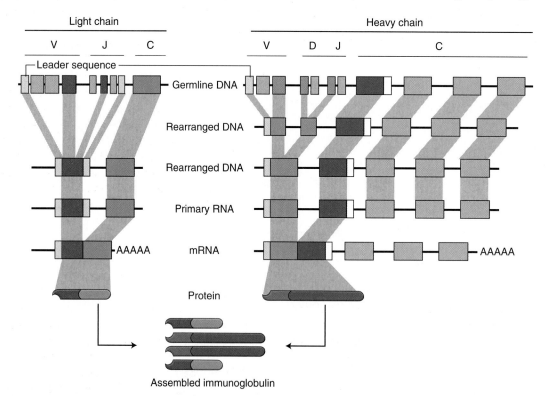

FIGURE 7-2 ▪ **Immunoglobulins, genes, rearrangement and synthesis.** Immunoglobulin-diverse regions result from DNA chromosomal rearrangement. Light chains are generated by the random selection one of 35 $V_L\kappa$ (30 $V_K\lambda$) and its accompanying leader sequence, one of 5 $J_L\kappa$ (4 $J_L\lambda$), and one constant ($C_H\kappa$ or $C_H\lambda$) region gene segment. Heavy chains are generated by the random selection of one of 45 V_H and its accompanying leader sequence, one of 23 D_H, and one of 6 J_H gene segments. Rearranged DNA is transcribed into primary RNA, intervening sequences are edited out of messenger RNA (mRNA), and polypeptides are synthesized and assembled within the Golgi apparatus.

J_H). Both the V_L and V_H regions of the immunoglobulin molecule contribute to the epitope-binding site so that 1.8×10^6 ($295 \times 6,210$) binding specificities can be generated by recombination alone. Diversity of several orders of magnitude are also added by an enzyme, **terminal deoxyribonucleotidyl transferase (TdT)**, that removes or adds nucleotides between the V, D, and J genes in a process known as **junctional diversity.** The net effect is that junctional diversity greatly increases V region diversity so that at least 10^{10} specificities can be generated. While undergoing rapid proliferation following activation, B cells can also accumulate small mutations in the V, D, and J genes of their light and heavy-chain genes.

Because of its particular combination of V_L and V_H regions and allelic exclusion, an individual B cell synthesizes immunoglobulin of only a single specificity. Initially, B cells synthesize and display monomeric IgM (and IgD) on their cell surfaces. B cells, however, have the ability to change the immunoglobulin isotype they produce to IgG, IgE, or IgA, a process known as the **isotype switch,** and by doing so influence the ultimate nature of the humoral immune response. Immunoglobulins may be likened to the "ballistic missiles" of the adaptive immune system: their V regions form a specific "warhead," and their constant regions constitute the "rocket" portion of the molecule. Although a single B cell can manufacture a single type of warhead, it can be placed on different rockets. As we will see, often T cells stimulate B cells to proliferate, switch isotype, and differentiate into immunoglobulin-secreting (plasma) cells. The intracellular machinery of the stimulated B cell is such that immunoglobulins of only a single isotype can be produced at a given time. The isotype ultimately determines whether an antibody activates complement, is secreted into a lumen or onto a mucous membrane, or is immobilized by certain tissues of the body. Isotype switching permits the adaptive immune system to direct antibodies with identical specificity toward a variety of immune responses.

The immunoglobulin heavy chains encoded by C_H genes (μ, δ, γ, ε, or α) determine the isotype (IgM, IgD, IgG, IgE, or IgA, respectively) of the immunoglobulin monomer. The nature of the constant region (particularly the Fc region) of the immunoglobulin determines what type of interaction will occur with other cells and molecules of the immune system. Large-sized immunoglobulins (e.g., IgM) are confined to the bloodstream, while those of lower molecular weight (IgG and IgE) can leave the vasculature and enter the tissues. IgG is the only isotype that can cross the placenta and enter the fetal circulation. Maternally derived IgG provides the primary immunologic protection for newborns until their own immune systems become sufficient at about 6 months of age. IgM and IgG can activate the complement system. IgA can dimerize, and specialized secretory epithelial cells can internalize dimeric IgA, transport it across the cell, and release it to the exterior in saliva,

tears, breast milk, and mucus secretions. Secreted IgA (sIgA) is extremely important in immunologic functions involving the alimentary and respiratory tracts and can provide some immunologic protection to nursing infants.

T Cell–Associated Molecules

As distinct cell surface antigen-specific receptors, TCRs are members of the immunoglobulin supergene family. The TCR is a heterodimer composed of an $\alpha\beta$ or $\gamma\delta$ polypeptide pair. Similar to immunoglobulin, each membrane-bound polypeptide contains a single variable domain but only a single constant region domain. In addition, an $\alpha\beta$ TCR associates with transmembrane molecules (CD4 or CD8) that stabilize the interaction of the TCR with its ligand and with the CD3 complex responsible for transmembrane signal transduction once the variable region of the TCR is engaged. Unlike antibodies that can readily bind soluble or particulate antigen, TCRs can only bind enzymatically cleaved fragments of larger peptides presented as peptide–MHC (pMHC) complexes. This is discussed later in the chapter when antigen presentation is considered.

TCRs are generated by gene rearrangement and recombination, in a manner similar to that seen in immunoglobulins, to produce heterodimers consisting either of a smaller α chain and a larger β chain ($\alpha\beta$ TCR), or a smaller γ chain and a larger δ chain ($\gamma\delta$ TCR). The variable regions of the TCR α and δ chains are encoded by uniting V_H and J_H genes. The variable regions of β and δ chains are encoded by uniting V_H, D_H, and J_H genes (Fig. 7-3). The constant region genes ($C\alpha$ and $C\beta$ or $C\gamma$ and $C\delta$) encode the constant domains for each TCR heterodimer. Junctional diversity, a process mediated by TdT, contributes greatly to the number of possible specificities, similar to that seen for immunoglobulins. However, unlike immunoglobulins, TCRs do not increase their diversity by incorporation of small mutations during T-cell proliferation.

Cell Surface and Soluble Molecules

Molecules encoded by the MHC, also known as HLA, are important to immune function (Table 7-3). Small proteolytic cleavage peptides (p) are loaded by the cell into MHC class I or class II molecules (pMHC class I or class II) for display at the cell surface. The display of pMHC complexes is "scrutinized" by the TCRs.

MHC class I molecules are found on the surfaces of all nucleated cells (Fig. 7-4). These single-chain, 45-kDa glycoproteins are found on the cell surface in association with 12-kDa $\beta2$ microglobulin. Codominantly expressed genes at each of the three MHC class I loci—**HLA-A, HLA-B,** and **HLA-C**—are highly polymorphic, with more than 100 possible alleles at each locus. Up to six MHC class I molecules (if all three loci are heterozy-

FIGURE 7-3 ▪ **T-cell receptor: genes, rearrangement, and synthesis.** The α and β polypeptides of the T-cell receptor (TCR) complex contain a single variable (Vα and Vβ) and a single constant (Cα and Cβ) region. A V-region gene segment combines with a joining (J) segment and a C region to be transcribed into messenger RNA (mRNA) and translated into an α polypeptide chain within the endoplasmic reticulum. Recombination of the β-chain DNA is similar to that of the α chain but also includes a diversity (D) gene segment. The γδ TCR has a similar construction but uses distinct gene sets for the γ and δ chains. The cell surface TCR complex is composed of an αβ heterodimer pair, associated CD3 (γ, δ, and ε) and a CD247 ξ-chain homodimer, and CD4 or CD8 molecules. The short cytoplasmic tail of the TCR lacks signaling sequence or immunoreceptor tyrosine activation motifs (ITAMs). The CD3 and CD247 molecules supply these.

gous) are displayed on the surface of each nucleated cell. All MHC class I molecules fold to produce a cleft that holds a peptide of eight to nine amino acids in length. Peptides, the fragments resulting from proteasome degradation of cytoplasmic proteins, are transported into the endoplasmic reticulum, where some are loaded into nascent MHC class I molecules. MHC class I molecules, peptides, and β2 microglobulin are exported via exocytotic vesicles, where they are displayed on the cell surface. This combination of peptide, MHC class I, and β2 microglobulin is often termed **pMHC class I.** In general, endogenous peptides such as intracellular bacterial or viral proteins synthesized within the cell's cytoplasm are loaded into MHC class I molecules.

MHC class II molecules are αβ heterodimers (see Fig. 7-4) displayed on the surfaces of a relatively small

table **7-3**	Molecules of the Major Histocompatibility Complex[a]		
HLA CLASS	**NOMENCLATURE**	**DISTRIBUTION**	**FUNCTIONS**
I	HLA-A, HLA-B, HLA-C	All nucleated cells	Presentation of intracellularly derived antigens
II[b]	DPα, DPβ, DQα, DQβ, DRα, DRβ1, DRβ2, DRβ4	Dendritic cells, macrophages, B cells, and some activated T cells	Presentation of extracellularly derived antigens
III	C2, C4, Bf	Secreted, not expressed on cell surfaces	Some components of the complement system

[a]Also known as human leukocyte antigen (HLA) molecules.

[b]Class II molecules α and β are encoded by the α and β loci, respectively. Thus, DPA encodes the DPα chain, DPB the DPβ chain, DQA the DQα chain, and so on. Bf, regulatory factor B.

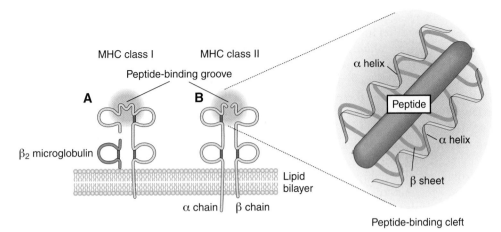

FIGURE 7-4 ▪ Hallmarks of major histocompatability complex (MHC) class I and class II molecules. Molecules of the human MHC are also known as human leukocyte antigens (HLA). **A.** MHC class I molecules are single-chain 45-kDa polypeptides displayed on the surfaces of all nucleated cells in association with 12-kDa β2 microglobulin. MHC class I molecules contain three immunoglobulin-like domains, two of which have intrachain disulfide bonds. A peptide-binding cleft is formed between the first and second domains (see insert). **B.** MHC class II molecules are expressed as α and β heterodimers. Each polypeptide contains two immunoglobulin-like domains. The amino terminus portion of each molecule contributes to the peptide-binding portion of the heterodimer (see insert).

number of cells: dendritic cells, macrophages, B cells, thymic epithelial cells, and some activated T cells. It needs to be stressed that the use of the terms α and β for MHC class II molecules is distinct from the use of α and β for TCRs, and the two should not be confused with one another. Human MHC class II polypeptides are encoded by genes within the HLA-DP, HLA-DQ, and HLA-DR regions. Contained within each region are α and β loci (DPα, DPβ, DQα, DQβ, etc.). MHC class II polypeptides only associate with other class II peptides encoded within the same region. The combination of α (32- to 38-kDa) and β (29- to 32-kDa) chains forms a peptide-binding grove that can accommodate peptides of 18 to 20 amino acids or more in length (**pMHC class II**). Like MHC class I genes, a large number of allelic forms are known to exist for each locus. Genetic variation among MHC class II molecules, as well as αβ association, creates a wide range of subtly varying binding grooves for which peptides compete. Peptides that load into MHC class II molecules are generally of exogenous origin. Antigens (microbes or their products) present in the extracellular fluid are engulfed (phagocytosis), contained within phagocytic vesicles that fuse with lysosomal vesicles to form phagolysosomes that enzymatically degrade the ingested material to produce peptides that may be loaded into nascent MHC class II molecules.

MHC class III molecules are several components of the complement system—namely, C2, C4, and regulatory factor B (Bf).

Cluster of differentiation (CD) molecules populate the surfaces of a wide variety of cell types and serve as indication of the functional capacities of leukocytes and a number of other cells. It is beyond the scope of this book to describe more than just a few of the more than 250

CD molecules that have been so far identified. Fortunately, a basic understanding of the underlying mechanisms of the adaptive immune response requires knowing only a few of these:

- **CD3 complex** contains several molecules associated with the TCR (see Fig. 7-3). It is composed of six polypeptides (2 CD3ε + 1 CD3γ + 1 CD3δ + 1 CD247 ζ–ζ homodimer) that function to both support the TCR and is involved in transmembrane signaling when the TCR is engaged.
- **CD4** is a single-chain member of the immunoglobulin supergene family and is expressed on the surfaces of approximately two thirds of mature T cells. CD4 molecules recognize a nonpeptide-binding portion of MHC class II molecules. CD4$^+$ T cells, also known as helper T (Th) cells, are "restricted" to the recognition of pMHC class II complexes.
- **CD8** is a two-chain cell surface molecule composed of homodimers (αα) or heterodimers (αβ) and expressed by about one third of mature T cells. CD8 molecules recognize the nonpeptide-binding portion of MHC class I molecules. CD8$^+$ T cells, "restricted" to the recognition of pMHC class I complexes, are also known as cytotoxic T (Tc) and suppressor T (Ts) cells.

Mature αβ T cells express CD4 or CD8 cell surface molecules. A useful mnemonic to use to remember CD4/CD8 MHC restriction is the **rule of eight:**

CD4 × MHC class II = 8, and CD8 × MHC class I = 8

T cells of the γδ lineage often express neither CD4 nor CD8, and their restriction, if any, is unclear.

Cytokines are chemical messengers. Involved in all aspects of innate and adaptive immune responses, cytokines are low-molecular-weight soluble molecules that function to initiate growth, differentiation, and maturation of cells and to promote or inhibit inflammation and tissue repair. Originally termed lymphokines and monokines to reflect their production by lymphocytes or monocytes, it is now recognized that these same substances may be produced by a wide variety of leukocytes and nonleukocytes. Chemoattractant cytokines known as **chemokines** stimulate leukocyte movement and migration. Whether or not certain cytokines or chemokines are expressed on microbial encounter strongly influences the nature and strength of the immune response.

Various cell surface molecules, called **adhesion molecules,** provide stable cell-to-cell contact. Because the immune system polices the body for invaders, adhesion molecules establish a temporary, yet stable, contact that allows leukocytes to scrutinize other cells, leukocytes and nonleukocytes alike. Stable contact for a period between cells, provided by adhesion molecules, is critical to the ability of cell surface receptors and ligands to interact. They are classified as widely distributed **integrins** that initiate adhesion interactions, and **selectins** and **addressins** that have a limited leukocyte distribution and function to activate leukocytes and facilitate leukocyte migration.

Lymphocyte Development and Receptor Selection

The immune system must be able to distinguish its own molecules, cells, and organs—**self**—from those of foreign origin—**nonself.** The innate immune system does this elegantly by expressing germline-encoded pattern recognition receptors on cell surfaces, receptors that have been selected over time to recognize structures on potentially invasive organisms (see Chapter 6). The adaptive immune system, on the other hand, uses antigen-specific receptors (TCRs and BCRs) that are somatically created anew and randomly within each individual (indeed, within each lymphocyte) by gene recombination *prior to* encounter with an antigen. This also means that no two individuals, even identical twins, have identical adaptive immune systems. Three distinct categories of receptors are randomly generated: those that recognize peptide epitopes that will never be encountered, those that recognize peptides produced by potential pathogens or peptides of nonself origin, and those that recognize peptides produced by the self. Recognition of self peptides by the immune system could lead to a "coup," with the immune system attacking the very body it is intended to protect and defend. Fortunately, the adaptive immune system has developed an elegant solution against this threat, and

it occurs within the thymus where self- and nonself-recognizing TCRs are sorted out.

T Cells

T-cell precursors have their embryological origin in the hematopoietic tissues of bone marrow from which they migrate by the circulation to the thymus. These thymocytes, as they are now called, do not express a TCR, nor do they express either CD4 or CD8 molecules; thus, they are called **double-negative (DN) cells.** DN cells proliferate in the thymic subcapsular region, where most differentiate and express low levels of newly generated αβ TCR and *both* CD4 and CD8 molecules, and are termed **double-positive (DP) cells.** Some cells develop γδ TCRs and may or may not express CD4 and CD8 molecules. Thymocytes that generate a γδ TCR appear to exit from the thymus early, before undergoing any selection. Their functions are not well understood. On the other hand, the αβ DP cells migrate deeper within the thymus, fated to die within 3 to 4 days unless their TCRs recognize an MHC class I or class II molecule on thymic dendritic cells, a process known as **positive selection.** Thymocytes that generate a γδ TCRs appear to exit from the thymus early, before undergoing this selection.

Although the mechanism of positive selection is not fully understood, it is known that partial recognition of MHC class I by CD8 molecules or MHC class II by CD4 molecules must occur. Cells that "pass muster" and recognize self MHC molecules will survive, and those that do not will die. A DP thymocyte that engages MHC class I may become a CD8$^+$ T cell, and one that recognizes MHC class II may become a CD4$^+$ T cell. Because MHC class I and class II molecules are not displayed on cell surfaces unless their binding cleft contains a peptide (pMHC), only peptides of self origin are seen by the DP thymocytes. Thymocytes that show strong interaction with pMHC complexes are selectively rejected and undergo programmed cell death or **apoptosis,** a process known as **negative selection.** Thymocytes that survive both positive and negative selection migrate from the thymus as T cells and are destined to populate the lymphoid tissues and organs.

It is a tough military academy: less than 2% of all thymocytes are estimated to "graduate" as T cells. By applying both positive and negative selection of thymocytes, the adaptive immune system is assured of a population of naive T cells that will react with nonself peptides presented by self MHC molecules and in which T cells reactive to self peptides have been eliminated.

B Cells

Only B cells and plasma cells synthesize immunoglobulins. Arising from pluripotent hematopoietic stem cells in the fetal liver and bone marrow, B cells are divided into two distinct lineages, B-1 and B-2 cells. They do not migrate to the thymus but remain in the bone marrow during development.

Because they are the first to embryologically develop, B-1 cells are a self-renewing population that predominate the plural and peritoneal cavities. Although the function of B-1 cells is not fully understood, as a population they constitutively secrete IgM antibodies of limited diversity that react strongly with carbohydrates. A large portion of serum IgM in normal individuals is of B-1 origin and is often referred to as "natural antibodies." As a cellular class, B-1 cells may bridge innate and adaptive immunity by producing antibodies that react with carbohydrates expressed by infectious organisms.

In contrast, conventional or B-2 cells arise during and after the neonatal period, are continuously replaced from the bone marrow, and are widely distributed throughout the lymphoid organs and tissues. Somatic gene rearrangements are more extensive in B-2 cells than in B-1 cells, giving them a broader repertoire of immunoglobulin specificities and affinities. Unstimulated B-2 cells, unlike B-1 cells, produce low levels of immunoglobulins that increase only when they are activated by helper T cells that cause them to differentiate into antibody-secreting cells. B-2 pathway-committed cell precursors graduate though several levels that involve changes in gene activity (Fig. 7-5):

- **Pro-B cells produce recombination activation genes, Rag-1 and Rag-2.** Rag-1 and Rag-2 are responsible for chromosomal rearrangement of V, D, and J genes to form the V_H domain. Following union with the μ heavy-chain gene, the cytoplasmically confined immunoglobulin μ heavy chain is synthesized.
- **Early-stage pre-B cells synthesize a transitional or surrogate non-κ, non-λ light chain.** The surrogate light

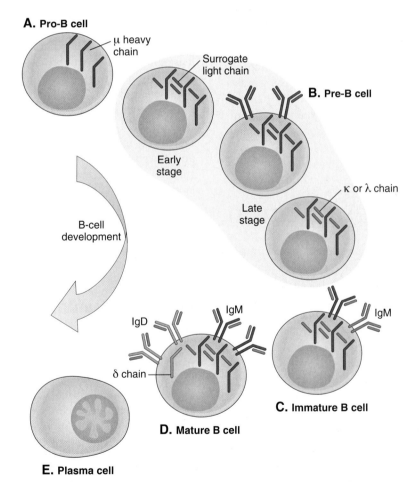

FIGURE 7-5 ▪ **B-cell developmental stages.** The stages of B-cell development reflect changes in gene activity within the cell and its ability to synthesize, display, and secrete immunoglobulin. **A.** A pro-B cell synthesizes μ heavy chains; this polypeptide is confined within the cell. **B.** Pre-B cells are the next developmental stage (shaded), beginning with an early stage in which μ and surrogate light chains are synthesized and the μ-surrogate light chain monomer may be displayed on the cell surface. The final pre-B cell stage occurs when κ or λ light chains replace surrogate light chains. **C.** Immature B cells synthesize and display IgM monomers on their cell surfaces. **D.** Each mature B cell displays both IgM and IgD of *identical specificity* on its cell surface. **E.** Plasma cells represent the end stage of differentiation of B-lineage cells and function as "factories," synthesizing and secreting large amounts of immunoglobulin.

chain associates with the μ heavy chain to form a monomer-like structure that decorates the surface of the cell. **Late-stage pre-B cells** synthesize κ or λ light chains that replace the surrogate light chain and the cell expresses true IgM monomers.

- **Immature, or naive, B cells are so called because their BCRs (IgM monomers) have not engaged the appropriate epitope.** If the BCR of a naive B cell engages an epitope within the bone marrow environment, the cell is destroyed by apoptosis. Surviving cells exit the bone marrow and enter the circulation. On leaving the bone marrow, the naive B cells are fated to have a short half-life unless they receive additional signals from lymph node stromal cells that allow them to further develop. Within the lymph node, B cells begin to synthesize both δ heavy chains and μ heavy chains and display both IgD and IgM monomers with identical specificity on their cell surface.

- **Mature B cells coexpress IgM and IgD cell surface monomers.** Activation for the vast majority of mature B-2 cells requires both epitope binding and T-cell interaction for further differentiation.

- **Plasma cells are derived from differentiated mature B cells and secrete immunoglobulin.** All the immunoglobulin secreted is exported, and the cells cease using it as a membrane receptor. Plasma cells can be viewed as "munitions factories," producing large quantities of immunoglobulin during their short lifespan of less than 30 days.

Lymphocyte Activation

Unlike the innate immune system, the adaptive immune system recognizes epitopes using a very diverse array of randomly generated TCRs and BCRs. Because of the initial paucity of lymphocytes bearing the appropriate epitope-specific TCR or BCR, epitope-specific lymphocytes must clonally proliferate to make enough cells and cell products to deal with a perceived threat. Consequently, adaptive immune responses develop slowly compared with responses of the innate system. In the process of randomly generating receptors, the adaptive immune system can make receptors that recognize nonpathogens or receptors that recognize self molecules. A system of checks and balances minimizes the potential for adverse immune responses that rely on different cell types for recognition, regulation, and effector function. T cells play a central role as arbiters of immune function; therefore, the manner in which T cells recognize and are activated by epitopes is highly regulated.

Cells of the innate immune system are the gatekeepers of the adaptive immune response. In large part, adaptive immune responses are initiated by components of the innate system resulting in T-cell activation and clonal expansion. Effector responses of the adaptive immune system often end by activating and focusing the cells and/or molecules of the innate system on targets selected by lymphocytes.

Self Recognition

"Who are you, friend or foe?" A simple question, you would think, but one that is critical to our survival in the microbial world in which we live. The body must be able to distinguish self molecules and cells from those of non-self or foreign origin. This is not a problem for the innate immune system, in which genomically encoded pattern recognition receptors have been selected over evolutionary time to recognize a limited number of epitopes widely expressed by microbes, but not by cells of the body. For the adaptive immune system, it is another matter altogether. In large part, self-reactive TCRs fail to "graduate" from the thymus (occasional self-reactive T cells "slip by" to become autoreactive). However, this only begs the question, "How do you recognize an epitope that you have never seen?" Enormous numbers of TCRs and BCRs are generated in anticipation that at least some of them will be specific for an epitope of non-self origin. But the peril with this approach is that without some means of identification, molecules of self origin that were not seen during lymphocyte development could possibly trigger a response. The adaptive immune system's solution is elegant. This is also where the innate and adaptive immune systems interact. Phagocytic cells, such as dendritic cells and macrophages, sample their environment by phagocytosis and pinocytosis, proteolytically degrade what they find, and load the peptide fragments into MHC class I (forming pMHC class I) or MHC class II (forming pMHC class II) molecules in a process that immunologists call **antigen presentation.**

Antigen Presentation

Specialized cells located at potential microbial portals of entry into the body (e.g., skin and mucous membranes) serve as sentinels. These are **dendritic cells** named for their elongated, branchlike projections and comprise less than 1% of the cells in these tissues. Known at this stage as immature dendritic cells, they are voracious eaters, ingesting large amounts of soluble and particulate matter by phagocytosis or macropinocytosis. **Phagocytosis** involves the engagement of cell surface receptors (e.g., Fc receptors, heat shock proteins, and low-density lipoprotein-binding scavenger receptors; see Chapter 6) associated with specialized regions of the plasma membrane called **clathrin-coated pits.** Receptor engagement induces actin-dependent phagocytosis and receptor internalization to form small **phagosomes** or endocytic vesicles.

Immature dendritic cells also sample large amounts of soluble molecules present in the extracellular fluids by **macropinocytosis,** a process in which cytoplasmic projections (**cytoplasmic ruffles**) encircle and enclose extra-cellular fluids to form endocytotic vesicles. Macropinocy-tosis does not require clathrin-associated receptor en-gagement. Enzyme-containing cytoplasmic vesicles (**lyso-somes**) fuse with the endocytic vesicles derived from phagocytosis or macropinocytosis (Fig. 7-6). Within this newly formed **phagolysosome**, ingested material is enzy-matically degraded into short peptides. For the most part the process of ingestion and enzymatic degradation has little consequence immunologically, but that can rapidly change.

If an immature dendritic cell senses an invasive threat, it begins to mature, and maturation comes rapidly.

Dendritic cells detect threats either directly or indirectly through the same cell surface receptors used by the innate immune system. **Direct sensing** occurs through engage-ment of pattern recognition receptors, which recognize **pathogen-associated molecular patterns** (**PAMPs**) on viruses, bacteria, fungi, and protozoa (see Chapter 6). Engagement of other receptors (e.g., those that detect antibodies or complement molecules bound to microbes) are responsible for **indirect sensing** of perceived threats. Although the physiological mechanisms for dendritic cell maturation remain to be clarified, threat sensing is known to cause the dendritic cells to migrate to nearby lymph nodes, decrease their phagocytic and macropinocytic ac-

FIGURE 7-6 ▪ **Antigen presentation pathways.** The manner by which a microbe or its products enter an antigen-presenting cell strongly influences the nature of the immune response. **A.** Antigen-presenting cells capture microbes or their products from the extracellular environment by phagocytosis or macropinocytosis and contain them within endocytic vesicles (phagosomes). Phagosomes fuse with enzyme-laden lysosomes to form a phagolysosome for degra-dation of the microbial material into proteolytic fragments. Vesicles containing the MHC class II–invariant chain complex bud off from the endoplasmic reticulum to fuse with the peptide-containing phagolysosome. The invariant chain disintegrates within the acidic environment, allowing the peptide to load into the vacated peptide-binding groove of the MHC class II molecule. Exocytotic vesicles containing peptide-loaded MHC (pMHC) class II are trans-ported to the cell surface for display and recognition by the TCRs of CD4+ T cells. **B.** Some microbes avoid endo-cytic vesicles altogether to enter the cytoplasm. Ubiquitin covalently attaches to many of these proteins, marking them for enzymatic degradation by the proteasome. Proteolytic peptide fragments are transported into the endoplas-mic reticulum by a heterodimer composed of transporters associated with antigen processing (TAP-1 or TAP-2) for possible loading into nascent MHC class I complexes. Exocytotic vesicles containing pMHC class I are transported to the cell surface for display and recognition by the TCRs of CD8+ T cells.

tivity, and upregulate MHC class II synthetic activity. MHC class II α and β polypeptides, together with an invariant chain, are assembled as a complex within the endoplasmic reticulum. Vesicles bud off from the endoplasmic reticulum to fuse with the peptide-containing, acidic phagolysosomes. The invariant chain disintegrates in the acidic environment of the newly formed vesicle, allowing phagolysosome-derived peptides to possibly occupy the peptide-binding groove of the MHC class II molecule. The pMHC class II complex is transported to the cell surface for display and possible recognition by CD4$^+$ T cells.

Not all pathogens enter cells through phagocytosis or macropinocytosis. Some avoid phagocytes and endocytic vesicles entirely. Pathogens such as intracellular microbes and viruses bind to cell membranes (see Chapter 6) and directly enter the cytoplasm of the host cell (see Fig. 7-6). As part of normal physiological processes, nucleated cells constantly degrade and recycle cytoplasmic proteins. Cytoplasmic proteins targeted for destruction are covalently tagged with **ubiquitin,** a highly conserved protein with 76 amino acids. The underlying mechanisms for selecting molecules for ubiquitination are not known. The binding of one or more ubiquitin molecules to a protein targets it for destruction by the **proteasome,** a large proteolytic complex with the cytoplasm. Postproteasome peptides of 6 to 24 amino acids are transported to the endoplasmic reticulum by a heterodimer, composed of **transporter associated with antigen processing (TAP-1** and **TAP-2).** The TAP heterodimers allow peptides to load into MHC class I (pMHC class I). Special transport exocytotic vesicles containing pMHC class I molecules bud from the Golgi and are rapidly transported to the cell surface for display to CD8$^+$ T cells.

T-Cell Activation

T cells largely direct the adaptive immune response. Unlike receptors within the innate immune system, TCRs cannot recognize soluble molecules. The nature of the adaptive immune response is strongly influenced by how epitopes are presented by antigen-presenting cells (APCs). The interface between an APC and a naive T cell is called the **immunologic synapse.**

The initial step in building the immunologic synapse occurs when the TCR recognizes pMHC. The weak interaction of the TCR with pMHC is stabilized by the interaction of CD4 or CD8 molecules. CD4 and CD8 molecules bind to the "constant" nonpeptide-binding portions of pMHC class II and class I, respectively (remember the **rule of eight).** Formation of the pMHC–TCR–CD4 (or CD8) complex provides an initial or first signal through the TCR-associated CD3 complex to the T cell. This first signal is necessary, but not sufficient, to stimulate a naive T cell to proliferate and differentiate. A second signal provided by one or more **costimulatory molecules** is required for T-cell activation. The first and second signals initiate intracellular signal-

ing cascades that cause the activation of one or more transcription factors leading to specific gene transcription. Without costimulation, T cells either become selectively unresponsive, a condition known as **anergy,** or undergo apoptosis.

The immunologic synapse both stabilizes T cell–APC interaction and promotes the migration of molecules within the T-cell membrane. The cytoplasmic tails of certain of those molecules contain **immunoreceptor tyrosine-based activation motifs (ITAMs),** which initiate a signaling cascade on close proximity. The CD3 (2 CD3ε + 1 CD3γ + 1 CD3δ + 1 CD247 ζ–ζ homodimer) complex contains ITAM-bearing molecules. The cytoplasmic tails of the TCR lack ITAMs. TCR engagement leads to signal transduction through the CD3 complex, and the activation of transcriptional factors leads to cytokine synthesis, T-cell proliferation, and differentiation. The nature of the immune response largely depends on the manner in which the APCs initiate the immunologic synapse.

The initial encounter of T cells with antigen is called **priming,** and the nature of this encounter is crucial to the development of the subsequent adaptive immune response. As shown earlier, CD8$^+$ T cells interact with pMHC class I and CD4$^+$ T cells recognize pMHC class II. Primed CD4$^+$ T cells are called **T helper** cells because they are instrumental in "helping" other leukocytes respond (Fig. 7-7). CD4$^+$ Th cells can mature along one of two pathways. In one developmental pathway, CD4$^+$ T cells generally respond to intracellular pathogens by recruiting and activating phagocytic cells. These T cells are known as **Th1 cells.** To avoid detection by cells of the adaptive immune response, some pathogens circumvent phagolysosomes either by directly entering the cytoplasm (e.g., viruses) or by exiting the phagolysosome before they can be enzymatically harmed (e.g., *Listeria monocytogenes* or *Legionella pneumophila*). But the microbial ruse is not perfect, because some infected cells die, prompting dendritic cells to scavenge their cellular debris and display the proteolytic peptides, including those derived from microbes displayed by MHC class II molecules. T cells that develop along the other pathway are known as **Th2 cells,** and they generally respond to extracellular pathogens by stimulating B cells to differentiate into antibody-secreting plasma cells.

Antigen naive CD4$^+$ **Th precursor (Thp) cells,** on activation by engagement of an epitope through the immunologic synapse, are stimulated to secrete a variety of cytokines and express cell surface cytokine receptors, thus becoming pathway uncommitted **Th0 cells.** The developmental pathway that the Th0 cell follows depends primarily on the nature of signals provided by the APC. In the presence of microbe-derived lipopolysaccharide (LPS), the APC may secrete interleukin 12 (IL-12). Consequently, Th0 causes cells to further differentiate into Th1 cells, of which some actively secrete cytokines such as IFN-γ and others increase leukocyte recruitment and activation. In some cases the presence of IL-4 may lead

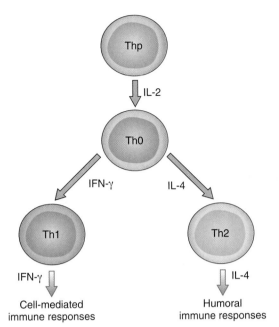

FIGURE 7-7 ▪ **Th1 and Th2 maturational pathways.** Initial epitope engagement through the immunologic synapse induces naive CD4$^+$ T cells to undergo several rounds of proliferation, resulting in their maturation into pathway-uncommitted Th0 cells. Cytokine and costimulatory signals from antigen-presenting and other cells determine whether Th0 cells will differentiate along a Th1 or Th2 pathway. In the presence of interleukin-12 (IL-12), Th0 will differentiate into interferon-γ (IFN-γ)–secreting Th1 cells. Th1 cells are mediators of cell-mediated immune responses. If Th0 cells initially encounter IL-4, they will differentiate into Th2 cells and secrete IL-4, which mediates B cell differentiation, isotype switching, and transformation into plasma cells. Animal models show polarization of Th1 and Th2 cytokine secretion and cellular function. Human Th1 and Th2 cells show cytokine polarization, but the degree of polarization of Th1-Th2 function is less dramatic.

Th0 to follow the Th2 differentiation pathway. Among the functional roles of Th2 cells is the production of cytokines responsible for the growth and stimulation of B cells as well as their differentiation into plasma cells.

Some pathogens, such as viruses, avoid contact with endocytic vesicles entirely by directly entering and replicating within the host cell's cytoplasm. Naive CD8$^+$ T cells recognize pMHC class I (first signal) displayed on the surface of an infected cell. On encountering an appropriate pMHC class I on an infected cell, CD8$^+$ cells proliferate and differentiate into cytolytic effector cells called **cytotoxic T lymphocytes (CTL)**. Fully differentiated CTLs contain two types of cytolytic granules, **perforin** (a pore-forming protein) and **granzymes** (serine proteases), which are used to deliver a fatal blow to a cell expressing the appropriate pMHC class I complex.

B-Cell Activation

In contrast to TCRs, BCRs recognize and bind soluble molecules. The BCR complex of mature B cells contains membrane-bound IgM and IgD monomers associated with Igα and Igβ molecules (Fig. 7-8). Similar to CD3 complex, the cytoplasmic tails of Igα and Igβ molecules contain ITAM motifs. Cross-linking of BCRs leads to the initiation of the downstream intracellular-signaling cascade. Because all the immunoglobulins on a given B cell have the same specificity, an antigen must contain multiple identical epitopes for cross-linking to occur. A microbe may bind to a BCR, but additional copies of that epitope may not be present. B cells use a fail-safe mechanism that requires signaling by both the BCR and a C3b complement receptor. Engagement of the C3b receptor serves as a second signal for B-cell activation.

BCR binding initiates endocytosis, enzymatic degradation, and subsequent display of peptide fragments as pMHC class II complexes. In addition, the B cell expresses costimulatory molecules, thus allowing the B cell to function as an APC for TCR recognition by a CD4$^+$ T cell. T–B cell communication is necessary for the B cell will gear up its cellular machinery for the production of antibodies. T cell signaling induces the B cell to proliferate, differentiate, and in the presence of additional T cell–derived cytokines (such as IL-4), differentiate into an antibody-secreting plasma cell.

Functions of the Adaptive Immune System

Not only must the adaptive immune system recognize invasive organisms or their products as nonself, but also it is critically important for host survival that action be taken to minimize the microbial threat. As in any state of war, it is important first and foremost to prevent microbial spread. The innate immune system does this by surrounding, phagocytizing, and enzymatically degrading or otherwise preventing the spread of would-be invaders throughout the body. Two arms of the adaptive immune system also are dedicated to preventing microbial dissemination.

One arm is called the **humoral immune response,** named for the fluids or humors of the body that prevent or defend against microbial attack. Humoral responses can be likened to the arrows or missiles of the immune system. Locally produced by B cells and plasma cells, they may travel great distances to reach their target epitopes. Antibodies recognize and bind to microbial epitopes to prevent microbial spread by immobilization (**agglutination**), prevention of microbial attachment to host cells (**neutralization**), promotion of microbial

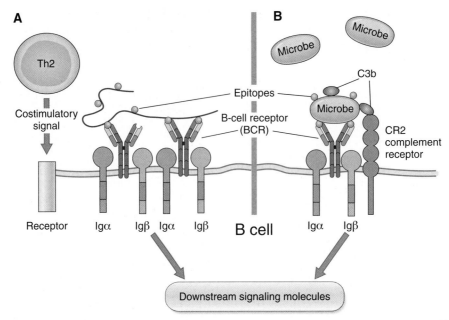

FIGURE 7-8 ▪ **B-cell activation.** B cells recognize soluble or cell-bound epitopes through their B-cell receptors (BCRs) without antigen presentation. **A.** Multiple epitopes on an antigen engage and cross-link several BCRs. Immunoreceptor tyrosine-based activation motifs (ITAMs) present on BCR-associated molecules Igα and Igβ phosphorylate and provide a first signal to the B cell. A second (cytokine) signal is provided by a CD4$^+$ Th2 cell that, together with the first signal, begins a downstream signaling cascade that leads to B-cell activation. **B.** Microbes recognized by the innate immune system may also trigger B-cell activation. Activated fragments of the third component of complement (C3b) bind to a microbe. Bound C3b fragments are themselves bound by a CR2 complement receptor on the surface of the B cell to provide a first signal. Binding of microbe epitopes by the BCR provides a second signal through the Igα and Igβ BCR-associated molecules. Both signals combine to initiate a downstream signaling cascade leading to B-cell activation.

phagocytosis and clearance (**opsonization**), and targeting of microbial destruction by soluble molecules (complement) or by leukocytes (antibody-dependent cell-mediated cytotoxicity).

The other arm of the adaptive immune response is called **cell-mediated immunity.** Like hand-to-hand combat, leukocytes encounter invaders "face-to-face" to destroy invading cells. Cell-mediated adaptive immune responses are controlled and regulated by T cells either to directly cause the destruction of invading cytotoxic T lymphocytes or to direct other leukocytes to perform the deed; the latter action is called delayed-type hypersensitivity (DTH).

Humoral Immunity

Humoral immunity is based on the actions of two sets of soluble molecules, antibodies and complement. Although the production of both depends on cellular activity, it is the binding of these soluble molecules that initiates the humoral immune responses of the adaptive immune system. One response, neutralization, is a direct result of the binding by antibodies, while the other responses—opsonization, complement activation (more specifically, the classical pathway of complement activation), and an-

tibody-dependent cell-mediated cytotoxicity—involve the use of antibodies to "tag" cells or molecules for destruction by other elements of the immune system.

Antibody–Antigen Reactions

Antigen–antibody (Ag–Ab) interactions are some of the most specific noncovalent biochemical reactions known and can be represented by the following simple formula:

$$\text{Ag} + \text{Ab} \rightleftarrows \text{AgAb}$$

Although the reaction is driven to the right, notice that **antigen–antibody interactions are reversible.** The strength of interaction (i.e., how far the reaction is driven to the right) is termed its **affinity.** Immunoglobulin populations within an individual show a wide range of affinity. **Valence** (the number of epitope-binding sites on an immunoglobulin molecule) varies from 2 for monomeric forms of all isotypes, to 4 for secretory IgA, to 10 for pentameric IgM. The term **avidity** is often used to describe the collective affinity of multiple binding sites on an antibody molecule.

The **precipitin reaction** is the term applied to the interaction of soluble antigen with soluble antibody, resulting in a precipitate. Although discovered in the late nineteenth century, it was not until the 1930s that scientists were able to quantify the amount of antibody present in serum using this reaction. Understanding antigen–antibody reactions requires an understanding of the **quantitative precipitin reaction.**

In the classical series of experiments by Heidelberger and Kendall, rabbits were immunized with capsular polysaccharide (antigen) from *Streptococcus pneumoniae*. Several weeks later the sera from the immunized rabbits were prepared and used as the antibody source (antisera). Known amounts of antigen (in a constant volume) were mixed with an equal, constant volume of antiserum and incubated (Fig. 7-9). Precipitate formed in several tubes and was separated (by centrifugation) from the supernatant, and the amount of total nitrogen in the precipitate was determined. In these experiments a polysaccharide antigen was used, and because the antigen did not contain nitrogen, any nitrogen detected had to originate from the antibody (i.e., protein). This experiment demonstrated that an **antibody is a protein** and that antigens and antibodies react in a **predictable** manner. The degree of antigen–antibody cross-linking results in lattice formation and can be used to describe the three distinct zones of the quantitative precipitin curve.

- **Zone of antigen excess:** The antigen–antibody complexes are too small to precipitate. The net result is the formation of soluble complexes.
- **Equivalence zone:** Optimal precipitation occurs in this area of the curve. Large, visible precipitating complexes are formed. It is this property, the formation of a visible precipitate, that is the basis for many immunologically based diagnostic tests.
- **Zone of antibody excess:** Not enough antigen is present to form a precipitate. The net result is formation of soluble complexes.

The principles of the quantitative precipitin curve apply to all antigen–antibody reactions and form the basis for many modern clinical diagnostic tests.

Agglutination

Antibodies can also bind to and cross-link cells or particles, causing an aggregate formation in a reaction known as **agglutination.** Agglutination has the effect of throwing a molecular net over microbial invaders, greatly hindering their mobility and spread throughout the body before they encounter the tissue, cells, and fluids of the body

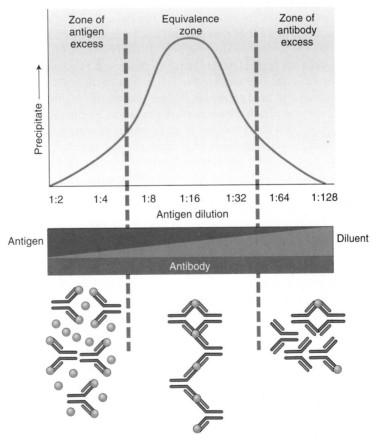

FIGURE 7-9 ■ **Quantitative precipitin curve.** Antigen composed of multiple epitopes (green spheres) is diluted in a mild salt solution (diluent) in a test tube and expressed as a ratio (1:2, 1:4, 1:8, etc.). Identical amounts of antibody are added to each test tube. After a brief incubation period, precipitation is seen in some of the tubes. Optimal precipitation (equivalence zone) occurs when antigen and antibody react to form large latticelike complexes. Much smaller complexes, too small to precipitate, are formed where there is a relative abundance of antigen to antibody (zone of antigen excess) or a relative abundance of antibody to antigen (zone of antibody excess).

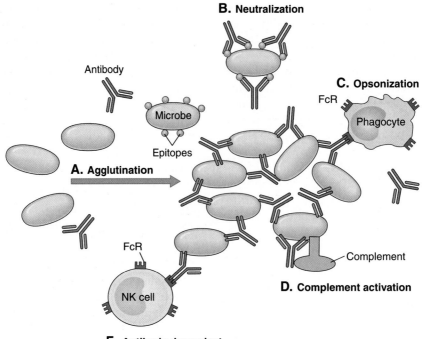

FIGURE 7-10 ▪ **Humoral immune effector functions. A.** Agglutination: Recognition of microbial surface epitopes by antibodies causes a cross-linked lattice formation analogous to the equivalence zone of the quantitative precipitin curve (see Fig. 7-9). This process prevents systemwide spread of the microbes. The order of efficacy is IgM >> IgA > IgG. **B.** Neutralization: In some instances antibodies are specific for epitopes on the microbe, epitopes that would normally interact with molecules on the surface of the host cell. Antibodies that prevent molecule-to-molecule interaction between microbe and host cells are termed neutralizing antibodies. **C.** Opsonization: Antibody binding to microbial epitopes causes a conformational alteration in the Fc portion of the antibody molecule. Specialized Fc receptors (FcR) on phagocytes recognize and bind to the altered Fc portion of the antibody molecule, initiating phagocytosis of the FcR–antibody–microbe complex for enzymatic degradation by the phagolysosome. A fragment of the third component of complement (C3b) can also function as an opsonin, binding both to a microbial surface and to a specialized complement receptor (CR2) on the surfaces of phagocytes and signaling enzymatic destruction by phagocytosis and the phagolysosome. **D.** Complement activation: Antibody binding to a microbial surface may initiate the classical pathway of complement activation to initiate complement-mediated lysis and/or the binding of C3b as an opsonin. **E.** Antibody-dependent cell-mediated cytotoxicity (ADCC): Antibody binding to microbial epitopes causes a conformational alteration in the Fc portion of the antibody molecule. FcRs on natural killer (NK) cells recognize and bind to these altered Fcs on the antibody. The microbe-antibody-FcR complex triggers the NK cell to release perforin and granzymes that facilitate the pore formation in the microbe, leading to its death.

(Fig. 7-10A). Antibodies of the IgM and IgA isotypes are particularly adept at this because they contain 10 and 4 binding sites, respectively; but sufficient concentrations of IgG isotype antibodies will also agglutinate particles. Antibodies can also agglutinate nonmicrobial cells, as demonstrated by the agglutination seen when antibodies are used for ABO typing of erythrocytes.

Neutralization

Neutralization describes the process of antibodies binding to microbial epitopes or soluble molecules (e.g., toxins) in a manner that inhibits the ability of the microbes or molecules to bind to host cell surfaces. Many microbes and all viruses inflict damage when they bind to host cell surfaces to facilitate entry. Likewise, most toxin molecules bind to host cell surface structures before en-

try and exertion of their toxic effects. In both cases, the binding to host cell surfaces is specific. The binding structures on the microbe or toxin are shaped to fit together with specific host cell surface structures. For example, rhinoviruses (the common cold viruses) bind to the intracellular adhesion molecule 1 (ICAM-1) found on the surfaces of respiratory epithelium.

Antibodies generated against the microbes (or toxins) often include some that can bind and block the microbial structures that interact with the host cell surface, effectively preventing the microbe (or toxin) from entering the cell (see Fig. 7-10B). This form of immunoglobulin-mediated protection is called neutralization because it neutralizes the infective capacity of the invader. Neutralizing antibodies are usually of the IgG and IgA isotypes. It is the presence of neutralizing antibodies generated during the initial infection that provides the greatest protection against subsequent reinfection by the same organism.

Opsonization

Sometimes the binding of an antibody (usually IgG) to a microbial surface is enough to "whet the appetite" of a phagocyte, making the microbe an attractive "meal." In essence, antibodies bind to structures and mark them for subsequent destruction by phagocytic cells. Phagocytic cells such as macrophages, dendritic cells, and neutrophils bear surface receptors (FcRs) for the Fc portion of immunoglobulin. By binding an epitope, an antibody molecule makes several conformational changes that include changes in the Fc region (see Fig. 7-1). The FcRs on phagocytic cells recognize and bind conformationally changed Fcs but not immunoglobulins that have not bound an epitope. The binding of a microbe-associated epitope–antibody complex by the FcRs tethers the bound invader to the phagocytic cell and stimulates it to engulf and destroy the microbe (see Fig. 7-10C). In fact, initial microbe binding and engulfment stimulates the phagocytic cell to increase its search for other such "tagged" microbes. The immunoglobulin serves as an **opsonin** (an agent that stimulates phagocytosis), and the increased phagocytic activity that ensues is termed **opsonization.**

Complement Activation

The **classical pathway of complement activation** is one in which antibodies mark a structure for destruction by facilitating the attraction and subsequent binding of components of the complement system. Unlike the alternative pathway of complement activation, the classical pathway must be initiated by the action of a product unique to the adaptive immune system. In this case the antibodies (usually of the IgM and IgG isotypes) facilitate the sequential binding of the C1, C2, C3 and, C4 components of the complement system (see Fig. 6-1). As with the alternative pathway, completion of the classical complement pathway produces **C3b,** a "sticky" fragment of C3 that readily binds to a microbial surface and serves as an opsonin (see Fig. 7-10D), the release of small proinflammatory fragments **C2b** and **C4a** (in contemporary nomenclature, the small fragment of C2 is designated as **C2a**) and in the assembly of the **membrane attack complex** (see Fig. 6-1).

Antibody-Dependent Cell-Mediated Cytotoxicity

The binding of an antibody to an invasive organism can act as a "tag" to attract not only phagocytic cells but also cytolytic cells. Cells such as **natural killer (NK) cells** and **eosinophils** bear FcRs that aid in the detection of infectious organisms as large as worms. Like phagocytic cells, they use these receptors to identify invasive organisms identified by IgG or IgA antibodies; but rather than engulfing them, they use cytolytic and inflammatory mechanisms to kill the tagged organisms (see Fig. 7-10E). These cytolytic mechanisms are discussed later in this chapter. The process is termed **antibody-dependent cell-mediated cytotoxicity (ADCC).**

Cell-Mediated Immunity

The actions of both the innate and adaptive immune systems are like warfare waged against (potentially) invasive organisms. Humoral immune responses, both antibodies and complement activation pathways, may be viewed as the arrows and missiles of the immune system that are aimed or lobbed at a distant enemy. Often these responses are used as preemptive strikes, attacking a potential enemy before it has the ability to breach epithelial, endothelial, or cell membrane barriers. Agglutination, neutralization, opsonization, complement-mediated lysis, and ADCC all serve to curtail the potential spread of an infectious organism once it has established a beachhead. Yet, as Sun-tzu said, "Warfare is the Way of deception," and microbes are not beyond employing pathogenic stealth.

Cell-mediated immune responses are directed to curtail microbial stealth by determining whether infectious agents are sheltered within host cells and thus are beyond the "reach" of humoral immunity. Cell-mediated responses resemble "hand-to-hand combat" and take two basic forms: delayed-type hypersensitivity mediated by CD4$^+$ Th1 cells and cell-mediated lysis mediated by CD8$^+$ CTLs. Cell-mediated immunity is a life-or-death struggle at close quarters. In the case of DTH, some T cells act as scouts and senior officers, identifying sites of infection, calling in reinforcements (mostly macrophages and other leukocytes), and ordering them to kill the infectious foe or the host cell that harbors the foe. CTLs, on the other hand, directly engage in cell-to-cell combat to actively destroy their infectious opponent or the host cell in which it is hiding.

Delayed-Type Hypersensitivity

Previously activated CD4$^+$ Th1 cells patrol the body, looking for host cells displaying the same pMHC class II combination that originally triggered their activation (e.g., a *Mycobacterium tuberculosis* peptide-bearing MHC class II complex). If, during its recirculation through body tissues, a previously activated Th1 cell reencounters the appropriate pMHC class II displayed on a host cell, it reactivates to synthesize and secrete cytokines that attract and activate macrophages (Fig. 7-11). Thus, the T cells from the adaptive immune system can recruit, direct, and activate elements of the innate immune system. Activated macrophages become blind, enraged killers that attack not only infectious agents and infected cells but also normal uninfected cells in the

FIGURE 7-11 ▪ **Delayed-type hypersensitivity (DTH).** Previously activated CD4$^+$ Th1 cells on recognition of pMHC class II on antigen-presenting cells (phagocytes) become reactivated (1). Reactivated Th1 secrete cytokines and chemokines that increase MHC class II expression, degradative enzymes, and reactive oxygen species in macrophages (2). **3.** The activated macrophage becomes a killing machine, destroying everything that comes within its "grasp (3)."

vicinity. When activated by Th1 cells, macrophages increase their production and release of destructive enzymes and reactive oxygen intermediates that injure adjacent cells. They also begin to secrete cytokines that attract other leukocytes, especially neutrophils, to the site of infection. Together the activated macrophages and neutrophils rampage through the site of infection, assaulting both infected and normal cells, and removing cellular debris.

DTH responses can be a double-edged sword. Because the activated macrophages are not "antigen-specific," they are perfectly capable of destroying friend and foe alike, normal tissue along with infected cells. Excessively active or chronic DTH responses can create permanent damage that impairs normal function and, in some cases, is fatal. For example, much or most of the injury to the lungs of tuberculosis patients stems from the damage inflicted by the activated macrophages of the DTH response against *M. tuberculosis* rather than by the infectious agent itself.

Cytotoxic T Lymphocytes

Only a small proportion of the cells of the body express MHC class II molecules, although all nucleated cells express MHC class I molecules. Previously activated CD8$^+$ CTLs circulate throughout the body "sampling" for the initial activating pMHC class I combination. If the CTL encounters that combination on the surface of another cell, it recognizes that it has contacted an infected cell (Fig. 7-12). CTLs bind directly to infected cells and destroy them using one or more mechanisms. They release perforins that puncture the cell membranes, effectively lysing them. CTLs also release granzymes that enter the cyto-

plasm through the perforin-created holes. Granzymes induce the infected cell to commit suicide by destroying its own DNA, a process known as apoptosis. CTLs alter their membranes in the area of contact to make themselves resistant to the perforins and granzymes being released. Finally, CTLs may engage receptors on the surfaces of the infected cells, inducing the infected cells to undergo apoptosis. Apoptosis is an important protective mechanism because, in destroying its own DNA, the infected cells also destroy the nucleic acids of the infectious organisms within it, thus preventing the spread of infection.

Immunologic Memory

An important feature that distinguishes the adaptive immune system from the innate immune system is the presence of **immunologic memory.** Simply put, once an infectious organism stimulates an adaptive response, subsequent encounters with that organism produce mild or even unapparent effects because of the rapid and enhanced action of antibodies or effector T cells. Antigen-specific cells that have been clonally expanded and have undergone some activation during previous encounters with antigen (**memory cells**) can be rapidly mobilized in much greater numbers, thus shortening the response time to antigen. Whether generated against infectious organisms or other types of antigens, these **secondary responses** are typically faster and more vigorous than the primary responses stimulated by the initial exposure (Fig. 7-13). In addition, the antibody isotypes generated against a repeatedly encountered antigen change over

FIGURE 7-12 ▪ **Cytotoxic T lymphocyte (CTL) activation.** Activated CD8$^+$ T cells circulate throughout the tissues of the body as CTLs, scrutinizing the pMHC class I molecules displayed by nucleated cells (1). On recognition of the appropriate pMHC class I complex, a series of events are initiated by the CTL that ultimately leads to the lysis of the infected "target cell (2)." Although contact between the CTL and the target cell lasts only a few minutes, the CTL delivers a fatal "kiss of death" to the target cell in the form of perforin granules and granzymes (3). The perforin granules polymerize to form pores in the cell, creating an electrolyte imbalance and through which granzymes enter. Both perforins and granzymes conspire in the demise of the target cell by osmotic lysis and apoptosis, respectively.

time. IgM is the predominant isotype seen in primary responses, while secondary responses include mostly IgG, with IgA and IgE also present. As the antibody isotypes change with repeated stimulation by a given antigen, the binding affinity of the antibodies also increases because of the incorporation of small mutations in the DNA encoding the variable regions of the light and heavy chains. B cells with mutations that result in tighter binding actually proliferate more rapidly and come to dominate the response. The deliberate initial exposure to an infectious

organism, in a form unable to cause full-blown disease, can thus provide protection against a subsequent exposure with a fully virulent form of that organism. This, of course, is the basis of **vaccination.**

Although immunological memory is primarily associated with enhancing the response against subsequent exposures to an infectious organism or other antigen, that is not always the case. In some cases, responses to future exposures can be diminished, a state known as **tolerance.** This phenomenon is important in preventing

FIGURE 7-13 ▪ **Immunologic memory.** The hallmark of the adaptive immune response is its ability to recall a previous encounter with a microbe and mount an accelerated, enhanced response against it. Initial activation of antigen-naive lymphocytes with microbe A results in their activation, proliferation, and response of microbe-specific lymphocytes. This process requires time, hence the lag time between initial encounter and a discernible immune response. Reencountering the same microbe days, months, or years later results in a robust, rapid response with a significantly shorter lag time—a heightened and persistent immune response. Encountering the antigenically distinct microbe B at the time of the reencounter with microbe A results in a primary response similar to that seen for the initial encounter with microbe A.

the immune system from producing superfluous (and potentially injurious) responses against harmless organisms and molecules in the environment, as well as against the body's own cells and molecules.

What Happens If a Good System Goes Awry?

The function of the innate and adaptive immune systems is to recognize and attack the nonself while leaving the self relatively undisturbed. The innate immune system readily makes this distinction by expressing a finite number of receptors expressed by a wide variety of potentially pathogenic organisms. Because its receptors are somatically generated, the adaptive immune system is faced with a much more daunting task of distinguishing nonself from self. Selection mechanisms eliminate overtly self-reactive T and B cells during lymphocyte development. However, the adaptive immune system often encounters self molecules that were not present at the time of receptor selection, such as molecules that arise during and after puberty. If these mechanisms fail to distinguish self from nonself, serious and potentially fatal consequences may result. Fortunately, the adaptive immune system has evolved several mechanisms to deal with potentially self-reactive lymphocytes.

Tolerance and T-Cell Regulation

Normally, the immune system's offensive machinery is reserved for use against external threats. Part of the selection process during T-cell development (i.e., positive selection) requires that a thymocyte recognize self. Selective nonresponsiveness or **tolerance** requires that when recognizing self, the adaptive immune system must adopt a nondestructive strategy. Several tolerance mechanisms have evolved to minimize potential harm caused by post-developmental selection-autoreactive cells.

One mechanism, anergy, has already been discussed briefly. Basically, anergy is a state of lymphocyte nonresponsiveness that occurs following pMHC engagement (T cells) or free epitope engagement (B cells). T cells require interaction with both pMHC *and* a costimulatory second signal. B cells, too, require a second signal following BCR engagement. Failing to receive a second signal, lymphocytes become unresponsive to the combined restimulation by both first *and* second signals. Anergized cells are not killed but remain in circulation and cannot, under normal circumstances, be reactivated.

Regulatory T (Treg) cells can also maintain tolerance. Characteristically, they inhibit the activity of autoreactive lymphocytes. The molecular basis for their regulatory action is still unclear, but they appear to fall into one of two categories. Treg cells express both CD4 and CD25 molecules and are thought to be important inhibitors of immune-mediated inflammatory diseases, such as inflammatory bowel disease. Suppressor T cells are $CD8^+$ and inhibit the activation and proliferation of $CD4^+$ T cells, including Th1 cells. Both $CD8^+$ and $CD4^+$ T-cell subpopulations inhibit specific antibody production by B cells. One possible mechanism for minimizing unwanted reactivity might be apparent in the cytokines produced by Th1 and Th2 cells. Th1-produced IFN-γ inhibits the maturation of Th0 cells into Th2 cells, and Th2-produced IL-4 inhibits the differentiation of Th0 cells along the Th1 pathway.

Immunodeficiency

Unlike the nervous, visual, olfactory, and similar systems, the immune system is one of the few systems in the body that humans do not directly sense. No one wakes up in the morning and says, "My immune system feels great!" or "My immune system is feeling a little out of sorts." We generally perceive that something is wrong with our immune systems only when we are subjected to multiple, recurrent infections or when our immune systems overtly misperceive self and nonself. The immune system employs a great deal of redundancy, with a number of mechanisms available to fight a given threat. As a result, should one mechanism be ineffective or fail altogether, others can still clear the infections. Under these normal circumstances the immune system functions reliably.

Sometimes, however, the system fails dramatically, leaving the individual open to potentially fatal infection or to the consequences of an imbalanced immune system. Such defects in the immune system—**immune deficiencies, or immunodeficiencies**—occur infrequently but can have severe consequences. Although some are extremely dramatic in their effects, those tend to be relatively rare; subtle immune deficiencies with less dramatic effects are more common. **Primary immune deficiencies** occur as intrinsic defects, usually genetically inherited but sometimes also due to random errors during development. Thus, although individual immunodeficiency diseases are rare, there are so many of them that collectively they represent a significant health problem. **Secondary immune deficiencies** are cases of reduced immune function caused by environmental factors (e.g., malnutrition, infection, malignancy, and therapeutic treatments for other diseases). Individuals with secondary immune deficiencies are more susceptible to infectious disease and may also suffer from other health problems associated with the immune deficiencies.

Immune deficiency diseases have several characteristics. Some are common to numerous forms of immunodeficiency, while others are associated with only a few such deficiencies. Among the most common are unusually frequent infections, chronic infections, an inability to clear infectious agents from the body, and diminished responses to standard treatments.

The types of responses that are affected usually categorize primary immunodeficiencies, and each such category can include several defective mechanisms. Among the best known of these diseases are those that cause the many different forms of **severe combined immunodeficiency disease (SCID)**. Most of these diseases involve defects in the stem cells that give rise to most or all of the cellular elements of the immune system, including T and B cells. Individuals with SCID display varying degrees of reduced antibody-mediated and cell-mediated responses.

Defects in antibody-dependent responses may result from defective development of B cells (e.g., Bruton hypogammaglobulinemia), an inability to undergo the isotype switch (e.g., immunodeficiency with hyper-IgM), an inability to interact with T cells (common variable immunodeficiency), or a variety of defects in the genes encoding the immunoglobulin light or heavy chains or other molecules critical to normal function. However, individuals with B cell defects typically have normal cell-mediated immunity. Deficiencies in T-cell function include defects in T-cell development (e.g., DiGeorge syndrome), an inability to express MHC class I or class II molecules (e.g., bare lymphocyte syndrome), an inability to load antigenic peptides into MHC class I (e.g., TAP-2 deficiency), and a variety of other defective molecules involved in specific T-cell functions. Because T cells are critical to the normal function of B cells, individuals with T-cell defects often also display defective antibody-mediated responses.

Defects in cells other than lymphocytes can also diminish immune function. Defects in phagocytic cells, for example, can reduce their ability to ingest and destroy microbes (e.g., chronic granulomatous disease). As a result, innate immunity is lessened, as is the ability of the phagocytes to interact with T cells for initiation of adaptive responses. In addition, individuals bearing defects in the genes encoding various components of the complement system may face severe infectious problems because of the importance of these molecules in both innate and adaptive immunity.

In most cases, attempts at therapy of immunodeficient patients involve protection, appropriate antibiotic treatments, and an attempt to replace the missing molecules or cells on a repeating basis. More recently, however, attempts have been made to replace defective cells with cells from the patients that have been genetically engineered to function normally and provide a self-sustaining population that does not need regular replacement.

Hypersensitivity Reactions

Like any weapon or tool, the immune system can harm its user if not properly controlled. Its destructive capacity, meant to be directed against infectious agents or intruding toxins, can damage the body when it becomes too vigorous, too sustained, or misdirected. The state of having an immune system that inflicts damage on the body is called **hypersensitivity.** Unlike autoimmunity, hypersensitivity need not be a response against the self but often results from an "innocent bystander" destroying normal cells and tissues in the vicinity of a "free fire zone," where the immune system is aggressively battling infectious agents. The four recognized types of hypersensitivities are described in the following paragraphs and in Table 7-4.

Type I or immediate-type hypersensitivity manifests itself seconds to a few hours after an appropriate stimulus. Commonly known as **allergy,** this hypersensitivity state results from cross-linking surface-bound IgE antibodies on

table 7-4   Hypersensitivity Reactions

TYPE	COMMON NAME	INITIATED BY	IMMUNE RESPONSE	INFLAMMATORY MECHANISM(S)	REACTION TIME
I	Immediate hypersensitivity or allergy	Allergens: pollens, parasites (e.g., dust mites), etc.	IgE-mediated degranulation of mast cells or basophils	Histamine and vasoactive amine release	Seconds to a few hours
II	Antibody-dependent cytotoxicity	Antibodies binding to molecules displayed on host cell surfaces, membranes, or extracellular matrices	Conformational change in Fc portion of antibody activates complement or FcR binding by phagocytes	Complement or cell-mediated lysis of cells	Hours to days
III	Immune-complex disease	Antibodies binding to soluble molecules	Extracellular deposition of antigen–antibody complexes	Activation of the classical complement pathway	Hours to days
IV	Delayed(-type) hypersensitivity	Intracellular microbes (e.g., *Mycobacterium tuberculosis*, *Leishmania* spp.)	Cell-mediated immune response to intracellular organisms	Macrophage and neutrophil activation and infiltration in infected tissues	1 to 4 days

mast cells (and some basophils), triggering the release of vasoactive amines. Humoral immune responses against relatively harmless substances (e.g., pollens, food, etc.) lead to the secretion of specific IgE antibodies by plasma cells. Mast cells and some basophils express an ε-specific heavy-chain Fc receptor (FcR$_\varepsilon$). Unlike other FcRs specific to other heavy chains, the FcR$_\varepsilon$ binds epitope-free IgE molecules. Mast cells and some basophils decorate their cell surfaces with IgE molecules of various specificities. These IgE molecules then serve as epitope-specific receptors. Encounter with the appropriate antigen containing multiple recognized epitopes causes IgE cross-linking, triggering the release of cytoplasmic granules from the cell. The granules contain various pharmaceutical mediators that trigger the changes in the skin, vasculature, airways, or gut that are associated with allergy. Severe, life-threatening manifestations of allergy can lead to asthma.

Type II hypersensitivities are those caused by the activation of complement, via the classical pathway, by antibodies (usually IgG but sometimes also IgM) bound to cell surfaces, membranes, or intracellular matrices. The antibodies may be directed against normal self molecules (autoimmunity) or against nonself molecules that attach themselves to membranes or matrices in the body. In either case the location of the bound antibodies focuses the inflammatory response initiated by complement activation to that site and can lead to temporary or permanent damage (e.g., Goodpasture syndrome). Damage can also be incurred by the interaction of the bound antibodies with FcRs of phagocytic cells or cells capable of ADCC.

Type III hypersensitivities, like those of type II, are caused by the activation of complement via the classical pathway. However, the antibodies involved are binding to soluble molecules rather than surfaces. As a result, antigen–antibody complexes can form, and if they become large enough, they can precipitate out of solution (see Fig. 7-9) and become deposited on tissues. The most common sites of deposition are the kidney glomeruli (the filtering apparatus of the kidney), the endothelial surfaces of blood vessels, the skin, and the synovial membranes of joints. Once deposited in tissues, the antibodies bound within the complexes interact with and activate complement, leading to inflammation focused on the site of deposition. Again, the damage inflicted may be temporary or permanent (e.g., rheumatoid arthritis).

Type IV hypersensitivities do not involve antibodies, but are due to inflammatory reactions arising from purely cell-mediated immune responses. Usually, these are CD4$^+$-mediated DTH responses, but sometimes they also involve the action of CD8$^+$ CTLs. Among the most common examples of this hypersensitivity type are positive skin tests for tuberculosis (the Mantoux test); inflammations caused by contact with poison ivy, poison sumac, and other plants; and the inflammations (contact sensitivity) resulting from contact with metals or chemicals.

Autoimmunity

Despite the checks and balances that are built into the adaptive immune system, it sometimes mistakes self epitopes for nonself. The loss of self-tolerance mechanisms leads to a condition known as **autoimmunity,** a state in which the immune system attacks the body's own normal molecules, the very cells and tissues that it was designed to protect. Unfortunately, autoimmune diseases occur all too frequently.

Microbial epitopes sometimes bear structural similarities to molecules expressed by host cells. In attempting to curtail the spread of an infectious organism, the adaptive immune system may respond to these structurally similar epitopes, a process known as **molecular mimicry.** Strong host defenses to a particular microbial epitope can also inflict damage to host cells that display similar epitope-bearing structures. A classic example of this mechanism is **rheumatic fever,** which can lead to life-threatening heart disease. Pharyngeal infection with *Streptococcus pyogenes* is the common cause of "strep throat." Group A β-hemolytic stains of *S. pyogenes* produce large quantities of **M protein.** The adaptive immune response readily makes IgM and IgG antibodies to M protein. Unfortunately, antibodies to M protein can cross-react with similar structures found on the sarcolemma of cardiac muscle and on the heart valves. Antibody binding to the sarcolemma and heart valves initiates inflammation of these tissues that can result in fatal damage to the tissues. Chronic strep throat infections can be life threatening. This is the main reason that pediatricians promptly treat children with strep throat with antibiotics, thereby minimizing the adaptive immune response to this organism and preventing autoimmune sequelae. Autoimmune type 1 diabetes mellitus is another example of molecular mimicry. T cells of individuals infected with *Coxsackie virus* or *cytomegalovirus* may develop responsiveness to glutamate decarboxylase responses, a pancreatic islet β-cell enzyme that is a major target for autoreactive T cells.

Other autoimmune diseases that collectively are known as **reactive arthritis** may be attributable to molecular mimicry. These include **ankylosing spondylitis,** an inflammatory disease of the lower spine, in which prior *Klebsiella* infection leads to immune cross-reactivity with a certain MHC class I (HLA-B27) molecule in susceptible individuals. *Klebsiella* have also been implicated as the causative agent in **Reiter disease,** marked by arthritis in the lower-limb joints and involving the gastrointestinal, genital, and urinary tracts. Molecular mimicry has also been implicated in **myasthenia gravis,** a disease in which the nerve ending–muscle junction is impaired, and **hypoglycemia,** which affects the insulin receptor is affected.

In some cases autoimmune disease results from the loss of regulatory T or suppressor T cells. Evidence suggests that the ability of Treg and Ts cells to prevent responses by self-reactive cells is lost with time. Therefore, as people age, the opportunity for self-reactive lymphocytes to escape regulation also increases. Autoimmune diseases such as **systemic lupus erythematosus (SLE)** are thought to result from impaired regulation, and affected individuals produce antibodies against nucleic acids and chromosomal proteins.

Some autoimmune diseases result from an altered immune response to an initial infection. Initial infection can expose normally sequestered antigens to immune scrutiny. The phenomenon, called **epitope spreading,** appears to originate with an immune response to an infectious disease, and the collateral damage to normal tissues makes sequestered antigens available to the adaptive immune system. Epitope spreading has been suggested as a contributing mechanism to SLE, inflammatory bowel disease, multiple sclerosis, and some forms of diabetes.

Well Patients; or, How Innate and Adaptive Immune Responses Maintain Health

Immune system responses to microbial infection are vital for the protection of the body. The adaptive immune system is designed to attack infectious organisms that enter the body. Often microorganisms resist attack by the immune system by evading or subverting and redirecting the immune response. Sometimes it is just as important that the immune system not respond to an antigen. For instance, the mucosal surfaces are constantly awash in nonself molecules and microorganisms associated with our environment and with the food and fluids that we consume. Immune defenses must focus on potentially infectious microorganisms and their products but ignore or selectively diminish responses to others.

From the human perspective, the microbial world has four classes of citizens: (1) those that do not inhabit the human body; (2) those that live on or in the body, benefiting one or both partners and harming neither; (3) those that that live on or in the body in a state of truce, neither benefiting nor harming either partner; and (4) those with the potential for causing harm to the human body. Members of the fourth category are known as **pathogens.** The disease-causing potential for a pathogen often depends on circumstances. Some pathogens invade the human body as part of their life cycle. Others are **opportunistic** pathogens and become a threat only when the immune system is weakened. Products of some microbes, such as the *Vibrio cholera* toxin, can be life threatening, and the development of specific, neutralizing antibodies against the toxin are crucial for protection. Many people enjoy a healthy, active life, unaware of the critical, life-sustaining role played by their immune systems. In fact, most of us become aware of immune dysfunction by the inability of our bodies to resist infection.

Effective Immune Responses to Pathogens

Immune responses vary in their effectiveness against particular types of pathogens. Which responses will be effective in providing protection is determined by the physical nature of the pathogen in question as well as its "lifestyle." Pathogens or their toxic products vary in the ways that they enter the body, the cells or tissues that they infect once they are within the body, and the ways in which they move through the body and reproduce. All these factors participate in determining which types of immune responses will be most effective against them.

Viral infections trigger both innate and adaptive immune responses. Infected cells synthesize and secrete cytokines that heighten the resistance of neighboring uninfected cells, while rendering themselves more "available" to the immune system to trigger the initiation of protective responses by NK cells and phagocytic cells. NK cells are lymphocytes that bridge both the innate and adaptive immune systems able to detect cells that have subnormal expression of MHC class I molecules and to kill them by direct contact. This is an important ability because, as will be seen shortly, some viruses attempt to escape the notice of the immune system (especially CTLs) by reducing the number of MHC class I molecules on the surface of the cells they infect. Following the activation of the innate immune system by viral infection, humoral and cellular adaptive responses arise.

During **primary infections** (the initial exposure to a particular virus), adaptive cell-mediated responses, primarily involving CTLs, clear the viral infection by destroying the cells within which the viruses are replicating. The generation of antiviral antibodies, although not effective in clearing active infections (because replicating viruses are sequestered within cells and not accessible to antibodies), is extremely important because antibodies minimize or prevent reinfection through neutralization. Even if reinfection is not completely prevented by neutralizing antibodies, the infected cells remain few and can be destroyed readily by increased cell-mediated responses. These reinfections may be dealt with so rapidly that symptoms do not become evident.

Extracellular bacteria remain in the body fluids and intercellular spaces, while intracellular bacteria enter and reproduce within cells. Various immune responses are effective against each of these two categories of bacteria. Free-living extracellular bacteria, such as *Staphylococci* and *Streptococci*, are readily exposed to antibodies and complement. As a result they are vulnerable to destruction and clearance by phagocytic cells (via recognition and binding by pattern recognition receptors) and by all the pathways of complement activation. Recognition and binding of the bacteria by antibodies also increases their clearance through opsonization.

Intracellular bacteria (e.g., *Mycobacterium* spp. and *Legionella pneumophila*) are exposed to complement and antibodies en route to the cells they are to infect. Once inside the cell, they are no longer available to the actions of antibodies and complement. The portal of entry for many intracellular bacteria is the phagosome. Thus, destruction of these intracellular bacteria often requires activation of the infected phagocytes by CD4$^+$ T cells through DTH. Because CD4$^+$ T cells can only recognize pMHC class II complexes, this is only effective if the infected cells express MHC class II molecules. This activation causes the phagocytes to increase their metabolic activity and synthesis of bactericidal molecules, allowing them to kill or inhibit the growth of the microbes residing in the phagosomes.

Cells infected by intracellular bacteria can sometimes also be killed by CTLs. Some intracellular bacteria (e.g., *Listeria monocytogenes* and *Rickettsia* spp.) can escape from phagosomes and move into the cytoplasm. Once in the cytoplasm, some of the bacterial proteins are degraded by proteasomes; their proteolytic fragments are loaded onto MHC class I molecules and displayed on the cell surface as pMHC class I complexes. These pMHC class I complexes can be recognized by CTLs that go on to destroy the infected cell.

Immune responses to infectious **protozoa** are much like those seen for bacteria. Free-living protozoa are sometimes vulnerable to antibody-mediated opsonization or antibody-initiated complement lysis, while intracellular protozoa are destroyed primarily by cell-mediated responses (usually DTH). While fungal infections trigger both antibody and DTH responses, it is the latter that are responsible for resistance and clearance of infectious **fungi.** Immune responses can even be generated against larger pathogenic invaders such as flatworms (flukes and tapeworms) and roundworms (such as nematodes, hookworms, and *Ascaris* spp.). Tapeworms are generally localized in the gastrointestinal tract, while various species of flukes infect a variety of tissues such as blood, liver, lung, and intestine. Roundworms usually infect either the blood or the gastrointestinal tract. Infections by flatworms and roundworms can trigger inflammatory responses involving IgE and DTH that may provide some degree of protection against subsequent reinfection, although not as effectively as is seen against bacteria or viruses.

Evasion and Subversion of the Immune Response

Infectious organisms do not lie down and surrender when confronted by the immune system. After millions of years of interactions with their hosts, they have developed numerous methods for countering immune responses, ranging from simple evasion ("camouflage") to deliberately destroying cells and molecules of the immune response ("assassination").

Various forms of camouflage allow some microbes to sneak beneath the radar of the immune system. For example, the larval and adult forms of some blood flukes (*Schistosoma*) can cover themselves with molecules from host cells, passing themselves off as the self. Others (e.g., *Plasmodium* spp.) practice a form of invisibility by entering erythrocytes. Mature erythrocytes, being enucleate and lacking MHC class I or class II molecules on their surface, are ignored by T lymphocytes. Finally, many microbes can reduce the expression of some of their surface molecules, making them less visible to the immune system.

Many infectious organisms evade the immune response by altering the antigen molecules on their surfaces. In some cases (e.g., bacteria such as *Neisseria gonorrhoeae* and protozoa such as *Trypanosoma* spp.), the organisms carry numerous, slightly varying, copies of genes to encode some of their critical surface antigens. Periodically, they alter their surface antigens by changing the gene being used for transcription. Some organisms (e.g., influenza virus and HIV) use error-prone polymerases to replicate their DNA, leading to an elevated rate of accumulated small mutations—a process known as **antigenic drift.** Influenza and HIV are also representative of organisms that can change their surface antigens in more drastic ways through a process known as **antigenic shift.** Antigenic shift occurs when viruses from different sources infect the same cell and recombine. For example, in regions of the world where domestic birds and mammals are in close contact, an avian influenza virus (e.g., from a duck) and a mammalian influenza virus (e.g., from a pig) can infect a single cell (e.g., in the pig). Once within the same cell, the duck-derived and pig-derived influenza genomes can recombine to form hybrid progeny containing parts of the two genomes. These hybrid forms may infect not only the parental avian and mammalian species but other species as well (e.g., humans). Often the hybrid viruses are so different from their progenitors that individuals with strong immune responses against the original forms have little protection against the new hybrid forms. Thus, in all these cases the immune system must start anew, developing responses to the newly expressed antigens, only to find that by the time they become effective, the organism has generated yet other new antigens.

Some infectious organisms have developed the ability to interfere with the immune responses generated

FIGURE 7-14 ▪ **Viral evasion of pMHC class I presentation.** Some viruses (e.g., some herpesviruses, adenoviruses, cytomegaloviruses, and HIV) are able to disrupt different stages of the normal MHC class I presentation pathway (light blue arrows). Points of viral intervention (dark blue arrows) include the following: **A.** Prevention of peptide entry into the endoplasmic reticulum via TAP-1 and TAP-2. **B.** Inhibition of peptide exit from TAP-1 and TAP-2 into the endoplasmic reticulum. **C.** Diversion of pMHC class I complexes from the endoplasmic reticulum back into the cytoplasm. **D.** Return of pMHC class I complexes from the Golgi to the endoplasmic reticulum. **E.** Diversion of pMHC class I complexes from exocytotic vesicles to the lysosomes. **F.** Diversion of cell surface pMHC class I complexes to the lysosomes.

against them. For example, *Chlamydia*, an intracellular bacterium, can prevent fusion between the phagosome in which it resides and lysosomes containing the enzymes that would otherwise kill and degrade it. Some pathogens secrete factors that interfere with the proliferation of nearby lymphocytes, while others produce enzymes that degrade complement molecules or immunoglobulins in their vicinity. Even organisms as small as viruses have developed several means to protect themselves from the immune system by inhibiting the presentation of virus-derived peptide fragments into MHC class I molecules and their expression on the surface of the infected cell (Fig. 7-14). Finally, some infectious organisms can trick the immune system into generating immune responses that are least detrimental to the organism. Organisms that are susceptible primarily to cellular responses may promote antibody-dominated responses, or vice versa.

Conclusion

The adaptive immune system builds and amplifies upon the defensive foundation established by the innate immune system. It adds several defensive features including (1) the random generation of antigen-specific receptors with far greater variety than is available in the innate system; (2) the ability to intensely focus a variety of destructive mechanisms (including those of the innate system) narrowly defined targets that vary among different infectious agents; and (3) the property of memory that allows the adaptive system to modify its response to stimuli that are encountered repeatedly. In concert with the innate immune system, the adaptive immune system provides a versatile and coordinated set of defensive responses capable of dealing with the invasive styles of a broad array of infectious agents.

chapter 8

The Parasite's Way of Life

Victor J. DiRita

In view of our long acquaintance with infectious diseases, it is not surprising that we tend to take an anthropomorphic view of our relationship with our microbial neighbors. Analogies to war are common, as in references to a microbial "attack" or "invasion" repelled by host "defense systems." In reality, what drives microbes is not aggression but survival and reproduction. To succeed, many microbes have evolved the ability to persist in the body, only incidentally causing disease, making them more analogous to unwanted houseguests than to invaders. Whether as aggressive pathogens or harmless commensals, microbial agents face many problems in their association with the host. To survive, microbes must do the following:

- Avoid being washed away (colonize the surfaces of host cells)
- Find a nutritionally compatible niche
- Survive the constitutive and induced defenses
- Transfer to a new host

Every successful commensal or pathogen has evolved a specific repertoire of strategies to face these challenges. Those strategies are discussed in detail in the chapters on individual agents. This chapter presents an overview of the mechanisms involved.

Surface Colonization

Picture a microbe entering the mouth and imagine the obstacles it faces trying to remain there. Strong liquid currents will wash it away unless the organism can adhere to the surface of the teeth or mucous membranes. At places not exposed to the flushing action of saliva, such as the crevices of the gums, the organism encounters a large **resident flora** that already occupies potential adherence sites outmaneuvering the resident microbes of the normal flora.

Colonization of microbes to host surfaces involves both microbial and host factors. Microbes elaborate substances or organelles that are involved in the adherence and are known as **adhesins** (Table 8-1). In many cases adhesins bind to special **receptors** on host surfaces. Both adhesins and receptors are usually highly specific for the species of microbes and the host.

Some Gram-negative bacteria position their adhesive molecules on the tips of long, slender structures—fimbriae or pili—as if "reaching out" for the host cell surface. **Fimbrial adhesins** interact with structural constituents of host epithelial cells, often

table **8-1**	Bacterial Adhesins
GRAM-NEGATIVE BACTERIA	**GRAM-POSITIVE BACTERIA**
Pili (fimbriae)	Surface proteins
Surface proteins (nonfimbrial)	Capsules
Capsules	

glycolipids. In other Gram-negative bacteria, adhesins are found directly on the cell surface and not on protrusions. An example of such an adhesin is **invasin,** a protein that recognizes normal cellular receptors on host cells called **integrins.** Integrins are receptors primarily involved in other processes, such as the adherence of white blood cells to endothelial surfaces, but at that site bacteria usurp the integrins for another use. Binding of bacteria by integrins results in an intimate association between the bacteria and the host cell membrane. Such an appropriation of normal host functions by microbes is a recurrent theme in pathogenic microbiology. The interplay between adhesins and host cell receptors is different in Gram-positive bacteria. A receptor for certain Gram-positive bacteria is the protein **fibronectin,** which normally coats the mucosal surfaces of epithelial cells. Fibronectin plays an important role in selecting the kind of bacterial flora in the mouth and pharynx, as suggested by the finding that the oropharynx of individuals in poor general health, including many hospitalized patients, is deficient in fibronectin. When levels of this protein are low, Gram-negative organisms tend to displace Gram-positive bacteria, in part because the fibronectin-denuded mucosal cells reveal the receptors for Gram-negative fimbrial adhesins. The greater incidence of pneumonia caused by Gram-negative bacteria in hospitalized patients can be explained in part by such adherence specificity.

The mouth, large intestine, vagina, perineum, skin, and other sites are normally laden with bacteria. Because the bacterial populations at these sites are fairly stable, it follows that colonization by new organisms is an unlikely event. The successful colonizer must be adept at outmaneuvering the resident microbes. On the other hand, microbial competition is not an important factor in colonization of sites that are normally sterile or carry a sparse load of microbes, such as all the deep tissues or the small intestine.

Obviously, in our long history of coexistence and coevolution with the microbial world, our bodies have learned what territory is safe to share and what is off limits; and we have managed to share this space preferentially with well-behaved guests. Foreign devices, like plastic catheters inserted into arteries and veins, may upset the delicate ecological balance between microbes and host tissues, partly because they allow bacteria and fungi to bypass the normal defenses and partly because they potentiate growth by organisms with the special ability to stick well to plastics (e.g., strains of *Staphylococcus epidermidis,* which are otherwise harmless skin residents; see Chapter 11).

Finding a Nutritionally Compatible Niche

To microbes, the human body would seem to be a rich nutritional environment. Body fluids such as plasma contain sugars, vitamins, minerals, and other substances that bacteria, fungi, and animal parasites can use for growth. Still, bacteria grow sparsely on fresh plasma in a test tube, primarily because of the presence of antimicrobial substances, such as lysozyme, constituents of the complement system, and antibodies. In addition, some nutrients are in short supply in body fluids. Plasma and most other body fluids, for example, contain very little **free iron.** The metal is highly insoluble and must be combined with avid iron-binding proteins for transport. The lack of free iron significantly limits the growth of bacteria in the body, because bacteria need iron for the synthesis of their cytochromes and other enzymes. The body may sequester iron even further in response to microbial invasion. When a sufficient number of organisms enters the body, iron-binding proteins are poured into plasma and tissue fluids, and the normally low amount of available iron is further reduced. Many bacteria respond to this challenge by excreting highly iron-avid compounds (chelators). After capturing an iron molecule, these compounds may contact another bacterium and deliver the iron to specific bacterial receptors (Chapter 3). Other bacteria possess surface molecules that can "steal" iron from the host's iron-binding proteins. Certain bacteria (e.g., some streptococci) scavenge intracellular iron by making toxins that destroy host cells, such as red blood cells.

Some microbes use specific nutrients found only in certain sites of the body. Thus, mouth strains of streptococci are adept at using dietary sucrose, which gives them a growth (and colonization) advantage over bacteria that do not have that ability. Even more startling is the example of brucellosis in cattle, which is caused by the microbe *Brucella abortus.* Brucellosis is a systemic disease in humans and other animals. In addition, brucellosis causes abortion in cattle and a few other animal species. The reason for this species-specific abortion is that the placentas of cattle and some other animals, but not humans, contain a 4-carbon sugar, erythritol, for which the organisms have a special affinity. An example of how finely tuned the physiology of *B. abortus* is to the presence of erythritol in the placenta is that this sugar increases the production of iron-scavenging molecules, which are also critical for growth in the animal, more than does any other sugar on which the microbe is capable of growing.

The spectrum of nutritional requirements of microbes that live in the body reflects their ecological habits. For instance, many of the bacteria found mainly in the human body, such as staphylococci or certain streptococci, have complex nutritional requirements and need several amino acids and vitamins for growth. Organisms found both in the body and in soil or water are usually much less picky and can fulfill their organic requirements with simple carbon compounds. Examples are *Escherichia coli* and many pseudomonads that can grow in the laboratory in "minimal media." Another connection between physiology and ecology is illustrated by a bacterium's oxygen requirements. Many of our most heavily colonized sites—for instance, the periodontal spaces and the colon—are anaerobic. Not surprisingly, the bacteria found in those sites are overwhelmingly anaerobic, with very few strict aerobes present.

Surviving the Constitutive and Induced Defenses

Many bacteria that enter the body do not survive because of the physical barriers and inhospitable microenvironments that they encounter. These factors are the host's first lines of defense against infection. However, over millennia of coevolution with their bacterial neighbors, mammals have also developed second lines of defense to deal with microbes that manage to evade the first-line defenses. How do microbial agents overcome these powerful defense mechanisms? How do they avoid the action of complement and phagocytosis or evade antigenic recognition by the host immune system?

Defending Against Complement

The most effective way to protect against the antimicrobial action of complement is to prevent its activation. Bacteria prevent complement activation in several ways (Table 8-2). One is by **masking** surface components that activate the alternative pathway. Lipopolysaccharides of Gram-negative bacteria, teichoic acids of Gram-positive bacteria, and other structural components of microbes are potential complement activators. Meningococci and pneumococci are examples of bacteria that prevent complement activation by secreting capsules that cover these activators (Fig. 8-1).

Some organisms take advantage of the host's own mechanism for avoiding complement activation. Most host cells incorporate **sialic acid,** a sugar that inhibits complement activation into their surface molecules. Many bacteria achieve the same protection by incorporating sialic acid into their capsular polysaccharides. When they grow in tissues, gonococci add sialic acid to the terminal sugar of their lipopolysaccharide, which makes them resistant to complement lysis. Meningococci employ a different strategy to avoid complement activation: they become coated with **circulating IgA antibodies,** a class of immunoglobulins that do not

table **8-2**	**Some Microbial Anticomplement Strategies**

1. Activate masking substances
   a. Coat with capsule (e.g., staphylococci)
   b. Coat with IgA antibodies (e.g., meningococci)
2. Apply appropriate inhibitor of activation to surface: bind factor H (e.g., *E. coli, Borrelia,* group B streptococci); bind decay-accelerating factors (e.g., schistosome); mimic component C4bp (e.g., vaccinia virus)
3. Cover up target of membrane attack complex (e.g., *E. coli,* salmonellae)
4. Inactivate complement chemotaxin C5a (e.g., group A streptococcus, *Pseudomonas aeruginosa*); activate surface of plasminogen to plasmin and cleave of C3b (e.g., *Staphylococcus aureus*)

activate the complement cascade (a "wolf in sheep's clothing" strategy). The IgA coating prevents other kinds of antibodies capable of setting off complement activation by the classical pathway from reaching the surface of the organisms.

Certain viruses have also evolved mechanisms to prevent complement activation. For example, herpes simplex virus has an **envelope glycoprotein** that binds **complement component C3b,** thus inhibiting activation by the alternative pathway (see Chapter 41). Cells infected with vaccinia virus secrete a virally encoded protein that shares amino acid homology with a complement control protein (C4bp). C4bp binds to the C4b fragment. By mimicking the action of the host C4bp, the

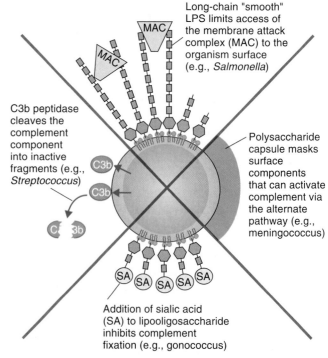

FIGURE 8-1 ■ **Mechanisms microbes use to prevent harmful effects of complement.**

virus limits complement activation by the classical pathway and causes the accelerated decay of C3 convertase. Mutants of vaccinia virus that lack the protein produce smaller, more rapidly healing skin lesions in experimental animals.

Some Gram-negative bacteria, such as *Salmonella* and *E. coli*, do not prevent formation of the complement **membrane attack complex** but rather hinder its access to its target, the bacterial outer membrane. "**Smooth**" **strains**, which have a long O-antigen polysaccharide chain, do not allow access of the membrane attack complex to their outer membrane, while "**rough**" **mutants**, which have little or no O antigen, are readily killed by it. The presence or absence of the O antigen correlates well with pathogenicity. Smooth strains tend to be virulent, while rough strains are not. However, capsules and other protective surface structures come with a price: most of them are highly antigenic and in time elicit the production of anticapsular antibodies that enable the activation of complement by the classical pathway. Notice that these organisms defend themselves better against the more immediate host defense, activation of complement by the alternative pathway, than against later events, the formation of antibodies.

Subverting Phagocytosis

Microbes employ a number of strategies to avoid being killed by phagocytes. The host attempts to overcome these microbial countermeasures, and in turn those efforts are answered by yet other microbial tactics. A point must be made at the outset: being phagocytized by a cell is not necessarily a bad thing from the microbe's point of view. Some microbes are able to grow within host cells, where they are shielded from antibodies and certain antimicrobial drugs. Such is the allure of intracellular growth that some microbes have evolved mechanisms to induce their uptake into cells of the host.

The following paragraphs present a few examples of strategies used by microbes to withstand the killing power of phagocytic cells. Various aspects of phagocytosis are affected, from the arrival of the phagocytes at the scene to the killing powers of phagocytic cells (Table 8-3).

Inhibiting Phagocyte Recruitment and Function

As previously discussed, some microbes prevent the activation of complement. In doing so they prevent the secondary release of neutrophil chemotaxins and opsonins, thus reducing the risk of encountering those cells as well as their function. Other organisms (e.g., *Bordetella pertussis*; see Chapter 19) directly inhibit neutrophil motility and chemotaxis by producing a toxin that increases cyclic adenosine monophosphate (AMP) to inhibitory levels. Group A streptococci produce a **C5a peptidase**

that specifically inactivates this chemotactic product of the complement cascade.

Microbial Killing of Phagocytes

Some pathogenic bacteria produce exotoxins called **leukocidins** to kill neutrophils and macrophages. Leukocidins are soluble products that work at a distance and thus may protect bacteria before the phagocytes come near them. In many cases, however, microbes kill after they are ingested. In this strategy the phagocyte commits suicide by carrying out phagocytosis (see Chapter 9). Typical leukocidin producers are highly invasive bacteria, such as pseudomonads, staphylococci, group A streptococci, and the clostridia that cause gas gangrene. Yersiniae produce proteins that are injected directly into host cells and interfere with cellular activation (see Chapter 17 paradigm), and through a similar injection mechanism, shigellae kill phagocytic cells.

Escaping Ingestion

A notable microbial counterdefense to phagocytosis is the capsule. One of the more captivating visual experiences in microbiology is to watch a preparation of live neutrophils and encapsulated pneumococci under the microscope: each time a neutrophil attempts to embrace a pneumococcus, the slimy bacterium squeezes away with what looks like total indifference, and repeated attempts are no more successful. The picture changes when a small amount of capsule-specific antiserum is added: the neutrophils have no trouble engulfing the opsonized pneumococci. Anticapsular antibodies thus provide protective immunity against infection by encapsulated bacteria. However, bacteria have evolved measures to counter opsonization, either by complement components or by specific antibodies. Any mechanism that inhibits activation of complement or synthesis or activity of antibodies will reduce the probability of opsonization.

Staphylococci, streptococci, and probably other bacteria have evolved a mechanism to reduce opsonization even when antibodies are present: they make a surface component, **protein A**, that binds to IgG molecules by the "wrong" end, the Fc portion. These antibodies therefore cannot act as opsonins because their orientation on the surface of the bacteria is reversed from what is required to bind to the Fc receptors on phagocytic cells. It is not known to what extent this antiphagocytic mechanism plays a role in actual infections.

How Microbes Survive Inside Phagocytes

Microbes have many ways to survive once they are taken up by host cells:

- **Inhibition of lysosome fusion with phagosomes:** When lysosomes fuse with phagosomes, they release powerful

table 8-3   Microbial Strategies to Evade Phagocyte Function

ANTIPHAGOCYTE ACTIVITY	MECHANISM	EXAMPLE
Avoid being phagocytized		
Diversion (to nonproductive use)	Activate complement C5a Leucoaggregation Pulmonary sequestration	Streptococci Gram-negative enterics
"Playing hard to get"	Slimy capsule on organisms M protein Pili	Pneumococci, meningococci, *Haemophilus influenzae*, *Bacteroides fragilis*, many others Group A streptococci Gonococci
Humiliation	Release adenylate cyclase, leading to high levels of cyclic adenosine monophosphate; all phagocyte functions depressed	*Bordetella pertussis* (toxin)
Paralysis	Make cells unresponsive to chemotactic factors Induce inhibitors of migration Inactivate chemotaxins (C5a)	*Capnocytophaga* Tubercle bacilli Leprosy bacilli *Pseudomonas* (elastase)
After being phagocytized		
Murder	Membrane lysis	Streptococci (streptolysins O and S) *Pseudomonas* (exotoxin A) *Staphylococcus aureus* (α-toxin)
Indifference (resist lysosomal enzymes)	 Protection by surface lipophosphoglycan	*Salmonella enterica* var. *typhimurium* mycobacteria spp. *Leishmania* spp.
Disablement (inhibit phagosome–lysosome fusion)	? Redirect phagosomal trafficking Remove host proteins from the phagosomal membrane	Tubercle bacilli *Legionella pneumophila* *Toxoplasma gondii*
Disablement (inhibit oxidative killing)	Inhibit respiratory burst Catalase breaks down H$_2$O$_2$	Virulent salmonellae *Legionella pneumophila* *Listeria monocytogenes* *Staphylococcus aureus*
Escape (from phagosome into cytoplasm)	Pore-forming hemolysins? Phospholipase (?)	*Listeria monocytogenes* *Shigella* Rickettsiae Influenza viruses

Modified from a table by Mark Klempner.

microbicidal substances (see Chapter 6). Inhibiting this fusion clearly benefits intraphagosomal microbes, such as the agents of tuberculosis, psittacosis, and legionnaires disease. How this inhibition is accomplished is an active area of investigation, and it is likely that compounds secreted or present on the surface of the microbes modify the phagosome membrane and alter the trafficking processes that would normally fuse the phagosome with the lysosome.

■ **Escape into the cytoplasm:** The shigellae, *Listeria monocytogenes*, and the rickettsiae cross the membrane of the phagocytic vesicle, the phagosome, and enter the cytoplasm. Because lysosomes do not release their contents in the cytoplasm, the microbes are protected from lysosomal enzymes in that site.

This escape is accomplished by destroying the phagosomal membrane. *L. monocytogenes* secretes a pore-forming toxin, **listeriolysin,** which is required for the phagosomal escape. A surface-bound phospholipase may also be responsible for weakening the phagosomal membrane.

■ **Resistance to lysosomal enzymes:** Some microbes are innately resistant to the lysosomal enzymes and survive in the phagolysosome, the vesicle formed by fusion of the lysosomes with the phagosomes. An example is the protozoa called *Leishmania*, which causes several severe tropical diseases. Resistance of *Leishmania* to lysosomal enzymes may be a result of resistant cell surfaces and to the excretion of enzyme inhibitors. Note that the pH of the phagolysosome may be as low as 4, which means that leishmaniae can thrive in an extreme environment.

- **Inhibition of the phagocytes' oxidative pathway:** Some microbes, such as *Legionella*, inhibit the hexose-monophosphate shunt and oxygen consumption in neutrophils, thus reducing the respiratory burst used by these cells for killing engulfed microbes. Others, such as some staphylococci, produce a powerful catalase that breaks down the hydrogen peroxide necessary for oxidative killing.

Intracellular Life

Many bacteria, protozoa, and fungi have adapted to intracellular existence within the host. This lifestyle is obviously obligatory for viruses but not for organisms capable of free existence. The advantages of a free existence are clear: while inside host cells, the organisms are protected from antibodies and some antimicrobial drugs. However, intracellular residence is not without peril and requires ingenious forms of adaptation. An intense subject of current research, intracellular existence requires the expression of specific microbial genes and the usurpation of normal cell functions. The following paragraphs describe some issues associated with intracellular existence.

Penetration

Penetration of the host cell by a microbe is not a problem when the cell is a professional phagocyte, such as a neutrophil or macrophage. However, taking up microbes is not a normal activity for other types of cells. Thus, penetration is often induced by microbial activities, including binding to specific receptors and sending signals to the interior of the cell that stimulate uptake by rearrangements of the cellular cytoskeleton.

Surviving Host Cell Defenses

As previously mentioned, microbes have developed a repertoire of strategies to avoid or resist antimicrobial factors such as the lysosomal contents. So successful are some parasites that they grow within dedicated antimicrobial cells, such as macrophages. Members of *Ehrlichia* thrive even within the most powerfully antimicrobial of cells, the neutrophils.

Transmission to Other Cells

When the growth of microbes results in the lysis of the host cell, transmission through the blood or body fluids can take place directly. Other organisms do not impair the cell's integrity, but they can spread from cell to cell directly, without exposing themselves to the extracellular environment. Several viruses spread by causing infected cells to fuse with uninfected, neighboring cells. The histopathology associated with these viral infections (e.g., herpes simplex virus, varicella zoster virus, and respiratory syncytial virus) are notable for the formation of **syncytia** and **multinucleated giant cells**.

Some bacteria can also spread directly from one cell to another. This type of spread is accomplished by making intricate use of the host cytoskeleton. For example, *Shigella* species and *L. monocytogenes* induce polymerization of actin at one of their ends, which results in the formation of a cytoskeletal scaffold at that end (Fig. 8-2). In the electron microscope, this scaffold can be visualized as a cometlike trail behind the bacterium, with actin polymerizing at the "head" and depolymerizing throughout the "tail." As more actin polymers are formed at the bacterial surface, the organisms are pushed ahead and can be observed microscopically to be moving through the host cell cytoplasm. If the bacteria reach the cell membrane,

FIGURE 8-2 ▪ **Actin-dependent intracellular motility and intercellular spread. A.** The bacterium is ingested by conventional phagocytosis and resides briefly in a membrane-bound phagosome. **B** and **C.** The ingested bacterium lyses the phagosomal membrane surrounding it. **D.** After escaping into the cytoplasm, the organism may divide. **E.** Actin polymerizes at one pole of each bacterium. **F.** Continued actin polymerization forms scaffolding that propels the bacteria through the cytoplasm in random directions. **G.** Both bacteria encounter the cell membrane and continue to move outward; one is pushing toward a second cell, the other into an extracellular space. **H.** The second cell has ingested one of the bacteria, its actin tail, and some of the cell membrane and cytoplasm from its neighbor. Eventually, this bacterium will be released into the cytoplasm of the second host cell.

they push out fingerlike projections, each containing one bacterium. These projections extend into adjacent cells, where they are eventually engulfed and snipped off. The microbes are now within two sets of membranes: one from the original cell and the other from the neighboring cell. Through production of membrane-damaging enzymes, they cross these membranes into the cytoplasm of a new host cell.

Subverting the Immune Responses

As with their ability to evade phagocytosis, microbes have many ways to avoid clearance by other arms of the immune system. Some of these are aimed broadly at the general immune responsiveness of the host, whereas others more specifically target the precise host response to a specific pathogen.

Immunosuppression

Some infectious agents protect themselves by inducing a general suppression of the host's immune responses. The outcome is that the host becomes susceptible to all kinds of agents and the threat to survival is heightened. Patients infected by immunosupressive agents may suffer from several concurrent infections, which expands considerably the complexities of their clinical problems. The ability of infectious agents to cause immunodeficiency has reached its known limit with AIDS. Immunodeficiency in this disease is especially profound because HIV, the AIDS virus, infects the CD4+ (inducer-helper) subset of lymphocytes (see Chapter 6), leading to the collapse of the immune system (see Chapter 38).

The regulatory interactions of the immunocompetent cells may go awry even when lesser changes are introduced into the network. Long before AIDS, it was known that infection with measles virus is immunosuppressive. It had been noticed, for example, that tuberculosis was more common in a community after a widespread measles outbreak. Immunosuppression has been found to follow other viral infections as well, like hepatitis B and influenza. These viruses function more subtly than HIV, impairing the function of lymphoid or myeloid cells without causing major structural changes.

In some cases immune suppression results from inhibition of the synthesis or of the function of selected cytokines, which stimulate the proliferation and differentiation of lymphocytes. Cytokines, themselves the secreted products of inflammatory and immunodirected cells, act to amplify the inflammatory response (see Chapter 6). Mycobacteria, certain viruses, and some multicellular parasites have been shown to affect different steps in the cytokine cascade, perhaps thereby enhancing the pathogen's persistence in the host.

Another mechanism for immune suppression carried out by some bacteria and many viruses is to target the process of antigen presentation carried out by infected cells. To revisit the mechanism of antibody formation or

stimulation of a cellular response (see Chapter 7), recall that antigen-presenting cells display on their surfaces the peptides derived from antigens they engulfed. Such peptides are "presented"—that is, reach the cell surface—in association with major histocompatibility complex (MHC) class I or class II molecules. These complexes are recognized by T cells, setting in motion the processes of cell-mediated immunity or specific helper functions to enhance antibody production. Some pathogens specifically disarm MHC class I or class II function, thereby removing a major process for amplifying the immune response.

Diversion of Lymphocyte Function: Superantigens

Certain bacteria and viruses have evolved a particularly insidious strategy to subvert the immune response. Instead of suppressing immune functions, they actually stimulate them, but in a manner that squanders these important defensive tools in a nonproductive way. An example are toxins made by certain streptococci, called **superantigens**, which stimulate a **nonspecific T-cell response**. A large subpopulation of T cells is stimulated by superantigens, but these cells have specificities that are mostly unrelated to streptococcal antigens. This misdirection of the immune response not only keeps the host from mounting a proper response but also unleashes a toxic cascade of cytokines.

FIGURE 8-3 ■ **A comparison of antigen-mediated and superantigen-mediated T-cell activation.** Both antigens and superantigens bring antigen-presenting cells and T cells together. Antigens, in conjunction with major histocompatibility complex (MHC) class II molecules, interact with the specific antigen-binding domain of the T-cell receptor (TCR). In contrast, superantigens form a bridge between the two molecules that does not involve the antigen-binding groove. Instead, they bind to a portion of the TCR, the Vβ domain. Every T cell has a TCR with one of numerous Vβ types. Each superantigen binds preferentially to one Vβ type and can activate any T cell carrying that type, regardless of the specificity of the TCR for antigen.

Superantigens take a shortcut, binding directly to both the MHC molecule (but not at the antigen-binding groove) and the T-cell receptor (but not at the antigen recognition sites; Fig. 8-3). Because it is not dependent on specific antigen recognition, superantigen binding occurs on the surface of many more antigen-presenting cells than is usual and thus leads to the diversion of these cells to nonproductive uses. As an example of why these compounds are known as superantigens, consider that normally 1 in 10,000 antigen-presenting cells is stimulated by processed antigens, whereas the figure for superantigens is as high as 1 in 5. The result is an overwhelming, but wholly inappropriate, immune response that can be lethal. The advantage, if any, to the microbe that produces such a response is unclear.

Masquerading by Changing Antigenic Coats

Certain bacteria, viruses, and protozoa are unusually adept at frustrating immune recognition by changing their surface antigens. The classical cases are trypanosomes, gonococci (the agents of relapsing fever), and influenza viruses (see Chapter 14 paradigm).

Trypanosomes One of the best-studied examples of antigenic variation is seen with the protozoan that causes sleeping sickness, *Trypanosoma brucei*. The organism affects humans and domestic animals and infects the blood and interstitial fluids. Thus, the organisms are exposed to circulating antibodies. Trypanosomes are covered with a thick protein coat called **variable surface glycoprotein,** which undergoes periodic antigenic changes during the infection. These parasites have several hundred genes that encode for various antigens, but they express only one at a time (see Chapter 50). When antibodies against one type are made, the number of parasites in the blood of an infected host drops, but they are soon replaced by a new antigenic type. There can be many successive waves of antigenically different parasites in a single host. Thus, protective immunity does not function in the long term against this master of disguise.

Gonococci Like the trypanosomes, some bacteria can also switch their surface antigens. For example. gonococcus undergoes periodic changes in **pilin,** which is the protein that makes up its pili, the apparent means of attachment of host cells (see Chapters 3 and 14). This enables multiple new gonococcal infections, because the immune response an infected individual may raise to one antigenic type does not protect against a variant that may cause a subsequent infection. The borreliae also undergo antigenic variation of their major surface antigen in a manner that is analogous to the trypanosomes (Fig. 8-4). Thus, the surface of these organisms displays a highly variable antigenic profile to the host immune system, causing relapsing fever every time a new antigenic type emerges.

Influenza viruses The tendency of influenza to reappear in a population on a regular basis is due in part to the great ability of the influenza virus to change its antigenic composition. This is also the major obstacle to developing a

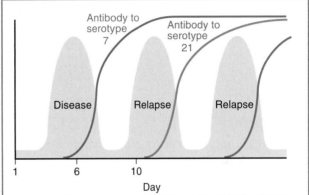

FIGURE 8-4 ▪ **An experimental infection in which the development of type-specific antibodies against *Borrelia* sp. is associated with the emergence of new antigenic types.** The emergence of each new type is associated with a relapse of disease; thus, the common name for these *Borrelia* infections—"relapsing fever." The rapid emergence of the new antigenic types is mediated by successive DNA rearrangement.

truly effective vaccine against this pathogen. Unlike the processes of antigenic variation in trypanosomes and gonococci, antigenic changes in influenza viruses do not emerge repeatedly within individual hosts. Instead, the novel antigenic types develop gradually in a population of viruses over the course of an epidemic season. Minor changes are called **antigenic drift** and occur every 2 or 3 years. Major antigenic changes, called **antigenic shifts,** take place every 10 years or so. These changes involve two surface proteins: a **hemagglutinin** that serves to bind to cell surface receptors and a **neuraminidase** that changes these receptors. How these proteins are involved in attachment and penetration of the virus is discussed in Chapter 36.

Proteolysis of Antibodies

Certain bacteria—gonococci, meningococci, and *Haemophilus influenzae*—and some dental pathogenic streptococci make extracellular proteases that specifically inactivate antibodies of the secretory IgA class. They cleave IgA molecules at the hinge region to yield complete but relatively ineffective fragments. The proteases are present in active form in tissues and fluids infected by the bacteria that produce them. Nonpathogenic relatives of these organisms are protease-negative. The absence of proteases in nonpathogenic bacteria suggests, although it does not prove, a role for IgA proteases in pathogenesis. Other mechanisms, perhaps more subtle, exist for destroying immunoglobulins. For example, staphylococci produce **staphylokinase,** which cleaves host plasminogen into plasmin at the bacterial cell surface. This serine protease then degrades both immunoglobulin G and the complement protein C3b (see Table 8-2), which enables the microbe to avoid opsonization and phagocytosis.

In some instances it is known that when an organism cleaves IgA, the antigen-binding fragment (Fab) remains attached. The attached Fab fragment makes the antigens unavailable for binding by intact antibody molecules. This phenomenon has been called **fabulation** (after "Fab") and may serve to protect organisms from antibodies. Fabulation may be more widely used by pathogens than is currently known.

Viral Latency

The more chronic an infection, the more lasting must be the mechanisms for microbial evasion of host defenses. This tenet is well illustrated in herpes infection. To limit access from circulating defenses, herpes viruses do not usually enter the extracellular fluid but pass from cell to cell over cytoplasmic bridges. Intracellular herpesviruses reside within certain cells but do not proliferate; therefore, such a virus can avoid a host response and remain in a state called **latency** (see Chapters 41 and 42). A latent virus is not affected by antibodies, cell-mediated immunity, or interferon and can survive for a long time in an immunocompetent host. Later, often when the host's defenses have subsided, the virus may reactivate to cause disease and perhaps even cancer.

Latent infections are not unique to viruses; many pathogenic bacteria remain in chronic association with the host, either asymptomatically or with limited host response that is insufficient for clearing the infection. Important examples are *Helicobacter pylori*, which causes gastric ulcers and probably is responsible for gastric adenocarcinomas (see Chapter 22), and the tubercle bacillus *Mycobacterium tuberculosis* (see Chapter 23).

Transmission to a New Host

Infectious agents are carried into a new host through food, drinks, aerosols, bites, or sexual contact or by introduction into a wound from the skin or soil. Although these modes of transmission may seem passive, many infectious agents contribute actively to their transmission to new hosts. They do this by taking on traits specific for transmission, or by producing molecules that cause the host to participate in transmissions.

Many microbes **differentiate** into a **transit form,** a stage in their life cycle that helps them survive in the environment and in reservoirs or, if vectorborne, in insects. Among the animal parasites, transit forms usually differ greatly in structure and function from those that cause disease in the host, as in the case of worms or the protozoa that cause malaria. Note that living reservoirs and vectors shield infectious agents from deleterious environmental factors and obviate the need for the transit form to be highly resistant. In certain bacteria, such as the chlamydiae, the transit form (in this case called the elementary body) becomes encased in a tough envelope composed of highly cross-linked proteins (see Chapter 27). The chlamydiae elemental body is thus reminiscent of the bacterial spore, the environmentally tough life form par excellence. In other bacteria—for instance, the enterics—changes are more subtle and are revealed at the level of selective expression of certain genes, such as those involved in entering the stationary phase of growth.

An active area of investigation is how infectious agents know where they are—that is, how they express different sets of genes outside and inside the body. The problems of transit are minimized when contact between hosts is direct and the agent is not subjected to prolonged exposure to the environment. In this context it is logical that many sexually transmitted agents do not appear to have developed tough transit forms. For example, the gonococci, the treponemes of syphilis, and HIV are particularly sensitive to drying and chemicals (chlamydiae may be an exception).

Microbes can actively **potentiate** their spread from one host to another, thus providing themselves with new feeding grounds. Examples are organisms that cause diarrhea (e.g., *Vibrio cholerae* and pathogenic strains of *E. coli* or *Shigella*), which is an effective way of spreading large amounts of bacteria-laden intestinal contents in the environment. Agents that induce coughing (e.g., *M. tuberculosis*) lead to their dispersal via aerosols, and those that produce exudative lesions on the skin (e.g., *Streptococcus pyogenes*) are transmitted through the contamination of objects or skin.

Some of the mechanisms developed by microbes for actively enhancing their transmission seem fiendishly clever. For example, the agent of plague, *Yersinia pestis*, is transmitted from an infected human to another by a flea bite. These bacteria greatly increase the efficiency of this transmission by making the flea feel hungry. How do the bacteria enhance the flea's appetite? The plague bacilli reproduce within the digestive tract of infected fleas, eventually causing blockage. To ward off starvation, the "blocked fleas" feed repeatedly and, during each feeding, regurgitate some of the contaminated material, thus increasing the chances of infecting a new host. Not all pathogens that are transmitted by insects use such a mechanism, but it should not be surprising that many microbes alter an arthropod vector's behavior to enhance their own survival and transmissibility.

Conclusion

The ways of microbes that must make a living by interacting with hosts are as complex and varied as the mechanisms that have evolved in hosts to avoid infection. The story of microbial diseases is one of progressively escalating rounds of response and counterresponse from each side, the microbe and the host. The measures taken by each can be general or very specific; for every constitutive immune mechanism that hosts have to protect themselves, there is a microbe out there with the capacity to avoid it. Likewise, although the development of specific immunity is generally very effective for protecting against second infection, some microbes have developed impressive ways to steer clear of that response. The exquisite specificity of these responses points to coevolution of hosts and microbes. Given that microbes can go through multiple generations in a very short time and that they are constantly subject to new selection pressures, it is not surprising to find remarkable variation among pathogenic species.

Damage by Microbial Toxins

Joseph T. Barbieri

Infectious diseases inflict many kinds of damage to host tissues and organs. Advances in our understanding of the action of microbial toxins, coupled with our progress in understanding the molecular biology of the human cell, provide a framework to understand the molecular basis for microbial pathogenesis and the host response to infection. Damage during the infectious processes may be caused by the direct action of the microbial pathogen or by the host's response to infection. These actions are often interrelated, and both are usually active during an infection. This chapter presents an overview of the cellular damage that occurs during infection and provides detailed descriptions of the major classes of microbial toxins.

Mechanisms That Damage the Host During Infections

Cell Death

The most dramatic effect of a microbial infection is the death of cells in host tissues. The pathology associated with cell death depends on the type and number of cells involved and the speed of the infectious process. If the infected cells are a component of an essential organ, such as the heart or the brain, the outcome is likely to be serious and could be fatal. For example, myocarditis, an infection of the heart muscle, is a fulminating and deadly disease when caused by the coxsackievirus. This virus is also thought to kill the insulin-producing cells of the islets of the pancreas and may be one cause of infantile diabetes. During a microbial infection, two mechanisms lead to cell death: cell lysis and programmed cell death.

Lysis of Host Cells

Lysis of host cells occurs in three ways:

- The microorganism produces a toxin that affects the integrity of the cell membranes. In patients with **gas gangrene,** membrane-damaging toxins produced by one of the anaerobic clostridia lyse red blood cells.
- The microorganism multiplies within the host cell, leading to cell lysis. This is seen in **Rocky Mountain spotted fever,** which derives its name from the skin rash produced when endothelial cells of small vessels are killed by the intracellular growth of the infecting rickettsiae. The infected cells are eradicated by killer lymphocytes as the

result of cell-mediated immunity. This is observed when microorganisms such as viruses or the tubercle bacilli grow intracellularly without directly causing lysis.

Programmed Cell Death (Apoptosis) of Infected Cells

Programmed cell death, or **apoptosis**, is a normal part of the mammalian cell cycle that ensures the maintenance of healthy cells. Some microorganisms, such as *Shigella* (the agent of dysentery), usurp this process when invading the host cell. That might explain why *Shigella* survives after being taken up by phagocytes. Some viruses, such as herpes simplex virus and HIV, may stimulate cells to undergo premature apoptosis. In contrast, viruses like the Epstein-Barr virus, block apoptosis and thereby immortalize the host cell.

Pharmacologic Alterations of Metabolism

Certain infections do not kill cells directly but result in some of the most severe diseases, such as **tetanus, botulism, cholera,** and **whooping cough.** The pathology of each of these diseases is the result of a bacterium-produced toxin that alters a key aspect of metabolism in ways that resemble the action of hormones or other pharmacological effectors.

Mechanical Causes of Cell Death

If present in sufficient numbers, infectious agents can obstruct vital passages. Although rare, such mechanical obstructions do occur in children with an overload of worms in their intestines. A heavy infestation with the large roundworm *Ascaris* (15 to 35 cm long and about 0.5 cm thick) can cause occlusion of the intestinal lumen. A single worm may also migrate into the common bile duct and obstruct the passage of bile.

Often mechanical obstruction results not from the microorganism but from the inflammatory response of the host. In **elephantiasis,** an enormous swelling of limbs or the scrotum is caused when small worms, called filariae, become lodged in lymphatics. The worms stimulate a tissue reaction that occludes the vessels, causing swelling and tissue hypertrophy. Almost any duct or tubelike organ, thick or thin, can be obstructed during an infection, sometimes with life-threatening consequences. Inflammation of the epiglottis may impede the passage of air; infection of the meninges can cause hydrocephalus (a dilatation of the cerebral ventricles resulting from obstruction of the flow of cerebrospinal fluid); infection of the prostate can obstruct the flow of urine from the bladder; and an inflammatory reaction to the eggs of the liver fluke may result in severe disturbances of the portal circulation.

Damage Caused by Host Responses

The symptoms of infectious diseases are typically the product of the microbial pathogen and the host's response to infection. The host response is rarely so finely tuned that only the infection is controlled. In gonorrhea, the gonococci set off the host response, an inflammation that accompanies copious pus production and swelling and accounts for disease symptoms. Likewise, in many chronic infections, like tuberculosis, damage to tissues is caused by chronic inflammation.

The host response to infection is often owing to both **inflammation** and the **immune response.** The importance of these mechanisms cannot be overemphasized. Both operate in acute and chronic diseases and can manifest either locally or systemically. The mechanisms involved in inflammation are discussed in detail in Chapter 6, and those involved in immunopathology are discussed in Chapter 7. The role of inflammation and the immune response on cell damage will be further emphasized in chapters on individual diseases, where they may occupy center stage.

Examples of host responses to infection leading to harmful outcomes for the host include (1) the accentuated inflammatory response that places patients with a brain abscess at risk of dying, (2) the overwhelming activation of the **complement** system that kills patients suffering from septicemia, (3) an autoimmune response that causes rheumatic fever, and (4) cell-mediated immunity responsible for manifestations of chronic tuberculosis. In circumstances like these, medical intervention is required to attenuate the inflammatory response to infectious disease. Although the overemphatic expression of the host response contributes greatly to the immediate signs and symptoms of disease, it also helps the host survive. This is illustrated by tuberculosis, a chronic disease that some patients live with for many years. However, if the host response is defective, as in AIDS, tuberculosis can progress rapidly to a lethal infection.

Bacterial Toxins

Bacterial **toxins** alter the normal metabolism of host cells with deleterious effects on the host. Toxins are often responsible for the major symptoms of a bacterial infection. Knowledge of how toxins work fosters an understanding of the pathophysiology of many infectious diseases and, in some instances, reveals important information about normal cellular processes of the host. The role of many toxins in causing disease has been studied in detail and will be described in the chapters on specific bacterial pathogens. Here the discussion focuses on the basic concept of how bacterial toxins damage the host. Although many toxins have been associated with bacterial diseases, toxins have not been implicated as important compo-

Exotoxins (AB)   **Type III cytotoxins**

FIGURE 9-1 ▪ **Bacterial toxins that modify intracellular host proteins.** Most bacterial exotoxins bind to receptors on the surface of host cells and travel into the intracellular environment using the host's endocytotic pathway. After it matures, the endosome acidifies, stimulating a conformational change in the B domain, which inserts into the endosome membranes to generate a pore that is involved in the translocation of the A domain into the cytosol. Type III cytotoxins are synthesized in the cytosol of the bacterium and are delivered into the host cell by the type III secretion system. Thus, the bacterium provides the B domain function. Once inside the cell, type III cytotoxins subvert host cell physiology by direct cytotoxicity or by modulation of the host actin cytoskeleton.

nents of diseases caused by fungi, protozoa, or worms. Bacterial toxins are categorized by their site of action in the host. **Exotoxins and type III cytotoxins** modulate intracellular targets (Fig. 9-1); **endotoxin, membrane-damaging toxins,** and **superantigens** act on the cell surface (Fig. 9-2); and **exoenzymes** modulate targets in the extracellular matrix.

Toxins that Modulate Intracellular Targets

Toxins that modulate intracellular targets possess enter cells and modify host targets through covalent mechanisms. Exotoxins are organized into three distinct domains that can bind surface receptors and stimulate the

FIGURE 9-2 ▪ **Toxins that act on the surface of host cells.** Pattern recognition receptors include lipoteichoic acid (TCA), the endotoxin lipopolysaccharide (LPS), and flagella (FLA), which bind to specific toll-like receptor (TLR) proteins. Binding to the TLR stimulates intracellular signal transduction, which results in the production of cytokines that activate both the innate and adaptive immune systems. Pore-forming toxins bind to the host's cell membrane and polymerize to form a pore that allows ions and water to pass. Superantigens bind to the MHC and T-cell receptor (TCR) to stimulate an antigen-independent production of antibodies and cytokines.

anthrax = dangerous infectious disease of cattle & sheep, which can passed to humans.

CHAPTER 9 Damage by Microbial Toxins **129**

change of position

translocation of a catalytic domain into the cytosol of the host cell. In contrast, bacteria directly inject type-III cytotoxins into the host cell.

Exotoxins

Exotoxins are proteins usually secreted by the bacterium into the surrounding medium by the type I secretion system (an autotransport system built into the toxin) or the type II secretion system (an apparatus within the bacterial cell membrane), which transport toxins out of the bacterial cell. Occasionally, exotoxins are bound to the surface or synthesized in the cytoplasm of the bacterium and released on lysis of the cell. Exotoxins circulate throughout the host, attach to receptors on the surface of sensitive cells, and possess the ability to become internalized into the host cell and then delivered into the intracellular compartment of the host cell (see Fig. 9-1). Bacterial exotoxins vary in their specificity; some act only on specific cells, while others affect a wide range of cells and tissues. Some bacteria make a single toxin, while other bacteria produce numerous toxins (Table 9-1). Some bacteria, like the pneumococci, make no known toxins and probably cause disease by toxin-independent mechanisms.

For each toxin-producing pathogen, it is ideal to know whether the toxin is important in the infectious process. Answering the following questions can help make that determination:

- Does the toxin alone, in purified form, damage the host, using animals or cultured cells as experimental hosts?
- Is virulence quantitatively correlated with toxin production?
- Can a specific antibody (antitoxin) prevent or alleviate [*v relief*] the manifestations of the disease? [*expression*]
- If toxin production is impaired in the pathogen, is the disease process affected?

When a toxin contributes to the infectious process, the following questions need to be answered:

- What is the toxin's mechanism of action?
- Why does the toxin damage certain cells or tissues?
- Does the pathogen make other toxins? Do these toxins interact during an infection?

These questions are easiest to answer when a single toxin is responsible for the symptoms of the disease, which is the case in cholera, diphtheria, tetanus, and botulism. In contrast, many pathogenic bacteria, such as staphylococci, streptococci, and bordetellae, make several toxins. In such multifactorial situations, the importance of any one toxin is difficult to assess. [*uncertain*]

Toxins share with antibiotics an ambivalent position in the life of the pathogen that produces them. On the one hand, toxins are dispensable because they are not required [*pump*] for bacterial growth. On the other hand, toxins may be essential for the survival and spread of the bacteria within the host. Reflecting their dispensability, the genes that encode toxins are frequently contained within DNA elements that are themselves dispensable: **plasmids** and **temperate bacteriophages**. The locations of these genes on mobile DNA molecules ensure that the ability to produce toxin can rapidly spread to nontoxigenic bacteria. Conversely, these genetic elements may be lost by "curing" the bacteria of [*recovery*] plasmids or prophages. Some toxins are produced continuously by growing bacteria; others are synthesized when the bacteria enter the **stationary phase**. The latter is often also true for antibiotics and other "secondary metabolites," which are produced as growth stops or slows down. In some instances, producing toxin only when the growth rate slows makes sense, because the toxin helps the bacterium obtain nutrients that have become scarce. Thus, high levels of diphtheria toxin are produced only when the diphtheria bacilli are iron starved. Because little free iron exists in normal tissues, it is believed that pathogenic bacteria obtain iron from cells killed by the toxin.

Sporulating bacteria sometimes release toxins during spore formation. In this process the bacterial cells in which the spores are formed eventually lyse, leading to the liberation of cytoplasmic proteins—including accumulated toxins. Sporulating bacteria that make potent exotoxins include the organisms that cause botulism, gas gangrene, and tetanus, which are of the genus *Clostridium*, and the organisms that cause anthrax, which are of the genus *Bacillus*. In a heterogeneous environment, such as a contaminated wound, some organisms are growing and others are sporulating. In such an environment, toxins will be produced continuously during the course of the infection.

Bacterial toxins work at extraordinarily low concentrations and are among the strongest poisons for humans. One gram of tetanus, botulinum, or shiga toxin can kill about 10 million people; thus, 1 pound could theoretically kill all humankind. In contrast, humans are about a hundredfold more resistant to the action of diphtheria toxin.

Structure-function organization of exotoxins Most exotoxins are proteins with an **A domain** and a **B domain** (Fig. 9-3). The B domain binds to the cell membrane and delivers the A domain into the host cell. The A domain possesses enzymatic activity that is specific for each toxin. One example of an enzymatic reaction catalyzed by bacteria toxins is the adenosine diphosphate (ADP) ribosylation of host proteins, resulting from the covalent transfer of ADP ribose from the coenzyme nicotinamide adenine dinucleotide (NAD) to target proteins. These **ADP ribosyltransferases** are exemplified by diphtheria toxin, cholera toxin, and exotoxin A of *Pseudomonas aeruginosa*. Other exotoxins express different enzymatic activities and may act as proteases, glucosyltransferases, or deamidases.

Exotoxins are organized in various ways. An exotoxin can be a single AB protein in which the A and B domains are covalently joined, as observed in diphtheria toxin, or it can be a complex of six proteins noncovalently bound with the stoichiometry of A:5B, as seen in cholera toxin. Some exotoxins, such as anthrax toxin, are synthesized by bacteria as independent proteins that associate on the host cell membrane (2A + B). Anthrax

table 9-1   Major Toxinogenic Organisms

ORGANISM (TOXIN AND AB ORGANIZATION COMPONENT)	EFFECT	MECHANISM
Bacillus anthracis		
Anthrax toxin 2A+B	Required for other toxins	Receptor binding domain
Protective antigen B		
Edema factor A	Edema	Adenylate cyclase
Lethal factor A	Pulmonary edema	Protease
Bordetella pertussis		
Adenylate cyclase toxin AB	Inhibits, kills white cells	Adenylate cyclase
Pertussis toxin AB5	Many hormonal effects	ADP ribosylation of G protein
Tracheal cytotoxin	Kills cilia-bearing cells	Unknown
Campylobacter jejuni		
Enterotoxin AB5	Diarrhea	ADP ribosylates G protein
Clostridium botulinum		
Botulinum toxin AB	Neurotoxin	Blocks neuromuscular presynaptic junctions; flaccid paralysis
Clostridium difficile		
Enterotoxin	Hemorrhagic diarrhea	Acts at membrane
Cytotoxin AB	Cytoplasmic; cells lose filaments	Deamidation of RhoGTPase
Clostridia spp.		
α-toxin	Necrosis in gas gangrene; cytolytic, lethal	Phospholipase C
β-toxin	Necrotic enteritis	Unknown
Enterotoxin	Food poisoning; diarrhea	Cytotoxin; damages membranes
Clostridium tetani		
Tetanus toxin AB	Neurotoxin	Inhibits GABA and glycine release from nerve terminals at inhibitor synapses; spastic paralysis
Corynebacterium diphtheriae		
Diphtheria toxin AB	Kills cells	ADP ribosylates elongation factor 2
***Escherichia coli* (enterics)**		
Heat-labile enterotoxin AB5	Diarrhea	Identical to cholera toxin
Cytotoxin	Hemorrhagic colitis	Like shiga toxin
Heat-stable enterotoxin	Diarrhea	Actives host guanylate cyclase
Legionella pneumophila		
Cytotoxin	Lyses cells	Unknown
Listeria monocytogenes		
Listeriolysin	Membrane damage	Like streptolysin O
Pseudomonas aeruginosa		
Exotoxin A	Kills cells	Like diphtheria toxin
Type III cytotoxins	Modulate host cell physiology	Inhibit actin cytoskeleton
Salmonella		
Type III cytotoxins	Modulate host cell physiology	Alter actin cytoskeleton

(continued)

table **9-1**	**Major Toxinogenic Organisms** *(Continued)*	
ORGANISM (TOXIN AND AB ORGANIZATION COMPONENT)	**EFFECT**	**MECHANISM**
Shigella dysenteriae		
Shiga toxin	Kills cells	Inactivates 60S ribosomes
Staphylococcus aureus		
α-toxin	Hemolytic, leukocytic, paralysis of smooth muscle	Pore-forming toxin
β-toxin	Cytolytic	Sphingomyelinase
δ-lysin	Cytolytic	Detergent-like action
Superantigens		
Enterotoxins	Food poisoning (emesis, diarrhea)	Activate host antibody and cytokine synthesis by an antigen independent mechanism
Toxic shock syndrome toxin	Fever, headache, arthralgia, neutropenia, rash	Activate host antibody and cytokine synthesis by an antigen independent mechanism
Exfoliating toxin	Sloughing of skin ("scalded skin syndrome")	Protease
Streptococcus pneumoniae		
Pneumolysin	Cytolysin	Similar to streptolysin O
Streptococcus pyogenes		
Streptolysin O	Cytolysin	Pore-forming toxin
Erythrogenic toxin	Fever, neutropenia, rash of scarlet fever	Mediated through IL-1
Vibrio cholerae		
Cholera toxin AB5	Diarrhea	Hormone-independent activation of adenyl cyclase
Yersinia enterocolitica		
Heat-stable enterotoxin	Diarrhea	Activate host guanylate cyclase
Type III cytotoxins	Modulate host cell physiology	Regulate actin cytoskeleton

ADP, adenosine diphosphate; GABA, gamma-aminobutyric acid; IL, interleukin.

[handwritten: edema = excessive accumula of serum-like fluid in tissue spaces or body cavity]
[handwritten: lethal = capable cause death]

toxin is a tripartite toxin with two A domains produced: A1 is an adenylate cyclase (termed the edema factor), and A2 is a protease (termed the lethal factor).

Exotoxins are synthesized as protoxins that must be activated on binding to the host cell membrane. Diphtheria, cholera, tetanus, and shiga toxins must be activated to become toxic. Activation usually involves a proteolytic cleavage and reduction of a disulfide bond that often holds the A and B domains together.

After binding to the cell membrane, exotoxins are typically internalized into the cell by a **receptor-mediated endocytosis** mechanism. During this process the A domain is translocated across the cell membrane and into the intracellular compartment of the host cell, where it modifies host components. Although host proteins are the typical targets for modification, shiga toxin inhibits host protein synthesis by modifying RNA.

While diphtheria and cholera toxins are members of the ADP-ribosylating family of exotoxins, the botulinum and tetanus toxins are neurotoxins, which are zinc proteases. The molecular aspects of theses exotoxins are described in the following paragraphs.

Diphtheria toxin. The diphtheria toxin inhibits cell physiology by blocking host cell protein synthesis. After binding to a cell membrane receptor, diphtheria toxin is cleaved at a protease-sensitive site between the A and B domains, which remain covalently associated by disulfide linkage. The diphtheria toxin–receptor complex then enters the cell by receptor-mediated endocytosis, just like hormones and many enveloped viruses. Once inside the endosomal vesicle, reduction of the disulfide bond separates the toxin into its A and B domains. The acidic conditions within the vesicle promote insertion of a portion of the B domain into the endosomal membrane, which forms a pore to facilitate passage of the A domain into the cytosol. Thus, the B domain contributes three functions for the delivery of the A domain into the cytosol: receptor binding, transport into the endosome, and a translocation function for the A domain into the cytosol. Once internalized, the A domain ADP ribosylates elongation factor 2 (EF-2), a factor in eukaryotic protein synthesis that catalyzes the hydrolysis of GTP required for the movement of ribosomes on messenger RNA. The A domain remains active for a long time inside cells, which in part accounts for

A

Diphtheria
toxin
AB

Cholera
toxin
A+5B

Anthrax
toxin
2A+B

B

A

B

Diphtheria toxin

FIGURE 9-3 ▪ **AB organizations of bacterial exotoxins.**
A. The three common structural organizations of bacterial exotoxins, in which the A domain is the catalytic domain and the B domain is the binding domain. Diphtheria toxin is an AB toxin, with the A and B domains covalently aligned within a single protein. Cholera toxin is an AB5 toxin, with six peptides noncovalently bound in a complex. Anthrax toxin is a 2A+B toxin, in which the proteins are expressed as independent proteins that associate on the host cell membrane. **B.** Diphtheria toxin has a three-dimensional structure. The B domain is divided into two domains, which are involved in two sequential steps in the intoxication process: receptor binding and translocation of the A domain into the host cell. Image obtained from Protein Data Base: 1SGK. Bell CE, Eisenberg D. Crystal structure of nucleotide-free diphtheria toxin. Biochemistry. 1997;36:481.

ADP ribosyla = posttransla modifica of prot tat involves addition one or more ADP & ribose moieties

its potency, because internalization of a single A domain is sufficient to kill a cell.

ADP ribosylation of EF-2 by diphtheria toxin

$$\text{EF-2} + \text{NAD}^+ \rightarrow \text{ADP-ribosylated EF-2}$$
$$+ \text{ nicotinamide} + \text{H}^+$$

EF-2 is the only known substrate for diphtheria toxin. The reason for this specificity is that EF-2 contains a rare modification in one of its histidine residues, and this is the site at which diphtheria toxin ADP ribosylates EF-2. Mutant mammalian cells lacking this modified histidine are resistant to diphtheria toxin. The addition of ADP ribose inactivates EF-2 and kills cells by irreversibly blocking protein synthesis.

Cholera toxin. The cholera toxin modulates normal cell functions by elevating the intracellular level of cyclic

adenosine monophosphate (**cAMP**) but does not kill the target cell. As a secondary messenger, cAMP regulates numerous cellular functions. The target tissue for cholera toxin is the epithelium of the small intestine. Cholera toxin is composed of six noncovalently associated proteins comprising one A protein and five identical B proteins (AB5). The B pentamer binds specifically to the intestinal epithelial mucosa. On internalization, the A domain of cholera toxin ADP ribosylates a G protein, which upregulates host adenylate cyclase and produces more intracellular cAMP.

ADP ribosylation of G-protein by cholera toxin

$$\text{G protein} + \text{NAD}^+ \rightarrow \text{ADP-ribosylated G protein}$$
$$+ \text{ nicotinamide} + \text{H}^+$$

The adenylate cyclase complex is membrane bound in intestinal cells and includes the G protein and the adenylate cyclase. G proteins exist in two conformations: a GTP-bound form that binds and activates adenylate cyclase and a guanosine 5′-diphosphate (GDP)–bound form that is inactive. The guanosine 5′-triphosphate (GTP)–bound form has a short half-life because the G protein possesses GTPase activity that cleaves GTP to GDP. The activity of adenyl cyclase is determined by the nucleotide state of the G protein. Cholera toxin promotes the "active" GTP-bound form of the G protein by the ADP ribosylation of one of its arginine residues. ADP-ribosylated G protein is locked in the active conformation that stimulates adenylate cyclase. The elevated intracellular synthesis of cAMP provokes the movement of massive quantities of fluid across the intestinal membrane and into the lumen of the gut that is characteristic of cholera.

Activation of adenylate cyclase by ADP ribosylation of G proteins is a strategy adopted by a number of other diarrhea-producing pathogens, including the heat-labile enterotoxin of *Escherichia coli*. Other toxins, such as pertussis toxin produced by *Bordetella pertussis*, the agent of whooping cough, raise cAMP in leukocytes through the ADP ribosylation of a G protein that is different from the G protein ADP ribosylated by cholera toxin. The different effects of cholera toxin and pertussis toxin on the host illustrate the importance of the site of bacterial colonization.

Numerous bacterial toxins possess the ability to ADP ribosylate host proteins. The specificity of toxins is realized by the observation that each toxin ADP ribosylates a unique host protein. Thus, while diphtheria toxin and cholera toxin both catalyze the ADP ribosylation reaction, the pathology that each toxin elicits is unique because each toxin ADP ribosylates a unique host protein: diphtheria toxin targets EF-2, and cholera toxin targets a G protein.

Botulinum and tetanus toxins. Because they act on the nervous system, the botulinum and tetanus toxins are collectively called **neurotoxins.** Botulinum toxin is the most potent protein toxin to humans and recently has been implicated as a potential agent of **bioterrorism.**

[handwritten margin notes: "involuntary muscle contractions", "lacking muscle tone, vigor or energy"]

Tetanus toxin produces irreversible muscle contraction, yielding spastic paralysis, while botulinum toxin blocks muscle contraction, yielding flaccid paralysis. These neurotoxins are produced by anaerobic spore-forming bacteria of the genus *Clostridium*. Tetanus and botulinum toxins, like diphtheria toxin, are single proteins that contain A and B domains. Their actions as neurotoxins are based on the specific binding of the B domain to receptors on the surface of neurons. The A domain is a protease that cleaves intracellular proteins responsible for the fusion of intracellular vesicles with the plasma membrane. The specific pathology associated with each neurotoxin is based on its ability to migrate to unique locations in the nervous system to inactivate specific steps in neuronal signaling. Both neurotoxins enter peripheral nerve cells through receptor-mediated endocytosis. Once inside the endosome, the A domain of botulinum toxin is delivered into the cytoplasm to inactive vesicle fusion at the peripheral nerve ending, which inhibits the release of **stimulatory neurotransmitters,** resulting in flaccid paralysis. Tetanus toxin migrates up the axon, across the interneuronal junction, and into the internal neuron, where its A domain inactivates vesicle fusion at the interneuronal junction to inhibit the release of **inhibitory neurotransmitters,** resulting in spastic paralysis. In tetanus and botulism, the excitatory and inhibitory effects of motor neurons become increasingly unbalanced, which can lead to death from decreased ventilation.

[handwritten margin notes: "mechanism botulinum toxin", "mechanism"]

Tetanus is caused by the introduction of the **tetanus bacilli** into the host, typically through the penetration of a foreign object, such as a rusty nail. Although the bacillus rarely moves from its location in a wound, tetanus toxin is released by the bacterium and travels to the central nervous system to produce the symptoms of tetanus, which are distanced from the site of infection. Thus, tetanus is a good example of a disease that results from a single toxin acting on a distant target. Botulism occurs from the production of botulinum toxin on the infection of the intestine of an infant by *Clostridium botulinum* (**infant botulism**), or from the ingestion of botulinum toxin made in food contaminated by *C. botulinum* and stored under anaerobic conditions, such as improperly sterilized canned foods. The latter is therefore a true intoxication; it does not require the presence of the bacterium to cause symptoms and pathology.

✱ Type III Cytotoxins

Some pathogenic bacteria have the ability to secrete **type III cytotoxins** (see Fig. 9-1) directly into the host cell by a **contact-dependent** mechanism when the bacterium directly contacts the host cell. The stimulus provided by the host cell is not well characterized but may include temperature, oxygen tension, and salt concentration. On contact with the mammalian cells, the bacterium uses a type III secretion apparatus to generate a pore in the host cell membrane that delivers the type III cytotoxin directly into the cytosol of the host cell. Type III cytotoxins are delivered efficiently and are not likely to contact

neutralizing antibodies. Numerous bacteria, including *Salmonella, Shigella, Pseudomonas,* the cholera bacilli, and the plague bacilli, deliver type III cytotoxins into host cells (see Chapter 17 paradigm). Type III cytotoxins vary in their mechanism of action but often interfere with the ability of the host to respond to infection by direct cell killing or through the modulation of the actin cytoskeleton. A functional actin cytoskeleton is required for the efficient phagocytosis of pathogens by macrophages and other phagocytes.

Toxins that Act at the Host Cell Surface

Surface-acting toxins bind to the cell membrane and modulate host cell physiology without having to enter the intracellular compartment of the cell. Modulation can affect host cell signaling or through the direct damage to the cell membrane.

Endotoxin

[handwritten note: "mannans = any of gp of plant polysaccharides tat r polymers of mannose."]

Endotoxin is the **lipopolysaccharide (LPS)** of the outer membrane of Gram-negative bacteria (see Fig. 3-2) and plays an important role in the diseases caused by those organisms. At low concentrations endotoxin elicits a series of **alarm reactions:** fever, activation of complement by the alternative pathway, activation of macrophages, and stimulation of B lymphocytes. At high concentrations it produces **shock** and even death. The term *endotoxin* is misleading on two counts: endotoxin is not internalized, and it exerts a toxic effect only at high concentrations. Recent studies have highlighted the importance of endotoxin in the host response to infection. Endotoxin is one of several structural components of microorganisms that stimulate our innate immune system as an early indication of infection. These structural components have been referred to as **pattern recognition receptors** (see Fig. 9-2) and are highly conserved among microorganisms. Pattern recognition receptors include endotoxin from Gram-negative bacteria, lipoteichoic acid from Gram-positive bacteria, lipoglycans from the mycobacteria, and mannans from yeast. Early activation of our **innate immune system** by pattern recognition receptors provide us with a rapid and effective response to infection and is the catalyst for activating our **adaptive immune system**, which is responsible for long-term resistance to infection.

Chemistry of endotoxin As discussed in Chapter 3, bacterial lipopolysaccharide is composed of three parts: a glycolipid called **lipid A**; a **core** of sugars, ethanolamine, and phosphate; and the **O antigen**, a long side chain of species-specific, often unusual sugars (see Fig. 3-6). Lipid A is the biologically active component, while the other components serve as carriers. Lipid A alone is water insoluble and inert, but its activity is restored when complexed with large-molecular-weight carriers, such as proteins. The

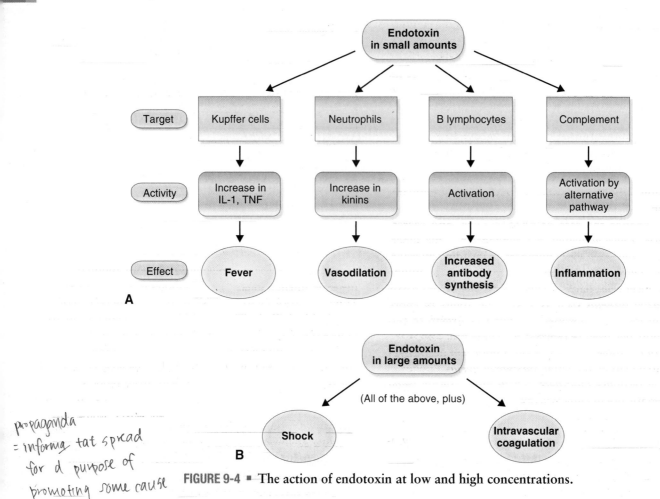

FIGURE 9-4 ▪ The action of endotoxin at low and high concentrations.

[handwritten left margin: propaganda = informa tat spread for d purpose of promoting some cause]

structure of lipid A is unusual: it contains uniquely short fatty acids (12, 14, and 16 carbons in length).

Endotoxin has different pharmacological effects when delivered at low or high concentrations (Fig. 9-4): In small amounts, endotoxin sets off a series of alarm reactions, and in large amounts, shock is induced. The extent to which these complex events overlap depends not only on the amount of endotoxin but also on the route of injection and the previous exposure of the host to this substance.

The primary targets for endotoxin are mononuclear phagocytes (peripheral blood monocytes, macrophages of the spleen, bone marrow, lung alveoli, peritoneal cavity, and Kupffer cells), **neutrophils, platelets,** and **B lymphocytes.** These cells possess specific endotoxin receptors, called **toll-like receptors (TLRs).** There are several TLRs that recognize different pattern recognition receptors. The binding of the pattern recognition receptors to TLRs stimulates a signal transduction cascade within the cell. This results in the production of proteins known as **cytokines,** which induce "alarm reactions" such as fever, activation of complement, activation of macrophages, and stimulation of B lymphocytes (see Fig. 9-2).

Fever   In the words of the pioneering immunopathologist Lewis Thomas, endotoxin acts like propaganda: it tells the body that bacteria are present. Endotoxin in small amounts is **pyrogenic;** that is, it elicits **fever,** a common sign

[handwritten: produced by fever]

of infection. About 100 ng (0.1 μg) of endotoxin injected intravenously in an adult human volunteer will produce a measurable pyrogenic response. Note that this amount comes from about 10 million *[handwritten: within intestine]* enteric bacteria, which is not a particularly large number of microbes; the normal intestinal flora contains perhaps 1 million times more bacteria. If all the endotoxin in the intestine were to enter the bloodstream, and if fever followed an absurdly linear response, body temperature would rise to about 1 million degrees. Obviously, the amount of endotoxin that spills over from the intestine into the circulation is quite small. Nonetheless, endotoxin serves as a constant low-level stimulation of the immune response in healthy people, without pathological manifestations. Low titers of antibodies to endotoxin are found in most healthy persons.

Fever induced by endotoxin during activation of the innate immune system is caused by the release of cytokines from mononuclear phagocytes. The best-characterized cytokines are **interleukin-1 (IL-1)** and **tumor necrosis factor (TNF-α),** which set off a complex series of events known as the **acute phase response** (see Chapter 6). Lipoteichoic acids of Gram-positive bacteria also stimulate the innate immune system with the subsequent release of IL-1 and TNF.

Activation of complement   Endotoxin activates complement by the alternative pathway (see Chapter 6). At a low complement ⇒ a gp of prot in blood serum fat interact systematically as part of d body's immune response to destroy disease-causing antigens, esp bact. Complement prot interact wif antibodies & other chemical substances to cause disintegra of foreign cells & enhance other immune func such as phagocytosis.

CHAPTER 9 Damage by Microbial Toxins **135**

endotoxin concentration, the most likely consequence to bacteria is the production of the **membrane attack complex (MAC)**, plus phagocyte chemotaxis and opsonization. Neutrophils are activated and, because of the opsonizing effect of C3b, become available for phagocytosis. Complement activation also leads to the production of **anaphylatoxins** (C3a, C5a), which increase capillary permeability and release of lysosomal enzymes from neutrophils (degranulation). Thus, endotoxin elicits an inflammatory response. opsonizg = make (bact or other cells) > susceptible to act of phagocytes.

Activation of macrophages Endotoxin activates **macrophages** to increase the production of lysosomal enzymes, enhance the rate of phagocytosis, and secrete hydrolases. Once activated, macrophages become superscavengers, ingesting large numbers of invading microorganisms. Their high activation state extends to killing certain cancer cells, partly by direct attachment and partly by releasing proteins such as TNF. The ability of endotoxin, through macrophages, to limit the growth of certain tumors has been recognized for some time and is the subject of continued investigation. Endotoxin derivatives belong to a class of potential anticancer agents known as **biological response modifiers,** which are currently being evaluated for use in clinical work.

Stimulation of B lymphocytes By inducing the release of IL-1, endotoxin induces B lymphocytes (but not T lymphocytes) to divide. B lymphocytes mature into antibody-producing cells, thus adding to long-term resistance to infection by increasing the concentration of antibodies in circulation. In this capacity, endotoxin is an **immunological adjuvant.** an additive fat enhance d effectiveness of medical treatment.

Shock The full panoply of endotoxin activity is more array emphatically displayed when it is administered in large amounts. Fully activated endotoxin produces a condition known as **bacterial sepsis** (Fig. 9-5). Fortunately rarely seen, bacterial sepsis overwhelms the body with bacteria, often Gram-negative bacteria such as *E. coli, P. aeruginosa,* or meningococci (see Chapters 14, 19, and 64). The result is a frequently lethal condition known as **endotoxic shock,** which manifests as a serious drop in blood pressure (**hypotension**) and **disseminated intravascular coagulation.** spread abroad. TNF and IL-1 appear to be key mediators in endotoxin-induced hypotension, since hypotension is considerably reduced by the administration of antisera against TNF or IL-1 prior to the injection of endotoxin. An earlier view was that decreased resistance of peripheral vessels results from a buildup of vasoactive amines (histamine and kinins). Considerable work is being carried out to clarify the situation and to understand the molecular basis for endotoxic shock.

Disseminated intravascular coagulation (DIC) is the deposition of thrombi in small vessels, with consequent damage to the areas deprived of blood supply. The effect is most severe in the kidneys and leads to cortical necrosis. Other organs affected include the brain, lungs, and adrenals. In some cases of meningococcal infection,

Summary of endotoxin

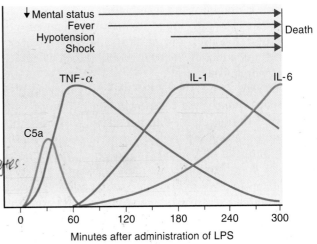

FIGURE 9-5 ▪ **Release of mediators of sepsis following the experimental injection of lipopolysaccharide (LPS).** Tumor necrosis factor α (TNF-α) triggers the release of interleukin 1 (IL-1). These cytokines act synergistically to induce the damaging effects of sepsis. Other cytokines, such as IL-6, are released as a consequence of this synergy. IL-6 does not produce shock, but the level of IL-6 release is highly correlated with death from septic shock.

⇒ a condi which a localized area of muscular tissue die becuz insuff blood supply

adrenal insufficiency due to infarction leads to rapid death, a condition known as the **Waterhouse-Friderichsen syndrome.** Endotoxin contributes to coagulation of blood in three ways: clotting factor XII (the so-called Hageman factor) is activated to set off the intrinsic clotting cascade; platelets release the contents of their granules, which are involved in clotting; and neutrophils release proteins known to stabilize fibrin clots.

Endotoxin represents the calling card of Gram-negative bacteria. The binding of endotoxin to the TLRs on macrophages stimulates the production of a series of alarm reactions that rapidly help to fend off the invading pathogen. These include the mobilization of neutrophils, the activation of macrophages, and the stimulation of B lymphocytes. Stimulation by the pattern recognition receptors also initiates the adaptive immune system of the host, leading to long-term resistance to microbial infections. In large amounts, endotoxin is deserving of its name and induces shock and widespread coagulation. Thus, recognition of endotoxin is a mechanism our bodies use to activate our immune response against Gram-negative bacterial pathogens, but we have not developed ways to regulate this response to prevent some of the detrimental effects of exposure to this agent.

Membrane-Damaging Toxins

A large number of toxins harm the host cell as membrane-damaging toxins. They act either as **lipases** or by inserting themselves in the membrane to form pores. **Lecithinase** is a lipase toxin produced by the clostridium of gas gangrene. Lecithinase lyses cells indiscriminately because its main substrate, phosphatidylcholine undistingu

sepsis: the presence pathogenic organism or their toxins blood or tissues.

(lecithin), is ubiquitous in mammalian membranes. Microbes that elaborate lipase toxins thus eliminate potential host defenses and at the same time create a necrotic, nutritionally rich anaerobic milieu in which the microorganisms thrive.

One class of membrane-damaging toxins comprises **hemolysins,** which lyse cells, including red blood cells and white blood cells. Another class of membrane-damaging toxins are **pore-forming toxins,** which insert directly into the host membrane to generate pores (see Fig. 9-2). Pore-forming toxins make the membranes permeable to water, which flows into the cytoplasm to swell the cell and, if excessive, lyse the cell. Even at toxin concentrations too low to cause cell lysis, cellular functions are damaged by perturbations of the permeability barrier that allow leakage of potassium ions needed for protein synthesis and cell viability. Thus, pore-forming toxins effectively inhibit the function of the phagocytes, the host's first line of defense.

The pattern of ion leakage and subsequent damage is the same for many pore-forming toxins. Working nonenzymatically, these toxins use a mechanism similar to the MAC of complement (see Chapter 6). The pores formed by the complement complex as well as by the pore-forming bacterial toxins consist of fortified protein structures unusually resistant to proteases and detergents. This resistance likely contributes to the stability of the toxin at the cell surface. An example of a toxin that works in this manner is the α-toxin of *Staphylococcus aureus.* This toxin is a **homogeneous pore former;** that is, each pore has the same number of protein molecules (see Fig. 6.5 for similar-looking channels produced by the MAC of complement).

The **heterogeneous pore-forming toxins** constitute another class of membrane-damaging toxin. These toxins make pores that vary in size and number of monomer toxin molecules. The prototype of this class is **streptolysin O,** a toxin produced by certain streptococci. Streptolysin O (O stands for "oxygen labile") binds to cholesterol in the cell membrane. Streptolysin O lyses red blood cells but not neutrophils or macrophages. Nevertheless, this toxin contributes indirectly to white blood cell death because it acts preferentially on the membranes of lysosomes, releasing their hydrolytic enzymes. This results in damage to the cytoplasmic contents of the white blood cell, leading to a suicidal type of cell death. In addition, the lysosomal enzymes released from killed neutrophils damage the surrounding tissue. The heterogeneous pore formers demonstrate that pores made by toxins need not be well defined to cause widespread damage.

Superantigens

A unique aspect of the action of several virulence factors is their ability to subvert the normal antibody response of the host. Acting as so-called **superantigens,** some toxins stimulate the production of large amounts of antibodies, not directed against the superantigen, by complexing MHC molecules of an antigen-presenting cell with the T-cell receptor on lymphocytes to stimulate antigen-independent activation of the lymphocyte (see Fig. 9-2). Such antibody production is wasteful and inefficient in combating infection. This intriguing aspect of how microbes can "twist" a normal body response is described in Chapter 8.

Toxins that Act in the Extracellular Matrix

In contrast to toxins that modify proteins in the intracellular compartment of the host cell or act on the cell surface, numerous virulence factors, **exoenzymes,** act in the extracellular matrix of the cell. These toxins include degradative enzymes that function as **spreading factors** by facilitating the dispersal of infecting organisms. Some Gram-positive bacteria secrete a **hyaluronidase** that breaks down hyaluronic acid, the ground substance of connective tissue and also secrete **deoxyribonuclease (DNase),** which thins pus made viscous by the DNA released from dead white blood cells. Other bacteria make proteins that bind and activate host plasminogen. For example, **streptokinase** produced by *Streptococcus pyogenes* is an enzyme that activates plasminogen and converts it to plasmin, a serum protease that in turn attacks fibrin clots. In this way, streptokinase eliminates fibrin barriers that might interfere with invading streptococci. Similar roles have been suggested for the **collagenases and elastases** produced by other organisms. Such "meat tenderizer" forms of these enzymes also exist in the uninfected host, but their activities are normally under control.

Immune Protection Against Exotoxins

Because exotoxins are foreign proteins and stimulate an immune response when produced in the host, **immune protection** is a possible response to the toxin. For some diseases, such as tetanus, the clinical disease itself does not confer immunity to subsequent infections, probably because the toxin is produced in amounts too small to be an effective immunogen. On the other hand, vaccination and treatment with **antitoxins** have been used successfully against tetanus and other diseases. Of course, injecting the toxin itself is dangerous and does not result in active immunization. Fortunately, some exotoxins can be chemically modified to eliminate their intrinsic toxicity while retaining immunogenicity. These chemically inactivated toxins are termed **toxoids** and are commonly used to vaccinate against several diseases, including diphtheria and tetanus (as part of the widely used DTP vaccine). Undergoing a series of vaccinations through the first 5 years of life and boosters every 10 years enables humans to mount an immune response that is sufficient to maintain immunity to natural infection caused by the diphtheria and tetanus bacilli. As may be anticipated, infection by the bacilli can occur in individuals immune only to the toxin, but serious clinical symptoms of the diseases are not observed.

to cause to happen in advance

Passive immunization involves administration of an antitoxin, usually produced in horses or other animals, to individuals who have been exposed to toxin-producing pathogens, like the diphtheria and tetanus bacilli. One problem with antitoxin administration is the possibility of **serum sickness**, an immune reaction against foreign proteins. In the nonimmune individual, antitoxin must be administered rapidly to be effective against infection resulting from the tetanus or diphtheria bacilli, because once exotoxins are bound to host cell, they are rapidly internalized and become unavailable to antibody molecules.

Recombinant DNA technology may refine some of the vaccination procedures used to generate an immunogen that elicits a protective immune response to an exotoxin. And it may soon be possible to immunize using tailor-made domains of the exotoxin. The B domains of AB exotoxins seem to be particularly promising candidates, because antibodies which prevent binding of a toxin block the initial steps of toxin action. In the absence of the A domain, the B domains are innocuous *harmless* and can be administered with little risk to the host. Vaccination with a recombinant form of the B domain of anthrax toxin is an approach being pursued to develop a safe and effective vaccine against intoxication by the bacillus responsible for anthrax.

Not all toxin-mediated diseases respond to vaccination. In particular, some of the approved vaccines against cholera elicit only limited protection. An effective cholera vaccine must elicit secreted IgA antibodies in the intestine that are active against the microbe, blocking its ability to colonize and intoxicate the host. Cholera vaccines administered by injection give poor or short-lived protection, in part because an effective IgA antibody response is not achieved. However, live strains of oral vaccine, made of the disarmed pathogen, stimulate intestinal antibody production of the IgA class similar to what natural infection does. These strains hold promise for generating long-lived protection against cholera.

Bacterial exotoxins are also being used in systems to target drugs to specific cell populations, such as coupling a specific antibody to an A domain of an exotoxin. The antibody seeks out the specific cells, and the A domain is delivered to kill the cell. Although there have been specific successes in treating cancers this way, nonspecific toxicity and potential adverse side effects are issues that have to be addressed with this therapeutic approach. Nonetheless, the idea of using toxins to this advantage remains appealing.

Conclusion

Advances in our knowledge of toxin action and host cell physiology provide a foundation for understanding the molecular basis of infectious disease. Pathology associated with disease is often a combination of the toxicity of the toxin and the host response to the infectious agent. Toxins are categorized based on their site of action, targeting the intracellular compartment of the host, the host cell surface, or the extracellular matrix. Toxins have specific modes of action that are responsible for the unique pathology associated with an individual infectious agent, such as cell death caused by the action of diphtheria toxin or elevated cAMP resulting from the action of cholera toxin. Often toxins can be detoxified (toxoids) and administered as protective vaccines.

part **2**

Infectious Agents

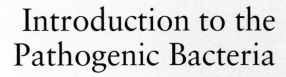

chapter **10**

Introduction to the Pathogenic Bacteria

Victor J. DiRita

Thousands of species of bacteria, both harmless and pathogenic, are found in association with the human body. Although you need to know only the principal bacteria, even they make up a long list. However, knowing the taxonomy of bacteria may help you make important diagnostic and treatment decisions. For example, among other things, it is helpful to know that staphylococci and streptococci both belong to a group called the Gram-positive cocci, that *Escherichia coli* is classified among the Gram-negative enteric bacteria, and that the tubercle bacillus belongs to the acid-fast bacteria.

This chapter uses a simplified, practical scheme to divide the main pathogenic bacteria, rather than the organizational scheme used in the science of bacterial taxonomy (Fig. 10-1). In broad terms, medically interesting bacteria belong to one of two large categories:

1. The "typical" bacteria—the rods and cocci (spheres) that lack unusual morphological features. These "garden variety" bacteria can be subdivided into the Gram-positive and Gram-negative bacteria, and each of those categories can be further divided into rods and cocci.
2. Those that do not fall in the first category.

Like all other forms of life, every bacterium is named by its genus, as in *Escherichia,* and species, as in *coli.* Conventionally, after its first use in a text, the genus name is shortened to the first letter, as in *E. coli.* Many bacteria also have common names, usually related to the main disease they cause—for example, the cholera bacillus (*Vibrio cholerae*) and the tubercle bacillus (*Mycobacterium tuberculosis*). Sometimes the origin of the genus and species names is interesting and useful to know. Many bacterial names honor famous microbiologists; for instance, *Escherichia* is named after the German pediatrician Theodor Escherich and *Salmonella* after the American veterinarian Daniel Elmer Salmon. Other names are descriptive; *pyogenes* (as in *Streptococcus pyogenes*), for example, indicates that the bacteria promote pus production.

A confusing aspect of bacterial taxonomy is that considerable variety usually exists within a species. Thus, a *Staphylococcus aureus* isolated from one patient may be distinctly virulent, whereas another strain of the same bacterium may not be. These isolates are called **strains.** This point is well illustrated by the many strains of *E. coli,* which include the strain commonly used in molecular biology research, known as K12, as well as less benevolent strains that cause infection of the intestine, the urinary bladder, or the meninges. All are *E. coli,* but each is a different strain expressing different pathogenic factors.

FIGURE 10-1 ■ **The major groups of medically important bacteria.** This illustration is a practical representation of the principal groups of pathogenic bacteria. It is meant to be a study aid, not a taxonomic or phylogenetic tree.

"Typical" Bacteria

The **Gram stain** property reflects fundamental differences among bacteria; these differences lie mainly in their permeability properties and surface components. The chief differences that the Gram stain illustrates are the presence of an outer membrane in the Gram-negative bacteria and of a thick **murein** layer in the Gram-positive bacteria (see Chapter 2). These organisms can also be divided into rods and cocci, yielding four categories in which to classify them (Fig. 10-2).

Because the Gram stain reflects such fundamental differences among bacteria, Gram-positive bacteria differ more from Gram-negative bacteria than cocci differ from rods. For instance, the Gram-positive streptococci are closely related to the lactobacilli, which are Gram-positive rods; however, the streptococci are quite distinct from Gram-negative cocci, such as the gonococci. Gram-positive bacteria accept the Gram stain and appear dark violet, whereas Gram-negative bacteria do

Gram-positive cocci

Gram-positive rods

Gram-negative cocci

Gram-negative rods

FIGURE 10-2 ■ **The "Big Four" typical bacteria.** Many of the chapters on individual infectious agents include sections called paradigms. These sections highlight points of general relevance to the understanding of microbial pathogenesis.

not accept the stain and appear red (see Chapter 3 and Table 3-2).

The four categories presented in Figure 10-2 are fairly evenly represented in the normal flora of the mouth, the pharynx, and the large intestine; major pathogens, however, are represented in fewer numbers. The Gram-positive cocci and the Gram-negative rods are the most common agents of infection, followed by the Gram-negative cocci and the Gram-positive rods.

Gram-Positive Cocci

The two most medically relevant genera of Gram-positive cocci are *Streptococcus* and *Staphyloccus*. Species within each genus are among the most successful human pathogens and, consequently, are the targets of vigorous research efforts to understand and combat them.

Streptococci

Streptococci grow in chains of spherical cells—like strings of pearls—and constitute a large and diverse group. Streptococci are subdivided according to the changes they produce when grown on agar-containing blood. Thus, β-**hemolytic** streptococci (or "beta strep"), which cause most streptococcal infections, lyse red blood cells signified by a clear area around the colonies. The α-**hemolytic** streptococci produce a different change and cause blood-containing media around the colony to turn green. Other streptococci do not change the blood at all. Many streptococci strains are nonpathogenic and are found in the environment as well as in the normal human intestine. Some strains are associated with dairy products and contribute to the production of cheese.

Streptococci do not carry out respiration, only fermentation. Fermentation is characteristic of anaerobic bacteria, and indeed some streptococci are strict anaerobes. However, most of the pathogenic species of streptococci grow in air and are thus described as **oxygen-tolerant anaerobes.** Streptococci usually grow in small colonies on agar. Streptococci produce many extracellular proteins, some of which are virulence factors that confer on the organisms the ability to destroy tissues and damage host cells.

The main pathogens in the *Streptococcus* genus are the β-hemolytic strains. These strains are further subclassified into groups by the presence of different cell wall polysaccharides. Of all the groups (A through T), the most important strains in human disease are those of group A. The full taxonomic name of these organisms is *S. pyogenes,* but they are often referred to as "group A strep." They cause "strep throat," infections of soft tissues, and other serious infections. These infections can cause serious complications, such as rheumatic fever or glomerulonephritis. α-Hemolytic streptococci include one important pathogen, *S. pneumoniae* (the main agent of bacterial pneumonia), and other, mainly opportunistic species.

Staphylococci

The two main pathogenic species of *Staphylococcus* are *S. aureus* and *S. saprophyticus;* however, opportunistic infections by staphylococci that are part of the normal flora, such as *S. epidermidis,* can also occur. Under the microscope, staphylococci look like arrays of buckshot or bunches of grapes (*staphylo* comes from the Greek word for grapes). They are more robust than streptococci and are able to withstand many chemical and physical agents; these qualities make it difficult to eradicate them from the human environment. Their colonies on agar are larger than those of the streptococci, and they are aerobes.

Staphylococci are found in many sites of the body, especially on the skin. They are the most likely organisms to cause pus in wounds and may produce serious infections in deep tissues, such as osteomyelitis (infection of the bone marrow) or endocarditis (infection of the heart valves). Like the streptococci, they also secrete a large number of extracellular enzymes and toxins. One enzyme, **coagulase,** clots plasma and is useful in classification because only the most pathogenic species of the genus, *S. aureus,* produces the enzyme.

Gram-Negative Cocci

Gram-negative cocci include several genera of medical importance, the most significant of which is the *Neisseria*. This genus includes many organisms found in the mouth and pharynx of healthy people and two important pathogens, the **gonococcus** and the **meningococcus.** Like all Gram-negative bacteria, their outer membranes contain endotoxin (lipopolysaccharide). The gonococcus causes gonorrhea, and the meningococcus causes meningitis and severe septicemia.

Gram-Positive Rods

Abundant in the environment, this group includes bacteria that only infrequently cause diseases, at least in the developed regions of the world. One disease, diphtheria, was deadly among children until vaccination nearly eradicated it. The agent of diphtheria is called *Corynebacterium diphtheriae* and has many relatives called the **diphtheroids.** The diphtheroids are common inhabitants of the skin and mucous membranes and can cause opportunistic infections. (Notice that *diphtheria* has two *h*'s.)

In the human environment, the most common Gram-positive rods are the **spore-forming rods.** They are the largest of the typical bacteria, with 5 to 10 times the volume of an average *E. coli,* and can measure 3 to 5 μm in length. They are divided into two genera: the **aerobic** *Bacillus,* containing only one important pathogenic species, *B. anthracis,* which causes anthrax; and the **strict anaerobes,** which are members of the genus *Clostridium.* This genus includes several medically important species such as *C. bo-*

tulinum, which cause botulism; *C. tetani,* the agent of tetanus; and several other species that produce gas gangrene (most commonly *C. perfringens*). Symptoms of these diseases are caused by powerful exotoxins. Among the most commonly encountered clostridial disease is one associated with antibiotic use: pseudomembranous colitis caused by *C. difficile.* Another important pathogen among the Gram-positive rods is *Listeria monocytogenes,* which occasionally causes serious infections in infants and in adults who are immunocompromised and in pregnant women.

Gram-Negative Rods

Enteric Bacteria

The Gram-negative rods are a large group of bacteria that includes many important pathogens. The **enteric bacteria** are among the most clinically important of the Gram-negative rods. The exemplar is *Escherichia coli,* the typical bacterium *par excellence.* The enteric bacteria (or family Enterobacteriaceae) comprise many genera, including *Salmonella,* species of which cause typhoid fever and food poisoning, and *Shigella,* which causes bacillary dysentery. All enteric bacteria grow readily on laboratory media, make middle-sized colonies (usually less than 1 mm across) on agar and do not form spores or have special cell arrangements. Many, but not all, are motile. They are divided into two main groups: those that ferment lactose (*E. coli* and others) and those that do not (*Salmonella* and *Shigella*). Although many pathogens are not lactose fermenters, the characteristic is not universal, and many exceptions exist. Relatives of the enteric bacteria include the yersiniae, which cause plague and certain intestinal infections.

Among their more distant relatives are Gram-negative rods that differ in metabolism and somewhat in morphology. These are in various families outside the Enterobacteriaceae, including the genus *Vibrio* (containing *V. cholerae,* the cholera bacillus) and the genus *Pseudomonas.* Pseudomonads, as the members of the *Pseudomonas* genus are sometimes called, are often found in aqueous environments, such as rivers, lakes, swimming pools, and tap water; these environments are thus frequent sources of human infection. Other clinically important Gram-negative rods outside the Enterobacteriaceae are *Campylobacter jejuni,* a common agent of infectious diarrhea, and *Helicobacter pylori,* an organism implicated in gastritis, gastric ulcers, and gastric cancer.

"Fastidious" and Small Gram-Negative Rods

Besides the organisms already mentioned, the Gram-negative rods include an important and heterogeneous group of genera. They can be lumped, somewhat arbitrarily, into a group that may be awkwardly described as the "fastidious" and small Gram-negative rods because they have complex nutritional requirements and tend to be smaller than, for example, *E. coli.* Included in this group are the following genera: *Haemophilus* (which causes pneumonia and meningitis), *Bordetella*

(whooping cough), *Brucella* (brucellosis), *Francisella* (tularemia), *Bartonella* (cat scratch fever), and others. *Legionella,* the genus of the legionnaires disease agent *L. pneumophila,* is also a small Gram-negative rod but varies considerably from the others in its habitat (soil, water) and chemical composition.

Strictly Anaerobic Gram-Negative Rods

Lastly, an important group of Gram-negative rods is distinguished by its strictly anaerobic way of life. Clinically, the most noteworthy of these organisms belongs to the genus *Bacteroides.* These bacteria are common in the human body and are the most frequent members of the intestinal flora, a critical stimulus for proper tissue development within the intestine. They are also found in the gingival pockets that surround the teeth. Although the bacteria are usually harmless, members of this genus may cause serious disease when deposited in deep tissues, such as when they are associated with peritonitis, the abdominal infection that results from the outpouring of intestinal contents into the peritoneum. These organisms usually do not cause disease alone but are found in association with other bacteria, thereby causing mixed or polymicrobial infections. They will not reproduce if incubated aerobically, and their growth requires special anaerobic techniques.

"Not So Typical" Bacteria

A taxonomic hodgepodge, the "not so typical" bacteria include organisms that have special shapes, sizes, or staining properties. They do not have many features in common, other than their medical importance. Thus, each group stands alone.

Acid-Fast Bacteria

This group is almost synonymous with the genus *Mycobacterium,* which includes the **tubercle bacillus,** **M. tuberculosis,** and the **leprosy bacillus,** **M. leprae.** Acid fastness refers to the ability of these organisms to withstand many chemicals; as such, they must be stained by a special procedure (see Chapter 3). They are surrounded by a waxy envelope that can only be penetrated by dyes if the bacteria are heated or treated with detergents. The Gram stain is irrelevant for these bacteria because they do not take up the Gram stain dyes.

The special staining procedure used for acid-fast bacteria is called the **Ziehl-Neelsen technique.** Its most frequently used modification consists of treating smears with a solution of a red dye (fuchsin) that contains detergents. After washing, the smear is treated with a solution of 3% hydrochloric acid that removes the dye from all bacteria except the acid-fast organisms. The preparation is then exposed to a blue dye that counterstains all other bacteria, white blood cells, and so on. Tubercle or leprosy bacilli, the "red bugs," are clearly visible against the blue background.

Several species of mycobacteria found free living in the environment can cause opportunistic infections, especially in immunocompromised patients. These environmental species used to be called **atypical acid-fast bacilli.** Among the most commonly encountered of these bacteria are members of a complex known as *Mycobacterium avium-intracellulare.* All mycobacteria grow slowly and are resistant to chemical agents, but not to heat.

The name of this genus contains the root word for fungus (*myco*) because the organisms sometimes form branches that vaguely suggest the fungi. Even more akin to fungi in morphology are relatives of the mycobacteria called the actinomycetes. These organisms take up the Gram stain and are Gram-positive. Some are also weakly acid-fast. They form true branches and long filaments with complex structures, a feature that places them among the most highly differentiated of the prokaryotes. There are two pathogenic genera: *Nocardia,* which are aerobic, and *Actinomyces,* which are strict anaerobes. Bacteria of these genera cause certain forms of pneumonia and soft tissue infections. A generally nonpathogenic genus, *Streptomyces,* includes organisms that make important antibiotics (streptomycin, tetracycline, etc.)

Spirochetes

These bacteria are helical, shaped like a spring (not a screw). They include the agent of syphilis, *Treponema pallidum,* the species name of which refers to the fact that these organisms are so thin ("pale") that they do not take up enough dye to be readily seen under the microscope. Unstained, they can be seen with a phase contrast or a darkfield microscope. The spirochetes of syphilis are not readily cultivated in the laboratory.

Other spirochetes include the genus *Leptospira,* which cause a disease called icterohemorrhagic fever, and *Borrelia recurrentis,* the agent of relapsing fever. Another spirochete in the *Borrelia* genus, *B. burgdorferi,* causes Lyme disease (named after a town in Connecticut), which is one of the most important spirochetoses in both eastern and western United States.

Chlamydiae

The chlamydiae are small, strictly intracellular bacteria that cannot be grown in artificial media. They are among the smallest cellular forms of life but have a fairly complex life cycle. Their morphological form when they are growing inside cells differs from their form when they are in transit between cells. *Chlamydia trachomatis* is the most common cause of sexually transmitted disease (chlamydial urethritis) and other more unusual infections. *C. pneumoniae* is an agent of pneumonia in young adults and has been linked to atherosclerosis. These organisms set up housekeeping within phagocytic vesicles of their host cells and obtain their energy from them.

Rickettsiae

Like the chlamydiae, the rickettsiae are small, intracellular bacteria that are also obligate parasites. Among the diseases these bacteria cause are epidemic typhus and Rocky Mountain spotted fever. Included in this group is the genus *Ehrlichia,* bacteria that infect white blood cells in humans and animals. Each species is transmitted by the bite of different arthropod species (lice, fleas, ticks, etc.), with the exception of *Coxiella burnetii,* the agent of Q fever, which may also be acquired by inhalation. Rickettsiae are small, rod-shaped bacteria that lack distinctive growth cycle stages.

Mycoplasmas

Perhaps most evolutionarily distant from all other bacteria, mycoplasmas lack a rigid cell wall. They are almost plastic in structure, grow slowly on laboratory media, and have special nutritional requirements. The most unique of these requirements is the need for sterols, which are not required by any other group of bacteria. Mycoplasmas lack murein and consequently are resistant to penicillin and other cell wall antibiotics. The oldest known human pathogenic mycoplasma is *Mycoplasma pneumoniae,* which causes a form of pneumonia. Others, such as *Ureaplasma ureae,* have been implicated in various diseases.

Mycoplasmas resemble the laboratory-produced forms of regular bacteria—the so-called L forms—which lack cell walls. Regular bacteria take on the same amorphous appearance as the mycoplasma when their cell walls are removed with lysozyme or when murein synthesis is inhibited with penicillin. Cell lysis usually occurs, but if the L forms are placed in a hypertonic medium, they can be grown in colonies that resemble those of the mycoplasmas. However, the similarity is only superficial. L forms usually revert to the regular bacterial form when they are removed from lysozyme or penicillin. Mycoplasmas, on the other hand, do not. Mycoplasmas also differ in terms of their degree of relatedness to all other bacteria as measured by DNA hybridization.

Current Concepts Regarding the Microbial Flora

Many microorganisms can be seen under the microscope but cannot be cultured. Some are suspected of causing important diseases, but the point has been difficult to establish without pure cultures. New technologies have allowed scientists to make some progress in this area. For example, *Tropheryma whipplei*—the agent of the rare Whipple disease, which is characterized by diarrhea and intestinal bleeding but can have systemic manifestations such as lymphadenopathy—was identified by PCR and 16S rRNA sequence analysis several years before it could be cultured in the laboratory (see Chapter 58).

Cloning techniques have been useful in studies of bacteria that are well known but cannot be cultivated, such as the treponeme of syphilis or the mycobacterium of leprosy. The genes of these agents have been introduced into surrogate organisms, such as *E. coli*, and many of the protein gene products have been studied, especially with regard to their immunological properties.

More and more possible agents of disease are being recognized and studied because of the disruption in immune system function caused by HIV and other agents of immunosuppression. Bacteria, viruses, fungi, protozoa, and worms that were previously unknown or known to be present only in animals or the environment have now joined the list of potential or known human pathogens. The combination of new technologies and the changes in the human immune condition will undoubtedly lead to the discovery of many more agents of infectious diseases. At the same time, with progress in sanitation and vaccination, the importance of many of the classic infectious pathogens is waning. The list of important pathogens is constantly changing.

Conclusion

Over the hundred or so years that microorganisms have been studied in the laboratory, they have exhibited remarkable genetic constancy. The staphylococci or streptococci of today fit their original descriptions from the end of the nineteenth century. Likewise, a microbiologist from Robert Koch's laboratory would have no problem correctly identifying a modern strain of *Vibrio cholerae* or tubercle bacilli. On the other hand, important changes have occurred with alarming speed. Virtually all the pathogenic bacteria have become significantly more resistant to every new antibiotic that has been introduced in the last five decades. For example, pathogenic staphylococci are now almost universally resistant to penicillin, although in the 1950s, when the drug came into general use, their ancestors were sensitive to it. Furthermore, we are now in an era in which the threat of biological weapons based on human pathogens is very real, and our understanding of how some of those microbes cause disease and how to protect populations from them is scant. Thus, the study of microbial pathogens remains a rich target area for innovations that will have a significant impact on human health.

Staphylococci: Abscesses and Toxin-Mediated Diseases

Patrick M. Schlievert and Marnie L. Peterson

key **concepts**

Staphylococci:

- Are considered pyogenic ("pus-forming") bacteria, except toxic shock syndrome staphylococci, which may not appear pyogenic.

- Cause many different diseases, including furuncles and abscesses, food poisoning, and toxin-induced diseases (toxic shock and scalded skin syndromes). If the organisms enter the bloodstream, they may cause osteomyelitis, kidney abscesses, and endocarditis.

- Include *Staphylococcus aureus, S. epidermidis, S. saprophyticus* (which almost exclusively causes urinary tract infections), and numerous others.

- Possess a variety of virulence factors: *S. aureus* produces cell wall factors (peptidoglycan, teichoic acids, protein A, clumping factor, and other **microbial components recognizing adhesive matrix molecules [MSCRAMMs]**); and secreted factors (free coagulase, hemolysins, leukocidins, and other exotoxins). Some strains produce β-lactamase (an enzyme that breaks down penicillin) and penicillin-binding protein 2a (which makes the organism methicillin resistant).

- Infections are treated with antibiotics, although antibiotic resistance to penicillin and other antibiotics is a problem, draining abscesses, and supportive therapy for hypotension and shock.

*S*taphylococcus aureus* (Gram-positive cocci) are the most common of the **pyogenic,** or pus-producing, bacteria that cause human diseases. They colonize the anterior nares of 30 to 40% of individuals and may be present on other mucous membranes and the skin. The organism also causes more-frequent and varied types of diseases than perhaps any other human pathogen (see box, *Diseases Caused by Staphylococci*). The bacteria can produce focal abscesses at almost any site in the body, from the skin (furuncles, or "boils") to the lungs, bones (osteomyelitis), kidneys, and heart. In addition, many strains of the bacterium secrete potent exotoxins that can cause signs of illness at sites distant from the bacteria themselves. These illnesses include **toxic shock syndrome (TSS),** caused by toxic shock syndrome toxin-1 (**TSST-1**) and staphylococcal enterotoxin serotypes A through T; **staphylococcal scalded skin syndrome (SSSS),** caused by exfoliative toxin serotypes

Diseases Caused by *Staphylococcus aureus*

Skin and soft tissue infections
    Furuncles, carbuncles, paronychia (nail infections)
    Wound infections (traumatic, surgical)
    Cellulitis
    Impetigo (also caused by streptococci)
    Bacteremia (frequently with metastatic abscesses)
Endocarditis
Central nervous system infections
    Brain abscess
    Meningitis (rare)
    Epidural abscess
Pulmonary infections
    Embolic
    Aspiration

Musculoskeletal infections
    Osteomyelitis
    Arthritis
Genitourinary tract infections
    Renal abscess
    Lower urinary tract infection
Toxin-related diseases
    Toxic shock syndrome
    Scalded skin syndrome
Food poisoning (gastroenteritis)

A and B; and **staphylococcal food poisoning (SFP)**, caused by ingestion of staphylococcal enterotoxin serotypes A through E. Staphylococcal enterotoxin F was renamed TSST-1 because of its association with TSS and its lack of ability to cause food poisoning. TSS is a serious condition that results from focal infections at any body site by toxin-producing *S. aureus*, but vaginal mucosal and respiratory infections are most likely to lead to the illness. SSSS, another serious illness, occurs most often in neonates who have acquired focal infections, often of the upper respiratory tract, by exfoliative toxin-producing staphylococci.

    S. aureus can persist in the human host and cause illness because it produces numerous cell surface virulence factors, exotoxins, and enzymes. The secreted and cell surface virulence factors produced by staphylococci act locally mainly to help them withstand phagocytosis by neutrophils. For example, **clumping factor** (also known as bound coagulase) binds fibrin and helps the organism form walled-off abscesses protected from phagocytes. In addition, some factors act systemically to interfere with normal immune system function (for example, TSST-1). As a result, staphylococci are among the most adaptable of the pathogenic bacteria. They are difficult to eliminate from the human environment, and they are responsible for many community- and hospital-associated infections.

Case

Skin Infection, Osteomyelitis, and Food Poisoning

Mr. B., a 45-year-old pastry chef, abraded his left forearm while working. Over the next week he noticed swelling, redness, and warmth at the site. He thought his symptoms were a reaction to the abrasion, but after 4 more days, the initial site was larger and clearly more inflamed, and he developed fever with shaking chills. When he came to the emergency department, he also had severe low-back pain.

    Physical examination revealed a fever of 39.4°C and a swollen left forearm with an area of central softness, indicating an abscess. He had tenderness to pressure over his lower spine. The laboratory reported that he had a high white blood cell count. A Gram stain of organisms grown on blood agar plates from the forearm showed Gram-positive cocci in clusters (Fig. 11-1). *Staphylococcus aureus* was cultured from the pus. Blood cultures were positive for the same organism. A nuclear bone scan showed increased uptake of the third lumbar vertebra, suggesting osteomyelitis (Fig. 11-2). The organism was resistant to penicillin but sensitive to nafcillin, which was used to treat Mr. B. with good results.

    The day after Mr. B. was admitted to the hospital, the local public health department was notified that eight customers at the restaurant where he worked had developed severe vomiting and diarrhea 4 to 6 hours after eating there. Health department investigators learned that 6 of the 8 persons who had diarrhea had eaten cream pie, whereas only 1 of 15 patrons who were well ate pie. Cultures of the remaining cream pies in the restaurant refrigerator were positive for *S. aureus*. A preformed staphylococcal toxin called enterotoxin A was detected in the cream pies. The organisms from the contaminated food belonged to the same pulsed field gel electrophoresis type as those isolated from the patient's abscess and blood and were therefore likely to be the same.

FIGURE 11-1 ▪ **Gram stain of *Staphylococcus aureus*.**

This case raises several questions:

1. What was the source of the organisms that infected Mr. B.?
2. What contributed to the development of the abscess in the skin?
3. How did *S. aureus* invade his bloodstream?
4. How did *S. aureus* cause infection in the bone?
5. What caused the food poisoning in the restaurant patrons?
6. What are the properties of *S. aureus* that allow it to cause such different types of disease?

The case of Mr. B. illustrates several features typical of *S. aureus* infections. The initial lesion, what might be referred to as a boil, was mild and localized. Boils are the most common manifestation of *S. aureus* disease. Although boils are usually self-terminating, in Mr. B.'s case the infection moved to the bloodstream, a complication that can be life threatening. The only apparent metastatic focus of Mr. B.'s infection was a

FIGURE 11-2 ▪ **X-ray of the lumbar vertebrae showing destruction of bone associated with staphylococcal osteomyelitis.**

vertebral bone infection (osteomyelitis), a localized form of *S. aureus* infection. Ha metastatic infection of the heart valve (endo brain or kidney abscess, he would have been at and serious risk.

Case

Toxic Shock Syndrome

A 20-year-old college athlete, Ms. G., had arthroscopic knee surgery. Over the next week she noticed mild swelling, increasing pain, and a small amount of redness at the incision site. Within three weeks the incision site had nearly completely healed, but the patient's knee remained swollen and painful. In addition, she was febrile (41.3°C) and had developed vomiting and diarrhea. She came to the emergency department for treatment. Examination revealed a "toxic-appearing" young woman who had a sunburnlike rash on her face, mild skin peeling above the eyes, and red eyes and lips (Fig. 11-3A). Her blood pressure was 70/50 mm Hg, indicating she was hypotensive, and she had elevated white cells in the blood and a significantly reduced number of platelets.

Ms. G. was admitted to the intensive care unit for management of her fever and hypotension. Throat, anterior nares, and vaginal cultures were negative for *S. aureus* and *Streptococcus pyogenes*, but because the surgical incision site had healed, it was not cultured originally. Over the next day her condition worsened, despite being treated with oxacillin and supportive care (fluid and electrolytes and vasopressors to maintain blood pressure), and she developed gangrenous toes (Fig. 11-3B). A needle was inserted into the site of the previous knee surgery, and 300 ml of serous fluid was removed that cultured positive for *S. aureus* (a strain that made

FIGURE 11-3 ▪ **Toxic shock syndrome. A.** Appearance of the rash associated with staphylococcal toxic shock syndrome (TSS). **B.** Gangrenous toes associated with prolonged hypotension in TSS. **C.** Desquamation of the skin that occurs during the resolution of TSS.

slowly progressive,
d he developed
carditis) or a
immediate

...hicillin resistant. The
...nclude vancomycin,
...ulin (which contains
...eeks after recovery
...ling (Fig. 11-3C).

...s that infected

...of the subcuta-

...why is the incision site not highly inflamed?
4. What properties of TSST-1 led to the patient's symptoms?
5. What are the properties of the organism that prevented it from being cleared by oxacillin?

The case of Ms. G. illustrates several features typical of *S. aureus* toxin-mediated diseases. The initial lesion was a subcutaneous abscess that was overlooked because of its minimal inflammatory features. This is not surprising, because the primary site of *S. aureus* infection is often trivial or inapparent in TSS. The lack of inflammation makes it difficult to identify the infection site, but the clinical features are clearly typical of staphylococcal TSS. It is important in such patients to maintain blood pressure adequately to prevent development of gangrene, as happened with Ms. G.'s toes. She lost the tips of two toes as a consequence of her prolonged hypotension. The patient's causative bacterium was methicillin resistant, which emphasizes the need to find the infection site and determine antibiotic susceptibility. Intravenous immunoglobulin has been shown experimentally to reduce the case fatality rate of streptococcal TSS, and it is being used to treat both staphylococcal and streptococcal TSS. Its mechanism of action is likely to be neutralization of the causative exotoxins.

■ ■ ■ ■ ■

Staphylococcus aureus is a large (1 μm in diameter) Gram-positive coccus that grows in grapelike clusters. It is one of the hardiest of the non–spore-forming bacteria and can survive for long periods on dry, inanimate objects. It is also relatively heat resistant. These properties permit *S. aureus* to survive in almost any environment in which humans coexist.

The genus *Staphylococcus* includes several species (Table 11-1). The most ubiquitous *Staphylococcus* species is *S. epidermidis*, which is found on the skin of most people and only infrequently causes disease in otherwise healthy individuals. The organism causes numerous infections in hospitals and in patients with implanted artificial devices (e.g., intravenous catheters, vascular grafts, and artificial joints). *S. aureus* is less common but generally more pathogenic. The species name *aureus* means "golden" and refers to carotenoid pigmentation of *S. aureus* colonies (other species colonies are white, but occasionally *S. aureus* colonies are also white). *S. saprophyticus* is unique in that it apparently causes only urinary tract infections. A fourth species, *S. lugdunensis*, is an uncommon cause of aggressive endocarditis. The genus *Staphylococcus* contains other species that occasionally cause disease; those species are described in standard microbiological texts. The four species specified here suffice for the purposes of this book.

It is relatively easy to identify staphylococci in the laboratory. All members make large, creamy colonies on nutrient agar, and in a Gram stain they look like clusters of grapes (*staphylo* is derived from the Greek word for grape clusters). *S. aureus* is best distinguished from other species of the genus by using the **coagulase test.** Free coagulase, a secreted enzyme that clots plasma, is made by *S. aureus* but not by the other staphylococci. Occasional strains fail to produce free coagulase, but *S. aureus* also makes clumping factor (bound coagulase) that causes plasma to clump around the organisms in a slide test.

Within a species of staphylococci, individual strains can be identified by differences in their resistance to a panel of antibiotics, using a procedure called phage typing, or more commonly, pulsed field gel electrophoresis. Phage typing, which is rarely done today, involves determining the sensitivity of a strain to a variety of standard bacteriophages. **Pulsed field gel electrophoresis** involves isolating staphylococcal DNA, treating the DNA with restriction enzymes that cut the DNA only rarely, and then resolving those DNA fragments in agarose gels. The newer molecular techniques for typing staphylococci based on the DNA sequence of the bacterial chromosome provide greater discrimination than phage typing

table **11-1**	Properties of Various Species of *Staphylococcus*				
SPECIES	FREQUENCY OF DISEASE	COAGULASE	COLOR OF COLONIES	MANNITOL FERMENTATION	NOVOBIOCIN RESISTANCE
S. aureus	Common	+	White to Gold	+	−
S. epidermidis	Common	−	White	−	−
S. saprophyticus	Occasional	−	White	−	+
S. lugdunensis	Uncommon	−	White	−	−
Others	Different responses by individual species				

between outbreak-related and non–outbreak-related strains, and as shown in the cases cited in this chapter, showed the relatedness of the organisms.

Staphylococci

ENCOUNTER

Staphylococci share their environment with that of human beings. They live on people and survive on inanimate objects and surfaces (fomites), such as bedding, clothing, and doorknobs. Humans are the major reservoir for *S. aureus*. The organisms frequently colonize the anterior nares and are found in approximately 30% of healthy individuals. However, studies of individuals over time have found that up to 90% of people are eventually colonized in the nares with *S. aureus* at some point in their lives. The organisms can also be found transiently on the skin, oropharynx, vagina, and in feces. Staphylococci are well equipped to colonize the skin because they grow at high salt and lipid concentrations. They make enzymes, referred to as **lipases** and **glycerol ester hydrolases,** that degrade skin lipids.

The ability of *S. aureus* to colonize the skin and mucosal surfaces has been associated with bacterial cell surface proteins—the MSCRAMMs—that bind to a variety of extracellular matrix proteins. **Fibronectin-binding proteins (FnbpA and FnbpB)** have been identified on the surface of *S. aureus*. Fnbp's allow the bacteria to invade epithelial and endothelial cells and to attach to exposed fibronectin in wounds, which may make FnbpA and FnbpB important virulence factors for the invasion of deeper tissues. *S aureus* also has MSCRAMMs for **collagen binding;** called CNAs. they are important components of connective tissue, bones, and joints. Other MSCRAMMs, called clumping factors A and B, are present for **fibrinogen binding,** and experimentally have been shown to be important in clot formation and endocarditis. These proteins are responsible for the clumping seen in the slide coagulase test.

Staphylococci spread from person to person, usually through direct contact or aerosols associated with upper respiratory viral or bacterial infections. It is important to remember that *S. aureus* is an important secondary pathogen associated with patients recovering from influenza and parainfluenza (croup) infections. Infants may become colonized with *S. aureus* shortly after birth, acquiring the organism from people in their immediate surroundings. Some people will become carriers for prolonged periods, while others will harbor the organisms only intermittently. For unknown reasons people in certain occupations, including physicians, nurses, and other hospital workers, are more prone to colonization. Also, certain patient groups, including diabetics, patients on hemodialysis, and chronic intravenous drug abusers, have a higher carriage rate than does the general population.

ENTRY

S. aureus and most other bacteria do not usually penetrate into deep tissues unless the skin or the mucous membranes are damaged or actually cut. Skin damage may be caused by burns, accidental wounds, lacerations, insect bites, surgical intervention, or associated skin diseases. In Mr. B.'s case, the organisms penetrated through a skin abrasion. If present in very large numbers, some bacteria, including *S. aureus*, are able to enter spontaneously and cause disease. This scenario occurs in cases of poor hygiene or prolonged moisture of the skin, which permit the growth of large numbers of organisms. It is not known if these infections are caused by spontaneous penetration or if the organisms enter through inapparent cuts and abrasions.

SPREAD AND MULTIPLICATION

The survival of *S. aureus* in tissues depends on several factors: the number of entering organisms, the site involved, the speed with which the body mounts an inflammatory response, and the immunological history of the host. When the inoculum is small and the host is immunologically competent, infections by these and other organisms are usually stopped. Nonetheless, staphylococci possess a particularly complex but effective pathogenic strategy, and even healthy persons may be unable to combat *S. aureus*. Luckily, the area of inflammation most often remains localized, and the organisms can be contained.

DAMAGE

Most local staphylococcal infections lead to the formation of a collection of pus called an **abscess**. Abscesses in the skin are called boils or, in medical parlance, **furuncles.** Multiple interconnected abscesses are called **carbuncles.** Alternatively, staphylococci can spread in the subcutaneous or submucosal tissue and cause a diffuse inflammation called **cellulitis.** In most cases these skin infections are caused by *S. aureus* and not by the other staphylococcal species.

The development of an abscess is a complex process that involves both bacterial and host factors (Fig. 11-4). The early events are characteristic of an **acute inflammatory reaction,** with a rapid and extensive influx of neutrophils. Chemotactic factors, derived both from bacteria and complement, are made in large amounts. However, some staphylococci not only survive this onslaught but are even capable of killing and lysing many of the neutrophils that have entered the infection area. The lysed neutrophils pour out large amounts of lysosomal enzymes, which damage surrounding tissue.

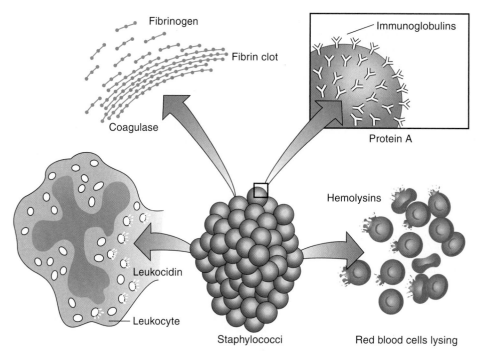

FIGURE 11-4 ■ Virulence properties of *S. aureus* in pus and abscess formation.

The combination of MSCRAMMs and an intense host response to the organisms results in the area being surrounded with a thick-walled fibrin capsule. The center of the abscess is usually necrotic and contains debris consisting of dead neutrophils and epithelial cells, dead and live bacteria, and edema fluid. An abscess, then, is a well-defined area in tissue that contains pus. From the point of view of the host, it represents a containment of invading organisms in one site. However, from the point of view of the staphylococci, it represents a walled-off site protected from the host immune attack. The site may also be the source of toxins such as toxic shock syndrome toxin-1 and staphylococcal enterotoxins that can result in TSS.

Staphylococcal infection involves a massive struggle between the white blood cells and the invading organisms (see Fig. 11-4). Despite an impressive array of virulence factors, *S. aureus* does not always win the struggle; neutrophils usually gain the upper hand. The importance of neutrophils in containing staphylococcal infections is evident in children with the hereditary defect in phagocyte function called **chronic granulomatous disease.** This potentially fatal disease is characterized by frequent and serious infections with *S. aureus.* Neutrophils of these patients are unable to make sufficient hydrogen peroxide to set off the oxidative killing pathway. In these children the balance between staphylococci and phagocytes is clearly shifted toward the microorganisms.

S. aureus produces an unusually large number of virulence factors that either prevent the bacteria from being phagocytized or help them to survive in phagocytes after they are ingested. These factors include soluble enzymes, toxins, and cell envelope constituents. This formidable list invites speculation: why are so many virulence factors needed? Perhaps these factors do not individually impart virulence but act in concert to permit the pathogen to cause disease. Or perhaps different factors are important in different sites of infection. More detailed study of these molecules is needed to answer these puzzling questions.

What are the main factors that allow staphylococci to defend themselves against neutrophils? First, the cell surface of staphylococci plays an important defensive role. More than 90% of *S. aureus* strains that cause disease are surrounded by a **capsule** that may inhibit phagocytosis, but its role in virulence is far less clear than the capsules of meningococcus or pneumococcus. By far the most common capsular serotypes are 5 and 8. Staphylococci also make a slime layer that provides protection from host neutrophils. **Peptidoglycan** in the cell wall of *S. aureus* activates complement by the alternative pathway, thus contributing to the inflammatory response. Peptidoglycan also interacts with toll-like receptors (particularly **toll-like receptor-2**) on the surface of macrophages, causing these phagocytic cells to release proinflammatory cytokines. Note that in this regard staphylococcal peptidoglycan resembles the endotoxin of Gram-negative bacteria. Endotoxin activates the alternative pathway of complement and interacts with toll-like receptor 4 on macrophages to cause proinflammatory cytokine release. Another important cell wall constituent is **teichoic acid,** a polymer of ribitol and glycerophosphates (see Chapter 3), which also appears to be involved in complement activation and possibly in the adherence of these organisms to mucosal cells.

A fourth wall component, **protein A,** has an unexpected property: it binds to the Fc terminus of immunoglobulin G. This binding incapacitates the antibody function of these molecules because their antigen-binding end, the Fab portion, is dangling away from the surface of the organisms. As a result, the number of Fc residues available for attachment to phagocytes is reduced, thereby reducing opsonization. Protein A is also released into the environment surrounding bacterial growth, where it may bind free antibodies in the same manner (see Fig. 11-4).

In addition to these components, *S. aureus* secretes many enzymes and toxins that are almost certainly directed toward the struggle with phagocytes. **Catalase** converts hydrogen peroxide to water and may help counteract the neutrophils' ability to kill bacteria by the production of oxygen free radicals. **Coagulases** convert fibrinogen to fibrin and may help prevent the organisms from being phagocytized, since white cells penetrate fibrin clots poorly.

Several **pore-forming toxins** are important virulence factors of *S. aureus*. The molecules damage not only phagocytic cells but also other cells (e.g., vascular endothelium, renal endothelium, neurons, and myocardial cells). These toxins exert their effect by creating channels in cell membranes that significantly disturb cellular homeostasis. The α-, γ-, and δ-toxins have been traditionally referred to as **hemolysins** because they lyse red blood cells contained in blood agar plates. However, this effect on red cells does not appear to play a role in human infection. γ-Toxin and a related toxin called **Panton-Valentine leukocidin** are particularly effective in damaging neutrophils. Another non–pore-forming hemolysin is called β-toxin; this protein toxin is a sphingomyelinase (also called hot-cold hemolysin) that prepares red blood cells at 37°C for lysis at 4°C. The role of β-toxin in human disease is unclear.

Several other proteins made by *S. aureus* probably enhance its virulence by damaging tissues. Many strains make a **hyaluronidase,** which hydrolyzes the matrix of connective tissue and perhaps facilitates bacterial spread along tissue planes. Most strains also make lipases, proteases, deoxyribonucleases (DNases), and other enzymes that may also act as **virulence enhancers.**

In addition to tissue-damaging factors, *S. aureus* produces substances that make them difficult to treat with antibiotics. Two highly clinically significant examples of these substances are β-**lactamase,** a powerful enzyme that hydrolyzes the classical penicillins, and production of **penicillin-binding protein 2a (PBP2a),** which confers resistance to all penicillin- and cephalosporin-class antibiotics (referred to as **methicillin resistant**). β-lactamase is found in about 90% of *S. aureus* strains and is responsible for the resistance to penicillins that was identified in the late 1940s and spread rapidly around the world. PBP2a mediates continued peptidoglycan synthesis in the presence of all types of penicillin and cephalosporin antibiotics as a result of an alteration in the binding site and decreased affinity for these antibiotics. Today as many as 50% of hospital-associated *S. aureus* strains and 20% of community-associated strains may be methicillin resistant owing to PBP2a. PBP2a is encoded by as many as four staphylococcal cassette chromosome (SCC) methicillin resistance (*mec*) DNAs contained within the chromosome. All four SCC *mec* DNAs code for PBP2a.

In Mr. B.'s case the organisms escaped from the abscess in the skin and entered the bloodstream. This outcome is somewhat unusual because most local staphylococcal diseases are self-limiting by spontaneously draining through the skin; they do not typically result in metastatic infections. In healthy individuals, organisms that escape from a local abscess are usually destroyed by the clearance mechanisms of the blood and the lymphatics. Mr. B. did not appear to have impaired defenses, although impairment could have been temporary. On the other hand, the "shower" of organisms from the skin lesion could have been so great that it overwhelmed the capacity of the body to destroy them. When staphylococci become implanted in deep tissues, they tend to colonize tissues that have been previously damaged by physical trauma, disease, or surgical intervention. Otherwise, the site of metastatic infection seems random and is probably dictated by the clearing capacity of the organ and the amount of blood flowing through it. The main sites of metastatic abscesses are the highly vascularized organs: bones, joints, lungs, and kidneys. Immunocompromised patients frequently have multiple staphylococcal metastases, which can lead to serious and often fatal diseases.

Once implanted in deep tissue and able to survive, *S. aureus* elicits an inflammatory reaction similar to that of a skin abscess. In the words of Pasteur, osteomyelitis is a "boil of the bone." The consequences of abscess formation in deep sites depend on their location. Nowhere is it more devastating than in the heart, lung, or brain. However, if the function of the organ is not directly compromised, staphylococcal abscesses can persist for a considerable period and cause relatively mild symptoms. These symptoms may tax the diagnostic acumen of the physician.

Damage Caused by Other Species of Staphylococci

S. epidermidis, the common inhabitant of the normal skin, rarely causes disease. However, infections with *S. epidermidis* and other coagulase-negative staphylococci are found with increasing frequency in patients with implanted artificial devices, such as prosthetic joints or intravenous catheters. When defense mechanisms are impaired, *S. epidermidis* can cause serious infections, like septicemia and endocarditis. A potential virulence factor of these organisms is the peptidoglycan, and the same exopolysaccharide **slime layer** that is present in *S. aureus* has been found in more than 80% of disease-causing isolates of *S. epidermidis*. It is thought that this slime layer allows the organisms to stick to the surface of plastics used in various devices.

S. saprophyticus, another coagulase negative organism, may be the most highly specialized of the staphylococci in terms of pathogenicity because it is almost entirely associated with urinary tract infections, particularly cystitis in young women. The reason for this specialization is not yet known, but it seems likely that this organism has unique properties that allow it to bind the epithelium of the urethra or the bladder. Uncommonly, the coagulase-negative *S. lugdunensis* is now recognized as the cause of an aggressive endocarditis. The virulence properties of the organism that lead to this infection are unclear.

Staphylococcal Toxin Diseases

In contrast to the classical complicated infections already discussed, staphylococci cause three definite toxin-related diseases. The symptoms of each of these diseases are clearly caused by toxins, even in the absence of bacteria. The first disease is called **staphylococcal scalded skin syndrome (SSSS)**, a life-threatening disease that mainly affects neonates. SSSS is characterized by extensive sloughing of the skin. Two exotoxins, known as **exfoliative toxins A** and **B,** cause these symptoms. Their role in human disease has been clearly established because the administration of specific antitoxin prevents the skin lesions in humans or mice. Exfoliative toxins are highly tissue-specific serine proteases that cause separation of the layers of the epidermis at the **desmosomes.** Exfoliative toxin production by *S. aureus* does not contribute to systemic infections by the bacteria.

A second disease definitively caused by exotoxins, called **toxic shock syndrome (TSS),** is characterized by fever, skin rash, hypotension, peeling of the skin on recovery, and the dysfunction of several essential systems as was the case in Ms. G's illness (see Fig. 11-3). However, TSS can occur in the absence of one or more of those defining symptoms. The disease was originally associated with the use of highly absorbent tampons, which appear to introduce oxygen into the vagina and stimulate toxin production by the organisms. Oxygen is absolutely essential to the production of TSS-inducing toxins, and the vagina in the absence of tampons is anaerobic. TSS still occurs in association with tampon use, though less frequently as a result of the use of lower-absorbency tampons, but also commonly follows staphylococcal infections of any other type, and it occurs in men as well as women. Ms. G presented with the typical signs of TSS; she was of menstrual age, and also used tampons. However, her case of TSS was associated with an abscess associated with recent arthroscopic knee surgery. Of particular importance is the increasing association of TSS with lung infections and necrotizing pneumonia, particularly in strains of bacteria that are methicillin resistant.

The exotoxins involved include **toxic shock syndrome toxin-1,** the cause of all menstrual TSS cases and one half of nonmenstrual cases, and **staphylococcal enterotoxins,** particularly enterotoxin serotypes B and C. These three exotoxins are produced by the bacteria in high concentrations, and that may be why they cause TSS. The toxins have recently been referred to as **superantigens** because of their novel way of interacting with T lymphocytes and macrophages (see Fig. 8-3). Superantigens cross-link one chain (β-chain) of the T-cell antigen receptor with major histocompatibility complex class II molecules on macrophages. The effect of this interaction is a massive release of cytokines from macrophages and T cells that mediate TSS. For example, interleukin 1 (endogenous pyrogen) released from macrophages causes the fever of TSS. Tumor necrosis factor-α released from macrophages and tumor necrosis factor-β released from T cells cause capillary leak and therefore hypotension. Finally, interferon-γ and interleukin 2 release from T cells accounts for the rash of TSS patients. It is also important to remember that the massive release of interferon-γ in TSS appears to prevent formation of protective neutralizing antibodies against the superantigens. Thus, TSS patients mostly remain susceptible to recurrent TSS, particularly women who continue to use tampons after TSS episodes. In addition, superantigens appear to subvert the formation of inflammation through an undefined mechanism when the organism is in abscesses. Thus, for example, surgical incision sites may not show the characteristic inflammation associated with staphylococcal infections. The staphylococcal superantigens are structurally related to the streptococcal scarlet fever toxins, which also cause TSS.

Finally, **staphylococcal enterotoxins serotypes A through E** are major causes of **food poisoning** when ingested, as in the cases of the people who ate the pies Mr. B. baked. These exotoxins can cause disease even in the absence of the organism. They cause intensive intestinal peristalsis, apparently by working directly on the vomiting control center of the brain. They are heat stable, resist proteases, and are not necessarily destroyed by cooking, even though the staphylococci that produced them are killed. These toxins cause signs and symptoms that mimic the disease when administered to laboratory animals. Note that the same strain of *S. aureus* can cause several of the diseases mentioned. In the case described here, a single strain was responsible for Mr. B.'s bone and soft tissue infection, as well as for food poisoning in the people who ate the pastries prepared by him.

All of the virulence factors, whether cell associated or secreted, are under the control of global genetic regulators. As in many other bacteria, these regulators include two-component regulatory systems, such as **accessory gene regulator (Agr)**, **staphylococcal respiratory response (Srr)**, and others (see Chapter 19 paradigm).

Diagnosis

Recognizing staphylococcal infections is not usually a difficult diagnostic problem, and they are among the most frequent infections seen both in the community and in the hospital. A localized abscess in a seriously ill patient should be aspirated and the contents examined by Gram stain and culture to identify the staphylococcal species as well as the antibiotic susceptibility patterns. Clusters of large Gram-positive cocci point to staphylococcal infection. The patient's blood should also be cultured to determine if the organisms have invaded the bloodstream. Both *S. aureus* and coagulase-negative staphylococci are commonly isolated in blood cultures; however, the latter is most often a contaminant and is considered pathogenic only under special circumstances. The coagulase test serves to distinguish the two species.

Treatment

A staphylococcal abscess, such as those seen in Mr. B., should be drained and an appropriate antibiotic should be administered. The bacteria will probably be resistant to penicillin but sensitive to semisynthetic penicillins— that is, **methicillin-sensitive *S. aureus* (MSSA)**. Semisynthetic penicillins and cephalosporins that are resistant to staphylococcal β-lactamase will kill these bacteria. **Methicillin-resistant *S. aureus* (MRSA)** has appeared with increasing frequency, first in hospitals and more recently in the community. Infections with MRSA require treatment with vancomycin, which until recently was the last available drug for some highly resistant strains.

Other antibiotics (e.g., aminoglycosides, macrolides, trimethoprim/sulfamethoxazole, clindamycin, and tetracyclines) may be useful second-line agents in the treatment of certain kinds of staphylococcal infections (particularly in penicillin allergic patients), although some strains are resistant to them as well. Fluoroquinolones had been used to treat MRSA infections. Unfortunately, resistance to these antibiotics has also developed rapidly; 60 to 70% of MRSA isolates are also quinolone-resistant. One antibiotic that deserves special mention is clindamycin. This inhibitor of protein synthesis has become a useful antibiotic in the treatment of exotoxin diseases of both staphylococci and streptococci because of its ability to prevent exotoxin synthesis prior to inhibiting

the growth of the organisms. The choice of drugs should be based on the antibiotic sensitivity of the infecting strain and the special characteristics of the patient.

Unfortunately, in the last few years, a handful of patients in the United States have been identified with high-level vancomycin resistance in the presence of methicillin resistance. **Vancomycin-resistant *S. Aureus* (VRSA)** has acquired the genes that encode vancomycin resistance from resistant *Enterococcus* species in patients infected with both pathogens. Newer antimicrobial agents, such as linezolid, Synercid, and daptomycin, generally have activity against staphylococci that are resistant to multiple antibiotics. These newer antibiotics are generally reserved for such cases and when vancomycin cannot be used. Nevertheless, if multidrug-resistant staphylococci emerge as major clinical entities, we may one day face the daunting problem of common and potentially dangerous staphylococcal infections with no effective antibiotics at our disposal.

Some physicians have advocated the use of intravenous immunoglobulin in the treatment of superantigen-mediated TSS. These antibody preparations are obtained from large pools of human volunteers, many of whom have preexistent antibodies to superantigens. There is published evidence of reductions in fatality rates with use of intravenous immunoglobulins for the treatment of streptococcal TSS.

Over the years, vaccines have been developed for the treatment of recurrent, recalcitrant staphylococcal infections and to prevent the carrier state. Success has been limited, probably because circulating antibodies play a relatively minor role in these infections. Attempts to develop vaccines continue today.

Conclusion

Staphylococci are potent pathogens, are widely found in the human environment, and may cause a variety of infections. They are hardy organisms that can survive under adverse conditions. They possess a large number of virulence factors that allow them to cause serious diseases by various mechanisms. The most common diseases caused by these versatile pathogens are pyogenic infections, sometimes leading to the formation of abscesses in deep tissues. They can also cause distinct disease entities by making specific toxins. Staphylococci have acquired antimicrobial resistance promptly after the introduction of new antibiotics. Currently, many strains are resistant to all but one or two available antibiotics, and the prospect of the emergence of a strain resistant to all available antibiotics is a serious concern.

chapter **12**

Streptococci and Enterococci: Sore Throats and Beyond

George C. Fogg

key **concepts**

Streptococci:

■ Are Gram-positive cocci that grow in pairs or chains.

■ Are classified by their characteristic hemolytic patterns, serologic reaction of cell wall antigens, and speciation based on metabolic or biochemical profiles and DNA sequence differences.

■ Group A streptococci (GAS) elaborate several extracellular proteins that allow them to cause extensive tissue damage and spread from the local site of infection. This results in a wide range of clinical manifestations of infection.

■ GAS infection can result in immune-related disease, even after the organism has been cleared from the body.

■ Group B streptococci (GBS) are a leading cause of neonatal sepsis and meningitis.

Enterococci:

■ Are intrinsically resistant to many antibiotics and often require synergistic antibiotic combinations to successfully treat infection.

■ Vancomycin-resistant enterococci are an increasing problem in hospitals because physicians are running out of effective antibiotics to treat them.

The streptococci and enterococci are a heterogeneous group of bacteria that colonize and infect humans and animals. In humans they cause diseases as diverse as streptococcal pharyngitis ("strep throat"), cellulitis, neonatal meningitis, brain abscesses, endocarditis, and life-threatening necrotizing fasciitis (the "flesh eating" bacteria). For humans the most significant member of this diverse family is *Streptococcus pyogenes,* also known as **Group A streptococcus (GAS),** because they cause the most widespread disease in humans, cause a wide variety of clinical manifestations as a result of infection, and are the best understood in terms of mechanisms of disease. The pneumococcus (*Streptococcus pneumoniae*) is another important bacteria within the streptococcal family that is covered in detail in Chapter 13.

Case

V., a 5-year-old girl, had a sore throat, headache, and fever for 5 days. Her mother then brought her to the pediatrician because she developed a red, rough "sandpaper-like" rash on her arms. She had swollen, tender cervical lymph nodes, and her oropharynx was red with a grayish-white exudate covering both tonsils. Her throat swab was positive for presence of GAS antigen on the rapid enzyme immunoassay (rapid strep test), and the culture subsequently grew a β-hemolytic streptococcus. A 10-day course of penicillin was prescribed. After the second day on antibiotics, V. felt much better, and her mother decided to stop giving her the penicillin so she could have it for other illnesses in the future. Three weeks later, V. was having trouble keeping up with her classmates on the playground, had pain in her knees, and was again having fevers. After hearing a loud heart murmur on physical examination, her pediatrician obtained an echocardiogram that demonstrated mitral valve regurgitation and extensive damage to the valve leaflets.

This case raises several questions:

1. Streptococcal pharyngitis is a common self-limited disease. Why do physicians always treat this disease?
2. What bacterial process caused the rash?
3. Why were 2 days of antibiotics insufficient treatment, even though V. felt better?
4. Did the GAS directly spread to the heart and cause the damage to the heart valves?

Classification of Streptococci and Enterococci

The nomenclature for the streptococci and enterococci is confusing because there are three different methods of classification:

- **Hemolytic pattern:** When streptococci are grown on blood agar media in the clinical laboratory, the colonies may be surrounded by an area of partial hemolysis that appears greenish (α-hemolysis), or a clear zone of complete hemolysis (β-hemolysis). Nonhemolytic colonies have no zone surrounding them and are called γ-hemolytic.
- **Group-specific antigens (Lancefield classification):** Rebecca Lancefield used **serological reactivity** to extracted cell wall antigens from various streptococci to divide them into groups lettered A through U. Many streptococcal species cannot be assigned to any group because there are no antisera that react to their cell wall antigens.
- **Species:** Various species of streptococci can be determined by performing a battery of **biochemical tests** that analyze the metabolism and presence of enzymes in the bacterium. Newer molecular techniques that differentiate species on the basis of **DNA sequences** can also be used.

In the clinical laboratory all three methods may be employed to characterize an isolated streptococcus. Figure 12-1 shows a simplified scheme used clinically to classify the streptococci and enterococci. Although they react with group D antisera, the enterococci have recently been assigned their own genus.

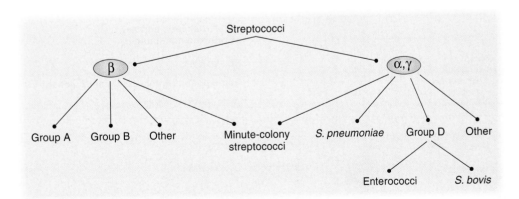

FIGURE 12-1 ▪ A classification of streptococci. β-Hemolytic streptococci are sometimes simply called hemolytic streptococci. α-Hemolytic and γ-hemolytic streptococci are lumped together because most species or groups shown on the right side of the diagram include strains of both hemolytic patterns. Often such organisms are called viridans ("greening") streptococci after the greenish color seen in α-hemolysis.

Group A Streptococci

Historically, group A streptococci (GAS) have been the most important pathogenic organisms in the streptococcal family. Serious GAS infections have become less common in the developed world, but recently the sporadic emergence of highly virulent strains reminds us that this bacterium has the potential to be a significant reemerging pathogen. Morbidity and mortality as a result of GAS infection is still common in the developing world. The spectrum of diseases caused by GAS is influenced by the strain type, host factors, and portal of entry. Some of the most important clinical manifestations of GAS infection are shown in Figure 12-2.

EPIDEMIOLOGY

GAS is ubiquitous in the human population and is distributed worldwide. Disease is most common in school-aged children more than 3 years old, and like V., presents as **acute pharyngitis,** or **"strep throat."** The other common site of infection is in the skin and soft tissues, where a group of infections called **pyoderma** occurs. Pyoderma is most prevalent in preschool children and is seen more frequently in tropical climates or during periods of hot, humid weather. The occurrence of an invasive skin disease following a varicella infection has also been described. GAS also occasionally causes foodborne outbreaks but is not usually associated with gastrointestinal disease. The late nonsuppurative sequelae of GAS infection, acute glomerulonephritis and acute rheumatic fever, are more commonly encountered in tropical regions and developing countries, probably because of more frequent disease and poor access to medical care.

ENCOUNTER

GAS are usually found on the skin and in the nasopharynx of humans. As many as 20% of school-aged children may carry GAS in their pharynxes during the winter months, although many do not have symptoms of infection. V. probably acquired her infection from a schoolmate who may have had a clinical, subclinical, or asymptomatic infection. Person-to-person spread is mediated by **respiratory droplets** or by **direct contact** in the case of skin transmission. GAS carriers are usually asymptomatic and may be colonized for months at a time. People with nasal colonization are able to transmit the organisms more efficiently than are people with skin or pharyngeal colonization.

ENTRY

For streptococcal pyoderma infections, the bacterium must gain entry into deeper layers of skin through direct implantation after a break occurs in the skin (e.g.,

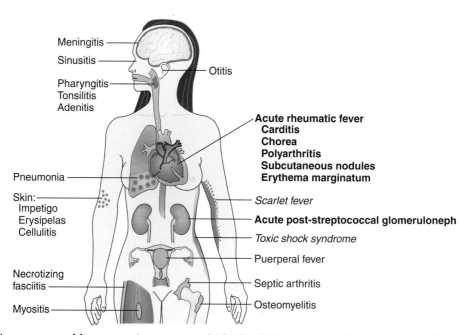

FIGURE 12-2 ▪ **Diseases caused by group A streptococci (GAS).** GAS cause a wide spectrum of diseases throughout the human body. The suppurative diseases (labeled in black) are caused by direct damage by the organism and the secreted enzymes of GAS. The nonsuppurative sequelae of GAS infection (labeled in bold) are late manifestations caused by a self-directed immune response. The toxin-mediated diseases (labeled in italics) are caused by streptococcal exotoxins that are secreted into the bloodstream.

abrasions, chickenpox lesions, bites, wounds, and eczema) because GAS cannot penetrate intact skin. In many cases the damage to the skin can be quite subtle, and even a minor scratch can serve as a portal of entry for GAS. In streptococcal pharyngeal infections, the bacterium is thought to bind to the mucous membranes of the pharynx using **adhesins** on the bacterial cell surface to prevent it from being swept away by fluid secretions. The first adhesin described in GAS was **lipoteichoic acid (LTA),** which is a constituent of the Gram-positive cell envelope. LTA has been shown to bind to the human protein **fibronectin,** which is a protein that coats the cells of the oropharynx. In addition to LTA, several other adhesins have been described in GAS. **Protein F** is another surface protein that binds to fibronectin with high affinity, and its expression seems to be regulated to allow the protein to be expressed under appropriate environmental conditions. **M protein,** one of the most studied streptococcal virulence factors, has been implicated as an important adhesin to keratinocytes, the main cell type in the outer layers of the skin.

SPREAD AND MULTIPLICATION

Most strains of GAS remain localized to the site of initial infection, but an increase in aggressive strains that invade deeper tissues and cause life-threatening diseases was noted in the 1990s. In the oropharynx, infections are usually localized to the pharynx and tonsils, which results in the erythema and exudate associated with strep throat. Rarely, the infection can cause a peritonsillar abscess (quinsy), or spread to adjacent structures such as the mastoids and middle ear. GAS infection of the superficial layers of skin results in crusty lesions called **impetigo,** which are most common in children living in hot, humid climates. Infections in deeper layers of skin cause **erysipelas** and **cellulitis.**

On rare occasions GAS reaches deeper tissues (such as traumatic implantation at a wound site or through an infected insect bite) and rapidly spreads laterally from the initial site of infection. GAS secretes several enzymes that may promote spread along tissue planes resulting in life-threatening diseases such as **necrotizing fasciitis** and **myositis.** These enzymes include proteases, hyaluronidase, deoxyribonucleases (DNases), and **streptokinase.** Streptokinase must bind to the human protein **plasminogen** to form a catalytic complex that converts plasminogen to plasmin, which in turn degrades fibrin, one of the major constituents of blood clots. GAS also secretes **streptolysins S and O,** which form pores in the membranes of various host cells. It is their ability to lyse red blood cells that is the basis for the β-hemolysis pattern seen on blood agar media. Their precise role in the pathogenesis of GAS infection

is unclear, but conceptually they could contribute to the extensive tissue damage seen in invasive GAS infections. With this armamentarium of secreted products, GAS can digest proteins in the extracellular matrix and other large molecules that may hinder spread.

Once GAS enters a host, it must avoid phagocytosis to multiply and establish an effective infection. Two of the most important antiphagocytic factors of GAS are M protein and a hyaluronic acid capsule.

M Protein

M protein is the best-studied virulence factor in GAS and is a central player in streptococcal pathogenesis (Fig. 12-3). In addition to its previously described role in adhesion to keratinocytes, M protein also prevents opsonization by complement through two mechanisms. First, M protein binds the host cell plasma protein, **fibrinogen,** which interferes with the alternative pathway of complement deposition by forming a dense layer on the bacterial surface (Fig 12-4). Second, M protein binds host **complement control proteins.** The complement control proteins inhibit the formation of opsonins by the complement cascade. Despite all these antiphagocytic properties, antibodies formed against the hypervariable regions of M protein (see Fig. 12-3) are able to effectively opsonize the organism and are protective against infection. Unfortunately, there are more than 100 M protein serotypes, and protective immunity is type specific. Although this was probably not the first GAS infection for V., the strains of her previous infections had M proteins different from those of her current infection, so antibodies generated from her previous exposures would not protect her during any subsequent infection. Finally, M protein has characteristics that mimic aspects of human proteins that may contribute to the immune-mediated diseases described later in the chapter.

Hyaluronic Acid Capsule

The hyaluronic acid capsule is another **antiphagocytic structure** on the streptococcal surface. Hyaluronic acid is found in great abundance in human connective tissue. Therefore, streptococci enveloped in a hyaluronic acid capsule have camouflaged themselves in a host antigen that does not elicit an immune response. Indeed, outbreaks of severe GAS infections are often associated with highly encapsulated strains of bacteria that appear mucoid when cultured on blood agar media. Interestingly, this capsule interferes with adherence of GAS to epithelial cells, and the organism may need to shed the capsule during the early stages of infection. This may be achieved by digesting the capsule with hyaluronidase secreted by the bacteria. Hyaluronidase has also been suggested as a spreading factor.

damage. GAS also secrete several toxins that can enter the bloodstream and cause systemic effects.

Streptococcal Toxins

V. had a localized infection in her throat but developed a rash in distant parts of her body. This rash is the hallmark of **scarlet fever,** a toxin-mediated phenomenon usually associated with pharyngeal infections (scarlet fever is rarely associated with pyoderma). The three toxins responsible for scarlet fever are the **streptococcal pyrogenic exotoxins (SPE) A, B,** and **C.** In addition to causing a rash, SPE-A and SPE-C are also bacterial **superantigens** that can nonspecifically activate a large subset of T cells. The resulting massive release of proinflammatory cytokines by the activated T cells results in a sepsislike clinical picture with shock and multiorgan failure. This **streptococcal toxic shock syndrome** has a similar presentation and mechanism as the toxic shock

FIGURE 12-3 ▪ **M protein of GAS.** M protein molecules are typically 500 amino acids long. They are anchored in the cell membrane by a hydrophobic sequence near the C terminus of the protein. They then traverse the cell wall through a sequence rich in glycine and proline and finally emerge to project from the cell wall as fibrils. The fibrils are mostly α-helical and contain two or three blocks of repeating amino acid sequences. Two α-helical fibrils of M protein are wound around each other in a coiled coil conformation. The proximal portion of the molecule binds the complement control protein factor H. The amino-terminal halves, despite their structural heterogeneity, retain the ability to bind fibrinogen, which protects GAS from nonspecific opsonization by the alternative pathway of complement.

DAMAGE

GAS characteristically evokes an intense inflammatory response in tissues. Although it has mechanisms to avoid the immune response, the large variety of secreted substances cause considerable damage to host tissues. The digestive enzymes that enable the GAS to spread to deeper tissues and along tissue planes do much of the

FIGURE 12-4 ▪ **Electron micrographs of GAS. A.** After growth in liquid culture, the organisms have a fuzzy layer on the surface, which is composed of M protein and lipoteichoic acid. The hyaluronic acid capsule cannot be seen because it is in a dehydrated and collapsed state resulting from the fixation process. **B.** After exposure to blood plasma, the fuzzy layer of the same organisms appears dense owing to fibrinogen bound to M protein. Because streptococci grow in chains, the division planes are parallel to each other. Cross walls begin to form in preparation for the next cell division.

syndrome caused by *Staphylococcus aureus* (see Chapter 11). Epidemiologically, SPE-A has been most closely linked with streptococcal toxic shock syndrome, but GAS also make several other superantigens.

Immunologically Mediated Disease

Although most GAS infections are mild, self-limited diseases, the immune system's intense inflammatory reaction to an infection may cause a group of diseases called the **nonsuppurative sequelae** (non–pus-forming secondary results of infection). The most feared nonsuppurative sequela of GAS infection is **acute rheumatic fever (ARF)**, a significant cause of valvular heart disease in the preantibiotic era. Streptococcal pharyngitis is the only type of infection that can lead to ARF. The clinical manifestations of ARF appear 1 to 4 weeks following strep throat and include **carditis, polyarthritis, chorea** (a neurological disorder resulting in uncontrollable dancelike movements), **subcutaneous nodules,** and a distinctive rash called **erythema marginatum.** The most common manifestations are carditis and polyarthritis. Eventually, all these manifestations except the carditis resolve.

The primary reason streptococcal pharyngitis is treated with antibiotics is to prevent ARF and the subsequent heart disease. The ongoing inflammation in the heart can lead to extensive **valvular scarring,** which affects the function of the heart. People with ARF may ultimately die from heart failure. Furthermore, the turbulent flow of blood across the scarred valves can predispose people to bacterial endocarditis. People who have had ARF are susceptible to further exacerbations when they get streptococcal pharyngitis. To protect the heart from additional damage, these people are given **prophylactic antibiotics** until well into adulthood or even for life. Fortunately, ARF can be prevented by eradicating the bacteria with antibiotics before a fulminant immunological response is mounted. Studies have shown that treatment with penicillin can be initiated up to 9 days after the onset of sore throat, but a full course of antibiotics must be completed to prevent ARF. Therefore, the 2-day course that V. received may have attenuated the symptoms but did not eliminate the organism. Three weeks later she developed arthritis and mitral valve regurgitation, which are manifestations of ARF.

The precise pathogenic mechanism of ARF remains incompletely understood, but the most compelling evidence suggests that ARF may be an **autoimmune disease** in which the body's own tissues are attacked by the immune system in a misguided attempt to eradicate the streptococci. GAS possess a number of cell wall and surface constituents that immunologically appear identical to host tissue components when presented to the immune system. In particular, there is immunological cross-reaction between GAS antigens (including M proteins from certain serotypes of GAS) and tissues in the heart, synovium, and neurons in the brain. Some serotypes (called **rheumatogenic strains**) are considered more likely to produce ARF than others; however; only small subsets of people infected by a rheumatogenic strain of GAS go on to develop ARF. It is interesting that only one organism that infects only one body site can produce ARF. As generations of scientists who have tried and failed to elucidate the basis of ARF can attest, the development of the disease is probably a complex process that depends on both human and bacterial factors we currently do not fully understand.

The other important nonsuppurative sequela of GAS infection is **acute post-streptococcal glomerulonephritis (APSGN)**. This disease is caused by only a few M serotypes and probably only certain strains within those serotypes. Unlike ARF, APSGN may follow either a pharyngitis or pyodermal infection. In some outbreaks the attack rate is as high as 40%, suggesting that susceptibility is common, if not universal. Treatment with antibiotics does not affect the risk of APSGN. The pathogenic mechanism of APSGN is also incompletely understood, but it is thought that **immune complexes** are deposited in the glomerular basement membrane, leading to complement fixation and subsequent renal injury. Like ARF, APSGN usually occurs one to four weeks after an infection, and several streptococcal antigens have been found to cross-react with renal tissue. Patients with APSGN have blood and elevated protein in their urine and may go on to renal failure and dialysis.

DIAGNOSIS

The diagnosis of streptococcal skin infections is usually straightforward and can be made on clinical grounds. **Impetigo** presents as a cluster of small vesicles on a pink base that breaks down to honey-colored crusts. **Erysipelas** is a raised, bright red patch of skin with a sharply demarcated but rapidly advancing margin. Deep infections such as **necrotizing fasciitis** should be treated aggressively with both antibiotics and surgery without delay, because culture results will not be available in time to make an impact on therapy.

The diagnosis of streptococcal pharyngitis, on the other hand, is more problematic. Despite efforts to develop clinical criteria specific for strep throat, the condition cannot be reliably distinguished from viral pharyngitis, which is also extremely common in children. To determine the cause of pharyngitis, physicians collect a throat swab, perform **rapid strep tests** in the office, and culture the organism on blood agar plates. The rapid strep tests rely on detection of a group A carbohydrate antigen from organisms obtained from the throat swab. They are very specific, so a positive test indicates the presence of GAS, but they are not as sensitive as throat cultures. Therefore, streptococcal pharyngitis is not ruled out until the results of the throat culture are also negative. This may take up to 3 days. Neither one of these tests can distinguish asymptomatic GAS carriage in the oropharynx with a concurrent viral pharyngitis from a true GAS infection. In a case of ARF, APSGN, or streptococcal toxic shock syndrome, diagnosis requires evidence of a preceding GAS infection. Because the organism may not be present by the time some of the late non-suppurative sequelae present themselves, serologic titers to GAS antigens can be used to establish a previous infection. The most common serologic tests are the **anti-streptolysin O (ASO) titer, anti-DNase B titer,** and **Streptozyme® screen** (an agglutination test that detects a mixture of five secreted streptococcal enzymes).

TREATMENT AND PREVENTION

Fortunately, resistance to **penicillin** has never been detected in GAS, so penicillin remains the antibiotic of choice for patients who are not allergic to it. A course of 10 days of oral penicillin therapy is standard therapy. As V.'s case demonstrates, compliance with the full course of therapy is a major problem, and shorter courses are not sufficient therapy to prevent ARF. An alternative therapy is a single-dose injection of long-acting penicillin (**benzathine penicillin**) that persists in the bloodstream for an adequate period. Although this prevents the compliance issue, the injection is painful. A repeat throat swab at the end of therapy is usually not necessary. For individuals allergic to penicillin, **erythromycin** or other **macrolide antibiotics** are appropriate. A caveat is that there have been isolates of erythromycin-resistant GAS found in the community.

Prevention of GAS infection is difficult because it is continuously circulating in the human population. Avoiding crowded living conditions and practicing good hygiene are the most effective public health measures to prevent GAS infections. In the school-aged population, early recognition and treatment of pharyngeal and skin infections can decrease spread to other children. At least 24 hours of antibiotic therapy should be completed before a child is allowed to return to school. There is active research to develop a vaccine against GAS, but currently there is no such vaccine available to physicians.

Group B Streptococci

Group B streptococci (GBS; *Streptococcus agalactiae*) are aerobic Gram-positive diplococci that are β-hemolytic on blood agar plates. Common inhabitants of the lower gastrointestinal and female genital tracts, GBS generally do not cause significant disease in healthy people. Because GBS are particularly pathogenic organisms in **newborn infants**, colonization

of the bacteria in a pregnant woman can lead to a life-threatening infection if the baby acquires the organism during the delivery. The colonization rate ranges from 15 to 40% in pregnant women, and currently pregnant women are screened for GBS at **35 to 37 weeks gestation** by the collection of vaginal and rectal swabs. If a woman has a positive GBS screen, **intrapartum antibiotics** are given to the mother to reduce the transmission of bacteria to the infant. Despite these measures, GBS is still a leading cause of **neonatal sepsis** and **meningitis.** The mortality rate in infants is approximately 5%, and many surviving infants with neonatal infection have long-term problems such as seizures, deafness, developmental delay, and motor deficits. In pregnant women GBS can cause urinary tract infection, endometriosis, and amnionitis. The other major population susceptible to severe GBS infection is the elderly, especially those with chronic diseases such as diabetes mellitus, liver disease, renal disease, or malignancy. Fortunately, like GAS, GBS are still susceptible to penicillin, the first-line therapy for these organisms.

The main mechanism GBS uses to avoid the host immune system is to prevent opsonization and phagocytosis with a **polysaccharide capsule.** There are nine capsular serotypes, and type III is responsible for the majority of the cases of neonatal sepsis and meningitis in the United States. In general, the capsular polysaccharides are poor antigens for stimulating a protective immune response. Therefore, there has been great interest in developing a protein-carbohydrate conjugate vaccine similar to the vaccine for *Haemophilus influenzae* type B, for use in females of childbearing age.

Other Streptococci

There are many other streptococcal species that on occasion cause diseases in humans. **Groups C, G,** and **F streptococci** are **hemolytic** on blood agar plates and can cause several of the same infections as GAS. They have also been associated with the nonsuppurative sequela of acute glomerulonephritis, but not ARF.

The members of this diverse *Streptococcus* group are called the **viridans streptococci** because they are α-hemolytic with a greenish discoloration of blood agar. This group of organisms includes medically important species such as *S. mutans* and *S. sanguis*. Both organisms are important components of **dental plaque** and production of lactic acid during metabolism of sugars causing dental caries. They also intermittently seed the bloodstream after activities such as toothbrushing and can cause endocarditis in people with defective heart valves, including patients with ARF. *S. milleri* is another viridans streptococci that is anaerobic and has a propensity of being involved in abscesses. The brain, liver, and abdominal cavity are frequent sites of infection, and the abscesses tend to be **polymicrobial,** with several other bacterial species present in addition to *S. milleri.*

Another medically significant group comprises **nutritionally variant streptococci** that are difficult to grow in the laboratory because they require supplemental cofactors in their growth media. They can cause a destructive form of endocarditis that results in more complications than do infections with other streptococci.

Enterococci

Initially characterized as group D streptococci, the enterococci are currently in their own genus, *Enterococcus.* In humans, two species, *E. faecalis* and *E. faecium,* are medically important because they cause urinary tract infections, wound infections, endocarditis, intraabdominal abscesses, and bacteremia. Enterococci are part of the normal flora of the gastrointestinal and genitourinary tracts, and they are distinguished from the streptococci by their resistance to bile and the high salt concentrations found in the intestine. For years they were regarded as harmless colonizing bacteria. However, as various antibiotic classes were used with much more frequency, the enterococci demonstrated their amazing adaptability by developing resistance to every type of antibiotic. Thus, in the 1990s this usually harmless commensal bacterium became one of the most feared **nosocomial (hospital-acquired) infections** because it had developed resistance to the last-line antibiotic against Gram-positive organisms, vancomycin.

Despite having low virulence, **vancomycin-resistant enterococci (VRE)** were untreatable because physicians had no effective antibiotics to use against them. One of the reasons enterococci emerged after being subjected to antibiotic selection was that they have remarkable **intrinsic resistance** to several classes of antibiotics. Antibiotics like penicillins usually kill bacteria because they disrupt their cell wall synthesis. In enterococci, however, penicillins are merely **bacteriostatic** (i.e., they inhibit growth but do not kill the bacteria), and cephalosporins are generally not active at all. Enterococci are also intrinsically resistant to aminoglycosides.

Effective killing can be achieved by using a combination treatment of a β-lactam and an aminoglycoside. Using a combination of antibiotics that works much better than either antibiotic alone is called **antibiotic synergy.** Unfortunately, VRE strains are so highly resistant that even antibiotic synergy is not sufficient to kill them. Recently, three antibiotics have been developed that are currently effective against VRE. **Dalfopristin–Quinupristin** is a combination of two synergistic agents that inhibit bacterial protein synthesis. It is effective against vancomycin-resistant strains of *E. faecium,* but not active against *E. faecalis. E. faecalis* infections are clinically more common but are less likely to have vancomycin resistance. **Linezolid** is an antibiotic from a new class of drugs called the oxazolidinones, which inhibit bacterial protein synthesis by preventing formation of the translational initiation complex. It is effective against vancomycin-resistant strains of both *E. faecalis* and *E. faecium.* Lastly, **daptomycin** is a novel lipopeptide that inserts into the bacterial membrane and causes the cell to undergo a metabolic death. Daptomycin appears to be bactericidal against both species of enterococci.

Although all these drugs are welcome additions to the antimicrobial armamentarium, there are already reports of bacteria developing resistance to the first two mentioned in the previous paragraph. Good infection control measures and prudent antibiotic use in hospitals are the best ways to prevent the proliferation of VRE strains in medical centers.

Conclusion

Streptococci are a diverse group of Gram-positive pathogens that cause a wide variety of infections in humans. GAS can cause disease by direct damage, by elaborating potent toxins, and by causing the immune system to direct its attack against itself. GBS is an important pathogen to both mother and child in the peripartum period. While both organisms remain susceptible to penicillins, the previously innocuous enterococci have emerged as significant pathogens, not because of an increase in virulence but because of their ability to acquire antibiotic resistance traits as new classes of antibiotics are used and abused in hospital settings.

chapter 13

Pneumococcus and Bacterial Pneumonia

Jeffrey N. Weiser

key concepts

Pneumococcus:

- Is an α-hemolytic streptococcus that commonly colonizes the human nasopharynx.

- Is a frequent etiologic agent of respiratory tract infections, including otitis media, sinusitis, chronic bronchitis, and pneumonia, as well as invasive infections such as bacteremia and meningitis.

- Causes infection characterized by an acute inflammatory response.

- Resists phagocytic clearance through expression of a polysaccharide capsule.

- Expresses multiple capsular types that are antigenic and combined for use in vaccines.

- Has developed increased resistance to penicillin and other commonly used antibiotics.

*S*treptococcus pneumoniae, the pneumococcus, referred to by Sir William Osler as "the captain of the men of death," remains a leading cause of serious infection, particularly bacterial pneumonia, worldwide. It commonly colonizes the mucosal surface of the nasopharynx without causing disease, unless host factors allow it to gain access to normally sterile sites such as the lung, where it is able to trigger an acute inflammatory response. The presence of a thick layer of surface polysaccharide, however, inhibits otherwise effective host clearance functions involving complement and antibody-mediated phagocytosis. Progress in treating disease caused by this major pathogen is now being eroded by the acquisition and widespread dissemination of antibiotic resistance.

Case

In January Mr. P., a 68-year-old retired salesman and a heavy smoker, noted that he had nasal congestion, muscle aches, and a low-grade fever. He felt that his symptoms were resolving until he abruptly developed a shaking chill, cough, and severe pain on the right side of his chest that worsened with breathing. The cough was productive of rust-colored (blood-tinged) sputum. When he was seen in the emergency department 2 days later, he appeared acutely ill and had a temperature of 40°C. His respiratory rate was rapid at 30 breaths per minute. His breathing was shallow, with diminished breath sounds over the right side of the thorax, indicating consolidation of the air spaces of the lung. This pattern of breathing, in which the patient is reluctant to move one side of the chest because of inspiratory pain, is a condition known as splinting and indicates inflammation of the pleura (lining of the thoracic cavity and lungs) or pleurisy.

The laboratory reported that Mr. P.'s white blood cell count was 23,000/μL^3, indicative of a leukocytosis (an increase in the number of circulating white blood cells that often characterizes bacterial infection). A chest radiograph revealed a dense infiltrate in the right lung (Fig. 13-1). A Gram stain of the sputum showed many neutrophils and lancet-shaped Gram-positive diplococci (Fig. 13-2). Blood was obtained for culture, and treatment for a **community-acquired pneumonia** was begun with a fluoroquinolone antibiotic, levofloxacin. Both the blood cultures and sputum cultures were positive for the pneumococcus, *Streptococcus pneumoniae*. Because the isolate was found to be sensitive to penicillin, the antibiotic regimen was revised. Two days later Mr. P. was much improved, and after eight more days of penicillin therapy, he recovered completely.

Mr. P.'s case illustrates many of the classical features of pneumococcal pneumonia: abrupt onset of severe symptoms, ill appearance of the patient, rust-colored sputum,

FIGURE 13-1 ▪ **Chest radiograph showing homogeneous consolidation involving the right upper and middle lobes.** The air spaces of the lobes are filled with liquid.

FIGURE 13-2 ▪ **Gram stain of sputum revealing many neutrophils and lancet-shaped Gram-positive diplococci.**

homogeneous involvement of an entire lobe of a lung (lobar consolidation), leukocytosis, and rapid response to antibiotics. **Bacteremia,** the presence of bacteria in the bloodstream, occurs in about 25% of the cases and is indicative of more severe illness. Pneumococcal pneumonia is a dramatic illness that can be life threatening in a patient who may have been well only a few days earlier. It was one of the most common causes of death in the preantibiotic era.

Today, as a result of penicillin (and other antibiotics), it is less often fatal. However, penicillin, once considered a "miracle," must now be used in much higher doses and is ineffective for some strains and some manifestation of pneumococcal disease. Nevertheless, pneumococcal pneumonia remains the most common form of community-acquired bacterial pneumonia and continues to be fatal in up to 5% of all patients, with higher mortality rates in elderly or debilitated patients and those with bacteremia, even when they are treated with an antibiotic to which their organism is sensitive. Pneumococcal disease frequently follows a viral infection of the upper respiratory tract, particularly influenza, as illustrated in Mr. P.'s case by the preceding "flulike" illness that was resolving as his pneumonia began. Because of his age, Mr. P. should have previously received immunization against both influenza and the pneumococcus. Either of these might have prevented the development of pneumococcal pneumonia.

This case raises several questions:

1. Where did Mr. P. acquire this organism? What host factors might have contributed to the pneumococcus gaining entry into his lungs?
2. What possibilities should be considered if the initial antibiotic treatment was not effective in this case?
3. If Mr. P.'s own immune response was not sufficient to control this infection, why might immunization have ameliorated or prevented these events?

Streptococcus pneumoniae

CHARACTERISTICS

The pneumococcus is classified in the genus *Streptococcus*, based on its morphology and purely fermentative energy metabolism. It is one of many species of aerobic streptococci that tolerate ambient levels of oxygen, a characteristic that is critical to its niche on the surface of the airway. Other closely related species such as *S. oralis, S. sanguis,* and *S. mitis* coinhabit the same environment in the human nasopharynx, but compared with the pneumococcus are uncommon causes of infection. The pneumococcus, like other streptococci, lacks the enzyme catalase; therefore, its normal metabolism generates copious amounts of **hydrogen peroxide**. This substance inhibits the growth of competitive members of the microflora and, together with the cholesterol-dependent toxin **pneumolysin**, accounts for much of its ability to damage host tissue and inhibit effective clearance by the infected host. In addition, like other Gram-positive bacteria, pneumococcal cells are surrounded by a thick cell wall, fragments of which are recognized by the innate immune system and are responsible for stimulating much of the inflammatory response associated with pneumococcal infection. In the stationary phase of growth, pneumococci express the enzyme **autolysin**, which degrades its own cell wall. The continuous self-destruction, or autolysis, further contributes to the release of these inflammatory mediators.

Exterior to the cell wall is a **capsule** that imparts a mucoid or "smooth" appearance to colonies on agar. (In 1944 Avery, McCarty, and MacLeod reported that an extract consisting of DNA derived from smooth pneumococcal strains was able to transform "rough," to smooth strains. This was among the earliest evidence that DNA is the carrier of genetic information.) Capsules are composed of porous, noncovalently attached zones of polysaccharide that completely envelop the cell (Fig. 13-3). Thick polysaccharide capsules, much like carbohydrate O antigens on the surface of the lipopolysaccharide of some Gram-negative bacteria, do not activate complement efficiently in the absence of a specific antipolysaccharide antibody and thus serve to obscure the underlying components of the bacterial cell surface (see the paradigm).

Expression of a capsule is particularly important for an organism to survive in the bloodstream, where the activity of complement is most pervasive (see Chapter 6). The presence of a capsule therefore enables the pneumococcus to cause infection beyond where it normally resides in the respiratory tract. For bacteria to pass through the blood-brain barrier and reach the central nervous system, for example, it generally requires a

FIGURE 13-3 ▪ **Immunoelectron micrograph showing a diplococcus.** The arrow points to the thick layer of capsular polysaccharide surrounding the cell. (Original magnification, × 41,200.) Modified from Kim JO et al. Infect Immun 1999;67:2327–2333.

sustained (rather than transient) presence of bacteria in the bloodstream or bacteremia. This is what occurs in **meningitis**, which is inflammation in the meninges, the three membranes that envelop the brain and spinal cord. The importance of capsule is demonstrated by the pathogens that are the most common causes of this life-threatening infection: like the pneumococcus, all are encapsulated. Nonencapsulated pneumococci rarely cause disease and are seldom found in nature.

Capsular polysaccharides tend to be highly immunogenic and are often the dominant or serotype-determining antigen on the organism. Because they are the target of selective pressures from the immune response, there is often considerable structural and thus antigenic variation among pneumococcal capsular polysaccharides. The basis for antigenic differences among serotypes lies in the chemical structure of the capsular polysaccharide. Various pneumococcal strains express capsules with distinct sugar constituents or the same array of sugars linked in various ways. There are 90 known pneumococcal capsule structures or types. Even though these structures are antigenic, they allow for extracellular bacterial survival in the nonimmune host until a specific bactericidal and/or opsonic antibody to these polysaccharides can be generated to enhance clearance of the pathogen. Capsules can be visualized by the addition of an antibody that causes an antigen–antibody precipitation in the normally transparent zone occupied by the capsule (Quellung reaction). This has been used in the past for selection of type-specific serum therapy and is currently used for epidemiological studies. Antibodies to the capsules play a major role in protection against subsequent infections by pneumococci of the same serotype but have minimal impact on pneumococci of different capsular types.

Bacterial Capsules as Defenses Against Opsonization and Phagocytosis

The antiphagocytic capsule that characterizes virulent strains of pneumococcus is also found in a number of other extracellular pathogens. Examples of encapsulated organisms include the following:

Bacteria
- *Streptococcus pneumoniae* (pneumococcus)
- *Streptococcus pyogenes* (group A streptococcus)
- *Streptococcus agalactiae* (group B streptococcus)
- *Staphylococcus aureus*
- *Neisseria meningitidis* (meningococcus)
- *Haemophilus influenzae* (except nontypable strains)
- *Klebsiella pneumoniae*
- *Escherichia coli* (some strains)
- *Bacteroides fragilis*

Fungi
- *Cryptococcus neoformans*

Prominent examples of encapsulated bacteria are *Haemophilus influenzae* type B and *Neisseria meningitidis* (the meningococcus), which, together with the pneumococcus, are the most frequent causes of bacterial meningitis after the newborn period. Nonencapsulated pneumococci are readily opsonized and phagocytized; consequently, they are avirulent. More than 10,000 nonencapsulated pneumococci must be injected into the peritoneal cavity to kill a mouse, but only about 10 encapsulated bacteria are required—a thousandfold difference in virulence.

How does encapsulation protect the pathogen from antibacterial defenses? One of the main host defense mechanisms against bacterial infection involves the complement system, which can be directly bactericidal through the generation of the lytic membrane attack complex. The complement system is highly efficient in eliminating most extracellular bacteria. Other organisms, like the pneumococcus, are not killed by complement alone but require phagocytosis by neutrophils or macrophages, the professional phagocytes. Recognition by professional phagocytic cells, however, requires signaling through opsonization, a process whereby complement components with or without antibodies are activated on the bacterial cell surface. A successful pathogen circumvents these mechanisms by completely enveloping its cell surface in a thick layer of hydrophilic polysaccharide, or capsule. The polysaccharide does not activate complement efficiently in the absence of a specific antibody and thus serves to protect the underlying components of the bacterial cell surface. In other words, the capsule provides the pneumococcus with "stealthlike" capability.

How then is the host able to vanquish this formidable opponent? Not all capsular polysaccharides are totally effective in shielding underlying structures from recognition by complement and antibodies. Moreover, other components of the innate immune system contribute to host defense and to opsonizing pneumococci. Eventually, the capsular material, itself antigenic, will elicit a specific anticapsular antibody response that promotes opsonophagocytic clearance and tips the balance in favor of the host.

Streptococcus pneumoniae

EPIDEMIOLOGY

Pneumococcal pneumonia is the most common form of **bacterial pneumonia** acquired in the community (as opposed to hospital-acquired pneumonias; see Chapter 59). It is estimated that approximately 500,000 cases of pneumococcal pneumonia occur each year in the United States. Worldwide it is estimated that more than a million deaths occur annually as a result of this disease, making it one of the leading infectious causes of mortality. The incidence is highest in certain subgroups, including children younger than 5 years, adults older than 40 years, African Americans, and Native Americans. Although the reason for this distribution is not known, poverty and a debilitated state of health are risk factors. Certain diseases also predispose to pneumococcal infections, including sickle cell anemia, alcoholism, Hodgkin disease, multiple myeloma, HIV infection, and the absence of a functional spleen. Pneumococcal infections are also distinctly seasonal, with the highest incidence occurring in the winter and early spring, often in the setting of recent upper respiratory viral infection, as illustrated in the case of Mr. P. Most cases are sporadic, but outbreaks do occur, particularly in residential institutions, army barracks, and work camps, where people live in crowded conditions. In addition, the pneumococcus is a leading cause of other infections involving the respiratory tract, including acute otitis media (infection of the middle ear space), acute sinusitis, and chronic bronchitis. Several million cases of otitis media occur each year in the United States, making the disease the single most common reason for medical visits among children. It is estimated that 40% of acute bacterial otitis media is caused by the pneumococcus. Bacteremic infection can also introduce the organism into other normally sterile sites, resulting in pneumococcal infections of the peritoneal cavity (in the presence of increased fluid, called ascites), joints, or heart valves that cause peritonitis, septic arthritis, and endocarditis, respectively. As previously noted, the pneumococcus is one of the encapsulated pathogens that causes meningitis, an especially devastating disease. There are several thousand cases of pneumococcal meningitis per year in the United States.

ENCOUNTER

The environmental **reservoir** of *S. pneumoniae* is humans colonized by the organism, rather than animals or the inanimate environment. Interestingly, if the physician had asked Mr. P. whether he had been exposed recently to another person with pneumonia, the answer would probably have been "no." By far the majority of individuals who harbor pneumococci never experience symptoms, because the organism most often exists in a commensal relationship with its human host. Pneumococci have a particular predilection for the human respiratory tract, although the precise reasons for this marked tropism is unknown. The initial step in the host–pathogen interaction is **colonization** on the mucosal surface of the nasopharynx. The outcome of colonization can be clearance of the organism, asymptomatic persistence for several months (the **carrier state**), or progression to disease. The outcome is determined by the intrinsic virulence of the colonizing strain and the efficiency of host defense mechanisms. Some serotypes of *S. pneumoniae* are more virulent than others. Certain serotypes can cause severe disease, whereas others colonize the nasopharynx of asymptomatic persons but seldom are responsible for disease. The interval between colonization and the onset of disease is variable (and ordinarily undefinable in clinical practice), but there is some evidence to suggest that disease is most likely to occur shortly after colonization.

Several aspects of *S. pneumoniae* colonization have been elucidated by longitudinal studies in which nasopharyngeal cultures were obtained at regular intervals from healthy individuals. Pneumococci are carried by up to two thirds of normal preschool children. In general, the incidence of colonization declines with increasing age; rates of colonization in adults average only 10%, although close contact with children increases its frequency. One individual may become colonized many times, usually with different serotypes. This occurs because in immunocompetent individuals, colonization generates a serotype-specific immune response that limits reacquisition of an isolate of the same serotype. Sometimes one individual is simultaneously colonized by more than one pneumococcal serotype.

Transmission from a sick person, or more commonly from an asymptomatic carrier, occurs through **droplets** of respiratory secretions that remain airborne over distances of a few feet. Infecting organisms can also be carried on hands contaminated with secretions. Transmission occurs directly from person to person and appears to be highly efficient considering the high rates of colonization in settings such as family groups and day care centers. Because healthy carriers far outnumber symptomatic individuals, most of the links in the chain of person-to-person transmission are invisible. In contrast, an agent such as measles is also transmitted person to person by a respiratory route, but asymptomatic colonization does not take place, and each link in the chain is evident as disease.

ENTRY

Disease occurs when the organism spreads from its site of residence in the nasopharynx and becomes established in normally sterile parts of the airway, usually as a consequence of multiple host factors. Ordinarily, the lungs are protected by elaborate mechanisms, including the tortuous pathway that air and inhaled particles must follow to reach the lungs, the **epiglottis** that protects the airway from aspiration, the **cough reflex,** the presence of a layer of sticky **mucus** that is continuously swept upward by the **cilia** of the respiratory epithelium, and **alveolar macrophages** that phagocytose bacteria and foreign particles. These mechanisms are highly effective in preventing progression from colonization of the upper respiratory tract to infection of the lower respiratory tract. However, a number of factors can interfere with these mechanisms, including aspiration that can occur with loss of consciousness, cigarette smoking, alcohol consumption, viral infections, or excess fluid in the lungs. Likewise, otitis media is often a consequence of eustachian tube dysfunction leading to aspiration of nasopharyngeal contents into the normally sterile middle ear space.

How do these considerations relate to the case of Mr. P.? The source of the infecting organisms was certainly another individual who may have been entirely healthy. His smoking history and recent viral infection may have depressed his defense mechanisms by weakening his cough reflex, damaging the mucociliary escalator, and decreasing the activity of alveolar macrophages. It is possible that Mr. P. had the misfortune to acquire one of the more virulent pneumococcal serotypes.

SPREAD, MULTIPLICATION, AND DAMAGE

Much of the current understanding of the pathogenesis of pneumococcal pneumonia is derived from studies carried out in the 1940s by W. Barry Wood and his colleagues, who produced pneumonia by injecting pneumococci suspended in mucin into the bronchi of anesthetized mice. These animals were sacrificed at various intervals, and histological sections of the lungs were examined. Four zones of the pneumonic process were identified, corresponding to four stages of the inflammatory process (Fig. 13-4).

In the first stage the alveoli fill with **serous fluid** containing many organisms but few inflammatory cells. Recent studies suggest that components of the pneumococcal cell wall stimulate the outpouring of fluid and the subsequent inflammatory response. The fluid that fills the alveoli serves as a culture medium for multiplying organisms and a means of spreading the infection, both into adjacent alveoli through the pores of Kohn and to

nearby areas of the lung via the small airways. While this outpouring of fluid may have minimal effects in some organs, it threatens the basic function of the lung—namely, gas exchange.

In the second stage, called **early consolidation,** the alveoli are infiltrated by neutrophils and red blood cells. Strong **chemotactic signals,** produced by the pneumococci and by the alternative pathway of **complement,** lead to the recruitment of large numbers of neutrophils and a typical acute inflammatory process. The stage is now set for the classic struggle between bacteria and phagocytes. On the one hand, pneumococci resist phagocytosis because of the presence of capsules. On the other hand, if the pneumococci are ingested by the neutrophils or macrophages, they are rapidly killed. The extent of successful phagocytosis determines the outcome of the infection.

Fortunately, the immune system employs various mechanisms that make even the heavily encapsulated pneumococci more "ingestible" to the neutrophils. If the patient has had previous contact with pneumococci of the invading serotype, he or she will have developed type-specific anticapsular antibodies that interact with complement to opsonize the organisms and facilitate their uptake. If the individual lacks specific adaptive immunity, the organisms may be opsonized by nonspecific or innate immunity. Complement components that bind to the bacterial surface in the absence of

FIGURE 13-4 ▪ **Four zones or stages of lung involvement in pneumococcal pneumonia.** Pneumonia was induced in rats by intrabronchial installation of live pneumococci suspended in mucin. **A.** Alveoli filled with clear exudate (original magnification, × 430). **B.** Early consolidation: organisms are plentiful, and some are engulfed by neutrophils (original magnification, × 430). **C.** Late consolidation: a closely packed cellular infiltrate is present, and phagocytosis of organisms has occurred (original magnification, × 530). **D.** Resolution found at center of lesion: macrophages are present, and the exudate is beginning to clear (× 430). From Wood WB Jr. Studies on the mechanism of recovery in pneumococcal pneumonia: I. The action of type specific antibody upon the pulmonary lesion of experimental pneumonia. J Exp Med. 1941 Feb; 73:201–222.]

antibodies (activated mostly by the alternative pathway) are particularly important in protecting the host. Binding of complement components differs among pneumococcal serotypes, which may explain in part why some serotypes are more virulent than others.

An additional protective mechanism of the innate immune system involves interaction of a serum component, **C-reactive protein (CRP)**, with cell surface phosphorylcholine, a conserved feature on pneumococcal teichoic acid (C substance or C polysaccharide). Binding of CRP to the bacterial surface leads to activation of the complement cascade through the classical pathway. Because levels of CRP rise dramatically in the sera of patients with many inflammatory diseases, not just pneumococcal infection, it is referred to as an **acute phase reactant.** Individuals with lower-baseline unstimulated serum levels of CRP appear to have an increased risk of invasive pneumococcal disease.

In the case of Mr. P., phagocytic cells, mainly neutrophils, failed to contain the pneumococci early on, and the infection progressed to adjacent areas until it involved an entire lobe of his right lung. What accounted for his fever and ill appearance? Although Mr. P.'s lung involvement was serious, the resulting impairment of gas exchange does not fully explain why he became so sick. It is likely that the systemic manifestations were the result of the host inflammatory response triggered by pneumococcal components, particularly cell wall fragments produced locally or entering the circulation, rather than being a direct effect of any bacterial toxin or other secreted product.

The third stage of pneumococcal pneumonia is called **late consolidation.** At this stage the alveoli are packed with victorious neutrophils and only a few remaining pneumococci. On a macroscopic level the affected areas of the lungs are heavy and resemble the liver in appearance, a state that early pathologists called **hepatization.** In the fourth and final stage, or **resolution,** neutrophils are replaced by scavenging macrophages, which clear the debris resulting from the inflammatory process. One of the remarkable aspects of pneumococcal pneumonia is that in most cases the architecture of the lung is eventually restored to its normal condition. This restoration is different from what takes place in many other forms of pneumonia, in which recovery is accompanied by necrosis and normal lung tissue is replaced by fibrous scar tissue.

Pneumococcal pneumonia may lead to both local and distant complications. The most common local complication is **pleural effusion**—the outpouring of fluid into the pleural space—which occurs in about one quarter of all cases. Usually, the pleural fluid effused is a sterile exudate, stimulated by the adjacent inflammation. However, in about 1% of cases, pneumococci can be isolated from this site. Infection of the pleural space is called **empyema** and is a purulent condition that may require drainage of the infected fluid.

Distant complications of pneumococcal pneumonia result from spread of the organisms via the bloodstream. In the early stages of pneumonia, the organisms may enter the lymphatic vessels that drain the infected area of the lungs, pass into the thoracic duct, and from there enter the bloodstream. The organism can be documented by positive blood cultures in about 25% of all cases of pneumococcal pneumonia. However, transient pneumococcemia probably occurs much more often. When bacteremia is present, the organisms may cause infection at secondary sites such as the meninges, as discussed earlier. Had Mr. P. not responded quickly to antibiotic therapy, he would have been at risk for such complications. Spread to the bloodstream is usually a complication of pneumonia, although in young children there may also be direct seeding of the bloodstream by organisms resident in the nasopharynx (a process called occult bacteremia).

Host defenses against pneumococcal bacteremia depend largely on the lymphoreticular system to remove circulating bacteria from the bloodstream. **Humoral factors,** including antibodies, complement, and perhaps C-reactive protein, assist macrophages in the spleen, liver, and lymph nodes in carrying out their filtering function. The critical filtering function of the spleen is demonstrated by the fulminant, rapidly progressive pneumococcal bacteremia that sometimes strikes individuals with anatomic or functional asplenia (e.g., postsplenectomy or sickle cell disease).

DIAGNOSIS

Pneumococcal infection is often suspected because of the clinical scenario, because it is a leading cause of lobar pneumonia, acute otitis media, chronic bronchitis, and acute sinusitis. In the case of pneumonia, the first step in obtaining a microbiological diagnosis is the examination of expectorated sputum. When **Gram stain** of sputum contains neutrophils and more than 10 lancet-shaped Gram-positive diplococci per oil immersion field, the diagnosis of pneumococcal pneumonia is likely (Fig. 13-5). In the case of Mr. P., the results of the Gram stain of sputum confirmed the clinical suspicion and justified the use of initial therapy with an antipneumococcal antibiotic, such as levofloxacin.

In Mr. P.'s case final identification was made by a culture of his sputum, purulent material expectorated from his lungs. The culture was performed by streaking the specimen on **blood agar.** Pneumococcal colonies are surrounded by an area of α-**hemolysis,** a green-brownish discoloration caused by hydrogen peroxide production without the clearing from lysis of the red blood cells that characterizes β-hemolysis. Because most of the other streptococcal species normally present in the heavily colonized upper respiratory tract are also α-hemolytic,

FIGURE 13-5 ▪ **Classic appearance of a Gram stain of sputum from a patient with pneumococcal pneumonia.** The smear shows lancet-shaped diplococci with polymorphonuclear leukocytes, and no other prominent bacterial morphology is present.

pneumococci must be differentiated from less pathogenic contaminants by other properties. These properties include sensitivity to a compound called **Optochin** and solubility in bile salts. Because pneumococci are fastidious organisms with exacting growth requirements, they are not always cultured from sputum of patients with pneumococcal pneumonia. Thus, a negative sputum culture does not rule out pneumococcal pneumonia.

Unfortunately, the interpretation of a positive sputum culture is not always straightforward. A positive finding may indicate the cause of the patient's pneumonia. However, it may also be the result of contamination of the sputum specimen as it passes through the mouth of a colonized individual, in which case the clinical context is important and therapy is often empiric. In contrast to sputum cultures, growth of *S. pneumoniae* from Mr. P.'s blood could be considered definitive proof of the etiology of the disease. In recent years, interest has increased in the use of specific antisera to detect the capsular antigen directly in sputum, blood, or urine, thus obviating the need for culture. Unfortunately, these techniques tend to be positive in no more than 50% of the cases of pneumococcal pneumonia.

TREATMENT AND PREVENTION

Penicillin revolutionized the treatment of pneumococcal infection. Other antibiotics, such as erythromycin, are available for patients who are allergic to penicillin. Despite the dramatic effectiveness of penicillin, the mortality rate in pneumococcal pneumonia remains

unacceptably high. Treatment fails because of rapid progression of the infection or underlying debility of the patient. Recent work on the pneumococcal cell wall has suggested another possible explanation. Lysis of pneumococcal cells by antibiotics releases breakdown products of the cell wall that stimulate an abrupt increase in inflammation. The ultimate effect of antibiotic therapy is to cure the infection, but the short-term effect of increased inflammation may be deleterious to some patients.

Recently, the worldwide spread of antibiotic resistance in pneumococci has emerged as a major concern. Resistance to penicillin was first recognized in the 1960s. During the 1980s, antibiotic resistance became widespread in a number of European countries, and by the 1990s a major increase in antibiotic-resistant pneumococci in North America was apparent. Rates of resistance vary widely among communities but are generally highest where antibiotics are used most frequently. Approximately three fourths of the penicillin-resistant strains have only an intermediate level of resistance and can still be treated with penicillin or related drugs unless the infection occurs in the central nervous system, where the penetration of penicillin is insufficient. The remaining one fourth of strains, however, have high-level resistance (minimum inhibitory concentration greater than or equal to 2 μg/ml) and must be treated with other antibiotics. Unfortunately, the penicillin-resistant strains are often also resistant to other β-lactams, as well as unrelated antibiotics that might have served as alternatives. In particular, rates of resistance to other common classes of oral antibiotics, such as macrolides and sulfas, are now generally high.

The mechanism of penicillin resistance does not involve the production of β-lactamase, an enzyme that breaks down penicillin and accounts for penicillin resistance among staphylococci. Instead, the resistant pneumococci have accumulated mutations in the enzymes that cross-link the cell wall and are normally bound and inactivated by penicillin. These altered **penicillin-binding proteins** allow for continued cell wall synthesis but no longer bind or are affected by penicillin. Moreover, pneumococci with altered penicillin-binding proteins become more resistant to other β-lactam antibiotics, including cephalosporins, so that these modified forms of penicillin may be no more effective than penicillin itself. The genetic information encoding these altered proteins appears to have been acquired from other species of streptococci that may reside in the oropharynx. The emergence of resistance, therefore, appears to be a result of the strong selective pressure caused by the presence of antibiotics coupled with the natural ability of the organism to adapt by taking up and integrating DNA found in its environment in a process known as **transformation.**

The physicians caring for Mr. P. initially selected treatment with levofloxacin, because of the currently low rates of resistance to this agent and the possibility of a high level of a penicillin-resistant strain in the clinical setting of a life-threatening community-acquired pneumonia. Once the microbiology laboratory excluded the possibility of a high level of resistance to penicillin, it was appropriate to complete his therapy with penicillin.

The adaptability of the pneumococcus, as demonstrated by its ability to develop drug resistance, has also made it a challenging target for vaccine development. A vaccine would be especially useful for people at highest risk for pneumococcal disease, such as young children, the elderly, and individuals with underlying conditions that predispose them to infection or severe disease. The antigenic diversity of the pneumococcus, however, is a significant barrier to developing a vaccine based on the polysaccharide capsular antigens. Nonetheless, most cases of pneumococcal pneumonia are caused by a limited number of serotypes. Accordingly, a vaccine based on those serotypes was approved for use in 1977. This vaccine now contains the capsular polysaccharides of the 23 most common serotypes and is recommended for the elderly and individuals with predisposing conditions. Unfortunately, patients with Hodgkin disease or multiple myeloma, who are especially at risk, often do not make an adequate antibody response to the vaccine. Because it is a complex vaccine targeting a population with highly variable and often complicated health problems, the impact on the overall morbidity and mortality caused by this organism remains controversial. Likewise, young children respond poorly to polysaccharide vaccines (see Chapter 45 for a discussion of vaccination of children against *H. influenzae*).

Rising rates of antibiotic resistance have spurred efforts at improving prevention, particularly among children. In 2000 a **pneumococcal conjugate vaccine**, based on the successful approach for *H. influenzae* type B, was introduced in the United States for use in children. This vaccine contains the seven most common serotypes found in that age group linked to a protein carrier that results in a more effective antibody response because, unlike vaccines consisting strictly of polysaccharide antigens, the presence of a protein recruits T cells to help. The pneumococcal conjugate vaccine reduces carriage of the serotypes in its formulation and has thus far been shown to be highly efficacious against invasive pneumococcal disease and somewhat effective at preventing overall cases of pneumonia and otitis media. Interestingly, parents and grandparents of vaccinated children also appear to have a lower incidence of pneumococcal pneumonia, presumably because of decreased transmission. There is concern that selective pressure will result in an increasing prevalence of nonvaccine serotypes and over time render the conjugate vaccine less effective in preventing pneumococcal infection.

Conclusion

The pneumococcus is a Gram-positive streptococcus that commonly colonizes the human nasopharynx and is a leading infectious cause of morbidity and mortality. The expression of a capsule makes the organism more resistant to opsonization and phagocytosis by antibodies and complement. In susceptible hosts, this characteristic enables the pneumococcus to overcome the acute inflammatory response when it gains access to normally sterile sites such as the lung. Antibiotics continue to have a major impact on pneumococcal disease, although rising rates of resistance are increasingly limiting treatment options. Prevention is currently based on vaccines made from the capsular polysaccharide of the most common serotypes.

Neisseriae: Gonococcus and Meningococcus

David Stephens and Peter Dull

key **concepts**

Neisseria gonorrhoeae (the gonococcus):

- Is a Gram-negative diplococcus.

- Causes the sexually transmitted infection gonorrhea in men and women, which can lead to pelvic inflammatory disease (PID) in women and epididymitis in men.

- Can be carried asymptomatically by both men and women in the genital tract.

- Exhibits phase variation and antigenic variation.

- Can cause disseminated infections (serum-resistant strains).

- Infections are treated with antibiotics, although many strains can be resistant to penicillin and other antibiotics.

Neisseria meningitidis (the meningococcus):

- Is a Gram-negative diplococcus.

- Causes septicemia and meningitis.

- Is often carried asymptomatically in the nasopharynx.

- Can be heavily encapsulated, which allows them to multiply and disseminate in the bloodstream and can lead to disseminated intravascular coagulation (DIC).

- Can be prevented with vaccines containing capsular polysaccharide, except for serogroup B strains.

The Gram-negative cocci, in contrast with the great variety of pathogenic Gram-negative bacilli, contain only one genus of organisms that frequently cause disease. This genus, *Neisseria*, has two important species that are pathogenic for humans: *N. gonorrhoeae*, the agent of **gonorrhea**, and *N. meningitidis*, a major cause of **septicemia** and **meningitis**.

The gonococcus (*N. gonorrhoeae*) usually causes an uncomplicated, localized **cervicitis** and **urethritis**. In addition, it can cause PID and disseminated gonococcal infection (DGI). About 700,000 new cases of gonorrhea occur every year in the United States. Of the infectious diseases that must legally be reported to the U.S. Public Health Service,

Gonococcal Infections: Sites and Types

Lower tract infections
  Cervicitis
  Urethritis (male and female)
  Abscess formation in glands adjacent to the vagina,
    such as Skene duct or Bartholin glands
Upper tract infections
  Endometritis (uterine infection)
  Epididymitis
  Pelvic inflammatory disease (PID; infection of the
    fallopian tube [salpingitis], the ovary, or adnexal
    tissues)
Other (nonreproductive tract) localized sites
  Proctitis (rectal gonorrhea)
  Pharyngitis

Ophthalmia neonatorum (bilateral conjunctivitis in
  infants born of mothers infected with gonococci)
Extension of the infection to areas contiguous with
  the pelvis causing peritonitis or perihepatitis (Fitz-
  Hugh-Curtis syndrome)
Disseminated gonococcal infection (DGI)
  Dermatitis–arthritis–tenosynovitis syndrome: fever,
    polyarthritis, and tenosynodermatitis (vesicles or
    pustules on a hemorrhagic base) caused either by
    immune complexes or by whole gonococci
  Monoarticular septic arthritis (one infected joint)
  Rarely, endocarditis (infection involves heart valves)
    or meningitis (infection of the central nervous
    system)

only genital chlamydial infections are identified more frequently. Gonococcal infections and their complications are responsible for more than $1 billion per year in direct and indirect health care costs in the United States.

The gonococcus attaches through pili and other adherence ligands to the mucosal epithelia of the male urethra or female cervix, where it can elicit a brisk inflammatory response. Ascent of the organism into the female upper reproductive tract results in infection and inflammation of the uterus and fallopian tubes, called **pelvic inflammatory disease (PID)**. This condition may result in scarring of the upper female genital tract and adjacent organs and chronic pelvic pain. Tubal scarring can lead to **ectopic pregnancy** (development of the embryo in the fallopian tube rather than the uterus) and/or infertility. In men, ascent of the gonococcus into the upper reproductive tract is less frequent but can cause **epididymitis**. Rarely, a localized gonococcal infection can invade the bloodstream and cause an acute dermatitis–arthritis–tenosynovitis syndrome called **disseminated gonococcal infection (DGI)**. Individuals with complement deficiencies are predisposed to such systemic spread because the membrane attack complex consisting of the late complement components can lyse most neisseriae. Nevertheless, DGI and gonococcal arthritis can be seen in patients without complement deficiency.

Meningococci are also piliated and colonize human upper respiratory mucosal surfaces. Meningococci are surrounded by a capsule that enhances the ability of the organism to resist host defense mechanisms, such as complement-mediated killing in the bloodstream. This allows meningococci to grow to high numbers in the blood. Meningococci also shed large amounts of outer membrane material. These membrane blebs contain lipopolysaccharide (**endotoxin**), also called

lipooligosaccharide (**LOS**) because of the absent O antigen. Lipopolysaccharide is a major inducer of release into the bloodstream or cerebrospinal fluid of potent biological mediators, such as tumor necrosis factor-α (TNF-α), that elicit the systemic signs of meningococcemia, disseminated intravascular coagulation, and shock. Meningococci have a predilection for the central nervous system, where they can cause the serious complication of bacterial meningitis.

Neisseriae

BIOLOGY

The gonococcus and the meningococcus belong to the genus *Neisseria*, the main group of Gram-negative cocci associated with human disease. The neisseriae include a number of nonpathogenic organisms often found on the mucous membranes of healthy people, especially in the nasopharynx. Another Gram-negative coccus, *Moraxella catarrhalis*, causes upper respiratory tract infections, especially in immunocompromised patients. Neisseriae are aerobes but can grow anaerobically. They have typical Gram-negative cell envelopes containing outer membrane proteins and endotoxin. These organisms are fragile and may not survive for long outside of their human hosts. The only source of infection for Ms. C. is another infected person (not objects such as a toilet seat).

When initially cultured from patients, neisseriae grow best in an atmosphere with increased CO_2 (which can be provided by a "candle jar," a closed canister that uses a burning candle to convert O_2 to CO_2). A complex

Case

Pelvic Inflammatory Disease

Ms. C., a 14-year-old female, came to the emergency room with an acutely painful abdomen. Her temperature was 38.5°C, and laboratory tests indicated an elevated white blood cell count and sedimentation rate. Before results of the urinalysis and a pregnancy test were returned, a pelvic examination revealed a purulent cervical discharge. A culture was sent, and a Gram stain of the discharge was prepared and examined (Fig. 14-1). Abdominal tenderness was apparent during the bimanual examination.

Ms. C. reported that her last menses was 4 days ago. When asked about her sexual behavior, she told the resident physician that she had intercourse for the first time 2 years ago. That relationship ended a few months ago, and she recently began "going steady" with a new friend. She and her partners have never used condoms or any other form of birth control.

This case raises several questions:

1. What test should be ordered for the cervical specimen? What will the stained preparation most likely reveal?
2. Assuming that Ms. C. has PID, how did she acquire the infection?
3. Is it significant that this patient has just finished her menses?
4. If the patient has PID, what other causative organisms, other than gonococci, should be considered?
5. If the patient has PID, would the proper use of male condoms have prevented the infection? Could any other forms of birth control and/or disease prevention have prevented transmission?
6. What other benefits would Ms. C. realize if she and her partner used condoms consistently and correctly? (See Chapter 69 for additional discussion of PID.)

FIGURE 14-1 ▪ Gram stain of urethral pus. Notice the neutrophils with associated gonococci.

medium containing boiled blood, iron, and vitamins ("chocolate agar") also facilitates optimal growth.

Substantial differences exist in the pathogenic potential of various strains of gonococci. A given strain may cause uncomplicated **cervicitis** or **urethritis,** complications such as PID, or DGI. Host factors like complement are also thought to be important in the severity and clinical presentation of the disease. Likewise, strains of meningococci differ in their pathogenic potential.

ENCOUNTER AND ENTRY

Gonococci are obligate human pathogens. They do not spontaneously infect other animals, cause disease in any convenient experimental animal, or persist free in the environment. Thus, humans serve as the reservoir for these organisms. Both men and women can carry gonococci without demonstrating symptoms, although the prevalence of **asymptomatic carriers** is greater among women. Asymptomatic carriers of either sex are a major problem in the control of gonorrhea because, without symptoms, they are unlikely to be diagnosed or receive treatment.

As part of its insidious pathogenic profile, the gonococcus has evolved to maximize its transmissibility. Consequently, it is important to test and treat the known sexual contacts of a patient with gonorrhea. Such **case-contact tracing** and treatment is especially important in PID because the male sexual partners of PID patients are more likely to be asymptomatic and may not seek therapy on their own. Thus, a cured PID patient may be discharged from the hospital only to return to an infected sexual partner and become infected again.

Once gonococci are introduced into the vagina or the urethral mucosa of either gender, they attach to epithelial cells of the distal urethra or cervix. There they attach to the surface of the cells and multiply. Several surface structures of the gonococcus facilitate attachment and anchor the organisms to the urethral or vaginal epithelial cells. Gonococci possess **pili** (Fig. 14-2), other **surface proteins,** and **lipooligosaccharide** that help them attach to host cells. Sophisticated genetic mechanisms enable the bacteria to express or not express these adherence components

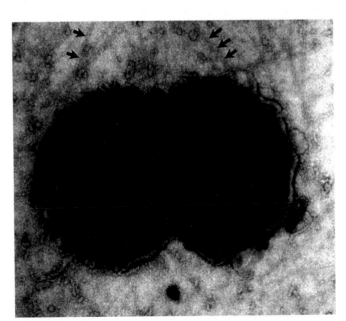

FIGURE 14-2 ▪ **Transmission electron micrograph of** *Neisseria gonorrhoeae.* Notice the presence of pili—long, thin strands of protein—emanating from the surface of the organisms and outer membrane blebs.

Paradigm **Box**

Alteration of Gene Expression by DNA Rearrangements

The basic strategies that pathogenic microbes employ in immune avoidance, subversion, or disruption are found in highly unrelated species. In some cases immune evasion involves activities or molecules that are expressed continuously. Examples include **sialylation of lipopolysaccharide,** capsule structures that mimic host structures, production of **IgA1 protease,** and occupancy of an intracellular environment. In other cases evasion of specific host immune responses (e.g., antibodies) involves a process called **antigenic variation.** Antigenic variation results in changes in the composition or structure of predominant surface molecules. These changes allow an organism to avoid recognition by specific antibodies arising during the course of infection. Rather than occurring in response to specific antibodies, variation is generated by genetic rearrangements that take place at a high frequency within the bacterial population. Consequently, new variants are selected for and emerge by virtue of their escape from antibody-mediated immune mechanisms. In many cases the repertoire of new antigenic types that can be expressed is so great that protective immunity rarely develops. Thus, chronic and repeated infections are hallmarks of diseases such as gonorrhea caused by these agents.

Antigenic variation occurs in microorganisms as diverse as African trypanosomes (which cause African sleeping sickness), *Borrelia* species (which cause relapsing fever), and *N. gonorrhoeae.* In all these microbes, antigenic variation can result from the reassortment and recombination of duplicated gene segments. This mechanism is analogous (but not identical) to the way in which diversity is generated within immunoglobulins of animals. Variation in *Neisseria* species also results from horizontal transfer of DNA between strains by transformation and homologous recombination.

Having evolved to grow exclusively within human hosts, gonococci are a paradigm for organisms that have evolved special mechanisms to adjust to life in immunocompetent individuals. Efforts to develop a gonococcal vaccine have involved a great deal of work to understand the molecular mechanisms of gonococcal antigenic variation. For example, the gonococcal chromosome contains a single copy of the complete **pilin** gene (pilin is the structural protein that is polymerized to form pili). This gene is called *pilE,* for "pilin expression locus." In addition, the gonococcal chromosome contains 10 to 15 copies of variant-encoding pilin genes. All of these copies are truncated at their 5' ends

FIGURE 14-3 ▪ Antigenic variation of pili in *N. gonorrhoeae.*

and lack transcriptional promoter elements, as well as the sequences specifying the N-terminus part of pilin. These copies are called *pilS* loci, for "silent (nonfunctional) loci." Antigenic variation occurs when the genetic information from the nonfunctional alleles is transferred to the complete pilin gene locus by homologous recombination. Figure 14-3 depicts this process as an antigenic switch from a β-pilin type to an α-pilin type.

Pilin diversification depends not only on the mere number of *pilS* genes but also on the fact that small stretches of *pilS* sequence can be recombined into the expression locus resulting in chimeric pilin types. Such an event is depicted in Figure 14-3 as the formation of a *pilE* hybrid between the α- and γ-alleles Note that the *pilS* alleles always act as donors of new genetic information but are not altered themselves by the process. The result is a virtually infinite variety of pilin serotypes that can be expressed using only a limited number of *pilS* alleles.

Another form of altered gene expression arising from DNA rearrangements results in **phase variation.** In this process the expression of a particular gene product is turned on or off at high frequency. Oscillation between on and off states occurs by two basic mechanisms. One mechanism involves the site-specific **inversion** of a DNA segment that bears a transcriptional promoter. An example of this mechanism is the phase variation of type I fimbriae expression in *E. coli* (Fig. 14-4). In the "on" state, the promoter element is

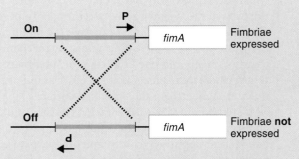

FIGURE 14-4 ▪ **Phase variation of *Escherichia coli* fimbriae by inversion of a DNA segment containing a promoter.**

oriented so that transcription of the fimbrial subunit gene, *fimA,* can take place. Inversion of the element (shown in blue) orients the promoter in a direction divergent to that of *fimA* (i.e., the off state). Analogous inversion systems control the expression of flagellar types in *Salmonella* and pilus expression in other Gram-negative pathogens.

The second mechanism of phase variation is associated with the somewhat unusual occurrence of short nucleotide repeats at the 5′ ends of genes. Such repeats can readily be gained or lost as a consequence of strand misalignment during normal DNA replication and repair. Events of this sort, termed **slipped strand mispairing,** occur at frequencies much higher than point mutations and disrupt the integrity of the gene's translational reading frame. *N. gonorrhoeae* employs this mechanism to change the expression of its virulence-associated Opa proteins. Multiple copies of complete *opa* genes (which each encode different Opa antigenic variants) are scattered throughout the genome. Each gene copy contains

repeats of the sequence CTCTT within the 5′ end of its reading frame. Gain or loss of these elements alters the translational reading frame of the gene and determines whether the intact protein can be made. For example, Figure 14-5 shows a protein expressed from a gene carrying six copies of the element. If a CTCTT sequence is gained or lost within this stretch, the reading frame is altered and translation is terminated prematurely. In this way, gonococci can turn on or off the expression of any of *opa* genes independently.

A similar mechanism is known to control the expression of many other gonococcal and meningococcal surface proteins and to oscillate expression of the biosynthetic genes for gonococcal and meningococcal lipopolysaccharide, resulting in its structural variability. Analogous phase variation mechanisms have been shown to operate in a number of important surface molecules in other Gram-negative pathogens. In each of these other instances, different repetitive elements are found. The only common feature is that the number of nucleotides of the repeat element is not three, nor is it divisible by three. Because the genetic code operates through trinucleotide codons, deletion or addition of a three base pair repeat would not change the reading frame.

The biological significance of phase variation can represent a simplified form of antigenic variation, but gain or loss of the molecules also has important functional consequences unrelated to immune pressure. The widespread distribution of this form of phase variation among microbes suggests that it is biologically important and that pathogens find advantages in existing in heterogeneous populations.

FIGURE 14-5 ▪ **Representation of the phase variation mechanism of the gonococcal *opa* genes.** The sequences have been modified and shortened to demonstrate the mechanism succinctly.

(a phenomenon called **phase variation;** see the paradigm) or to control their structure (**antigenic variation**). Pili and gonococcal surface proteins are immunodominant; that is, they are well recognized by the immune system. However, they are also highly variable in structure, which makes them ineffective targets. It is not surprising that antibodies to these components do not protect against various gonococcal strains.

Gonococci may or may not be taken up by neutrophils, depending on the type of outer membrane proteins they possess. Some of the outer membrane proteins are called **colony opacity-associated (Opa) proteins**. Organisms that lack these proteins are not engulfed by neutrophils. Gonococci lacking Opa proteins are commonly associated with PID, DGI, and arthritis.

SPREAD AND MULTIPLICATION

After colonizing the mucosal cell surface, gonococci multiply rapidly and are shed in large numbers into the genital secretions of infected men and women. Gonococci do not have flagella but have twitching motility related to the expression of pili. Movement into the urethra or through the cervix can be aided by menses, secretions, or urethral or uterine contractions.

Genital mucosal secretions contain three types of IgG and both IgA1 and IgA2. IgG found in secretions may indicate leakage of the antibody from serum onto the mucosal surface, whereas most of the IgA is actively secreted into the lumen of the genital tract. Gonococci produce an extracellular **protease** that specifically cleaves IgA1 but not IgA2 in the hinge region. This property is also present in other bacteria that inhabit mucosal epithelia, such as *Haemophilus influenzae* and certain streptococci. How this protease contributes to pathogenicity is not known. The protease also may have activity on gonococcal surface proteins and may help the organisms escape phagocytosis by removing the Fc end of the immunoglobulin from gonococcus-bound IgA molecules. Because the Fc region is the portion recognized by phagocytes, the organisms may be less likely to be taken up by white blood cells when this portion of the immunoglobulin molecule is removed.

Gonococci also can enter epithelial cells. What is known about invasion of epithelial cells by gonococci is assumed from studies with in vitro organ culture of human fallopian tubes. Two major types of cells compose the epithelial mucosal surface of human fallopian tubes: ciliated cells and nonciliated cells. The nonciliated cells have fingerlike processes, called microvilli, on their luminal surface. When gonococci are exposed to fallopian tube sections, several events occur:

- **Attachment:** Gonococci attach to the microvilli of nonciliated cells.

- **Ciliary stasis:** Motility of the ciliated cells slows and ultimately ceases. Ciliary activity is thought to be important in moving the fertilized egg from the fallopian tube to the uterus and in providing a flushing mechanism for clearing mucus and bacteria from the mucosal surface.
- **Death of ciliated cells:** Ciliated cells die and are selectively sloughed from the epithelial surface (Fig. 14-6). This step does not require intact organisms and can be elicited by gonococcal lipopolysaccharide (LPS) or gonococcal peptidoglycan fragments (parts of the cell wall).
- **Internalization:** Through a cascade of events initiated by the gonococcus, the microvilli of nonciliated cells, acting as pseudopodia, engulf the bacteria. Gonococci are then internalized by these "nonprofessional" phagocytes by a process termed parasite-directed endocytosis.
- **Intracellular replication:** Gonococci are transported to the interior of the cell within phagocytic vacuoles. These vacuoles coalesce to form larger vacuoles, within which gonococci multiply. Inside the nonciliated cells, gonococci are sheltered from antibodies, professional phagocytes, and antibiotics that do not enter human cells well.
- **Intracellular traffic:** The gonococci can be transported to the base of the nonciliated cells where the bacteria-laden vacuoles fuse with the basement membrane.
- **Exocytosis:** The phagocytic vacuoles discharge gonococci into the subepithelial connective tissue. From there the organisms probably either cause local inflammation or enter blood vessels to cause disseminated disease.

FIGURE 14-6. ▪ Scanning electron micrograph of human fallopian tube tissue 20 hours after infection with *Neisseria gonorrhoeae*. Notice that gonococci attach almost exclusively to the surface of nonciliated cells. The damage occurs to ciliated cells. Ciliated cells sloughed from the surface of the mucosa appear at the left and center of the photomicrograph, whereas intact ciliated cells are seen at the top and right.

DAMAGE

Gonococci are not known to secrete exotoxins; thus, damage to host tissues is most likely caused by LPS and other components of the bacterial cell wall, such as peptidoglycan. Both LPS and peptidoglycan are known to induce the production of tumor necrosis factor-α (TNF-α) by a variety of human cells, and TNF-α has been shown to cause the sloughing of ciliated cells from human fallopian tube mucosa. In addition to the death of ciliated cells, as demonstrated in the fallopian tube model, nonciliated epithelial cells containing gonococci may lyse, releasing cellular tissue factors that mediate further inflammation. The inflammatory response in the male urethra is probably responsible for local symptoms such as pain on urination (**dysuria**) and urethral discharge of pus. It is noteworthy that these symptoms do not distinguish gonococcal urethritis from that caused by other genital pathogens, like the chlamydiae (see Chapter 27). However, the urethral discharge in gonorrhea tends to be more copious, thick, and greenish yellow, and the pain is more intense. Although women with gonococcal cervicitis are more often asymptomatic than are men with urethritis, women can experience dysuria, dyspareunia (pain on intercourse), discharge, or genital discomfort.

Survival of Gonococci in the Bloodstream

Normal human serum is capable of killing circulating organisms of many Gram-negative species, including *N. gonorrhoeae*. This natural protective effect depends on complement activation and IgG and IgM antibodies. In the case of the gonococcus, the targets for antibodies are LPS; the major outer membrane protein, called **protein I**; and other proteins exposed on the surface of the organisms. Thus, for gonococci to survive in the bloodstream, they must be able to evade this defense mechanism.

However, gonococci, and especially those strains associated with DGI, can be serum resistant. Gonococci can become serum resistant when LOS is altered by the addition of a terminal sialic acid molecule on the short, core carbohydrate chain (unlike enteric bacilli such as *E. coli,* gonococci and meningococcal LPS does not have O side chains). Because sialic acid is a negatively charged molecule and a surface component of cells, it is believed that this modification camouflages the organisms and protects them from the antibodies responsible for serum killing. The surface constituents of DGI strains are different from those of their serum-sensitive counterparts. However, the serum-resistant strains may be more sensitive to penicillin and have specific nutritional requirements. It is not clear whether these properties directly contribute to the ability of the organisms to disseminate or whether these properties are closely linked genetically.

Host factors also affect the outcome of gonococcal infections. For example, individuals deficient in the final components of the complement cascade that form the membrane attack complex are predisposed to recurrent systemic infections with both gonococci and meningococci.

The manifestations of disseminated gonococcal infection include pustular skin lesions with a surrounding red areola, inflammation of the tendons and joints (**tenosynovitis**), and frank infections of the joints (**suppurative arthritis**). Often, despite appropriate diagnostic attempts, cultures of blood, joint fluid, or skin lesions are sterile. There are several reasons for this phenomenon. First, gonococci may be present but in numbers too low to be detectable in culture. Second, the nutritional requirements of these organisms may be unusual, and they may be inhibited or not grow using normal culture conditions. Third, in cases of tenosynovitis, fragments of cell wall peptidoglycan (murein) or perhaps immune complexes consisting of gonococcal antigens and host antibodies, rather than viable gonococci, may be deposited in synovial tissue and cause local inflammation. The latter possibility is supported by experiments in rats showing that purified gonococcal peptidoglycan, when injected into joints, induces arthritis. If this phenomenon were to apply to humans, active joint infection need not be present at the site of intense inflammation.

Outcome of Gonococcal Infection

What is the outcome of gonorrhea? Data from the preantibiotic era suggest that the symptoms of urethral infection in males usually subside in several weeks without treatment. However, repeated infections, if untreated, can lead to scarring and stricture of the urethra. Such sequelae of gonococcal infection are now relatively unusual, because most men seek medical attention once urethritis becomes apparent. Symptoms of cervicitis include cervical discharge (reported as vaginal discharge), bleeding, and pain. Paradoxically, local urogenital infections are asymptomatic in approximately 30% of women and are often heralded by the complications of the infection. Chronic fallopian tube inflammation can lead to scarring and stricture, resulting in such long-term sequelae as chronic pelvic pain; ectopic pregnancy; recurrent PID caused by chlamydiae, anaerobes, and other organisms; and infertility. For unknown reasons, DGI occurs predominantly in women. Gonococcal arthritis remains a common type of joint infection in sexually active adults.

The outcome of gonococcal infection depends not only on the gender of the patient but also on the timeliness of medical attention. Prompt treatment decreases the risk of ascending or disseminated infection and the resulting sequelae.

Meningococcal Infections

Meningococcal meningitis
Meningococcal bacteremia
Meningococcemia (purpura fulminans and the Water-
    house-Friderichsen syndrome)
Respiratory tract infection
Pneumonia
Epiglottitis

Otitis media
Focal infection
Conjunctivitis
Septic arthritis
Urethritis
Purulent pericarditis
Chronic meningococcemia

Meningococcal Infections

Gonococci and meningococci are close taxonomic cousins; the two organisms share about 90% of their DNA base sequences as measured by DNA hybridization and genome sequencing, and both possess similar virulence factors including pili, outer membrane proteins, and lipopolysaccharide. However, only N. *meningitidis* expresses a capsule. Both organisms can colonize mucous membranes without causing symptoms. (It is estimated that in endemic areas, 5 to 10% of the population are meningococcal carriers.) Both gonococci and meningococci cause purulent infections. Nevertheless, they usually cause a contrasting spectrum of diseases. Whereas gonococci most often produce a localized infection and, even when the gonococci spread to the bloodstream, the infection is rarely lethal, meningococcal infection of the bloodstream is a systemic and life-threatening disease. Why do these two species cause such different illnesses? As previously mentioned, a major factor is that the meningococcus is heavily **encapsulated,** which plays an important role in the pathogenicity of this organism.

While isolated cases, case clusters, or large epidemics of meningococcal disease can occur, the more usual outcome of exposure to the meningococcus is colonization of the nasopharynx with no local symptoms or systemic consequences. Based on organ cultures of nasopharyngeal epithelium, the cascade of events (attachment, ciliary stasis, death of ciliated cells, etc.) at upper respiratory mucous membranes appear to be similar for the meningococcus in the nasopharynx and the gonococcus in the fallopian tube (as described earlier). Patients susceptible to meningococcemia or meningococcal meningitis are often deficient in bactericidal anticapsular antibodies or in activity of the complement cascade. Individuals with capsule-specific antibodies or antibodies directed at other surface components, presumably produced in response to cross-reacting antigens or past colonization, resist the ability of the meningococcus to invade and multiply in the bloodstream. By providing a serologic correlate of protection, these observations were instrumental in developing the currently licensed vaccines made of purified capsular polysaccharide or capsular polysaccharide conjugated to protein.

If they are not killed by bactericidal activity or phagocytes in the bloodstream, meningococci multiply rapidly, reaching blood titers that are among the highest known for any bacterium. It is possible, for example, to observe the organisms directly on a smear of the buffy coat of blood (the layer containing the white cells when whole blood is centrifuged). Other bacterial septicemias rarely result in bacteria visible in buffy coat stains.

The entry of meningococci into the human bloodstream can lead to devastating systemic disease marked by **purpura fulminans** and **disseminated intravascular coagulation (DIC)** with generalized skin manifestations (petechiae and ecchymoses), meningitis, shock, and death. These systemic signs are the direct result of the ability of the meningococcus to survive and multiply in the bloodstream. DIC is accompanied by shock, fever, and other responses to endotoxin or other cell components mediated by cytokines such as TNF-α and interleukin 1. In meningococcal sepsis and meningitis, the likelihood of death or neurologic damage is proportional to levels of endotoxin and the elevation in serum and cerebrospinal fluid of TNF-α concentrations. Because TNF-α is a chemical mediator of our host defense system, this observation gives weight to Lewis Thomas' observation: "Our arsenals for fighting off bacteria are so powerful . . . that we are in more danger from them than from the invaders. We live in the midst of explosive devices. We are mined."

As mentioned earlier, meningococcal disease is effectively prevented by vaccines containing capsular polysaccharide. A notable exception is disease caused by serogroup B meningococci. The capsule of serogroup B strains is a homopolymer of sialic acid that is identical to human sialic acid polymers, is poorly immunogenic, and does not normally elicit protective antibodies.

In contrast, when gonococci reach the bloodstream of most individuals, they are usually killed by host defense mechanisms. Even serum-resistant strains do not grow appreciably in the circulation, although they may survive long enough to reach other organs. Although gonococcal meningitis is reported on rare occasions and gonococcal endocarditis was common in the preantibiotic era, gonococcal bacteremia is now seldom fatal.

DIAGNOSIS

The finding of neutrophils containing Gram-negative diplococci in cervical or urethral secretions is presumptive evidence of gonococcal infection. Positive microscopic findings justify beginning antibiotic therapy before the results of cultures are known in the appropriate clinical setting. The Gram stain of urethral exudate of men is more sensitive than the Gram stain of cervical exudate in women. A cervical Gram stain may be negative, despite a positive culture result. A positive Gram stain of cervical secretions is confirmatory evidence of active gonorrhea in a symptomatic woman, but routine Gram stains of secretions from asymptomatic women are not clinically useful.

Because the social implications of gonorrhea can be as serious as the medical consequences, the physician must confirm the clinical findings by culturing or using genetic probes. It is also important to monitor how the laboratory identifies these organisms. There are three reasons to culture: (1) to be completely certain of the identity of the infecting microorganism, (2) to identify infection in asymptomatic individuals, and (3) to deal with public health and the legal ramifications of gonococcal infection. Nucleic acid-based detection tests are increasingly used and are both sensitive and specific for diagnosis; however, cultured bacteria are needed to characterize potential antimicrobial resistance.

Gonococci grow on several kinds of media that allow presumptive identification within a day. The most commonly used medium is called "chocolate agar" because it contains heated blood and has the appearance of milk chocolate. Special varieties of this medium are known as **Thayer-Martin medium** and **Martin-Lewis medium;** each contains unique antibiotics to inhibit other bacterial species and yeasts. Specimens taken from the cervix, urethra, and other sites that contain other bacteria should always be cultured on chocolate agar with antibiotics (e.g., Thayer-Martin or Martin-Lewis medium) to inhibit the normal flora. It is noteworthy that an occasional strain of gonococci is sensitive to the antibiotics used in the Thayer-Martin medium. For this reason, fluids that are normally sterile (e.g., cerebrospinal fluid, blood, and synovial fluid) should be cultured on chocolate agar without antibiotics to allow recovery of antibiotic-sensitive gonococcal strains.

All members of the genus *Neisseria* and related genera possess an oxidative enzyme that makes the colonies turn purple when flooded with a so-called **oxidase reagent.** If a Gram-negative diplococcus is oxidase-positive, it is a member of *Neisseria* or a close relative. To distinguish *N. gonorrhoeae* from the other species of this genus, the microbiological laboratory determines the pattern of fermentation of various sugars. Unlike other neisseriae, gonococci utilize glucose but not maltose or sucrose, and meningococci utilize both glucose and maltose. Although Gram stain and culture remain the mainstays of diagnostics for meningococcal infection, polymerase chain reaction (PCR)–based testing has begun to move from the research to the clinical lab as well.

TREATMENT

A relatively high proportion of gonococci now bear a plasmid that encodes a β-lactamase, an enzyme that destroys penicillin. Gonococci bearing the resistance plasmids can cause serious locally invasive diseases, like PID, as well as disseminated gonococcal infections. As a consequence of widespread penicillin resistance, the recommended initial therapy for gonorrhea is no longer penicillin but a β-lactamase-resistant cephalosporin—cefixime or ceftriaxone—given orally or intramuscularly, respectively. Single-dose oral therapy is effective and offers the distinct advantage of observed therapy. Both quinolones (ciprofloxacin, ofloxacin, and levofloxacin) and cefixime are available for this purpose, but gonococci resistant to quinolones have become a serious problem in Southeast Asia, and resistant strains are being reported with increasing frequency in Hawaii, California, and elsewhere among men who have sex with men.

Patients infected with *N. gonorrhoeae* are often coinfected with *Chlamydia trachomatis*. This has led to the recommendation that patients treated for gonococcal infection should also receive an antichlamydial agent such as azithromycin or doxycycline. Treatment of meningococcal infection by intravenously administered antibiotics, such as ceftriaxone or penicillin, and other supportive therapy is indicated. Although reports of meningococcal isolates with decreased susceptibility to penicillin have been reported, the clinical significance of this level of resistance remains uncertain.

PREVENTION

Despite effective antimicrobials and active public health measures, an estimated 700,000 cases of gonococcal infection occur annually in the United States. Prevention efforts must be based on a multipronged approach that includes the following:

- Behavioral interventions, including condom use and decreasing the number of sexual partners
- Early diagnosis and treatment
- Partner notification
- Screening and case finding
- Vaccine development and use

Vaccine development has proven to be difficult because gonococci, as solely human pathogens, have a longstanding and sophisticated relationship with their hosts. These organisms have managed to survive the host immune response, as discussed in the paradigm, by antigenic variation, phase variation, and the occupation of protective intracellular environments. Acquired immunity following infection is inadequate, and repeat infections are common among individuals with repeat exposures. New approaches to prevention are being actively pursued. Topical microbicides for intravaginal and intrarectal use are being developed to safely and effectively prevent sexually transmitted diseases, including HIV.

Prevention of meningococcal infections is primarily approached with two strategies: treatment with antibiotics such as rifampin or ciprofloxacin of close contacts of cases and targeted mass vaccination in outbreak settings where indicated. A new polysaccharide conjugate vaccine for prevention of meningococcal disease resulting from serogroups A, C, Y, and W-135 has recently been licensed and recommended for adolescents. Efforts are ongoing to develop a broadly protective serogroup B meningococcal vaccine based on noncapsular antigens.

Conclusion

Gonococci and meningococci are found only in humans and are often carried asymptomatically. Both gonococci and meningococci have developed mechanisms to attach to and avoid loss from host cells, cause ciliary stasis, and invade cells. They are able to traverse epithelial cells and either cause local inflammation or disseminate to other parts of the body. Meningococci have an exceptional ability to survive in the bloodstream and cause systemic infections that often have disastrous consequences. In principle, effective vaccines may be developed which could control and prevent disease. Recent progress has been made in vaccine development against meningococcal infection, but the challenges remain for prevention of infection by *N. gonorrhoeae*.

Bacteroides and Abscesses

Laurie Comstock

key concepts

Bacteroides:

■ Is a dominant genus of bacteria found in the human colon, comprising up to 25% of the organisms in that site.

■ Consists of strict anaerobic Gram-negative rods that play a causative role in intraabdominal abscess formation following contamination of the peritoneal cavity with colonic content.

■ Includes *Bacteroides fragilis,* a bacterium that can tolerate exposure to oxygen and has a nontoxic lipopolysaccharide and a capsular polysaccharide complex (CPC) involved in abscess formation.

■ Is resistant to many antibiotics and able to transfer antibiotic resistance genes to other species through conjugation.

Abscess formation in the peritoneal cavity:

■ Begins when the colon wall is breached by a ruptured bowel, a ruptured appendix, or abdominal surgery and a large number of bacteria enter the otherwise sterile peritoneal cavity.

■ Is caused by a mixture of facultative and strict anaerobes (including *Escherichia coli, B. fragilis,* clostridia, and anaerobic streptococci).

■ Is facilitated by the alternating positive and negative charges of the CPC of *B. fragilis* that initiates a host response contributing to abscess formation.

■ Is treated with abscess drainage and antibiotics; a combination of antibiotics effective against both facultative anaerobes and strict anaerobes is necessary, with particular attention paid to the resistance profile of *Bacteroides* species.

Spillage of microbe-laden content of the colon into the peritoneal cavity initiates an infection that often begins with peritonitis and bacteremia, followed in some cases by intra-abdominal abscess formation. These infections are polymicrobial and include **strict anaerobes** and **facultative anaerobes** (such as members of the Enterobacteriaceae family), probably interacting in complex metabolic ways. This chapter focuses on one of the most frequently isolated genera of bacteria from intra-abdominal abscesses, the *Bacteroides*. These strictly anaerobic Gram-negative rods are common members of the normal colonic microbiota. The main opportunistic pathogen of the genus, *B. fragilis*, synthesizes a capsular polysaccharide complex (CPC) with a structural motif that facilitates the formation of abscesses when introduced into the peritoneal cavity.

No other place in the body is more prone to contamination by a large number of endogenous bacteria than the peritoneal cavity. The resulting intra-abdominal infection dramatically illustrates what happens when microorganisms are introduced in large numbers into the wrong place. The spillage of a few milliliters of intestinal content into the peritoneal cavity delivers many billions of bacteria to a customarily sterile site. Left untreated, peritonitis is often fatal. Physicians must be aware of the need for the proper antibiotic regimen, including effective treatment for *Bacteroides,* at the time of the contamination to reduce the likelihood of subsequent abscess formation.

Case

Ms. A., an 18-year-old college freshman, was admitted to the hospital with diffuse abdominal pain, diarrhea, and nausea without vomiting. Her pain was localized to the right side of the abdomen. Physical examination revealed tenderness in the lower quadrant of her abdomen, principally over McBurney point. She received a first-generation cephalosporin antibiotic (cefazolin) and was taken to the operating room, where her ruptured appendix was removed. Cultures of the peritoneal cavity in the neighborhood of the appendix grew a mixture of bacteria, typical of those found in stool. On the second day after the operation, her temperature spiked to 38.6°C. Blood cultures obtained preoperatively grew *Escherichia coli.*

Ms. A. improved postoperatively and completed a 7-day course of cephalosporin. Because she had no further symptoms and her blood cultures were negative, the antibiotic was stopped. However, 36 hours later her temperature was 38.8°C and she felt diffuse pain over the site of the appendectomy. A CAT scan of her abdomen revealed a retroperitoneal abscess. Cultures obtained after drainage of the abscess grew *B. fragilis.* She was again treated with antibiotics. This time metronidazole was used for 14 days, and Ms. A. had an uneventful recovery.

This case raises several questions:

1. How did the two episodes of Ms. A.'s disease differ with regard to pathogenesis and the kind of bacteria involved?
2. Why did *B. fragilis* survive the first course of antibiotic treatment?
3. Was Ms. A. treated properly? What could have been done to lessen the likelihood of abscess formation?
4. How does *B. fragilis* facilitate intra-abdominal abscess formation?

Two points should be emphasized. First, intra-abdominal infections typically result in **biphasic diseases,** as in the case of Ms. A. They start with an acute inflammation and progress to the formation of localized abscesses. Second, of the hundreds of species contained in the colonic inoculum, a few are most commonly isolated from abscesses. *B. fragilis* is found in the majority of cases and is the most important of the anaerobic bacteria associated with abscess formation. Although it can be isolated in pure culture from an abscess, it is typically cultured with a variety of other bacteria.

The majority of intra-abdominal infections result from the rupture of **infected appendices** or **intestinal diverticula,** the abnormal outpouchings of the colon. In the United States more than 250,000 cases of appendicitis and some 350,000 cases of diverticulitis are reported each year. Of these infections about 15% perforate and result in peritonitis, and many produce abscesses as a late complication. The prevalence of diverticula increases with aging, as does diverticulitis as the cause of intra-abdominal infection.

Bacteroides
CHARACTERISTICS

Organisms of the genus *Bacteroides* are anaerobic, Gram-negative rods present in high concentrations in the large intestine of humans and other vertebrates. They number 10^{10} or more per gram of human feces and are one of the dominant organisms of this niche. The *Bacteroides* group comprises many species (Table 15-1), of which *B. fragilis* is the most prominent opportunistic pathogen.

Two other frequently isolated genera of anaerobic Gram-negative rods were originally classified as *Bacteroides.* Unlike the *Bacteroides,* however, *Porphyromonas* and *Prevotella* form characteristically pigmented colonies on blood agar. *Prevotella melaninogenica,* named for its production of a black pigment, is commonly found in the human gingival flora and is often associated with periodontal diseases. Although this organism is also found in other sites, it is most commonly associated with infections of oral origin, including aspiration pneumonia (see Chapter 62) and rather serious infections following human bites. In contrast, *Prevotella bivius* and *Prevotella disiens* are common vaginal flora associated with pelvic infections and peritonitis. Table 15-1 includes the major strict anaerobes of clinical significance, except the clostridia, which are described in Chapter 20.

In addition to the phylogenetic reclassifications just mentioned, molecular phylogenetic techniques have revealed that two species previously designated as *Bacteroides* species, *B. distasonis* and *B. forsythus,* are more appropriately grouped within other genera (*Porphy-*

Paradigm Box

Polymicrobial Infections

The contamination of deep tissues with endogenous microbial residents, such as that of the intestine or the oropharynx, often results in infection caused by a mixture of bacteria that are part of the normal flora of the original site. Examples are **peritonitis** caused by a ruptured appendix and a **pulmonary abscess** caused by aspiration of oropharyngeal bacteria. From such sites it is usually possible to isolate many different combinations of bacteria. These infections are exceptions to a "one germ, one disease" concept. That is, they are usually **polymicrobial** rather than monomicrobial.

Peritonitis in the Preantibiotic Era

The magician Houdini died of peritonitis. Houdini was known for his astounding feats of escape while enchained and enclosed in containers submerged in water. He possessed amazing physical strength and could control many muscles, including, it is said, some normally not under voluntary control. His fame was the cause of his demise. Houdini received an unexpected blow to his abdomen from a bystander intent on testing his legendary muscular powers. The magician's large intestine ruptured, and he died a few days later. Had Houdini lived today and been in the hands of a competent physician, he would have been treated with antibiotics and surgical repair and would have had a good chance of surviving.

table 15-1	Major Clinically Significant Non–Spore-Forming Anaerobic Bacteria		
GROUP	**GENUS**	**TYPICAL SPECIES**	**TYPICAL DISEASES**
Gram-negative			
Rods	*Bacteroides*	*fragilis, thetaiotamicron, vulgatus*	Intra-abdominal infection
	Fusobacterium	*nucleatum, necrophorum*	Oral, dental, pleuropulmonary infections
	Porphyromonas	*asaccharolytica, gingivalis*	Oral and dental infections
	Bacteroide (Porphyromonas)	*distasonis[a]*	Intra-abdominal infection
	Prevotella	*bivius, disiens melaninogenicus*	Pelvic infection
			Oral, dental, and pleuropulmonary infections
	Tannerella	*forsythensis*	Oral and dental infections
Gram-positive			
Rods	*Actinomyces*	*israeli*	Actinomycosis (lumpy jaw)
	Propionibacterium	*acnes*	Infections of prosthetic devices
Cocci	*Peptostreptococcus*	*magnus, asaccharolyticus, anaerobius*	Intra-abdominal, soft tissue, bone, and joint infections

[a]Phylogenetic reclassification not yet finalized.

romonas and *Tannerella*, respectively). Like *B. fragilis*, *B. distasonis* is a normal resident of the colon and is an opportunistic pathogen if released into the peritoneal cavity. *T. forsythensis* is a periodontal pathogen isolated from subgingival plaque of diseased periodontal pockets.

The *Bacteroides* obtain energy by fermenting carbohydrates. They are able to use the complex plant polysaccharides that the host cannot digest. Thus, the *Bacteroides* have a symbiotic relationship with the host, providing it with a digestive function that contributes significantly to the host's caloric intake. The ability of the *Bacteroides* to use a diverse array of the complex polysaccharides present in the colonic environment is one of the important factors contributing to its abundance in that ecosystem.

The *Bacteroides* are also able to cleave host-derived glycans present in the colon such as mucin, hyaluronate, chondroitin sulfate, and sialylated glycans. Neuraminidase, an enzyme that cleaves terminal sialic acid from host carbohydrates, is required for *Bacteroides* to produce abscesses in an animal model. It is not known if enzymes involved in cleaving host products contribute to the virulence of the *Bacteroides* when they are released to the peritoneal cavity. Like the staphylococci, streptococci, and pseudomonads, *B. fragilis* probably has multiple virulence factors that act in concert.

Although *Bacteroides* are strict anaerobes, they are not killed by exposure to oxygen and can grow in extremely reduced (nanomolar) concentrations of oxygen. *B. fragilis* has an extensive, highly regulated oxidative stress response system, including several enzymes typically absent from strict anaerobic organisms that protect the organism from oxygen radicals. These include a **superoxide dismutase,** which detoxifies oxygen radicals, and a **catalase,** which breaks down hydrogen peroxide. The organism synthesizes as many as 28 products in response to oxidative stress. As the peritoneal cavity has a higher P_{O_2} than the colon, products contributing to the organism's tolerance of air are likely important for survival of *B. fragilis* when it is initially released into the peritoneal cavity.

The outer membrane of *B. fragilis* contains a **lipopolysaccharide (LPS)** with a lipid A component that has a significantly different structure compared with that of *Escherichia coli*. This structural difference accounts for the **low endotoxicity** of *B. fragilis* LPS compared with that of *E. coli* and many other Gram-negative organisms.

A very important virulence factor in the ability of *B. fragilis* to facilitate the formation of abscesses is the **capsular polysaccharide complex.** The CPC is composed of at least nine distinct polysaccharides, the most described for a bacterium to date. The expression of these polysaccharides undergoes an on-off phenotype known as **phase variation.** Phase variation of these polysaccharides is regulated at the transcriptional level by DNA inversion of promoter regions that drive expression of the polysaccharide biosynthesis genes.

Whether the synthesis of such an extensive number of phase variable surface polysaccharides contributes to the virulence of this organism is not known. What is clear is that the structural motif present on at least one of these polysaccharides, **polysaccharide A (PSA),** is essential for the ability of *B. fragilis* to induce abscesses in animal models. The repeating unit of PSA is **zwitterionic** in that it contains residues with **both positive and negative charges.** This structural motif induces a host immune response, mediated by the activation of $CD4^+$ T lymphocytes, which leads to abscess formation in the peritoneal cavity. In addition, the CPC has been shown to be involved in the attachment of *B. fragilis* to the peritoneal mesothelium, the first cell boundary likely encountered in the peritoneal cavity following release from the colon.

Although several antibiotics are still effective treatments for *Bacteroides* infections, antibiotic resistance continues to be a significant problem. Members of *Bacteroides* possess sophisticated genetic systems that transfer genes for drug resistance not only among the *Bacteroides* species but also to species of other genera. These antibiotic resistance genes are often encoded on mobile genetic elements such as **conjugative transposons** or conjugative plasmids, enabling their transfer to other organisms. The transfer of these elements is likely facilitated in their natural colonic environment because the organisms are present in high numbers. The gene conferring resistance to clindamycin is harbored on conjugative elements of *Bacteroides*. Clindamycin, once the drug of choice against *Bacteroides,* is now reported to be ineffective in as many as 42% of clinical isolates.

ENTRY, SPREAD, AND ABSCESS FORMATION

The colon wall can be breached as a result of blunt trauma, intestinal disease, a penetrating wound, abdominal surgery, a ruptured appendix, or other causes. In the case of Ms. A., obstruction of outflow from the appendix led to inflammation and eventually to perforation. Whatever the mechanism, the number of organisms contaminating the peritoneal cavity is enormous when a breach occurs.

Because the bacterial inoculum is potentially diverse, a large number of factors are involved in determining which species become dominant in the infection. Many intestinal bacteria can grow in the peritoneal fluid, which is not particularly antibacterial. Before the content of the colon spills, the peritoneal cavity is well oxygenated, and highly oxygen-sensitive anaerobes are killed. After the spillage, the first organisms that become numerically dominant are facultative anaerobes, especially *E. coli*. However, many of the less oxygen-sensitive strict anaerobes survive and can be isolated from both the fluid and surface of mesothelial cells. Eventually, the site of infection becomes increasingly anaerobic, in part because facultative anaerobes metabolize what oxygen is present. The surviving strict anaerobes then take over. Animal studies have documented a need for synergy between various microorganisms for abscess formation. The inoculation of a single species of intestinal bacteria seldom leads to infection, but infection by a mixture of facultative and strict anaerobes produces acute inflammation and abscess formation.

DAMAGE

Organisms that enter the peritoneal cavity find themselves first in a liquid environment that could, in principle, lead to their dissemination throughout the cavity. However, the omentum and the loops of the small intestine drape themselves around areas of inflammation and serve to contain the infection. Although this takes time, the abscesses that eventually develop are usually well localized. Lymphatic drainage and the effect of gravity also influence the location of abscesses. These factors likely influenced the location of Ms. A.'s abscess at a retroperitoneal site, even though the original bacterial spill was near her appendix.

Following bacteria leakage, an immediate host response is mounted. Much of the contaminating bacteria are removed by the diaphragmatic lymphatics. Phagocytes are mobilized rapidly to the infected site and, to a point, dispose of large numbers of bacteria and debris. Because of the many phagocytes that migrate to the site of peritoneal contamination, the minimal infecting dose that results in disease in humans is possibly quite high, perhaps several milliliters of intestinal content, judging from experiments with laboratory animals.

If the peritoneal defenses are unable to eradicate spilled intestinal content, an abscess usually develops. Bacterial contamination triggers an increase in vascular permeability, resulting in the influx of plasma and **fibrin deposition.** Fibrin accumulation is enhanced as a result of reduced abdominal fibrinolytic activity during intra-abdominal infection. Bacteria that are adherent to or near the peritoneal mesothelium become trapped in fibrin matrices that develop to delimit the necrotic material and residual bacteria. These areas become surrounded by a thick, fibrous collagen-containing capsule (Fig. 15-1). Inside the capsule are live and dead white blood cells, bacteria, and cell debris. In general, these abscesses resemble those caused by the staphylococci (see Chapter 11). Inside peritoneal abscesses, the dominant *B. fragilis* is often accompanied not only by facultative anaerobes but also by other strict anae-robes, such as clostridia or anaerobic streptococci (i.e., *Peptostreptococcus*).

Intra-abdominal abscesses exact a high toll on the host because they can extend to nearby sites and cause necrosis of adjacent tissue. In addition, they serve as a fo-

FIGURE 15-1. ▪ **Intra-abdominal abscesses of the mouse abdominal wall following intraabdominal challenge with *B. fragilis*.** This photograph, taken 6 days after infection, shows fully formed abscesses that have become extensively vascularized. Photo by A. Tzianabos.

cus of bacterial contamination from which organisms can enter the bloodstream. The resulting bacteremia may produce septic shock or cause metastatic infections and abscesses at distant sites.

Other *Bacteroides*-Associated Diseases

In addition to intra-abdominal abscesses, *Bacteroides* can also be isolated from other clinical sites, usually as part of a polymicrobial infection. These include the blood of patients with intra-abdominal infection, secondary abscesses resulting from the hematogenous spread from a primary intra-abdominal abscess, infections of the diabetic foot, soft tissue infections, and suppurative infections of the genital tract.

An increasing number of *B. fragilis* strains have been demonstrated to express an enterotoxin termed *BFT*, a metalloprotease that disrupts the tight junctions of epithelial cells by cleaving E-cadherin. Although *B. fragilis* strains that harbor *bft* are part of the normal flora of apparently healthy individuals, these strains are associated with acute diarrheal disease of livestock and humans. Recent data show that Bft induces cellular proliferation that may contribute to oncogenic transformation and colon cancer.

DIAGNOSIS

Intra-abdominal abscesses should be suspected in patients with prior history of appendicitis, diverticulitis, or other predisposing conditions who present with abdom-

FIGURE 15-2 ▪ An anaerobic glove box used for the culture of strictly anaerobic bacteria. This device is used for large-scale work and for experimentation. The port on the right is used to introduce and remove material from the chamber. It has two doors (not visible) and can be independently flushed free of oxygen.

inal pain. Various imaging procedures, including computed tomography and ultrasonography, are used to confirm and localize the abscesses.

Proper chemotherapy of mixed bacterial infections requires the determination of the bacterial species involved and their antibiotic sensitivity. Specialized techniques are required for growing members of the genus *Bacteroides* and other anaerobes. Clinical specimens must be protected from air using special collecting devices and transported to the laboratory without delay. The most convenient way to handle and culture clinical specimens is with the use of an incubator in the form of a glove box, a device in which the atmosphere can be made anaerobic by flushing with a mixture of nitrogen, carbon dioxide, and hydrogen (Fig. 15-2). This equipment is specialized and costly, and not all hospital laboratories have it. However, it is possible to carry out anaerobic microbiological work with smaller but less convenient glass jars.

TREATMENT AND PREVENTION

Measures can be taken to minimize the risk of intra-abdominal infection and abscess formation if contamination from the colon is suspected. In Ms. A.'s case, the appendix had perforated and bacterial contamination of the peritoneal cavity was confirmed. When contamination is known or even suspected, appropriate antibiotic therapy is necessary. The antibiotics should be broad spectrum and designed to prevent bacteremia resulting from facultative anaerobes and abscesses caused by *Bacteroides*. Several antibiotics, including **metronidazole, β-lactam–β-lactamase inhibitor combinations,** and the **carbapenems** have good activity against *Bacteroides*. However, the target in these infections is seldom a single bacterial species but a mixed population with different sensitivities. Thus, a combination of antibiotics or an antibiotic effective against both aerobes and anaerobes is indicated. For Ms. A., the cephalosporin first administered was effective against *E. coli* but not against *B. fragilis*. Her second treatment recognized the need for an appropriate choice, and she also received metronidazole, an effective drug against this organism.

If intra-abdominal abscesses do form because either antibiotic treatment was not effective or leakage from the bowel was not previously identified, dual therapy—namely, drainage of the abscess and administration of antibiotics—is usually required. In addition, the anatomical defect that allowed spillage from the intestine must be repaired. Thus, a combined medical and surgical approach is often necessary in cases of intra-abdominal infection. Percutaneous drainage of intra-abdominal abscesses, guided by computed tomography, is a viable alternative to surgical drainage when the abscess is localized with no evidence of generalized peritonitis.

Conclusion

The *Bacteroides* species are abundant members of the colonic microbiota of humans and other mammals and can become opportunistic pathogens if they gain access to the peritoneal cavity or other normally sterile body sites. The predominant pathogen of the genera, *B. fragilis*, possesses a CPC containing both positive and negative charges. This zwitterionic motif stimulates an immune response in the host that leads to intra-abdominal abscess formation. Although the diseases caused by *Bacteroides* can be cured, the organisms still present challenges to therapy and, above all, to prevention. Although mechanisms are in place to reduce intra-abdominal abscess formation, none presently available can totally prevent these infections.

chapter **16**

Enteric Bacteria:
Secretory Diarrhea

Victor J. DiRita

key **concepts**

Enteric bacteria that cause secretory (watery) diarrhea:

- Include members of Enterobacteriaceae and Vibrionaceae.

- Are usually transmitted to humans in contaminated food and water.

- Face formidable defenses in the gastrointestinal tract; they adhere to the epithelial cells of the tract via pili (fimbriae) or surface adhesins.

- Can elaborate toxins (*Vibrio cholerae* and enterotoxigenic *Escherichia coli*) that reduce sodium absorption and increase chloride secretion of the intestinal cells, which leads to watery diarrhea.

- Can be treated with oral rehydration therapy.

Diarrhea, usually no more than a bothersome but brief illness in industrialized nations, is one of the leading causes of infant and childhood mortality in developing countries. Diarrheal diseases kill more than 5 million children annually and contribute to malnutrition and growth retardation in those who survive the illnesses. Thus, diarrheal disease control remains a major goal for the World Health Organization.

Secretory or watery diarrhea is caused by the loss of electrolytes and fluids from the small intestine. An extreme example is cholera, which can cause fatal dehydration in hours, usually in small children. Travelers diarrhea is a generally milder form of watery diarrhea. It most commonly affects adults. Infections of the intestinal tract can lead to local tissue damage or inflammation and cause **bloody diarrhea** or **dysentery** (see Chapter 17).

Bacteria, viruses, and protozoa that cause diarrheal disease are grouped together as **enteric pathogens.** Several traits endow these agents with the ability to cause secretory diarrhea, and these virulence factors vary in their mode of action. The array of factors particular to each organism determines the characteristics of the clinical illness.

Case

Mr. D., a 33-year-old fully immunized, rather nervous accountant who is blood group O positive and taking H_2 blockers for ulcer disease; his 29-year-old healthy wife; and their 10-month-old baby boy returned from a 2-week trip to South America. The next morning Mr. D. passed a semisolid stool, which was quickly followed by a large watery bowel movement. Within an hour he passed another large watery stool, now opaque gray–white in color. He vomited several times and became slightly sweaty. After passing another large watery stool, Mr. D. called his physician, who advised him to go to the emergency department. When he arrived there Mr. D. was afebrile but had a rapid heart rate with a feeble pulse and low blood pressure. He complained of muscle cramps and dizziness. All these signs and symptoms were consistent with a significant loss of extracellular fluids. Laboratory studies showed a normal leukocyte count, a slightly elevated level of serum sodium, a normal serum potassium level, and an elevated blood urea nitrogen level, also consistent with dehydration.

A diagnosis of cholera was suspected. Mr. D. was immediately given 2 liters of fluid intravenously and then started on oral rehydration solution. His stool volumes progressively diminished over 48 hours, and he was discharged. Because of the suspected diagnosis, special media were used, and the stool culture grew *Vibrio cholerae*, serogroup O1, biotype E1 Tor. Mrs. D., a native Peruvian, had two loose bowel movements on the second day of her husband's illness. Her stool culture grew only *Escherichia coli*.

Two weeks later, Baby D. stopped feeding and developed watery diarrhea. His rectal temperature was 38°C. His parents brought the infant to the pediatrician. The baby had signs and symptoms of dehydration, with fluid loss estimated at approximately 7% of body weight. He was admitted to the hospital. Neither leukocytes nor red blood cells were seen in the stool. Baby D. was rehydrated with an oral rehydration solution. His fever abated and appetite returned, although the diarrhea persisted. The preliminary laboratory report stated that the stool cultures contained "normal fecal flora"; 2 days later the laboratory identified enteropathogenic *E. coli* (EPEC) by polymerase chain reaction (PCR) test for the characteristic adherence factor. Baby D. improved and was discharged after 4 days, having lost 1 lb in weight. One month later he returned to his normal growth curve.

This case raises several questions:

1. Why did the physician caring for Mr. D. think of cholera?
2. Are all enteric bacteria capable of causing disease, or are some more frequently pathogenic than others? Which enteric pathogens cause diarrhea, and where do they come from?
3. What are the clinical manifestations caused by enteric pathogens? Why do the organisms cause different intensity of symptoms in individuals?
4. What factors are involved in colonization? What factors are involved in causing symptoms?
5. What is the proper therapy for watery diarrhea?
6. Can these diseases be prevented?

Mr. D. and his son developed two different secretory diarrheal diseases. Mr. D. had acquired cholera during travel; Baby D. was infected with an enteropathogenic *Escherichia coli* (EPEC), probably acquired after returning home. Among the most common bacterial pathogens in the United States are strains of *E. coli* present in the intestine of humans or animals. Other important causes of watery diarrhea include *Shigella sonnei* and *Salmonella* (see Chapter 17). In addition, viruses (most commonly, rotavirus) and protozoa (*Giardia*, *Cryptosporidium*, and *Cyclospora*) can cause watery diarrhea.

Diarrheal Diseases

Most diarrhea episodes can be traced to a specific pathogen; however, clinical laboratories do not routinely use all available diagnostic methods. The predominant isolate under aerobic culture conditions, *E. coli*, cannot usually be classified as either pathogenic or nonpathogenic strains by the usual laboratory studies. As many as 40% of patients under 2 years of age have rotavirus (see Chapter 37), and many preschool children in day care are infected with *S. sonnei* or protozoa (see Chapter 53).

Although infants in the United States may have 1 or 2 readily treated diarrhea episodes per year, infants and children in developing countries may have as many as 10 or more. Many of these infants and children advance to life-threatening dehydration. Limited access to medical care in some countries means that many potentially treatable cases end in death.

Most of the bacteria that cause diarrheal disease belong to a large family of Gram-negative rods, the **Enterobacteriaceae**; some belong to the **Vibrionaceae** family (Tables 16-1 and 16-2). The Enterobacteriaceae include members of the normal flora of the intestine as well as frank pathogens. Members of both families may cause a wide spectrum of disease including diarrhea, urinary and respiratory tract infection, sepsis, and meningitis. Members of the Enterobacteriaceae family are differentiated on the basis of serological and metabolic properties. The family Vibrionaceae also includes many nonpathogenic species as well as organisms that cause epidemic cholera, sporadic diarrhea, and local skin or bacteremic infections.

table **16-1**	Main Genera of Pathogenic Enterobacteriaceae and Vibrionaceae	
GENUS	**MAIN RESERVOIRS**	**PRINCIPAL DISEASES**
Enterobacteriaceae		
Escherichia	Ileum and colon of vertebrates	Diarrhea, dysentery, urinary tract infections, septicemia, neonatal meningitis, others
Shigella	Human colon	Diarrhea, dysentery
Salmonella	Gastrointestinal system of animals and humans	Diarrhea, bloody diarrhea, typhoid (enteric) fever, aortitis, osteomyelitis, other focal infections
Proteus	Colon of vertebrates, water, soil	Urinary tract infections, septicemia, pneumonia
Klebsiella, Enterobacter, Serratia, Citrobacter	Colon of vertebrates, water, sewage	Pneumonia, septicemia; special problems in debilitated or immunocompromised patients
Yersinia	Rodents, pigs, water	Plague, bloody diarrhea, diarrhea, pseudoappendicitis, mesenteric adenitis syndrome
Vibrionaceae		
Vibrio (alginolyticus, vulnificus)	Marine water ecosystems	Watery diarrhea (certain species associated with phytoplankton); can cause skin infections or septicemia
Campylobacter	Gastrointestinal system of animals	Diarrhea, bloody diarrhea, septicemia (certain species only)

+ - principal manifestation
± - occasional manifestation

Cholera is the paradigm of secretory diarrhea and is caused by *Vibrio cholerae*, a member of the Vibrionaceae. One particular serological type, *V. cholerae* O1, has been responsible for yearly epidemics in the Indian subcontinent for centuries and, for at least the last two centuries, periodic global pandemics. The O1 in its name indicates that it contains a **lipopolysaccharide (LPS)** antigen that belongs to the O1 serogroup. The O1 group contains two biotypes, the **classical** and **El Tor** types. Until 1961 the El Tor type was considered an avirulent commensal when it was found to cause the seventh recorded pandemic in the early twentieth century. Beginning in Indonesia, El Tor

table **16-2**	Gram-Negative Rods That Cause Diarrhea, Bloody Diarrhea, and Dysentery			
			INFLAMMATORY DIARRHEA OR DYSENTERY	
ROD	**DIARRHEA**	**BLOODY DIARRHEA**	**ILEITIS**	**COLITIS**
Enterobacteriaceae				
ETEC	+			
EPEC	+		±	
EaggEC	+			
EIEC		+		+
EHEC		+		+
Shigella		+	±	+
Nontyphoidal *Salmonella*	+	±	+	±
Salmonella typhi			±	
Yersinia enterocolitica	+	+	+	
Others	+			
Vibrionaceae				
Vibrio cholerae	+			
Vibrio parahaemolyticus	+	+	±	±
Campylobacter jejuni	+	+	±	+

EAggEC, enteroaggregative *E. coli*; EHEC, enterohemorrhagic *E. coli*; EIEC, enteroinvasive *E. coli*; EPEC, enteropathogenic *E. coli*; ETEC, enterotoxigenic *E. coli*.

FIGURE 16-1 ▪ The spread of the seventh cholera pandemic from Southeast Asia. This pandemic was caused by the El Tor biotype of *Vibrio cholerae*, which has a higher asymptomatic carriage rate than the classical biotype. In the 1990s a new type emerged from El Tor by acquiring a novel lipopolysaccharide antigen, O139, instead of O1. Prior infection with El Tor provides no immunity to *V. cholerae* O139 (Bengal). Infections with this new strain appeared in Bangladesh in the 1990s and have spread to India and other countries; this may represent the beginning of the eighth pandemic of cholera.

cholera rapidly spread in Asia, reaching Europe and Africa in the early 1970s and Latin America in 1991. Although the disease rapidly disappeared from Europe, it has become endemic in Africa and Latin America (Fig. 16-1).

A small endemic focus of cholera, known since 1973, exists along the Gulf Coast of the United States, and a few cases of cholera occur yearly as a result of eating shellfish harboring the organism. In the United States cholera is transmitted primarily by eating contaminated raw or partially cooked shellfish harvested from that area of the Gulf of Mexico. Cholera rarely occurs in other areas of the United States because of the high level of environmental sanitation and protected drinking water supplies.

In contrast to *V. cholerae*, which is never a member of the normal human flora, *E. coli* is the most abundant **facultative anaerobe** in normal human feces. However, it is outnumbered by at least 1000 to 1 by **strict anaerobes** like the *Bacteroides* (see Chapter 15). Most fecal *E. coli* are avirulent and do not cause disease; some human strains have been cultivated in the laboratory for so long that they have lost the ability to colonize humans. These strains include *E. coli* K12, the strain that occupies center stage in molecular biology and gene cloning and is perhaps the best understood cellular form of life.

E. coli is an umbrella designation for a number of rather varied pathogenic and nonpathogenic strains. There are at least five distinguishable groups of *E. coli* now known to cause enteric disease (Table 16-3). With one exception (the non–sorbitol-fermenting *E. coli* serotype O157:H7), routine stool cultures cannot

table 16-3 Classification of Pathogenic *Escherichia coli* and Representative Serotypes

GROUP	SYMPTOMS	EPIDEMIOLOGY
Enterotoxigenic (ETEC)	Watery diarrhea (travelers diarrhea)	Worldwide, adults and children
Enteropathogenic (EPEC)	Watery diarrhea	Infants < 1 year of age
Enteroaggregative (EAggEC)	Watery diarrhea, persistent diarrhea	Infants < 6 months of age, AIDS patients
Enteroinvasive (EIEC)	Bloody diarrhea	Uncommon, often foodborne
Enterohemorrhagic (EHEC)	Bloody diarrhea, hemorrhagic colitis, hemolytic–uremic syndrome, thrombotic thrombocytopenic purpura	Western nations

distinguish pathogenic from nonpathogenic *E. coli.* The problem in distinguishing "bad" *E. coli* from "good" *E. coli* is that all strains share the same basic taxonomic and biochemical features, although they may have different virulence factors. How then are these strains distinguished? The classic way is to determine the antigenic reactivity of the **O antigen** of the outer membrane lipopolysaccharide (see Chapter 3). There are 173 different *E. coli* O antigens. These O antigens can associate with the 60 different H antigens, resulting in a vast number of combinations. In addition, some strains have a capsular polysaccharide antigen called K. Determining the combination of O and H antigens helps identify certain virulent clones (see Table 16-3). Similar tests are also used to distinguish the cholera vibrios and the many distinct *Salmonella* serotypes.

Enteric Pathogens

ENCOUNTER

Some enteric pathogens are well adapted to the external environment and only incidentally cause disease. *V. cholerae* is a normal inhabitant of coastal estuarine waters, where it lives in close association with phytoplankton. Humans are incidentally infected when they enter this ecosystem or when the organisms contaminate drinking water or food. Seasonal variation in the *Vibrio* population can also occur, perhaps as a result of the action of vibriophages that live in the same water as the bacteria. High temperatures, algal blooms, or changes in the local phage population can lead to *Vibrio* blooms, thereby increasing the likelihood of transmission to humans. If the organisms reach the drinking water and food supplies, epidemic spread can occur. The diarrhea that is so characteristic of this disease can be viewed as an evolutionary mechanism facilitating dispersal of the organisms and their transfer to new hosts.

Certain enteric pathogens (for example *Salmonella* and *Campylobacter*) are seldom found in the environment but are usually associated with humans or animals. Although these organisms display considerable host specificity, species barriers are often crossed. The diseases caused in humans by animal-specific strains are called **zoonoses** (see Chapter 73).

The route for transmission of enteric pathogens is from feces to mouth; however, many intermediary vehicles intervene, characterized as the "seven Fs": feces, food, fluids, fingers, flies, fomites (inanimate objects), and fornication. The number of organisms required to cause disease (**inoculum size**) is probably better known for enteric bacteria than for most other organisms. Experimental infections have been induced in human volunteers who agree to drink buffered solutions containing a known number of living bacteria. A few hundred *Shigella dysenteriae* type 1 are sufficient to cause disease in many volunteers. In contrast, 1,000 to 10,000 *Shigella flexneri* and more than 100 million enterotoxigenic *E. coli* are required to cause the same attack rate. A direct consequence of a small infective dose is that, under the same conditions, *Shigella* are generally transmitted from person to person, because small inocula are readily passed by fingers or objects after contact with stool or soiled diapers. Directly transferring an infectious dose of enterotoxigenic *E. coli* is more difficult because transmission requires a visible lump of feces. It is more likely that large numbers of *E. coli* enter humans when they ingest contaminated food or water in which the organisms have already multiplied.

Despite the high standards of modern hygiene, we are in constant contact with enteric bacteria. Feces are an approximate 20% suspension of bacteria in water. Each day we are in contact with and ingest fecal microorganisms to a greater or lesser extent, depending on our age (which determines behavior) and the state of environmental sanitation. Because potential pathogens are so common, why do we not get diarrhea every day? The answer to this question requires an understanding of the mechanisms of pathogenesis of these diseases and host defenses, both specific and nonspecific.

ENTRY

Having arrived at the mouth, microorganisms face a perilous journey along the alimentary canal to their final destination. The gastrointestinal tract is a tube lined with differentiated epithelial cells that keep bacteria "outside" the body and deliver them to the environment through the anus. The journey is perilous because the microorganisms face host defenses and hostile conditions. The pH of the stomach may be less than 1, a condition that is lethal to most microorganisms. In the duodenum near the ampulla of Vater, surviving organisms are bathed in bicarbonate-buffered pancreatic juice with a pH that can be as high as 9. In the small intestine, microorganisms are smothered in mucus; rolled up in sticky polysaccharide balls; and kneaded, squeezed, and swept distally toward the anus by **peristaltic motions** of the bowel, unless they find a way to hold on. Throughout the journey, they encounter soluble proteins such as lysozyme, proteases, lipases, and secretory IgA, as well as bile salts and phagocytic and lymphoid cells. If they pause in the large intestine, they meet the populous normal flora that resists implantation by new species, in part by previous occupancy of adhesion sites on the gut wall and in part by producing inhibitory substances (e.g., bacteriocins).

The efficiency of these host defenses is the reason why the infectious dose of most noninvasive enteric pathogens is high and that disease is not common. Some conditions, however, may be advantageous to the pathogen. For example, pathogens mixed with food are protected from stomach acid, and the infectious dose is therefore diminished. In some patients the ability to secrete gastric acid is seriously impaired by intrinsic disease (pernicious anemia), infections (e.g., *Helicobacter pylori* or gastritis; see Chapter 22), prior surgery (gastric resection, diversions, or transections of the vagus nerve), or antiulcer drugs that inhibit or buffer gastric acid. These patients are at greater risk for infection with acid-sensitive bacteria like *V. cholerae* or *Salmonella*.

Mr. D. was at risk of developing clinical cholera on exposure to the organism for two reasons: he was an ulcer patient receiving H_2 blockers to reduce gastric acid secretion, and he was blood group O positive. For unknown reasons, O-positive persons are predisposed to develop more severe cholera, presumably because certain oligosaccharides on cells or in secretions enhance binding of the organism or cholera toxin production, or cause other altered responses of the mucosa.

SPREAD AND MULTIPLICATION

Cholera vibrios have several features that may help them reach the epithelial surface of the small intestine. Their flagella make them actively mobile, and they produce a protease that hydrolyses mucus. They colonize the intestine by adhering to the epithelial surface. **Adherence** is not a simple feat because the surfaces of both microbe and host are negatively charged (for optimal adherence, the surfaces should not be mutually repulsive). Cholera vibrios have specific **pili** or **fimbriae** (see Chapter 4) that serve in part to increase the distance between the host cell surface and the bacterium and diminish the electrostatic repulsion. The complex system of macromolecular assembly for producing these organelles involves synthesis of appendage proteins, chaperones to deliver them to the bacterial cell surface, and usher proteins to assist in proper assembly.

Examples of nonpilus adhesins are also known. Virtually all Gram-negative bacteria possess type 1 or **common pili**, which are protein rods that help the bacteria stick to the mucosal surfaces of the gastrointestinal tract. Common pili have a special affinity for mannose-containing proteins and lipids in mucosal membranes. Despite their frequency, common pili are rarely involved in adherence of pathogenic microorganisms, which are endowed with more specialized adhesins. For example, cholera bacilli stick to one another using a specific adherence pilus called the **toxin-coregulated pilus (TCP)**. It is so named because its synthesis is regulated by the same system that controls the production of cholera toxin (Fig 16-2).

FIGURE 16-2 ■ **The pathogenesis of cholera and enterotoxigenic *Escherichia coli* (ETEC) infections.** The organisms colonize the mucosal surface via microbial adhesins—for example, colonization factor antigen (Cfa) of enterotoxigenic *E. coli*. The factor that binds *V. cholerae* to cells is not clearly defined, but a toxin coregulated pilus (Tcp) causes the organisms to adhere to one another and form microcolonies on the epithelial surface. Once colonization has occurred, cholera toxin (Ctx) or labile toxin (LT) binds to a receptor, is taken up in vesicles, and an active subunit of each (CtxA or LTA) is transported to the basolateral membrane to the adenylate cyclase (AC) complex. The toxins transfer ADP ribose to the guanosine 5'-triphosphate (GTP)–binding protein of AC, elevating cAMP. ETEC also produces a heat-stable (ST) toxin that binds to the membrane guanylate cyclase (GC) and increases cyclic guanosine 5'-monophosphate (cGMP) levels. Both cAMP and cGMP reduce sodium absorption in villus cells and increase chlorine secretion in crypt cells, leading to watery diarrhea.

After colonizing the intestinal brush border through the action of their pili, neither the cholera vibrios of Mr. D. or the *E. coli* of the baby were able to invade the mucosa. These vibrios can readily multiply because the resident flora at the level of the jejunum and upper ileum is scanty and thus pose no significant competition.

DAMAGE

V. cholerae and Enterotoxigenic *E. coli*

Mr. D.'s diarrhea was caused by colonization of the small bowel by organisms that survived their passage across the stomach. If the small bowel mucosa had been examined, no visible damage would have been noted. Instead, the pathology occurs at the biochemical level; that is, the increase in **adenylate cyclase** activity is caused by cholera toxin. In the small intestine, cholera bacilli make **cholera toxin,** the TCP, and several accessory virulence genes. Proving that nature is both parsimonious and creative, the genes for cholera toxin are encoded on the genome of a bacteriophage that is integrated into the chromosome and uses TCP as its receptor on the surface of the organism.

How do cholera bacilli "know" that they are in the small intestine? A number of their virulence genes, including the one for cholera toxin and TCP, are regulated by the activity of a complex but logical regulatory cascade that responds to cues within the human host. By switching on the virulence genes only when they are in a host, these pathogens do not waste energy making products not required in their natural aquatic environment. The switching occurs rapidly within the intestine and results in an ordered expression of the adherence organelle TCP followed by expression of cholera toxin. **Sensory mechanisms** of this sort that coordinate regulation of virulence are a common theme in bacterial pathogens (see Chapter 19 paradigm).

Once it is made, cholera toxin binds to a cell surface receptor (the **GM1 ganglioside**) and is internalized within a vesicle. The active subunit A of the toxin is routed to the basolateral membrane of the intestinal epithelial cell where the specific target of the cholera toxin, the **G$_S$ regulatory protein of the adenylate cyclase complex,** is located. Cholera toxin is an enzyme capable of modifying G$_S$ by **adenosine diphosphate (ADP) ribosylation** (the transfer of the ADP-ribosyl moiety of nicotinamide adenine dinucleotide [NAD] to substrate proteins; see Chapter 9). The modification of G$_S$ protein results in permanent activation of adenylate cyclase and an increase in intracellular **cyclic adenosine monophosphate (cAMP)**. Increased concentrations of cAMP inhibit sodium absorption by small bowel villous cells and increase chloride secretion by crypt cells. Because the amount of sodium chloride in the gut lumen increases, passive secretion of water occurs by osmotic force and generates watery, diarrheal stool. In a case of cholera like Mr. D.'s, the volume of water lost can be so prodigious that the patient is rapidly dehydrated, may go into shock, and if not quickly treated, may die.

In endemic regions of Asia, Africa, and Latin America, cholera occurs primarily in children less than 10 years old, because older adolescents and adults are usually protected by adaptive immunity. During epidemics in previously cholera-free areas, all age groups are susceptible. This age-specific pattern is typical of endemic infections, not epidemic infections. Mortality is caused by electrolyte and water losses; therefore, with proper fluid replacement, no patient should die of cholera. Without therapy as many as 50% of patients may die.

Related to cholera are infections caused by **enterotoxigenic *E. coli* (ETEC)**. These strains produce one or both **enterotoxins,** called **LT** and **ST,** that act by changing the net fluid transport in the gut from absorption to secretion. LT is structurally identical to cholera toxin and activates the adenylate cyclase–cAMP system in the same manner and for the life of that cell (Chapter 9). However, cholera is usually more serious as it leads to the secretion of much greater amounts of liquid stools.

Unlike ETEC, *V. cholerae* has a very efficient mechanism for secreting toxin into its milieu, which may account for the different severities of two diseases caused by very similar toxins. In neither case is the intestinal mucosa visibly damaged; the watery stool does not contain white or red blood cells, and no inflammatory process occurs in the gut wall. ST interacts with and activates the **guanylate cyclase** of intestinal cells. This interaction leads to an increase in the **cyclic guanosine monophosphate (GMP)** and altered sodium and chloride transport, much like LT and cholera toxin. However, effects on guanylate cyclase are turned off if the toxin is washed away from the cell. Toxins related to cholera or ST toxins have also been found in a number of other diarrheal pathogens such as *Salmonella, Yersinia, Aeromonas,* and the enteroaggregative *E. coli.*

Enteropathogenic E. coli

Baby D. was infected with an enteropathogenic *E. coli* (EPEC), one of a small group of specific serotypes originally recognized because they cause outbreaks of diarrhea in the newborn nursery (see Table 16-3). This kind of diarrhea is caused by complex mechanisms that result in disruption of the microvillus surface and alteration of host cellular signaling processes by the action of a specialized mechanism, called a type III secretion system, that is elaborated by EPEC (for more on type III secretion, see Chapter 17 paradigm). Multiple steps in this pathogenesis have been uncovered. In the earliest stage, organisms adhere to target epithelial cells in a relatively distant ("nonintimate") manner. Binding occurs by means of a so-called **bundle-forming pilus** (Fig. 16-3), which is structurally similar to the TCP of *V. cholerae.* Subsequently, the type III secretion system is assembled and delivers some of its effector molecules into the host cells. The precise role of many of these **effector proteins** is the subject of ongoing research, but one of them is well

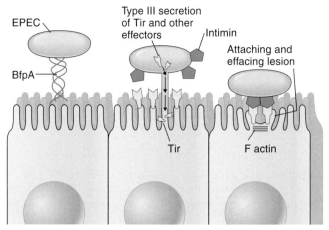

FIGURE 16-3 ■ **The pathogenesis of enteropathogenic** *Escherichia coli* (EPEC). First, the organism attaches to the small bowel epithelial cell via a bundle-forming pilus (BfpA). Subsequently, a type III secretion system bridges to the cell and delivers a membrane receptor protein, Tir, and other effectors to the host cell. In a third stage, intimin on the bacterial surface mediates intimate adherence to the cell by binding to the newly deployed Tir receptors. Polymerization of actin to filamentous actin (F actin) and other host cytoskeletal proteins is induced, and rearrangements of the cytoskeletal structure occur. Together these processes result in the characteristic EPEC pedestal with the intimately adherent organism (the attaching and effacing lesion).

understood to play a critical step in the next phase of the pathogenesis. This step is characterized by intimate attachment and damage of the host enterocytes, and the critical type III effector protein is called **Tir.**

Serving as the receptor for the bacteria, Tir enables the close attachment and subsequent enterocyte effacement. In essence, EPEC sends over its own receptor, which assembles into the host cell membrane. The microbes also produce a protein called **intimin** on their surfaces, and interaction between intimin and Tir serves to establish the intimate adherence of the microbes. Once this has occurred, Tir-mediated reorganization of the host actin cytoskeleton follows, and the surface of the enterocyte rearranges to form an actin-based 10 nm "**pedestal**" underneath the EPEC. These pedestals and the disruption they cause to the host enterocyte surface represent the characteristic **attaching and effacing EPEC lesion.** How does this lesion cause diarrhea? The mechanism of this is an active area of investigation, but it likely includes malabsorption from the villus rearrangement and disruption of epithelial tight junctions that results in intestinal permeability. The production of a classic enterotoxin like LT or cholera toxin does not appear to be involved.

Other Infections Caused by Vibrios and *E. coli*

In late 1992 an unprecedented event occurred. Epidemic cholera caused by a non-O1 *V. cholerae* strain was detected in South India, rapidly spreading to Bangladesh and neighboring countries in Asia and displacing the resident O1 strain. Individuals immune to *V. cholerae* O1 were not immune to the new strain, *V. cholerae* O139. Thus, a new epidemic began that involved all ages in the endemic countries of Asia, not just younger children as before. This event is an example of the continuing emergence of new disease pathogens with extended virulence.

The appearance of the new strain was traced to exchange of the O-antigen synthesizing genes from another *V. cholerae* serogroup into an O1 El Tor strain. The precise source of the new DNA is not clear, but the outcome of the exchange was expression of a previously unknown lipopolysaccharide somatic antigen, O139. In addition, the organism acquired at least one new gene involved in making a capsule, an unusual feature in *V. cholerae* O1. The new organism traveled to Europe and the United States, although early concerns that a new pandemic, which would have been the eighth recorded cholera pandemic, were not borne out. In 1995 the classic *V. cholerae* O1 displaced O139 as the dominant cholera organism in Dhaka, Bangladesh, whereas *V. cholerae* O139 has persisted in nearby Calcutta, India.

Other marine vibrios lacking the characteristic virulence attributes of *V. cholerae,* such as *V. parahaemolyticus,* cause a bloody diarrhea associated with ingestion of sushi or raw shellfish, especially in Japan. Other vibrio species, such as *V. vulnificus* and *V. alginolyticus,* are often acquired through an injury or a break in the skin and may cause severe subcutaneous and invasive illnesses.

EPEC and ETEC strains of *E. coli* represent only the earliest described diarrhea-causing *E. coli* species (see Table 16-3). The repertoire is already large and consists of a veritable alphabet soup of pathogenic groups—EPEC, ETEC, EIEC (enteroinvasive), EHEC (enterohemorrhagic), and EAggEC (enteroaggregative)—and more may be waiting in the wings. Each group is associated with identifiable genetic traits and characteristic epidemiology and causes distinctive conditions. EIEC and EHEC are discussed in Chapter 17. EAggEC autoagglutinate (aggregate) in tissue culture and are associated with diarrhea in children less than 6 months old, often persisting for weeks with marked nutritional consequences. EAggEC may also be the agent of persistent diarrhea in some adults with HIV infection.

Other strains of *E. coli* involved in invasive disease in infants and young children and which cause bacteremia and systemic diseases such as meningitis or urinary tract infections in children and adults are discussed in Chapters 62 and 64, respectively. In every case, specific virulence factors are critical in determining the nature of the resulting disease. Many of these factors are known, others are being investigated, and still others remain to be discovered.

DIAGNOSIS

Mr. D. was diagnosed with cholera because his physician knew about the ongoing epidemic in the country Mr. D. visited and alerted the laboratory to use special media not routinely employed. On the usual media for bacterial diarrhea, *V. cholerae* is similar to commensals in its sugar fermentation patterns and is not picked for further diagnostic studies. On special media, however, the distinctive *V. cholerae* colonies are easily identified. Further analysis of the isolate from Mr. D. at the Centers for Disease Control and Prevention in Atlanta, Georgia, revealed it to be genetically identical to the Latin American epidemic and not to the Gulf Coast endemic strain. This information indicated that Mr. D.'s was an imported case and constituted no threat to the local population. The case was not attributed to contaminated seafood that could cause a local outbreak, nor was excretion of viable organisms a problem because of the effective water sanitation in Mr. D.'s hometown.

The stool from Baby D. was grown on cholera-selective media (because of the father's diagnosis) as well as on other media designed for both selection and differentiation of possible pathogens. By incubating the culture in air, the numerically dominant strict anaerobes in normal feces were eliminated. The media used permit the growth of enteric bacteria and not others by inclusion of inhibitors, such as dyes (e.g., eosin and methylene blue, as in the so-called EMB agar) or bile salts (as in MacConkey lactose agar), which selectively inhibit growth of Gram-positives. Because these media are not especially rich, they also exclude fastidious Gram-negatives (such as *Haemophilus influenzae*).

The diagnosis of Baby D. was not as simple as that of Mr. D. All the pathogenic groups of *E. coli* described look alike on agar plates and under the microscope, as do most other enteric Gram-negative rods. They must be further classified on the basis of their biochemical and nutritional properties, such as which sugars they ferment and other biochemical reactions. Because some of the classical intestinal pathogens, like *Salmonella* and *Shigella*, do not ferment lactose, inclusion of the sugar in the medium, together with a colored pH indicator, allows rapid selection of possible non–lactose-fermenting pathogens; the lactose-fermenting colonies turn a distinctive color because they produce acid. The lactose negatives are picked for further determinative work. Other pathogens cannot be selected by this method and must be sought by different techniques. Probes and polymerase chain reaction (PCR)

primers against the components of the adherence system are the gold standard for diagnosis. However, it is virtually never used in clinical practice because the tests are not available in most laboratories and because the diagnosis rarely affects management. In the case of the remaining member of the D. family, Mrs. D., it is likely that she had an ETEC infection, but no lab studies were carried out.

TREATMENT AND PREVENTION

The therapeutic needs of Mr. D. and his son were to replace electrolyte and fluid losses and correct metabolic imbalances. Luckily, secretory diarrheas are usually self-limiting and terminate without specific antibiotics, as long as the patient is well hydrated and prevented from going into shock. Mr. D. was so severely dehydrated that he required intravenous fluids. Baby D. did well with only an **oral electrolyte–glucose solution** designed to enhance a physiological sodium and glucose cotransport system in the small bowel epithelial cell. Mrs. D. had such a mild and self-limited disease that no specific therapy was needed.

Oral rehydration is a simple form of therapy that, if universally applied, could save the lives of millions of children every year throughout the developing world. Effective solutions can be made in the community by mixing salt, table sugar, and water. Unfortunately, it is not easy to ensure that such a simple solution is available in every country and household. Experience has shown that practical problems occur in ensuring that the solution is made correctly and that adequate amounts are given at the right times. The key is education of mothers, caretakers, and medical practitioners. Much effort is now being devoted to determining how to teach the methodology. Given access to isotonic replacement fluids, no one should succumb to cholera. Mortality rates in cholera epidemics exceeding 1% point to a lack of public health resources and/or inappropriate case management by inexperienced clinical personnel.

For most enteric diseases, the best preventive measures are those that interrupt the fecal-oral route of transmission. These may take the form of basic public sanitation efforts, water purification, or attention to proper food preparation (see Chapter 76). Nevertheless, infectious diarrhea continues to occur in societies where these efforts are maximized. Thus, other methods of personal protection, such as immunization, have also been considered.

Considerable efforts have been devoted to **vaccine** development for cholera as a prototype enteric infection. The challenge has been twofold: identify and prepare protective antigens, and find a way to present the antigen in a way that leads to a local immune response in the intestine. So far, partial success has been achieved using live oral vaccines with attenuated genetically engineered strains or killed cholera vibrios given by mouth. The attenuated live vaccines have the most promise because they most closely mimic natural infection, which is known to confer long-lasting immunity. With the exception of a first-generation live oral cholera vaccine, it is important to note that no vaccines for secretory diarrhea pathogens have become available for routine use in endemic areas; current vaccines are approved and used for travelers. However, improved live vaccine strains for cholera are on the horizon and will likely be available in the next few years for use in endemic areas.

Conclusion

Diarrhea is not simply a trivial bother that besets all of us occasionally. It is a major cause of infant death in the developing world. Symptomatic treatment by fluid replacement requires widespread educational efforts.

In every instance, local defenses of the gastrointestinal tract must be overcome for disease to occur. The efficacy of these defense mechanisms is best demonstrated by the relative rarity of intestinal infections in developed countries, even though the gut is a tube open to the exterior. Disease is seen when the load of pathogens in the environment and their opportunity for transmittal are high and when predisposing causes like malnutrition, which impair host defenses, are also present.

chapter 17

Invasive and Tissue-Damaging Enteric Bacterial Pathogens: Bloody Diarrhea and Dysentery

Victor J. DiRita

key **concepts**

Primary invasive enteric pathogens:

- *Shigella,* which causes dysentery and bloody diarrhea. *Shigella* is closely related to enteroinvasive *Escherichia coli* (EIEC).

- Enterohemorrhagic *E. coli* (EHEC), which causes hemorrhagic colitis. The most common serotype is O157:H7.

- *Salmonella,* which can cause nontyphoidal gastroenteritis and typhoid fever, a systemic infection of mononuclear phagocytes sometimes characterized by relapses and a carrier state caused by bacterial survival in the gallbladder.

This chapter describes a group of intestinal pathogens that cause structural damage to the distal portions of the intestine, most commonly the large bowel. These organisms invade and damage the mucosa, leading to **bloody diarrhea,** or **dysentery.** Dysentery is characterized by the frequent passage of stools (often more than 30 per day) that typically contain small volumes of blood, mucus, and pus. Other symptoms include cramps and pain caused by straining to pass stool (Table 17-1).

These serious, sometimes life-threatening infections frequently require antibiotics. The use of antibiotics causes problems in some developing countries where antibiotic resistance is common and effective new drugs are either unavailable or too expensive. Rehydration therapies so useful in secretory diarrhea have little impact on dysentery.

The chapter focuses on *Shigella,* the prototypic invasive enteric pathogen and the closely related **enteroinvasive *Escherichia coli* (EIEC).** These organisms are contrasted with other tissue-damaging pathogens, including *Salmonella* and **enterohemorrhagic *E. coli* (EHEC).** Also discussed in the chapter is the agent of typhoid fever, *Salmonella typhi,* because it too enters the host by crossing the intestinal mucosa. However, typhoid fever, a systemic infection of mononuclear phagocytes, is a unique syndrome.

table **17-1**	Definitions of Clinical Types of Intestinal Infection		
INFECTION	**STOOLS**	**SITE**	**EXAMPLES**
Secretory or watery diarrhea	Copious, watery, no blood, no pus Tissue invasion: absent	Small intestine	*Vibrio cholerae,* ETEC strains
Dysentery	Scant volume, blood, mucus, pus Tissue invasion: present	Large intestine	Shigellae, *Entamoeba histolytica* (leukocytes absent in stool)
Hemorrhagic colitis	Copious, liquid-like, bloody, no leukocytes Tissue invasion: absent	Large intestine	EHEC strains
Bloody, watery diarrhea	Copious, liquid-like, bloody or blood-tinged, pus (sometimes) Tissue invasion: present	Ileum, colon	Salmonellae, *Campylobacter jejuni, Yersinia enterocolitica*

Enterohemorrhagic *Escherichia coli* (EHEC); enterotoxigenic *E. coli* (ETEC).

Shigellae

The classic causes of **dysentery** are bacteria of the genus *Shigella* but also include the **ameba** *Entamoeba histolytica* (see Chapter 52). Approximately 15,000 to 20,000 cases of **shigellosis** are reported to the U.S. Centers for Disease Control and Prevention (CDC) each year. Because fecal cultures are infrequently obtained, it is estimated that the real number of cases is at least ten times greater. Children less than 5 years old are 10 times more likely to contract this disease than the rest of the population. Severe and fatal cases are uncommon in industrialized countries.

The genus *Shigella* consists of **four species,** which are distinguished serologically by the **O antigen** of their lipopolysaccharide (LPS). The species are named *S. dysenteriae* (serogroup A), *S. flexneri* (group B), *S. boydii* (group C), and *S. sonnei* (group D). Each group is further divided into subgroups. *S. dysenteriae* type 1 (which is now encountered primarily in developing countries) causes the most serious illness (dysentery), and *S. sonnei,* the predominant isolate in industrialized countries, causes the mildest one (watery diarrhea). *Shigella* species cannot be readily distinguished from *E. coli* by DNA hybridization and are actually differentiated pathogenic clones of *E. coli.*

Case

Infant T., a 22-month-old girl living in a low-income section of a Texas city near the Mexican border, became febrile, lost her appetite, and developed watery diarrhea. By the next day her diarrhea had abated, but her parents noticed that her stools contained mucus and were blood tinged. The number of stools and the bloody appearance increased, and the baby began to vomit. The parents brought T. to a hospital emergency department. Her temperature was found to be 40°C. Shortly after arrival, she had a generalized seizure. Physical examination revealed an ill-appearing, somnolent infant with mild dehydration and hyperactive bowel sounds. Laboratory results showed leukocytosis and a mild decrease in serum sodium and glucose. T. was given fluids and an antibiotic. Several days later, *Shigella flexneri* grew from her stool culture. No further seizures occurred, and over the next few days, the dysentery subsided. The child had lost 2 lb in weight but caught up to her growth curve 2 months later.

This case raises several questions:

1. What is the likely source of the shigellae?
2. How did these organisms enter into T.'s intestinal tract?
3. What bacterial properties were involved in producing the bloody diarrhea?
4. How should this disease have been treated?

ENCOUNTER

Shigellae are highly host specific, causing natural infections in humans and only occasionally in other higher primates. Encounter is most commonly by direct person-to-person contact, although transmission through food or water contaminated with feces also occurs. In contrast to cholera, enterotoxigenic *Escherichia coli* (ETEC), and enteropathogenic *E. coli* (EPEC) strains (see Chapter 16), the inoculum needed for *Shigella* infection is very small—a few hundred to a few thousand organisms. The small size of the effective inoculum allows the organisms to be easily transmitted from one person to another.

ENTRY, SPREAD, AND MULTIPLICATION

How do shigellae survive in the low pH environment of the stomach? These organisms are relatively acid resistant

Changing Nature of Infections by Shigellae

The known history of shigellosis has followed an interesting course. Originally described in 1898, *Shigella dysenteriae* was the major isolate until it was replaced by *S. flexneri* after World War I, which was in turn supplanted by *S. sonnei* in industrialized countries following World War II. Beginning in 1969, however, epidemic *S. dysenteriae* reappeared in Latin America, Asia, and Africa. The reasons for these changes in prevalence over time are not known. *S. flexneri* increased again in the United States among young adult males, apparently related to homosexual practices, but not in the rest of the population.

during certain phases of their growth, significantly more so than many other enteropathogenic bacteria. The organisms sense the acid environment and adapt to it because they possess a global regulatory system of genes whose expression requires a **sigma factor** of **RNA polymerase (RpoS)** that is made only in the stationary phase of growth. When exposed to acid, the organisms survive but are less able to invade cells, at least in cell culture. Once they reach the small bowel (an alkaline or neutral environment) and begin to grow again, their acid resistance is repressed and the invasive phenotype is restored. **Acid resistance** is also enhanced by anaerobiosis, the condition the organisms later encounter in the colon. It is likely, therefore, that when shigellae are excreted in the stool, they express the acid resistance phenotype. This phenotype is useful because the bacteria are already prepared to survive passage through the stomach when a new host ingests them. Thus, acid resistance may well contribute to the shigellae's success as pathogens.

After passing the stomach, the organisms go through the small bowel and enter the colon. Bacterial multiplication occurs mainly in the intracellular environment of the intestinal epithelial cell. Invasion and survival of shigellae within gut cells is a complex process that involves multiple genes present on both a large virulence plasmid and the chromosome. This is an interesting story and makes a good model for understanding the invasive properties of other enteric bacteria. Several steps are involved:

1. The shigellae approach the mucosal surface by an as yet unknown mechanism (they have no flagella and are nonmotile). Intestinal epithelial cells are resistant to invasion by *Shigella* at their luminal surface, although they are susceptible at their basal surface.
2. How do the shigellae reach the lower portion of the intestinal cells? By stealth, first entering specialized **M cells,** which are antigen-sampling cells that overlie the lymphoid follicles (Fig. 17-1). Invasion of M cells, and subsequent invasion of epithelial cells, is effected by plasmid-encoded proteins (**invasion plasmid antigens,** or Ipa proteins) delivered by a type III secretion system, which is also plasmid encoded (see paradigm).
3. The bacteria are released into the **lamina propria,** where they are ingested by macrophages that may

FIGURE 17-1 ▪ **Invasion strategies of *Shigella* compared with *Salmonella* in the intestinal epithelium. A.** Shigellae cannot invade intact epithelial cells from the luminal surface. Instead, they initially enter the mucosa overlaying intestinal lymphoid follicles through specialized M cells (1). Having transited through the M cells (2), some bacteria enter underlying macrophages (3). There cytokines IL-1 and IL-8 are induced by the action of proteins secreted by the *Shigella* type III system (see paradigm). A cascade of additional cytokines generates an influx of polymorphonuclear leukocytes (3), which migrate through the mucosa and cause separation of tight junctions between columnar epithelial cells (4). This separation subsequently permits the organisms to penetrate the disturbed epithelium. Once in the lamina propria, shigellae can invade the basal surface of epithelial cells (3). Internalized bacteria escape from phagosomes and travel from an infected cell to adjacent ones, using a mechanism that depends on actin and other host cytoskeletal proteins (4). Cell death results in a focal ulcer and exudation of inflammatory cells into the lumen, along with red blood cells to produce the dysentery stool (5). **B.** In *Salmonella* infection, organisms approach the mucosal surface (1), where they induce MAP-kinase (MAP-K), PLA-2 activity, production of leukotriene LTD4, and mobilization of intracellular Ca^{++} (2). These events induce surface ruffles (3, and see Figure 17-3), leading to uptake of organisms within host cell membrane-bounded vesicles (4). These mediators result in electrolyte accumulation in the lumen (4) and an inflammatory exudate (5), to produce the diarrhea of *Salmonella* gastroenteritis. Bacteria are captured from the lumen by dendritic cells and transported to mesenteric lymph nodes. Some bacteria transit to the lymph nodes and are taken up by macrophages. Some escape to the bloodstream, resulting in transient bacteremia (5).

undergo apoptosis as a result. Macrophages release interleukin 1 (IL-1), causing a marked inflammatory response with recruitment of neutrophils (the process can be inhibited by IL-1 antagonists or by an antibody to CD18, a surface determinant that mediates migration of neutrophils in inflammation). This initial inflammatory response to small numbers of invading shigellae markedly increases the subsequent invasion—which itself leads to further release of proinflammatory cytokines—and is essential to causing clinical illness. The host leukocytic response is thus a key part of pathogenesis. At this stage the invading organisms are near the susceptible basal surface of the epithelial cells.

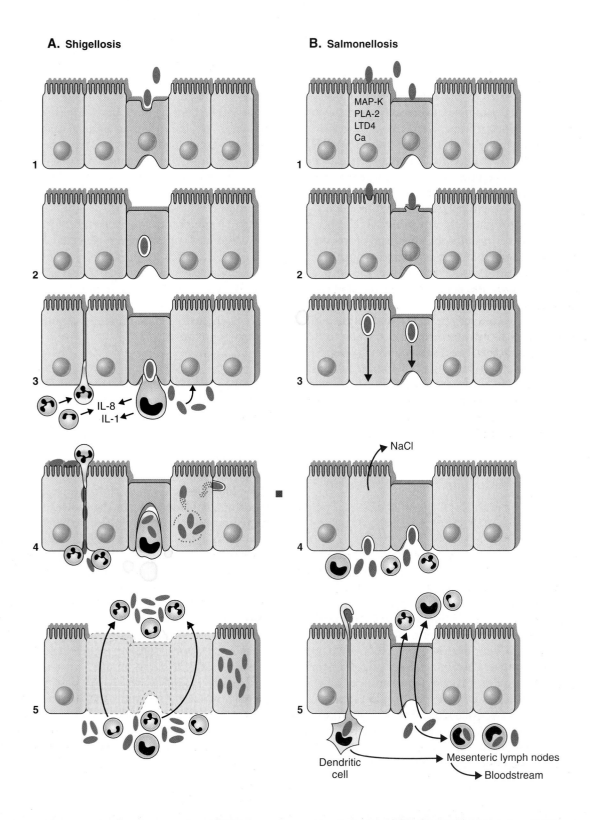

A. Shigellosis

B. Salmonellosis

4. Like so many other pathogens, shigellae can stimulate their uptake into epithelial cells. Unlike M cells, typical mucosal epithelial cells are not "professional phagocytes" and usually do not ingest large particles. *Shigella*-induced entry requires major reorganization of actin and cytoskeletal elements, just as occurs in typical phagocytosis. These changes are elicited by the *Shigella* type III secretion effectors.

5. Once inside the epithelial cells, the organisms escape the **phagosomal vesicle,** assisted by a microbial protein that lyses the phagosome membrane. They then enter the cytoplasm where they multiply.

6. Having successfully invaded an epithelial cell, how do the organisms infect other epithelial cells? Rather than starting over from the intestinal lumen, they invoke a particular example of **molecular parasitism** that involves appropriating elements of the host cell's cytoskeleton. As they multiply, the shigellae make a protein called **IcsA** (*Ics* stands for "intracellular spread") at one pole of the rod-shaped organisms. IcsA induces polymerization of host cell **actin** (see Fig. 8-2). The rapid polymerization and depolymerization of actin filaments at one end of the bacterium (the "rear") propels the organisms forward. The force exerted is strong enough to push the organism and the overlying cell membrane into a fingerlike projection that pokes into the adjacent cell (see Figs. 8-2 and 17-1). The bacterium is now surrounded by two cell membranes: one from the old (previously invaded) cell, and one from the new cell. When these membranes lyse, the organism is released in the cytoplasm of the new host cell and the process can begin again. In this manner, **cell-to-cell spread** occurs without the need to reenter the extracellular milieu. The mechanism used by *Shigella* for cell-to-cell spread is remarkably similar to a process put to similar use by the Gram-positive pathogen *Listeria monocytogenes*, a foodborne pathogen that causes abortions, septicemia, and meningitis (see Chapter 21 paradigm).

DAMAGE

When a sufficient number of contiguous invaded cells die and slough off, the result is surface erosion in the gut wall, or an **ulcer.** Neutrophils that accumulate in large numbers in the mucosa are shed in the stool, where they are easily detected by light microscopy.

The bloody and pus-containing stools and the pain associated with bowel movements (**tenesmus**) are characteristic of *Shigella* dysentery. Despite the ulcers and the inflammatory response, bacteremia is uncommon, except for *S. dysenteriae* type 1 infection. Bacteremia is most often encountered in poorly nourished infants in developing countries and is promoted by defects in host defenses associated with malnutrition, such as depressed complement activity.

One species, *S. dysenteriae* type 1, produces **shiga toxin,** a cytotoxin that kills intestinal epithelial and endothelial cells. Shiga toxin cleaves the mammalian 60S ribosomal subunit, thereby stopping protein synthesis. The action of shiga toxin has two effects: First, by targeting the sodium-absorptive villus cell and decreasing sodium absorption, it leads to an excess of fluid in the lumen. Second, effects of the toxin on mucosal endothelial cells contribute to the bloody diarrhea that follows.

Experimental infections in monkeys have shown that strains with inactivated Shiga toxin gene still cause disease but with much less damage to the mucosa and less bleeding. Thus, both invasion and toxin production are important in pathogenesis, which may explain why the highly toxigenic *S. dysenteriae* type 1 causes the most severe clinical illness of all *Shigella* species. *S. flexneri* also causes severe illness, dysentery, and bloody diarrhea, despite its lack of the genes for shiga toxin.

It is curious that *S. sonnei* uses the same mechanisms of invasion as *S. dysenteriae* type 1 and *S. flexneri* but only rarely causes the dysentery syndrome; most commonly, it leads to a self-limited watery diarrhea. The basis for these differences is not understood but is probably related to the fact that these organisms do not induce as intense an inflammatory response and do not make shiga toxin.

DIAGNOSIS

When patients develop bloody diarrhea or dysentery, *Shigella* must obviously be included in the list of possible causes. In some parts of the world, up to 50% of patients with bloody diarrhea or dysentery are culture positive for *Shigella*. In contrast, this diagnosis may escape consideration in the mild watery diarrhea caused by *S. sonnei,* which grossly resembles that of other pathogens such as ETEC, EPEC, or even rotavirus. The presence of leukocytes in diarrheal stool is a simple indicator of an invasive pathogen, and their detection provides immediately useful diagnostic information.

The specific diagnosis of shigellosis relies on culturing the organisms. Because shigellae die off rapidly when excreted in stool, isolation rates depend on rapid processing of the stool sample, by either streaking directly onto isolation agar or, in field studies, into a transport medium to maintain viability until the sample can be processed. As with other enteric bacteria, media have been designed to detect the lactose-negative phenotype characteristic of *Shigella*. A rapid presumptive diagnosis can be made by suspending suspicious

Paradigm Box

Bacterial–Host Communication Using Specialized Secretion Mechanisms

Microbes have evolved a variety of mechanisms for secretion of proteins into the environment. Often this ability allows microbes to survive within a host because the secreted molecules aid in microbial survival or dissemination. The challenge for microbes is how to transmit water-soluble proteins across their own membranes and the host's lipid membranes. Complex and incompletely understood mechanisms operate in these processes. In Gram-negative cells, toxins are typically delivered extracellularly in a two-step process. The toxin is first secreted into the periplasmic space—through the standard secretory pathway also used by many other (non–toxin-related) molecules—where it assembles into its final quaternary structure. In a second step the toxin is transferred across the outer membrane, apparently without unfolding. Translocation across the outer membrane may require a dedicated protein pore through which the toxin, but not other proteins, can pass. Once extracellular, the secreted toxins gain access to the host cell by first binding to host surface molecules. This process of extracellular secretion is sometimes termed **type II secretion** and is the subject of intense study. The cholera toxin is secreted from *Vibrio cholerae* by this mechanism.

Another mechanism for transmitting proteins from the microbe to the host cell that has received a great deal of attention in recent years is called **contact-dependent** or **type III secretion**. In contrast to the process described in the previous paragraph, there is no detectable periplasmic form of the protein secreted in this system. In some examples of type III secretion, there is no detectable extracellular form. Rather, the secreted protein is delivered directly from the microbe into the host cell by a process that has been likened to injection with a syringe.

Type III secretion systems have been studied in a wide range of pathogens, including some that cause disease in animals and plants. Examples are *Yersinia* (responsible for mild diseases such as food poisoning as well as the more notorious and life-threatening plague), *Shigella,* and EPEC. The type of molecule delivered into the host cell differs in each case. In the case of *Yersinia,* type III secretion is used to translocate toxin molecules that disrupt the monocyte signaling pathways, thereby eliminating a major arm of the immune system. For *Shigella* the system is used to transfer proteins that cause the host cell to take up the microbe. Host cell invasion by shigellae is the first step in its eventual intracellular survival and cell-to-cell spread. EPEC transfers its own receptor, called Tir, which assembles into the host membrane and binds another EPEC protein, intimin.

How type III systems function is the focus of much current research. Each type III system that has been studied consists of several proteins that are genetically conserved; that is, they share sequence similarity and therefore are likely to have similar functions. Many proteins of the type III secretion system from one organism can functionally replace those of another. Some of the conserved proteins appear to form a pore within the host cell membrane, through which other proteins can pass into the cytosol of the host. In addition, in the *Yersinia* type III system, an outer membrane protein has biochemical and sequence similarity to the proposed outer membrane pore of the type II system described earlier. This suggests that the protein of the two systems may share common functions. Type III systems are structurally and evolutionarily related to the apparatus that some Gram-negatives use for assembling their flagella proteins. In fact, some pathogens use the flagellar pore to secrete virulence proteins, instead of a dedicated type III system. Once the flagellum is finished being assembled, secretion of the other proteins then ceases.

In these days of rapidly diminishing antibiotic choices, the possibility that type III secretion systems may prove useful targets for antimicrobial drug design has captured the imaginations of investigators. Another possibility for exploiting type III secretion lies in the notion of using suitably engineered microbes to deliver therapeutic molecules into eukaryotic cells with the same efficiency that they currently deliver toxins and invasion proteins. Both of these fanciful possibilities will likely be much closer to reality after more basic research is done to fully define how type III secretion can so efficiently accomplish the challenging task of moving proteins across membranes.

colonies in saline and carrying out **agglutination reactions** with antisera to group antigens of *Shigella*. Testing for biochemical and fermentation patterns allows genus and species identification.

Now that many genes characteristic of *Shigella* and EIEC strains have been cloned and sequenced, it has become possible to identify the organism more rapidly by looking for specific genes using **DNA probes** or **amplification methods** such as polymerase chain reaction (PCR; see Chapter 58). These methods can be used on stool samples or environmental samples such as food or water for quick diagnosis or to trace transmission routes.

TREATMENT AND PREVENTION

Shigellosis does not usually cause severely dehydrating diarrhea; therefore, intravenous fluids are rarely needed to treat the infection. Oral fluids usually suffice to correct the mild-to-moderate degree of dehydration and electrolyte abnormality. In more severe cases that involve bloody diarrhea or dysentery and high fever, the use of effective antibiotics reduces the duration of illness and the period of infectivity to others. Reducing the infective period is particularly important because the small inoculum needed for infection with *Shigella* frequently results in transmission to other household members.

The use of antibiotics is complicated by the ease with which the organisms acquire **antibiotic resistance;** it is not pure chance that transferable antibiotic resistance was first discovered in *Shigella*. The problem is greatest in developing countries where multiresistant *S. dysenteriae* type 1 is most commonly found, and where cost and availability of the newest antimicrobials are limiting factors. The most reliably effective drugs at present are the **fluoroquinolones.** However, fluoroquinolone resistance is emerging. Some β-lactam and cephalosporin antibiotics are also effective. To make educated empiric decisions on which drug to use, clinicians should be aware of the drug susceptibility pattern of pathogens encountered in their communities and institutions.

No vaccine for shigellosis has been licensed, but many studies are under way using virulence molecules as candidate antigens. These antigens are being altered and packaged in various ways; the goal is to produce living attenuated vaccines that can be administered by mouth and will immunize the gut itself. There is also renewed interest in the possibility of using nonliving antigens for the same purpose. Various gene fusions and chemically conjugated vaccine antigens are being made and tested in experimental systems. Ultimately, however, these vaccines must be tested in humans because no animal model truly mimics human shigellosis.

Enterohemorrhagic *E. coli*

Case

Mr. R., an 85-year-old resident of a nursing home, was awakened by the onset of severe abdominal cramps, primarily in the right lower quadrant of the abdomen. Later that morning he had a watery diarrhea every 15 to 30 minutes, initially with small amounts of visible blood. Later that day bright red stools consisting of what seemed to be pure blood appeared. He was nauseated but did not vomit. When seen the next morning by the physician on call, he did not have a fever. However, clinical examination of the abdomen revealed tenderness over the colon.

Because of the clinical findings, Mr. R. was hospitalized. Frankly bloody stools continued. A barium enema revealed edema of the ascending and transverse colon with areas of spasm. Routine stool cultures were negative for *Salmonella* and *Shigella*. However, **sorbitol nonfermenting** *E. coli* were subsequently identified by the state public health laboratory as serotype O157:H7, an EHEC strain. The patient was treated with intravenous fluids and gradually recovered over the next 7 days. By the time he was discharged and returned to the nursing home, his stool was negative for that particular *E. coli* strain.

The day before he became ill, Mr. R. was visited by E., his 3-year-old granddaughter. The two shared a fast-food hamburger for lunch. Two days after Mr. R. fell ill, E. developed watery diarrhea. The diarrhea increased over the next 2 days and then became tinged with blood. When E. began to vomit and her urine output appeared to diminish, her parents took her to the pediatrician. E. was somewhat pale and lethargic, with a fluctuating level of consciousness. The laboratory reported a significant decrease in platelets and red blood cells, many of which looked abnormal. A diagnosis of diarrhea-associated hemolytic–uremic syndrome (HUS) was made, and the child was hospitalized. A stool culture was negative. E. was treated conservatively, and no antibiotics were given. No hypertension developed, the renal failure and hemolytic anemia did not progress, and dialysis was not performed. She was discharged 1 week later with no further diarrhea and improvement in the blood count.

This case raises several questions:

1. What is the likely source of the organisms that caused these diseases?
2. Why do only certain strains of *E. coli* cause the clinical manifestations seen in these cases?
3. By what mechanism does the etiological agent responsible cause these diseases?
4. What are the principal therapeutic concerns in such cases?

The EHEC strains include a number of *E. coli* serotypes that can cause a characteristic nonfebrile bloody diarrhea known as **hemorrhagic colitis.** The most commonly identified serotype in the United States is **O157:H7.** It is estimated that EHEC strains cause at least 20,000 to 40,000 infections annually in the United States. Approximately 250 to 500 deaths are caused by the **hemolytic–uremic syndrome (HUS),** a complication of hemorrhagic colitis consisting of a particular form of hemolytic anemia, thrombocytopenia, and renal failure. Death from HUS occurs most commonly in young children, and the disease is the most frequent cause of acute renal failure in children in the United States. EHEC produces one or two related but antigenically distinguishable toxins that share the same enzymatic specificity and binding site as shiga toxin of *S. dysenteriae* type 1. These constitute a family of protein toxins; the *E. coli* versions are known as shiga toxins 1 and 2 (also called shigalike or vero toxins). Less often in the United States, bloody watery diarrhea is caused by other pathogens, including *Shigella, Salmonella, Campylobacter jejuni,* or more uncommonly, *Yersinia enterocolitica.*

ENCOUNTER

We know the most about *E. coli* O157:H7 because the organism can be easily identified in the clinical laboratory. These strains have a convenient distinguishing laboratory characteristic: the inability to ferment sorbitol. However, their real prevalence compared with other EHEC serotypes has not been determined. O157:H7 clearly causes both outbreaks and sporadic disease, primarily as a **zoonosis** transmitted from animals to humans. Under-cooked hamburger is the principal vehicle, but other food vehicles have been described. Groundwater contaminated in the vicinity of cattle farms can transmit infection as well. The organism appears to be acid resistant, and the estimated infectious dose is tiny, approximately 50 organisms per gram of hamburger. As in *Shigella* infections, person-to-person transmission of *E. coli* O157:H7 in day care centers has been documented.

ENTRY, MULTIPLICATION, AND DAMAGE

Once past the stomach, EHEC colonize the terminal regions of the bowel where they remain confined to the surface of the gut mucosa and multiply locally. They do not invade the bloodstream. EHEC possess a homologue of the EPEC genes (see Chapter 16) that mediate the same dramatic rearrangements of actin and cytoskeletal elements leading to characteristic **attaching and effacing** lesion of the brush border (see Fig. 17-2A). Production of shigalike toxins by EHEC may be responsible for a local cytokine response in the colonic mucosa. It is currently believed that profuse bleeding is caused by the interaction of inflammatory cytokines and shigalike toxins, which damages blood vessels in the lamina propria.

The major complication of EHEC, which occurs in approximately 5% of severe clinical cases, is damage to small blood vessels. When this occurs, predominantly in renal glomeruli and usually in small children, HUS results. When the target is the brain, commonly in older adults, the syndrome is called **thrombotic**

FIGURE 17-2 ■ *Escherichia coli* with distinctive interactions with host cells. **A.** Electron micrograph of colon infected with the EHEC strain O157:H7. Notice the attaching bacteria and the altered epithelial cell membrane beneath them showing intimate attachment and "pedestal" formation. This attaching and effacing lesion is associated with EHEC and EPEC expressing the *eae* gene complex. (Original magnification, × 28,526.) **B.** Enteroinvasive *E. coli* within host cells.

thrombocytopenic purpura. It is quite clear from various studies that the toxin causes these clinical pictures. HUS resulting from EHEC is the most common cause of acute renal failure in children in the United States. It is estimated that as many as 5 to 10% of HUS-affected children will die promptly, and an unknown number may require dialysis or, eventually, kidney transplants. Shiga toxin is cytotoxic, suggesting that direct damage to glomerular endothelial cells may be the initiating factor of these diseases. Endothelial cell products (including von Willebrand factor, plasminogen activator inhibitor, prostacyclin, nitric oxide, and others) can mediate local pathophysiology leading to **platelet thrombi,** the characteristic feature of the disease.

Enterohemorrhagic *E. coli* species are lysogens, carrying on their chromosomes a temperate bacteriophage that encodes the shigalike toxin (see Chapter 4 for a discussion of bacteriophage biology and other examples of phage-encoded virulence factors). In the lysogenic state, the phage genes—including the toxin gene—are not expressed or are expressed to low levels. The phage is induced to undergo **lytic growth** when the DNA of the EHEC lysogen is damaged. During lytic growth, toxin is expressed at high levels from the phage, and its release is the result of phage-mediated lysis of the host bacteria that occurs after induction. Spontaneous lysis occurs at a very low frequency, thereby maintaining a low rate of toxin expression and release in infected people. However, phage-mediated toxin liberation can be dramatically increased when DNA-damaging antibiotics are used against the bacteria, because these can cause phage induction.

DIAGNOSIS

The classic syndrome of hemorrhagic colitis is sufficiently characteristic to be recognized clinically (as in the cases of Mr. R. and his granddaughter). Less severe bloody diarrhea is not so revealing, and diagnosis depends on detecting the organism in stool. Culture methods using MacConkey lactose agar identify just O157:H7 but miss the occasional sorbitol-positive O157:H7 and other EHEC strains, which, like most *E. coli,* ferment sorbitol. An enzyme immunoassay to detect shiga toxins 1 and 2 is commercially available to detect toxin or any toxin-producing organisms in stool and is both highly sensitive and specific. Methods using PCR to detect specific DNA are also useful for detection.

TREATMENT

Treating EHEC infections is controversial. Some clinicians have suggested that antibiotic therapy may increase the likelihood of the hemolytic–uremic syndrome, and

epidemiological data bear this out. This may not be strictly related to antibiotic-induced lytic growth of toxin-encoding phage in EHEC, because even antibiotics not known to significantly damage DNA appear to be associated with HUS. One explanation for this association may be that patients with more severe diarrheal disease are more likely to be treated with antibiotics and will thus fare worse than patients with less severe disease, with or without the drugs. Fluid therapy is relatively simple because EHEC strains do not typically cause large volume losses and severe dehydration. The major challenge is to treat complications of EHEC by supportive measures, including dialysis for renal failure if needed. Thrombotic thrombocytopenic purpura usually responds rapidly to exchange transfusion, for unknown reasons.

Nontyphoidal *Salmonella* and Typhoid Fever: Introduction to the Agents

Case

Ms. J., an Asian exchange student in the United States, returned home for a 3-month visit. Near the end of her visit, she cared for her aunt, who had high fevers and some diarrhea. Three weeks later, when she returned to the United States, Ms. J. had a shaking chill and fever to 38.5°C, with headache, muscle pain, and loss of appetite. The fever continued and progressively increased over the next several days. When seen at the student health service, she appeared ill and confused. Her abdomen was diffusely tender, and her liver and spleen were enlarged, although she did not have jaundice. In spite of the high fever, her pulse was relatively low at 90 beats per minute. Her white blood cell count was low, only 3,000/mm³, with a moderate monocytosis. An astute clinician made the presumptive diagnosis of typhoid fever, and therapy with ceftriaxone was initiated and continued for 14 days.

Admission blood cultures subsequently grew *Salmonella typhi,* thus confirming the diagnosis. The fever gradually abated over the next 3 days, and Ms. J. made an uneventful recovery. However, 6 weeks later all her symptoms recurred, including a maximum fever of 38.5°C. *S. typhi* was again isolated from blood culture and was found to still be sensitive to trimethoprim–sulfamethoxazole. She was treated again for 2 weeks with the same drug with a rapid response. She experienced no further recurrence.

This case raises several questions:

1. Do the same salmonellae cause diarrhea, dysentery, and typhoid fever?
2. Can the epidemiology of typhoid fever be distinguished from that of other salmonelloses?
3. Why were organs other than those of the digestive system involved in Ms. J.'s disease?
4. Why is it particularly important to treat cases of typhoid fever with antibiotics?

Four clinical syndromes, plus the carrier state, are associated with the genus *Salmonella:*

- Gastroenteritis: nausea, vomiting, and diarrhea, caused mainly by *S. enterica* subspecies *enterica*. This disease resembles some of those described in Chapter 16.
- **Focal infection of vascular endothelium:** caused by serovars Choleraesuis and Typhimurium.
- **Infections of particular organ systems:** osteomyelitis in patients with sickle cell disease, most commonly caused by *S. typhimurium*.
- **Typhoid fever:** caused mainly by serovars *S. typhi* and *S. paratyphi* A and B.

Some salmonellae are specific to animals and do not cause human disease; some, such as *S. typhi* and *S. paratyphi* subspecies A or B, are human specific and cause typhoid fever. A large number can cross host species. These are the most common causes of *Salmonella* diarrhea.

The genus *Salmonella* is vast, comprising more than 2,300 serological varieties (**serovars**), and the number is growing. The main antigens of *Salmonella* that distinguish its serovars are **somatic (O)**, **flagellar (H)**, and **capsular (K)**. Individual isolates express more than one O and H antigen at a time, and each strain is defined by a particular combination. The tremendous diversity of the genus stems from the ability of *Salmonella* to undergo **antigenic variation**, the ability to create mosaics of genes for their antigens through recombination, alterations in length, gene duplications, and point mutations. Only two species of *Salmonella* are now recognized: *S. enterica* and *S. bongori*. *S. enterica* consists of six subspecies, each of which contains multiple serovars (Table 17-2). Most human pathogens are grouped within a subdivision of *S. enterica* called subspecies *enterica* (subsp. I). However, it is still clinically useful to sort serovars into groups designated by the letters *A, B, C,* and so on. Serogrouping is usually the first information available from the clinical laboratory regarding a *Salmonella* isolate and provides a tentative clue to identification of the organisms likely to be involved.

table 17-2	Classification and Serogroup of Some Human Pathogenic Salmonellae	
SPECIES	**GROUP**	**SEROVAR**
Salmonella enterica	A	Paratyphi A
	B	Typhimurium
		Derby
		Heidelberg
	C1	Choleraesuis
		Infantis
		Virchow
	C2	Muenchen
		Newport
	D1	Dublin
		Enteritidis
		Typhi
S. bongori		

ENCOUNTER

Salmonellae are common members of the normal flora of many animals, including chickens, cattle, and reptiles (e.g., pet turtles). The strains that cause **gastroenteritis** are usually transmitted by chicken meat, eggs, and dairy products. Unless care is taken in poultry farms, chicken eggs often become contaminated, both on their surface and within. Outbreaks are most frequent in summer months and are often related to contaminated egg or chicken salads. **Typhoid fever,** on the other hand, is traceable to a human carrier (such as the infamous Typhoid Mary), although the routes of transmission often involve contaminated water or food. It is interesting that, because its host range is strictly limited to humans, *S. typhi* could potentially be eradicated, whereas organisms that colonize many other species cannot.

Like other enteric pathogens, salmonellae must travel from feces, whether human or animal, to the mouth. Significant changes and adaptations in the organisms are required for survival of this trip. The organism must use its genetic potential for attachment, replication, and survival. In addition, it must be able to disperse in the environment and infect new hosts.

ENTRY

Salmonellae are more acid sensitive than shigellae; therefore, susceptible individuals are often those who produce little or no stomach acid (a condition called **hypochlorhydria** or **achlorhydria**). A relatively large inoculum is required to infect human volunteers with normal gastric acid secretion (10 million to 100 million organisms), but the inoculum size is reduced 10 to 100 times when bicarbonate, which buffers the acidic pH of the stomach, is given along with the inoculum. Salmonellae also sense the acid environment of the stomach and at low pH express at least 40 proteins of possible importance in pathogenesis.

Organisms that successfully escape being killed in the stomach pass through the small bowel to the distal ileum and colon. There, like shigellae, they penetrate the mucosal barrier (see Fig. 17-1). Bacteria can enter M cells and the apical membrane of the gut epithelial cells. Contact of salmonellae with cells in culture induces a dramatic "ruffling" of the plasma membrane, a visual harbinger of cytoskeletal rearrangements that lead to uptake of the organisms within phagocytic vesicles (Fig. 17-3). Thus, the entry of salmonellae into cells is an example of **bacterial-mediated endocytosis (BME)**.

The process of BME in *Salmonella* is directed by a type III secretion system encoded on a large (more than 40 kilobase pairs) region of the genome called *Salmonella* **pathogenicity island 1 (SPI1)**. Pathogenicity islands are found in many microbes and, as the name implies, typically encode features required for virulence. They often have a G + C content distinct from the overall G + C content of the genome and, curiously, are frequently inserted into genes that encode transfer RNA molecules. Pathogenicity islands are thought to be evidence of horizontally acquired genetic information that converts an otherwise nonpathogenic strain into a pathogen through acquisition of virulence genes en bloc. Within 30 minutes of contact with host epithelial cells in vitro, ruffles form on the host cell, and the microbe is taken up (see Fig. 17-3). Some experiments demonstrated the presence of nonpili appendages on the surface of the bacteria before host cell ruffling, and these appendages were shown to require genes of the type III system called *inv* genes, although the relevance of those structures is unclear.

In contrast to the shigellae, which escape to the cytoplasm and multiply intracellularly, salmonellae remain within vesicles. Salmonellae are unusually resistant to the lysosomal contents of cells and to the antibacterial peptides made by intestinal epithelial cells called **cryptins**. The bacteria-containing vesicles eventually travel to the basal membrane, and the organisms are released into the lamina propria. Thus, gut epithelial cells are not the main habitat for multiplication of salmonellae but rather are barriers to be crossed. After the alterations in the brush border are reversed, the gut cells are apparently not harmed.

FIGURE 17-3 ■ **Ruffling of host cell membranes during intracellular *Salmonella* infection.** A mouse pathogenic *Salmonella* (var. *typhimurium*) was inoculated into ligated loops of mouse ileum and samples for electron microscopy taken after 30 minutes. At that time the bacteria were associated exclusively with M cells. **A.** A bacterium in contact with an M cell and the initial phase of a ruffle response on the M-cell surface. **B.** Pronounced ruffling. The arrows point to two bacteria seen in a vesicle inside the M cell. (Original magnification, × 12,000.)

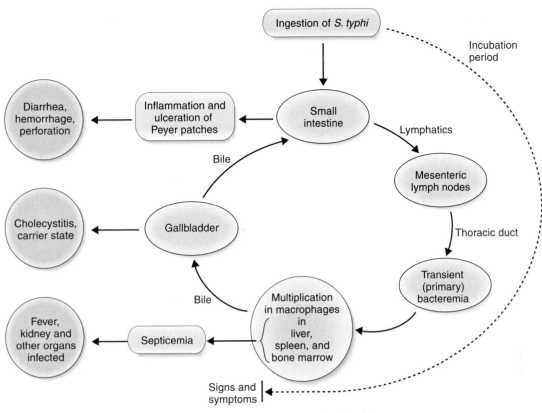

FIGURE 17-4 ▪ Pathogenesis of typhoid fever.

The mechanisms determining whether *Salmonella* causes gastroenteritis or typhoid fever are not clear. The former is associated with production of inflammatory mediators and influx of neutrophils into the intestinal lumen, and bacteria are generally contained within the follicle-associated epithelium. In contrast, typhoid fever is marked by dissemination of the bacteria from the intestine to the reticuloendothelial system (Fig. 17-4). After salmonellae reach the lamina propria, they often enter the bloodstream and may be recovered in blood cultures early in the course of the disease. They normally do not cause sustained **bacteremia** because they are rapidly taken up by the phagocytic cell system and are effectively killed. Exceptions to this rule include some serovars (Typhimurium, Enteritidis, and Dublin) that spread systemically more often than the others and frequently cause focal systemic infections. Clinical conditions that impair mononuclear cells enhance susceptibility to *Salmonella* bacteremia. For example, patients with sickle cell anemia have a tenfold higher incidence of invasive salmonellosis. A marked increase in incidence and severity of infection is also observed in patients with AIDS, leukemia, lymphoma, and chronic granulomatous disease.

The hallmark of typhoid-causing serovars is their ability to survive and grow within these phagocytes (see Fig. 17-4), in contrast to the salmonellae that cause gastritis. Macrophage survival is associated with a second type III secretion system encoded on a pathogenicity

island called **SPI2**. Systemic spread of bacteria in typhoid fever is clinically silent and brief. As the organisms multiply in macrophages of liver, spleen, and mesenteric lymph nodes, patients are also clinically asymptomatic. When the number of intracellular organisms reaches a threshold, they are released into the bloodstream, initiating the continuous bacteremia characteristic of typhoid fever. This event signals the start of clinical illness, manifested by daily high fevers that continue for 4 to 8 weeks in untreated cases. This **second bacteremia** leads to invasion of the **gallbladder** and **kidney** and reinvasion of the **gut mucosa**, especially at the Peyer patches. At that stage the organism can be isolated not only from blood but also from stool and urine (Fig. 17-5). Uptake of organisms by monocytes or macrophages in bone marrow makes this site a useful source of culture material when other sites are negative, because the organisms can actually be enriched at this site.

Salmonella entering M cells likely facilitates uptake by underlying macrophages, which leads to dissemination. However, *Salmonella* can also disseminate into deeper tissue beyond the intestine by virtue of **intestinal dendritic cells**. These phagocytic cells of the innate immune system (see Chapter 6) can directly sample luminal contents by extending dendrites through the epithelial layer in such a way as not to disrupt the tight junctions between the enterocytes. Once ingested this way, the

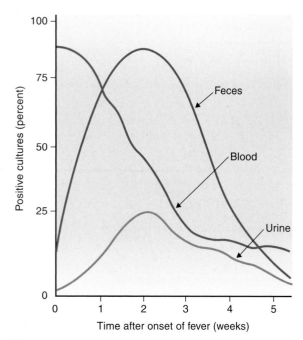

FIGURE 17-5 ▪ **The isolation of typhoid bacilli from various sources in the course of untreated typhoid fever.** The late rise in positive stool cultures is caused by secondary invasion of the gut by organisms from the gallbladder.

Salmonella can be disseminated by the bloodstream to deeper tissue. This pathway of dendritic cell-dependent dissemination does not require the SPI1 invasion genes required for epithelial cell invasion.

DAMAGE

The interaction of gastroenteritis-producing salmonellae with epithelial cells activates the inflammatory response and results in damage to the intestinal mucosa. Many biochemical events are activated by signals during invasion. Activation of the **mitogen-activated protein kinase (MAP kinase)** may be the first signal. MAP kinase is linked to a receptor on the cell surface. Binding of the organisms leads to activation of phospholipase A_2, release of arachidonic acid, production of prostaglandins and leukotrienes, and a sharp increase in intracellular calcium concentration. As yet, the mechanism by which fluid secretion is induced by *Salmonella* remains uncertain. Invasion induces production of inflammatory cytokines, such as IL-8, leading to local leukocyte infiltration, particularly migration of neutrophils. This ability to invade and cause inflammation is known to be necessary but not sufficient to cause diarrhea in experimental animals. Thus, additional traits need to be expressed. It is known that the disease is dependent on **transepithelial signals,** probably cytokines, elicited by the organism to recruit neutrophils.

The microbial contribution to macrophage survival has been extensively studied in *S. typhimurium* infection of mice. This organism typically causes a typhoidlike syndrome in mice and diarrhea in humans, whereas the human typhoid bacillus is not a mouse pathogen. Virulence of *S. typhimurium* is regulated by **two-component regulator or signal system** (see Chapter 19 paradigm), consisting of two genes, **PhoP** and **PhoQ**. These genes regulate a number of genes in *Salmonella,* most notably those whose products act to modify the bacterial lipopolysaccharide. The result of PhoP-PhoQ-regulated modification is microbial resistance to innate killing mechanisms of the host immune system, particularly killing by cationic peptides. This type of surface remodeling is seen in both Gram-negative and Gram-positive pathogens.

Invasive nontyphoidal salmonellae (such as serovar Dublin) possess a virulence plasmid that shares a conserved 8–kilobase pair region of DNA containing *spv* (for *Salmonella* plasmid virulence) genes. This region encodes genes that are turned on when salmonellae enter eukaryotic cells. Other plasmid genes encode resistance to complement by blocking assembly of the terminal attack complex on the cell surface, thus enabling the organisms to resist that host defense mechanism.

In addition to microbial factors, host genes also regulate survival of salmonellae within macrophages. The susceptibility of some inbred strains of mice to several intracellular pathogens, including *Salmonella,* the protozoan *Leishmania,* and the attenuated vaccine strain for tuberculosis, BCG, led to discovery of the gene *NRAMP1.* Susceptibility to all three microbes is a result of a mutation at amino acid 169 of this gene. *NRAMP1* localizes to the membranes of phagosomes and may regulate availability of the iron or other cations to phagosomes. A human homologue of this gene has been identified and was found to be part of a family of at least three genes that control a natural macrophage-specific membrane transport protein.

Invasion of the gallbladder by typhoid bacilli may be temporary or may result in the long-term colonization that characterizes the **typhoid carrier state,** especially in the presence of gallstones. Occasionally, acute necrotizing cholecystitis may result. Typhoid bacilli survive well in gallstones and can be recovered from the center of a stone; viable organisms may still be obtained after dipping stones in antibiotics. Gallstones are a source of prolonged asymptomatic carriage and excretion of the organism in stool.

The source of secondary gut invasion may be bacteria from the bloodstream during the prolonged secondary bacteremia or bacteria shed in the bile that penetrate M cells. Such secondary reinvasion leads to severe bleeding and/or perforation attributable to the marked inflammatory response induced in the **Peyer** patches. We do not know why the invasion of the gut at this stage results in more extensive damage to the intestinal mucosa than the primary invasion, but severity could be immunologically mediated. Invasion of the liver, spleen, or kidney can result in hepatitis, splenitis that makes the spleen prone to rupture, or glomerulonephritis. The clinical prognosis is much worse when those events occur.

Endocarditis and **vascular infection** are caused by specific *Salmonella* serovars capable of adhering to endovascular surfaces. *S. choleraesuis* and *S. typhimurium* adhere well to endothelial cells and may cause aortitis or endocarditis. These conditions are difficult to treat and often require surgical intervention. *S. typhimurium* also causes osteomyelitis in individuals with hemoglobinopathies (e.g., sickle cell anemia), trauma, and underlying bony abnormalities. Despite its predilection to cause continuous bacteremia, *S. typhi* only rarely adheres to vascular epithelia and is an uncommon cause of endocarditis.

DIAGNOSIS

Salmonellosis is generally diagnosed in the laboratory by culture on selective media and a combination of serological and biochemical tests to identify individual serovars. The salmonellae are nonlactose fermenters, and the same media used for shigellae allow them to be selected for further testing as well. Most clinical laboratories can identify *S. typhi,* determine the O serogroup for other isolates (A through E for human *Salmonella*) and deduce the most likely serovars, but they are not usually equipped for more detailed diagnoses. Further identification is most useful for epidemiological purposes and usually requires the assistance of a state public health laboratory or the CDC.

Typhoid fever is not recognized in the asymptomatic incubation period. The specific diagnosis is usually made by blood culture, which becomes positive early in the course of clinical illness (see Fig. 17-5). Isolation of *S. typhi* is helped by their resistance to bile salts (the organisms survive in bile itself within the gallbladder). *S. typhi* is one of just three organisms that produce a capsular antigen called **Vi,** an antiphagocytic virulence factor.

Typhoid fever can also be diagnosed by **serology.** A rising titer or a single very high anti-O antigen titer is suggestive. The Vi antigen also elicits an antibody response; however, because other organisms produce that antigen as well, the response is suggestive but not definitive for *S. typhi*. These tests rely on **agglutination** of the organisms by antibodies present in patient sera. In a positive test the bacteria make clumps visible to the naked eye. The highest dilution of serum that results in agglutination is the antibody titer.

TREATMENT AND PREVENTION

In the past, *Salmonella* **gastroenteritis** was not usually treated with antibiotics, because the drugs did not shorten the duration of the disease but rather prolonged carriage of the organisms in the stool. This is not the case with new fluoroquinolones, which both eradicate the organism and decrease the period of illness. A concern exists that excessive use of fluoroquinolones will eventually select for widespread resistance—reports of resistance have already been made—and that they may therefore no longer be effective in the future.

Systemic nontyphoidal *Salmonella* infections require antimicrobial therapy. A number of drugs may be used, depending on antibiotic resistance patterns. Prevention of salmonellosis relies on avoiding potentially contaminated water or foods that contain raw eggs or unpasteurized milk or milk products, or cooking these foods enough to kill the organisms. Preventive measures are especially important for people with diminished gastric acid or an immunodeficiency disease, such as HIV infection. However, it is neither easy nor foolproof. Considerable work is currently under way to develop attenuated vaccine strains for immunization.

The morbidity and mortality from typhoid fever have been significantly reduced by antibiotic therapy. Most cases in the United States are now imported. It must be remembered that therapy does not eradicate the organism. Oddly, the relapse rate is higher in treated individuals, possibly because early therapy aborts the immune responses necessary for preventing relapse. Without effective cell-mediated immunity, surviving bacteria can multiply to the point where they again cause clinical symptoms.

Progress has been made in developing a **typhoid vaccine.** Live, attenuated vaccines are under investigation, and one, Ty21a, is approved and used for travelers, with the standard exception of those who are immunocompromised. Several other live, attenuated strains are being investigated for possible use, including those with mutations in the *galE* gene required for LPS synthesis, or in genes for aromatic amino acid biosynthesis, or in the *phoP* and *phoQ* regulatory genes. Each class of mutant is immunogenic but sufficiently growth-impaired in vivo to render them unable to cause systemic infection. Thus, natural immunity can develop while the organism self-destructs. A cell-free Vi polysaccharide vaccine is available that induces protection in older children and adults, and a Vi–protein conjugate vaccine is being developed to immunize infants too young to respond to the polysaccharide alone, and this has shown early promise.

Typhoid carriers are a public health concern because they are often asymptomatic shedders; they not only carry the organism but constantly spread them through their feces. Treatment of typhoid carriers has been difficult but also represents a social imperative. Because no successful treatment was available in her day, Typhoid Mary was jailed. Today the recommended course of action is prolonged antibiotic therapy (a new fluoroquinolone may be the most effective form) with removal of the gallbladder if gallstones are present.

Conclusion

Bacterial pathogens may damage the intestinal mucosa and lead to bloody and/or inflammatory enteritis. Damage results from the invasion or intimate interaction with the surface of the intestinal mucosa, the elicitation of an inflammatory response alone or in concert with the production of cytotoxins that alter gut epithelial cells or endothelial cells, or production of bacterial protein toxins. Multiple genes encoded by chromosomal or plasmid DNA are required for virulence. The inflammatory response may not only be a response to injury but also, as in the example of *Shigella*, be required for pathogenesis.

Watery diarrhea appears the same, on the clinical level, whether it is caused by nontyphoidal *Salmonella*, ETEC strains, certain *Shigella* species, or rotavirus. Shigellae and occasionally certain salmonellae may produce frankly bloody diarrhea or dysentery. The non-invasive EHEC typically cause nonfebrile grossly bloody diarrhea known as hemorrhagic colitis, with the potentially fatal sequela of hemolytic-uremic syndrome. These organisms share virulence traits with EPEC and *Shigella*. The differences in clinical manifestations can be ascribed to the specific virulence factors these organisms express, but this extrapolation is less than perfect.

Typhoid bacilli are highly human-specific organisms that enter the host through the fecal–oral route and invade the intestinal mucosa. However, unlike nontyphoidal *Salmonella*, they produce typhoid fever, a fundamentally different infection in which the organism behaves as an intracellular pathogen of mononuclear phagocytes. Both microbial and host genes affect this interaction. The identification of these genes has yielded new information about the basic pathogenic mechanisms involved.

Pseudomonas aeruginosa:
A Ubiquitous Pathogen

Joanna B. Goldberg

key concepts

Pseudomonas aeruginosa:

- Is a ubiquitous, opportunistic pathogen found in soil and water.
- Has minimal nutritional requirements and survives in a variety of environments.
- Is a frequent cause of nosocomial (hospital-acquired) infection.
- Is an important pathogen in individuals with cancer, cystic fibrosis, and burns.

Pseudomonads are Gram-negative bacteria that inhabit the soil and water; contact with healthy humans is widespread but usually insignificant. As a group, pseudomonads have flexible nutritional requirements and are capable of using a wide variety of carbon and nitrogen sources to grow in diverse environments. Among this group, *Pseudomonas aeruginosa* is the most prevalent **opportunistic pathogen** that causes a variety of infections in immunocompromised patients, such as burn victims, cancer patients, and persons with cystic fibrosis.

Because of its adaptability and intrinsic and acquired resistance to many common antibiotics, *P. aeruginosa* finds the hospital environment accommodating. Equipment that requires a wet, body-temperature environment, such as dialysis tubing and respiratory therapy equipment, is particularly susceptible to contamination by this organism. In the hospital *P. aeruginosa* can be cultured from hand-washing sinks, hand creams, and even certain cleaning solutions. Although few healthy humans are colonized with *P. aeruginosa,* admission to the hospital increases the carriage rate.

P. aeruginosa generally causes disease in humans only when a local or systemic breach occurs in the immune system (Table 18-1). Local lesions are often seen in people with corneal abrasions, burns, and surgical wounds. Puncture wounds of the foot, such as those caused by stepping on a nail while wearing tennis shoes, can give rise to *P. aeruginosa* infections. *P. aeruginosa* infects chronic cutaneous ulcers in persons with impaired local circulation, such as diabetics. Once the organism has gained entry, dissemination through the bloodstream and sepsis are possible. Patients with severe defects in immunity, such as those induced by malignancies, diabetes, or chemotherapeutic or other immunosuppressive agents, are at greatest risk from

table 18-1　Relationship Between Various *P. aeruginosa* Infection and Predisposing Factors

TYPE OF INFECTION	PREDISPOSING FACTORS
Localized infections	
Respiratory tract	Cystic fibrosis
	Congestive heart failure
Urinary tract	Indwelling catheter
	Kidney stone
Gastrointestinal tract	Compromised immunity
Central nervous system	Trauma
	Surgery
Corneal	Eye injury
	Extended wear contact lenses
Mild otitis externa	No obvious predisposing factor
Necrotizing otitis externa	Diabetes
Dermatitis and folliculitis	Hot tubs
	Skin abrasions
Bone and joint	Trauma
Systemic infections	
Respiratory tract	Compromised immunity
	Ventilator-associated pneumonia
Surgical operations	
Tracheostomy	
Bacteremia and septicemia	Compromised immunity
Diabetes	
Surgical wounds	
Burns	
Endocarditis	Intravenous drug users
Bone and joint	Intravenous drug users
	Other infections
Central nervous system	Compromised immunity

systemic pseudomonal infections. Infections in these patients are most often caused by the bacteria with which they are colonized. Therefore, acquisition of *P. aeruginosa* and other Gram-negatives in the hospital is an important problem.

Case

Infection of an Immunocompromised Patient

H., a 4-year-old Caucasian boy on maintenance chemotherapy for acute lymphocytic leukemia (in remission), was brought by his parents to the emergency room because of fevers as high as 41°C over the preceding 24 hours. In the emergency room, he was alert but appeared ill and preferred to sit on his mother's lap. His skin was pale, his breath and pulse were rapid, and he was in mild respiratory distress with clear lung fields. Despite his fever, his extremities were cool and clammy. A central venous catheter had been surgically implanted because of the many intravenous medications he required. The site where the catheter entered the skin was intact and dry without any redness.

Blood analysis revealed that he had a white blood count of 2,000/mm^3, of which 30% were neutrophils (an absolute neutrophil count of 600, normal being >1,000). A third-generation cephalosporin (ceftazidime) and an aminoglycoside (tobramycin) were started intravenously. Within the next few hours, H.'s status deteriorated, with worsening respiratory distress requiring intubation and mechanical ventilation and circulatory failure requiring fluid therapy and drugs to increase his blood pressure. He was tentatively diagnosed with shock probably caused by sepsis (bacterial infection of the bloodstream).

The initial blood cultures were positive for *Pseudomonas aeruginosa*, but those obtained during fevers the second and third days of hospitalization were negative. H. gradually improved and he was slowly weaned from the drugs used to increase his blood pressure and from ventilatory support. His next course of cancer chemotherapy was delayed because his blood counts remained low, but eventually they did improve and his therapy was continued.

This case raises several questions:

1. What was the main predisposing factor for H.'s illness?
2. Where did *P. aeruginosa* come from? How did it gain entry into H.'s bloodstream?
3. What caused the symptoms of the infection?
4. What other sites could become infected in such a patient?

H.'s impaired host defenses, a consequence of his cancer and treatment, put him at increased risk for infection. Although not a factor in this case, an endotracheal tube or an indwelling catheter in the bladder or a vein increases risk by serving as a portal for infection.

Case

Infection of a Cystic Fibrosis Patient

The parents of Z., a 2-year-old girl with a chronic cough, became alarmed because her cough worsened over a week's time and her color "became poor." Her parents told the pediatrician that they could not remember when she was last cough free and that she would sometimes spit yellow–green mucus after forceful coughing, most often on arising in the morning.

On examination, Z. was an alert but pasty and pale-looking child with increased respiratory effort and rapid breathing. On inspiration, crackles were heard throughout the lung fields. Her extremities showed moderate clubbing with mild cyanosis. A chest radiograph showed increased

FIGURE 18-1 ▪ **Chest radiograph of a patient before and after antibiotic treatment. A.** X-ray shows interstitial and peribronchial markings. **B.** X-ray of the same patient after 2 weeks of intravenously administered ceftazidime and tobramycin.

(abnormal) interstitial and peribronchial markings (Fig. 18-1A). By gagging the child with a sterile swab, a specimen of the green mucus was obtained and sent for Gram stain and culture.

Based on the history, physical examination, and radiograph, a tentative diagnosis of cystic fibrosis was made. Intravenous ceftazidime and tobramycin were administered while awaiting the results of a sweat chloride test (diagnostic of cystic fibrosis) and sputum culture. The sputum Gram stain showed many Gram-negative bacilli. In culture the bacteria were initially described as non–lactose-fermenting Gram-negative rods and then identified as *P. aeruginosa*. Z. gradually improved, and after 2 weeks of therapy her radiograph showed improvement (Fig. 18-1B).

This case raises several questions:

1. How does the *P. aeruginosa* infection in Z.'s case differ from that of H.?
2. Is the strain of *Pseudomonas* that infects patients with cystic fibrosis the same that infects other people?
3. What was the route of entry of the organism in Z.'s case?
4. Would antibiotics help in Z.'s case?

This case illustrates an early episode in the course of *P. aeruginosa* infection in cystic fibrosis. Cystic fibrosis is an autosomal recessive disease affecting many organs, including the gastrointestinal and respiratory tracts and the pancreas. Patients can be identified by their difficulty in feeding and failure to gain weight. These patients also have high concentrations of sweat electrolytes. Many of the

clinical manifestations can be treated with pancreatic enzymes. However, the lung is the site of infection, and chronic respiratory infections, particularly with *P. aeruginosa*, are the major cause of morbidity and mortality in cystic fibrosis patients. Bronchopulmonary *P. aeruginosa* infection in this disease is characterized by exacerbations and remissions. Although the organism is probably never completely eradicated, antipseudomonal antibiotic therapy leads to a decrease in the number of organisms in the sputum and improved pulmonary function.

Interestingly, some antibiotics with little in vitro antipseudomonal activity often appear to improve the clinical status of patients with cystic fibrosis. It is possible that these antibiotics down-regulate the production of virulence factors by *P. aeruginosa* in the cystic fibrosis lung. In vitro, subinhibitory concentrations of antibiotics have been shown to have this effect.

In chronic infections in the cystic fibrosis lung, the appearance and characteristics of *P. aeruginosa* is different from that in other infections; mucoid strains are associated almost exclusively with this disease. Overproduction of polysaccharide alginate, responsible for the mucoid phenotype, does not by itself cause tissue destruction, but it can enable the organism to evade host defenses and persist in the lung.

P. aeruginosa infection in cystic fibrosis is unique because of its exceptionally chronic course. Individuals can become infected in childhood and, despite continued infection, live into the fourth or fifth decade of life with ongoing therapy. Although the infection is never cleared and lung function progressively declines, sepsis as a result of this organism virtually never occurs in cystic fibrosis.

Pseudomonas aeruginosa

CHARACTERISTICS

The members of the genus *Pseudomonas*, colloquially called the pseudomonads, belong to a large group of aerobic nonfermenting, actively motile Gram-negative rods. Pseudomonads produce indophenol oxidase, an enzyme that renders them positive in the "oxidase test" frequently used in diagnostic microbiology to discriminate them from other Gram-negative bacteria. They share this characteristic with the neisseriae; but few other clinically important bacteria are oxidase positive. Pseudomonads often produce water-soluble pigments, giving them distinctive colors on solid media. They are motile bacteria owing to the presence of one or several polar flagella. Rapidly growing, robust organisms, pseudomonads can persist in marginal environments. Consequently, they are difficult to eradicate from contaminated areas, such as hospital rooms, clinics, operating rooms, and medical equipment, including respiratory support devices. They may even survive in some antiseptic solutions used to disinfect instruments and endoscopes.

These organisms do not carry out fermentations; rather, they obtain energy from the oxidation of sugars. Many strains can grow anaerobically using nitrate as a terminal electron acceptor. Pseudomonads have minimal nutritional requirements, needing only acetate and ammonia as sources of carbon and nitrogen, respectively. In addition, these simple needs are met by a large number of organic compounds, so they grow well on relatively simple minimal media in addition to common complex laboratory media. However, pseudomonads generally cannot break down polymers into monomers and thus cannot use lactose or sucrose as their sole source of carbon.

Medically, the most important species of this genus is *P. aeruginosa*, but others also cause disease, albeit infrequently. Colonies of *P. aeruginosa* are distinguished from other bacteria of this genus by the production of the water-soluble pigments **pyocyanin** and **pyoverdin,** giving them a characteristic blue–green color on agar media (Fig. 18-2). On agar plates, colonies of the organism have a characteristic fruity or grapelike odor, which is sometimes noticed near wounds or other sites that are heavily colonized. *P. aeruginosa* can grow between 20°C and 43°C; growth at the higher temperature can distinguish it from other pseudomonads.

P. aeruginosa is resistant to many commonly used antibiotics, including first- and second-generation penicillins and cephalosporins, tetracyclines, chloramphenicol, and vancomycin. The aminoglycosides, fluoroquinolones, and some newer β-lactams are usually effective. Because the resistance pattern among *P. aeruginosa* varies from hospital to hospital and changes from year to year,

FIGURE 18-2 ▪ **Appearance of *Pseudomonas aeruginosa* growing on a colorless media.** Notice the straining of the media with pyoverdin, the green pigment produced by this organism.

the proper choice of antibiotics for empiric therapy of hospital-acquired infection must be based on continuous surveillance of drug sensitivity.

A large number of cell-associated and secreted molecules participate in the pathogenesis of *P. aeruginosa* infections (Table 18-2). As discussed in the case of Z., some strains associated with lung infections in cystic fibrosis patients make a polysaccharide capsule consisting of a compound called alginate that gives colonies a distinctive mucoid phenotype. To analyze the importance of potential virulence factors as well as to test new therapeutic strategies to combat *P. aeruginosa,* animal models of infection have been developed. Models that involve injury of epithelium or immune suppression before exposure to the organism have proven particularly informative. These models are attractive because they take into account the clinical observation that *P. aeruginosa* infections occur when the immune system—local or systemic—is breached.

Although appropriate animal models have been developed to study the pathogenesis of acute *P. aeruginosa* infections such as those occurring after corneal injury, burns, or administration of cytoxins as chemotherapeutic agents, developing an animal model of the chronic, persistent lung infection seen in cystic fibrosis is more difficult. When *P. aeruginosa* is instilled intratracheally in an animal, the organism is either cleared or the animal dies of acute pneumonia. To overcome this problem and establish experimental chronic infection, bacteria are embedded in agar beads before instillation. Histological changes resembling those seen in cystic fibrosis lung infection then occur. These models are useful for studying therapeutic interventions or, by the use of isogenic strains (only mutated in a single gene), the role of specific bacterial gene products, that function during infection. Epidemiological and animal studies demonstrate the importance of various virulence factors (see Table 18-2).

table 18-2	Notable Virulence Factors of *Pseudomonas aeruginosa*		
PRODUCT	**LOCATION**	**MECHANISM OF ACTION**	**POSSIBLE CONTRIBUTION TO VIRULENCE**
Pili	Polar	Adherence, twitching motility	Biofilm formation, colonization
Lipopolysaccharide	Outer membrane	Lipid A is endotoxic; core interacts CFTR	Sepsis, internalization, serum resistance
Flagellum	Polar	Motility, adherence	Dissemination and initiation of the innate immune response
Siderophores	Secreted	Scavenge iron	Acquisition of iron
Exotoxin A	Secreted	ADP-ribosylation of EF-2	Inhibits host cell protein synthesis
Exoenzymes S, U, T, Y	Secreted via type III secretion system	Interaction with components of the host cell cytoskeleton	Cytotoxicity, tissue damage, antiphagocytosis
Elastase	Secreted	Proteolysis of proteins such as elastin, collagen, immunoglobulins, complement components	Tissue damage
Proteases	Secreted	Proteolysis	Tissue damage
Phospholipases	Secreted	Hydrolysis of phospholipids, especially in eukaryotic membranes	Tissue damage, obtaining phosphate
Alginate	Cell associated	Adherence, protection from dehydration, and immune evasion	Antiphagocytic, biofilm formation

ENCOUNTER AND ENTRY

Because *P. aeruginosa* lives in the water and soil, it can be found on vegetables and living plants as well as in water taps, drains, and other wet surfaces. Humans can ingest the *P. aeruginosa* from such sources. Splashed water from a contaminated sink or droplets suctioned from a colonized endotracheal tube can spread the organism. This is generally not a cause for worry because, for the most part, *P. aeruginosa* relies on a breakdown of normal human defenses before it can cause infection. In fact, while it can be found in normal intestinal flora and on the skin, *P. aeruginosa* does not adhere well to normal intact epithelium. However, if present in large enough numbers, *P. aeruginosa* can enter the skin, possibly through insignificant abrasions. Infections involving the hair follicles (**folliculitis**) can occur as a result of bathing in contaminated hot tubs. The temperature in hot tubs favors *Pseudomonas* reproduction: a hot tub can contain up to 100 million organisms per milliliter. Such large inocula can overwhelm normal defenses and result in infections, even in immunocompetent people. In swimmers *P. aeruginosa* can cause **otitis externa** that may be benign or serious and is often recurrent. In the case of immune-suppressed or otherwise compromised people, *P. aeruginosa* can cause infections that initiate at the site of compromise. Particularly in hospitalized patients, these localized infections can lead to more severe disease. For example, gastrointestinal colonization or **catheter-related infections** can lead to bacteremia or aspiration into the respiratory tract and serious **pneumonia.**

ADHERENCE

To cause disease *P. aeruginosa* must get to and establish itself at the site of infection. *P. aeruginosa* has at least two distinct modes of motility. It has the typical **flagella-mediated motility**, whereby the bacteria swim, and a second system of **twitching motility**. This latter form of motility results from the extension and retraction of the organism's polar pili.

Aside from their functions in motility, both these factors have other roles with respect to virulence. Flagella and pili have been shown to mediate adherence to epithelial cells. It has been suggested this capability is a result of their interactions with the glycolipid **asialo GM1** on the host cell surface. In addition, flagella interact with one of the components of the innate immune system, the toll-like receptor TLR5, to initiate an inflammatory response. **Type IV pili** have been shown to be important for the formation of structures called **biofilms.** These complex structures house bacteria held together by polysaccharides and are thought to be responsible for adherence to surfaces, protection from dehydration, and increased antibiotic resistance. The so-called biofilm mode of growth is distinct from how bacteria grow in culture and in blood infections and may aid in attachment to cells and avoidance of immune cell recognition. The polysaccharide **alginate** can also act as an adhesin that offers protection. Alginate is one of the major components of the biofilm in isolates from the lungs of cystic fibrosis patients.

Lipopolysaccharide (LPS) can act as an adhesin. LPS is composed of three parts. The lipid A portion (also known as endotoxin) is the biologically active component of LPS that interacts with the host cell receptor TLR4 to initiate the inflammatory response. This interaction is responsible for inducing many inflammatory effectors that lead to the production of acute-phase proteins, fever, hypotension, and other effects generally known as Gram-negative sepsis. In the case of *P. aeruginosa*, lipid A is generally less inflammatory than that of other typical Gram-negative bacteria, such as *Escherichia coli* and *Salmonella typhimurium*. However, in susceptible patients like H., *P. aeruginosa* can cause hypotension and shock, likely because of lipid A. The core oligosaccharide portion of LPS interacts with the cystic fibrosis transmembrane conductance regulator (CFTR) on epithelial cells. This interaction leads to bacterial internalization and initiation of innate immune resistance to the pathogen. Expression of long O-antigen side chains is responsible for resistance to normal human serum, detergents, and some antibiotics (see Chapter 3); strains without O antigen can be killed by normal human serum. Interestingly, strains of *P. aeruginosa* isolated from chronic lung infections in cystic fibrosis patients often have an O-antigen defect and thus are serum sensitive and cannot be serotyped.

SPREAD AND MULTIPLICATION

P. aeruginosa are typical extracellular pathogens. Their growth in tissue depends largely on their ability to resist ingestion by neutrophils. The low frequency of *P. aeruginosa* infections in healthy persons shows that the phagocytes usually have the upper hand. Patients with reduced numbers of circulating neutrophils, like H. in the case presented earlier, are at high risk for *P. aeruginosa* infection.

What determines whether colonization, local infection, or systemic infection occurs after contact with *P. aeruginosa*? The use of isogenic strains of *P. aeruginosa* in animal models has allowed the role of a given gene product to be studied. Animals are infected with strains differing only in one gene, and thus any pathogenic differences can be attributed to the product of this gene. In a burned mouse model, strains deficient in any of a number of products (exotoxin A, elastase, or ExoS; see Table 18-2) persist in the wound but do not disseminate. Strains lacking flagella are also less virulent than wild-type strains. In an experimental model of ulcerative keratitis, ExoU and ExoT are virulence factors and pili and flagella act as adhesins. In this model, LPS–CFTR-mediated internalization leads to survival within buried epithelial cells and increased corneal injury.

P. aeruginosa employs several strategies to obtain scarce nutrients during infection. Obtaining iron is vital

and difficult; virtually all the iron in human serum is tightly bound to transferrin. *P. aeruginosa* produces iron-binding **siderophores** (see Chapter 3), which compete with transferrin for iron. Iron limitation increases the production of secreted products of *P. aeruginosa*, including siderophores, exotoxin A, proteases, and hemolysins. In turn, these proteins may damage tissues, making iron more accessible to the organism. When another necessary nutrient, phosphate, is limited, *P. aeruginosa* increases production of phospholipase C. This enzyme can hydrolyze phospholipids from host cell membranes to release phosphate in an available form.

As discussed in the next section, *P. aeruginosa* elaborates a wide variety of exotoxins that can cause local inflammation and tissue destruction. This damage can degrade tissues and enable *P. aeruginosa* to obtain the nutrients it needs to persist. Damage may also be necessary for dissemination; as mentioned previously, strains lacking exotoxins and elastase persist locally in burn wounds but fail to disseminate.

To survive in the host, *Pseudomonas* must not only obtain nutrition but also be able to evade host defenses. In the bloodstream the organisms do not usually survive and only cause sepsis in immunocompromised patients, as in the case of H. **Neutrophils are clearly involved in curbing the proliferation of the organism,** as seen by the increased incidence of *P. aeruginosa* sepsis in persons with severe neutropenia.

P. aeruginosa specifically colonizes the lungs of patients with cystic fibrosis, like Z., even though these individuals have an apparently functional immune system. Several independent, although not completely mutually exclusive, theories explain the hypersusceptibility of cystic fibrosis patients to chronic *P. aeruginosa* lung infections. In this disease, ion transport across the respiratory epithelium is abnormal because of a defect in CFTR. Persistence of the organism may be attributable, in part, to dehydration of respiratory secretions resulting in impairment of the mucociliary system, which normally rids the lungs of inhaled particles and bacteria. It has also been suggested that the cystic fibrosis lung environment inhibits the effectiveness of antimicrobial peptides; however, this theory is controversial. One finding suggests that *P. aeruginosa* binds to asialo GM1 and the expression of this glycolipid is increased on epithelial cells from cystic fibrosis patients. On the other hand, *P. aeruginosa* can activate and be internalized into CFTR-expressing cells; internalization, which may be responsible for clearance, is defective in cystic fibrosis. Moreover, although high levels of antibodies to *P. aeruginosa* antigens have been found in serum from cystic fibrosis patients, they appear to be ineffective at clearing the infection. This may be a result of specificity of the antibodies, particularly in their ability to opsonize *P. aeruginosa*.

P. aeruginosa also changes in character during the chronic lung infections in cystic fibrosis patients.

As mentioned earlier, the production of alginate is increased, resulting in a mucoid appearance. In addition, strains express an altered LPS with a modified lipid A structure. These cystic fibrosis isolates also express fewer proteases and toxins and become non-motile, all of which may serve to hide the organism from the immune system. The switch to a chronically infecting strain is under complex regulation. The release of the complete sequence of the *P. aeruginosa* genome has allowed investigations into the regulation of virulence factor production and the similarities and differences between clinical and environmental isolates of this ubiquitous opportunist.

DAMAGE

For a generally innocuous bacterium, *P. aeruginosa* strains produce a wide variety of damage-causing factors. It secretes a toxin, **exotoxin A,** whose activity is identical to that of the diphtheria toxin, ADP-ribosylating elongation factor 2 of the host, which is required for protein synthesis. *P. aeruginosa* also secretes a number of extracellular proteases of varying specificities. **Elastase,** as its name suggests, can degrade elastin in host cells. However, it is actually a zinc metalloprotease that degrades a myriad of other proteins as well. Another protease, **LasA,** is a serine protease that acts synergistically with elastase to degrade elastin. Other proteases, including alkaline protease and protease IV, have activities on components of host cells. **Phospholipases** hydrolyze phospholipids and cause membrane perturbation. While strains lacking or mutated in the genes encoding these enzymes are often defective in animal models of infection, they often have overlapping specificities, making it difficult to conclude the exact functions of any of these in a natural infectious process. Injury of host cells and tissues by these bacterial factors may also lead to increased attachment and colonization. In fact, *P. aeruginosa* appears to bind much more avidly to damaged epithelium.

P. aeruginosa also inserts a number of virulence factors directly into host cells. These proteins are delivered using a **type III secretion** system. With a structure similar to flagella, the type III secretion system targets specific proteins from the cytosol of the bacteria into the cytoplasm of the host cell, thereby avoiding diffusion during secretion and recognition by the immune system. Secretion is induced by host cell contact, or environmental signals such as low calcium that apparently mimic this situation. In the case of P. aeruginosa, secretion of the effectors ExoS, ExoT, ExoU, and ExoY is controlled by the transcriptional activator ExsA. ExoS and ExoT have similar activities: both can ADP-ribosylate target proteins. However, each also has unique functions: ExoS causes rounding of cells and ExoT interferes with

internalization of *P. aeruginosa* by epithelial cells and macrophages. ExoY has adenyl cyclase activity. ExoU is a phospholipase that readily causes lysis of host cells. The production of this latter cytotoxin is associated with more severe disease; strains isolated from lung infections in cystic fibrosis patients rarely produce ExoU.

In addition to the detection of and response to host cells, *P. aeruginosa* can sense and react to the presence of other bacteria in their environment. This "**quorum-sensing**" activity results from the production of **autoinducers,** of which *P. aeruginosa* can synthesize at least three: two that are derivatives of the molecule **homoserine lactone** and one that is similar to quinolones. These molecules readily diffuse out of the bacteria. With increasing cell density, the autoinducers can accumulate inside the bacteria and, once they reach a threshold level, can bind to a regulatory protein and together activate transcription of a number of genes. **Up to 10% of *P. aeruginosa* genes may be regulated by quorum sensing,** and many of these encode known or potential virulence factors. In fact, biofilm formation is regulated by one of the autoinducers. The use of quorum sensing to control expression of these factors has been proposed to allow *P. aeruginosa* to accumulate in the host before the expression of immunoactivating factors. *P. aeruginosa* quorum-sensing mutants are less virulent in many animal models of infection. In addition, *P. aeruginosa* can likely sense and respond to molecules released by other species of bacteria in their environment. Aside from its role in regulation, one of these *P. aeruginosa* autoinducers itself can induce a potent immune response.

The antimicrobial resistance of *P. aeruginosa* is a predisposing factor in treatment failure. This resistance of *P. aeruginosa* is the result of the limited permeability of the outer membrane as well as the presence of numerous multidrug resistance efflux pumps. As is typical for all bacteria, *P. aeruginosa* can also readily acquire antibiotic resistance genes from other bacteria by transformation, conjugation, and transduction. In addition, the biofilm mode of growth provides protection from antibiotics.

DIAGNOSIS, TREATMENT, AND PREVENTION

P. aeruginosa is easily cultured and identified by the clinical microbiology laboratory. Knowledge of prevailing patterns of susceptibility and resistance in a given hospital allows for empiric therapy while awaiting culture and sensitivity results. Because *P. aeruginosa* is relatively resistant to most antimicrobials, serious infections are usually treated with two antibiotics in combination to achieve an additive or synergistic effect. Clearly, the ability to develop and acquire antibiotic resistance contributes to the success of *P. aeruginosa* in the hospital environment, as does the resistance of the organism to many commonly used disinfecting agents.

The outcome of *P. aeruginosa* infection depends on the nature and severity of the infection, the state of host defenses, and the promptness and efficacy of treatment. A high-grade bacteremia in a neutropenic patient carries a 50 to 70% mortality rate. Attention to infection control measures may allow prevention of some *P. aeruginosa* nosocomial infections.

Conclusion

P. aeruginosa represents the paradigm of an opportunistic environmental pathogen. It is abundant in our environment and causes diseases mainly in patients who have impaired defenses. Occasionally, if the inoculum size is very large, it overcomes the defenses of healthy persons. Preventing and treating *P. aeruginosa* infection in patients debilitated by major underlying diseases, by developing either new antimicrobials or vaccines, is an important goal in modern medicine.

chapter 19

Bordetella pertussis and Whooping Cough

Victor J. DiRita

key concepts

Bordetella pertussis:

- Causes whooping cough, or pertussis, a disease that causes characteristic paroxysmal cough in infants.

- Can be prevented with DPT or DTaP vaccines containing *B. pertussis* antigens, along with diphtheria and tetanus antigens.

- Is extremely contagious.

- Involves several virulence factors, including adhesins and toxins.

The agent of whooping cough, *Bordetella pertussis*, is found on epithelial cells of the trachea, bronchi, and bronchioles of patients. These **Gram-negative coccobacilli** make powerful toxins that penetrate tissues, kill cells, immobilize the ciliary elevator, and cause the accumulation of thick mucus in the airway. The characteristic **whooping cough** is thought to be caused by sensitization of cough receptors in the trachea by a toxin and to the patient's effort to expectorate the accumulated mucus and cell debris. Killed whole *B. pertussis*, added to diphtheria and tetanus toxoids, yields the **DPT vaccine** given to infants for many years. Rare but unpleasant adverse effects of that vaccine compelled the development of a widely used **acellular** vaccine consisting of inactivated toxins and adhesins. Along with the diphtheria and tetanus toxoids, the triple vaccine is called DTaP.

Whooping cough, or **pertussis,** is a severe childhood disease that has been nearly eradicated by vaccination. In the early part of the twentieth century, hundreds of thousands of cases occurred each year, peaking in 1938 with 260,000. The vaccine originally developed for pertussis (the *P* in DPT) contained killed *Bordetella pertussis*, was very effective in preventing the disease, and caused a steady decline in disease incidence after its introduction in 1949. However, in recent years the number of infants who have not received the vaccine has increased. As a result, the number of cases of whooping cough in the United States has risen sharply. In 1981 the childhood incidence of whooping cough was 0.5 per 100,000 population. This number

223

Case

Eight weeks after her birth, L. was taken to her family doctor for a checkup and her first baby shot. The immunization was postponed for a month because she had a slight cold and a runny nose. The baby may have acquired her cold from one of her three siblings or a grandfather living with the family, who all had colds recently. Subsequently, L. began sneezing and coughing. Any loud noise would bring on a coughing spell. L.'s mother became concerned when the baby turned blue after a series of coughing spells that ended with vomiting. Later, during an examination of the infant by a physician, L. had a series of "barky" coughs, after which she vomited and could not catch her breath. L.'s mother was told that her baby had whooping cough and needed to be hospitalized.

The laboratory report showed an elevated white blood cell count, chiefly owing to a large increase in the number of lymphocytes. A nasopharyngeal specimen contained *Bordetella pertussis* by fluorescent antibody detection, the causative agent of whooping cough.

This case raises several questions:

1. How dangerous is whooping cough?
2. Why was the physician sure of the diagnosis?
3. Where did L. catch the "bug"?
4. Will antibiotics make L. better?
5. When can L. start getting her vaccinations?

■ ■ ■ ■

increased threefold to 1.5 per 100,000 children by 1985, and by 2002 the incidence was 3.01 per 100,000, with 8,296 reported cases.

Whooping cough is an important disease for four reasons:

1. Adults with mild disease, indistinguishable from a cold, are the reservoir.
2. It is highly communicable among susceptible infants less than 1 year old.
3. It is life threatening in infants with underlying cardiac or pulmonary disease.
4. It can lead to neurological sequelae.

The local manifestations of whooping cough are **tracheitis** and **bronchitis,** with accumulation of mucus, inflammatory cells, bacteria, and dead epithelial cells in the airway lumen. The **mucociliary elevator** is impaired by damage to the ciliary epithelial cells, and the cough is easily triggered because cough receptors are sensitized. The intense straining against the closed vocal cords (known as a **Valsalva maneuver**) in an effort to expel the mucus and debris in the lower airway can lead to hemorrhages in the brain, conjunctiva, and beneath the tongue. The result is the violent cough that gives the disease its name. In addition, infants with whooping cough have systemic manifestations, such as low-grade fever,

malaise, and lymphocytosis. Feeding can precipitate a coughing attack in an infant, precluding adequate oral intake and leading to dehydration.

Bordetella pertussis

PATHOBIOLOGY

Bordetella species are small, Gram-negative, strictly aerobic coccobacilli belonging to a group of nutritionally fastidious organisms that includes the genus *Haemophilus*. Bordetellae grow in complex media containing blood, which fulfills their nutritional requirements, plus other additives to neutralize fatty acids and other inhibitory compounds. The organisms are also very sensitive to chemical and physical agents in the environment and do not survive outside the body for appreciable amounts of time.

B. pertussis organisms have specific adhesins that permit them to attach to epithelial cells of the respiratory tract. They also manufacture exotoxins that penetrate into host cells and ultimately produce the signs and symptoms of the disease. Like other Gram-negatives, *B. pertussis* possesses **endotoxin,** which is probably responsible for some of the signs of the disease, including fever.

ENCOUNTER

B. pertussis is thought to be an exclusively human pathogen because it does not have a known environmental reservoir and is not known to infect other animal species. Its reservoir is suspected to be older adults with chronic bronchitis or bronchiectasis, or young adults with symptoms of a mild upper respiratory tract infection; however, *B. pertussis* is rarely recovered from the nasopharynx of healthy persons. The failure to recover the organisms may be the result of their ability to enter respiratory epithelial cells of carriers. The turnover of epithelial cells would then make the sequestered bacteria available for transmission. The organisms are exceptionally contagious and may infect more than 90% of the exposed members of a nonimmune family.

Not all people will recognize that they have been infected by *B. pertussis* because the classic symptoms of whooping cough are dependent on the state of immunity. Young infants have whooping, paroxysmal cough with vomiting and respiratory distress. In people older than 15 years, the disease may be indistinguishable from a mild "viral" upper respiratory tract disease without cough. This milder manifestation of *B. pertussis* disease may be attributed to host resistance resulting from previous immunization or infection. Thus, it becomes important for a physician treating a baby like L. to take a complete history of all family members and to alert them to the possibility that they may contract or already have whooping cough. In addition, the epidemiology of this disease is not always clear because vaccination records for childhood diseases are often poorly kept.

ENTRY

B. pertussis enters the trachea and bronchi by inhalation. The organisms attach to the cilia of epithelial cells of the large airways and are seldom found anywhere else (Fig. 19-1). Whooping cough is entirely a superficial infection, which means that the organisms do not invade tissue but remain on the mucosal surface: other important bacterial diseases with this characteristic include diphtheria and cholera. *B. pertussis* shows a strong **tissue tropism** for the ciliated epithelial cells of the respiratory tract.

The reason for this tropism is not clearly understood, but it may be the result of the specific interaction between pertussis adhesins and receptors on the cilia of these cells. *B. pertussis* has specific adhesins for ciliated respiratory epithelial cells as well as adhesins for phagocytic cells. **Filamentous hemagglutinin (Fha)** is a surface structure without a distinct organization that mediates binding to the galactose residues of ciliated cell glycolipids called **sulfatides.** Another ciliated cell glycolipid, lactosylceramide, is the target for binding of an adhesin, the bacterial cell–associated **pertussin** toxin. When secreted, pertussin also functions as a toxin by a mechanism similar to that of cholera toxin, by adenosine diphosphate (ADP) ribosylating Ga protein bound to the inner membrane of the

FIGURE 19-1 ■ *Bordetella pertussis* **adhering to dilated respiratory epithelial cells seen in the scanning electron microscope.** The arrow points to the clump of bacteria attached to the partially extruded epithelial cell.

host cell (see Chapter 9). In addition to Fha, other surface components, **pili** (or fimbriae) and a protein called **pertactin,** also facilitate binding of *B. pertussis* to mammalian cells. The possession of multiple, if not redundant, mechanisms for adherence emphasizes the importance of this step in the infectious process. Many of the *B. pertussis* virulence factors are coordinately regulated by a system called BvgAS (see the paradigm box).

SPREAD AND MULTIPLICATION

The first stages of whooping cough result in a mild inflammatory response in the submucosa, which is manifested clinically by infrequent coughing, a runny nose, and a low-grade fever. At this so-called **catarrhal stage,** the organisms multiply rapidly and spread to contiguous mucosa of the lower respiratory tract. Within a few days, masses of bacteria are entrapped in the cilia and thick mucus. The epithelium remains intact, but the submucosa beneath it becomes increasingly inflamed and the peribronchial lymph nodes enlarge. Reactive hyperplasia in the lymph nodes indicates that bacteria, their toxins, or other products have moved to those sites from their superficial origin in the bronchial lumen. Destruction of respiratory epithelial cells, which also evokes subepithelial inflammation, may also occur in prolonged infections.

Approximately 3 weeks after entry of the organisms, the cough becomes intense and uncontrollable (**paroxysmal stage**). At the end of a series of coughs (a **paroxysm**), deep inspiration and a "forced" expiration—which make up the "whoop"—occur. In infants with poor systemic oxygenation, either from chronic pulmonary disease (such as bronchopulmonary dysplasia) or congenital heart disease, the decreased cardiac output (resulting from the increased intrathoracic pressure) can cause severe systemic hypoxia and death. The cough persists with varying severity for another 2 months. It results from attempts by the body to clear the airways of the large amount of material that accumulates on the epithelium when the mucociliary elevator is impaired and sensitivity of the cough receptors increases.

DAMAGE

B. pertussis has an impressive array of virulence factors (Table 19-2). One of its most important, pertussis toxin, resembles many other bacterial toxins (e.g., cholera toxin, diphtheria toxin, and *Pseudomonas* exotoxin A) by affecting **cyclic adenosine monophosphate (cAMP) metabolism.** Also like other toxins, it is an A-B toxin, consisting of an A (active) subunit and a B (binding) domain composed of five nonidentical subunits (see Chapter 9). The toxin attaches to host cells via the B domain allowing the A fragment to enter and act in the cytoplasm. Toxins like pertussis toxin are **ADP–ribosyl**

Paradigm **Box**

Regulation of Virulence Properties

Microbial factors that affect normal host physiology and thereby result in disease are often under rigorous control by the microorganism. It is not advantageous to a microbe to produce a toxin or an invasion protein, for example, if a host environment lacks the proper receptor for such factors. Consequently, microbes have evolved sophisticated regulatory systems to control expression of virulence factors and thereby optimize their effectiveness.

One of the most widely observed schemes used by bacteria to control production of virulence factors is the two-component regulatory system. In this system, two gene products interact to control transcription of other genes whose expression is presumed to be required in a specific host environment (Fig. 19-2). The two factors that make up this system are a **sensor kinase** (called BvgS in *B. pertussis*, for "*Bordetella* virulence genes") and a **response regulator** (BvgA in *B. pertussis*) that activates transcription after being phosphorylated by the sensor kinase. A single bacterial species may have several such systems that allow the microbes to adapt to the various environments they

may encounter, ranging from systems that respond to the level of available nitrogen to those that control the response to changes in the osmolarity of the growth environment.

Sensor kinase and response regulator proteins contain conserved domains that are important for the basic function of each type of protein. It is therefore possible to identify genes encoding potential two-component systems by sequence analysis tools that can recognize the conserved domains. A single microbe may have several two-component systems, each controlling a specific trait. From the genome sequence of *Escherichia coli*, for instance, 62 genes are considered to be part of two-component regulatory systems. Because of the modular nature of these proteins and the conservation of functional domains, cross-regulation—in which a response regulator of one system is phosphorylated by the sensor kinase of another two-component system—has been observed.

Two-component systems that regulate a variety of phenotypes in pathogenic microbes have been identified (Table 19-1). With the genome sequences for many pathogens now available, the clear prevalence of these highly conserved systems in so many species has generated interest and some limited success in designing new classes of broad-spectrum antimicrobials that can block these systems.

The possibility that strains of pathogenic bacteria with mutations in specific two-component systems may be good candidates for vaccine use has also been tested. The rationale for this approach is that some two-component systems may regulate gene expression only during certain stages of microbe interaction with a human host. Mutants deficient for such systems might survive within the host long enough to elicit an immune response before becoming growth-limited because of the mutation. *Salmonella typhi*, the agent of typhoid fever, was mutated by deletion of the *phoP–phoQ* two-component system that regulates survival of this organism within macrophages. When tested in human volunteers, a single dose of the resulting strain, Ty800, induced greater intestinal and humoral immune responses than did four doses of the approved oral typhoid vaccine strain, Ty21a. This work establishes a precedent for studying the use of two-component mutants as vaccines against other important pathogens.

FIGURE 19-2 ▪ **The two-component regulatory system for signal transduction.** The sensor/transmitter is activated by a signal to become an active protein kinase capable of phosphorylating a response regulator. In the phosphorylated form, the regulator protein acts on DNA to either allow or prevent the expression of a specific set of genes.

table 19-1   Examples of Two-Component Regulatory Systems in Pathogenic Bacteria

ORGANISM AND MANIFESTATION	SENSOR/REGULATOR	SIGNALS	REGULATED VIRULENCE PROPERTIES
Bordetella pertussis Whooping cough	BvgS/BvgA	Mg^{+2} SO_4^{-2}, temperature	Pertussis toxin, adenylate cyclase Toxin/hemolysin, filamentous hemagglutinin
Pseudomonas aeruginosa Lung infections in cystic fibrosis patients	PilS/PilR ?/A1gR	? ?	Pilus colonization factor, Alginate biosynthesis; mucoidy
Salmonella Gastroenteritis, typhoid fever, bacteremia	PhoQ/PhoP	Mg^{+2}, cationic antimicrobial peptides	Macrophage survival, invasion of epithelial cells, resistance to innate immune mechanisms
Staphylococcus aureus Abscesses	AgrC/AgrA	Peptide Pheromone	Exoprotein production, including activation of hemolysins, proteases, and toxins; repression of coagulase and protein A
Enterococcus faecalis Urinary, biliary, cardiovascular infections	VanS/VanR	Vancomycin	Enzymes for vancomycin resistance
Streptococcus pyogenes Invasive skin infection; necrotizing fasciitis	CsrS/CsrR (CovR/CovS)	Mg^{+2}	Repression of hylaruronic acid capsule and other virulence factors; activation of some genes associated with pathogenicity

transferases, which means they split the nicotinamide portion from nicotinamide adenine dinucleotide (NAD) and attach the remaining ADP ribose to specific host cell proteins. One of the target proteins is a **G protein,** which is involved in the regulation of adenylate cyclase. ADP ribosylation of this enzyme results in an increase in cAMP, which inhibits several functions of neutrophils, such as chemotaxis and the oxidative burst.

Another cAMP-enhancing mechanism that *B. pertussis* uses is the secretion of an extracellular adenylate cyclase. This enzyme enters host cells and increases their content of cAMP. Why *B. pertussis* has two mechanisms to increase intracellular cAMP is not certain. It must be important to the bacterium, because *B. pertussis* adenyl-cyclase requires mammalian calmodulin to become active. Adenylcyclase is actually a **bifunctional molecule** because its amino terminus has the catalytic activity and its carboxyl terminus, in addition to acting to allow the catalytic domain into the cell, can form cation-selective channels in membranes and has weak hemolytic activity.

Local damage is probably caused by another toxin, a **tracheal cytotoxin,** which kills ciliated cells specifi-

table 19-2   Major Toxins and Virulence Factors of *B. pertussis*

NAME	CHEMICAL NATURE	SITE OF ACTION	BIOCHEMICAL ACTIVITIES	PHYSIOLOGICAL EFFECTS
Pertussis toxin	Protein	Local and systemic	ADP ribosylates protein	Impairs neutrophil chemotaxis, phagocytosis, and bactericidal activity; encephalopathy; lymphocytosis; hypoglycemia
Adenylate cyclase/hemolysin	Protein	Local	Converts ATP to cAMP Membrane insertion	Histamine sensitization mimics pertussis toxin activity on neutrophils; increases capillary permeability leading to edema Hemolytic activity
Tracheal cytotoxin	Murein	Local	Stimulates nitric oxide production	Cytopathological damage to tracheal epithelia Kills ciliated respiratory epithelial cells; adjuvant
Endotoxin	Lipopolysaccharide	Systemic	?	Fever; adjuvant
Pili (fimbriae)	Protein	Local	?	Facilitating adherence to respiratory epithelium
Filamentous hemagglutinin	Protein	Local	Heparin binding; agglutinates red blood cells	Binds bacteria to cilia

ADP, adenosine diphosphate; ATP, adenosine triphosphate; cAMP, cyclic adenosine monophosphate (cAMP).

FIGURE 19-3 ▪ Portion of cell wall murein that corresponds to the structure of tracheal cytotoxin. ala, alanine; GlcNac, N acetylglucosamine; DAP, di-aminopimelic acid; glu, glutamic acid; MurNac, N acetylmuramic acid.

cally and causes their extrusion from the epithelium. Curiously, this exotoxin is not a protein but consists of a **peptidoglycan fragment** called 1,6 anhydromuramic acid–N–acetylglucosamine tetrapeptide (Fig. 19-3). A similar compound is made by gonococci and acts in an analogous fashion by killing ciliated epithelial cells in the fallopian tubes (see Chapter 14). It is likely that tracheal cytotoxin is not the only one involved in local damage. *B. pertussis* also produces a **heat-labile toxin** that can inflict cytotoxicity on nucleated human cells. Thus, there are many mechanisms by which the organism can inflict local damage.

Given the nature of the local damage, is it likely that antibodies will have a significant effect on the cause of the disease? Preexisting antibodies produced by previous infections or by vaccination prevent the disease, especially if they are of the IgA type. However, once the disease is established, antibodies may play a lesser role. When the exotoxins have entered their target cells, they become inaccessible to antibodies.

DIAGNOSIS

Whooping cough is an uncommon disease in countries where the vaccine is widely used. Although the clinical signs and symptoms are usually quite distinctive, neither clinicians nor the laboratory are always alert to this particular diagnosis. It is also important to remember that laboratory diagnosis of *B. pertussis* is difficult because the number of organisms decreases as the severity of symptoms increases. Thus, *B. pertussis* can be cultured only from a small number of patients.

To culture *B. pertussis*, a small swab is placed in the posterior wall of the pharynx, which usually makes the patient cough. The swab is often treated with a drop of penicillin solution to kill other normally occurring bacteria that are sensitive to the drug (to which *B. pertussis* is intrinsically resistant). The swab is then applied to the surface of a plate containing a medium called **Bordet-Gengou**, which is incubated for 2 to 3 days. Positive identification of the organisms may then be carried out using specific antisera. An alternative to culture is a direct fluorescent antibody test to visualize bacteria in mucus specimens. Serology for *B. pertussis* antibodies can be done but is of little value for individual patients.

TREATMENT AND PREVENTION

Macrolides and tetracyclines are active against *B. pertussis* but are most beneficial if given early in the course of illness. In general, antibiotic treatment will reduce the shedding of bacteria, and it may shorten the course of disease and lessen symptoms, but the beneficial effects of treatment are not as dramatic as they are with pneumococcal pneumonia.

It is well established by now that vaccination should be widespread. Countries that suspended pertussis vaccination requirements in response to public concern about adverse effects, or because sufficient high-quality vaccine was unavailable or undeliverable, have seen dramatic increases in cases of whooping cough. All states in the United States require children to be immunized against pertussis prior to enrollment in schools or, in some areas, day care centers.

The traditional **vaccine** against pertussis consists of a killed suspension of *B. pertussis* cells mixed with purified diphtheria and tetanus toxoid proteins (DPT). As a consequence of real adverse effects, such as pain at the site of injection, fever, and malaise, and of erroneously attributed effects, such as severe neurological damage from the whole-cell pertussis component of DPT, acellular pertussis vaccines have been developed and have largely replaced the whole-cell vaccine.

The acellular vaccines are also included as a combination with vaccines against diphtheria and tetanus (DTaP), and typically contain detoxified pertussis toxin in combination with other proteins. The formulations differ depending on the manufacturer, but most approved acellular vaccines include filamentous hemagglutinin and pertactin. Like the older DPT vaccine, they are given at 2, 4, and 6 months of age, and some have been approved for up to two booster applications. It is not yet clear whether administration of acellular pertussis vaccines to adolescents and adults can reduce the burden of disease in younger children.

Conclusion

Much has been learned about basic mechanisms general to many bacterial pathogens by studying specific aspects of *B. pertussis* pathogenicity. As a superficial pathogen, *B. pertussis* does not penetrate into deep tissues. It produces a number of powerful toxins, most of which function to counteract the defense mechanisms of the lower respiratory tract. The disease it produces, whooping cough, can be virtually eliminated by vaccination. Effective acellular vaccines have been developed and are given in combination with vaccines for diphtheria and tetanus.

chapter 20

Clostridia: Diarrheal Disease, Tissue Infection, Botulism, and Tetanus

Stephen Melville

key concepts

Clostridia:

- Are Gram-positive, anaerobic, spore-forming rods responsible for several unrelated diseases including pseudomembranous colitis, gas gangrene, cellulitis, tetanus, and botulism.

- Often cause disease by producing toxins.

- Includes pathogens such as *Clostridium difficile*, a cause of antibiotic-associated diarrhea and pseudomembranous colitis; *C. perfringens*, the cause of gas gangrene; *C. botulinum*, the cause of botulism; and *C. tetani*, the cause of tetanus.

The many species of *Clostridium* are strictly anaerobic Gram-positive rods responsible for several unrelated diseases with various clinical manifestations. These include **pseudomembranous colitis** (an inflammatory disease of the colon); soft tissue infections, including muscle invasion (**gas gangrene**) and **cellulitis** (an infection of subcutaneous connective tissue); **tetanus; botulism;** and food poisoning. Many of the clostridial diseases are serious and life threatening. All are caused by exotoxins secreted by the clostridia. In the case of botulism, the disease is acquired by eating toxin-contaminated food; the clinical symptoms are produced by the toxin without colonization or invasion by the organism.

Production of protein toxins by at least 14 clostridial species is associated with a range of diseases, including botulism, tetanus, gas gangrene, food poisoning, diarrhea, and pseudomembranous colitis (PMC). The toxins responsible for botulism and tetanus are **neurotoxins,** whereas those causing gas gangrene and intestinal infections are **cytotoxins;** that is, they cause direct damage to cells. **Botulism** is caused by preformed botulinum toxin in contaminated food; thus, the *Clostridium botulinum* organism itself need not be present in the victim. In tetanus and PMC, the organisms are ensconced in the host, either in a wound (in the case of tetanus) or in the bowel lumen (in PMC). However, the organism itself does not invade the tissues; it merely produces toxins that cause the disease. The organism that causes gas gangrene, *Clostridium perfringens,* produces multiple virulence factors and is highly tissue invasive. Clostridia

Case

Mr. F., who is 81 years old, was hospitalized after 5 days of having fevers reaching 38.5°C. Because of confusion and inability to care for himself, he had been a resident of a local nursing home for 3 years. However, he had been able to dress himself and move about the home until a week before his hospital admission, when he complained of weakness and could not get out of bed. Except for a urinary tract infection 4 weeks previously, for which he was treated with a 10-day course of ampicillin, he had experienced no recent illness.

On physical examination, he was resting comfortably in bed but appeared confused and rather unhappy about his change of surroundings. His temperature was 39°C; other vital signs were normal. There were no localized physical findings, and an abdominal examination was unremarkable.

As the hospital staff and attending physician pondered the diagnostic possibilities at Mr. F.'s bedside the next morning, their deliberations were interrupted by one of the nurses, who informed the group that the patient had passed two loose bowel movements during the night. Indeed, the attending physician's olfaction, perhaps heightened by the new information, now recognized the occurrence of another such event, no doubt triggered by his deep palpation of Mr. F.'s abdomen.

A stool specimen was sent to the laboratory, which within 24 hours yielded a positive result for the toxin of *Clostridium difficile*. Specific treatment for antibiotic-associated diarrhea caused by *C. difficile* was begun with oral metronidazole. Mr. F. became afebrile within 36 hours, and he returned to his nursing home without further laboratory investigations within 72 hours.

This case raises several questions:

1. Where do the causative organisms come from?
2. Is the history of previous treatment with ampicillin pertinent to *C. difficile* infection?
3. What is the role of the spores of *C. difficile* in the disease process?
4. What caused the patient's symptoms?

table 20-1	Major Clostridial Diseases	
DISEASE	**TOXIN PRODUCTION**	**TISSUE INVASIVENESS**
Botulism		
Botulinum food poisoning	+	−
Infant botulism	+	−
Wound botulism	+	±
Tetanus	+	±
Pseudomembranous colitis	+	±
Gas gangrene	+	+
Suppurative wounds and abscesses	−	+

Clostridium difficile and Diarrheal Disease

An anaerobic, Gram-positive, spore-forming rod, *C. difficile* was first identified in 1935. As the name implies, it has fastidious growth requirements. Although isolated occasionally in blood cultures and in wounds, it went unrecognized as a cause of diarrheal disease until 1977, when it was identified as the organism responsible for a severe ulcerating disease of the large bowel known as **pseudomembranous colitis** (**PMC**; *pseudomembranous* refers to the yellowish plaques composed of fibrin with cellular debris that overlay the ulcerations in the colonic mucosa). Since then the organism has been linked to a spectrum of intestinal disorders associated with antibiotic treatment, ranging from an asymptomatic carrier state, to mild or moderate diarrhea, to fulminating, life-threatening PMC.

ENCOUNTER, ENTRY, SPREAD, AND MULTIPLICATION

can also produce **suppurative wounds** and **tissue abscesses,** in which the organism acts as a simple invader, without systemic signs of toxin production (Table 20-1).

In addition to the 30 clostridial species encountered in human infections, another 50 or more species are found in the environment, particularly in soil and in animal wastes. Clostridia are highly active metabolically, and many strains have important industrial uses. Clostridial fermentation of crude substrates produces useful chemicals like alcohols and acetone, and some species are used in the production of fermented foods and cheese. The clostridia used for these purposes, like most members of the genus, are not ordinarily pathogenic.

C. difficile is harbored in the large intestine of a small percentage of healthy humans, where it tends to remain in low numbers. It can also be found in environmental sources, particularly hospitals in its highly resistant spore form. The spores can be cultured from the floor, bedpan, and toilet in a hospital room occupied by a patient with *C. difficile,* as well as from the hands and clothing of medical and nursing personnel. The mode of transmission is via the spore form, which is extremely difficult to eradicate from the environment and is often carried on the hands of health care personnel who are caring for multiple patients. *C. difficile* is currently the major cause of diarrhea acquired in a hospital. In nursing homes, where patients tend to stay for prolonged periods, 20 to 30% of the residents are asymptomatic carriers of *C. difficile*.

A remarkable feature of *C. difficile* diarrhea is its association with antimicrobial drugs. Most symptomatic patients have received an antimicrobial agent in the recent past. Virtually all antimicrobial drugs have been implicated; however, the most common antimicrobial drugs associated with *C. difficile* diarrhea are cephalosporins, ampicillin, and clindamycin. (This order reflects the frequency of use of the drugs in clinical practice; actually, clindamycin is associated with a higher incidence of disease per administration.)

The risk associated with use of a particular antimicrobial drug is not necessarily related to its in vitro activity against *C. difficile* but rather to the relative resistance of the spore form of *C. difficile* to almost all antimicrobial drugs. The sequence of events in antibiotic-associated *C. difficile* diarrhea begins with suppression of normal flora by the antimicrobial drug, with persistence of the spore form of *C. difficile*. Clindamycin suppresses the most common type of bacteria in the flora, the anaerobic bacteria; this suppression may explain the strong association of its use with *C. difficile* diarrhea. *C. difficile* is either present already in the flora or is acquired from the hospital environment during antibiotic treatment.

At some time during or after antibiotic administration, the spores germinate and the vegetative form of *C. difficile* grows in large numbers, producing its toxins. When toxin production achieves a critical level in the large bowel, diarrhea begins. As the disease progresses, PMC may develop. Sigmoidoscopy of the patient's colon is the most reliable way to diagnose PMC, since the lesions are readily visible in the sigmoidoscope. Because 10 to 20% of patients will suffer a relapse of the disease, they should be closely monitored for symptoms.

DAMAGE

Like other toxin-related gastrointestinal infections (notably, diarrhea caused by *Vibrio cholerae* and toxigenic *Escherichia coli*), bacterial invasion of the bowel wall is not found in *C. difficile* diarrhea. Instead, the organism produces its toxins in the intestinal lumen, and the toxins cause damage to the epithelial lining of the bowel wall. The major toxins are designated A and B. **Toxin A** causes both fluid production and damage to the mucosa of the large bowel. **Toxin B** is a cytotoxin that causes rounding up of tissue-culture cells. Toxin B is thought to work in conjunction with toxin A to cause the symptoms associated with the clinical disease. Toxins A and B are enzymes, which act in the cytoplasm of the host cell to glycosylate small guanosine 5'-triphosphate (GTP)–binding proteins such as **Rho** and **Rac,** using UDP-glucose as the substrate. Glucosylated Rho and Rac are inactive and the cell loses its cytoskeletal structure and

can die as a result. The standard laboratory diagnosis of the disease detects toxin A in the feces of patients using an immunological test called an **enzyme-linked immunosorbent assay** (**ELISA**; see Chapter 58).

TREATMENT AND PREVENTION

Clostridium perfringens and Tissue Infections

Traumatic wounds are commonly contaminated with clostridial spores other than those of *C. botulinum* and *C. tetani*. These other clostridial spores are widespread in soil. In contrast to *C. tetani* and *C. botulinum,* which have little or no invasive properties, the other clostridia in wound infections cause local damage in addition to systemic effects. The major pathogen of wound infections, *C. perfringens,* produces a variety of toxins that act both locally and systemically. The more common form of clostridial wound infections is a localized cellulitis that can usually be cured with surgical management and antibiotics. More severe trauma can be associated with gas gangrene, a necrotizing, gas-forming infection of muscle associated with systemic signs of shock. Cessation of the original antibiotic treatment that led to the development of *C. difficile* diarrhea can limit the duration of the infection and associated symptoms. The antibiotics metronidazole and vancomycin can be used to successfully treat the overgrowth of *C. difficile* in the intestine (see Case Study).

Preventing *C. difficile* diarrhea and PMC can be achieved using a variety of strategies. Antibiotics most commonly associated with the disease (cephalosporins, ampicillin, and clindamycin) should not be used on susceptible populations of patients if other antibiotics are available. Transmission of the disease most often occurs when health care personnel carry the heat resistant spores from patient to patient. Proper education about disease transmission and frequent changes of gloves and outer clothing can reduce the spread of the spores. Extensive disinfection of the rooms of patients with the disease can lower the number of spores in the environment. In some cases, isolation of infected patients may be called for.

ENCOUNTER, ENTRY, SPREAD, AND MULTIPLICATION

C. perfringens and a variety of other clostridia are found in soil and in the intestinal tract of many animals. In wartime, 20 to 30% of wounds are contaminated by these organisms. The physiological condition of the

FIGURE 20-1 ▪ **Gram stain of *Clostridium perfringens* in exudate from gas gangrene.** Notice the absence of neutrophils.

wound site is critical in allowing the organism to germinate and to produce its toxins. The proper conditions are a low oxidation reduction potential (anaerobic conditions), compromised blood supply, calcium ions, and the availability of various peptides and amino acids. All these conditions are characteristic of damaged tissue.

DAMAGE

C. perfringens produces 12 toxins, but the α-toxin, a **lecithinase** that damages cell membranes, is the toxin most responsible for the symptoms of gas gangrene. A phospholipase type C, it interacts with eukaryotic cell membranes and **hydrolyzes phosphatidylcholine and sphingomyelin,** leading to cell death. Because the muscle tissue is destroyed (myonecrosis), it no longer reacts to stimuli. The muscle tissue appears reddish-blue to black. Large Gram-positive bacteria can be readily detected in the infected area (Fig. 20-1), and there is nearly a complete absence of leukocytes in the infected region. Abundant gas is produced by the organism, resulting in crepitus, which can be palpated as small gas bubbles under the skin. Systemically, the patient develops fever, sweating, low blood pressure, and decreased urinary output. The mortality rate for untreated gas gangrene approaches 100%; the patient generally succumbs to shock and renal failure within a few days of onset.

TREATMENT AND PREVENTION

Treatment of gas gangrene should be administered promptly because the organism can spread rapidly through healthy tissue. Treatment involves surgical removal of the involved muscle, which may necessitate extensive resection and even amputation of the affected limb. Antibiotics such as penicillin are administered to control the wound infection, but they are ineffective without adequate surgical debridement and drainage. Antitoxin, which is produced in

horses, has had a negligible effect in this disease and is not recommended for treatment. Oxygen administered under high pressure (hyperbaric) is used in centers with appropriate chambers but appears to work in only a subset of cases. Milder forms of clostridial wound infection, without evidence of myonecrosis or systemic effects, can be managed with more conservative surgical intervention and appropriate antibiotics.

Prevention of gas gangrene and other clostridial wound infections involves prompt and appropriate attention to traumatic injuries. Under war conditions, frontline hospitals and evacuation facilities have ameliorated the damage caused by gunshot and shrapnel. Trauma units, now available in most U.S. cities, have reduced the incidence of clostridial soft tissue infections by initiating prompt attention to injured wounds. Restoration of the arterial blood supply to the affected area is the most effective means of preventing gangrene from developing in traumatic wounds.

Clostridium perfringens and Food Poisoning

Food poisoning is unrelated to gas gangrene but is caused by sporulating *C. perfringens* cells that produce an **enterotoxin** in the intestines of people who have consumed contaminated food, usually a substance containing meat. The enterotoxin causes diarrhea about 12 to 24 hours after the contaminated food is eaten. The disease is self-limiting, and the symptoms disappear after 1 to 3 days. *C. perfringens* food poisoning is the third most common type of bacterial food poisoning in the United States.

Clostridium botulinum and Botulism

Although rarely seen in the United States, botulism is one of the most feared diseases because of the incredible potency of the botulinum toxin. The toxin has frequently been identified as a potential weapon of bioterrorism because of its potency and means of ingestion by contaminated food or water. Methods to detect the bacterium and the toxin in the food supply are becoming a high priority to prevent both the natural form of the disease and the use of the toxin as a biological weapon.

ENCOUNTER, ENTRY, SPREAD, AND MULTIPLICATION

C. botulinum spores found in soil or marine sediments contaminate meats, vegetables, and fish. Because the spores are relatively heat resistant, they survive food processing and canning when the temperatures are insufficiently high. Under anaerobic conditions, as found in canned foods, the spores germinate and release potent toxins. Proteolytic enzymes produced by some strains of the organism cause spoilage of the food; however, in many cases the food has a normal appearance and taste. Even an experimental nibble of such food can contain enough toxin to cause lethal disease.

DAMAGE

C. botulinum produces eight immunologically distinct neurotoxins (types A, B, Cα, Cβ, D, E, F, and G). Human cases are associated mostly with types A and B and occasionally with type E, which is formed in fish products. As the interest in home canning and prepared foods has increased, cases of foodborne botulism have risen concomitantly. Among the most potent poisons known, botulinum toxins are protein **neurotoxins.** One microgram is sufficient to kill a large family, and 0.4 kg could kill all the people on Earth.

Botulism is an intoxication caused by the ingestion of a preformed toxin. The toxin prevents the release of the neurotransmitter acetylcholine, thereby interfering with neurotransmission at **peripheral cholinergic synapses.** The toxin is a zinc metalloprotease that cleaves proteins involved in the docking of neurotransmitter-filled vesicles with the cytoplasmic membrane of neurons, thereby preventing transmission of the neurological signal to muscles to contract. This accounts for the symptoms of the clinical disease, **flaccid paralysis** of muscle, which occurs within 12 to 36 hours after ingestion of the toxin. Cranial nerves are affected first, particularly those involving the eyes, producing diplopia (double vision) and blurred vision. Difficulty swallowing is an early sign. The paralysis descends, and striated muscle groups weaken, especially those in the neck and extremities, with subsequent involvement of respiratory muscles. The toxin does not produce systemic signs of fever or sepsis. Patients generally succumb to paralysis and respiratory failure.

Infant botulism is a paralytic disease occurring in infants between 3 and 20 weeks of age. It produces a generalized hypotonic ("floppy") state. The infant's cry becomes feeble and the suck reflex weakens. In this disease, *C. botulinum* colonizes the large intestine, where it produces toxin. Infant botulism differs from the classic botulinum food poisoning in three ways: (1) the toxin is not found in food but rather is produced in the infant's intestinal tract; (2) the condition has a slow onset, probably because the toxin is absorbed more slowly from the large intestine; and (3) the disease has a favorable outcome in most cases, without specific treatment.

Wound botulism is a very rare form of the disease in which a traumatic wound is contaminated by spores of *C. botulinum,* which can multiply in the wound if the tissue is anaerobic. Toxins are produced at the wound site and absorbed into the tissues, causing a severe neurological disease similar to that of foodborne botulism.

TREATMENT AND PREVENTION

Specific **antitoxin** is available for types A, B, and E intoxication. The trivalent antitoxin should be administered as soon as possible to bind any circulating toxin. Because this antitoxin is acquired from horses, a high incidence of hypersensitivity reactions is associated with its use. The most important aspect of treatment is supportive care, including placement on a respirator, which is necessary to maintain breathing and other vital functions. Patients should be given parenteral nutrition. The illness may last for many weeks, and individual muscles may be paralyzed for months or even permanently. With good supportive care, the mortality from botulism is currently 25%.

Botulism can be prevented by proper canning methods. Although the spores are heat-resistant, the toxins are heat labile, and terminal heating of contaminated food can kill *C. botulinum* spores. As a result of improvements in the canning industry, outbreaks associated with commercial foods are quite rare, and most cases of botulism are now associated with home canning.

Clostridium tetani and Tetanus

Tetanus, which is caused by *C. tetani,* is a tragic disease, not only because of its severity but also because it can be completely prevented by appropriate immunization. Indeed, prevention of tetanus by active immunization has been one of the triumphs of modern bacteriology. Experience with tetanus in the two world wars of the past century demonstrated beyond doubt the benefits of the tetanus toxoid vaccine. Universal immunization of the American forces in World War II virtually eliminated the disease as a complication of traumatic injuries in soldiers. In developing countries where immunization is not widely practiced, tetanus remains a serious public health problem.

ENCOUNTER, ENTRY, SPREAD, AND MULTIPLICATION

C. tetani is ubiquitous in the gastrointestinal tract of humans and animals and in soil samples. Because of their resistance to environmental conditions, tetanus spores contaminate wounds of trauma victims.

Most cases of tetanus are associated with a **traumatic wound.** Tissue necrosis, anoxia, and other bacterial contaminants in the wound provide an optimal environment for germination of tetanus spores and production of toxin. Neonatal tetanus results from contamination of the umbilical cord at the time of delivery, either through unsanitary procedures or local customs of wrapping the cord in dung or mud.

DAMAGE

The major toxin, known as **tetanospasmin,** accounts for all the symptoms of tetanus. Tetanospasmin is a 150-kilodalton protein molecule composed of a heavy chain and a light chain held together by a disulfide bridge. Like other A-B two-chain toxins, the individual heavy and light chains are nontoxic (see Chapter 9). The complete toxin attaches to peripheral nerves in the region of the wound, where it is transmitted to **cranial nerve nuclei** either through intraspinal transmission among involved motor neurons or bloodstream delivery of toxin to other neuromuscular junctions. The major action of tetanus toxin is **inhibition of neurotransmitter release** and **normal inhibitory input,** thereby causing the lower motor neuron to increase resting tone and producing the characteristic **reflex spasms** (see Chapter 9). Several types of neurotransmitters are blocked, including γ-aminobutyric acid (GABA). Clinically, the disease presents as a **spastic paralysis.** Despite causing symptoms exactly opposite that of botulinum toxin, tetanus toxin works in the same manner as botulinum toxin by cleaving proteins involved in neurotransmitter-filled vesicular secretion. Like botulinum toxin, it is also a zinc metalloprotease but it acts on a different set of neurons (as described earlier), resulting in a spastic paralysis, unlike botulism, which is characterized by a flaccid paralysis.

Generalized tetanus, responsible for about 80% of cases, usually begins with trismus, or "lockjaw." Trismus is caused by tetanic spasm of the masseter muscles and prevents opening of the mouth. The disease typically descends, initially involving the neck and back muscles, progressing to produce boardlike rigidity of the abdominal musculature, eventually causing stiffness of the extremities. Individual muscle groups spasm, leading to a generalized spasm that is characterized by a tonic seizure, adduction of the arms, arching of the neck and back, extension of the legs and clenching of the fists (Fig. 20-2). Death usually results from respiratory failure caused by paralysis of chest muscles.

TREATMENT AND PREVENTION

The treatment of tetanus is mainly a physiological exercise in preventing complications. Antitoxin should be given at the earliest possible moment, but it is often a fu-

FIGURE 20-2 ▪ **Advanced tetanus may lead to opisthotonos, the bending backward of the body caused by spastic paralysis of the strong extensors of the back.** This classic painting of a British soldier wounded in 1809 in the Napoleonic Wars portrays this condition, as well as the "sardonic smile" and lockjaw caused by spasms of facial muscles.

tile gesture because any toxin that has been produced is already irreversibly fixed to the nerve cells. Antibiotic treatment, particularly penicillin G, is directed at the organism because it may continue to produce toxin in the wound. In addition, surgical debridement of the involved wound should be performed to eliminate the environmental niche of the organism.

Prevention of tetanus is achieved through immunization. Active immunization should be carried out in all infants and children and in pregnant women who have not been previously immunized. The vaccine consists of **tetanus toxoid,** a form of the toxin that has been inactivated in formalin but retains its antigenicity. Tetanus toxoid is the *T* of the DPT vaccine given to infants and children. Passive immunization in the form of human globulin is administered to people with a "tetanus-prone wound." Because the disease itself does not produce sufficient antibody reaction for subsequent protection, it is necessary to immunize tetanus patients with the toxoid as well. Antibodies are insufficiently produced during the disease state because the amount of toxin present in the patient is too small to be immunogenic. It is a testament to the enormous potency of tetanus toxin that such a small amount is still sufficient to produce severe symptoms.

Conclusion

The pathogenic clostridia have a broad spectrum of colonization and invasiveness features. In botulism, the organisms do not invade the body at all; in tetanus, they barely set up housekeeping in tissues; and in clostridial gangrene, they show considerable invasiveness. The production of a wide range of toxins is a key feature of clostridial infections.

chapter 21

Legionella: Parasite of Amebas and Macrophages

Michele Swanson and Cary Engleberg

key **concepts**

Legionella:

- Grow slowly on specialized medium
- Natural reservoir is fresh water or soil, where they multiply within parasitic ameba
- Cycle between replication and transmission in response to the nutrient supply
- *L. pneumophila* is genetically diverse

Clinical disease:

- Opportunistic pathogens acquired from contaminated water or soil
- A disease of technological progress, managed by monitoring water supplies
- Replicates within vacuoles of macrophages
- Tissue damage likely due to host inflammatory response
- To be effective, antibiotics must cross macrophage membranes

The legionellae are aerobic Gram-negative bacilli and are opportunistic pathogens of macrophages in humans. These bacteria reside within protozoa in natural aquatic habitats and occasionally inhabit man-made water distribution systems. Humans acquire infection by inhalation. In the absence of robust host defenses, patients may develop a severe form of pneumonia called legionnaires disease. Because this infection is often associated with contaminated water systems, large institutional outbreaks of legionnaires disease can occur (e.g., in hospitals and hotels).

Case

Mrs. R., a 59-year-old schoolteacher, was admitted to the hospital with high fever and altered mental status. Eight days earlier she had developed a "flulike" illness with fever, anorexia, malaise, headache, and muscle aches. These symptoms were followed by a cough that became progressively worse but was productive of only scanty, clear sputum. Five days before admission, she saw a local physician who ordered a chest radiograph. The radiograph showed a small left upper lobe infiltrate, consistent with pneumonia. She was treated with an oral cephalosporin. In spite of the antibiotic treatment, her fever and chills increased steadily, she developed watery diarrhea, and she became confused and lethargic. Mrs. R.'s past medical history was unremarkable, but she had smoked one pack of cigarettes a day for 40 years. Two weeks earlier, Mrs. R. had returned from a 2-week holiday at a resort in southern Florida. None of Mrs. R.'s family members, coworkers, or students had a similar illness.

On admission to the hospital, her temperature was 40°C, her heart rate was 88 beats/minute. The patient was severely hypoxic, and her white cell count was 13,700/mm³. A Gram stain of the sputum showed numerous neutrophils but no bacteria. A chest radiograph showed extension of her left upper lobe infiltrate and a new right middle lobe infiltrate.

High-dose erythromycin was added to Mrs. R.'s antibiotic regimen on suspicion of legionnaires disease. She was intubated and placed on mechanical ventilation in the intensive care unit (ICU). After a stormy ICU course, Mrs. R. began to improve slowly and eventually recovered. A culture of respiratory secretions obtained by aspiration through the endotracheal tube grew *Legionella pneumophila* after 4 days of incubation.

This case raises several questions:

1. How did Mrs. R. acquire *L. pneumophila*, and why wasn't anyone in her family or workplace also infected?
2. Why was the diagnosis of legionnaires disease initially overlooked in this case?
3. Why did Mrs. R.'s pneumonia worsen during treatment with an antibiotic that kills *L. pneumophila* growing in a laboratory culture?

Epidemiology of Legionellae

Legionella was first recognized as a bacterial genus when researchers from the Centers for Disease Control and Prevention investigated a highly publicized outbreak of pneumonia at an American Legion convention in Philadelphia in 1976. In all, 182 attendees became ill and 29 died. Once the bacterium (*Legionella pneumophila*) was isolated, culture and serological methods were developed to facilitate the clinical diagnosis of legionnaires disease. We now know that many species of *Legionella* are ubiquitous in aquatic environments, and a few are significant causes of pneumonia. Although outbreaks of legionellosis continue to attract the most attention from the general public, by far the more typical form of infection is sporadic, community-acquired pneumonia. Most severe is nosocomial legionellosis, which especially affects vulnerable hospitalized patients.

Characteristics of Legionellae

Legionella species do not grow on routine bacteriological media. Instead, the microbes are cultured on a special medium that contains a source of amino acids to supply carbon and energy, inorganic iron, high levels of cysteine, activated charcoal to absorb inhibitory substances in the agar, and low sodium, which avoids inhibiting virulent forms. Some species do not grow on this special media and can be cultured only in amebas; these are known as *Legionella*-like amebal pathogens (LLAP).

More than 40 species of *Legionella* have been identified. In nature, the legionellae are found in ponds, lakes, and hot springs, where they are thought to make complex, adherent microbial communities and biofilms. Like other bacteria in these environments, they are preyed upon by **protozoa.** However, legionellae actually profit from ingestion by protozoa. Instead of being killed and digested like other bacteria, they grow to large numbers inside these unicellular organisms. When nutrients inside the cell are depleted and limit continued growth, the intracellular bacteria differentiate to a motile, resilient, and infectious form suited for transmission to another protozoan host.

Legionella pneumophila

ENCOUNTER

Numerous outbreaks have established a link between the occurrence of legionnaires disease and the **colonization of plumbing systems** with *L. pneumophila.* In hospitals and hotels where epidemics have occurred, the *L. pneumophila* strain isolated from respiratory cultures of patients can usually be found in tap water or in sediments from hot water tanks. Nonpathogenic protozoans are also common inhabitants of potable water supplies, and they may serve to amplify the population of infectious microbes and perhaps to promote *L. pneumophila* infection of human lungs when inhaled with bacteria. In some respects, *Legionella* is particularly well-adapted to water supply systems of buildings. The bacterium grows at temperatures up to 46°C and tolerates much higher temperatures. It is **relatively chlorine resistant** compared with enteric bacteria. In addition, bacterial biofilm communities are notoriously resistant to biocides.

Legionnaires disease is nearly always a **primary pulmonary infection** and is never transmitted from person to person. Humans acquire the infection from an **environmental source**, usually a water distribution system colonized with the microorganism (Fig. 21-1). Showers, humidifiers, water fountains, respiratory therapy equipment, or evaporative cooling towers associated with institutional central air conditioning systems can produce **infectious aerosols**. An alternative mode of entry is by microaspiration of bacteria from the oropharynx or mouth into the lower respiratory airways, during or after the ingestion of contaminated water or ice. The circumstances of Mrs. R.'s exposure are unknown, but if water was the likely source, she may have acquired the infection at home, at work, or at any place where tap water is available.

In outbreak situations, the risk of infection depends not only on the size of the inhaled inoculum but also on the susceptibility of the host. Several **host factors** are known to predispose individuals to infection. These include cigarette smoking, advanced age, chronic pulmonary disease, and immunosuppression (e.g., transplant patients and patients on corticosteroid therapy). Mrs. R. may have been particularly susceptible to infection because of her age and significant smoking history.

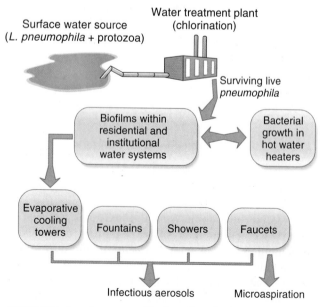

FIGURE 21-1 ▪ **Sources of legionellae for human disease.**

Although the source of her infection is unknown, it is possible that other less susceptible individuals were exposed to the same source as Mrs. R. but did not become infected. Because she was vacationing at the time of her likely exposure, the water system at the Florida resort became suspect and was investigated.

ENTRY

In the air spaces of the lung, *L. pneumophila* is ingested by resident alveolar macrophages. These phagocytic cells, which are normally regarded as a front line of defense against invaders, **fail to kill** or even inhibit the growth of *L. pneumophila* in the lung. In the laboratory, the organism grows faster in human macrophage cultures than in artificial media. In the lung, inhaled *L. pneumophila* must be able to grow in phagocytic cells; bacterial strains that lack this capacity will not cause disease.

SPREAD AND MULTIPLICATION

After ingestion of most bacteria by phagocytes, intracellular killing occurs after **acidification of the phagosome and fusion with lysosomes.** In contrast, after uptake of *L. pneumophila,* a very different sequence of events occurs (Fig. 21-2). The *L. pneumophila* phagosome is first surrounded by smooth vesicles and mitochondria. It is then enveloped in **endoplasmic reticulum** by a process that resembles **autophagy**—a process used by eukaryotic cells to sequester and digest cytoplasmic components in the lysosome. Within this specialized compartment, *L. pneumophila* differentiates into a **replicative form.** Eventually, the host cell becomes literally packed with bacteria. When nutrients become scarce, the organisms stop replicating and differentiate to the transmissible form. Thus, the life cycle of *L. pneumophila* is governed by the nutrient supply of its host.

A variety of factors dictate the intracellular fate of transmissive *L. pneumophila,* including those that initially inhibit phagosome-lysosome fusion and others that later lyse host membranes. Many of these factors appear to be exported into the host cell by a mechanism related to plasmid conjugation, known as Type IV secretion (similar in principle to type III secretion reviewed in the paradigm of Chapter 17). In particular, when conditions deteriorate, *L. pneumophila* not only become resistant to a variety of stresses, but also express a pore-forming toxin to escape from its host cell, flagella to disperse in the environment, and factors that block phagosome maturation to establish a protective niche within the next host cell.

Many of the same phenomena that occur when *L. pneumophila* infect macrophages have also been

FIGURE 21-2 ■ **Electron micrographs. A.** Uptake of *Legionella pneumophila* by a macrophage. **B.** At 4 hours after infection, a dividing organism is seen within an endosome that has associated with rough endoplasmic reticulum. **C.** *L. pneumophila* organisms begin to multiply within membrane-bound phagosomes of the host macrophage.

observed within ameba. Also, epidemiologists have established that this microbe is not transmitted from one human to another. Accordingly, pathogenic *L. pneumophila* most likely emerged from the environment as a consequence of the selective pressures exerted by parasitic ameba. In essence, *L. pneumophila* responds to alveolar macrophages in the lung as if it were encountering an ameba in a pond.

The host may be able to inhibit the intracellular growth of *L. pneumophila* by innate immune mechanisms. On contact with *L. pneumophila*, macrophages secrete **tumor necrosis factor-α** (**TNF-α**), which inhibits intracellular growth of the bacteria. Thus, healthy hosts may be able to limit *L. pneumophila* without ever inducing a specific immune response. Perhaps this explains why most healthy humans are resistant to legionnaires disease.

Once infection is established, its outcome depends on the specific immune response. Experience with animal models suggests that antibodies play a minor role in containing *L. pneumophila* infection. Antibodies produced during infection bind to the surface of *L. pneumophila* and enhance uptake by neutrophils, cells that neither kill nor support the growth of the bacteria. A cell-mediated immune response is required for recovery from infection. By cellular immune processes described in Chapter 7, *Legionella*-immune lymphocytes proliferate and secrete **cytokines** after contact with cells presenting *Legionella* antigens with major histocompatibility complex (MHC) class II molecules. One of the most important of these lymphokines, **interferon-γ**, can suppress the growth of *L. pneumophila* in macrophages by inducing cells to sequester **iron** from the intracellular bacteria. Limiting access to this essential nutrient may be the critical function of the immune system in controlling *L. pneumophila* infection.

DAMAGE

Macrophages infected with *L. pneumophila* release **cytokines** that contribute to the influx of blood monocytes and neutrophils into the air spaces of the lung. As nodular areas of infection enlarge, they become visible as infiltrates on a chest radiograph. These areas typically evolve into microabscesses and may coalesce to form cavities. The bronchi and bronchioles are not affected. Occasionally, *L. pneumophila* can be isolated from the blood or from organ tissues.

Much of the local damage produced by the infection is attributable to the vigor of the host inflammatory response. The source of toxic bacterial products is still a topic some debate. *L. pneumophila* possesses a lipopolysaccharide endotoxin that is weakly toxic. The microbe does produce an abundant extracellular protease with cytolytic and hemolytic activities. Although the purified protease can damage the lungs of experimental animals, protease-deficient mutants of *L. pneumophila* are as virulent as wild-type strains. Another microbial product likely to contribute to inflammation and damage is **flagellin**. This broadly conserved protein is essential for *L. pneumophila* motility; when recognized by the innate immune system of mammalian cells, flagellin can induce a cell death that is accompanied by release of the proinflammatory cytokine IL-1β. In mouse models of legionellosis, detection of cytosolic flagellin by macrophages appears to be critical step for clearance of the infection.

Legionnaires disease usually begins with flulike complaints, as in the case of Mrs. R. Virtually all patients have **fever** and develop clinical features of pneumonia: **cough, shortness of breath,** and possibly **chest pain.** Patients rarely have the grossly purulent (thick yellow or green)

Paradigm **Box**

Intracellular Parasitism

To grow in phagocytic cells, pathogens must be able to outmaneuver their host. They must evade the antimicrobial defenses of phagocytic cells and satisfy their nutritional requirements by competing successfully with the host cells for essential nutrients. To meet these necessities, bacterial and eukaryotic pathogens have evolved various strategies for intracellular growth and survival, as depicted in Figure 21-3. Often phylogenetically unrelated organisms use a common strategy. The precise mechanisms and virulence factors that mediate these events in any one species are usually very unique and have evolved independently.

The ability to survive phagosome-lysosome fusion may involve adaptation of the pathogen's surface, its metabolism, or both. *Leishmania* parasites adapt to the hostile environment of the acidified phagosome by possessing metabolic enzymes that function well at very low pH, and they deploy surface molecules that resist degradation by lysosomal enzymes (see Chapter 52). Similarly, mycobacteria may be protected by the waxy nature of their surfaces (see Chapter 23). Among *Salmonella* strains, those with smooth lipopolysaccharide are less susceptible to killing by lysosomal contents than are "rough" mutants that lack the long polysaccharide chains on their surface (see Chapter 17).

Some organisms evade intracellular killing by promptly escaping from the phagosome into the cytoplasm of the cell, where nutrients are abundant. The prototype for this intracellular lifestyle is *Listeria monocytogenes,* a Gram-positive bacillus that causes septicemia and meningitis. After ingestion by most cells, *L. monocytogenes* secretes a pore-forming cytotoxin, called **listeriolysin O,** that disrupts the phagosomal membrane. Mutant *L. monocytogenes* that cannot produce this cytotoxin cannot escape the phagosome and neither grow nor survive in the host cell. The *L. monocytogenes* promptly divide and, remarkably, begin moving within the cytosol. How do they do this? The bacteria have a surface protein at one of their poles that catalyzes the polymerization of cellular actin. The polymerized actin forms a growing scaffold that forcibly pushes the bacteria through the cytoplasm. Some of the organisms are pushed outward onto the plasma membrane, making long projections. Some can even push into neighboring cells, forcing ingestion of the bacteria at their tips. This process results in the direct spread of the infection to adjacent host cells. A very similar mechanism of cell-to-cell spread is employed by species of *Shigella, Rickettsia,* and the vaccinia virus.

Legionella and several other unrelated pathogens evade intracellular killing by avoiding the usual

FIGURE 21-3 ▪ **Three lifestyles of intracellular pathogens. A.** *Salmonella* species enter a cell by generating a membrane "ruffling" or "splash." The result is a large phagosome that may fuse with lysosomes; however, the bacterium survives and eventually grows within the phagolysosome. **B.** Intracellular life cycle of *Legionella pneumophila.* **C.** Intracellular survival, growth, and motility of *Listeria monocytogenes.*

endocytic pathway. A stealth strategy is employed by the eukaryotic parasite *Toxoplasma gondi* (see Chapter 52). This parasite enters mammalian cells by a mechanism that excludes all host membrane proteins from the phagosome, including those that target mediate the trafficking of the phagosome to the lysosome.

Regardless of the mechanism involved, intracellular parasitism has consequences in clinical medicine. Intracellular organisms are less accessible both to the host immune response and to antimicrobial agents. Recovery from infection may require a **cell-mediated immune response** that inhibits or kills intracellular organisms. Such a response generally takes longer to mount than an antibody response and is also more difficult to stimulate by standard vaccines. As a result, therapy of these infections is generally of longer duration, and **relapses,** presumably resulting from the reemergence of surviving intracellular organisms, are more common than with most extracellular infections. In selecting optimal antimicrobial therapy, the capacity of drugs to penetrate infected host cells must be considered. Antibiotics that penetrate poorly into host cells are generally less useful in treating these infections.

sputum associated with bacterial bronchopneumonias. **Watery diarrhea,** nausea, vomiting, or abdominal pain may also be present. Blood oxygen levels may become low, which might have contributed to Mrs. R.'s confusion and lethargy. Typically, blood counts show only moderate elevation of total leukocytes, without a preponderance of neutrophils. In many patients, other laboratory tests suggest dysfunction of the kidneys or liver. None of these clinical features is sufficiently specific to establish the diagnosis of legionnaires disease, because any of them can occur in association with other pneumonias.

DIAGNOSIS

A laboratory diagnosis of legionnaires disease can be difficult. The bacteria are not present in large numbers in the sputum, and they stain poorly. The Gram stain usually shows abundant neutrophils and no stainable bacteria. Several **rapid identification techniques** can be used to make a prompt diagnosis. They include examination of sputum by direct **fluorescent antibody staining** or detection of *L. pneumophila* serogroup 1 antigen in the urine by an **enzyme immunoassay.** Although these tests may be useful in guiding the initial therapy of the patient, none is sufficiently sensitive or specific to be relied on as the sole method of diagnosis. For example, diagnostic tests for serogroup 1 antigen in urine may miss as many as half of all *Legionella* infections. Culture is the most specific way to diagnose the infection, but it does have the drawback of requiring 3 to 5 days of incubation before *Legionella* colonies can be detected.

TREATMENT AND PREVENTION

Legionella grown in culture are sensitive to most antibiotics. However, successful antibiotic therapy requires drugs that can **penetrate** into infected cells where the bacteria grow. These include macrolides or ketolides, fluoroquinolones, and tetracyclines. As in Mrs. R.'s case, it is not unusual for patients to become worse while on treatment with a penicillin or cephalosporin antibiotic, because these antibiotics penetrate into eukaryotic cells poorly.

Because the laboratory diagnosis of legionnaires disease is imperfect and occasionally untimely, it is necessary to treat patients for this potentially fatal disease on suspicion alone. As a case in point, Mrs. R. was recognized as having a severe, atypical pneumonia that progressed in spite of treatment with an oral cephalosporin antibiotic. In the absence of an alternative etiological diagnosis, she was treated with an antibiotic that is known to be effective in legionnaires disease, pending the results of the culture. This clinical decision may have saved her life.

Prevention of legionnaires disease is presently practiced at an institutional level by monitoring water systems and by clinical surveillance for sentinel cases of legionellosis. In hospitals, hotels, and other large buildings where cases have occurred, water systems are checked regularly for *Legionella.* When found, the systems are flushed and decontaminated by superheating of the water to 60°C, ultraviolet irradiation, or treatment with copper and silver ions or monochloramine. Because a single case of legionellosis can reflect a larger outbreak, clinical diagnosis is often the critical first step in prevention. Following Mrs. R.'s case, *L. pneumophila* serogroup 1 was cultured from the water system of the Florida resort where she vacationed. Decontamination of that system probably prevented numerous subsequent cases.

Other *Legionella* Species and Their Associated Diseases

In addition to *L. pneumophila,* several other species of *Legionella* cause human disease. In general, these are also water-related infections, and they produce clinical features comparable to legionnaires disease. *L. micdadei* is one example.

Certain *Legionella* species have also been associated with an illness called Pontiac fever. The illness was first recognized during a 1968 outbreak at the county health department building in Pontiac, Michigan. In that outbreak 95% of the department's employees became ill with fever, muscle aches, headache, and dizziness that resolved spontaneously in 2 to 5 days. The cause of this flulike illness was not identified at the time, but serum samples from patients and lung tissue from guinea pigs exposed to the building air were kept frozen for future reference. After the identification of *L. pneumophila* 9 years later, the frozen specimens were retested. The Pontiac patients were found to have had a rise in specific *Legionella* antibodies, and the guinea pig lungs yielded growth of *L. pneumophila* in culture.

Like legionnaires disease, Pontiac fever is an airborne disease; but there the similarity ends. Unlike legionnaires disease, Pontiac fever typically affects a high proportion of exposed individuals, and it affects healthy as well as high-risk individuals. It does not produce pneumonia and is never fatal. It may not be an infection at all, because the microbe has not been cultured from any patient. How the same bacteria can produce two very different clinical syndromes is still a mystery. However, analysis of the genomes of three virulent serogroup 1 strains of *L. pneumophila* revealed extraordinary genetic diversity: More than 10% of each strain's genes were not encoded by the other two clinical isolates. Perhaps the ability of *L. pneumophila* to incorporate into its genome DNA obtained from the environment contributes to both the diversity of the species and the heterogeneity of clinical disease.

Conclusion

L. pneumophila is an opportunistic pathogen able to produce an airborne infection of the lungs that can develop into a life-threatening pneumonia. Infection depends on the capacity of the bacterium to grow within phagocytic cells of the host. Treatment and immune mechanisms are beneficial insofar as they can affect the bacteria that occupy this intracellular niche.

Helicobacter pylori: Pathogenesis of a "Slow" Bacterial Infection

Richard M. Peek Jr.

key concepts

Helicobacter pylori:

- Is a recently discovered bacterium that is the causative agent of most gastric and duodenal ulcers and gastric adenocarcinomas.

- Infects up to one third of the world's population.

- Causes clinical disease in only 10 to 15% of infected individuals.

- Can be detected by histologic examination, culture, rapid urease testing, stool antigen testing, serologic testing, and urease breath testing.

- Is treated with a combination of antibiotics and acid-reducing drugs.

*H*elicobacter pylori is a Gram-negative bacterium that resides in the mucus gel layer overlaying the gastric mucosa. In 1983 Barry J. Marshall and J. Robin Warren first identified curved bacilli adjacent to the gastric epithelium of patients with chronic gastritis (and in 2005 the two researchers won the Nobel Prize for their work). Since that discovery, a strong link has been established between *H. pylori* and a diverse spectrum of gastroduodenal diseases, including gastric and duodenal ulceration, gastric adenocarcinoma, mucosa-associated lymphoid tissue (MALT) lymphoma, and non-Hodgkin lymphoma of the stomach. The organism colonizes the stomach for years or decades, not days or weeks as is usually the case for bacterial pathogens. The longevity of colonization and persistent low-grade gastric inflammation with gradual progression to disease both suggest that *H. pylori* should be considered a prototypic "slow" bacterium. In that sense, *H. pylori* resembles the spirochetes of syphilis and Lyme disease and the leprosy bacillus, all of which can cause low-grade but persistent infection. Recent insights into *H. pylori* pathophysiology are beginning to answer perplexing questions raised by the bacterium's unique ecological niche, including why an organism that colonizes one third of the world's population leads to overt clinical disease in only 10 to 15% of infected individuals, and how *H. pylori* infection can cause such divergent clinical sequelae as ulcer disease and cancer.

Helicobacter pylori is the prototypic species of its genus. These organisms are Gram-negative, curved or spiral bacteria that live in the mucus layer above the gastric epithelium. They have multiple flagella at one pole and are nutritionally fastidious bacteria. They are also **microaerophilic,** which means they grow ideally in an atmosphere of reduced oxygen (approximately 5%), befitting their residence within the semipermeable mucus gel layer. *H. pylori* are robust producers of **urease,** which catalyzes the hydrolysis of urea into ammonia and carbon dioxide. Other *Helicobacter* species, such as *H. mustelae, H. muridarum,* and *H. nemestrinae,* natu-

Case

Forty-five-year-old Mr. K. was evaluated for recurrent burning epigastric pain. Seven years earlier he had noted abdominal pain that often awakened him from sleep, was associated with nausea, and improved with meals. He was initially treated with omeprazole, a **proton pump inhibitor,** to reduce the production of gastric acid, for 8 weeks, and his symptoms resolved. However, 4 months later his symptoms recurred. At endoscopy, a 1-cm ulcer was seen in the duodenal bulb. The patient was once again given omeprazole. However, four times in the ensuing 6 years, his burning epigastric pain recurred. Mr. K.'s mother and one of his two siblings also had a history of peptic ulcer disease. Another endoscopy showed that a duodenal ulcer was still present. Biopsies of two sites in the stomach were taken for histologic examination and culture. These specimens showed chronic active gastritis with elevated numbers of neutrophils and mononuclear cells in the lamina propria and the glandular epithelium (Fig. 22-1). Curved, Gram-negative, rod-shaped bacteria were identified on the gastric mucosal surfaces of all samples, and cultures grew *Helicobacter pylori.*

In addition to acid reduction therapy with omeprazole, Mr. K. began a 10-day course of amoxicillin and clarithromycin. A repeat endoscopy 6 weeks after completion of therapy showed healing of his ulcer, and biopsies of his stomach showed resolution of gastritis. No *H. pylori* was found on histologic examination or culture. Mr. K. remained symptom free after 6 months and required no further therapy.

This case raises a number of questions:

1. Was *H. pylori* the cause of Mr. K.'s 7-year bout of recurrent duodenal ulceration?
2. What features permit *H. pylori* to colonize the stomach when other bacteria are usually killed there?
3. What bacterial and/or host factors allow an infection with such high specificity for gastric epithelium to cause disease at an anatomically distinct site such as the duodenum?
4. How can *H. pylori* infection be detected in patients with disease?
5. How can *H. pylori* be eliminated from the stomach?

FIGURE 22-1 ▪ **Hematoxylin and eosin stain of** *Helicobacter pylori*–**associated gastritis. A.** Numerous neutrophils, lymphocytes, and plasma cells are present in the lamina propria. **B.** In another section of the tissue at higher magnification, a gastric gland with infiltration by neutrophils and lymphocytes is seen in the center of the image.

rally colonize the stomachs of other mammals and are strongly urease positive, suggesting that ammonia production is an important conserved survival mechanism for *Helicobacter* organisms within the acidic gastric environment.

Helicobacter pylori

ENCOUNTER, ENTRY, AND MULTIPLICATION

Present in at least one-third of the world's population, *H. pylori* remains one of the most common bacterial infections of humans. Although the prevalence of *H. pylori* is higher in developing countries than in developed countries (particularly among younger persons), in all locales, infection rates steadily increase with age among children and young adults, plateau at about middle age, and often decrease in old age.

The precise mechanism by which *H. pylori* is transmitted remains undefined, in part because of its long-term persistence within the stomach as well as the nonspecific nature of symptoms associated with acute infection. Risk factors for infection include poor socioeconomic status, familial overcrowding, ethnicity, and infection rates endemic to the country of origin. In developing countries, the incidence of *H. pylori* infection in children ranges between 3 to 10% per year. With socioeconomic development, however, fewer children are acquiring *H. pylori,* and this worldwide phenomenon preceded the introduction of antibiotics. The primary niche for *H. pylori* in humans is the stomach, although the bacteria can also be isolated from regions of gastric-type tissue (gastric metaplasia) in the duodenum. *H. pylori* has occasionally been cultured from saliva, dental plaque, and stools, but *H. pylori*–specific DNA has been detected more reliably from these sources, suggesting that the sites may contain only sparse concentrations of viable organisms.

Intrafamilial case clustering and the absence of a well-defined nonhuman reservoir suggest that transmission of *H. pylori* is likely to be person to person. This theory is supported by previous findings demonstrating an increased infection rate among patients residing in institutional settings with closed environments and close personal contact. Two ingestion experiments by human volunteers and several outbreaks of accidental infection have provided clues into the initial events that occur during acute *H. pylori* infection. One self-inoculation experiment resulted in severe gastrointestinal symptoms (abdominal pain, belching, regurgitation) and persistent gastritis. The fasting gastric pH on day 5 following ingestion was 1.2 (in the normal range of 1 to 2) and was accompanied by intense inflammation in the gastric antrum. By day 8, however, the fasting gastric pH rose to 7.6. Along with acute symptoms, specific IgM antibodies peaked early, and increased titers of both IgA and IgG developed later. These findings suggest that ingestion of organisms is followed by a period of intense bacterial proliferation and gastric inflammation with concomitant **hypochlorhydria,** which may last for weeks.

Ultimately, the inflammatory response equilibrates, and the host mounts a humoral immune response that is ineffective in eliminating *H. pylori* but may regulate the intensity of inflammation. Gastric pH values are also restored to within the normal range, and most infected persons remain asymptomatic for years or for life. Based on the presence of *H. pylori* in feces of African children and recent data showing that induction of vomiting and diarrhea in patients with preexisting *H. pylori* infection significantly increases the rate of bacterial culture positivity from vomitus, saliva, and diarrheal specimens, it is likely that *H. pylori* transmission increases during childhood episodes of gastroenteritis both by fecal shedding and/or oral–oral spread.

Damage

Essentially all persons who become infected with *H. pylori* develop **chronic superficial gastritis** involving the gastric antrum, fundus or corpus, and the cardia, and gastritis persists throughout their lifetimes, whether or not they have gastrointestinal symptoms. Long-term pathologic outcomes vary among infected persons (Fig. 22-2). Although the majority of colonized persons remain asymptomatic with only chronic gastritis, some develop **ulceration,** and in others the inflammatory process is associated with permanent loss of epithelial glands, termed **atrophic gastritis.** Atrophic gastritis occurs over the course of decades and is a well-recognized risk factor for **gastric cancer.**

H. pylori pathogenesis is complex, in keeping with the ability of the organism to cause a variety of clinical manifestations. Infection is invariably associated with chronic gastric inflammation, which may serve as a means for the organism to obtain a constant source of nutrients. In this model, *H. pylori* releases **effector molecules** that induce tissue inflammation, which causes

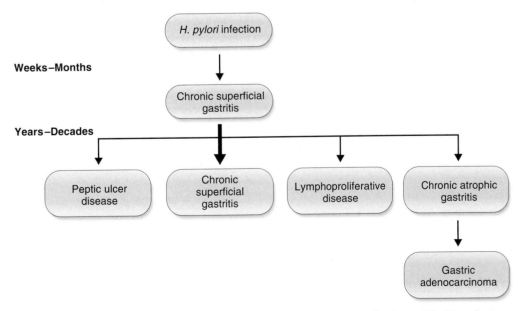

FIGURE 22-2 ■ Diversity of clinical consequences following infection with *H. pylori.*

release of nutrients that sustain the *H. pylori* population. One marker and effector of damage is CagA, a protein of 120 to 145 kilodaltons found in 60 to 70% of U.S. *H. pylori* strains. Serum and mucosal antibodies to CagA are present in approximately 90% of patients with duodenal ulceration, and expression of CagA in vivo is highly correlated with peptic ulcer disease and duodenitis. *H. pylori* isolates that are positive for CagA (*cagA*+ strains) induce higher degrees of inflammation and damage in the gastric mucosa than do *cagA*− strains. In addition, mucosal levels of **interleukin 8 (IL-8)**, a potent chemoattractant and neutrophil-activating host cytokine, are significantly higher in persons harboring *cagA*+ rather than *cagA*− strains, which may explain the link between *cagA*+ strains and peptic ulcer disease.

The gene (*cagA*) encoding CagA is a member of an entire cassette of linked *H. pylori* genes called the *cag* pathogenicity island, and some of these genes possess homology to components of the type IV bacterial secretion systems that export proteins. Befitting these homologies, CagA is translocated into host epithelial cells following *H. pylori* attachment, where it is modified by tyrosine phosphorylation; phospho-CagA then activates several host signaling pathways, leading to cellular morphological changes. In addition to stimulating cytoskeletal rearrangements, genes within the *H. pylori cag* island encode proteins that induce IL-8 secretion from gastric epithelial cells following bacterial attachment, which may explain the more intense inflammatory response that develops in persons harboring *cagA*+ strains.

Some *H. pylori* strains also secrete a **cytotoxin** (VacA), that induces **vacuolation** of cells in culture. *H. pylori* clinical isolates that produce the VacA cytotoxin are more frequently associated with peptic ulcer disease and increased infiltration of the gastric antrum by neutrophils. In addition to vacuolation, VacA exerts other effects that may influence clinical outcome. Inoculation of mice with either purified VacA or VacA-containing broth supernatants leads to epithelial cell injury, and VacA causes gastric epithelial cells in culture to undergo a specific form of cell death termed apoptosis. VacA also functions as a transmembrane pore, permeabilizing host epithelial cells to urea, which in turn may allow *H. pylori* to manipulate the pH of its environment by generating ammonia. When added to cultured epithelial cells, VacA increases paracellular permeability to organic molecules, iron, and nickel and causes cellular detachment. Collectively, these data indicate that VacA can induce multiple physiologic consequences that may contribute to pathogenesis.

The mechanism of ulcer development resulting from *H. pylori* infection is not completely understood. Continuous inflammation within the gastric mucosa may be sufficient to lead to mucosal breakdown, erosive gastritis, and ultimately gastric ulceration. A more perplexing question concerns the development of duodenal ulcers. *H. pylori* is found only in intimate association with

gastric epithelium. How then can this infection lead to disease in the duodenum? The answer most likely involves replacement of intestinal-type tissue with gastric tissue in the duodenum, a phenomenon that develops in patients with high acid secretion (as in a condition called the Zollinger-Ellison syndrome). *H. pylori* infection results in downregulation of **somatostatin-producing D cells** in the gastric mucosa, which in turn leads to inappropriately elevated **gastrin levels** and enhanced gastric acid secretion. *H. pylori* can then populate regions of gastric metaplasia in the duodenum, establish infection, cause inflammation, and in concert with elevated gastric acid levels, ultimately lead to ulceration at the site.

H. pylori infection is also associated with the development of **adenocarcinoma of the stomach.** The sequential progression of the disease is lengthy, from chronic superficial gastritis to chronic atrophic gastritis, through intestinal metaplasia to dysplasia, and finally to invasive adenocarcinoma. The entire process can take some 15 to 20 years after onset of superficial gastritis. Specifically, how does adenocarcinoma occur? Increased cell proliferation that develops secondary to chronic *H. pylori* infection may increase the likelihood of DNA damage in response to environmental mutagens such as **N nitrosamines** or **inflammation-related oxygen- or nitrogen-free radicals.** Persons infected with *H. pylori* have reduced gastric juice concentrations of ascorbic acid, an important defense mechanism against oxidative DNA damage (Fig. 22-3).

H. pylori infection has also been shown to decrease the rate of apoptosis within colonized tissue, leading to increased cell survival within an environment rich in inflammatory mediators and thus enhancing the possibility for mutagenesis. The risk of gastric cancer may also be related to certain strain characteristics of *H. pylori*. Infection with *cagA*+ toxigenic (as opposed to *cagA*− nontoxigenic) strains is associated with a significantly increased risk for gastric adenocarcinoma, perhaps caused by the heightened inflammatory response and/or alteration of host epithelial cell signaling that develops after infection with *cagA*+ toxigenic strains.

Host factors also contribute to oncogenesis within *H. pylori*–colonized gastric mucosa. One host determinant that may influence the development of gastric cancer is **gastrin.** Hypergastrinemia occurs early in the course of human *H. pylori* infection, precedes the development of atrophic gastritis, and often resolves after eradication. In vitro, gastrin stimulates gastric epithelial cell proliferation, and *Helicobacter*-infected mice that overexpress gastrin develop gastric cancer. Polymorphisms within the human IL-1β and TNF-α gene promoter sequences associated with increased expression of these proinflammatory, acid-inhibitory molecules also increase the risk for atrophic gastritis and distal gastric adenocarcinoma among *H. pylori*–infected persons. Thus, the seemingly divergent outcomes of peptic ulceration and gastric cancer can both be related to *H. pylori*

FIGURE 22-3 ▪ **Potential mechanisms of carcinogenesis following infection with *H. pylori*.**

infection. In its early stages, the infection induces sufficient inflammation to disrupt mucosal integrity, alter the acid homeostasis within the stomach, and potentially lead to ulcers, while in its later stage, it may promote the development of neoplasia on a pathologic background of atrophic gastritis.

In addition to ulcer disease and gastric adenocarcinoma, persons infected with *H. pylori* have an increased risk of developing mucosa-associated lymphoid tissue (MALT) lymphoma and **non-Hodgkin lymphoma of the stomach.** T cells that participate in the chronic inflammatory process can react with *H. pylori* antigens and produce cytokines supporting the uncontrolled growth and proliferation of B lymphocytes, leading to malignant lymphomatous degeneration. Although MALT lymphomas are rare in the United States with only 0.71 cases in 100,000 patients per year, elimination of *H. pylori* leads to complete regression of these tumors in more than 80% of cases, a remarkable demonstration that removal of a bacterium can affect a clonal lesion.

Although a signature feature of *H. pylori* colonization is induction of inflammation, the organism has also evolved mechanisms to ensure a prolonged existence within its host; for example, although both humoral and cellular recognition of *H. pylori* occur, the bacterium clearly evades immunologic clearance. *H. pylori* produces a protein called arginase, which confers protection against the host inflammatory molecule, nitric oxide. *H. pylori* has also evolved properties, such as an **endotoxin and flagellin that are less potent** than those in most other Gram-negative organisms. These properties lessen mucosal inflammation and injury, suggesting that it may be beneficial for the long-term

survival of the bacteria to tightly regulate the extent of damage to its host.

DIAGNOSIS

Several techniques are currently available to diagnose *H. pylori* and can be classified as either invasive or noninvasive (Table 22-1). All the tests are quite sensitive and specific, and the choice of which test to use depends on

table 22-1	Diagnosis of *Helicobacter pylori* Infection	
METHOD	**SPECIMEN**	**SENSITIVITY**
Invasive tests		
Urease test	Mucosal biopsy	High
Histology, Giemsa stain	Mucosal biopsies (2)	Very high
Culture	Mucosal biopsy	Very high
Noninvasive tests		
Serology (ELISA)	Serum	High
Urea breath test	Breath sample	Very high
Stool antigen test	Stool	Very high
Tests used in research		
Polymerase chain reaction	Stool sample, gastric juice, biopsy of stomach	High

ELISA, enzyme-linked immunosorbent assay.

FIGURE 22-4 ▪ **Warthin-Starry stain of *H. pylori*.** *H. pylori* stain black because they are impregnated with silver and are therefore easily detectable in biopsy specimens. Numerous bacteria can be seen on the surface of the gastric mucosa.

the laboratory resources available and the clinical situation—that is, diagnosing infection versus documenting eradication. Invasive methods involve obtaining gastric tissue specimens by endoscopy and include **histologic examination,** microbiological **culture,** and **rapid urease testing.** Most pathologists initially use the Giemsa stain because it is sensitive and inexpensive; the Warthin-Starry stain is more sensitive but more costly (Fig. 22-4). Detection of *H. pylori* by culture is less reliable than other available methods because of the fastidious growth of the organism. Biochemical confirmation of *H. pylori* includes positive tests for urease, catalase, and oxidase. A rapid urease test detects urease activity within a gastric biopsy sample. When a biopsy containing *H. pylori* is placed into a urea-containing indicator medium, ammonia is produced from urea, the pH increases, and the indicator turns red. The rapid urease test is less expensive than either histology or culture and is often the method of choice when endoscopy is used.

Noninvasive tests include **serology, urea breath tests,** and **stool antigen testing.** Serologic tests measure levels of circulating antibodies directed against a variety of *H. pylori* antigens and are very sensitive and specific for primary diagnosis of *H. pylori* infection. However, serological methods have limited utility in assessing posttreatment *H. pylori* status because titers fall gradually; it may be 6 months before a sufficient decrease is observed. Urea breath testing involves ingestion of radioactive carbon-labeled urea; if *H. pylori* (or other urease-containing gastric bacteria) are present, urea is metabolized to ammonia and bicarbonate, and radioactive carbon dioxide is detected in breath samples. The urea breath test is a convenient method to document *H. pylori* eradication because it does not require endoscopy and is easy to perform.

Recently, an enzymatic immunoassay (called HpSA and developed by Meridian Diagnostics, Cincinnati, Ohio) that detects the presence of bacterial antigens in feces has become available as an alternative noninvasive diagnostic technique for *H. pylori.* The *H. pylori* stool antigen test has now been determined to be both sensitive and specific, and the U.S. Food and Drug Administration has recently approved HpSA for initial diagnosis of *H. pylori* and for monitoring posttherapy responses. Following successful treatment of *H. pylori,* stool antigen levels rapidly decline and, in the majority of patients, are undetectable by 5 days after treatment. Stool samples can be stored for prolonged periods and multiple samples can be assayed at once. Testing stool for *H. pylori* antigens is cost-effective compared with both serologic testing before therapy and urea breath testing after therapy. Although data indicate that the *H. pylori* stool antigen test is a highly accurate technique that can identify the presence of *H. pylori* prior to and shortly following initiation of antimicrobial therapy, its place in the *H. pylori* diagnostic armamentarium in the United States remains to be determined.

TREATMENT

Physicians should only attempt to diagnose *H. pylori* if they are unequivocally committed to treating the infection. Currently, it is recommended that persons with a present or past history of peptic ulcer disease or gastric MALT lymphoma be tested for *H. pylori* and treated if positive. Less-clear indications exist for close family relatives of patients with gastric cancer, persons taking aspirin or nonsteroidal anti-inflammatory drugs (NSAIDs) that heighten the risk for peptic ulceration, or persons who have migrated from regions where the background prevalence of gastric cancer is high. An ideal treatment for *H. pylori* would be inexpensive, safe with minimal side effects, simple, effective, and short in duration. In addition, treatment should not induce significant resistance. All regimens used to date fall short of these parameters. Several factors that limit the effectiveness of therapy for *H. pylori* include (1) rapidly developing bacterial resistance to metronidazole, quinolones, and macrolides; (2) reduced efficacy of certain drugs, such as amoxicillin and clarithromycin, under acidic conditions; and (3) patient noncompliance owing to side effects or the burden of ingesting multiple pills for 7 to 10 days.

The goal of *H. pylori* therapy is to eliminate the organism from the stomach, and successful eradication is defined as a negative test for the bacterium 4 or more weeks after completion of therapy. In general, antisecretory agents such as H₂ blockers and proton pump inhibitors (PPIs) relieve ulcer symptoms and promote ulcer healing. In addition, the gastric pH is raised by these agents, which in turn increases the efficacy of antibiotics like **amoxicillin** and **clarithromycin.** Several large multicenter eradication trials have documented that eradication rates of more than 85% can be achieved with therapies lasting 7 to 10 days and consisting of a PPI and two antibiotics (usually **clarithromycin** and either **metronidazole** or **amoxicillin**; Table 22-2). There are no consistent advantages to using a particular PPI for *H. pylori* eradication; therefore, any agent in this class can be used as a component of triple therapy. The prevalence of antimicrobial resistance in *H. pylori* is increasing, particularly for metronidazole, which reduces treatment efficacy. Because the most effective second-line regimens contain metronidazole, it is advisable to use clarithromycin and amoxicillin instead of clarithromycin and metronidazole in first-line regimens to optimize results should subsequent therapy be required. Amoxicillin should be not be used in penicillin-allergic patients, and metronidazole should be avoided in persons consuming alcohol.

Second-line (rescue) therapies should be used if first-line regimens fail to eliminate *H. pylori*. The most effective rescue regimen is quadruple therapy combining a PPI, bismuth subsalicylate, metronidazole, and tetracycline for 14 days (see Table 22-2). Fixed combinations of anti–*H. pylori* agents, such as Prevpac (lansoprazole 30 mg, clarithromycin 500 mg, and amoxicillin 500 mg, each taken twice a day for 7 days) and Helidac (bismuth subsalicylate 262.4 mg, metronidazole 250 mg, and tetracycline 500 mg, each taken four times a day for 14 days), make treatment more tolerable and are currently being marketed. However, although these may be more convenient, they are not cost-effective, and the shorter duration (7 days) and lower dosage of amoxicillin (500 mg) in Prevpac compared with the standard triple therapy (see Table 22-2), as well as the need for combination therapy with a PPI (Helidac), preclude recommending these formulations as optimal first-line anti–*H. pylori* therapies.

Although eradication rates in controlled trials often exceed 90%, efficacy in clinical practice is usually lower, primarily because of differences in patient populations, differences in infecting *H. pylori* isolates, and/or antibiotic resistance patterns of strains in a particular geographic area. As a result of the current availability and accuracy of noninvasive diagnostic tests for *H. pylori*, it is recommended that urea breath testing or stool antigen tests be performed following intervention to confirm successful cure.

PREVENTION

The potential to prevent *H. pylori*–associated diseases with a vaccine is exciting. It is likely to be most appropriately applied in areas where childhood infection is endemic. To develop an effective vaccine against *H. pylori*, the factors important for its virulence must be identified, characterized, produced on a large scale, and then administered in an immunologically relevant way. In mice an oral vaccine consisting of *H. pylori* urease prevented chronic infection by the related species *H. felis*. Interestingly, infected mice that received an oral treatment with recombinant urease were able to eliminate a chronic *H. felis* infection and developed protection against subsequent *H. felis* challenge. Thus, therapeutic vaccination may be possible.

table **22-2**	Optimal Regimens for the Treatment of *Helicobacter pylori* Infection		
REGIMEN	**DRUG**	**DOSE**	**DURATION**
First line	Proton pump inhibitor[a] and	Twice a day[b]	7–10 days[c]
	clarithromycin and	250 or 500 mg twice a day[d]	7–10 days
	amoxicillin or	1,000 mg twice a day[e]	7–10 days
	metronidazole	500 mg twice a day	7–10 days
Second line	Proton pump inhibitor and	Twice a day	14 days
	bismuth subsalicylate and	120 mg four times a day	14 days
	tetracycline and	500 mg four times a day	14 days
	metronidazole	500 mg three times a day	14 days

[a] Proton pump inhibitors can be used interchangeably.
[b] Specific dose depends on proton pump inhibitor used.
[c] Ten days of therapy is preferable to 7 days.
[d] Lower dose is as effective as higher dose.
[e] Amoxicillin is preferable to metronidazole.

Conclusion

H. pylori infects approximately one third of the world's population, but in most individuals the infection is clinically silent. Transmission is probably via fecal–oral and/or oral–oral routes. *H. pylori*–induced gastritis is a necessary condition for the development of peptic ulceration in the absence of drug-induced disease. The infection is also linked with gastric adenocarcinoma and non-Hodgkin lymphoma of the stomach. Several excellent diagnostic tests are currently available, and effective therapeutic regimens now exist. The overwhelming evidence linking peptic ulcer disease to *H. pylori* infection indicates that ulcer patients infected with the organism should receive antimicrobial therapy directed toward *H. pylori* to decrease ulcer recurrence. In the future, vaccines may not only provide a means to prevent *H. pylori* infection but also offer a therapeutic intervention.

Mycobacteria: Tuberculosis and Leprosy

David Haas

key concepts

Tuberculosis:

- Is the disease caused by *Mycobacterium tuberculosis*, a slow-growing, acid-fast obligate aerobe that can replicate within host macrophages.

- Is usually acquired by inhaling aerosolized droplet nuclei.

- Elicits a cellular immune response that usually controls infection, the only sequelae being a positive tuberculin skin test.

- Can cause illness that begins soon after initial infection (primary disease) or can remain latent for years before reactivating and causing illness (endogenous reactivation).

- Tissue pathology is characterized by granulomas that may undergo caseous necrosis. In immunocompetent individuals, the lesions generally heal spontaneously. In immunocompromised individuals, infection may progress to miliary (disseminated) tuberculosis.

- Is characterized by delayed-type hypersensitivity that causes tissue damage during reactivation.

- Is usually diagnosed by microscopy and culture of sputum.

Leprosy:

- Is the disease caused by *Mycobacterium leprae*.

- Causes illness that ranges between two polar forms: tuberculoid (strong immune response with few organisms) and lepromatous (minimal immune response with immense numbers of organisms).

Tuberculosis is the illness caused by *Mycobacterium tuberculosis* (also called the **tubercle bacillus**). Worldwide the disease is **second only to HIV** as the most common cause of death from a single infectious agent. In 1993 tuberculosis was declared a global public health emergency by the World Health Organization. Tuberculosis can affect any organ, but the lungs are the most important site. The outcome of infection depends on factors that include a history of previous exposure to *M. tuberculosis*, the age of the individual, and overall immunocompetence. **At least 90% of healthy persons who become infected with M. tuberculosis never become ill.** The organism, however, can survive within macrophages and persist in tissues for many years.

251

In some individuals, previously dormant (**latent**) bacteria can cause illness months or years later, with tissue damage caused mostly by hypersensitivity of the sensitized host to bacterial products. In contrast, almost all persons with AIDS who are coinfected with *M. tuberculosis* eventually develop active tuberculosis. Already one of the most important infectious diseases in the world, tuberculosis has become even more significant since the rise of the **AIDS pandemic** and the spread of **multidrug-resistant** strains.

This chapter discusses the pathogenesis and selected clinical aspects of tuberculosis. Leprosy, a relatively common mycobacterial disease in some resource-limited countries, is also discussed. For clarification, the term *infection* describes entry, multiplication, and survival of an organism within the host, regardless of whether symptoms develop; the term *disease* indicates illness resulting from infection.

Mycobacterium tuberculosis

Epidemiology

Tuberculosis is an ancient disease; evidence of tuberculosis has been found in the bones of Neolithic, pre-Colombian, and early Egyptian remains. However, it became a major public health problem during the

Case

Ms. A., a 35-year-old child care worker, had been in good health until she began experiencing chronic cough and weight loss. Over two months she developed gradually worsening cough productive of yellow sputum. She also noted decreased appetite, a 15-lb weight loss, daily fever, and drenching night sweats. She did not improve despite being prescribed a routine antibiotic for one week. A chest radiograph revealed infiltrates in both lung apices (Fig. 23-1). On further questioning she described visiting South Africa several years earlier, where she worked briefly on an AIDS ward. She also recalled her mother having a positive tuberculin skin test about 20 years ago, but her mother was never ill.

Ms. A. had a tuberculin skin test placed (intradermal injection of tuberculin on the volar aspect of the forearm), but it showed no induration (thickening) when examined 48 hours later. She was referred to a local health department, where acid-fast staining and microscopy of her sputum showed acid-fast bacilli. She was placed on respiratory isolation at home and prescribed four antituberculous drugs. Within one week she felt much better, after two weeks was taken off respiratory isolation, and after one month was allowed to return to work. She was cured after receiving six months of therapy, with every dose administered under direct observation by a health department nurse, as required by local public health authorities.

This case raises several questions:

1. How and when did Ms. A. most likely become infected with *Mycobacterium tuberculosis*?
2. Why did it take so long for Ms. A. to develop active tuberculosis?
3. By what route did the tubercle bacilli most likely arrive at the apex of her lung?
4. Which individuals are most likely to develop active tuberculosis from contact with Ms. A.?
5. How would her illness have differed if she had had AIDS?

FIGURE 23-1 ▪ **Pulmonary tuberculosis. A.** Chest radiograph from a young adult with tuberculosis involving the apices of both lungs. **B.** The areas most affected are circled.

Industrial Revolution, when crowded living conditions favored its airborne spread. In the eighteenth century, tuberculosis killed one fourth of all adults in Europe. Major improvements began in the 1940s with effective antituberculous drugs. In the United States tuberculosis case rates have declined ever since accurate statistics became available, even before effective drugs were available. However, in the late 1980s rates in the United States increased sharply because of infections in individuals with AIDS and transmission from them to others. Inadequately funded tuberculosis control programs in some major cities could not manage this problem, and large outbreaks resulted. Because of incomplete adherence with therapy, there were epidemics of multidrug-resistant tuberculosis, especially in Miami and New York City. Fortunately, tuberculosis case rates in the United States have declined since 1992, and in 2002 the rates were the lowest in history (less than 10 cases per 100,000 population). Foreign-born persons account for one half of all cases in the United States (Fig. 23-2).

Mycobacterium tuberculosis infects one third of the world's population. Its rapid spread requires crowded living conditions and a population with little native resistance. In Europe case rates began declining before the turn of the century as those with less native resistance succumbed to the disease. The rate of decline doubled after chemotherapy became widespread, and epidemiologists once thought tuberculosis would eventually disappear. The prechemotherapy trend was the result of higher natural resistance in those who survived infection and improved living conditions. Currently, tuberculosis has its greatest impact in resource-limited countries (Table 23-1). With more than 40 million persons now

table **23-1**	Estimated Tuberculosis Case Rates Among Countries That Account for 70% of Cases Worldwide, 1997	
COUNTRY	**CASES**	**RATE PER 100,000 POPULATION**
India	1,799,000	187
China	1,402,000	113
Indonesia	583,000	285
Bangladesh	300,000	246
Pakistan	261,000	181
Nigeria	253,000	214
Philippines	222,000	314
South Africa	170,000	392
Russian Federation	156,000	106
Ethiopia	156,000	260
Vietnam	145,000	189
Democratic Republic of Congo	129,000	269

Adapted from Dye C, Scheele S, Dolin P, Pathania V, Raviglione M. Global burden of tuberculosis: estimated incidence, prevalence, and mortality by country. JAMA 1999;282:677–686.

living with HIV, the potential for interaction between AIDS and tuberculosis is immense (see the box titled "Mycobacteria and AIDS"). The situation is worst in Africa, where half of all HIV-infected adults also are infected with *M. tuberculosis*.

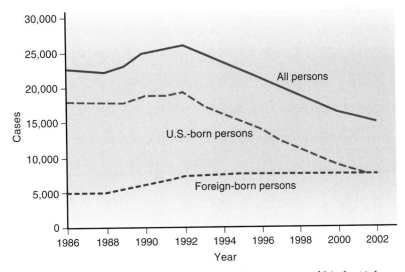

FIGURE 23-2 ■ **Reported cases of tuberculosis in the United States by country of birth.** (Adapted from Centers for Disease Control and Prevention. Tuberculosis morbidity—United States, 1997. Morb Mortal Wkly Rep. 1998;47: 253–257, and Centers for Disease Control and Prevention. Tuberculosis morbidity among U.S.-born and foreign-born populations—United States, 2000. Morb Mortal Wkly Rep. 2002;51:101–104.)

Mycobacteria and AIDS

The interaction between *M. tuberculosis* and HIV is causing global devastation. Nearly all persons coinfected with HIV and *M. tuberculosis* will eventually develop active tuberculosis unless the HIV or the tuberculous infection are effectively treated. Persons with AIDS are predisposed not only to reactivation of remote infection but also to rapid progression of recently acquired infection. Tuberculosis is somewhat unique among opportunistic infections in AIDS because of its person-to-person airborne spread. AIDS patients with tuberculosis are likely to develop widespread **extrapulmonary disease** as depletion of CD4$^+$ T cells impairs cell-mediated immunity. Fortunately, persons with AIDS respond well to antituberculous therapy.

Patients with advanced AIDS are also very susceptible to disease caused by *m. avium* complex (MAC).

This organism is often found in water and soil and is generally harmless to immunocompetent individuals. Before the AIDS epidemic, MAC occasionally caused chronic pneumonia in patients with underlying lung diseases, but disseminated infections were rare. In contrast, MAC frequently colonizes the gastrointestinal tract of patients with advanced AIDS before invading deeper tissues and causing disseminated disease. Patients with disseminated MAC may experience a nonspecific chronic illness with fever, malaise, and wasting, or patients may have local manifestations, such as diarrhea with involvement of the intestine or abdominal pain from involvement of the liver, spleen, and retroperitoneal lymph nodes. As with *M. tuberculosis,* effective therapy for MAC requires prolonged administration of multiple drugs.

DISTINGUISHING CHARACTERISTICS

The genus *Mycobacterium* includes closely related species of **obligate aerobes** (Table 23-2). Species other than *M. tuberculosis* are often called atypical mycobacteria. These organisms are usually acquired from the environment rather than from person-to-person spread and tend to cause diseases distinct from tuberculosis. This genus also includes the agent of leprosy, *M. leprae* (discussed later in the chapter). Many mycobacteria are harmless, and some live on the human body without causing disease (e.g., *M. smegmatis*), while some are found in soil and other niches in the environment. Mycobacteria are **acid fast,** are unusually **resistant to drying,** and **grow slowly** compared with most other bacteria.

table 23-2	Characteristics of Clinically Important Species of *Mycobacteria*[a]					
SPECIES	RESERVOIR	VIRULENCE FOR HUMANS	MAIN DISEASE CAUSED	CASE-TO-CASE TRANSMISSION	IN VITRO GROWTH RATE	OPTIMUM GROWTH TEMPERATURE (°C)
M. tuberculosis	Human	+ + +	Tuberculosis	Yes	S	37
M. bovis	Animals	+ + +	Tuberculosis	Rare	S	37
Bacillus Calmette-Guérin (BCG)	Artificial culture	±	Local lesion	Very rare	S	37
M. kansasii	Environment	+ +	Tuberculosis-like	No	S	37
M. scrofulaceum	Environment	+	Lymphadenitis	No	S	37
M. avium-intracellulare	Environment; birds	+	Tuberculosis-like *or* disseminated disease in AIDS	No	S	37
M. fortuitum	Environment	±	Skin abscesses	No	F	37
M. marinum	Water, fish	±	Skin granuloma	No	S	30
M. ulcerans	Probably environment; tropical	+	Skin ulcerations	No	S	30
M. leprae	Human	+ + +	Leprosy	Yes	None	Not applicable

[a]This table omits many essentially saprophytic mycobacteria.
S, slow; F, fast.

Acid Fastness: A Hallmark of Mycobacteria

Mycobacteria have the unusual property of retaining basic dyes when treated with acidic solutions. This property is a consequence of the mycobacterial envelope, which contains waxes composed of long-chain branched hydrocarbons. The most abundant wax, **mycolic acid,** is an α-alkyl-β-hydroxy fatty acid covalently linked to the cell wall. The name *Mycobacteria* reflects the presence of mycolic acid in the organisms. The waxy barrier greatly reduces permeability to many molecules, including Gram stain, and mycobacteria are neither Gram-positive nor Gram-negative. They can, however, be stained with special techniques such as briefly heating in the presence of a basic red dye called fuchsin. In some cases, detergent is added to the stain. The specimen is then treated with 3% hydrochloric acid in ethanol, which decolorizes nearly all organisms except mycobacteria (thus, they are **acid fast**). The smear is then counterstained with a blue dye to provide a contrasting background. Mycobacteria appear as slender red rods. **Fluorochrome dyes** are commonly used instead of fuchsin because they are more easily detected by fluorescence microscopy. The principle of staining with fluorochrome is otherwise similar to staining with fuchsin.

The waxy coat makes *M. tuberculosis* **resistant to drying** and to chemicals, which helps them survive both inside and outside the body. They are unusually resistant to killing by phagocytes. The resistance of mycobacteria to drying also facilitates airborne transmission. Their waxy coat does not, however, help them withstand heat.

For instance, in milk the bacteria are killed by **pasteurization** (heating to 60°C for 30 minutes).

Slow Growth

Mycobacteria grow much more slowly than most other bacterial pathogens. The generation time of *M. tuberculosis* is 15 to 20 hours compared with less than 1 hour for most bacterial pathogens. Because of this long generation time, visible growth on solid media may take up to 6 weeks. Some mycobacteria grow faster than *M. tuberculosis* but still more slowly than other bacteria. Slow growth may delay diagnosis by culture methods alone. Even using specialized liquid broth media, detection can take 2 weeks or longer. Testing for drug susceptibility requires additional time after the organism is recovered in culture. Thus, the patient who appropriately initiates therapy based on a positive sputum smear showing acid-fast organisms may wait many weeks before knowing whether the organism is susceptible to the prescribed antimicrobials.

ENCOUNTER AND ENTRY

Almost all tuberculous infections result from inhaling infectious particles that were aerosolized by coughing, sneezing, or talking. The initial source is the lung in almost all cases. These so-called **droplet nuclei** dry while airborne, can remain suspended for hours, and when inhaled can reach the terminal air passages (Fig. 23-3). A cough or sneeze can produce thousands of droplet nuclei, as can talking for several minutes. Accordingly, the **air in a room occupied by a person with pulmonary tuberculosis may remain infectious even after the person has left the room.** Fortunately, prolonged exposure and multiple aerosol inocula are generally required to establish infection. Brief contact carries little risk, and infection rarely occurs outdoors. Large drops of respiratory secretions or contaminated inanimate objects are unimportant in transmission. In the past, tuberculosis of the intestine or the tonsils was common from ingestion of contaminated milk. This was caused by *M. bovis,* an organism that is genetically similar to *M. tuberculosis* and causes infection in cattle.

Airborne spread of tuberculosis is efficient for several reasons. In source cases the host inflammatory response to tuberculosis creates open lung lesions (**pulmonary cavities**) that contain huge numbers of organisms. Coughing spreads the organisms from such lesions into the air. Contagiousness roughly correlates with the number of acid-fast bacilli visible by microscopy of sputum. Many new infections, however, are acquired from smear-negative but culture-positive cases, reflecting the limited sensitivity of acid-fast staining. The small size of droplet nuclei is also ideal for bypassing the mucociliary lining of large airways to reach the alveoli.

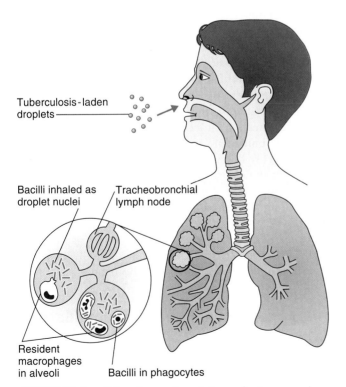

Tuberculosis-laden droplets

Bacilli inhaled as droplet nuclei

Tracheobronchial lymph node

Resident macrophages in alveoli

Bacilli in phagocytes

FIGURE 23-3 ▪ *Mycobacterium tuberculosis* transmission by inhalation of droplet nuclei.

SPREAD, MULTIPLICATION, AND DAMAGE

Tubercle bacilli do not produce exotoxins or endotoxin. Instead, the clinical manifestations of tuberculosis result largely from the host immune response. Damage is caused by chronic inflammation and survival of organisms within macrophages.

Primary Tuberculosis

In **primary infection,** airborne droplet nuclei reach the alveoli where multiplication begins. This primary infection usually involves the middle lung zone, where airflow is greatest. There the bacteria are ingested by alveolar macrophages, which may eliminate small numbers of bacilli. However, *M. tuberculosis* multiplies mostly unimpeded, destroying the macrophage (Fig. 23-4). Its ability to multiply both inside and outside cells makes *M. tuberculosis* a **facultative intracellular pathogen.** Lymphocytes and monocytes are attracted from the bloodstream, the latter differentiating into macrophages, which ingest bacilli released from dying cells. Infected macrophages are carried by lymphatics to regional lymph nodes. Some individuals develop the so-called **Ghon complex,** in which an area of lung inflammation is associated with enlarged hilar lymph nodes draining the area. In the nonimmune host, organisms may spread hematogenously throughout the body. During this early **lymphohematogenous dissemination,** the organisms preferentially localize in certain tissues, including lymph nodes, vertebral bodies, and meninges but most importantly the apices (upper parts) of the lungs. During the days and weeks before an effective cellular immune response develops, the organisms grow uninhibited in the initial pulmonary focus and the additional sites.

Primary infection can have various outcomes (Fig. 23-5). Cellular immunity and tissue hypersensitivity usually appear 3 to 8 weeks after infection and are marked by a positive tuberculin skin test (discussed later in the chapter). In most affected individuals this response controls infection (although viable organisms may persist in the tissues), no symptoms develop, and the only evidence of infection is a positive tuberculin skin test. However, in some cases the immune response does not control the primary infection, and progressive primary tuberculosis develops. This manifestation usually affects the very young, the elderly, and patients with advanced AIDS. In such individuals the primary focus directly progresses to worsening pneumonia, and the very young may develop tuberculous meningitis. The most important consequence of lymphohematogenous dissemination is seeding of the lung apices, where either progressive primary or secondary disease can occur.

In persons with immunity from previous exposure to *M. tuberculosis,* organisms in newly inhaled droplet nuclei are destroyed before significant multiplication occurs. Nearly all tuberculosis in previously infected patients is the result of endogenous reactivation. However, when the airborne inoculum is large, or when host defenses are compromised, exogenous reinfection can occur.

Age influences the course of infection. Infants and children younger than 5 years of age who become infected are at high risk for developing progressive primary disease. In contrast, from age 5 to puberty is a period of relative resistance to progressive disease, although not to infection. From puberty until young adulthood, formation of apical cavities soon after primary infection is common. Most disease in this age group is caused by relatively recent infection rather than reactivation of childhood infection. Infection in mid-adulthood has a much better immediate and probably long-term prognosis, presumably because of a reduced tendency to tissue necrosis. In the elderly, infection acquired years earlier can progress as age compromises immunity, leading to production of apical pulmonary cavities. In elderly persons who lack preexisting immunity to tuberculosis, new infection can cause progressive primary disease resembling primary infection in children, with involvement of lower or middle lobes and often without cavities.

Endogenous Reactivation (Secondary Tuberculosis)

Endogenous reactivation usually occurs within 2 years after initial infection but can occur any time thereafter (see Fig. 23-5). Clearly, any impairment of the cellular immune system can render a person vulnerable to

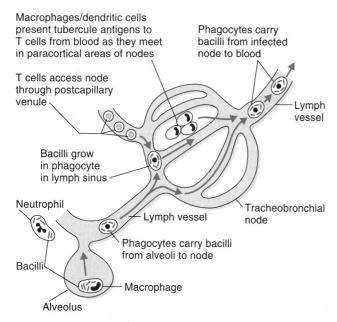

Macrophages/dendritic cells present tubercule antigens to T cells from blood as they meet in paracortical areas of nodes

T cells access node through postcapillary venule

Phagocytes carry bacilli from infected node to blood

Lymph vessel

Bacilli grow in phagocyte in lymph sinus

Neutrophil

Lymph vessel

Tracheobronchial node

Phagocytes carry bacilli from alveoli to node

Bacilli

Macrophage

Alveolus

FIGURE 23-4 ▪ *M. tuberculosis* multiplication in alveolar macrophages and spread to lymph nodes and beyond.

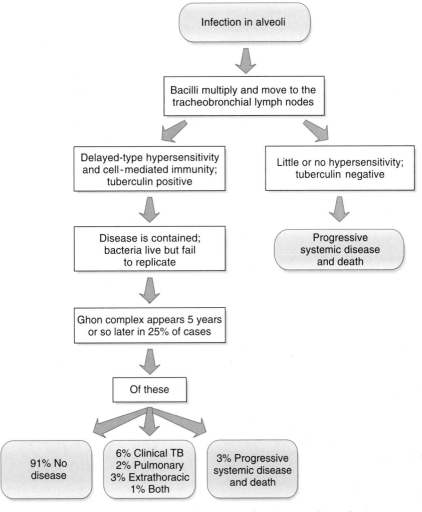

FIGURE 23-5 ▪ Outcomes of untreated primary tuberculosis.

reactivation of latent mycobacteria. Subtle depression of the immune system resulting from stress or hormonal factors may go undetected. Other factors include malnutrition, therapy with corticosteroids or other immunosuppressive drugs, malignancy, and end-stage renal disease. Worldwide the most important cause of reactivation is coinfection with HIV. The higher frequency of certain histocompatibility types (i.e., human leukocyte antigen, or HLA) in persons who develop active tuberculosis suggests a genetic predisposition. The disease may reactivate in the elderly because of poorly understood loss of immune competence that can occur with aging. In addition, local physical disturbance at the site of a latent focus can alter the balance between host and pathogen. For example, lung surgery can disturb quiescent pulmonary foci and cause active tuberculosis at that site.

The most common site of reactivation is **the apex of the lung** (see Fig. 23-1). Lesions slowly become necrotic, undergo **caseous necrosis** (named for its cheesy appearance), and eventually merge into larger lesions. With time the caseous lesions liquefy and discharge their contents into bronchi. This event has several major consequences. It creates a well-aerated cavity in which the organisms proliferate. The discharge of caseous material also distributes the organisms to other sites in the lung, which can lead to a rapidly progressive **tuberculous pneumonia.** In addition, the bacteria-laden contents of caseous lesions are coughed up and become infectious droplet nuclei. Although the reason for the apical pulmonary localization is not known with certainty, it is likely that deficient lymphatic flow at the apices, where the pumping effect of respiratory motion is minimal, favors retention of organisms. When hypersensitivity develops, tissue damage creates apical cavities characteristic of pulmonary tuberculosis in adults.

Immune Response

Tuberculosis requires a cellular immune response for control, with antibodies playing no apparent role. In the first few weeks after exposure, the host has almost no immune defense against *M. tuberculosis,* and small inhaled inocula multiply freely in alveolar spaces or within alveolar macrophages. Entry into macrophages involves interactions with complement receptors, mannose receptors, and Fc receptors. Once inside the cell, mycobacteria increase their chance of survival by preventing acidification of the phagolysosome. Unrestrained replication proceeds for weeks, both in the initial focus and in metastatic foci, until tissue hypersensitivity and cellular immunity supervene. This tissue hypersensitivity is florid compared with other intracellular infections.

All persons have CD4$^+$ lymphocytes that can recognize mycobacterial antigens if processed and presented by macrophages in the context of major histocompatibility complex class II proteins. When the lymphocyte encounters antigen in this manner, it is activated and proliferates, producing a clone of similarly reactive lymphocytes. These in turn produce many distinct lymphokines that attract, retain, and activate macrophages at the site of antigen. Activated macrophages accumulate lytic enzymes and reactive metabolites that increase their ability to kill mycobacteria, but if released into surrounding tissues, these macrophage products can cause necrosis.

When the population of activated lymphocytes reaches a certain size, cutaneous delayed-type hypersensitivity to tuberculin becomes manifest. This response generally takes 3 to 8 weeks. At the same time, enhanced macrophage microbicidal activity, or cellular immunity, appears.

The pathologic features of tuberculosis are the result of hypersensitivity to mycobacterial antigens. The classic tissue response involves organization of macrophages, Langhans giant cells, and lymphocytes resulting in formation of **granulomas** (sometimes called tubercles). This pattern constitutes a successful tissue reaction with containment of infection, healing with eventual fibrosis, encapsulation, and scar formation. However, with time the centers of the tubercles may become necrotic. Necrosis in tuberculosis tends to be incomplete, resulting in semisolid caseous material. Caseous necrosis is unstable, especially in the lungs, where it tends to liquefy and discharge through the bronchial tree, producing a cavity and providing conditions in which bacteria multiply to very high numbers.

Sustained immunity to new infection that follows natural infection is likely the result of persistent viable tubercle bacilli in the tissues with in vivo boosting. However, reactivation disease may arise from these sites. Activation of monocytes with tumor necrosis factor-α (TNF-α) effectively inhibits intracellular replication of *M. tuberculosis*. An effective response to *M. tuberculosis* tends to follow a Th1 CD4$^+$ T cell pattern with preferential expression of interferon-γ, interleukin 2 (IL-2), and IL-12 by mononuclear cells. Although activated macrophages usually kill intracellular bacteria, intracellular mycobacteria may persist. An uneasy equilibrium is reached; some macrophages kill the organisms, others are themselves killed and release their bacterial contents,

and still others harbor dormant bacteria for long periods. Proteolytic processing of killed bacteria leads to continued immunological stimulation.

Immunocompromised persons may not contain the primary infection, and organisms may invade the bloodstream and disseminate to cause a life-threatening infection known as **miliary tuberculosis.** The term *miliary* is derived from the resemblance of the tubercles to millet seeds (bird seed). Characteristic of the disease are tubercles found in many organs, including the liver, spleen, kidneys, brain, and meninges. Caseation and cavitation are less frequent than in secondary tuberculosis.

The involvement of macrophages in the containment of *M. tuberculosis* comes at a price. Two cytokines produced by these cells, **IL-1** and **TNF-α** (see Chapter 6), contribute to the symptoms of the disease. Among their various activities, these cytokines mediate **fever, weight loss, and night sweats.** In response to the carbohydrates, lipids, and proteins of the tubercle bacilli, macrophages also produce many other cytokines that modulate the immune response. In particular, increased production of IL-10 may suppress the immune response and promote disease progression. The net effects of these complex events are the local pathological manifestations of tuberculosis, including caseous necrosis and fibrosis with **calcification.**

Delayed-Type Hypersensitivity and the Tuberculin Skin Test

Immunological reactivity to tuberculosis can be demonstrated by tuberculin skin testing. This test involves the intradermal injection of proteins, or **tuberculin,** from tubercle bacilli. The material used is a poorly defined mixture known as **purified protein derivative (PPD).** A positive reaction is indicated by thickening (induration) of the skin several days after inoculation, which results from infiltration by mononuclear phagocytes and T cells. This **delayed-type hypersensitivity** reaction recapitulates the local events that take place in the lung and other infected tissue. Depending on the site of the reaction, delayed-type hypersensitivity may account for diverse manifestations, such as pleurisy with effusion (the sometimes massive accumulation of exudate in the pleural cavities) or the sudden inflammation of the meninges. Surprisingly few tubercle bacilli are present in the pleural fluid or cerebrospinal fluid during these infections, but they are able to cause considerable inflammation.

The tuberculin skin test is most useful for diagnosing latent tuberculous infection. It is especially useful in places like the United States where tuberculosis is relatively uncommon. The test is much less useful in countries where most of the population is tuberculin positive or has received the bacille Calmette-Guérin (BCG) vaccine (discussed later in the chapter). A newly positive test after a previous negative test (**tuberculin conversion**) indicates recent tuberculous infection and is an indication for chemoprophylaxis. Medical personnel who may have contact with infected patients are at increased risk of becoming infected and are regularly tested for skin test conversion.

There are caveats regarding the tuberculin test. About 15% of individuals with active tuberculosis have negative tuberculin tests. In some cases this tuberculin negativity appears to be specific for *M. tuberculosis* because reactivity to other skin test antigens (e.g., candida, mumps, or tetanus) is preserved. Soon after effective antituberculous therapy is initiated, the tuberculin test usually becomes positive as general overall health improves. Importantly, many immunocompromised patients with tuberculous infection (especially those with AIDS) have negative tuberculin tests. These individuals often lack skin test reactivity to other antigens. Thus, a negative tuberculin skin test does not exclude active tuberculosis. Conversely, a false-positive tuberculin test may be caused by exposure to atypical mycobacteria, although in such cases the diameter of induration is usually small.

CLINICAL MANIFESTATIONS

Tuberculosis is insidious. Most people are unaware of their initial encounter with the organism. However, some persons, particularly the very young, the elderly, and those who are immunocompromised, may not develop sufficient cellular immunity to contain the organisms and develop disseminated tuberculosis (see Fig. 23-5). This rampant infection differs from endogenous reactivation (although it sometimes occurs in patients with secondary tuberculosis).

Endogenous reactivation can affect virtually any organ in the body. However, the most common manifestation of tuberculosis in adults is a chronic pneumonia that characteristically forms cavities in the apex of the lung. Persistent fever, weight loss, and drenching night sweats are common during tuberculosis. *M. tuberculosis* also can affect vertebral bodies (**Pott disease**), in which patients present with chronic back pain. Failure to diagnose and treat Pott disease can result in destruction of vertebrae and permanent disability. Painless enlargement of lymph nodes resulting from infection by *M. tuberculosis* can affect virtually any region of the body. Less common manifestations include chronic inflammation of the meninges, pericardium, peritoneal cavity, or adrenal glands.

Considering that tissue damage is caused by the immune response to *M. tuberculosis,* one might ask which is worse: a robust cell-mediated immune response or no immune response at all. Effective immunologic control of tuberculosis is a matter of balance. Without cellular immunity and delayed hypersensitivity, caseous necrosis would not develop, but the tubercle bacilli would proliferate unchecked. The result could be miliary tuberculosis, a disease that can kill much more rapidly than chronic pulmonary tuberculosis. For example, the loss of CD4$^+$ T cells as a result of HIV infection leads to rapid progression of tuberculosis and death. In addition, persons with AIDS may not develop the lesions typical of reactivation tuberculosis. Thus, the immune response contains the disease, even if it eventually causes damage. In fact, the body relies on two defensive strategies: one involves the antimicrobial action of activated macrophages, and the other consists of walling off and containing the lesion by fibrosis and calcification. In short, defense mechanisms provide lifelong control of infection in most individuals.

DIAGNOSIS

The diagnosis of asymptomatic tuberculous infection is usually based on tuberculin skin test results. In contrast, active disease is usually diagnosed by acid-fast staining and culture of sputum or affected tissues.

The initial diagnostic approach includes a careful history, direct examination of sputum or exudates, and a chest radiograph (see Fig. 23-1). Direct examination of sputum can yield a rapid presumptive diagnosis. Importantly, contagiousness correlates with sputum smear positivity. Acid-fast stains are rapid and relatively sensitive, especially with cavitary pulmonary tuberculosis (Fig. 23-6). The yield increases by examining sputa collected on three separate days. Early morning sputa have the best yields because pulmonary secretions accumulate during sleep.

The **gold standard** for diagnosis of tuberculosis is **culture.** Sputum from some patients with active tuberculosis but too few organisms to detect microscopically may have positive cultures. Detection of colonies on solid media usually takes 3 to 6 weeks. **Radiometric culture techniques** accelerate the diagnosis by early

FIGURE 23-6 ▪ Acid-fast stain of *M. tuberculosis* from a pulmonary cavity.

detection of radioactive CO_2 released by organisms metabolizing ^{14}C-labeled palmitic acid, providing results within 7 to 14 days. If growth of tubercle bacilli occurs, it is important to test for antibiotic susceptibility. Overall, the process may take 6 or more weeks. More sensitive nucleic acid amplification methods for rapid diagnosis are occasionally used in practice but have not replaced smear and culture.

What other infections can resemble tuberculosis? There are many, as shown in Table 23-2. They include those caused by the atypical mycobacteria such as *Mycobacterium avium* complex (MAC) and *M. kansasii*. Disease caused by these organisms tends to be less severe and more indolent. MAC causes disseminated illness during advanced AIDS. Other diseases in the differential diagnosis of tuberculosis are those caused by actinomycetes, nocardia, and systemic fungi.

TREATMENT

Excellent drugs are available for treating tuberculosis. These include **isoniazid (INH)**, **rifampin**, **pyrazinamide (PZA)**, and **ethambutol**. Persons with pulmonary tuberculosis usually become noncontagious within 2 weeks of therapy if the organisms are sensitive to the drugs administered. Unlike most bacterial infections that can be cured with a single drug, **active tuberculosis requires multiple drugs for cure** because of the remarkable propensity of the organism to **develop resistance**. In any population of tubercle bacilli, chromosomal mutations associated with resistance to any single drug are already present in about one of every 10^6 to 10^7 bacteria, even though the organisms have never been exposed to the drug. Because tuberculous cavities can contain in excess of 10^{11} organisms, many of the bacteria present will be resistant to any single drug, even before treatment is begun. In fact, some organisms will be resistant to drugs that are yet to be developed.

Fortunately, the chance that one organism will become resistant to two drugs simultaneously is small. Prescribing multiple drugs in combination therefore prevents resistance. Unfortunately, adherence with complex and prolonged treatment regimens is difficult. If treatment is sporadic, **multidrug-resistant strains** can emerge, making treatment more difficult or impossible. Spread of such strains to other individuals can be catastrophic. For this reason, directly observed therapy for tuberculosis has become the standard of care, with every dose directly administered by a health care provider, usually a public health worker.

Prescribing multiple drugs also allows a shorter duration of therapy. In cases of drug-sensitive tuberculosis, 18 months of INH plus ethambutol was once required for cure. In the 1970s it was discovered that including rifampin in the regimen allowed therapy to be shortened to 9 months. Later it was discovered that adding PZA

allowed cure in 6 months. In the United States individuals at risk for exposure to tuberculosis (e.g., health care professionals as well as medical students, interns, and residents) are routinely screened for tuberculin conversion. INH is administered to persons who convert to a positive reaction, which indicates recent infection. Such treatment of latent infection is called **chemoprophylaxis**. Unlike treating active tuberculosis, chemoprophylaxis requires only a single drug (e.g., INH) because there are so few organisms that it is highly unlikely that resistant organisms will be present.

PREVENTION

The history of tuberculosis suggests that improving the standard of living decreases rates of disease. In many resource-limited countries, that is unfortunately not a reality. Currently, an effective vaccine made from killed *M. tuberculosis* does not exist. The immunology of tuberculosis tells us why: killed vaccines may generate antibodies, but humoral immunity does not protect against tuberculosis. Cell-mediated immune responses are best elicited when antigens are presented by live organisms.

The **bacille Calmette-Guérin (BCG) vaccine** is a strain of *M. bovis* made relatively avirulent (attenuated) by multiple passages in culture. It is routinely given to newborns and small children in many countries, including those with limited resources. Administering BCG vaccine causes tuberculin skin test positivity, a criterion for a successful "take" of the immunization. Long-term persistence of tuberculin positivity varies depending on the patient's age at BCG vaccination; the earlier the vaccination, the less durable the skin test positivity. Because BCG-induced tuberculin positivity would decrease the value of tuberculin skin testing to diagnose new infections, BCG is not used in the United States. The safety and immunogenicity of BCG also make it a potential vector to deliver protective antigens from other pathogenic organisms. Genes for such antigens have been introduced into BCG to generate "multivaccines" that might protect against multiple pathogens.

Mycobacterium leprae

Leprosy is the disease caused by *M. leprae*. It shares some pathobiological features with tuberculosis, but it differs in its clinical manifestations. Leprosy has historically been more feared and resulted in more social stigmatization than other infectious diseases. Because the skin lesions of leprosy are often obvious, persons with this disease were once vehemently shunned, even though leprosy is much less contagious than tuberculosis. Although rare in the United States, leprosy is still important worldwide. An estimated 6 million people have leprosy, mainly in tropical, resource-limited countries, where the disease causes economic loss and human suffering.

The mode of transmission of *M. leprae* is not certain. Leprosy is clearly communicable, and acquisition requires prolonged contact with infectious cases. With skin involvement as a major feature, leprosy was once thought to be transmitted by contact with skin lesions. However, persons with leprosy shed *M. leprae* in their nasal secretions, and it is now thought that the disease is transmitted by the airborne route. Because leprosy is primarily a rural and not an urban disease, transmission by soil also has been suggested.

The study of *M. leprae* is difficult because **the organism cannot be continuously grown in vitro.** *M. leprae* was one of the first microbes to be linked to a human disease. In 1873 G. A. Hansen discovered *M. leprae* in lesions of leprosy patients. In recognition of this discovery, leprosy is often called **Hansen disease.** It was not until 1960 that researchers discovered that *M. leprae* can grow in the footpads of mice. Even there, it grows very slowly (doubling once every 14 days), and yields of the organisms are low. In 1970 *M. leprae* was found to naturally infect the nine-banded armadillo, where it grows to more than 10^{10} bacilli per gram of tissue. In fact, 15% of wild armadillos in Louisiana and Texas are infected with *M. leprae.* This finding revolutionized leprosy research because it provided sufficient quantities of the organism for basic studies. Many genes encoding important *M. leprae* antigens have since been cloned and expressed in *Escherichia coli* and other organisms, providing novel reagents to study the host immune response.

M. leprae, like *M. tuberculosis* and MAC, survives and multiplies within macrophages. This mycobacterium has an arsenal of defenses to escape killing by phagocytes. For example, **phenolic glycolipid,** a surface lipid of *M. leprae,* has been implicated as a defense against oxidative killing. To exert their maximal killing potential, macrophages must be activated by cytokines produced by CD4$^+$ T cells.

Leprosy bacilli grow best at low temperatures. Accordingly, they multiply most rapidly in the skin, nose, and other superficial tissues. Clinical leprosy ranges between two polar forms, tuberculoid and lepromatous. The prognosis of leprosy has dramatically improved with the introduction of effective drugs like **dapsone, rifampin,** and **clofazimine.**

Tuberculoid Leprosy

Tuberculoid leprosy is often characterized by red blotchy lesions with localized anesthesia (loss of sensation) on the face, trunk, and extremities. The organisms grow and cause thickening in nerve sheaths. These thickened nerves can be felt through the skin, a characteristic of leprosy. Such patients usually demonstrate delayed-type hyper-

sensitivity to **lepromin** (the *M. leprae* equivalent of tuberculin) prepared from infected tissues. Patients with tuberculoid leprosy have a vigorous cell-mediated immune response to *M. leprae,* which mediates the nerve damage, but few acid-fast bacilli can be found in the tuberculoid lesion.

Tuberculoid leprosy is analogous to secondary tuberculosis in that it invokes a vigorous cell-mediated immune response and tissue hypersensitivity. The prognosis with tuberculoid leprosy is better than with lepromatous leprosy, and in some cases tuberculoid leprosy is a self-limiting disease.

Lepromatous Leprosy

M. leprae can reduce or suppress the number of specific T cells produced by the host that can activate the infected macrophages and provide cell-mediated immunity. **In lepromatous leprosy there is little or no delayed-type hypersensitivity to lepromin.** This lack of cellular immunity is associated with enormous numbers of *M. leprae* in the skin and superficial nerves. The number of bacilli harbored by a lepromatous patient (10^{15}) is far greater than in any other human disease. Both **skin and nerves may be involved.** With time, the loss of local sensation leads to inadvertent, traumatic lesions of the face and extremities. These may become secondarily infected, resulting in additional disfigurement.

Lepromatous leprosy is the more debilitating form of the disease. Pathogenically, it is analogous to systemic, progressive (miliary) tuberculosis, in which the organisms grow profusely. In both diseases the cell-mediated immune response is weak. It is not clear why cell-mediated immunity is decreased in persons with leprosy. The infecting organisms may play a role in this immunosuppression, and host genetic factors may also be involved. For example, it appears that persons belonging to the histocompatibility haplotype HLA-DR3 are more likely to develop tuberculoid leprosy, whereas those with the HLA-MT1 class are more likely to develop lepromatous leprosy.

Conclusion

Tuberculosis is one of the most important diseases in the world. Tissue damage occurs primarily because of exuberant hypersensitivity to the organism. The tubercle bacillus has a waxy coat, grows very slowly, and is a highly successful intracellular pathogen. Clinical manifestations differ between the initial and subsequent encounters with the organism. It may not cause illness in the infected individual for many years, if at all. In the absence of HIV infection or other immunocompromising illness, a pivotal event in the pathogenesis of tuberculosis is the formation of a pulmonary cavity, where organisms grow to huge numbers, ensuring airborne spread and increasing the chance of transmission. Although the availability of effective antituberculous drugs once raised hope of eliminating tuberculosis, the AIDS pandemic and increasing drug resistance has made this unrealistic in the foreseeable future.

Leprosy is rare in the United States but still a significant problem in many countries. Studying *M. leprae* is particularly difficult because it cannot be cultivated in vitro. The two polar forms of leprosy are tuberculoid and lepromatous. Tuberculoid leprosy is characterized by a vigorous cell-mediated immune response with few organisms present. In contrast, lepromatous leprosy is associated with diminished delayed-type hypersensitivity to *M. leprae* and enormous numbers of organisms. Fortunately, there are now effective drugs for treating leprosy.

Treponema palladium and Syphilis: A Disease With a History

John R. Ebright and Jack D. Sobel

key **concepts**

Syphilis:

■ Is caused by the spirochete *Treponema palladium.*

■ Is most commonly acquired by sexual contact.

■ Is characterized by three stages: primary syphilis, in which the organism is localized to a chancre, or skin lesion; secondary syphilis, in which the organism disseminates to distant sites; and tertiary syphilis, in which the immune response to the organisms leads to the destruction of tissue.

■ Can be transmitted from mother to fetus (congenital syphilis).

■ Is initially diagnosed by tests such as the Venereal Disease Reference Laboratory Test (VDRL); positive results should be confirmed with more specific tests.

■ Is readily treated with penicillin.

The agent of syphilis, *Treponema pallidum*, although most commonly acquired by sexual contact, can be transmitted from an infected mother to her fetus, causing congenital syphilis. The disease has often occupied center stage in the history of medicine (see box, "For One Small Pleasure I Suffer a Thousand Misfortunes"). A recent resurgence of syphilis in select populations within the United States has once again focused attention on this ancient infectious disease. Syphilis is a multistage disease, and each stage has a dramatically different clinical presentation. The first two stages (**primary and secondary**) manifest as acute and subacute disease respectively, whereas **tertiary syphilis** is a chronic disease that lasts many years.

T. pallidum, a **spirochete,** cannot be cultured in artificial media and does not produce toxins. In fact, it is not known how *T. pallidum* causes disease. Nevertheless, scientific observations are beginning to elucidate why the organism is able to escape the immune system and how it induces disease. Fortunately, *T. pallidum* remains sensitive to penicillin, which is why the disease is easily treatable today.

Case

Mr. W., a homosexual 24-year-old, came to the clinic with fever, swollen lymph nodes, and spotty discolorations of his skin, most notably on the palms of his hands and soles of his feet. He had recently noted a penny-sized, gray, translucent lesion on the inner aspect of his lower lip. The physician recognized the macular rash on the palms and soles and the lesion on his lip as characteristic of secondary syphilis. Mr. W. reported that he engages in oral sex as well as anal-receptive intercourse.

A scraping of Mr. W.'s lip lesion was examined under a darkfield microscope, revealing the presence of large numbers of corkscrew-shaped spirochetes. The laboratory reported positive serology, indicating the presence of the characteristic serum antibodies to *T. pallidum*. These laboratory findings confirmed the diagnosis of secondary syphilis. Because his sexual behavior put him at high risk of other sexually transmitted diseases, Mr. W. consented to a serum test for the presence of antibodies to HIV. He was serologically negative for HIV at that time. Mr. W. was treated with a course of penicillin, and his lesions and symptoms abated. He was considered cured because his syphilis serologic titers (the level of antibodies in serum) declined over months.

This case raises several questions:

1. Is it possible that Mr. W. was not aware of having had a chancre before presenting with secondary syphilis?
2. How did the spirochetes travel from the chancre to Mr. W.'s skin, lower lip, and lymph nodes?
3. Are the clinical features of secondary syphilis (rash, swollen lymph nodes, and mucous membrane lesions) fully explained by spirochetes invading Mr. W.'s skin, lymph nodes, and lower lip? What host factors may be contributing to the disease process?
4. Are the skin lesions and mouth lesions infective? Could another person acquire syphilis by touching them?
5. What would have happened to Mr. W.'s skin rash, lip lesion, and swollen lymph nodes if he had not received prompt treatment with antibiotics?

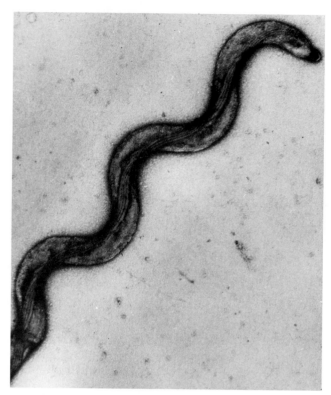

FIGURE 24-1 ■ **Electron photomicrograph of *Treponema pallidum*, negatively stained.** At the dark end of the organism are the insertion points of the periplasmic flagella (ropelike contractile structures), which enable the organisms to engage in their typical corkscrewlike motility.

diseases pose no medical problem in the United States, a person who acquires one of them in a tropical country may develop positive serologic tests for syphilis that remain positive for life.

T. pallidum is too narrow (0.1 to 0.2 μm) to be seen by standard microscopic techniques. It can be visualized by special stains (silver impregnation or immunofluorescence) or with special lighting (**darkfield microscopy**). When observed in a freshly prepared wet mount using a darkfield microscope, it exhibits a characteristic **corkscrewlike movement and flexion.** The organisms resemble Gram-negative bacteria in that they have an outer membrane that, although lipid rich, does not contain lipopolysaccharide. Unlike the flagella of other bacteria, which protrude freely into the medium, those of spirochetes are contained within the periplasm.

Understanding of the mechanisms by which *T. pallidum* causes disease has been limited both by the inability to cultivate the organisms serially in artificial media and by the lack of a suitable animal model. In artificial media, these bacteria can be kept alive for only short periods (a few divisions at most). To bypass these constraints, research efforts have focused on producing and characterizing specific proteins of *T. pallidum* using genes cloned into *Escherichia coli*.

The agent of syphilis belongs to the genus *Treponema* and is a **spirochete,** a type of bacteria with a highly characteristic appearance. Spirochetes are helical, slender, and relatively long cells (Fig. 24-1). They are widespread in nature, but only a few cause disease in humans and animals. The principal human spirochetoses are syphilis, Lyme disease (see Chapter 25), relapsing fever (caused by members of the genus *Borrelia*), and leptospirosis (caused by members of the genus *Leptospira*). Other organisms of the genus *Treponema* cause rare diseases such as yaws, pinta, and bejel found mostly in tropical countries. Although these exotic

Treponema pallidum

ENCOUNTER, ENTRY, SPREAD, AND MULTIPLICATION

T. pallidum is sensitive to drying, disinfectants, and heat (as low as 42°C). Therefore, the bacteria are unlikely to be acquired by means other than personal contact. The two major routes of transmission are **sexual** and **transplacental.** Sexual exposure to a person who has an active syphilitic chancre carries a high probability of acquiring syphilis.

The organisms enter a susceptible host through the mucous membranes or the minute abrasions in the skin surface that occur during sexual intercourse. Once in the subepithelial tissues, the organisms replicate locally in an extracellular location (Fig. 24-2). In culture, they adhere to cells by their tapered ends and probably stick to cells in tissue by the same means. Not all of them stick, and many are soon carried through lymphatic channels to the systemic circulation. Thus, even if the initial manifestation of the disease consists of an isolated skin lesion, syphilis is a systemic disease almost from the outset.

Treponemes can cross the placental barrier from the bloodstream of an infected mother and cause disease in the fetus. It is not known how the organisms cross this barrier (Chapter 72 provides a general discussion of this issue).

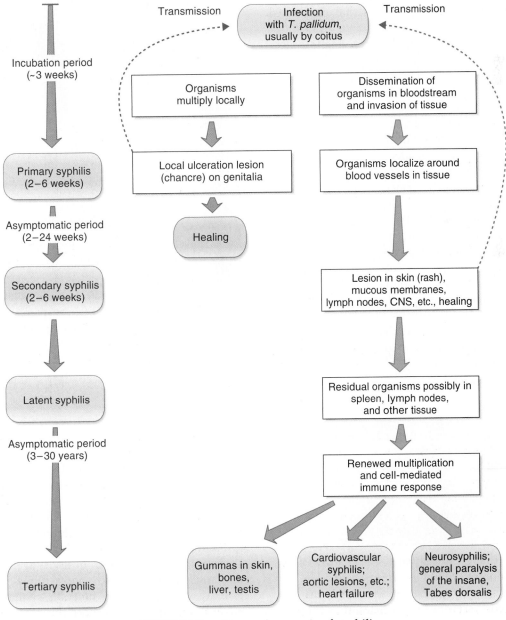

FIGURE 24-2 ■ **The pathogenesis of syphilis.**

DAMAGE

Primary Syphilis

Initially, neutrophils migrate to the area of inoculation and are later replaced by plasma cells, lymphocytes, and macrophages. The result of the battle between the locally replicating treponemes and the cellular defenses of the host is the lesion of primary syphilis, the **syphilitic chancre** (Fig. 24-3). The chancre is painless. The time between the initial introduction of the organisms and the appearance of the ulcer depends on the size of the inoculum. The larger the size of the inoculum, the earlier the chancre appears. This lesion heals spontaneously within 26 weeks, but by that time the spirochetes have spread through the bloodstream and may cause lesions in other parts of the body. These diverse lesions comprise the cluster of findings that characterize "secondary syphilis," such as that manifested in Mr. W.

The syphilitic chancre and other genital ulcer diseases are associated with increased risk of HIV transmission. Patients who have genital ulcers are estimated to have a three- to fivefold increased risk of acquiring HIV infection. Furthermore, recent studies have demonstrated that HIV can be isolated from genital ulcers, which increases the likelihood of transmitting the virus. The possible role of genital ulcers in facilitating the transmission of HIV underscores the importance of recognizing and promptly treating primary syphilis, chancroid, or herpes.

Three to six weeks after the ulcer heals, the secondary form of the disease occurs in about 50% of infected individuals. **Secondary syphilis** results from the systemic spread of the infection when treponemes replicate in the lymph nodes, liver, joints, muscles, skin, and mucous membranes distant from the site of the primary chancre (Fig 24-4). The signs and symptoms of secondary syphilis can be so varied and involve such varying tissues and organs that the disease has been called "the Great Imitator." The rash and other

FIGURE 24-4 ▪ **Cutaneous lesions of secondary syphilis.** In addition to fever, headache, lymph node enlargement, and oral lesions, a scaly papular eruption involving the trunk and extremities, including palms and soles, is characteristic of secondary syphilis.

FIGURE 24-3 ▪ **Chancre of the penis.** The chancre is the first manifestation of syphilis in some patients. The lesion is painless and, on darkfield examination, has many motile "corkscrewing" spirochetes, thus confirming the diagnosis of syphilis.

manifestations of secondary syphilis resolve within weeks to months, but one fourth of affected individuals experience a recurrence of the secondary stage (relapse) within approximately 1 year or so (see Fig. 24-2).

This biphasic course of the disease is puzzling for several reasons. Researchers do not understand how spirochetes kill so many epidermal cells to create a chancre or how the ulcer heals. Why do the defense mechanisms that are so successful in resolving the primary chancre fail to function systemically during secondary syphilis? How does the organism survive in the body for long periods? Where are the organisms located, intracellularly or extracellularly? What is the role of the specific immune response in the disease process? These questions and others regarding additional aspects of syphilis are yet unanswered. It remains one of the more fascinating and puzzling of infectious diseases. However, a few clues are available. Recently, it has been demonstrated that *T. pallidum* contains a hundredfold fewer membrane-spanning proteins than the outer membrane of typical Gram-negative bacteria. This finding suggests that, in the case of *T. pallidum,* antibodies against surface proteins may not play their usual antimicrobial role. In addition, when the organism is isolated from tissues, it has been found to be coated with plasma proteins, which may play a protective role against human host defense mechanisms.

Tertiary Syphilis

The mystery deepens with the resolution of the secondary stage. In about one third of individuals, the organisms disappear and the person is spontaneously cured. In the remaining two thirds of individuals, the treponemes persist without causing signs or symptoms for years (**latent syphilis;** see Fig. 24-2). In about one half of this group, the manifestations of tertiary syphilis eventually develop, sometimes years or even decades after the primary infection.

In adults, **tertiary syphilis** is responsible for a majority of the morbidity and mortality associated with the disease. Fortunately, tertiary syphilis is uncommon in the United States, where routine serological screening identifies most cases before the stage develops. The hallmark of tertiary syphilis is the destruction of tissue caused by a response to the presence of treponemal antigens. This change manifests as **vasculitis** and **chronic inflammation.** Soft masses, or **gummas,** composed of few treponemes and inflammatory cells, are lesions that may destroy bone and soft tissue (**late benign syphilis**). However, the lesions can also involve vital organs, such as the liver. In cardiovascular syphilis, vasculitis involves the arteries (vasa vasorum) supplying the thoracic aorta. Destruction of the elastic tissue in the aorta media leads to dilatation of the wall and **aortic valve insufficiency** or to the formation of **aortic aneurysms** with resultant **rupture of the aorta.**

The central nervous system may also be involved, either by direct invasion of the parenchyma by treponemes or by brain infarction caused by vasculitis. The clinical findings of **neurosyphilis** can be subtle. The severity of signs and symptoms depends on the location of the lesions. Involvement of the dorsal columns of the spinal cord results in loss of position sensation, a classic condition known as **tabes dorsalis.** It often manifests as a staggering or **ataxic gait.** In turn, the loss of position sensation causes trauma in the knee and occasionally the ankle joints, which results in bone overgrowth and instability known as **Charcot joint.** A generalized involvement of the brain leads to impaired motor function (paresis) as well as to gradual loss of higher integrative functions and personality changes. This clinical picture is known as **general paresis** or paralysis of the insane. A physical sign of neurosyphilis is the **Argyll-Robertson pupil:** the pupil does not react to light but does contract when an object is moved from far to near the eye. If untreated, neurosyphilis can be fatal.

The lesions of tertiary syphilis usually contain few or no treponemes. What then accounts for the presence of lesions in the tissues? Researchers have demonstrated that the immune system likely plays a deleterious role in the development of the syphilitic lesions. Human cells exposed to treponemes in culture elaborate intercellular adhesion molecules (ICAMs), which facilitate the chemotaxis and attachment of inflammatory cells. Does this mobilization of inflammatory cells contribute to the disease? Further elucidation of this complex process awaits more research.

Congenital Syphilis

Despite serological tests that are readily available to detect syphilis as well as antibiotics available to treat the disease, thousands of babies are born with congenital syphilis in the United States each year (the exact figure is hard to come by). This number actually underrepresents the problem because the majority of infected fetuses likely die in utero. The manifestations of congenital syphilis are varied and include life-threatening organ damage, silent infections, congenital malformations, and developmental abnormalities. Congenital anomalies include **premature birth, intrauterine growth retardation,** and **multiple organ failure** (e.g., central nervous system infection, pneumonia, and enlargement of the liver and spleen). The most common manifestations of syphilis become evident at about 2 years of age and include **facial and tooth deformities** (the so-called **Hutchinson incisors** and **"mulberry" molars**). Other less common manifestations include **deafness, arthritis,** and **"saber shins."** Congenital syphilis is especially tragic because it is completely preventable by penicillin therapy early in the pregnancies of women with a positive serological test for syphilis. Prevention of congenital syphilis is one reason why prenatal care is essential.

DIAGNOSIS

In the past, physicians relied on the clinical signs and symptoms of the disease to make a diagnosis of syphilis. Therefore, only individuals with obvious skin or mucosal lesions were considered to have syphilis and thus received therapy. Patients with asymptomatic or latent

"For One Small Pleasure I Suffer a Thousand Misfortunes"

The route of the global spread of syphilis is a controversial subject that is not likely to be resolved. One view is that Christopher Columbus brought the syphilis agent back to Spain from the New World, because the first documented outbreaks of syphilis occurred in Europe shortly after Columbus's return. Whether or not Columbus's crew was the source of the outbreak, the spread of the disease through Europe was rapid and initially was accompanied by a high mortality rate. In 1494 King Charles VIII of France invaded Italy with an army of mercenaries from many countries, including Spain. Because the mercenaries initially saw little fighting, much of the campaign was spent consorting with female camp followers. In returning to their home countries, the mercenaries carried syphilis to all of Europe. Understandably, no country wanted to claim syphilis as its own:

> The Italians called it the Spanish or the French disease; the French called it the Italian or Neapolitan disease; the English called it the French disease; the Russians called it the Polish disease. And . . . the first Spaniards who recognized the disease called it the disease of Espaniola, which meant, at that time, the disease of Haiti.
>
> —Ludovico Moscardo, 1672, Haiti

Interestingly, it was the poet Fracastorius who gave the disease the name by which we know it today. Fracastorius's poem, *Syphilis Sive Morbus Gallicus,* published in 1530, assigned a nonpolitical name to the "venereal pox," that of the shepherd Syphilos. In 1575 the Renaissance surgeon Ambroise Paré referred to it as "Lues Venerea," the lover's plague.

During the sixteenth and seventeenth centuries, many clinical manifestations of syphilis were observed and catalogued. One of the most puzzling aspects of the disease is that within a few years of its emergence, it ceased to be a rapid killer and acquired the complex clinical manifestations that today characterize the disease (Fig. 24-5). The change in the organism's virulence, from high to moderate, supports the notion that the most successful pathogens do not kill their host. In fact, the less severe the symptoms, the less likely the pathogen will be eliminated. The epitome of this principle is the organism that causes asymptomatic disease, because the host is neither diagnosed nor treated. An organism that goes undetected is able to reproduce, and it is this ability and not the ability to cause disease that is the main selective force in nature. *T. pallidum* is particularly successful as a human parasite because it possesses,

FIGURE 24-5 ▪ In previous years syphilis stirred the imagination to extremes of gloom and hysteria. This French illustration ascribes to syphilis a degree of mortality that has not been seen since the advent of serological testing and penicillin therapy in the twentieth century.

among others, the following traits: spread by sexual transmission, efficient transmission from one adult to another (horizontal transmission), a long infectious period, transmission from mother to child (vertical transmission), long persistence in the host, and lethality usually only after decades of infection.

In general, sexually transmitted diseases do not "travel alone." Thus, early physicians found it difficult to separate the manifestations of one disease (e.g., gonorrhea) from another (syphilis) because one person might have both diseases simultaneously. Many physicians who studied these diseases thought that they

"For One Small Pleasure I Suffer a Thousand Misfortunes" *(Continued)*

were separate entities. Unfortunately, however, John Hunter confused the issue for six decades. In 1767 Hunter, in a courageous but ill-conceived experiment, placed onto his skin pus taken from the urethra of a man with gonorrhea. A chancre developed. Undoubtedly, Hunter had taken pus from a man coinfected with both *Neisseria gonorrhoeae* and *T. pallidum*. It was not until 60 years later that Philippe Ricord correctly distinguished the two diseases. Ricord also recognized the three stages of syphilis.

The incidence of syphilis has changed in recent decades. Between 1947 and 1965 a dramatic decline in the cases of syphilis was reported in the United States. However, from 1986 through 1990 the nation experienced a syphilis epidemic. Although the incidence fell during the following decade, the rate of primary and secondary syphilis has again increased in 2001 and 2002, especially among men. This suggests the increase results primarily among men who have sex with men.

---

syphilis were undiagnosed and untreated. Early in the twentieth century Wassermann, Neisser, and Bruck discovered that the sera of patients with syphilis have antibodies that react with normal human tissue. The tissue component was found to be a lipid present in the membranes of mitochondria, called **cardiolipin**. Why patients with syphilis form these curious antibodies is not known. In fact, the antibodies are produced in patients with other diseases as well; **biological false-positive tests** for syphilis occur in patients with hemolytic anemia, systemic lupus erythematosus, leprosy, narcotics abuse, and aging.

The original test of Wassermann and colleagues led to the development of more rapid and reproducible tests. Several variations exist and are known by their acronyms (e.g., the Venereal Diseases Reference Laboratory test, or **VDRL**, and the rapid plasma reagin, or **RPR**). Although nonspecific, these tests are cheap and easy to perform, which makes them suitable for initial screening of large numbers of serum samples, as in premarital "blood tests." However, their relative lack of specificity makes it necessary to test all positive samples by more specific, technically demanding, and expensive tests directed against treponemal antigens. One such **treponeme-specific test** is the **fluorescent treponemal antibody test (FTA)**, an indirect fluorescent antibody test (see Chapter 58).

The diagnosis of syphilis can be established by one of two methods: (1) obtaining a positive specific serologic treponemal test, usually following a positive nonspecific screening test such as the RPR or VDRL, or (2) directly visualizing the organisms scraped from mucocutaneous lesions by darkfield or immunofluorescence microscopy (in primary, secondary, or early congenital syphilis only).

TREATMENT: "ONE NIGHT WITH VENUS, THE REST OF LIFE WITH MERCURY"

Two major advances in the diagnosis and management of syphilis have occurred during the twentieth century: the development of serological tests for diagnosing syphilis and the use of penicillin for treating the disease. Fortunately for Mr. W. and for the rest of the world, the organisms are still exquisitely sensitive to penicillin.

Before penicillin, treatment depended on an arsenic-containing compound synthesized by Ehrlich early in the twentieth century (it was the first effective synthetic chemotherapeutic agent). This compound was called 606, in recognition of the 605 previous failures in that laboratory. Before the introduction of penicillin, therapy consisted of the tedious, expensive, and dangerous administration of arsenic and **mercury** or **bismuth** for a minimum of 2 months and as long as 2 or 3 years. An alternative therapy was the induction of high fevers in individuals with neurosyphilis. The basis of the therapeutic use of fever was the known heat sensitivity of *T. pallidum*. Fever was first induced by the production of erysipelas (streptococcal skin infections). However, when the streptococcal infections spread to and killed others who did not have syphilis, this method was abandoned. Subsequent efforts focused on malaria as the fever-inducing agent. Deaths were not unexpected, especially when the extremely virulent and deadly *Plasmodium falciparum* was inadvertently used instead of the more innocuous *Plasmodium vivax*.

Currently, the treatment of all stages of syphilis relies on the continued sensitivity of *T. pallidum* to **penicillin.** The optimal strengths and types of penicillin (aqueous, procaine, or benzathine penicillin) and duration of therapy for each stage are still not known with certainty. In general, however, patients with primary and secondary syphilis are treated with an injection of penicillin (benzathine type) that provides effective tissue levels for at least 1 week. Patients with late latent or tertiary syphilis are treated with repeated injections to provide effective tissue levels for approximately 3 weeks.

Reports of treatment failures following accepted and standard regimens of penicillin have surfaced with increasing frequency. Treatment failure is believed to be the result of lack of penetration of penicillin into the central nervous system harboring treponemes. Known infection of the central nervous system (neurosyphilis) should be treated with high-dose intravenous penicillin for 10 days. Similarly, the lack of immunity in patients infected with HIV has also contributed to treatment failure. These failures have caused tremendous uncertainty. Accordingly, some experts recommend intensified treatment of patients with later stages of syphilis and of individuals coinfected with HIV. Although cases of treatment failure are dramatic, they are difficult to interpret without knowing how many individuals are successfully managed by the same regimen. Without further evidence to justify major changes in the approach to syphilis treatment, current recommendations by the Centers for Disease Control and Prevention have remained conservative.

Conclusion

From the mid-1980s to the mid-1990s, the largest single-year increase in infectious syphilis in more than a quarter of a century was reported in the United States. During that period, the incidence of congenital syphilis also increased. In addition, genital ulcer diseases, such as syphilis, increase the risk of HIV transmission, contributing to the epidemic of AIDS. Several factors are fueling the syphilis epidemic: drug use, high-risk sexual activity, a decline in socioeconomic and educational levels among groups at risk, and limited access to health care, owing in part to the overburdening of health care facilities by the AIDS epidemic.

Among all the sexually transmitted diseases, syphilis is one of the easiest to control for the following reasons:

- The cases are clustered. Most of the current increase is occurring among low-income, minority heterosexuals and their children.
- Good diagnostic tests are available. These tests are inexpensive and give accurate, fairly rapid results.
- Treatment is available. An inexpensive antibiotic, penicillin, is effective for primary and secondary syphilis in single doses. Moreover, antibiotic resistance is not a problem.

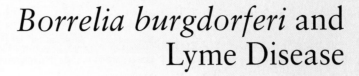

chapter 25

Borrelia burgdorferi and Lyme Disease

Jenifer Coburn and John Leong

key concepts

Borrelia species:

■ Are spiral-shaped bacteria (spirochetes).

■ Are transmitted to humans by arthropod bites.

■ Cause Lyme disease and relapsing fever.

Lyme disease

■ Is caused by *Borrelia burgdorferi* and is a multiphased disease treatable with antibiotics.

■ In stage 1 (acute, local) the skin is affected at the site of the tick bite (erythema migrans lesion).

■ In stage 2 (disseminated) the central nervous system, the skin, the heart, and other systems are affected.

■ In stage 3 (chronic) the joints and the central nervous system are affected; the organisms cannot usually be cultured from the lesions, but their DNA can sometimes be detected.

L yme disease, or **Lyme borreliosis,** is caused by the tickborne spirochete *Borrelia burgdorferi.* Prior to the recognition of this disorder in the 1970s (see box, "History of Lyme Disease"), *Borrelia* species were only known to cause an illness called **relapsing fever.** Although it differs from syphilis in the mode of transmission, Lyme disease is similar to syphilis in its multisystem involvement, occurrence in stages, and mimicry of other diseases (Fig. 25-1). As with syphilis, Lyme disease usually begins with localized infection of the skin. In Lyme disease a characteristic expanding skin lesion called **erythema migrans** usually occurs surrounding the site of the tick bite (stage 1). Within several days to weeks, the spirochete may spread to other sites (stage 2), particularly to other skin sites, the nervous system, joints, heart, or eyes. Symptoms change and are typically intermittent during this stage of the illness. After months to years, sometimes following long periods of latent infection, the spirochete may cause chronic disease manifestations (stage 3), most commonly of the joints, nervous system, or skin.

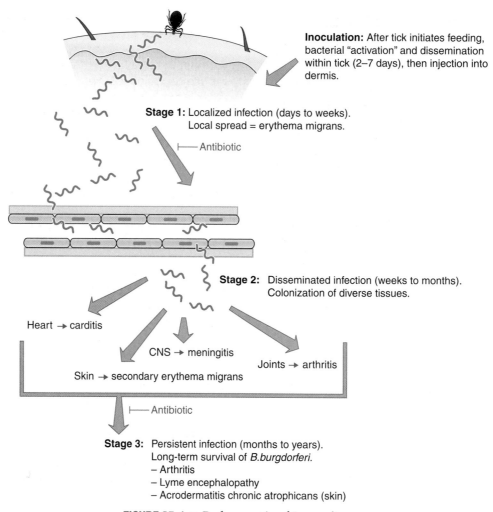

Inoculation: After tick initiates feeding, bacterial "activation" and dissemination within tick (2–7 days), then injection into dermis.

Stage 1: Localized infection (days to weeks). Local spread = erythema migrans.

├── Antibiotic

Stage 2: Disseminated infection (weeks to months). Colonization of diverse tissues.

Heart → carditis

CNS → meningitis

Joints → arthritis

Skin → secondary erythema migrans

├── Antibiotic

Stage 3: Persistent infection (months to years). Long-term survival of *B. burgdorferi*.
– Arthritis
– Lyme encephalopathy
– Acrodermatitis chronic atrophicans (skin)

FIGURE 25-1 ▪ Pathogenesis of Lyme disease.

Case

Mr. G., a 48-year-old resident of a suburb of Boston, Massachusetts, spent a weekend on Nantucket Island in June. Activities during the weekend included hiking through scrubby, grassy, and lightly wooded areas. When he returned home he felt well, but over the next few days his wife noticed a slowly expanding red rash on one shoulder blade. As the rash expanded, the outer margins stayed red but the center started clearing, giving a bull's eye appearance. Approximately two weeks later, while visiting Arizona, he developed a severe headache, fever, myalgia, and malaise. Mr. G. sought medical attention and was told that he probably had a viral infection. The symptoms gradually abated, but he later developed a somewhat droopy eyelid on one side and transient aches in multiple joints, which also spontaneously resolved with time. However, several months later at home in Boston he again sought medical attention because he had developed considerable pain and swelling in one knee. At that time, based on his medical history and current symptoms, he was tested for *Borrelia burgdorferi* infection (Lyme disease). Serological tests revealed a high IgG titer to *B. burgdorferi* antigens by

enzyme-linked immunosorbent assay (ELISA), and an IgG response to more than 10 different spirochetal proteins in an immunoblot. A polymerase chain reaction of joint fluid aspirated from the affected knee revealed the presence of *B. burgdorferi* DNA. He was treated with a one-month course of oral doxycycline and made a slow but complete recovery.

The case of Mr. G. raises several questions:

1. How did Mr. G. acquire the infection? What is the likely significance of his vacationing in Nantucket in June? Is he likely to transmit the infection to anyone else?

2. What early clinical feature did Mr. G. exhibit that might have provided his physician with the best diagnostic hint that he had Lyme disease? Why was the diagnosis of Lyme disease overlooked when he saw a doctor while visiting Arizona?

3. What feature(s) of the spirochete are responsible for Mr. G. suffering such diverse signs and symptoms, including headache, myalgia, facial droop, arthralgia, and arthritis?

4. Why was an immunoblot performed in addition to ELISA?

FIGURE 25-2 ▪ **Darkfield micrograph of *Borrelia burgdorferi*.** (Photograph taken by Dr. Roberta O'Connor.)

Borrelia species, along with the leptospires and treponemes, are **spirochetes.** Like all spirochetes, *Borrelia* structure consists of a long, thin corkscrew-shaped cell (Fig. 25-2) surrounded first by an inner (cytoplasmic) membrane, then by a thin peptidoglycan layer, and finally by an outer membrane that is only loosely associated with the underlying structures. Flagella, which provide spirochetes with the ability to swim rapidly through even viscous environments, are contained between the two membranes and determine the corkscrew shape of the cell. The *Borrelia* species are fastidious and grow best at 33°C in a complex liquid medium with a generation time of 10 to 24 hours. Three *Borrelia* species are known to cause human Lyme disease: *B. burgdorferi*, *B. garinii*, and *B. afzelii*. Infection in North America is caused solely by *B. burgdorferi*, but all three species are significant causes of human disease in Europe and Asia. All species cause similar but not identical clinical diseases and will generally be referred to as *B. burgdorferi* throughout this chapter.

The genome of *B. burgdorferi* is remarkably complex, consisting of a linear chromosome and about 22 linear and circular plasmids, depending on the particular strain. It encodes a large array of lipoproteins, many of which become localized in the outer membrane and are encoded by plasmid-borne genes, features that presumably facilitate rapid changes in the surface protein repertoire of the spirochete.

Borrelia burgdorferi

ENCOUNTER AND ENTRY

Humans are "accidental" hosts for *B. burgdorferi* because spirochetes from infected people are not trans-

mitted to other hosts. In most cases, rodents, such as the **white-footed mouse,** participate with the *Ixodes* (deer) tick to maintain the reservoir of *B. burgdorferi* in nature (Fig. 25-3). There is no vertical transmission of the spirochete from female tick to offspring, so rodents provide the critical means for the indirect transmission of spirochetes from one generation of deer tick to the next (Fig. 25-4). These rodents, typically after being fed upon for several days by nymphal-stage deer ticks, become chronically infected with *B. burgdorferi*, particularly in the skin, enabling them to efficiently pass the spirochete back to uninfected ticks months later when fed upon by the next generation of tick. Therefore, while deer are the most common hosts for adult stage ticks, it is the transmission of spirochetes between rodents, larval ticks, and nymphal ticks that is essential for the maintenance of *B. burgdorferi* within the tick population, and the nymphal tick is the major vector of transmission to humans.

The natural cycle of *B. burgdorferi* has significant implications for human disease. First, the geographic regions endemic for Lyme disease are restricted to those where all the essential elements of the natural cycle exist, and Lyme disease in the United States is concentrated in the northeastern and mid-Atlantic coastal states, and in the Great Lakes region, with more sporadic cases occurring elsewhere (Fig. 25-5). Second, most human infections occur in the spring and summer months, when outdoor activities bring people into contact with feeding nymphal ticks. These ticks are

FIGURE 25-3 ▪ **Deer ticks at the larval, nymphal, and adult stages.** Larval, nymphal, and adult ticks are approximately 0.5, 1, and 3 mm long (excluding legs), respectively. A sewing needle in the upper-left corner of the picture provides scale. (Photo provided by the American Lyme Disease Foundation.)

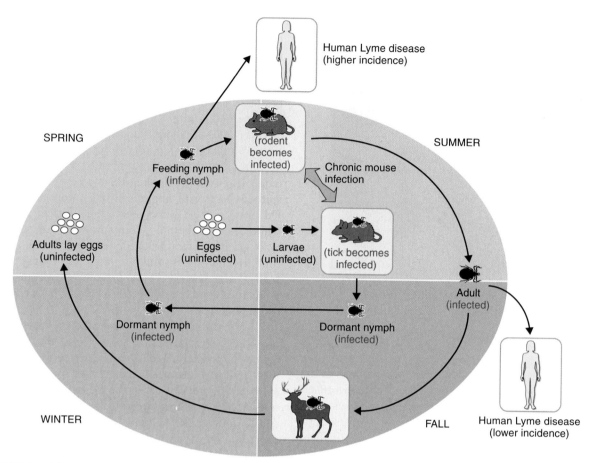

FIGURE 25-4 ▪ **The natural cycle of Lyme disease.** Deer ticks undergo a 2-year cycle that encompasses four stages: eggs, larvae, nymphs, and adults. In the summer larvae hatch in an uninfected state and then acquire *B. burgdorferi* by feeding on infected rodents. *B. burgdorferi* survives in the midgut as the larvae molt into nymphs in the fall and are dormant through the winter. Infected nymphs feed on rodents in the late spring and early summer, resulting in the chronic infection of this natural reservoir of *B. burgdorferi*. The population of chronically infected rodents transmits *B. burgdorferi* to the next generation of larval-stage ticks. Nymphal ticks can also feed on humans, giving rise to the peak of human Lyme disease in the late spring and summer. The ticks molt into adults in the fall, and while their preferred host is deer, they can occasionally feed on humans, giving rise to a smaller peak of human Lyme disease in the fall. (Adapted with permission from a figure from the Web site of the American Lyme Disease Foundation, http://www.aldf.com/DeerTickEcology.asp.)

extremely small (approximately 1 mm in length; see Fig. 25-3) and in many instances are not discovered by individuals that they feed on, a feature that allows the tick to remain attached for several days. Third, the ability of the spirochete to establish a chronic infection of rodents, with efficient colonization of the skin in particular, corresponds to important features of human Lyme disease.

While in the midgut of the *Ixodes* tick between feeding periods, the spirochetes of *B. burgdorferi* are in a dormant, nonreplicating state attached to epithelial cells. There they express a plasmid-encoded, major outer surface protein (OspA) that promotes attachment to tick cells and is required for tick midgut colonization. When the tick feeds on a mammalian host, the spirochetes are exposed to a higher temperature and to the content of mammalian blood. In response the spirochete undergoes

a number of phenotypic changes over the next two or three days. Most notably, expression of OspA decreases and expression of OspC, a second outer surface protein encoded on a different plasmid, increases. In addition, the host protease plasmin, present in ingested blood, binds to and becomes activated on the bacterial surface and is required for efficient dissemination through the tick.

The spirochete replicates and invades the gut wall to spread throughout the tick, including to the salivary glands, and are then injected into the skin of the mammalian host. Although the function of OspC is not entirely characterized, it is required for successful mammalian infection. The activation of spirochetes in response to tick feeding is essential, because if feeding ticks are removed within the first two days of feeding, before the spirochete can complete these events,

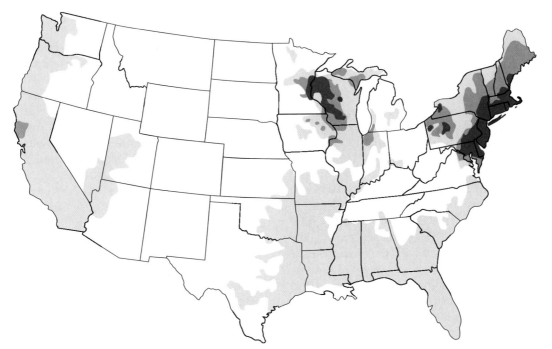

FIGURE 25-5 ■ **Risk areas for Lyme disease within the United States.** Areas colored dark blue have the highest risk. Risk is lowest in areas of pale blue and virtually nonexistent in uncolored areas.

History of Lyme Disease

Lyme disease was first described in 1975 as a distinct entity associated with a geographic clustering of children in Lyme, Connecticut, who were thought to have juvenile rheumatoid arthritis. The rural setting of the case clusters and the identification of the characteristic erythema migrans as a feature of the illness suggested that the disorder was transmitted by an arthropod. It soon became apparent that Lyme disease was a multisystem illness that affected primarily the skin, nervous system, heart, and joints. Epidemiologic studies implicated certain *Ixodes* ticks as vectors of the disease (see Chapter 56).

In addition to providing clues about the cause of the disease, erythema migrans helped link Lyme disease in the United States to certain syndromes in Europe. Early in the 20th century several European investigators described the characteristic expanding skin lesion of erythema migrans, which they attributed to *Ixodes* tick bites. Many years later it was recognized that erythema migrans was often followed by a chronic skin disease (acrodermatitis chronica atrophicans), which had already been described as a separate entity. In the 1940s a neurologic syndrome was described in Europe (called Bannwarth syndrome, meningopolyneuritis, or meningoradiculitis). That syndrome was sometimes preceded by an erythema.

The various syndromes were linked conclusively in 1982, when the causative agent, a previously unrecognized spirochete now called *B. burgdorferi*, was isolated from *Ixodes* (deer) ticks. The spirochete was then recovered from patients with Lyme disease in the United States, as well as from individuals in Europe with erythema migrans, Bannwarth syndrome, or acrodermatitis. The patients' immune responses were linked conclusively with this organism. Although regional variations exist, the basic outlines of the disease are similar worldwide, and its most common name is Lyme disease or Lyme borreliosis.

Whereas the various clinical manifestations of syphilis were brought together as a single entity in the nineteenth century, the many manifestations of Lyme disease were not recognized as parts of a single entity until the 1980s. As in syphilis, the causative spirochete in Lyme disease can survive for years and, after long periods of latency, can cause slowly progressive disease, particularly of the nervous system. Moreover, in both diseases the mechanisms of spirochetal attachment and survival and the ways in which the organism damages host tissues are not completely understood.

Why has Lyme disease become a major concern in certain parts of the world? The most obvious reason is the recent recognition of a disease that has escaped definition in the past. However, Lyme disease is now causing **focal epidemics** as it spreads in the northeastern and upper midwestern United States. These epidemics are thought to be the result of a large increase in the number of deer and, by extension, the deer ticks that transmit this disorder in those parts of the country. At the same time, rural areas where deer and the deer ticks live have become increasingly populated by susceptible suburbanites who have never been exposed to the spirochete.

transmission of the spirochete to the mammalian host is abrogated.

SPREAD AND MULTIPLICATION

The ability of *B. burgdorferi* to multiply and establish infection in the skin of the mammalian host is reflected in one of the characteristic signs of localized or stage 1 Lyme disease in humans, the erythema migrans rash (Fig. 25-6 and see Fig. 25-1). The spirochetes are highly motile and probably still coated with the host protease plasmin; thus, over a period of days, they are able to spread through the skin, resulting in expansion of the rash, leaving a blanched central area and a bulls-eye appearance. Some but not all strains of *B. burgdorferi* are capable of further multiplication and dissemination in humans in the following days to weeks, spreading to multiple tissues, including the nervous system, musculoskeletal tissues, and the heart. This stage is known as **early disseminated infection** or stage 2 Lyme disease. Later, in chronic or stage 3 Lyme disease, the rate of bacterial multiplication appears to be significantly reduced or is kept in check by the host defenses, resulting in the very low number of bacteria that can be found in tissues.

Although the bacterial properties that allow the spirochete to cause infection in a variety of tissues are still being defined, adherence of the spirochete to host cells and extracellular matrix is likely one critical factor in colonization of diverse tissues. Indeed, in vitro studies have demonstrated that *B. burgdorferi* adheres to many cell types and to extracellular matrix. To date, several classes of mammalian receptors that promote *B. burgdorferi* attachment have been identified. One pathway is mediated by a class of molecules called **proteoglycans,** which consist of long, linear polymers of repeating disaccharides linked to a protein. The proteoglycans are expressed both on the surface of mammalian cells and in extracellular matrix. A second component of extracellular matrix that is recognized is **fibronectin,** a protein to which mammalian cells bind. A third pathway is attachment to receptors that belong to the **integrin** family, which normally mediate attachment of mammalian cells to extracellular matrix proteins (including fibronectin). Whether each adhesion pathway contributes to the colonization of a specific tissue or, more likely, the adhesion pathways cooperate to promote colonization of multiple tissues is not yet known.

The ability to chronically infect the mammalian host that is essential for the ability of *B. burgdorferi* to complete the natural cycle is reflected in Lyme disease, because once human infection is established, the spirochete can survive for years, despite the development of a vigorous host immune response. Several mechanisms that promote long-term survival of the organism have been identified to date. First, *B. burgdorferi* is able to bind mammalian complement regulatory factors, which provides resistance to complement-mediated lysis and opsonization. Second, the pathogen appears to be quite adept at turning on and off the expression of many genes encoding surface proteins, thus presenting a

FIGURE 25-6 ▪ **Erythema migrans, the characteristic rash of Lyme disease.** The blanched central region that develops in many erythema migrans lesions is not apparent in this one. (Courtesy of the American Lyme Disease Foundation.)

"moving target" to the immune system. In addition, one particular *Borrelia* surface protein, **VlsE,** is subject to continual antigenic variation after the spirochete infects the mammalian host. Adjacent to the *vlsE* (the *E* stands for "expressed") gene are highly variant "cassettes" of nonexpressed DNA homologous to *vlsE,* and portions of the expressed *vlsE* gene are continually replaced with corresponding fragments of the nonexpressed cassettes by recombination. The *vls* locus can, in theory, generate on the order of 10^{30} variants of the protein and is likely to contribute to evasion of the immune response. VlsE, as well as bacterial factors that promote attachment to host tissues or resistance to complement, are plasmid encoded, a feature that may promote control of expression of proteins that interact with the host environment.

DAMAGE

Stages 1 and 2: Early Localized and Disseminated Infection

Evidence of damage is present at each stage of Lyme disease. Local skin infection results in erythema migrans, which reflects infiltration of primarily lymphocytes and macrophages (stage 1; see Fig. 25-1). Disseminated infection (stage 2) includes at least transient colonization of the bloodstream. At this stage some degree of vascular damage, including mild vasculitis or hypercellular vascular occlusion, may be seen in multiple sites, suggesting that the spirochetes colonize the vessel wall. This stage of disease is often heralded by signs and symptoms reflecting colonization of the skin, nervous system, heart, and musculoskeletal sites, such as secondary erythema migrans lesions, excruciating headache, mild neck stiffness, and migratory pain in joints, bursae, tendons, muscle, or bone. Neurologic abnormalities can include meningitis and neuritis. Inflammatory manifestations of ocular infection can include conjunctivitis, iritis, choroiditis, or panophthalmitis. Cardiac involvement may result in fluctuating degrees of atrioventricular block or myopericarditis. These clinical manifestations are likely to be a result of direct infection of the affected tissue, because spirochetes have been detected in or recovered from most of these sites during this stage of the illness.

B. burgdorferi is not known to produce toxins that directly damage any tissue. Rather, the spirochete persists in infected tissues and thereby elicits an immune response that causes "bystander" injury to the host. The spirochete does not produce lipopolysaccharide (LPS, also called endotoxin), but as mentioned earlier, its genome encodes an unusually large number of lipoproteins, which are potent stimulators of proinflammatory cytokine production via toll-like receptors. Consistent with this, affected tissues show an infiltra-tion of lymphocytes and macrophages, and sometimes plasma cells and/or neutrophils.

Stage 3: Chronic Infection

In untreated patients, diverse manifestations of disease can occur months to years after disease onset, reflecting the ability of the spirochete to establish chronic infection of many tissue sites. Patients, particularly those in the United States, may begin to suffer brief attacks of arthritis, especially in the knee. Although the pattern varies, episodes of arthritis often become longer during the second and third years of illness, and in a small percentage of patients, **chronic Lyme arthritis** begins during this period (see Fig. 25-1). This particular form of arthritis, which has become increasingly rare as Lyme disease has become better recognized and more frequently treated during the early stages of illness, does not always respond to antibiotic treatment, even when clearance of the organism from the joint is documented by polymerase chain reaction. Thus, as with a number of rheumatic diseases, treatment-resistant chronic Lyme arthritis appears to have an immunologic basis. For example, many patients with chronic arthritis have HLA-DR alleles that are also associated with rheumatoid arthritis, and the onset of prolonged episodes of joint involvement has been shown to often coincide with heightened immunoreactivity to the spirochete. In particular, IgG reactivity develops against OspA, a protein that usually is expressed when the spirochete is in the tick. It has been postulated that in genetically susceptible people, *B. burgdorferi* triggers a self-damaging immune response that continues even after the apparent eradication of the spirochete from the joint, perhaps owing to the presence of cross-reactive antigens.

Chronic neurologic involvement, affecting either the peripheral or central nervous system, may also occur in Lyme borreliosis, sometimes following years of latent infection. *B. burgdorferi* DNA has been detected in cerebrospinal fluid in patients with **Lyme encephalopathy** many years after disease onset, a finding that is analogous to the persistence of spirochetal DNA in tertiary neurosyphilis. However, the features of late neurologic involvement differ in the two diseases. In Lyme disease, the most common form of chronic central nervous system involvement affects memory, mood, or sleep, sometimes with subtle language disturbance.

Another example of prolonged latency followed by appearance of clinical signs of persistent infection in Lyme borreliosis is a late skin manifestation called **acrodermatitis chronica atrophicans,** which has been observed primarily in Europe after infection with *B. afzelii.* This skin lesion usually begins with bluish-red discoloration and swollen skin on an extremity. The lesion's inflammatory phase may persist for many years or decades, and it gradually leads to atrophy of the skin. *Borrelia* has been cultured from such lesions as much as 10 years after their onset.

DIAGNOSIS

The ability to culture the organism from infected sites is often the gold standard for diagnosis of bacterial infections. Unfortunately, except for erythema migrans skin lesions, it is generally not possible to culture *B. burgdorferi* from patients' specimens, and even then sophisticated culturing techniques and long incubation times are required. It is usually difficult to visualize the spirochete in histologic sections. Although it is possible to detect *B. burgdorferi* DNA in tissue biopsies from some of the affected sites, such as joints, technical challenges that limit the sensitivity and specificity of DNA-based tests have hindered the development of a widely available, routine, definitive diagnostic test for Lyme disease. Instead, the diagnosis is first and foremost a process of identifying clinical features, particularly erythema migrans, suggestive of Lyme disease coupled with a history that is compatible with exposure to infected deer ticks.

In cases in which the clinical assessment leads to the suspicion of Lyme disease, but not its definitive diagnosis, serologic testing, such as enzyme-linked immunosorbent assay (ELISA), to detect anti–*B. burgdorferi* antibodies can be employed to confirm the diagnosis. After the first several weeks of infection, particularly if the spirochete disseminates, most patients become seropositive. However, even these serologic tests have their limitations, and interpretation requires some experience and skill. As with syphilis, the specific immune response in Lyme disease is slow to develop, and patients with stage 1 infection are often seronegative. As with other serologic tests, false-positive and false-negative ELISA results can occur, but immunoblotting, which allows detection of antibodies against specific *B. burgdorferi* proteins, is often helpful in identifying false-positive ELISA results.

TREATMENT AND PREVENTION

Given the potential difficulties in diagnosis and treatment of Lyme disease, the prevention of infection has been emphasized. A Lyme vaccine based on OspA was available in the United States for several years but was withdrawn

Comparison of Various Spirochetoses

The spirochetoses that affect humans in the United States in addition to Lyme disease include **syphilis, relapsing fever,** and **leptospirosis** (Table 25-1). Except for syphilis, these are animal diseases that only incidentally affect humans when they are bitten by *Borrelia*-infected ticks or when they come in contact with animal urine contaminated with leptospires. All these spirochetes are highly motile, and all are capable of spreading from the initial site of infection. The initial phases of these infections have many similarities to Lyme disease, including the possible presence of fever, headache, muscle pain, meningitis, photophobia, malaise, or fatigue. However, each disease also has unique clinical features. Relapsing fever is associated with intermittent episodes of high fever, which are thought to occur because of variation of the major antigen, a surface protein of the spirochete. Leptospirosis often affects the kidney, but infection of many tissues is seen and can result in hemorrhage. Both Lyme disease and syphilis occur in stages over a period of years and typically cause neurologic abnormalities late in the illness. However, the neurologic syndromes of the two diseases are different. For syphilis and Lyme disease, diagnosis is usually made by recognition of a characteristic clinical picture with serologic confirmation. All the spirochetes are susceptible to a wide range of antibiotics.

table **25-1**	**Main Features of the Spirochetoses**		
NAME OF DISEASE	**CAUSATIVE AGENT**	**MODE OF TRANSMISSION**	**CHARACTERISTIC CLINICAL ASPECTS**
Lyme disease	*Borrelia burgdorferi*	Ticks of the *Ixodes ricinus* complex	Erythema migrans, recurrent arthritis
Relapsing fever	*B. hermsii, B. recurrentis,* others	*Ornithodoros* ticks, Human body louse	Recurrent high fever
Syphilis	*Treponema pallidum*	Sexual contact	Chancre, tabes dorsalis, aortitis
Leptospirosis	*Leptospira* spp.	Contact with infected animals or their urine	Jaundice, renal involvement

from the market for various reasons. The OspA vaccine was, however, interesting in light of *B. burgdorferi* biology. As discussed earlier, OspA is expressed while the spirochete is in the tick midgut but is not usually expressed while the spirochete is in the mammalian host. Thus, anti-OspA antibody does not promote clearance of bacteria in the mammalian host but rather is a "tick sterilizing" antibody. The anti-OspA antibody present in blood is ingested by the feeding tick and leads to killing of spirochetes in the tick midgut, thereby interrupting the activation and migration of spirochetes from the tick midgut to the salivary glands, a process required for mammalian infection. Currently, the best advice for prevention is behavioral: people should be warned to minimize the chances of tick bites by wearing long pants tucked into socks, spraying clothing with insect repellent, and performing careful checks for feeding ticks daily when engaging in outdoor activities in Lyme-endemic areas, particularly in the spring and summer.

The treatment of Lyme disease is guided by the stage and manifestation of the disease. For stage 1 or 2 the duration of therapy is generally 2 to 4 weeks and is guided by the clinical presentation of illness. In contrast to the agent of syphilis, *B. burgdorferi* is only moderately sensitive to penicillin; consequently, doxycycline is the most commonly prescribed antibiotic for adults and amoxicillin is the primary choice for children. For patients with arthritis, 1 to 2 months of the same antibiotics are recommended. Intravenous therapy is generally necessary for patients with objective neurologic involvement, and the third-generation cephalosporin drugs (e.g., ceftriaxone or cefotaxime) are used most often for this purpose.

Conclusion

Lyme disease is an insidious disease that can be readily treated if diagnosed in time. Untreated, the spirochete can cause a chronic, multisystemic illness that, like syphilis, can be divided into three stages based on the site(s) and duration of infection. Because diagnosis is still largely dependent on clinical suspicion and evaluation of the patient rather than on laboratory tests, physicians and other health personnel must be alert to the possibility of this disease among people living in affected areas, especially those who are frequently outdoors.

chapter 26

Cat Scratch Disease, Bacillary Angiomatosis, and Other Bartonelloses

David H. Walker

key concepts

Bartonella species:

- Include *Bartonella henselae,* which causes cat scratch disease (in immunocompetent persons), peliosis hepatis, and bacillary angiomatosis (in immunocompromised persons); *B. quintana*, which causes trench fever, bacteremia, and tumorlike proliferations in blood vessels; and *B. bacilliformis*, the agent of Oroya fever and verruga peruana.

- Are transmitted by a cat scratch or bite (*B. henselae*), the feces of a louse and possibly contaminated intravenous paraphernalia (*B. quintana*), and the bite of a South American sandfly (*B. bacilliformis*).

- Cause different diseases in immunocompetent and immunocompromised persons.

- Are diagnosed by prolonged culturing of the organisms, microscopic examination of biopsies using special stains, or the detection of specific antibodies in blood.

*B*artonella species can cause serious infections of both immunocompetent and immunocompromised persons, with markedly different consequences depending on the state of host defenses. *B. henselae* is the major cause of two diseases: **cat scratch disease,** a prevalent, self-limited infectious lymphadenitis transmitted by the scratch or bite of a healthy-appearing infected cat; and **bacillary angiomatosis,** cutaneous and visceral tumorlike proliferations of blood vessels principally in people with AIDS. In South America an endemic bartonellosis, caused by *B. bacilliformis*, is transmitted by sandflies and results in **Oroya fever,** a febrile illness with severe hemolytic anemia, and/or subsequent vasoproliferative skin lesions.

Cat scratch disease is a significant infection in the United States, with more than 20,000 cases reported annually. M. developed the typical clinical features and a self-limited course of cat scratch disease, whereas J. developed a more indolent and relapsing disease in the context of AIDS. In addition to cat scratch disease and bacillary angiomatosis, there are two other medically important *Bartonella* infections (Table 26-1).

In parts of Peru, Ecuador, and Colombia, a skin disorder called **verruga peruana** ("Peruvian wart") has been recognized since pre-Colombian times. The indolent angioma-like lesions of this condition resemble those seen in the case of J. In late nineteenth-century Peru, an epidemic of fever and anemia (**Oroya fever**) occurred among

Case

Two brothers, M. and J., became ill after having been scratched by a new kitten given to them by an aunt. M. is 5 years old and has been healthy all his life. He developed a 6-mm cutaneous papule on the right hand where the kitten had scratched him 1 week before. After another week, he developed numerous enlarged lymph nodes in the right axilla. Acute and convalescent sera collected by M.'s pediatrician showed an eightfold rise in titer of antibodies to *Bartonella henselae*. M.'s lymph nodes returned to normal size and consistency over a 3-month period without antimicrobial treatment.

J. is 3 years old. Unlike M., he acquired infection with HIV-1 congenitally from his mother and has AIDS. J. developed three painless, red protuberant skin lesions that resembled tumors. Biopsy of the largest of the lesions revealed proliferation of small blood vessels and numerous colonies of small bacteria. A diagnosis of bacillary angiomatosis was made. The lesions resolved after a month of continuous treatment with oral erythromycin. However, another crop of similar lesions developed 3 weeks after discontinuing the antibiotic. With the recurrence J. also developed fever and chills. Blood cultures for *Bartonella* organisms were obtained, and J. was treated with intravenous erythromycin until his fever resolved. Oral erythromycin was continued thereafter. His skin lesions disappeared on treatment, but he died of other complications of AIDS 4 months later. After 2 weeks of incubation, his blood culture grew *B. henselae*.

This case raises several questions:

1. Why did J. develop a different disease than M. when both were infected with the same organism, *B. henselae*?
2. Why did M. get well without treatment while J. suffered a relapse despite treatment with an appropriate antibiotic?
3. What was the source of the infection?
4. By what route(s) did the organisms travel to the skin papule, the lymph nodes, and the pseudoneoplastic skin lesions?

railroad construction workers. At that time a Peruvian medical student named Daniel Carrión demonstrated that the lesions of verruga peruana contain the same infectious agent responsible for Oroya fever. He injected himself with material from a skin lesion and unfortunately died of the acute febrile illness. His legacy was the important discovery that the two seemingly disparate diseases have a common etiology. It is now known that in the natural course of infection, the febrile illness occurs first and may resolve to be followed months later by the skin lesions. In honor of the medical student whose autoexperiment permitted this connection to be recognized, the disorder was renamed **Carrión disease.** The etiologic agent of Carrión disease, *B. bacilliformis*, was observed in 1913 by its discoverer, Alberto Barton, to infect red blood cells during the acute stage of infection. Blood infection leads to extreme anemia because of massive destruction of the red blood cells by the mononuclear phagocytes in lymphoreticular organs such as the spleen.

In the Northern Hemisphere **trench fever** caused by *B. quintana* was one of the major causes of morbidity in World War I. The disease has appeared again in new forms in people with AIDS and in homeless persons. Immunocompromised persons are particularly susceptible to this infection, which may manifest as febrile bacteremia or tumorlike proliferations in blood vessels of the skin and visceral organs, indistinguishable clinically or pathologically from *B. henselae* bacillary angiomatosis. Homeless persons in Europe and North America have been found to have *B. quintana* infections of the bloodstream and cardiac valves. The chronic bacteremia of this infection can extend for months beyond clinical recovery. Originally, the trench fever bacterium was believed to be a species of *Rickettsia*. In 1961 cell-free cultivation of this etiologic agent on blood agar demonstrated that it was not an obligate intracellular bacterium. For many years the trench fever agent was called *Rickettsia quintana* and later *Rochalimaea quintana* in honor of the Brazilian microbiologist da Rocha-Lima. However, contemporary molecular tools revealed that the bacterium, now known as *B. quintana*, is a close relative of *B. bacilliformis* and *B. henselae* (see paradigm).

table 26-1 Etiology and Epidemiology of *Bartonella* Infections

ORGANISMS	DISEASES	RESERVOIR IN NATURE	TRANSMISSION
B. henselae	Cat scratch disease, bacillary angiomatosis	Cats	Cat scratch or bite (cat to human), cat flea (cat to cat)
B. quintana	Trench fever, bacillary angiomatosis	Human	Louse feces, possibly other arthropods and contaminated drug paraphernalia
B. bacilliformis	Oroya fever (or Carrión disease), verruga peruana	Humans	Sandfly bite

New Methods and the Discovery of New Etiologic Agents

Ever since microscopy, microbial cultivation, and animal inoculation led to the concept that living things invisible to the naked eye could cause diseases, advances in technology have led to the discovery of new infectious agents. Cell culture has enabled the discovery of viruses and other etiologic agents that cannot be cultivated on agar or in broth. Electron microscopy allowed visualization of viruses and bacteria for which effective methods of growth had not been developed.

Recently, the application of molecular methods, particularly polymerase chain reaction (PCR) and amplification and sequencing of DNA derived from the infectious agent, has fostered the discovery of previously undetermined or undiscovered etiologic agents of infectious diseases. The major causative agent of bacillary angiomatosis, *Bartonella henselae*, was initially identified using this approach. Classic serologic, epidemiologic, and ecological investigations later revealed that it also causes cat scratch disease.

Other pathogens that had yet to be cultivated, including the agents that cause **human granulocytic anaplasmosis** and **Whipple disease,** have been identified by DNA analysis. Human granulocytic anaplasmosis is a life-threatening disease that was recognized as a veterinary pathogen in Great Britain in 1932 but was just recently discovered to pose a threat to humans. Whipple disease, on the other hand, has been known as a human disease since 1907. In both

instances, scientists obtained affected tissues from patients and used PCR to amplify a structural RNA gene known to be present in all bacteria—namely, **16S ribosomal RNA (16S rRNA).** The amplified RNA was sequenced and compared with the 16S rRNA sequences of other known bacteria stored in computerized data banks. Because certain variations in the 16S rRNA sequence are known to occur during the evolution of bacterial species, scientists can identify the closest relatives of the unknown pathogen even when an exact match is not available from the data bank. Subsequently, both *Anaplasma phagocytophilum* and *Tropheryma whippelii* have been propagated in cell culture.

Similarly, to identify the culprit causing the deadly, acute respiratory disease outbreak of 1993 in the Four Corners area of New Mexico, Arizona, Colorado, and Utah, researchers used a variation of this method. Based on serology, investigators suspected a Hantavirus-like agent. Consequently, researchers added a reverse transcription step to convert viral RNA in patient samples into DNA. Then primers for conserved Hantavirus sequences were used for PCR. These studies revealed that the etiologic agent was indeed a novel strain of Hantavirus. Many of the riddles of newly emerging and poorly understood infectious diseases will surely yield to the study of genomic sequences by ever-improving methods.

Bartonella species

ENCOUNTER AND ENTRY

Bartonella henselae is introduced into human skin by a scratch or bite from a cat with no apparent, prolonged infection. Transmission from cat to cat occurs through fleas. In contrast, *B. quintana* infections during World War I were transmitted among humans by the human body louse. Many affected individuals in modern times have not shown any signs of having lice. Other possible, but unproven, modes of transmission of *B. quintana* include contaminated intravenous drug paraphernalia or other arthropods. The third *Bartonella* species, *B. bacilliformis*, is transmitted through the bite of a phlebotomine **sandfly,**

which takes a blood meal from an infected host, possibly amplifies the quantity of organisms, and then transmits the organisms by feeding on a new susceptible host. Humans may be the only reservoir for *B. bacilliformis*, but other species of *Bartonella* infect a variety of mammals (e.g., rodents, felines, and canines) in endemic areas and throughout the world.

SPREAD, MULTIPLICATION, AND DAMAGE

In cat scratch disease, *B. henselae* causes a small papule at the site of inoculation. The organism then spreads via the lymphatic vessels to the draining regional lymph

FIGURE 26-1 ■ **Acquisition and courses of infection with *Bartonella henselae*.**

nodes where bacterial proliferation and a vigorous mixed **granulomatous** and **suppurative** host response occurs. This response typically limits the infection, and very few bacteria are found in infected lymph nodes (Fig. 26-1). In some patients, however, particularly people with AIDS, the host response is insufficient to control the infection. The organisms multiply freely and disseminate in large numbers through the bloodstream, often manifesting clinically as sepsis or as localized infection of the skin, liver, and other viscera. In infections of skin and other organs, the bacteria secrete substances and trigger cytokine production that stimulate proliferation of small blood vessels, resulting in the lesions of **bacillary angiomatosis** (Fig. 26-2).

B. quintana has been found to cause an indistinguishable angioproliferative lesion in people with AIDS, although the source of infection and mode of entry are not always clear. Both *B. quintana* and *B. henselae* are also frequent causes of culture-negative endocarditis, so called because routine cultures do not recover the organisms.

B. bacilliformis attaches to the erythrocyte, deforms the cell membrane as it enters the cell, and then multiplies within the erythrocyte cytoplasm. **Massive anemia** can then ensue from greatly enhanced erythrophagocytosis. This process can also alter host defenses. The pathogenesis of the ensuing chronic nodular skin lesions is similar to that of bacillary angiomatosis.

FIGURE 26-2 ■ **Multiple violaceous papules and nodules in a case of bacillary angiomatosis.**

DIAGNOSIS

Bartonella infections can be diagnosed by cultivation of the organisms from blood or skin lesions; however, growth is slow, and routine cultures are often discarded before organisms are detected. Alternatively, diagnosis of *B. henselae* or *B. quintana* infection can be made by detecting specific antibodies in patients with suspicious clinical signs and symptoms. *Bartonella* species can also be detected in biopsies with the use of special silver-staining methods. In people with AIDS, biopsies of lesions are often performed to rule out the similar-appearing, malignant angiomatous lesion of Kaposi sarcoma. Likewise, *B. bacilliformis* can be visualized diagnostically in Romanowsky-stained smears of peripheral blood of patients with Oroya fever.

TREATMENT

In cat scratch disease, the course of illness is only marginally affected by antibiotic treatment. Although various antibiotics (rifampin, ciprofloxacin, trimethoprim–sulfamethoxazole, and gentamicin) have been used, there is no established, effective antimicrobial therapy. The drug of choice for bacillary angiomatosis or bacteremia caused by either *B. henselae* or *B. quintana* is **erythromycin**; doxycycline and azithromycin also produce good results. Unfortunately, relapses requiring repeated or long-term maintenance treatment occur in patients with inadequate host defenses. For *B. bacilliformis* infection, **chloramphenicol** was traditionally given in the acute febrile stage (Oroya fever) because of the frequency of complications resulting from *Salmonella* superinfection. Currently, aprofloxacin is the drug of choice. **Rifampin** is used for the much less serious verrucous stage.

Conclusion

Organisms of the genus *Bartonella* belong to a large and heterogeneous group of fastidious Gram-negative bacilli that infect a variety of mammals. Decades of confusion passed before they were assigned a logical taxonomic home based on nucleic acid homology of evolutionarily conserved genes. The species that cause human disease, *B. henselae*, *B. quintana*, and *B. bacilliformis*, produce angiomatous skin lesions, sepsis, or visceral organ infection (e.g., peliosis hepatis and endocarditis), depending on the circumstances of infection and the immune status of the host. When the organisms proliferate in tissues or blood, treatment with an antibiotic is effective and warranted. In lymphadenopathic cat scratch disease, a vigorous host response limits bacterial growth but also produces lymphadenitis, which is a hallmark of the disease. Antimicrobial therapy is of minimal, if any, value in such situations.

chapter 27

Chlamydiae: Genital, Ocular, and Respiratory Pathogens

Priscilla B. Wyrick and Jane E. Raulston

key concepts

Chlamydiae:

- Are obligate intracellular Gram-negative bacteria.

- Undergo a unique developmental cycle within eukaryotic host cells.

- Exhibit two distinct morphological forms termed elementary bodies (EBs) and reticulate bodies (RBs).

- EBs are small (0.25-μm) extracellular infectious particles that attach to and enter into host cells but are metabolically inert; that is, they do not grow or divide.

- RBs are larger (0.6-μm to 0.8-μm) intracellular, noninfectious but metabolically active forms that divide by binary fission within a membrane-bound inclusion in eukaryotic host cells.

- Cause a wide variety of genital, ocular, and respiratory infections in humans; certain animal and avian isolates cause disease by zoonotic transmission.

The *Chlamydia* genus includes species of Gram-negative bacteria that have an obligatory requirement to grow and propagate within eukaryotic cells. They cannot be cultured in nutrient broth media or on agar plates. One evolutionary result of their restricted growth within eukaryotic cells is that chlamydiae are extremely isolated within their own phylogenetic grouping and are genetically distant from other eubacteria. Interestingly, these organisms have acquired several genes from eukaryotes that have never been found in other bacteria. The *Chlamydia* are widespread in humans, animals, and birds, and they have achieved a remarkably balanced relationship with their hosts. Thus, they are often referred to as "stealth pathogens." Although they cause many serious diseases with apparently immune-mediated complications, the organisms themselves have an extraordinary ability to evade host immune responses.

Case

Mr. C., who is 24, saw a physician because of a purulent discharge from his penis. A diagnosis of gonorrhea was made (see Chapter 14), and he was given a cephalosporin, ceftriaxone, by intramuscular injection and had to drink a slurry of a second antibiotic. Mr. C. improved but felt guilty when confessing the situation to his latest sexual partner, Ms. N. He urged her to make an appointment to be tested for the disease.

Ms. N. had no complaints of pain, vaginal irritation, or discharge. However, on physical examination she was found to have a mucopurulent discharge emanating from the mouth of her cervix. Her cervix was inflamed and bled easily when a swab was used to remove adherent secretions. Gram stain of the secretions revealed numerous neutrophils but no Gram-negative diplococci. Ms. N. was told she probably had a chlamydial infection, chlamydial cervicitis. An endocervical swab was collected for nucleic amplification assays for both chlamydiae and gonococci. Ms. N. was also given an intramuscular injection of ceftriaxone, as an added precaution against *Neisseria gonorrhoeae*, and drank the slurry of the second antibiotic in the presence of the physician. The physician then questioned Ms. N. about other sexual partners before releasing her.

These cases raise several questions:

1. What was the second antibiotic taken by Mr. C., and why was it given?
2. Why were nucleic acid amplification assays performed instead of culture on Ms. N.'s endocervical material?
3. If Ms. N. had not heeded Mr. C.'s advice and sought medical attention, what might have been the consequences for her? What are the pathophysiological mechanisms of such sequelae?

Chlamydiae

CLASSIFICATION AND TAXONOMY

Current, ongoing molecular analyses of a variety of chlamydial isolates confirm that the order Chlamydiales encompasses a wide range of pathogenic bacteria that share a unique biphasic developmental cycle within eukaryotic host cells. Presently, the taxonomical terms for human chlamydial pathogens that have been used since the early 1970s are most commonly used in the literature. In this nomenclature the order Chlamydiales contains one family, Chlamydiaceae; one genus, *Chlamydia;* and two species, *C. trachomatis* and *C. pneumoniae.* Organisms are also subdivided according to specific biological traits (i.e., biovariants, or biovars) as well as serology (i.e., serovariants, or serovars). Molecular studies do indicate that *C. pneumoniae* could be recategorized into a separate genus (*Chlamydiophila*); however, most investigators prefer to wait until significant biological properties are clearly delineated before adopting the new genus name. Analysis of 16S rRNA for the purpose of taxonomy has been particularly beneficial for speciation of chlamydiae associated with animal diseases. These animal pathogens are important in human medicine because accidental transmission to humans can produce acute, life-threatening illnesses. Table 27-1 briefly describes the chlamydial agents and associated illnesses.

EPIDEMIOLOGY

C. trachomatis and *C. pneumoniae* are among the most common bacterial disease agents observed in the human population in both developed and developing countries. The estimated annual incidence for genital infections by *C. trachomatis* serovars D through K is 4 million in the United States and 90 million worldwide. *C. trachomatis* is the leading bacterial agent of **sexually transmitted disease (STD)** and overall infections are perhaps second only to human papillomavirus as the most common STDs overall. Although actual numbers of reported cases are increasing (current rates are 275 to 300 cases per 100,000 overall population), possible reasons for the increase are improved detection methods and efficiency. For comparison, about 800,000 new cases of genital infections by *Neisseria gonorrhoeae,* the second most common bacterial STD agent, occur in the United States each year. Double infections are common; 55% of males and more than 65% of females with gonorrhea are concomitantly infected with chlamydiae. The most alarming observation is that the highest rates of chlamydial STDs are seen in adolescents and young adults between 15 and 24 years of age. *C. trachomatis* is also responsible for approximately one half of all cases of **pelvic inflammatory disease (PID)**.

Lymphogranuloma venereum (LGV, serovars L1 through L3), a genetically related biovariant of *C. trachomatis* serovars D through K, also causes STDs but with different clinical manifestations. LGV causes an invasive disease primarily of the lymph nodes and is more common in Africa, Asia, India, and South America. Although the disease occurs only sporadically in North America and Europe, the United States averages 200 to 400 cases of LGV infection each year, primarily among homosexual males residing in port cities. The LGV serovars are considered important as the agents of emerging infectious STDs.

Trachoma, caused by *C. trachomatis* serovars A through C, is an ocular disease of individuals living in poverty and rural areas with poor hygienic conditions; infection rates are highest among children. With a crude estimate of 400 million to 600 million cases, tra-

table 27-1 Chlamydial Agents and Diseases

AGENT	DISEASE MANIFESTATION
Agents of human chlamydial infections	
Chlamydia trachomatis biovar trachoma serovars A–C	Trachoma
C. trachomatis biovar trachoma serovars D–K	Sexually transmitted infections (urethritis, cervicitis, endometritis, salpingitis, pelvic inflammatory disease, epididymitis, prostatitis, proctitis, reactive arthritis, conjunctivitis, pneumonitis)
C. trachomatis biovar lymphogranuloma venereum (LGV) serovars L1–L3	Invasive sexually transmitted infections (lymphadenopathy, buboes)
C. pneumoniae	Pneumonia, bronchitis, pharyngitis, association with atherosclerosis
Agents of animal chlamydial infections	
C. muridarum	Pneumonitis in mice
C. suis	Sexually transmitted infections in pigs
C. pneumoniae biovar Koala	Pneumonitis in Koala bears
C. pneumoniae biovar equine	Pneumonitis in horses
C. psittaci serovars A–F[a]	Respiratory and gastrointestinal illnesses in wild and domesticated birds Acute respiratory disease (psittacosis) in humans
C. abortus[a]	Abortion in sheep, lambs Abortion in humans
C. felis[a]	Conjunctivitis in cats Conjunctivitis in humans
C. caviae	Guinea pig inclusion conjunctivitis
C. pecorum	Polyarthritis, encephalomyelitis, and pneumonia in sheep and cattle

[a]Agents for which zoonotic transmission to humans has been confirmed. The transmission of other nonhuman chlamydial pathogens is not known but is generally thought likely under opportunistic circumstances.

choma is considered the world's leading cause of preventable blindness. Trachoma is rare in developed countries but is endemic in tropical and subtropical regions such as Africa, India, the Middle and Far East, and Latin America.

C. pneumoniae was identified in 1989 as an agent of "walking pneumonia" of endemic proportions. Numerous serological studies indicate that 70 to 90% of all adults either have been or are infected with *C. pneumoniae*. Initial infections generally appear during the school-age years. In addition to **respiratory illness** and contributory roles in **asthma**, viable *C. pneumoniae* have also been directly isolated from human monocytes, foam cells, and smooth muscle cells in atherosclerotic lesions and likely participate in exacerbating the chronic inflammatory process of **atherogenesis** and **coronary artery disease**.

The most common **chlamydial zoonoses** involve accidental transmission of *C. psittaci* to humans. **Psittacosis** was recognized as early as 1879 and is primarily associated with ownership or care of exotic psittacine birds such as parrots, parakeets, cockatoos, cockatiels, and macaws. The term *ornithosis* is interchangeable with *psittacosis* in reference to the illness observed in humans but is indicative of infections originating from nonpsittacine birds such as turkeys and pigeons. Psittacosis

is frequent among workers in poultry processing plants in the United States, particularly preceding the holiday months of November and December. Unfortunately, this life-threatening illness is often not recognized; the reported cases from 1996 to 2001 of only 165 in the United States is severely underrepresented compared with 1,620 cases reported in Great Britain, where awareness of chlamydial zoonoses is heightened.

C. abortus infections represent a major economic burden for farmers of domestic sheep and lambs; although human infections are extremely rare, there are reports of human abortion among pregnant female farmers assisting with lambing. In recent years, *C. felis*, which is a common cause of conjunctivitis in cats, particularly kittens, has been recognized as a cause of conjunctivitis and atypical pneumonia in humans who have frequent and close contact with cats.

BIOLOGY

Chlamydiae are small in size (0.25 to 0.8 μm in diameter) compared with typical bacteria such as *Escherichia coli* (1.0 μm) and have small chromosomes ranging from

1.0 to 1.2 megabases in size. They are **Gram-negative** in architecture and composition, with an outer membrane containing lipopolysaccharide (LPS; truncated and not very endotoxic) and a cytoplasmic membrane. While the classic bacterial cell wall component peptidoglycan (murein) has not been confirmed by isolation and identification, chlamydiae are susceptible to penicillin and possess all the genes for murein synthesis and penicillin-binding proteins. A distinct layer located just beneath the outer membrane can be seen by freeze-fracture electron microscopy, suggesting a structure analogous to peptidoglycan. Chlamydiae also contain a plasmid, and bacteriophages have been identified in *C. pneumoniae* and *C. psittaci*, but the roles and consequences of the extra DNA and viral agents are unknown at this time.

These **obligate intracellular bacteria** parasitize their host epithelial cell for nutrients and are **auxotrophic** for several amino acids and three of the four nucleoside triphosphates; the demand for host cell adenosine triphosphate (ATP) has led to their designation as an "energy parasite." Although whole genome sequencing revealed that chlamydiae can produce limited ATP by glycolysis, their genomes contain two separate loci for the production of ATP/ADP (adenosine diphosphate) translocases that would function in taking ATP from the host to ensure sufficient quantities to drive their synthetic and metabolic needs.

ENTRY, SPREAD, AND MULTIPLICATION

Growth of chlamydiae in their target columnar epithelial cells is characterized by a unique developmental cycle (Fig. 27-1). Two forms of the organism are needed (or required) for growth to occur: the infectious, extracellular form called an **elementary body (EB)** and the noninfectious but metabolically active intracellular form called a **reticulate body (RB)**. Infection is initiated by attachment of EBs to the apical surfaces of epithelial cells of the conjunctiva, respiratory, gastrointestinal, or urogenital tracts, followed by entry by **receptor-mediated endocytosis** (Fig. 27-2A). The EBs quickly modify their early endosomal membrane to exit the endosomal pathway, thereby avoiding fusion with lysosomes, and traffic on microtubules to the peri-Golgi/nuclear hof region. The EB-containing endosomes of *C. trachomatis* then fuse homotypically with one another to form their one nascent microcolony called an **inclusion** (Fig. 27-3A); the EB-containing endosomes of *C. pneumoniae* and *C. psittaci* (Fig. 27-3B) develop independently and form multiple inclusions in each infected cell.

The EBs then transform into RBs, the chromosome becomes relaxed and transcriptionally active, and metabolic growth and binary fission ensue to generate

FIGURE 27-1 ■ The *Chlamydia* developmental cycle.

FIGURE 27-2 ■ **The *C. trachomatis* infectious process. A.** Infection is initiated by attachment of elementary bodies (EBs) to epithelial cells; notice projections facing down into the coated pit. **B.** Metabolically active reticulate bodies (RBs) in an early inclusion. **C and D.** Projections on an EB and RB penetrating through the inclusion membrane into epithelial cytoplasm. **E.** A single mature inclusion containing RBs and EBs.

progeny (Fig. 27-2B). Chlamydiae-directed modification of their inclusion membrane permits interception of trans-Golgi vesicles for transfer of sphingomyelin and glycerolphospholipids to the inclusion membrane, which can expand to accommodate some 200 to 1,000 progeny; this strategy of acquiring host cell markers for the inclusion also provides some degree of camouflage for the chlamydiae within.

It is speculated that RBs obtain their nutrients from the epithelial cytoplasm using at least two strategies: (1) insertion of chlamydial proteins (Incs) into the inclusion membrane, some of which likely have autotransporter functions; and (2) insertion of a unique appendage through the inclusion membrane. On the surface of chlamydiae are 18 to 23 projections arranged in a hexagonal array (Fig 27-2C); they span the envelope and can be seen passing through the inclusion membrane into the host cytoplasm (Fig. 27-2D). As the projections are hollow, they are thought to act as "drinking straws," allowing the prokaryotic chlamydiae to feed from their eukaryotic host without having to leave the confines of their protective inclusion vacuole. Isolated projections have a naillike morphology remarkably similar to that characterized for flagella. Even though the chlamydiae are not motile, information from the *C. trachomatis* D genome sequence revealed the existence of some flagella gene orthologues, including some basal body structural and flagella-associated transport functional equivalents.

More recently, some type III secretion homologues have been identified in chlamydiae, causing further speculation that the chlamydial projections might serve an alternative function as a type III secretion system. As with other Gram-negative bacteria, the projections might function during contact-dependent attachment to

FIGURE 27-3 ■ **Chlamydial inclusions and effect of antibiotic exposure. A.** Fluorescence photograph of *C. trachomatis* inclusions (yellow), one per infected epithelial cell (red); note few residual EBs (tiny yellow dots) attached to the host cells. **B.** Giemsa stain of multiple *C. psittaci* inclusions (arrows) per infected host cell. **C.** Disruption of chlamydial protein synthesis by azithromycin on growing RBs damages RBs.

prime the epithelial cell signal transduction and trafficking pathways for EB entry (from outside to inside; see Fig. 27-2A). A new, alternative concept is that they might function later in chlamydial development to deliver RB-secreted effector molecules into the host cytoplasm to further modulate host–pathogen interactions (from inside to outside), such as delayed apoptosis.

RBs are osmotically fragile and do not survive outside their inclusion, nor can they bind to epithelial cells. Thus, to perpetuate the infectious process, RBs must mature back into infectious EBs before escaping from infected cells (Fig. 27-2E). The signal for this conversion may be detachment from the inclusion membrane of the now replete RB. Numerous disulfide bonds are formed, cross-linking three major outer membrane proteins and helping to provide the rigidity and stability EBs need for their sojourn into the extracellular environment to find a fresh susceptible epithelial cell to infect. The inclusion membrane may then fuse with the host plasma membrane to release chlamydiae, or the host cell, depleted of nutrients and energy, may lyse. Luminal *C. trachomatis* progeny are released at the apical surfaces of polarized columnar epithelial cells to spread canalicularly to the upper genital tract, whereas the invasive LGV serovars are released at the basal domain into the submucosa en route to the regional lymph nodes. A chlamydia-specific protease is released early to shut down programmed epithelial cell death signals until late in the developmental cycle, after which apoptosis of the infected epithelial may factor in the release and spread of chlamydiae. This developmental cycle takes 2 to 3 days to complete, depending on the species.

Exposure of chlamydiae-infected cells in vitro to **interferon-γ** induces an altered state in RB known as **persistence** (see Fig. 27-1). Chlamydiae are auxotrophic for tryptophan, and interferon-γ activates a mammalian enzyme that catabolizes L-tryptophan. The persistent state is characterized by morphologically enlarged, aberrant RBs that are transcriptionally active but have lowered metabolic rates. The chromosome can be replicated and segregated, but some cell division gene transcription is halted, resulting in the lack of production of infectious EBs and a culture-negative scenario. It is believed that this persistent state is the more prevalent form of chlamydiae in vivo, where subinhibitory concentrations of interferon-γ occur through antigen-activated macrophages and CD4+ and CD8+ T cells; however, it is difficult to prove in vivo versus repeated reinfection. One convincing bit of evidence is the confirmed presence of persistent *C. trachomatis* serovar K RBs in monocytes in synovial tissues from patients with reactive arthritis who were previously culture positive.

The potential importance of the putative persistent state in vivo cannot be overstated, because it is postulated to be the key strategy by which chlamydiae avoid the host immune response and linger in tissues to cause chronic infection and/or reactivation disease. Interest-

ingly, while production of chlamydial antigens, such as the major outer membrane protein and LPS, are decreased in persistent RBs, the chlamydial heat-shock protein 60 (hsp60) antigen is dramatically increased and may be a stimulus for sustained inflammation. Chronic inflammation is thought to be one factor in the underlying pathology of disease sequelae.

DAMAGE

C. trachomatis serovars A through K initially infect and grow within epithelial cells of the ocular and genital mucosae; resident macrophages and dendritic cells are also exposed to released EBs but do not sufficiently support bacterial development. Inflammatory mediators and chemokines produced in infected epithelial cells serve as initial triggers for an influx of polymorphonuclear leukocytes and natural killer cells that eventually activate the phagocytes and antigen-presenting cells into programming and development of the cell-mediated immune response. As the host immune response develops, active sites of infection show an infiltration of plasma cells and macrophages. Lymphoid follicles containing macrophages, T cells, and B cells subsequently develop, and overall this continual chronic inflammatory process leads to necrosis, epithelial cell proliferation, and scar tissue formation. Thus, the serious sequelae of *C. trachomatis* infections are mediated by the host immune response. Evidence is accumulating for a delayed-type hypersensitivity response to the chlamydia-specific hsp60 antigen.

Clinically, the early stages of *C. trachomatis* serovars D through K genital infections are subtle. In women the endocervix is sometimes reddened and friable with a mucoid exudate that is less purulent than that observed for *N. gonorrhoeae*. In men there may be a scant amount of a mucoid urethral exudate. Depending on sexual practices and hygiene, the rectal and ocular mucosae of both men and women can become infected. Importantly, isolates of *C. trachomatis* serovars D through K are not invasive and do not penetrate or invade the submucosa but remain at the luminal surface of the epithelium and spread in an ascending manner in the genitourinary tracts. Infections in women progress from the cervix (**cervicitis**) to the endometrium (**endometritis**), then to the fallopian tubes (**salpingitis**), and eventually into the peritoneum. This canalicular ascension may be heightened in the estrogen-dominant phase of the menstrual cycle. In men with **urethritis,** the organisms can eventually colonize the epididymis (**epididymitis**) and the prostate (**prostatitis**) but rarely the testicles. Men are at particular risk for eventual development of **sexually acquired reactive arthritis** or **Reiter syndrome**, especially individuals with high levels of HLA-B27 histocompatibility antigen. Because the initial stages of the infectious process are often mild or asymptomatic, many patients do not seek treatment.

Persistent infections, as well as repeated exposures and reinfections, lead to more serious disease sequelae, such as **tubal factor infertility** and PID. When these later complications occur, patients can be treated for eradication of the organisms, but the tissue damage is generally irreversible, and women are at particular risk for life-threatening **ectopic pregnancies.**

Infants born vaginally to infected mothers acquire EBs in their eyes, ears, nose, and mouth and develop **mild conjunctivitis** and a **pneumonitis** that is characterized by a **chronic, repetitive cough without wheezing.** Untreated, approximately two thirds of these children suffer long-term respiratory abnormalities, including **asthma.**

The invasive LGV serovars of *C. trachomatis* can enter small breaks in the skin and initiate an inconspicuous genital papule or herpetic-like ulcer. Patients with these infrequent primary lesions are usually asymptomatic. They seek medical attention when infections have progressed to the secondary stage with **acute lymphadenitis,** perhaps accompanied by the appearance of inguinal buboes, and fever. Thus, **LGV infection is a disease primarily of the lymphatic tissue,** from which the organisms can spread to the bloodstream.

Similar to *C. trachomatis* infections, those with *C. pneumoniae,* a common agent of **atypical pneumonia,** can evolve into chronic inflammatory events mediated by the host immune response. *C. pneumoniae* EBs are spread by droplet aerosols and can remain viable for up to 30 hours on inert surfaces. Respiratory infections are generally mild or asymptomatic in healthy individuals and, in adults, symptoms are often clinically indistinguishable from those caused by *Mycoplasma pneumoniae.* Patients may present with pharyngitis, bronchitis, sinusitis, otitis media, or pneumonia that evolves over an extended number of weeks. Several individuals can be affected because *C. pneumoniae* is a frequent cause of **community-acquired pneumonia.** In more exacerbated cases of pneumonia, coinfections of *C. pneumoniae* with other respiratory pathogens such as *Streptococcus pneumoniae* or adenoviruses are common.

C. pneumoniae infects and multiplies within a wide range of host cells, including epithelial cells, endothelial cells, monocytes, macrophages, lymphocytes, and cells that participate in atherogenesis. Indeed, the ability to grow in various cells represents the likely vehicle in which *C. pneumoniae* is distributed from the lungs into circulation. The hypothesis that *C. pneumoniae* contributes to **coronary artery disease** is supported by several lines of evidence: adults with coronary artery disease have high titers of *C. pneumoniae*–specific antibodies; the organisms have been directly cultured from **atherosclerotic lesions;** and some, but not all, antimicrobial therapy trials suggest that a reduction in recurrent coronary events is attainable. In laboratory-grown host cells, the organisms stimulate inflammatory events consistent with atherosclerosis and can promote the development of coronary lesions in animal model studies.

C. trachomatis serovars A through K and *C. pneumoniae* are similar in that initial infections are often mild or asymptomatic and the organisms can enter into a nonculturable, persistent state within host tissues culminating in a chronic inflammatory pathobiology. Conversely, the **invasive and lymphotropic** sexually transmitted LGV biovariant of *C. trachomatis* and the zoonotic chlamydial animal pathogens generally cause acute, sometimes life-threatening, illnesses.

Inhalation of *C. psittaci,* present in fecal aerosols excreted by stressed or sick birds, initially causes an abrupt flulike illness in humans but can rapidly progress to endocarditis, central nervous system involvement, encephalitis, coma, or death. Pregnant female farmers that assist in the birthing of lambs are at risk of infection with *C. abortus,* which can cause abortion, renal failure, disseminated intravascular coagulation, or death. Because these illnesses are not common, a detailed patient history, including travel, recent sexual practices, pet ownership, and profession, is most often where an attentive physician derives a preliminary diagnosis.

DIAGNOSIS, TREATMENT, AND PREVENTION

Until recently, diagnosis of chlamydial infections was made following growth and culture of the organisms from patient specimens. This task was performed only by a limited number of experienced laboratories. Subsequently, antigen detection methods, either **direct fluorescence assay** or **enzyme immunoassay,** became popular and are still used in certain clinical studies. Currently, **nucleic acid amplification tests (NAAT),** such as polymerase chain reaction, ligase chain reaction, or transcription-mediated amplification, represent the most common and sensitive methods used for *C. trachomatis* detection and screening. One prominent advantage of NAAT is that specimens may be obtained by noninvasive procedures such as first-void urine; however, laboratories should be aware of the possibility that components in urine samples may interfere with or inhibit NAAT.

Because these organisms reside within epithelial cells, obtaining an appropriate specimen requires rotating a fibrous swab on affected mucosal epithelium. For suspected cases of genital *C. trachomatis* infection in women, any cervical exudate should be removed (and assayed for *N. gonorrhoeae*), and the sample to be tested for chlamydiae should be obtained by swabbing the endocervix at the squamocolumnar junction. Likewise, in men, excess discharge should first be removed and samples obtained by inserting a swab 3 to 4 cm into the urethra with rotation. Because of its high level of discomfort, this invasive procedure for men is rarely performed and is a primary reason for our lack of knowledge of prevalence of chlamydial genital infections among men. The adaptation of NAAT for first void urine samples, which contain infected epithelial cells, and self-collected vaginal swab material has been a major advance in diagnosing chlamydial STDs.

DNA amplification methods will be used in the near future for diagnosis of infections by *C. pneumoniae*. Culture and immunofluorescence microscopy are presently used by some laboratories, but commercially available *C. pneumoniae*–specific antibody reagents are limited. A confirmatory diagnosis requires an experienced laboratory to differentiate between *C. pneumoniae* and *C. trachomatis* or *C. psittaci*, all of which can cause respiratory illnesses. The optimal sample for the laboratory is obtained using a wire-shafted swab to obtain epithelial cells from the nasopharynx; throat swabs and sputum samples may not yield sufficient numbers of organisms. Because the clinical presentation of *C. pneumoniae* infections resemble those caused by *M. pneumoniae*, the cold hemagglutinin reaction can be used for a differential diagnosis (see Chapter 29). *C. pneumoniae* is agglutination negative, whereas *M. pneumoniae* is positive.

Antimicrobial therapy regimens for chlamydial infections require agents that have excellent tissue penetration properties; moreover, bactericidal concentrations should be maintained for an extended period because of the slow-growing and persistent nature of chlamydiae. Patients diagnosed with infections by *C. trachomatis* serovars A through K are prescribed azithromycin (Fig. 27-3C) or multiple doses of doxycycline over 7 days; erythromycin is an alternative for pregnant women and children where doxycycline is contraindicated. A prolonged course of therapy (3 weeks) is recommended for adults with flulike symptoms and suspected infection with *C. pneumoniae*; extended duration of treatment (3 weeks) is also recommended for LGV infections. Complete regimen compliance is important because most patients will show rapid clinical improvement even though the organisms persist, and noncompliance is one reason for the high annual rates of chlamydial infections. Sexual partners must also be treated for *C. trachomatis* genital infections, or therapy will likely be ineffective.

The development of a vaccine against human chlamydial infections represents a long-term objective requiring continual investigation. Numerous studies indicate that a CD4$^+$ Th1 cell-mediated immune response favors resolution of infection and protective immunity. Conversely, a CD4$^+$ Th2 response appears to drive destructive immune-mediated responses; Th2 cytokines are clearly associated with scarring and tissue damage. CD8$^+$ T cells are also induced during chlamydial infection, but whether their primary role is for lysis of chlamydiae-infected cells or in the secretion of cytokines requires further study. In patients with trachoma, decreased lymphoproliferative responses are associated with persistent ocular disease, whereas increased lymphoproliferative responses are associated with resolution of infection. Such observations resemble immune mechanisms in leishmaniasis and leprosy that have obligate intracellular pathogens as primary culprits of disease induction.

Chlamydiae-infected patients also produce a wide array of specific antibodies, and certain antibodies may limit spread of infectious EB. However, limited data indicate that protective humoral immune responses are strain-specific and of short duration. High serum antibody titers in general are also associated with complications of chlamydial disease. Because chlamydiae are adept at maintaining a persistent state of infection despite the development of an acquired immune response in patients, research efforts are focused on the innate immune mediators for development of a favorable adaptive response. The programming of T lymphocytes will be a central issue for vaccination, but it will be crucial to delineate those chlamydial antigens that evoke protective immunity over destructive immunopathology.

Conclusion

Chlamydiae are insidious pathogens. They sequester themselves inside host cells in vacuoles that protect them from the array of hostile armaments the host cell reserves for invading pathogens. The infected person mounts both humoral and cell-mediated responses that, in a subset of individuals, are destructive. Serious complications can occur, some of which are life threatening. Current research is focused on how chlamydiae behave inside eukaryotic cells and what the host response strategies are: What signals do chlamydiae induce in infected cells to thwart innate responses, and conversely, how does host surveillance, in animal models, prevail and protect us?

Rocky Mountain Spotted Fever and Other Rickettsioses

David H. Walker

key **concepts**

Rickettsiae:

- Are obligate intracellular bacteria (i.e., cannot be grown on artificial media).

- Are usually arthropodborne.

- Cause several severe diseases: Rocky Mountain spotted fever (*Rickettsia rickettsii*), typhus (*R. prowazekii*); murine typhus (*R. typhi*); scrub typhus *(Orientia tsutsugamushi)*, and others.

- Have a predilection for vascular endothelial cells, causing blood vessel damage and bleeding in various organs. In the skin, vascular damage results in rashes.

- Cause infections that can be treated with antibiotics that penetrate host cells.

The *Rickettsia* genus comprises a large number of bacteria that can only grow inside eukaryotic cells. With the chlamydiae, the rickettsiae are the principal medically important **obligate intracellular bacteria.** The other defining characteristic of these organisms is their epidemiology. Most rickettsioses are **zoonoses,** infections that are transmitted from animals to humans and are spread mainly through arthropod vectors (ticks, mites, fleas, lice, and chiggers). Table 28-1 outlines the etiology and epidemiology of the most common diseases caused by the *Rickettsia* bacteria.

The most important rickettsiosis in the United States, **Rocky Mountain spotted fever,** is a serious, life-threatening disease. Like many other species of rickettsiae, the causative agent invades vascular endothelial cells, resulting in generalized vascular damage. Other important rickettsioses are **Q fever** (which often manifests as pneumonia), **human monocytotropic ehrlichiosis,** and **human granulocytotropic anaplasmosis** (both of which infect leukocytes and cause thrombocytopenia). Some rickettsioses have played important roles in history, and some have appeared to emerge anew in people with AIDS.

table 28-1 Etiology and Epidemiology of Principal Rickettsioses

RICKETTSIAL AGENT	DISEASES	RESERVOIR IN NATURE	TRANSMISSION	GEOGRAPHIC DISTRIBUTION
Rickettsia rickettsii	Rocky Mountain spotted fever	Ticks (transovarian transmission)	Tick bite	North and South America
R. conorii	Boutonneuse fever	Tick (transovarian transmission)	Tick bite	Southern Europe, Africa, and Asia
R. prowazekii	Epidemic typhus Recrudescent typhus	Humans, flying squirrels Humans	Louse feces None	Potentially worldwide Potentially worldwide
R. typhi	Murine typhus	Fleas and rats	Flea feces	Worldwide, especially tropics and subtropics
Orientia tsutsugamushi	Scrub typhus	Chiggers (transovarian transmission)	Chigger bite	Asia, Oceania, and northern Australia
Ehrlichia chaffeensis	Human monocytotropic ehrlichiosis	Deer, goats, dogs	Tick bite	North America
Anaplasma phagocytophilum	Human granulocytotropic ehrlichiosis	Deer, elk, wild rodents	Tick bite	North America and Europe
Coxiella burnetii	Q fever	Cattle, sheep, goats, other livestock; cats	Aerosol from infected birth products; ticks	Worldwide

Case

S., a 9-year-old girl, was taken to her pediatrician on May 31, two days after the onset of fever reaching 40.5°C, severe headache, and muscle pains. The next day she developed nausea, vomiting, and abdominal pain and was admitted to the hospital for observation for possible appendicitis. On the second day following admission, an erythematous rash consisting of 2- to 4-mm macules (areas of discoloration) appeared on her wrists and ankles. Within 24 hours of its onset, the rash involved the arms, legs, and trunk, and many of the lesions had become maculopapular (discolored and raised) with petechiae (dark red spots caused by bleeding in the skin). A serological test for Rocky Mountain spotted fever and cultures of the blood, cerebrospinal fluid, and urine were negative. S. became stuporous and had edema in her face and extremities.

Treatment with intravenous doxycycline was begun for the suspected diagnosis of Rocky Mountain spotted fever. Within 72 hours, S. was alert and afebrile. She was sent home after 4 days in the hospital with instructions to take oral doxycycline for three more days. By the time of her discharge from the hospital, the rash had faded remarkably.

S. lived in a mobile home on the outskirts of Burlington, North Carolina, and played after school in the nearby high grass and weeds. Her mother had removed several ticks from her body nearly every day during the month of May before she became sick. When S. returned to her pediatrician at the end of June, she was completely recovered. A serum sample was collected and sent, along with one collected during the acute phase of her hospitalization, to the state public health laboratory. A dramatic rise in titer of antibody to *Rickettsia rickettsii* was detected in the convalescent sample.

This case raises several questions:

1. What caused the rash, stupor, and gastrointestinal symptoms?
2. Why was the serological test for Rocky Mountain spotted fever negative in the hospital?
3. Assuming that rickettsiae were circulating in the blood, why were the blood cultures negative?
4. How did a girl from an eastern state get "Rocky Mountain" spotted fever?

The classic rickettsiosis, epidemic **typhus,** has been one of the most significant infectious diseases in history because of its devastating effects on humanity, particularly in its influence on the outcome of most European wars between 1500 and 1900. During and immediately after World War I and the Russian Revolution, 30 million people suffered from epidemic typhus, and 3 million of them died. The human body louse transmits *Rickettsia prowazekii* by depositing its feces on the skin. With the discovery of effective insecticides, delousing interrupted the transmission of epidemic typhus in World War II and greatly reduced its incidence.

The most common rickettsiosis in the United States is **Rocky Mountain spotted fever.** It affects approximately 600 people annually, mostly in the eastern and southern states rather than in the Rocky Mountains

FIGURE 28-1 ▪ **Electron micrograph of a thin section of a human endothelial cell infected with *Rickettsia rickettsii*, the etiological agent of Rocky Mountain spotted fever.** The rickettsiae are the dark, rod-shaped bacteria in the nucleus, about the same size as the mitochondria and smaller than most other bacteria. These rickettsiae have invaded the nucleus. Although *R. rickettsii* organisms usually occupy the cytoplasm and few enter the nucleus, their presence in this location is characteristic of spotted fever rickettsiae and would be most unusual for other rickettsiae as well as *Mycobacteria, Salmonella,* and *Legionella* organisms.

where it was first described. This disease can be extremely serious and, if untreated, has a mortality rate of about 20%. Because the disease responds well to certain antibiotics, especially in the early stages, a speedy diagnosis is essential. The spotted fever group of rickettsioses as well as the typhus group are characterized by disseminated vascular infection. Injury in the lungs, central nervous system, and other systemic microcirculation may cause neurological signs, seizures, coma, acute respiratory failure, shock, and acute renal failure.

Q fever differs significantly from the typhus and spotted fever infections in that it has an acute form, manifested mainly as pneumonia, and a chronic form, in which the heart valves are usually affected. The causative agent, *Coxiella burnetii,* grows in the macrophages in the lung, liver, bone marrow, and spleen, where it stimulates granuloma formation. In another kind of rickettsiosis, called ehrlichiosis, the organisms grow in white blood cells. Ehrlichiosis is a tick-transmitted infection of monocytes and macrophages or neutrophils with systemic manifestations caused by the host response.

Rickettsiae are small Gram-negative rods that have an outer membrane and a thin murein layer (Fig. 28-1). However, they are not readily stainable by the Gram method. DNA homology studies reveal that spotted fever and typhus rickettsiae are relatively closely related to other strict intracellular parasites, the *Ehrlichia* and *Anaplasma,* as well as facultatively intracellular *Bartonella.* In contrast, *C. burnetii* is more closely related to *Legionella* and only distantly related to the other rickettsiae. Spotted fever and typhus rickettsiae have lipopolysaccharides that are antigenically distinct for each

group. *Ehrlichia* and *Orientia* lack both lipopolysaccharides and peptidoglycan.

Rickettsiae are highly adapted to the intracellular niche, where they propagate by binary fission with a generation time of 8 to 10 hours. Rickettsiae thrive in the high potassium environment of the eukaryotic cytosol and have specific membrane transport systems for acquiring adenosine triphosphate (ATP), amino acids, and other metabolites from the host cell. Unlike chlamydiae, rickettsiae are not strict energy parasites; they are also able to synthesize at least some of their required ATP. In addition, Rickettsiae are capable of **independent metabolism** (e.g., tricarboxylic acid cycle and electron transport system) and use their own biosynthetic machinery to make proteins and other complex components. However, they cannot be cultivated on artificial medium and in the laboratory they must be grown in animals, embryonated eggs, or cell cultures.

Rickettsia rickettsii: Rocky Mountain Spotted Fever

ENCOUNTER AND ENTRY

R. rickettsii organisms are transmitted from tick to tick by the transovarian route and usually cause little harm to that host. The ticks involved in Rocky Mountain spotted

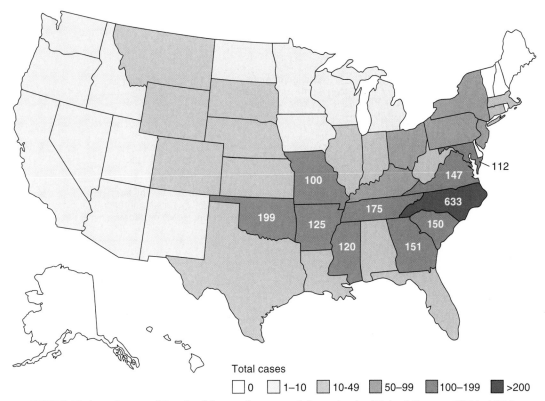

Total cases
☐ 0 ☐ 1–10 ☐ 10-49 ☐ 50–99 ☐ 100–199 ☐ >200

FIGURE 28-2 ▪ **Cases of Rocky Mountain spotted fever in the United States, 1994–1998.**

fever (*Dermacentor* species) are different from the *Ixodes* involved in Lyme disease (see Chapter 25). When some wild animals are bitten by *Dermacentor* ticks, they become transiently infected and a transient reservoir of the rickettsiae. Thus, the disease cannot be eradicated by public health measures. Risk of transmission can be reduced by the use of tick repellents and protective clothing. Individuals can prevent this illness by removing ticks from the skin before the bacteria are inoculated, usually between 6 and 24 hours after attachment (for a discussion of insectborne diseases, see Chapter 33 paradigm). The geographic distribution of cases of the disease occurring in the United States from 1994 to 1998 is shown in Figure 28-2.

SPREAD, MULTIPLICATION, AND DAMAGE

Signs and symptoms of Rocky Mountain spotted fever begin an average of 1 week after an infected adult tick inoculates *R. rickettsii* into the skin while taking a blood meal. The rickettsiae spread throughout the body via the bloodstream. On encountering vascular endothelial cells, rickettsiae attach to the cell membrane and induce the cells to engulf them (Fig. 28-3 and Table 28-2). Once inside the cells, rickettsiae rapidly escape

from the phagosome into the cytosol, apparently by lysis of the phagosomal membrane by a phospholipase.

Ensconced in the cytosol, *R. rickettsii* multiply and are propelled through the cytoplasm by polymerization of the host cell actin at one pole. The organisms then spread to other endothelial cells through long cellular projections of the cell membrane (see Chapter 17). Injury to the host cell correlates with the quantity of bacteria accumulated intracellularly. The subcellular target of injury appears to be the cell membrane, and the mechanism of damage to that structure appears to be the result of the action of free radical–induced membrane lipid peroxidation.

The effects of damage to foci of contiguous endothelial cells are visible in the skin, where dilation of the blood vessels first produces a pink rash. Later, leakage of red blood cells results in hemorrhagic spots (or **petechiae**), from which the name of the disease is derived (Fig. 28-4). Within the blood vessels of the brain, lung, heart, liver, and other visceral organs, these pinpoint hemorrhages lead to encephalitis, pneumonitis, cardiac arrhythmia, nausea, vomiting, and abdominal pain.

Even before the introduction of the effective antimicrobial treatment, 75% of patients with Rocky Mountain spotted fever survived. Clearance of intracellular rickettsiae from the endothelium is achieved through the strong effects of the immune system with important contributions by cell-mediated immunity, particularly

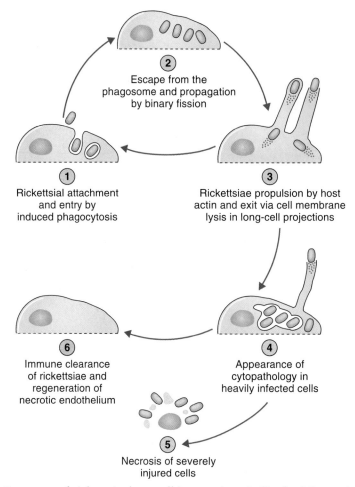

FIGURE 28-3 ▪ Sequence of rickettsia–host cell interactions in Rocky Mountain spotted fever.

T lymphocytes and their cytokines, such as interferon-γ and tumor necrosis factor. Older individuals are more likely to die from the disease.

Similar diseases are caused by antigenically related organisms. The geographic distribution of these diseases coincides with a population of infected ticks (e.g., in Southern Europe, Africa, and Asia, boutonneuse fever and **African tick bite fever;** in Australia, **Queensland tick typhus** and Flinders Island spotted fever; in northern Asia, Siberian tick typhus) or mites (in North America, Europe, and Asia, **rickettsialpox**). A substantial number of people become infected while traveling in Africa, where their activities expose them to ticks. On returning to North Amer-

ica or northern Europe, they seek medical attention for what is recognized by astute physicians as African tick bite fever. The prevalence of antibodies to spotted fever group rickettsiae among healthy subjects in the affected countries suggests that many infections are not diagnosed.

FIGURE 28-4 ▪ **Cross-section of a blood vessel from the dermis of a patient with Rocky Mountain spotted fever.** The rickettsiae are visualized within endothelial cells and vascular smooth muscle cells as tiny purple–red dots in clusters. Notice the infiltration of the vessel with lymphocytes and histiocytes.

table **28-2**	Cellular and Subcellular Locations	
RICKETTSIAL AGENT	**HOST TARGET CELL**	**CELLULAR LOCATION**
Rickettsia	Endothelium	Cytosol
Coxiella	Macrophages	Phagolysosome
Ehrlichia	Leukocytes	Cytoplasmic endosomal vacuole

Rickettsia prowazekii and *R. typhi*: Typhus Group Fevers

The classic epidemic disease, **typhus fever,** is spread among humans by the body **louse** and is associated with high mortality and dramatic epidemics. Epidemics begin with a single case of **recrudescent typhus (Brill-Zinsser disease)**, which is caused by reactivation of the agent, *R. prowazekii.* This agent can remain latent in the body for years or even decades after recovery from epidemic typhus or zoonotic typhus transmitted by fleas from flying squirrels. Recrudescent typhus was described in the late 1800s in New York City among immigrants from eastern Europe, where epidemics of typhus were notorious. It is presumed that typhus epidemics can be ignited from a patient with recrudescent typhus and body lice, which spread the infection to other persons. Absence of epidemic typhus in developed countries today is an effect of the socioeconomic conditions and low prevalence of human body lice. Where war, natural disasters, and famine occur, epidemic typhus has often followed; thus, the disease is associated with crowding, poverty, and "lousy" sanitary conditions. It is foolish to believe that epidemic typhus could never return.

The reservoir of the epidemic typhus rickettsiae is not only human beings but also flying squirrels and their fleas and lice. The infection has been transmitted from this source to humans in the eastern United States. Could an epidemic of typhus arise from one of these cases if it occurred among a louse-infested population? Possibly.

A more prevalent and widely dispersed rickettsiosis is **murine typhus.** This endemic disease is caused by *R. typhi,* which is transmitted in a natural cycle between rats and rat fleas. Humans become infected by the deposition of infected flea feces on their skin. Murine typhus occurs throughout the tropics and subtropics and was an important problem in the southern United States until the development of insecticides and intense rat control efforts.

Orientia tsutsugamushi: Scrub Typhus

Scrub typhus is a disease of major importance in parts of the world distant from the everyday lives of Americans and Europeans. However, during World War II and the Vietnam War, Americans and Europeans came into contact with the ecological conditions in the South Pacific, Burma, and China. As a result, *Orientia tsutsugamushi* infected 18,000 soldiers in World War II and was one of the major causes of undiagnosed febrile illness among soldiers in Vietnam. The indigenous populations of endemic areas in many countries of Asia are continuously exposed to the agent of this infection. In a study in rural Malaysia, scrub typhus was the most frequent reason for febrile hospitalization.

Several factors exacerbate the problem of scrub typhus. The organisms exist in various antigenic types, and immunity to one strain wanes over a period of a few years and to other strains after a few months. Subsequently, the patient becomes fully susceptible to reinfection. To make matters worse, clinical diagnosis is difficult because rash and eschar (a dry scab), considered the textbook hallmarks of the disease, are absent in most cases. In many endemic areas, medical care is suboptimal and laboratory diagnosis is virtually nonexistent. Scrub typhus is a neglected disease that, from time to time, rivets the attention of missionaries, the military, and medical examination committees.

Coxiella burnetii: Q fever

Q fever is short for "Query fever," referring to its unknown etiology when it was first described. The etiologic agent, *C. burnetii,* stands apart from other rickettsiae, and the disease differs from other rickettsioses in its clinical manifestations, pathological lesions, and epidemiology. Extracellularly, the organisms are much more resistant than the other rickettsiae to the many deleterious effects of the environment. Resistance may result from the formation of a sporelike structure that has been observed by electron microscopy. Consequently, this agent does not require the protection afforded by a living vector but may also be transmitted through aerosols. Q fever is distinctly zoonotic, and the main reservoirs are infected sheep and other animals. The organisms are present in large amounts in the placenta and fetal membranes and are spread in copious numbers when ewes give birth. The disease is most often seen among sheep farmers, veterinarians, and workers in laboratories that use sheep for experimentation.

The kind of disease produced by *C. burnetii* varies from acute pneumonia to chronic endocarditis. Acute infection may be asymptomatic or associated with nonspecific flulike febrile illness, atypical pneumonia, or granulomatous hepatitis. Chronic infection is usually diagnosed in patients with a long course, cardiac valvular infection, and negative routine blood cultures for bacteria. The pathogenic mechanisms appear to be largely immunopathological with T lymphocyte–mediated granulomas in self-limited disease and an immune complex–mediated component in some cases of chronic illness.

Ehrlichiae: Ehrlichiosis and Anaplasmosis

Previously unrecognized infectious diseases continue to be described; two human diseases caused by *Ehrlichia* species are among the newest to be discovered. *E. chaffeensis* and *E. ewingii* are transmitted by the Lone Star tick. They infect mainly monocytes and macrophages or neutrophils, respectively. Another intracellular pathogen of neutrophils, *Anaplasma phagocytophilum,* also infects rodents, ruminants, and deer and is transmitted by the same *Ixodes* ticks as Lyme disease. These obligate intracellular pathogens replicate intracellularly in membrane-bound vesicles. Occasionally, these vesicles can be seen by light microscopy of stained blood smears as round inclusions in either monocytes or neutrophils, depending on the species.

Most cases of ehrlichiosis and anaplasmosis are clinically similar to Rocky Mountain spotted fever and are characterized by fever, headache, and often severe multisystem involvement but with a lower incidence of rash. The spectrum of severity is quite broad and ranges from mild to fatal. Many patients with these infections have reduced numbers of circulating leukocytes as well as low platelet counts. Human granulocytic anaplasmosis is diagnosed much more readily than human monocytic ehrlichiosis because the organisms are visible more often in circulating leukocytes.

DIAGNOSIS OF RICKETTSIOSES

The clinical diagnosis of rickettsioses is difficult, particularly when the patient first visits a physician and treatment is most effective. At the time of presentation during the first 3 days of illness, only 3% of patients with Rocky Mountain spotted fever have the classic triad of fever, rash, and history of tick bite. In contrast to most infectious diseases, laboratory studies are seldom helpful in establishing a diagnosis of rickettsial disease in the acute stage of the illness. Very few laboratories attempt to isolate rickettsiae because of the technical requirements for inoculation of antibiotic-free cell culture. In addition, the handling of these agents is notoriously hazardous.

For these reasons the diagnosis of most rickettsioses requires considerable diagnostic acumen by physicians. Laboratory confirmation of rickettsioses is usually achieved in the convalescent stage by demonstrating a fourfold or greater rise in the titer of antibodies to rickettsial antigens. The only rickettsial disease that can be expected to have diagnostic levels of antibodies at the time the patient seeks medical attention is chronic Q fever. The serological methods usually employed are indirect fluorescent antibody assay or enzyme immunoassay (see Chapter 58); newer methods are currently being developed. The **Weil-Felix test,** an archaic test still in use in some laboratories, relies on the agglutination of certain strains of the enteric bacterium *Proteus vulgaris,* which shares cross-reactive antigens with certain rickettsiae. The results of the Weil-Felix test are nonspecific and insensitive, yet many

A Fraudulent Epidemic Saves Lives

Although it is now antiquated, it is worth recounting how the Weil-Felix test was put to a humanitarian use by two Polish physicians in World War II. These physicians were aware that the occupying Germans did not send people suspected of having epidemic typhus to labor camps. Ingeniously, these doctors inoculated the population of several villages with an innocuous vaccine consisting of killed *P. vulgaris.* The high Weil-Felix titer of these people's sera was taken by the German medical staff to indicate that these villages were hotbeds of epidemic typhus. The inhabitants were thus spared, thanks to the microbiological stratagem of the two physicians.

Serologic tests are not useful for making an early diagnosis of rickettsioses but are used to confirm the diagnosis in convalescing patients. An early diagnosis is sometimes possible, however, by taking a biopsy of a skin lesion and treating it with antirickettsial antibodies. Localization of these antibodies to endothelial cells by immunochemical staining is diagnostic of acute Rocky Mountain spotted fever (see Fig. 28-4).

hospitals persist in using it despite the availability of better methods.

TREATMENT OF RICKETTSIOSES

Rickettsial diseases generally respond well to antimicrobial agents that enter host cells and are active in the intracellular environment. Most of these diseases respond to oral or intravenous therapy with doxycycline (the drug of choice), tetracycline, or chloramphenicol, each of which has its advantages and disadvantages under particular circumstances. Fluoroquinolone antimicrobial drugs are becoming a popular treatment for some of the milder rickettsioses. Penicillins, aminoglycosides, and other antimicrobials do not affect the course of rickettsial diseases. Sulfa drugs actually seem to exacerbate both spotted and typhus fevers.

Conclusion

Although rickettsial infections are not common in the United States, some can be life threatening. The diseases must be diagnosed promptly, and antibiotic therapy must be instituted quickly. The most devastating disease caused by these organisms, epidemic typhus, has receded in importance as a result of louse control but could emerge among the homeless in the United States; an epidemic occurred in Burundi during its civil war, and outbreaks have been identified in Russia and the Andes.

Rickettsiae are delicate organisms (except that which causes Q fever) but are well adapted to intracellular life and to passage from reservoir to host via arthropods. Their localization in blood vessels causes vascular injury with increased permeability and hemorrhages, sometimes with severe consequences.

chapter 29

Mycoplasma: Curiosity and Pathogen

Joel B. Baseman and Joseph G. Tully

key **concepts**

Mycoplasmas:

- Are the smallest organisms capable of growth on cell-free media.

- Lack a rigid cell wall.

- Require sterols for growth.

- Include four species that cause human disease: *Mycoplasma pneumoniae, M. genitalium, M. hominis,* and *Ureaplasma urealyticum.*

M. pneumoniae:

- Causes tracheobronchitis and pneumonia limited to the respiratory mucosa that lines the airways.

- May cause a range of other extrapulmonary manifestations, including mild hemolytic anemia caused by production of a cold hemagglutinin IgM antibody.

- Is usually diagnosed by clinical features and serodiagnostic and polymerase chain reaction (PCR) testing.

- Is treated with erythromycin, tetracycline, or quinolones.

M. genitalium:

- Is transmitted through sexual contact.

- Causes urethritis, cervicitis, and endometritis.

- Is diagnosed by PCR testing.

M. hominis:

- Is transmitted through sexual contact as well as vertically.

- Causes pelvic inflammatory disease, chorioamnionitis, and postpartum fever.

- Has been isolated from the central nervous systems of newborns.

U. urealyticum:

- Is transmitted through sexual contact as well as vertically.

- Causes urethritis, pelvic inflammatory disease, chorioamnionitis, and postpartum fever.

- Is associated with chronic lung disease in premature infants with very low birth weights.

- Has been isolated from the central nervous systems of newborns.

Mycoplasmas belong to the class Mollicutes and are a highly distinct group of bacteria that **lack a cell wall,** are bounded by a plasma membrane, and **require sterols for growth.** Most of the species associated with the human body are innocuous members of the normal flora. One species, however, is a common cause of **tracheobronchitis** and **pneumonia,** and others cause infections in the genitourinary tracts of adults and in the respiratory tracts and central nervous systems of newborn infants. These infecting organisms are sensitive to broad-spectrum antibiotics that inhibit functions other than cell wall synthesis.

Case

B., a 7-year-old girl who previously had been in good health, developed fever, headache, and a dry cough. Her 12-year-old brother had had similar symptoms 2 weeks earlier. Over the next 2 days, her temperature increased and the cough worsened, producing small amounts of clear sputum. Her physician noted that she appeared slightly pale and had a temperature of 39.3°C and a respiratory rate of 40 breaths per minute. Scattered rales (abnormal respiratory sounds) were heard through the stethoscope over the left posterior lung.

Her white blood cell count was in the normal range, 8,600/μL, with a normal differential count. She was slightly anemic (hematocrit of 29%) and had an increased number of reticulocytes. A Gram stain of her sputum revealed only a few neutrophils and no bacteria. A chest radiograph showed an infiltrate of the left midlung field (Fig. 29-1). A test to detect so-called **cold hemagglutinins** was positive. This finding and the clinical picture allowed the tentative diagnosis of **primary atypical pneumonia** caused by *Mycoplasma pneumoniae.* B. was treated with erythromycin and made an uneventful recovery.

This case raises several questions:

1. How did B. acquire the organism?
2. What are distinguishing features of the organism and the treatment process?
3. How can a definitive diagnosis of mycoplasmal infection be made?

M. pneumoniae is a common cause of pneumonia in children and young adults. As in B.'s case, the illness usually has a less abrupt onset and a milder course than pneumococcal pneumonia. A rather imprecise term, "walking pneumonia," probably includes mycoplasmal infections. Occasionally, cases are quite severe in healthy and immunocompromised individuals and children with sickle cell disease. Headache and cough are prominent clinical features. Before the etiology of this disease became known, it was referred to as primary atypical pneumonia to distinguish it from "typical" cases of lobar pneumonia (usually caused by pneumococci). Clinicians knew that patients with typical pneumonia responded to penicillin but those with atypical pneumonia did not.

FIGURE 29-1 ▪ Chest radiograph reveals an infiltrate in left midlung field.

General Characteristics of Mycoplasmas

The mycoplasmas have a number of unusual features:

- They are the smallest prokaryotes capable of growth on cell-free media, although the highly fastidious nature of several pathogenic species, especially *Mycoplasma genitalium* and *M. pneumoniae,* frequently leads to failed laboratory culture.
- When successfully grown, these *Mycoplasma* colonies require 2 to 6 weeks of incubation before detection by dissecting microscope is possible. Therefore, clinical manifestations and serological and polymerase chain reaction (PCR) detection are used for decisions on diagnosis and treatment.
- Unlike any other bacteria, mycoplasmas lack a rigid cell wall (no murein) and can assume a variety of shapes. This characteristic has important implications for antibiotic therapy because many commonly used antibiotics (especially the β-lactams) act by inhibiting cell wall murein synthesis and thus are ineffective against mycoplasmas. Moreover, **the absence of a cell wall prevents the use of Gram stain for detection and classification.**
- Their cell membrane contains **sterols,** which must be supplied in the medium to support their growth.

table **29-1**	**Common Mycoplasmas and Diseases They Cause**	
ORGANISM	**DISEASE**	**SITE**
Mycoplasma pneumoniae	Primary atypical pneumonia, tracheobronchitis	Respiratory tract
M. genitalium	Urethritis, cervicitis, endometritis	Genitourinary tract
M. hominis	Pelvic inflammatory disease, neonatal infections	Genitourinary tract, oropharynx
Ureaplasma urealyticum	Urethritis, neonatal infections	Genitourinary tract
M. fermentans	Possibly HIV cofactor, arthritis	Possibly genitourinary tract, joint fluid
M. penetrans	Possibly HIV cofactor	Possibly genitourinary tract
M. salivarium, M. orale	None	Mouth, oropharynx
Others (less common)	None	Genitourinary tract, oropharynx

Mycoplasma species are common in nature and capable of causing disease in a wide range of animals, plants, and insects. Four species are known to cause human disease (Table 29-1): *M. pneumoniae*, a common cause of respiratory disease; *M. genitalium*, a frequent cause of genitourinary tract infections; and two species that account for some cases of infections of the genitourinary tract and joints, *M. hominis* and *Ureaplasma urealyticum*. The latter two organisms can also be isolated from many newborns, especially from the respiratory tract and central nervous system. *M. fermentans* and *M. penetrans* have been linked to a range of disease processes, including secondary complications in immunocompromised individuals, although their direct relationship to disease etiologies is not fully understood. Some believe that *M. fermentans* and *M. penetrans* contribute to the progression of AIDS, chronic fatigue, and malignant transformation. Other *Mycoplasma* species are commonly found as part of the normal human flora but have not been linked to disease. Still others cause severe disease in domestic animals.

Mycoplasmas can be readily cultivated in the laboratory, although most species require special media that contain sterols. *M. pneumoniae* grows slowly, and several weeks may be required for colonies to become evident. The colonies are much smaller than those of common bacteria and have a dense center that gives them a "fried egg" appearance, although this morphology occurs rarely during primary isolation and more often after serial passage (Fig. 29-2). *M. hominis* can be grown on the blood agar plates used in all clinical microbiology laboratories. However, this organism often goes undetected, probably because of its relatively small colonies and overgrowth by rapidly growing bacteria.

Mycoplasma Pneumoniae

ENCOUNTER AND ENTRY

Infected humans constitute the only known reservoir of *M. pneumoniae*. Patients become ill following exposure to the respiratory secretions of persons harboring the organism. As with the pneumococcus, prolonged asymptomatic colonization with *M. pneumoniae* occurs even after proper antibiotic therapy. In most cases the source of the infection is not recognized because the typical *Mycoplasma* infection is mild. However, *M. pneumoniae* infections are fairly contagious. Cases of spread within

FIGURE 29-2 ▪ Colonies of *Mycoplasma pneumoniae*. Notice their small size and "fried egg" appearance, especially in **B**.

households and residential institutions have been reported, some with intervals of 2 to 3 weeks between cases.

Mycoplasma infection begins with the binding of organisms to the respiratory epithelium. Microscopic studies of *M. pneumoniae* have revealed a unique terminal attachment structure. Specialized adhesin and adherence accessory proteins are part of this tip-mediated attachment organelle that helps the organisms bind to carbohydrate-containing receptors on the respiratory epithelium. Monoclonal antibodies to adhesin proteins inhibit the attachment of *M. pneumoniae*, and mutants lacking the proteins exhibit marked reduction in cytadherence and virulence in experimentally infected hamsters. Also, alternate adherence pathways that target fibronectin provide additional mechanisms for mycoplasma surface parasitism.

SPREAD, MULTIPLICATION, AND DAMAGE

The pathogenesis of *M. pneumoniae* infection differs markedly from other forms of pneumonia, such as that caused by the pneumococcus or *Legionella pneumophila*, mainly because its involvement is largely limited to the respiratory mucosa that lines the airways. There is no evidence of involvement of the lung alveoli. An infiltrate of mononuclear cells surrounds infected bronchi and bronchioles. The pattern of involvement is that of a **bronchopneumonia** rather than a lobar process.

In experimentally infected tracheal organ cultures, the organisms line up along the mucosa, with the terminal attachment structure in contact with the epithelium (Fig. 29-3). In this model, ciliary function is impaired and tissue cytopathology observed, probably as a result of local elaboration of tissue-toxic substances, including hydrogen peroxide. Also, cellular toxicity can arise from inflammatory mediators induced by *M. pneumoniae*. The main inflammatory response elicited by *M. pneumoniae* is characterized by perivascular and peribronchial infiltration of mononuclear leukocytes with very few neutrophils. These infections can lead to chronic lung damage and reduced lung function. Some immunocompromised patients with mycoplasmal infection do not have visible pulmonary infiltrates, suggesting that the immune response may play a role in causing disease pathogenesis.

The clinical manifestations of *M. pneumoniae* infections are generally limited to the respiratory tract, but other organs are occasionally involved. B. had a mild **hemolytic anemia,** which was caused by an antibody stimulated by mycoplasmal infection. An IgM antibody, it binds to red blood cells and, at reduced temperatures, causes them to agglutinate (stick together). The antibody is called a **cold hemagglutinin,** which is detectable in about 50% of severe *Mycoplasma* infections. Only a small number of patients with cold hemagglutinins actually experience clinically significant hemolysis. The reason *M. pneumoniae* infection stimulates the production of cold hemagglutinins is likely linked to a combination of molecular mimicry and shared antigens between *Mycoplasma* and mammalian proteins and autoimmunity.

Complications of *M. pneumoniae* infections include **encephalitis** and other pathologies of the central nervous system. Some patients develop a rash known as erythema multiforme, renal and cardiac disorders, or arthritis. The pathogenic mechanisms that account for these complications are not yet known.

DIAGNOSIS

Culturing *M. pneumoniae* from clinical specimens can take several weeks or more, requires special media and experienced personnel, and frequently fails. Consequently, the diagnosis of mycoplasmal pneumonia is usually suspected from clinical features and reinforced by serologic tests. Comparisons of *M. pneumoniae* or cold agglutinin antibody titers between acute and convalescent phase sera can be diagnostic. However, such results become available long after therapeutic decisions about the patient must be made. Rapid tests exist that do not involve culture, such as assays to directly detect mycoplasmal antigens or to amplify specific mycoplasmal nucleic acids, and this information, along with clinical signs and symptoms, is valuable in determining treatment modalities.

In contrast to pneumococcal pneumonia, sputum production is scanty and the sputum nonpurulent. The peripheral blood usually does not show the leukocytosis and marked increase in young leukocyte forms characteristic

FIGURE 29-3 ▪ Transmission electron photomicrograph of a hamster tracheal ring infected with M. pneumoniae. Notice the orientation of the mycoplasma (M) through its specialized tip-mediated attachment organelle, which permits close association with the respiratory epithelium (original magnification, × 50,000). m, microvillus; c, cilia.

of pneumococcal infection. The chest radiography in mycoplasmal pneumonia is highly variable but usually reveals a patchy infiltrate suggestive of bronchopneumonia. Cold hemagglutinins can be rapidly demonstrated at the bedside: blood drawn from the patient into a tube containing an anticoagulant will look clumpy when placed in an ice bucket. The clumps disappear when the tube is again warmed.

PREVENTION AND TREATMENT

No vaccine is currently available to prevent *Mycoplasma* infections. Treatment with erythromycin, tetracycline, or fluoroquinolones is effective, although it should be remembered that *M. hominis* is uniformly resistant to erythromycin.

Genital Mycoplasmas

In epidemiology and pathogenesis, *M. genitalium* is among the newest emerging pathogenic bacteria for humans. It is an important cause of chlamydia-negative, nongonococcal urethritis in men and has been directly linked to cervicitis, endometritis, and pelvic inflammatory disease in women. Also, this species of *Mycoplasma* has been isolated, along with *M. pneumoniae*, from the synovial and respiratory fluids of diseased individuals. As such, both *M. pneumoniae* and *M. genitalium* share common biological features, including tip-mediated attachment organelles and amino acid sequence–related adhesin and adherence-accessory protein homologues. Also, *M. genitalium* can be readily visualized extracellularly and intracellularly in vaginal cells of women, indicating that mycoplasmas are capable of invading cells and persisting and replicating for extended periods with high likelihood of transmission through sexual contact.

Infections caused by the genital mycoplasmas, *U. urealyticum* and *M. hominis*, differ considerably from infection by *M. pneumoniae* and *M. genitalium*. The former organisms are common residents of the genitourinary tract, especially of sexually active people. They are almost certainly transmitted through sexual contact among adults and are transmitted vertically, from mother to newborn infant, during pregnancy and birth. Not sur-

prisingly, most of the diseases caused by these organisms affect the respiratory tracts of newborns. *U. urealyticum* is clearly established as the cause of urethritis, and *M. hominis* as that of pelvic inflammatory disease (see Chapter 69). Both organisms can cause chorioamnionitis (inflammation of the fetal membranes) and postpartum fever. Spontaneous abortion and premature delivery have been linked to these organisms, although this association has not been definitively proven. Several provocative studies have demonstrated an association between *U. urealyticum* and chronic lung disease in premature infants with very low birth weights. Both organisms have also been isolated from the spinal fluid of newborn infants. This association is confusing because some infected infants have evidence of central nervous system inflammation, but others do not. It is possible that, at least in some cases, mycoplasmas are innocent bystanders in the central nervous system, whereas in other cases they are responsible for disease.

Conclusion

Mycoplasmas call attention to themselves because they lack a cell wall, require sterols for growth, and make characteristically small colonies on agar. These organisms show a marked tropism for mucous membranes and produce characteristic clinical manifestations.

M. pneumoniae is unequivocally responsible for a common form of pneumonia in humans, and *M. genitalium* is clearly emerging as a significant cause of genitourinary tract infections in men and women. Other mycoplasmas are commonly found in the genitourinary tracts of adults and in the respiratory tracts and central nervous systems of newborn infants. In those settings the presence of the organisms is not uniformly associated with disease.

Our knowledge about the mycoplasmas and their role in disease is accumulating at a rapid pace with the advent of new detection and diagnostic assays and genetic and molecular biological strategies in pathogenesis. However, only limited data exists concerning long-term antibiotic treatment and eradication of mycoplasmal infections. The association of mycoplasmas with a variety of clinical symptoms in humans suggests the need to clarify virulence determinants, host immune responsiveness, and effective therapies so that mycoplasmal disease transmission and progression can be controlled and prevented.

Strategies to Combat Bacterial Infections

Cary Engleberg

O ver the last two centuries, the health and longevity of people living in developed countries have taken a quantum jump forward. We take for granted that we, our relatives, and our acquaintances have survived infancy and will reach old age. Disease is an exceptional event for most people, and premature death is relatively uncommon. Two interrelated factors have contributed to this increased life expectancy: improvement in nutrition and control of infectious diseases. Initially, the most important factors in reducing the incidence of infectious disease were preventive measures, largely purification of the water supply and control of human wastes and disease vectors. Later, in the last hundred years, these measures were supplemented with effective medical interventions: vaccination and antimicrobial therapy. Clearly, preventive measures, not therapy, have played the greatest role in the control of infectious diseases.

This chapter discusses strategies that have been developed for prevention and therapy of infectious diseases. The emphasis here is on bacteria, but the basic principles apply to other infectious agents. Related topics also addressed in this text include the biological basis of antimicrobial activity and resistance (see Chapter 5), antiviral strategies (see Chapter 44), and immunization (see Chapter 45).

Antimicrobial Therapy

Despite the great advances in preventive medicine in the last century, little could be done to treat patients with infectious diseases until relatively recently. Medical literature from the early decades of the twentieth century is full of vivid descriptions of gruesome infections caused by streptococci, staphylococci, and clostridia. At the dawning of the age of antimicrobial therapy, with the introduction of the sulfonamides in the 1930s, physicians could finally cure many of those once-fatal infections. Here is a description of the first time penicillin was used clinically:

> *The time had now come to find a suitable patient for the first test of the therapeutic power of penicillin in man. . . . In the septic ward at the Radcliffe Infirmary (Oxford, England), there was an unfortunate policeman aged 43 who had a sore on his lip four months previously, from which he developed a combined staphylococcal and streptococcal septicaemia. He had multiple abscesses on his*

face and orbits: he also had osteomyelitis of his right humerus with discharging sinuses, and abscesses in his lungs. He was in great pain and was desperately ill. There was all to gain for him in a trial of penicillin and nothing to lose. Penicillin treatment was started on 12 February 1941, with 200 mg (10,000 units) intravenously initially and then 300 mg every three hours. . . . Four days later there was striking improvement, and after 5 days the patient was vastly better, afebrile and eating well, and there was obvious resolution of the abscesses on his face and scalp and in his right orbit.

Unfortunately, this first clinical trial of a β-lactam antibiotic ended abruptly because the total supply of the drug was exhausted by the 5-day course of treatment, despite efforts to recover the drug from the patient's urine. The patient died 4 weeks later.

Although the experiment ended tragically, it served to demonstrate the efficacy and superiority of the new therapy over any that was available until that time. Today it has become increasingly difficult to prove the superiority of new antibiotics over those already in use. In assessing new drugs, pharmaceutical companies must carry out complex and expensive trials that include laboratory work, experimental animals, and lengthy clinical studies. The practicing physician may often find it difficult to evaluate such intricate studies.

The selection of the most appropriate drug to treat a particular infection is also not a simple matter. For example, the carbepenem antimicrobial imipenem may be thought to be a true "wonder drug" because it has the widest antibacterial spectrum of any antibiotic presently available and is resistant to most inactivating β-lactamases. However, for some infections the preferred treatment is penicillin, which has neither of these desirable properties. Because of its broad spectrum, imipenem can wipe out other members of the normal bacterial flora and lead to colonization by resistant species. Moreover, imipenem is more likely than penicillin to cause seizures if the drug accumulates. Finally, imipenem is far more expensive than penicillin. Thus, pharmacological properties of the drugs, their adverse effects, their cost, and many other factors must be considered in making an appropriate therapeutic choice. When deciding which antibiotic to use for a patient, the clinician must consider the following questions:

- Which pathogens are causing the infection? If their identity cannot be determined at this time, what are the likely possibilities?
- What antibiotics are the suspected pathogens susceptible to?
- Will the drug penetrate the site of infection, and will it work under the conditions at that site?
- What is the toxicity of the drug to the patient?
- What is the effect of the drug on the microbial ecology? Will its use lead to the emergence of broadly based antibiotic resistance, thereby posing a threat to the patient being treated and to other infected patients in the community?
- Are other host factors relevant to the proposed therapy?

In some cases the proper conclusion will be that the patient should not be treated with antimicrobial drugs at all because the benefits of such treatment are not likely to outweigh the drawbacks.

Infecting Organisms

Choosing the proper antimicrobial drug depends on the identification of the infecting organisms. Consider, for example, patients with recurrent urinary tract infections. Often the infections are caused by *Escherichia coli*, but they can also be caused by *Enterococcus, Pseudomonas aeruginosa*, or one of the other Enterobacteriaceae, such as *Klebsiella, Enterobacter,* or *Serratia*. Each organism has a unique set of susceptibilities, and the determination of its antimicrobial susceptibility is mandatory.

Physicians treating first-time, uncomplicated urinary tract infections usually do not wait for the results of laboratory cultures and drug susceptibility testing. These infections are known to be almost always caused by *E. coli*. Other situations that require empiric therapy are those in which an adequate sample of infected material for direct analysis or culture cannot be obtained. In such cases **empiric treatment** is based on the clinician's knowledge of the usual causative agents in a particular clinical situation: factors pertinent to the individual patient and the local environment, large studies of similar cases in the medical literature, recent local experience with similar cases, and antibiotic susceptibility patterns in the local hospital or community. Failure to analyze the best empiric therapy invariably results in an attempt to treat all possible bacteria with one or several antibiotics. This "shotgun" approach to antibiotic therapy has several drawbacks:

- Failure to "cover" the pathogen
- Synergistic toxicity of multiple drugs
- Possible antagonism between drugs
- Increased likelihood of superinfection by resistant bacteria or fungi
- Increased cost of therapy

Obviously, these disadvantages are minimized when the identity of the infectious agent can be determined. In general, the more rapid the diagnosis, the sooner proper therapy can be instituted. Much effort is directed toward the development of rapid diagnostic methods, but most still require one or several days (see Chapter 58).

Antibiotic Susceptibility

Susceptibility to antibiotics varies among the many kinds of bacteria. Gram-positive bacteria, possibly because they lack an outer membrane, are potentially more susceptible than Gram-negative bacteria. For example, streptococci are generally about a thousandfold more susceptible to penicillin G than is *E. coli*. However, the exceptions are too numerous to make these generalizations very useful (mechanisms of bacterial resistance are outlined in Chapter 5). Much depends on the presence of antibiotic-resistant strains in a particular environment. Monitoring resistant strains nationwide and locally is helpful in providing general guidelines, but basically, each isolate should be tested for susceptibility.

Two fundamental shifts occurred in the 1990s in the spectrum of antibiotic resistance among clinically important pathogens. First, antibacterial resistance, which first appeared among Gram-negative bacteria, has become widespread in medically important Gram-positive bacteria. These include methicillin-resistant *Staphylococcus aureus* (MRSA), vancomycin-resistant enterococci (VRE), and penicillin-resistant *Streptococcus pneumoniae*. Organisms such as *S. aureus* and *S. pneumoniae*, which were among the most frequent killers in the preantibiotic era, are becoming increasingly serious clinical problems. Second, antimicrobial-resistant organisms have spread from hospitals into the community and now affect children in day care centers and elders in nursing homes.

It is extremely important that drug resistance be monitored both across the nation and on a local basis and that the information be readily available to medical personnel. The simplest and most widely used assay for microbial susceptibility is placing a disk containing an

FIGURE 30-2 ▪ **Antimicrobial susceptibility testing by measurement of the minimal inhibitory concentration (MIC) and minimal bactericidal concentration (MBC).** A series of tubes containing liquid media and decreasing concentrations of the antibiotic to be tested are inoculated with equal amounts of the bacterial isolate of interest. After incubation overnight, growth occurs in all tubes that have noninhibitory levels of the antibiotic. The first tube in the series in which no growth occurs contains the MIC of the antibiotic. To determine the MBC, 1/1,000 of the volume from each of the inhibited cultures is plated on agar media. The last tube from which no bacteria are isolated contains the MBC of the antibiotic.

antibiotic on an agar plate inoculated with the organisms (Fig. 30-1). As the antibiotic diffuses into the agar, it inhibits bacterial growth up to the limit of the effective concentration. This test is not a truly quantitative technique, however, because many factors influence the diffusion of the drug. Quantitative techniques require the use of dilutions of the drug in liquid media. These techniques provide an estimate of the **minimum inhibitory concentration (MIC)**, a parameter that is used to ascertain whether an effective antibiotic concentration is attainable in body fluids (Fig. 30-2).

Static Versus Cidal Drugs

The MIC indicates the **bacteriostatic** concentration of a drug but not the **bactericidal** one. The two concentrations are not usually the same: most agents that are bactericidal are bacteriostatic at lower concentrations. The **minimum bactericidal concentration (MBC)** is determined by subculturing the tubes or microtiter plates that have no visible growth into antibiotic-free media. This subculturing allows the bacteria that were inhibited from growing in the first culture, but are still alive, to replicate (see Fig. 30-2). Although this technique is time consuming and has some technical problems, it can yield important information because bactericidal and bacteriostatic drugs are not equally effective in all situations. A bacteriostatic therapy requires that the host clear the inhibited

FIGURE 30-1 ▪ **The disc diffusion method for determining antibiotic susceptibility.** Bacteria were uniformly seeded on the surface of a nutrient agar plate, and filter paper discs containing various antibiotics were placed at intervals over the surface. After incubation, susceptibility to some of the antibiotics becomes apparent as clear areas around the discs. The diameter of the clear area depends on the extent of diffusion of the drug throughout the agar. Resistance to other antibiotics is indicated by growth (turbidity) up to the edge of the discs.

bacteria. However, if host immune response is inadequate for this task, either because the effector cells are absent (as in neutropenia) or because the site of infection is inaccessible to effective immune clearance (as in endocarditis or meningitis), then bactericidal antibiotics are required.

Multiple-Drug Therapy

The use of combinations of antibiotics (usually two drugs) is clearly needed in a number of clinical situations. As discussed in Chapter 5, when drugs are combined, three results are possible:

1. **Synergism:** two drugs work better together than does either drug alone, simply because of the combination of their individual effects (e.g., penicillin and gentamicin against enterococci)
2. **Antagonism:** one drug prevents the full effect of the other (e.g., bacteriostatic drugs and penicillin)
3. **Indifference:** the actions of neither drug are affected by the presence of the other.

In some situations combined antibiotic therapy is desirable:

• **Treating severe infections when no single agent is sufficiently effective:** synergistic combinations of antibiotics could create a bactericidal effect at nontoxic concentrations (e.g., enterococcal endocarditis, *Pseudomonas aeruginosa* pneumonia).
• **Preventing the emergence of resistant organisms:** in active tuberculosis, for example, combination therapy is essential.
• **Treating polymicrobial infections, such as intra-abdominal abscesses:** each organism causing the infection could be susceptible to different drugs.
• Initiating empiric therapy to "cover" multiple potential pathogens.

Pharmacokinetics and Pharmodynamics

The pharmacokinetic factors that should be considered in the choice of drugs include absorption, distribution in tissues, and excretion. The **absorption** profile of a drug dictates its route of administration. The proportion of an administered dose of a drug that reaches the systemic circulation is referred to as its **bioavailability.** The most convenient route is usually by mouth, and this route is used with highly absorbable (or highly bioavailable) antibiotics like the fluoroquinolones, sulfamethoxazole–trimethoprim, linezolid, and rifampin. Of course, these medications cannot be given orally if the patient is vomiting, has impaired gastrointestinal absorption, or is in shock. Many antibiotics, such as vancomycin, the

aminoglycosides, and the newer β-lactams, are not absorbed in a normal gastrointestinal tract and must be given by parenteral injection. However, nonabsorbable antibiotics can be used to treat infections limited to the lumen of the gastrointestinal tract. An example is the use of oral vancomycin to treat diarrhea or colitis induced by *Clostridium difficile* (see Chapter 20).

Distribution of drugs takes place through the circulation and is followed by entry into tissues by passive diffusion. The diffusion and polarity properties of antibiotics are relevant in this process, as they are with all drugs. Some antibiotics bind to plasma proteins; this has a good and a bad side. On one hand, protein binding limits the amount of unbound drug available for diffusion. On the other hand, the drug remains available in the bloodstream for a much longer time.

Consideration must be given to the speed of **excretion** of the drug. Most drugs are excreted by the kidney, but some drugs (e.g., nafcillin, ceftriaxone) are excreted primary by the liver through the biliary tree and still others use both pathways. Patterns of excretion can be used to advantage in infections of the urinary tract or the biliary tree. However, the level of renal or hepatic function must also be taken into account because the excretion mechanisms must be working properly to achieve effective drug concentrations. If they are not, the drug could accumulate in the bloodstream with toxic consequences.

Antibiotics with similar activities against a particular bacterial pathogen and similar pharmacokinetics can nevertheless differ in their ability to clear an infection, depending on how they are administered. The **pharmacodynamic** profiles of the antibiotics—that is, their ability to clear infection—may differ because of their respective mechanisms of action. Antibiotics that kill bacteria slowly, such as the β-lactams, are most effective when given frequently or continuously. Larger doses to obtain higher levels of the antibiotic are not necessarily helpful, and the pharmacodynamic parameter that correlates best with therapeutic success is the time that the drug level exceeds the MIC (Fig. 30-3). In contrast, antibiotics that kill bacteria rapidly, such as fluoroquinolones and aminoglycosides, are most effective when administered at high doses at extended intervals. The pharmacodynamic parameters that best predict their effectiveness are the ratio of the maximum drug concentration to the MIC (**Cmax/MIC**) and the area under the drug-level curve that is above the MIC (**AUIC**).

Local Factors

Tissue inflammation, which occurs early in many infections, changes the environment in which an antibiotic is to work. If infection is not controlled, local tissue necrosis can alter conditions even further. In an abscess caused

FIGURE 30-3 ▪ **Pharmacodynamic properties of antibiotics.** A slowly bactericidal antibiotic is best administered to maximize the time that drug levels remain above the minimal inhibitory concentration (MIC) of the organism being treated. In contrast, rapidly bactericidal antibiotics are best administered so that the maximum drug concentration (C_{max}) is many multiples of the MIC, i.e., high C_{max}/MIC ratio, or the area under the inhibitory curve (AUIC) is maximized.

by staphylococci or a mixed anaerobic–aerobic flora, the environment becomes anaerobic and the pH may drop as low as 5.5. Antibiotics must be selected for their ability to function under those conditions. As shown in Table 30-1, the efficacy of aminoglycosides is diminished at low pH, at low redox potential, or in the presence of a high concentration of divalent cations.

The anatomical location of infection can dictate the choice of antibiotics if the drug must cross a natural barrier. For example, drugs that cross the blood-brain

barrier are nonpolar at neutral pH. This factor may be critical because of the seriousness of most central nervous system infections. Two other organs with important barriers are the eye and the prostate, and infections at these sites require careful selection of drugs. Infections of the interior of the eye may require direct injection of drugs into the tissue. Similar considerations apply to the placental barrier during pregnancy.

In the case of intracellular infections, the plasma membrane is a barrier to some antibiotics. Macrolides, fluoroquinolones, tetracyclines, and rifampin can efficiently penetrate host cells, a property that is highly desirable in treating infections caused by intracellular pathogens like chlamydiae or legionellae. In contrast, β-lactams and aminoglycosides are typically excluded by the plasma membrane and are not useful in treating intracellular infections.

Antibiotic Toxicity

Like any drug, an antibiotic can have both toxic and beneficial effects. Sometimes toxicity is so severe that it limits the drug's efficacy. For example, chloramphenicol, an antibiotic commonly prescribed in past decades, has virtually disappeared from clinical practice because of a rare and fatal aplastic anemia associated with its use. The following sections present a brief overview of the main types of toxicity. Practicing physicians need more detailed information and must constantly update it.

Allergy

Antimicrobial agents may be recognized as foreign substances by the immune system, resulting in sensitization of some individuals. The most common antibacterial drugs associated with severe allergic reactions are the penicillins, cephalosporins, and sulfonamides. A likely reason why penicillins lead this list is that they readily bind to proteins and function as haptens to elicit IgE antibody responses. The most severe reactions result in immediate hypersensitive responses—hives, angioneurotic edema, and anaphylactic shock—and can be fatal. Mild to fairly severe allergic reactions include rash, urticaria (hives), lymphadenopathy, asthma, and fever. In some cases fever confuses the clinical picture because it is attributed to the infection and not to the drug. Previous history of drug sensitivity often dictates the choice of other agents.

Other Systemic Reactions

All major organs of the body can be affected by toxicity from antimicrobial drugs. The most frequent reactions involve the **gastrointestinal tract.** Gastrointestinal distress

table **30-1**	**Physicochemical Conditions That Affect the Activity of Antimicrobial Agents**	
CONDITION	**DECREASE**	**INCREASE**
Low pH	Aminoglycosides	Tetracycline
	Some β-lactams (porin changes)	Chloramphenicol
	Erythromycin	
Low redox potential	Aminoglycosides	Metronidazole
High divalent cation concentration	Aminoglycosides tetracycline (Ca^{++})	

and diarrhea are the most common reactions and often require discontinuation of the drug. These manifestations are often caused by a direct stimulatory effect of the drug on the sympathetic nervous system. However, diarrhea can also result from changes in the intestinal flora. This form of toxicity usually occurs late in the course of treatment and may manifest only after treatment is stopped. About one third of the cases of antibiotic-associated diarrhea have been associated with the toxin produced by *C. difficile* (see Chapter 20). The spectrum of diseases caused by this organism ranges from a trivial and self-limiting diarrhea to a severe and life-threatening pseudomembranous colitis.

The **liver** is the major site of drug metabolism and is frequently affected. Many drugs induce mild alterations of function of the hepatic parenchyma, usually manifested by an increase in the serum level of certain transaminases. Some drugs affect biliary excretion. Most of these manifestations are mild and reversible, although cases of liver failure have been reported in pregnant women treated with tetracycline.

The **kidney** is also a frequent site of adverse reactions, resulting in decreased renal function. These reactions are caused by three general mechanisms: immunological damage to the glomeruli, which blocks filtration; damage to the tubules; and obstruction of the collecting system by crystals of the drug. Reactions in the kidney are an important problem because many drugs are excreted through the urinary tract. An unrecognized decrease in renal function could result not only in ineffective levels in the urine but also in toxic serum levels of the drug. The aminoglycosides are the most important class of drugs that cause these side effects. They also cause inner ear toxicity (hearing loss and imbalance). The frequency of toxic reactions in the kidney is so high that frequent monitoring of renal function and blood levels of the drug is required during aminoglycoside therapy.

The **skin** can also be affected by antimicrobial agents and is often the site of an allergic reaction. More serious skin reactions include exfoliative dermatitis and a disease known as Stevens-Johnson syndrome, which leads to the formation of bullae, large vesicles on the skin, and inflammation of the eyes and mucous membranes. The **hematopoietic system** can be adversely affected, leading to decreased production of red and white blood cells in the bone marrow. Further, peripheral red and white blood cells can become immunologically sensitized, resulting in their hemolysis or sequestration by fixed macrophages. Antibiotics can also affect the circulatory system, central nervous system, musculoskeletal system, and respiratory tract. Most reactions at these sites are specific to individual drugs. Information about the reactions caused by antibiotics is made available to physicians in reference manuals published periodically; physicians should consult this information before prescribing any medication.

Interactions With Nonantimicrobial Drugs

Antimicrobial drugs sometimes interact with other medications a patient is taking. The drugs can interact directly or by affecting enzymes that influence their pharmacology. The drugs most commonly involved are anticoagulants and anticonvulsants. The following case is an example.

Case

Mrs. O., a 67-year-old woman with recurrent thrombophlebitis and pulmonary embolism had been asymptomatic on an oral anticoagulant (warfarin), which maintained her prothrombin (clotting) time at 24 seconds, twice the normal value. Recently diagnosed with pulmonary tuberculosis, Mrs. O. began taking a four-drug regimen her physician prescribed. Several days later she required hospitalization for recurrence of her thrombophlebitis. Laboratory evaluation revealed that her prothrombin time was only 2 seconds above normal, despite taking the same amount of warfarin. Her physician then learned that rifampin, one of the four antituberculous drugs she was taking, induces the liver to accelerate the clearance of warfarin. Rifampin was stopped, and Mrs. O. was treated with intravenous heparin to raise her clotting time.

This case illustrates one of the numerous interactions that can occur between drugs. The potential consequences can be catastrophic for the patient, particularly if the therapy affected is life saving, as in this case. Imagine if Mrs. O. had required anticoagulation therapy to prevent clotting on an artificial heart valve. An opposite effect, prolongation of clotting time, could also occur with sulfonamides and metronidazole and lead to massive gastrointestinal bleeding. The severity of such complications cannot be overestimated, and the message must not be lost on the practitioner.

Prophylactic Use of Antimicrobial Drugs

Soon after the introduction of effective antibacterial agents in the 1930s, it became clear that they could be used not only to treat infections but to prevent them as well. However, prophylaxis is a complex and controversial subject because the use of antibiotics to prevent infections carries risks as well as benefits. Antimicrobial drugs can be used prophylactically for two purposes:

- **To prevent disease caused by exogenous pathogens:** An example is the administration of antibiotics to persons exposed to patients with meningococcal infections. The meningococcus spreads rapidly among susceptible individuals, but antibiotics such as rifampin can usually forestall its clinical manifestations. Likewise, the antituberculous drug isoniazid is given to persons who are at high risk of acquiring tuberculosis, such as children living in the same quarters as a patient with pulmonary tuberculosis (see Chapter 23).

- **To prevent commensal organisms from spreading from their usual residence to normally sterile sites of the body:** The use of antibiotics to prevent postoperative infections after certain high-risk surgical procedures also falls in this category. Another example is the administration of antibiotics to patients with damaged heart valves who are at risk of acquiring endocarditis. The drugs are used to prevent bacteremia and infection of damaged heart valves when such patients undergo dental or major or minor surgical procedures (see Chapter 12).

The risks involved in antibiotic prophylaxis must be clearly understood. They include allergy or other toxic reactions to the drugs, selection of resistant mutants, and masking or delaying the diagnosis of the infection. The following criteria should be met for the prophylactic use of antibiotics:

- A surgical or medical intervention carries a significant risk of microbial contamination. When a surgeon crosses a tissue plane that contains a rich microbial flora, such as the colon or the oral cavity, the risk of infection is unacceptably high, and the administration of prophylactic antibiotics is necessary. Antibiotic prophylaxis should also be used when infection is not extremely likely but could have disastrous effects—for instance, in surgery to implant a heart valve or hip prostheses. Antibiotic prophylaxis is not indicated when the risk of infection is low and the outcome trivial, such as in a hernia operation.
- The antibiotics used prophylactically should be directed against the most likely pathogens. Previous studies should suggest which infectious agents are likely to be involved and what drugs are likely to be effective. In operations involving the colon, antibiotics should cover the microflora of the intestine. When surgery crosses the oral mucosa, a prophylactic antibiotic with a narrow spectrum is indicated because most of the bacteria in the oral cavity are susceptible to penicillin.
- A suitable concentration of the drug must be achievable at the right time in the relevant tissues. Studies in experimental animals (which have also been confirmed in randomized human studies) have shown that prophylactic antibiotics are of no value when given after surgery is completed. However, their effectiveness is readily apparent when they are given just before surgery and adequate tissue levels are achieved. It makes sense that a drug should be present in the body when the wound is likely to be contaminated; once the wound is closed, it rapidly becomes impermeable to exogenous bacteria.
- Antimicrobial drugs should be used for a short time to minimize the emergence of drug resistance. Indications for the prophylactic use of antibiotics are expanding with the occurrence of new diseases, new drugs, and new therapeutic methods. The guidelines presented here should be applicable in the development of new indications.

Conclusion

Bacterial infections are no longer the inevitable threat to life they often were in the preantibiotic era. Today the clinician can choose from a vast array of antimicrobial agents with various kinetics, mechanisms, and spectra of activity against microbes. However, the wise clinician uses these agents judiciously, knowing that they pose risks of toxicity, allergy, drug interactions, and selection of resistant flora. Antibiotics can also be used to prevent infections, but the occasions when prophylaxis is appropriate are strictly limited.

chapter 31

Biology of Viruses

Terence S. Dermody and Jeffrey M. Bergelson

key concepts

Viruses:

- Are obligate intracellular parasites that use the machinery of the host cell to replicate.

- Contain a nucleic acid core surrounded by a protein capsid; the capsid of some viruses is surrounded by an envelope.

- Attach to host cells by binding to receptors expressed on the host cell surface; the virus then enters host cells by endocytosis or direct penetration of the host cell membrane.

- Have single- or double-stranded RNA or DNA genomes that, following entry of the virus into the host cell, are used as templates for synthesis of viral proteins and nucleic acids.

- Assemble new virus particles within the host cell, which are then released during cell lysis (nonenveloped viruses) or by budding (enveloped viruses).

Viral infection:

- Can be lytic, latent, or chronic.

- Can be acquired from other humans or from the environment; direct contact routes include sexual contact and vertical transmission, and environmental routes include respiratory (aerosols), gastrointestinal (fecal–oral contamination), and transcutaneous (inoculation) transmission.

- Is often characterized by an incubation period, during which the virus replicates within the host before disease symptoms become evident.

- Can spread through nerves to the central nervous system or through the blood to many organs. Some viruses use multiple pathways to spread.

- Is curtailed within the host primarily by cell-mediated immunity.

- Can be diagnosed by inoculation of cell cultures, immunocytochemical staining and identification of virus particles or antigens in tissue specimens, or detection of viral nucleic acids.

The fundamental difference between viruses and all other infectious agents is in their mechanism of reproduction. Unlike cellular forms of life, viruses do not simply divide. Virus replication is carried out by the host cell machinery, which synthesizes multiple copies of the viral genome and viral proteins. Those viral components assemble spontaneously within the host cell to form progeny virus particles. Viruses have no means to produce energy and contain a few enzymes at most. Thus, totally dependent on host cells, viruses are **obligate intracellular parasites.** They are important pathogens of virtually all forms of life, including humans and other animals, plants, and fungi. One type of virus, called bacteriophage, infects bacteria (see Chapter 4). Because they are relatively amenable to study, viruses serve as important models for examination of basic cellular processes.

Viruses are small, although the largest ones (e.g., smallpox virus) are barely visible with the light microscope and fall within the lower size range of bacteria (e.g., mycoplasmas and chlamydiae). Viruses vary in volume over a thousandfold range and in structure from relatively simple to very complex (Fig. 31-1). The genomic nucleic acid of a virus is either DNA or RNA, never both.

Structure and Classification of Viruses

A virus particle, called a **virion**, can be schematically represented as a delivery system that surrounds a payload (Fig. 31-2). The delivery system consists of structural components used by the virus to survive in the environment and bind to host cells. The payload contains the viral genome and often includes enzymes required for the initial steps in virus replication.

Viral genomes are incredibly diverse. The smallest viral genomes encode three or four proteins, and the largest encode more than 100 structural proteins and enzymes. The number of proteins encoded may be greater than predicted from the size of the nucleic acid because of the economical arrangement of some viral genomes. Thus, the same stretch of nucleic acid may contain multiple open reading frames or overlapping regions that can be transcribed into several distinct

FIGURE 31-1 ▪ Examples of virus morphology. These images of selected viruses were obtained using either cryoelectron microscopy and three-dimensional computer processing or transmission electron microscopy.

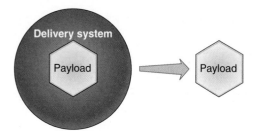

FIGURE 31-2 ▪ **Schematic diagram of a virus particle.** Viruses are simple structures consisting of a delivery system and a payload. The delivery system of a virus protects it against degradation in the environment and contains structures used to bind to target cells in the host. The payload of a virus contains the genome and enzymes necessary to initiate the first steps in virus replication.

messenger RNAs (mRNAs). The nucleotide sequences of most viruses known to infect humans have been determined.

The viral nucleic acid is surrounded by a **capsid,** a single- or double-layer protein shell. Together, the nucleic acid and the capsid are often referred to as the **nucleocapsid.** Capsids are composed of subunits (sometimes called "capsomers") arranged in symmetric patterns. The repeating subunits of viral proteins self-assemble into mature virions.

Viral capsid proteins are arranged in two basic patterns of capsid structural symmetry, **icosahedral** and **helical.** Viruses with icosahedral symmetry contain a defined number of structural subunits (20 triangular faces and 12 vertices), whereas the number of subunits varies in viruses with helical symmetry. Viruses with icosahedral symmetry usually have a spherical shape, with twofold, threefold, and fivefold axes of rotational symmetry (Fig. 31-3). In those viruses, the nucleic acid is packed inside the spherical core and is tightly associated with specific viral capsid proteins. A general feature of viruses with helical symmetry is that the protein subunits of the capsid are bound in a regular, periodic fashion along the nucleic acid. Human viruses with helical symmetry invariably have RNA genomes. Some of the largest viruses, such as the poxviruses, have complex structural arrangements.

Many viruses possess an **envelope** that surrounds the nucleocapsid (see Fig. 31-3). Those viruses are called **enveloped viruses;** viruses without an envelope are called **nonenveloped viruses.** The viral envelope is composed of virus-specific proteins plus lipids and carbohydrates derived from host cell membranes (e.g., the nuclear membrane, endoplasmic reticulum, Golgi apparatus, or plasma membrane). In some cases virus-specific envelope proteins include a **matrix (M) protein** that lines the inner surface of the envelope and is in contact with the nucleocapsid (Fig. 31-4). M proteins may stabilize the interaction between viral glycopro-

ICOSAHEDRAL SYMMETRY

HELICAL SYMMETRY

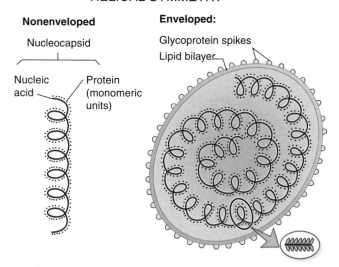

FIGURE 31-3 ▪ **Basic viral forms.** The inset depicts the nucleic acid–protein complex, often called the nucleocapsid.

teins and the lipid envelope, direct the viral genome to intracellular sites of virus assembly, or help in virus budding. Virus-specific envelope glycoproteins protrude from the outer surface of the envelope, forming structures known as **spikes.** The surface glycoproteins of some viruses agglutinate red blood cells (**hemagglutination**) by binding to receptors on the erythrocyte surface. Hemagglutination assays can be used in certain settings to diagnose viral infections.

A large number of viruses carry out **virion-associated enzymatic activities,** depending on the strategy used for replication of the nucleic acid. The viral enzyme that makes virus-specific mRNA, which is required for the synthesis of all viral proteins, is an RNA-dependent RNA polymerase if the genome is RNA, or a DNA-dependent RNA polymerase if the genome is DNA. Retroviruses contain an RNA-dependent DNA polymerase known as **reverse transcriptase.** Some viruses have mRNA processing enzymes such as "capping enzymes," which modify viral mRNAs at their 5′ end by adding a methylguanosine cap, or enzymes that

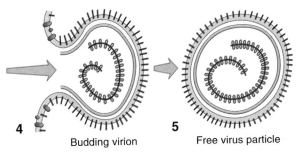

FIGURE 31-4 ▪ Virus budding through the cytoplasmic membrane. The host cell plasma membrane seen early in infection (1). Virus-encoded M proteins become associated with the plasma membrane (2). Viral glycoprotein spikes are incorporated into the membrane, the viral nucleocapsid is assembled near the membrane, and budding begins (3). Budding continues with further insertion of viral spikes in the membrane (4). Budding is completed, releasing a free virion (5).

polyadenylate the 3′ end of viral mRNA. Additional virus-encoded enzymes include protein kinases, nucleoside triphosphate phosphatases, endonucleases, and ribonucleases (RNases). Certain viruses, such as influenza virus, have enzymes on their surface (e.g., neuraminidase) that are involved in release of progeny virions from host cells.

The principal viruses that cause disease in humans belong to about a dozen families containing hundreds of species (Table 31-1, Fig. 31-5). Each species may contain many individual strains that differ in virulence and antigenic properties (serotypes). Viruses are classified using a combination of genetic, physicochemical, and biological factors. These factors include the type and structure of the viral nucleic acid (single- or double-stranded RNA or DNA); the ultrastructure of the virus particle (including size, type of capsid symmetry, and the presence or absence of an envelope); and the strategy for genome replication. In many instances, genomic sequence information is sufficient to identify both the family and the species to which a virus belongs. Subdivisions within the major taxonomic groups are usually based on immunologic, cytopathologic, pathogenetic, or epidemiologic features.

Virus Replication

The steps in virus replication include infection of a susceptible cell, reproduction of the nucleic acid and proteins, and assembly and release of infectious progeny. The structural and genetic diversity of viruses is reflected in the variety of replicative strategies that they employ.

Attachment and Penetration

The first step in viral infection of target cells is the attachment of the virus to the host cell surface. That step, which is also called **adsorption,** is initially reversible and results from random collisions between virions and target cells. Although attachment requires appropriate ionic and pH conditions, it is largely temperature-independent and does not require energy. The virion structure that mediates cell attachment has been identified for most viruses. For enveloped viruses, the attachment protein is usually one of the spikes inserted on the outer surface of the viral envelope, such as the hemagglutinin of influenza virus. Some enveloped viruses, such as the herpesviruses and poxviruses, have more than one type of attachment protein. For nonenveloped viruses, surface-exposed regions of capsid proteins function to mediate virus attachment.

Viruses have adapted to attach to a variety of molecules (receptors) on the cell surface. Viral receptors can be highly specialized proteins with limited tissue distribution, such as complement receptors, growth factor receptors, or neurotransmitter receptors, or they can be more ubiquitous components of cellular membranes, such as integrins and other intercellular adhesion molecules, complement regulatory proteins, phospholipids, or carbohydrates. Viruses of the same species but different serotypes can bind to the same receptors (e.g., poliovirus serotypes 1, 2, and 3) or different ones (e.g., human rhinovirus 2 and 14). In addition, viruses from widely divergent families can bind to the same receptor. Studies suggest that approximately 10^4 to 10^6 virus-binding sites (receptors) are present on any given cell.

Some viruses use multiple receptors, which may allow them to invade a variety of cell types as infection progresses. Many viruses use distinct molecules for attachment and internalization. For example, HIV binds to CD4 and one of several chemokine receptors. Utilization of multiple receptors may be important to ensure precise targeting of the virus to particular host cells.

Once adsorption has occurred, the entire virion or a component of the payload containing the viral genome and virion-associated polymerases must be translocated across the plasma membrane of the host cell. Some nonenveloped viruses, such as adenovirus, undergo re-

table 31-1   Classification of Viruses

FAMILY	EXAMPLE	NUCLEIC ACID POLARITY OR STRUCTURE	GENOME SIZE (KILOBASES OR KILOBASE PAIRS)	ENVELOPE	CAPSID SYMMETRY
RNA viruses					
Single stranded					
Picornaviridae	Poliovirus	(+) RNA	7–8	No	I
Caliciviridae	Norwalk virus	(+) RNA	8	No	I
Togaviridae	Rubella virus	(+) RNA	10–12	Yes	I
Flaviviridae	Yellow fever virus	(+) RNA	10–12	Yes	I
Coronaviridae	SARS-CoV	(+) RNA	20–33	Yes	H
Rhabdoviridae	Rabies virus	(−) RNA	11–15	Yes	H
Paramyxoviridae	Measles virus	(−) RNA	15–16	Yes	H
Arenaviridae	Lassa fever virus	Two circular (−) RNA segments	5–7	Yes	H
Bunyaviridae	Hantavirus	Three circular (−) RNA segments	10–23	Yes	H
Orthomyxoviridae	Influenza virus	8 (−) RNA segments[a]	12–15	Yes	H
Retroviridae	HIV	Two identical molecules (+) RNA	7–11	Yes	I (capsid), H (nucleocapsid)
Double stranded					
Reoviridae	Rotavirus	10–12 dsRNA segments[b]	18–30	No	I
DNA viruses					
Single stranded					
Parvoviridae	Human parvovirus B-19	(+) or (−)	5	No	I
Mixed strandedness					
Hepadnaviridae	Hepatitis B virus	Circular dsDNA with ss portions	3	Yes	Unknown
Double stranded					
Polyomaviridae	JC virus	Circular	5	No	I
Papillomaviridae	Human papillomavirus	Circular	8	No	I
Adenoviridae	Human adenoviruses	Linear	30–42	No	I
Herpesviridae	Herpes simplex virus	Linear	120–220	Yes	I
Poxviridae	Vaccinia virus	Linear with covalently closed ends	130–375	Yes	Ovoid

[a] Influenza C has 7 segments.
[b] Reovirus, orbivirus has 10 segments; rotavirus has 11 segments; Colorado tick fever has 12 segments.
(+) positive sense; (−) negative sense; ds, double-stranded; H, helical; I, icosahedral; SARS, severe acute respiratory syndrome; ss, single-stranded.
Adapted from Condit RC. Principles of virology. In: Knipe DM, Howley PM, eds. Fields Virology. 4th ed. Philadelphia: Lippincott-Raven Press; 2001:19–51.

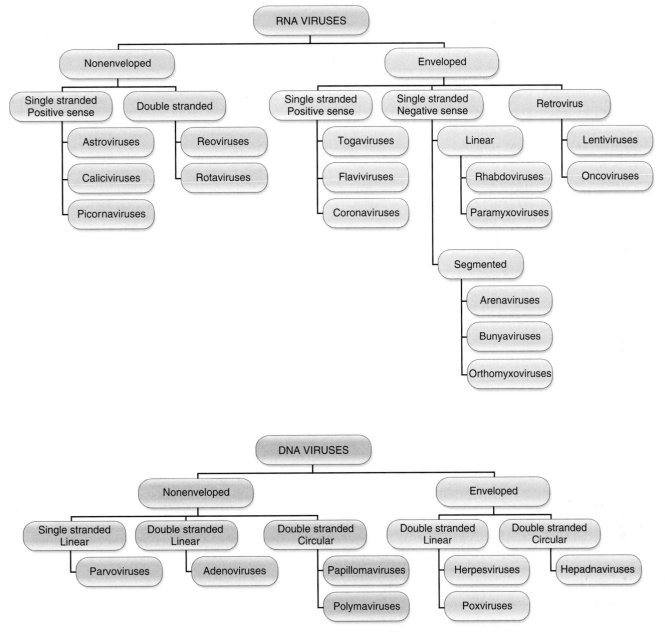

FIGURE 31-5 ▪ The main groups of human viruses.

ceptor-mediated endocytosis and appear in the cytoplasm within endocytic vesicles. Some nonenveloped viruses probably cross the plasma membrane directly and appear free in the cytoplasm in the absence of vesicle formation.

Enveloped viruses use at least two strategies for penetration. Influenza virus binds to cell surface receptors that aggregate at distinct sites on the plasma membrane (**clathrin-coated pits**). Virions are endocytosed within clathrin-coated vesicles and are delivered to endosomes (Fig. 31-6). Fusion between the viral envelope and the endosomal membrane releases the viral nucleocapsid into the cytoplasm. In contrast, most paramyxoviruses (such as measles virus) fuse directly with the plasma membrane.

The next step in virus replication is **uncoating**, the process in which the viral delivery system is removed to make the viral genome accessible to the cellular transcription and translation machinery. For many viruses, penetration and uncoating occur simultaneously. For certain viruses, contact with the receptor induces conformational changes in the capsid that facilitate release of the viral nucleic acid into the cytoplasm.

Some nonenveloped viruses require host cell enzymes for removal of their capsids. For certain reoviruses, proteases present in late endosomes and lysosomes sequentially remove the outer capsid proteins to produce a "subvirion particle." Those particles penetrate endosomal membranes, leading to activation of virus transcription in the cytoplasm.

Viral particle   Clathrin-coated pit

A

Penetration

B

Release

FIGURE 31-6 ▪ **Penetration and release of an enveloped virus (Semliki Forest virus). A.** The stages in the adsorption of the virus to clathrin-coated pits and the gradual invagination of the membrane carrying the virus into the interior within a clathrin-coated vesicle. **B.** The release of the virus by budding from the membrane.

Macromolecular Synthesis

The synthesis of all viral macromolecules first requires the translation of viral mRNA into virus-specific proteins. How is viral mRNA made? Viruses that contain double-stranded DNA synthesize mRNA just as the host cell does, using a DNA-dependent RNA polymerase. RNA viruses, however, must make their mRNA from RNA, which involves a different mechanism. Viruses have evolved several strategies to synthesize viral mRNA and translate it into protein (Fig. 31-7). The variations are described in more detail in the chapters covering the individual virus groups (see Chapters 32 to 43).

Single-Stranded Positive-Sense RNA Viruses

The simplest translation strategy is for the nucleic acid of the virion to function directly as mRNA. Examples of viruses that use that approach are the picornaviruses (e.g., poliovirus) and flaviviruses (e.g., West Nile virus). By convention, the genomes of those viruses are said to have **positive-sense polarity.** Following entry into the host cell, the viral genomic RNA acts as mRNA and is translated by cellular ribosomes to produce the various viral proteins. For certain viruses, such as poliovirus, mRNA is translated into a single large polyprotein that is sequentially cleaved by virus-encoded proteases to release the individual viral proteins; this process leads to expression of viral proteins in equimolar amounts.

For positive-sense RNA viruses, how is the viral RNA synthesized? A **virus-encoded RNA-dependent RNA polymerase** synthesizes a complementary **negative-sense** RNA using genomic RNA as a template. In turn, the newly synthesized negative-sense RNA serves as a template for the synthesis of additional copies of genomic positive-sense RNA. The newly produced genomic RNA may serve as mRNA or may be packaged into progeny virions.

FIGURE 31-7 ▪ Strategies for virus replication and the main enzymes involved.

Single-Stranded Negative-Sense RNA Viruses

The RNA of negative-sense viruses does not carry instructions for synthesis of viral proteins; only its complementary strand does. These viruses must therefore use a different strategy to make mRNA. The genomic negative-sense RNA is used as a template to produce mRNA transcripts corresponding to each viral gene. The transcripts differ in abundance, which allows the synthesis of each viral protein to be regulated independently. The genome is replicated by production of a full-length single-stranded positive-sense RNA intermediate, which then serves as a template to synthesize new copies of single-stranded negative-sense genomic RNA. Mammalian cells do not possess enzymes that use RNA as template for making

RNA. Therefore, viruses using that strategy must contain an RNA-dependent RNA polymerase in the virion, which is introduced into host cells during infection.

Some single-stranded negative-sense RNA viruses (e.g., influenza virus) have **segmented genomes,** which consist of more than one RNA molecule. As with the nonsegmented negative-sense RNA viruses, transcription results in unique mRNAs for each viral protein rather than a single large polycistronic mRNA molecule.

Double-Stranded RNA Viruses

The information encoded in double-stranded RNA (like that encoded in DNA), first must be copied into a positive-sense single strand of RNA to act as mRNA. Because of its double-stranded character, the virion RNA cannot function directly as mRNA (even though it contains a positive-sense strand). Viruses with double-stranded RNA genomes, such as the reoviruses and rotaviruses, contain a virus-encoded RNA-dependent RNA polymerase that transcribes single-stranded positive-sense RNAs using the negative-sense strands of the double-stranded RNA segments as templates. The double-stranded RNA genome is always found as segments, each of which is transcribed to produce a unique mRNA.

RNA Viruses That Replicate Through a DNA Intermediate

The retroviruses, such as HIV, contain single-stranded positive-sense RNA but employ a unique replicative strategy using a DNA intermediate. Viral positive-sense RNA serves as a template for a virion-associated RNA-dependent DNA polymerase (reverse transcriptase). The DNA is then integrated into host chromosomal DNA, where it resides for the life of the cell. Transcription of the integrated viral DNA, like transcription of host cell genes, is carried out be host cell DNA-dependent RNA polymerases.

DNA Viruses

In general, DNA-containing viruses make mRNA using strategies similar to those of host cells. In cells infected with adenoviruses, herpesviruses, papillomaviruses, and polyomaviruses, transcription of viral DNA into mRNA occurs in the host cell nucleus and depends on host cell enzymes. Transcription of most DNA-containing viruses is tightly regulated and results in synthesis of early and then late mRNA transcripts (Fig. 31-8). The early transcripts encode regulatory proteins and the proteins required for DNA replication, while the late transcripts encode mainly structural proteins of the virion. Several DNA-containing viruses, such as adenovirus and human papillomavirus (HPV), induce cells to express host proteins required for viral DNA replication by stimulating cell cycle progression. For example, the HPV E7 protein binds the retinoblastoma gene product pRB and liberates the transcription factor E2F, which drives the cell to progress through the cell cycle. To prevent programmed cell death in response to E7-mediated unscheduled cell cycle progression, the HPV E6 protein induces the ubiquitination and degradation of tumor suppressor protein p53.

The individual mRNAs for both early and late viral proteins often correspond to sequences of viral DNA

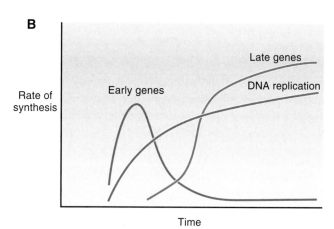

FIGURE 31-8 ▪ **Virus replication events during a single infectious cycle. A.** Viral titer. A single cycle of virus growth can be studied by determining the titer of infectious virus (e.g., by plaque assay) over time. Cells are adsorbed with virus, and at various intervals after adsorption, the cells are lysed, and viral titer is determined. Viral titer is stable during the brief period of virus attachment, indicating that removal of the virus after attachment but before internalization does not diminish infectivity. Following attachment, viral titer declines precipitously as the virus undergoes disassembly, transcription, translation, and genome replication. That interval is termed the eclipse. Viral titer begins to increase as progeny virions, which are fully infectious, are assembled. **B.** DNA virus transcription. Transcription of most DNA viruses results in synthesis of early and late mRNA transcripts. The early transcripts encode regulatory proteins and proteins required for DNA replication. The late transcripts encode mainly structural proteins of the virion. Initiation of DNA synthesis precedes transcription of the late genes.

called **exons**, separated by spacer sequences called **introns**. The products of transcription are RNA molecules with sequences identical to those of the DNA. The immature mRNA molecules are cut and then spliced back together to remove the intervening introns. For many viruses, mRNAs are synthesized from overlapping regions of the viral DNA. This redundancy reduces the amount of viral DNA required to encode some viral proteins and is another example of the genetic economy among the viruses.

Poxviruses are the most structurally intricate of the animal viruses, and their replicative cycle is correspondingly complex. The initial steps of transcription and translation occur in the host cell cytoplasm. Therefore, poxviruses viruses cannot use host RNA polymerases, which are located in the nucleus. Consequently, poxviruses carry their own DNA-dependent RNA polymerase to initiate transcription. One of the virus-encoded early proteins is responsible for a second stage of uncoating in which the viral DNA is made fully accessible for transcription and replication. Replication, transcription, and virus assembly all occur within virus-initiated organelles, known as "factories," located in the host cell cytoplasm. Early proteins include a number of enzymes (e.g., DNA polymerase and thymidine kinase) and some structural proteins. As infection proceeds, DNA replication begins, the synthesis of the early nonstructural proteins ceases, and the synthesis of late proteins takes place. Many of the late proteins are structural proteins, but other late proteins include enzymes and proteins that play roles in virus assembly.

Assembly of Progeny Virions and Release From the Host Cell

Once new viral genomes and proteins have been synthesized, intact virions are assembled and released from host cells. Assembly of the nonenveloped viruses and the nucleocapsids of enveloped viruses often occurs spontaneously, resulting in crystalline arrays of viral capsids. Once the capsid is formed, it becomes filled with viral nucleic acid resulting in the production of viable virions (see Fig. 31-8).

Nonenveloped viruses are usually released when the cell lyses. Events leading to cell disruption include inhibition of the synthesis of host cell macromolecules, disorganization of the host cell cytoskeleton, and alteration of host cell membrane structure. Membrane disruption may result in increased cell permeability and the release of proteolytic enzymes from lysosomes. Failure of the host cell to replenish energy-rich substrate molecules inhibits the function of ion transport pumps and disturbs transport of essential nutrients and cellular waste products.

Enveloped viruses are usually released from infected cells by budding. This process may or may not be lethal to the cell. In all cases virus-encoded proteins inserted into host cell membranes displace some of the normal protein components, which results in restructuring of the membrane. Viral capsids may then bind to virus-encoded M proteins lining the cytoplasmic surface of the altered patches of membrane (see Fig. 31-4). In the smallest enveloped viruses, the togaviruses, the nucleocapsids bind directly to intracytoplasmic domains of viral glycoproteins inserted into the host cell membrane rather than to M proteins.

Many viruses are capable of inducing the genetically programmed mechanism of cell death that leads to apoptosis of host cells. Apoptotic cell death is characterized by cell shrinkage, membrane blebbing, condensation of nuclear chromatin, and cleavage of cellular DNA. Those changes occur according to predetermined developmental programs or in response to certain environmental stimuli. In some cases apoptosis serves as an antiviral defense mechanism to limit virus replication by either the destruction of virus-infected cells or the reduction of potentially harmful inflammatory responses elicited by infection. In other cases apoptosis results from viral induction of cellular factors required for efficient virus replication.

Defective Viruses

Certain viruses cause disease even though they cannot replicate autonomously. To replicate, such **defective viruses** (e.g., hepatitis delta virus) require coinfection with a "helper" virus. Infection with hepatitis delta virus is dependent on coincident infection with hepatitis B virus (HBV) and does not occur in its absence. Coinfection with HBV and hepatitis delta virus frequently results in fulminant hepatitis, apparently by allowing increased multiplication of HBV. In contrast, the defective adeno-associated viruses do not significantly alter the disease caused by the helper adenovirus. Defective viruses can be detected by searching for their antigens or nucleic acids or by culture in the presence of helper viruses.

Prions

Prions are transmissible agents that defy a central tenet of biology. They consist of "infectious proteins" and are devoid of nucleic acid. How then do they transmit genetic information? The question has great clinical as well as biological importance because prions cause a number of fatal neurologic diseases, such as Creutzfeldt-Jakob disease (CJD) and kuru in humans, scrapie in sheep, and more recently, bovine spongiform encephalopathy (BSE or "mad cow disease") in cattle (see Chapter 56).

Prions consist of a single protein that is almost certainly the transmissible agent of disease. An understanding of the biological nature of prions came from the finding that the prion protein (called PrP^{sc}) has an amino acid sequence identical to that of a normal cellular protein (PrP^c), which is encoded by a cellular gene. The two forms of PrP differ only in their folded conformation. In the PrP^{sc} conformation, the protein is highly resistant to digestion by proteolytic enzymes, protein denaturing reagents, and high temperature. It appears that the two forms of the protein, PrP^{sc} and PrP^c, can combine in some way to generate the infectious agent. PrP^{sc} can function as a template, forcing PrP^c to assume the PrP^{sc} conformation. Once PrP^{sc} is formed, the process of conversion is continuous and results in an amplification of PrP^{sc} in neural tissue. Therefore, the transmissible agent (prion) does not transmit primary sequence information but instead serves as a template for improper molecular folding.

Prion-infected material can be transmitted by direct inoculation into the central nervous system (CNS), percutaneous exposure, or ingestion. In the case of kuru, the disease was transmitted and sustained by ritualistic cannibalism of human brains among certain New Guinea natives. Similarly, a recent epidemic of BSE in Great Britain was attributed to the practice of feeding offal from slaughterhouses (including neural tissues from slaughtered cows) to younger cattle as a source of protein. Transmission of CJD to humans has been associated with grafting of human tissues (e.g., corneal transplants and dura mater grafts) and treatment with human pituitary gland extracts. Cases of a novel form of the human disease (called variant CJD) have appeared in Great Britain in the wake of the BSE epidemic and may have been acquired by eating meat from cattle infected with BSE.

In all prion diseases the accumulation of nondegradable PrP in the brain and spinal cord eventually leads to neurological degeneration. The diseases caused by prions are referred to as **transmissible spongiform encephalopathies** because of the telltale pathological alterations—namely, spongy cavitations in the brain. With minor variations, all the known prion diseases manifest that pathology because they are associated with aberrantly folded PrP. How the abnormal forms of PrP contribute to the pathology is unknown. Fortunately, prion diseases are very rare, and transmission of prions from animals to humans occurs with less efficiency than between animals.

Viral Diseases

PATHOBIOLOGY

The signs and symptoms of viral disease are the culmination of a series of interactions between the virus and the host. After encountering a host cell, a virus must be able to enter it, undergo primary replication, and then spread to a final target tissue. Once a virus reaches its target organs, it must infect and successfully replicate in a susceptible population of host cells.

One of three possible outcomes follows infection of a host organism by a virus: acute infection, latent infection, or chronic infection (Fig. 31-9). In an **acute infection,** the virus undergoes multiple rounds of replication. Replication results in the death of the host cell, which is used as a factory for virus production. The number of virus particles produced in a single cell varies from a few for some viruses to thousands for others. Examples of acute infections are those caused by poliovirus or influenza virus.

At the opposite end of the spectrum is **latent infection,** which does not result in the production of progeny virus. Latent infections, which are caused by DNA viruses or retroviruses, reflect the persistence of viral DNA either as an extrachromosomal element (herpesviruses) or as an integrated sequence within the host genome (retroviruses). During cell growth the genome of the virus is replicated along with the chromosomes of the host cell. An example of latent infection is that produced by herpes simplex virus type 1 (HSV-1). The result of **reactivation** of HSV-1 is fever blisters or cold sores. Latent infection by some retroviruses may result in **transformation** of the cell, which leads to cancer.

Chronic infection differs from acute and latent infections in that virus particles continue to be shed after the period of acute illness. The mark of chronic infection is release of virus particles, sometimes without death of the host cell or overt cellular injury. Chronic infection is usually caused by RNA viruses. The amount of virus produced is usually less than in acute infections, and the viruses are often altered ("mutated") from the original ones. Chronic infections are associated with defective host immune responses that are insufficient to clear the infection. Some chronic infections do not result in overt disease, although they can produce disease after a prolonged interval. For example, HBV can cause a chronic infection in the liver that eventually leads to chronic hepatitis and even liver cancer.

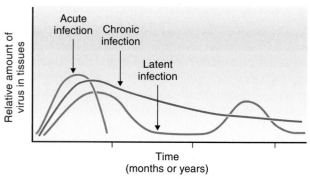

FIGURE 31-9 ▪ **The three types of viral infections.**

ENCOUNTER AND ENTRY

Transmission of a virus from an infected host to a susceptible individual can occur in various ways (Table 31-2). The sources of human-to-human transmission of viruses are acutely ill individuals or chronic carriers; pregnant women can also transmit viruses to their fetuses. Transmission is accomplished by direct contact, such as sexual contact (as in HIV/AIDS), or through the environment. Environmental spread may involve fecal–oral contamination (as in the diarrhea caused by rotaviruses), aerosols (as in chickenpox), or direct inoculation from infected needles or blood products (as in hepatitis B or C). Animal-to-human transmission usually occurs from the bite of a diseased animal (as in rabies) or the bite of an insect vector (as in many types of viral encephalitis).

For most viruses it is not known how many particles are required to initiate an infection. For adenovirus, coxsackie A21 virus, and influenza A virus, as few as 10 particles may suffice. In other cases the number is likely to be considerably larger.

Respiratory Route

Respiratory infection takes place by means of aerosol droplets, nasal secretions, or saliva. Respiratory aerosolization usually occurs from coughing or sneezing. A cough can generate up to 90,000 aerosol particles, and a sneeze up to 2 million. The fate of those particles depends on both ambient environmental conditions (e.g., humidity and wind currents) and particle size. Small particles remain airborne longer and may escape the filtering action of the nose, which traps particles larger than 6 μm in diameter; viruses transmitted in small droplets (e.g., varicella-zoster virus [VZV]) are highly contagious. Aerosolization is not the only possible route of respiratory transmission. Epstein-Barr virus (EBV) is usually spread by saliva, and some respiratory viruses can spread in child care facilities by persisting on contaminated toys. Rhinoviruses, which cause the common cold, are most efficiently spread not by aerosols but from contaminated hands to eyes, nose, or mouth—a cycle that can be interrupted by hand washing.

Entry via the respiratory route requires that the virus overcome a formidable series of host defenses. Respiratory epithelial cells are covered by a thick glycocalyx and tracheobronchial mucus that can trap virus particles. Ciliated respiratory epithelial cells continually sweep mucus up from the lower respiratory tract into the upper respiratory tract, where it is usually swallowed. In the lung, immunologic defenses include secretory IgA, natural killer (NK) cells, and macrophages.

Gastrointestinal Route

Gastrointestinal transmission occurs when viruses shed in feces contaminate the food or water subsequently ingested by a susceptible individual (fecal–oral spread). Stool-tainted hands, resulting from poor personal hygiene, provide another vehicle of spread for enteric viruses. The high incidence of enteric virus infections in child care centers reflects the difficulty of maintaining hygiene in those settings.

Gastrointestinal transmission is limited to viruses that can withstand the harsh environment of the gastrointestinal tract. The acidity of the stomach inactivates acid-labile viruses such as rhinoviruses. Bile salts, present in the lumen of the small intestine, can destroy the lipid envelopes of many viruses and may account for entry via the gastrointestinal route being limited largely to nonenveloped viruses. Proteolytic enzymes and secretory IgA also contribute to host antiviral defenses in the gastrointestinal tract. However, certain proteolysis-resistant viral

table **31-2**	Routes of Virus Transmission
ROUTE	**VIRUS**
Respiratory	
Airborne small droplet	Influenza virus Measles virus Smallpox virus (?) Varicella-zoster virus
Airborne large droplet	Adenovirus Parainfluenzavirus Parvovirus Smallpox virus
Direct contact with respiratory secretions	Respiratory syncytial virus Rhinovirus
Gastrointestinal	
Fecal–oral	Enteric adenovirus Hepatitis A virus Norwalk virus Poliovirus and other enteroviruses Rotavirus
Contact with lesions	Herpes simplex virus Smallpox virus Varicella-zoster virus
Blood and body fluids	Cytomegalovirus Epstein-Barr virus Hepatitis B virus Hepatitis C virus HIV
Insect bites	Dengue virus Eastern, western equine encephalitis virus La Crosse virus West Nile virus Yellow fever virus

capsid proteins allow some viruses to withstand digestion in the gut.

For some enteric viruses, passage across the mucosal barrier of the gut is mediated by **microfold (M) cells** overlying mucosal lymphoid tissues known as Peyer patches. M cells, and perhaps their analogs in bronchial lymphoid tissue, appear to facilitate transport of some viruses across the mucosal epithelium.

Transcutaneous Route

The stratum corneum of the skin provides both a physical and biological barrier against the entry of viruses. Some viruses overcome the skin barrier by direct inoculation from insect or animal bites or from mechanical devices such as needles.

In viral diseases in which the vector is an insect or an infected animal, the disease cycle may be complex. For example, transmission of dengue is characterized by a continuous cycle between humans and infected mosquitoes. Dengue viruses multiply in the gut of a mosquito, spread to its salivary glands, and are injected into a human as the mosquito takes a blood meal. Virus replication within the host leads to a high titer of virus in the bloodstream (**viremia**), which is sufficient to allow the virus to be picked up by an uninfected mosquito during biting. In other arthropodborne virus infections, humans are "dead-end" hosts because the degree of viremia in infected individuals is insufficient to transmit the infection to a new group of insect vectors. Examples of that type of cycle are found in the togaviruses, such as the various equine encephalitis viruses. The normal animal reservoirs for togaviruses include small birds and mammals. Horses, like humans, are also usually dead-end hosts, although in Venezuelan equine encephalitis, horses may be a reservoir of virus.

Some arthropodborne viruses do not require a viremic vertebrate intermediate host to maintain a transmission cycle in nature. The viruses are passed in transovarian fashion to the progeny of infected insects or by sexual transmission between males and females. Transovarian transmission may allow survival of arthropodborne viruses through the winter months.

Iatrogenic inoculation (caused by diagnostic or therapeutic procedures) sometimes allows the entry of viruses. Cytomegalovirus (CMV), HBV, and HIV may be present in contaminated blood products used for transfusion, although various screening procedures have diminished the risk of that means of transmission. Infected corneal transplants, instruments used in neurosurgical procedures, and pituitary tissues used to prepare growth hormone have been implicated as causes of Creutzfeldt-Jakob disease. Iatrogenic inoculation can be purposeful and benevolent, as in the case of vaccination using live-attenuated agents (e.g., the measles virus or Sabin poliovirus vaccines).

Sexual Route

Sexual transmission with entry across the genitourinary or rectal mucosa is important for CMV, HBV, HSV, and HIV. The virus can spread to other organs, but with some viruses, such as HSV, lesions are often found near the site of entry.

Endogenous and Exogenous Viruses

Most viral diseases result from exposure to **exogenous** virus. However, some viral diseases result from the reactivation of an **endogenous** virus that has been latent within specific host cells. Examples of infections caused by reactivated endogenous viruses include shingles (VZV), progressive multifocal leukoencephalopathy (caused by JC or BK polyomavirus), recurrent oral and genital herpes (HSV), and some types of CMV infections. Many latent viruses are held in check by the cellular immune system, and aging or immunosuppressive therapies can lead to virus reactivation.

For the majority of viral diseases, transmission of viruses occurs between members of a susceptible host population (**horizontal spread**). **Vertical spread** of infection occurs when the fetus becomes infected in utero through virus carried in the germ cell line, virus infecting the placenta, or virus in the maternal birth canal. CMV, HBV, HIV, HSV, rubella virus, and VZV can produce vertically transmitted congenital infections.

SPREAD AND REPLICATION

For some viruses, the processes of entry, primary replication, and tissue tropism all occur at the same anatomic site. Examples of that type of viral infection include the upper and lower respiratory infections caused by the orthomyxoviruses, paramyxoviruses, and rhinoviruses; the enteritis caused by rotaviruses; and the dermatologic lesions induced by HPV (warts). Other viruses enter at one site and, to produce disease, subsequently spread to a distant area, such as the CNS. In these diseases it is useful to distinguish between primary virus replication near the entry site and secondary replication at the eventual target organ or tissue. Enteroviruses enter via the gastrointestinal tract and spread to the CNS to produce meningitis, encephalitis, or poliomyelitis. Measles virus and VZV enter the body through the respiratory tract but then spread to produce skin disease (exanthem) and often generalized organ involvement. Neural, hematogenous, and lymphatic pathways are all used by viruses to spread to target tissues.

A great deal of virus replication can occur before any signs or symptoms of clinical illness are evident. The **incubation period** varies from a few days (influenza) to weeks (measles and varicella), months (hepatitis and rabies), or years (prions). Viral infection does not always lead to overt clinical disease. The percentage of infected people who develop overt disease ranges from 100% (measles and rabies) to nearly zero (BK and JC polyomaviruses). For many viral infections, symptomatic disease is less common in children than in adults (e.g., EBV mononucleosis, hepatitis A, and paralytic poliomyelitis).

Neural Spread

Examples of viruses that spread through nerves include HSV, rabies virus, and VZV. HSV is thought to enter nerves through receptors located primarily near synaptic endings rather than on the nerve cell body. Rabies virus accumulates at the motor end plate of the neuromuscular junction and may use the acetylcholine receptor or a closely related structure to enter the distal axons of motor neurons. Rabies virus also infects muscle and spreads through motor and sensory nerves to the spinal cord.

The kinetics of neural spread for HSV, poliovirus, and rabies virus suggest that these agents use intraneuronal mechanisms involved in fast axonal transport. Infection of Schwann cells may provide another pathway of dissemination to the CNS. Neural spread is important not only for entry into the CNS but also for spread within the CNS and from the CNS to the periphery (as in reactivation of latent HSV infections).

The olfactory system presents a special pathway for neural spread. The rod processes of olfactory receptor cells lie exposed in the olfactory mucosa and are the only place in the body where the nervous system is in direct contact with the environment. Experimental intranasal or aerosol inoculations of HSV, poliovirus, rabies virus, and some togaviruses have led to CNS infection via the olfactory route. That route may provide a pathway to the CNS in humans for rabies virus and possibly other viruses in circumstances where high-titer aerosols are present, such as in caves occupied by large numbers of rabid bats or in accidental laboratory-acquired infections. The olfactory route of spread might explain the localization of HSV in the orbitofrontal and medial temporal cortex in cases of HSV encephalitis.

Hematogenous Spread

Hematogenous spread is an important mechanism of dissemination for many viruses. A period of primary replication usually precedes the initial viremia and may be asymptomatic or result in prodromal symptoms. For enteric viruses, primary replication often occurs in Peyer patches and peritonsillar lymphatic tissue. For respiratory viruses, primary replication is thought to take place in epithelial or alveolar cells. In some cases virus travels through lymphatics, from the site of primary replication to regional lymph nodes before entering the bloodstream. The initial (primary) viremia often disseminates the virus to tissues like the spleen and liver, where continued replication in parenchymal cells leads to an amplified secondary viremia. Growth in endothelial cells may help sustain the viremic phase in some togavirus infections. Sustained secondary amplification of the viremia is required if the virus is to overcome clearance by lymphoreticular cells.

Bloodborne virus particles may travel free in the plasma or in association with cells. Enteroviruses, HBV, and togaviruses all travel free within plasma; Colorado tick fever virus and Rift Valley fever virus are associated with red blood cells; CMV, EBV, HIV, and rubella virus are associated with lymphocytes or monocytes.

Multiple Pathways for Spread

Some viruses use different pathways of spread at different stages in the infectious cycle. VZV disseminates to the skin by the hematogenous route to produce "chickenpox" (varicella) and then spreads centripetally along nerves from the skin to neurons in the dorsal root ganglion, where it becomes latent. Reactivation results in centrifugal spread of virus along sensory nerves to their skin dermatome and the production of "shingles" (zoster). Neural spread of virus accounts for recurrent episodes of oral and genital infections caused by HSV. Poliovirus is an example of a virus capable of spreading by both hematogenous and neural routes. The hematogenous route is generally accepted as the primary pathway to the CNS, although the virus may spread to the CNS from the gut through autonomic nerves or from infected muscle through peripheral nerves.

HOST FACTORS IN DEFENSE AND DAMAGE

A large number of innate and adaptive host defense mechanisms are involved in protection against viruses. The age and genetic makeup of the host have important implications for the outcome of certain viral infections. Newborns, for example, are particularly susceptible to severe disseminated HSV infections. In contrast, many of the exanthematous illnesses, EBV infection, and poliovirus infection are usually more severe in older individuals than in children. Specific host genes may help determine susceptibility to certain viral infections, acting through effects on the immune system or by altering viral receptors. Inadequate host nutritional status may increase susceptibility to some viruses such as measles virus, perhaps by depressing cell-mediated immunity; malnutrition accounts for the high mortality associated with measles in some developing countries. The host may influence viral infections in other ways that are still poorly understood. For example, stress can trigger recurrent fever blisters (herpes labialis), but how that occurs is unknown.

The most important adaptive defense mechanism against viral infections is cell-mediated immunity. Persons with defective cell-mediated immunity but normal capacity to make antibodies often have prolonged viral infections. That is most evident in persons with AIDS or in bone marrow transplant recipients, who may suffer fatal infections with herpesviruses and respiratory viruses that normally cause self-limited illnesses in immunocompetent persons. Antibody deficiency by itself usually does not change the outcome of viral infections, although antibody-deficient persons can suffer from severe and chronic infections caused by enteroviruses. Phagocytosis by neutrophils does not play an important role in defense against viral infections. Macrophages, on the other hand, are often involved in virus containment and can limit the spread of viruses in the body.

Innate Immune Responses

The innate immune system recognizes macromolecules likely to be expressed by microbial pathogens but not by host cells (pathogen-associated molecular patterns). Toll-like receptors expressed on a variety of cell types are activated by viral components such as double-stranded RNA and viral glycoproteins, triggering inflammatory responses, cytokine and interferon secretion, and activation of the adaptive immune system.

Cell-Mediated Immunity

Cell-mediated immunity is a major factor in both the termination of viral infections and the pathogenesis of viral diseases. Because of the viral intracellular habitat, infected cells are susceptible to the action of lymphocytes that recognize viral antigens bound to major histocompatibility complex (MHC) proteins on their surface (see Chapter 7). Virus-infected cells can be lysed by several types of lymphoid cells through antibody-independent and antibody-dependent pathways.

Cytotoxicity by **NK cells** provides one of the earliest host defenses against viral infection (peak activity at 2 to 3 days) and precedes the appearance of cytotoxic T lymphocytes (CTLs) and virus-specific antibody responses. NK cells are large granular lymphocytes that recognize and kill some virus-infected cells. Activation of NK cells is regulated by signals from a variety of cell-surface receptors that recognize the presence or absence of ligands, such as MHC antigens, on target cells. Viruses, by modulating expression of ligands, may render cells susceptible to NK-mediated lysis. NK cells appear to be particularly important for the control of CMV and other herpesvirus infections.

CTLs constitute a **specific** virus-induced defense mechanism because they must be activated by antigen presented by macrophages or other antigen-presenting cells. Lysis of infected cells mediated by CTLs is restricted to cells that express MHC class I proteins, although examples of MHC class II–restricted CTLs have been described (see Chapter 7). In contrast to neutralizing antibodies, which usually recognize epitopes on intact viral surface proteins, CTLs recognize protein fragments derived from both viral surface and internal proteins.

Antibody Response

Most viruses are sufficiently antigenic to stimulate a specific immune response. Viruses contain many foreign proteins, each of which may contain multiple antigenic sites. Although the amount of viral antigenic material may be initially quite small, it is amplified during virus replication. However, antibodies do not usually play a primary role in terminating acute viral infections. Instead, antibodies are important in preventing reinfection. In some cases antibodies may themselves be implicated in the pathogenesis of disease (e.g., in dengue hemorrhagic fever).

Antibodies that protect the host by destroying the infectivity of the virus are called **neutralizing antibodies.** They are usually directed against epitopes present on viral proteins located on the surface of the virus particle. Neutralizing antibodies are thought to reduce viral infectivity by inhibiting early steps of the replication cycle such as attachment, penetration, or uncoating of the virus. In addition, such antibodies may produce aggregation of virions, accelerate virus degradation in vesicles, or enhance viral opsonization and subsequent phagocytosis. If two isolates of a virus are neutralized by the same specific antibody, they are said to belong to a single **serotype.** Neutralizing antibodies directed against one member of a serotype protect against reinfection by other members of the same serotype but not against viruses belonging to a different serotype. There are nearly 100 serotypes of rhinovirus; therefore, after recovering from an upper respiratory infection caused by a rhinovirus, a person remains susceptible to many others. Although polioviruses, like rhinoviruses, belong to the picornavirus family, there are only three poliovirus serotypes. To provide protection against poliomyelitis, the poliovirus vaccine includes each of the three serotypes.

Antibodies also can participate in lysis of virus-infected cells via **antibody-dependent cell-mediated cytotoxicity (ADCC;** see Chapter 7). In ADCC immune responses, virus-specific antibodies bound to antigens on the surface of infected cells interact with receptors for the Fc portion of IgG on the surface of NK cells. Binding of IgG to Fc receptors activates the NK cells and results in target cell killing. Macrophages, lymphocytes, and neutrophils also have Fc receptors and also may participate in ADCC.

Interferons

In addition to the adaptive humoral and cellular defense mechanisms, viral infections elicit an inducible defense mechanism, the **interferons.** These are proteins encoded by host cells whose synthesis is induced by viruses and other proinflammatory agents. Interferons inhibit virus replication indirectly by inducing the synthesis of cellular proteins that inhibit the protein synthesis machinery. The discovery and practical applications of interferons are discussed in Chapter 44.

There are three main kinds of interferons, labeled α, β, and γ. Leukocytes produce more than a dozen types of interferon-α (leukocyte interferon), which share about 70% amino acid sequence homology. Interferon-β (fibroblast interferon) is produced by fibroblasts and epithelial cells and has 30% homology to interferons-α. Interferon-γ (immune interferon) is usually induced by the activation of T cells by specific antigens.

Interferon-α and interferon-β are induced by both viable and inactivated viruses, double-stranded RNA, and a number of other compounds. Newly produced interferon is released into the extracellular fluid and binds to specific interferon receptors on adjacent cells. Consequently, interferon tends to act locally rather than systemically. Binding of interferon to its receptor leads to a series of intracellular signaling events. Those events in turn lead to the expression of a large number of cellular genes that act in concert to create an "antiviral state." For example, interferon induces the expression of a protein kinase called **PKR** that phosphorylates a protein synthesis initiation factor. In the phosphorylated form, this factor cannot participate in the formation of the protein synthesis–initiation complex, thus leading to inhibition of viral protein synthesis. In addition, an induced 2,5-oligoisoadenylate synthetase produces 2,5-oligoadenylates, which in turn activate a cellular endonuclease (RNase L) that degrades viral mRNA. Interferons also increase the activity of NK cells, CTLs, and cells involved in ADCC.

Complement

Viruses can trigger the activation of both the classical and alternative pathways of complement in the absence of an antibody response. Activated complement components (e.g., C3b) may act as opsonins to enhance phagocytosis of viruses (see Chapter 6). Activation of the alternative complement pathway, in combination with antibodies, can lead to lysis of enveloped viruses or virus-infected cells. Although the complement system plays a role in protection against some viral infections in animals, human complement deficiency is not usually associated with an increase in the frequency or severity of viral illnesses. Thus, the complement system is not likely to be essential for defense against viral infections.

Virus-Induced Immunopathology

Immunological injury results from cell lysis elicited by one or more of the antiviral host defense mechanisms. Such damage is seen in children immunized with inactivated measles virus vaccine who experience severe disease when later infected with measles virus. The role of cell-mediated immunity is dramatically illustrated in mice infected with the virus that causes lymphocytic choriomeningitis. When inoculated intracerebrally with the virus, normal mice die within about a week. However, mice with defective cell-mediated immunity survive inoculation even though virus multiplication is unaffected. In humans, lymphocytic infiltrates are responsible for much of the myocardial damage that follows viral infections of the heart.

Virus-induced immunopathology can also result from antibody production. Viruses may combine with virus-specific antibodies to form circulating immune complexes to cause a variety of diseases. Immune complexes become trapped in basement membranes at various sites, including the skin, the kidney, the choroid plexus, and the walls of blood vessels. Accumulation of immune complexes results in tissue injury by attracting and activating a variety of inflammatory mediators. In addition, virus stimulation of B lymphocytes can induce cross-reacting antibodies to normal host structures that contain antigenic regions similar to those of the virus (**molecular mimicry**).

Virus Evasion of the Immune System

Viruses have evolved several mechanisms to evade the immune response. Perhaps the best adapted is HIV, which replicates and spreads within macrophages and T lymphocytes of the immune system itself. Other viruses avoid cytotoxic T lymphocyte responses by blocking antigen processing (CMV and HSV) or by inhibiting MHC expression (adenovirus and CMV). To prevent natural killer cell recognition of MHC-deficient cells, CMV encodes an MHC-like protein that engages inhibitory receptors on natural killer cells. HSV and some poxviruses express glycoproteins that interfere with complement activation, and a number of viruses encode cytokine homologs that interfere with normal immunologic functions. Other viruses express molecules that inhibit interferon responses or block effectors of apoptosis.

DIAGNOSIS

A reasonably accurate diagnosis of some viral illnesses, such as measles or varicella, can be made on clinical grounds alone. In other cases the best that can be done clinically is to identify the group of viruses that are the likely pathogens. More definitive diagnosis is often necessary because many of the available antiviral agents have activities that are limited to certain types of viruses. To make a definitive diagnosis, the clinician must isolate the virus in tissue culture, identify the virus or detect virus-specific antigens or viral nucleic acids in tissues or body fluids, or demonstrate specific serologic responses (Table 31-3). Appropriate specimens must be obtained for diagnostic studies during a suitable phase of the illness. Specimens must be rapidly transported to the diagnostic laboratory, and adequate clinical information must be provided.

Isolation of virus from clinical specimens is done in cell cultures, embryonated eggs, and occasionally animals, such as suckling mice. Cell culture techniques involve the use of primary cultures of cells prepared from organs (e.g., monkey kidney cells), human diploid cell lines, and continuous (heterodiploid) cell lines such as HeLa, HEp-2, BHK-21, and Vero. Some viruses grow better in certain cell lines than in others. Inoculation into the amniotic cavity or the allantoic cavity of embryonated chicken eggs is useful for the isolation of influenza virus.

Once cell cultures have been inoculated, the specimens are examined for distinctive patterns of **cytopathic effect**. Viruses such as HSV and many enteroviruses produce cytopathic effect within a few days, whereas cytopathic effect due to CMV, rubella virus, and some adenoviruses may take weeks to appear. Cultured cells are examined for cell lysis and vacuolization. The presence of syncytia suggests HSV, measles virus, mumps virus, or respiratory syncytial virus. Cytomegaly is seen with CMV, HSV, and VZV.

Immunocytochemical staining of cell cultures to detect viral antigens using fluorescein or enzyme-conjugated specific antiviral antibodies permits rapid detection and identification of many viruses. Orthomyxoviruses and paramyxoviruses may be detected by the capacity of infected cultures to adsorb certain red blood cells (**hemadsorption**).

Identification of virus particles or antigens in tissue specimens provides another important method of viral diagnosis. Skin scrapings from the base of vesicles can be stained for viral antigens to help identify HSV or VZV. Similar techniques are used to identify CMV-infected cells in the blood or measles-infected cells in scrapings from characteristic spots in the mouth (Koplik spots). In some cases examining specimens by electron microscopy can be of diagnostic value, especially in investigating outbreaks caused by new or poorly characterized pathogens, but only when viruses are present in high concentrations. Restriction enzyme analysis of the genomes of DNA viruses (e.g., CMV and HSV) and oligonucleotide fingerprinting of ribonuclease-cleaved genomes of RNA viruses (e.g., dengue virus, enteroviruses, and influenza virus) are valuable in epidemiologic studies and in establishing the origin of certain types of viral isolates. Nucleic acid detection techniques based on the polymerase chain reaction (or other nucleic acid–amplification methods) enable the detection of even single copies of viral genomes in tissue samples or cells from body fluids. These extremely sensitive methods are now used routinely in the diagnosis of infections caused by enteroviruses, hepatitis C virus, HIV, HSV, and parvovirus.

A fourfold or greater increase in the antibody titer to a specific viral agent in the serum of a patient taken in the convalescent phase of infection compared with that taken in the acute phase (over a period of 3 to 4 weeks) is usually considered diagnostic of acute infection. A single serum specimen is only occasionally useful in viral diagnosis. Several types of antibodies, including neutralizing, complement-fixing, and hemagglutination-inhibiting antibodies, are routinely assayed (see Chapter 58). The timing of antiviral antibody responses and their sensitivity and specificity differ greatly.

Treatment and prevention of viral diseases are discussed in detail in Chapters 44 and 45 and in the chapters describing the individual viruses.

table **31-3**	**Diagnostic Methods for Common Human Viruses**
VIRUS	**METHOD**
Adenovirus (gastrointestinal)	ELISA
Adenovirus (respiratory)	Antigen, PCR, culture
Cytomegalovirus	Antigen, PCR, culture
Enteroviruses (echo, coxsackie, polio)	PCR, culture
Epstein-Barr virus	PCR, serology
Hepatitis A virus	Serology
Hepatitis B virus	Antigen, PCR, serology
Hepatitis C virus	PCR, serology
Herpes simplex virus	Antigen, PCR, culture
HIV	Antigen, PCR, culture, serology
Influenza virus	ELISA, antigen, culture
Parainfluenza virus	Antigen, PCR, culture
Respiratory syncytial virus	ELISA, antigen, PCR, culture
Rotavirus	ELISA
Varicella-zoster virus	Antigen, PCR

ELISA, enzyme-linked immunosorbent assay; PCR, polymerase chain reaction.

Emerging Viruses

Within the last two decades many newly recognized viruses have come to the attention of clinicians throughout the world. In some cases new agents have been identified for well-characterized illnesses of unknown etiology. These include the identification of human herpesvirus 6 (HHV-6) as the cause of roseola (1986); the isolation of the agent for non-A, non-B hepatitis (1988); and the identification of human metapneumovirus as a common agent of pneumonia in young children (2002). More dramatically, the emergence of new illnesses—such as the AIDS epidemic first noted in 1981, the outbreak of hantavirus pulmonary syndrome in 1993, and the severe acute respiratory syndrome (SARS) epidemic of 2003—has led to the discovery of new viral agents. The ease of international travel and the threat of bioterrorism have caused concerns that relatively exotic pathogens (Ebola virus, Lassa fever virus, and West Nile virus), or viruses from the past (smallpox virus) may appear unexpectedly. The general principles discussed in this chapter may provide a framework for understanding the biology of these emerging pathogens, but each new virus is likely to have its own specific life cycle, evolutionary adaptations, and interactions with the immune system.

Conclusion

Viruses are simple structures that contain two components: a delivery system (the viral envelope and capsid) and a payload (the information contained in the viral genome). Viruses are obligate intracellular parasites that depend on the host cell for most essential enzymatic functions; depending on the virus replication strategy, the virus may need to encode some enzymes or incorporate an essential replication enzyme in the virion. Viral pathogenesis depends on an ordered series of interactions between a virus and its host: entry, uncoating, and primary replication; many viruses then spread to other target tissues within the body. Many components of innate and adaptive immunity act to defend against viral infections. Cell-meditated immunity is responsible for termination of acute viral infections, and humoral immunity is responsible for protection against reinfection. New viruses likely will continue to emerge, posing unique challenges for the development of antiviral drugs and vaccines.

chapter **32**

Picornaviruses and Coronaviruses

Vincent Racaniello and Mark Denison

key **concepts**

Picornaviruses:

■ Comprise a family of small, positive-sense RNA viruses.

■ Include the enteroviruses, rhinoviruses, and hepatitis A virus.

Enteroviruses:

■ Derive their name from their natural habitat, the gastrointestinal tract.

■ Include polioviruses, coxsackievirus, and echoviruses, among others.

Polioviruses:

■ Cause either asymptomatic infection or flaccid paralysis.

■ Replicate in the intestine and can be shed in the feces weeks to months after infection.

■ Can spread from the gastrointestinal tract to the central nervous system.

■ Infection can be prevented with either a killed vaccine (Salk) or a live, attenuated vaccine (Sabin).

Rhinoviruses:

■ Cause the common cold.

■ Comprise more than 100 serotypes, thereby impeding development of an effective vaccine.

■ Can be transmitted person-to-person through contamination or aerosols.

■ Bind to specific receptors on respiratory epithelial cells.

■ Probably cause damage by mechanisms other than virus-induced cytopathology.

The Picornaviridae (*pico* means "small," and *rna* stands for "RNA containing") is a family of small RNA viruses divided into six genera, four of which include human pathogens: the **enteroviruses**, such as **poliovirus, coxsackievirus, echovirus,** and others; the **parechoviruses; hepatitis A virus;** and the **rhinoviruses,** which are among the most common agents of the common cold (Fig. 32-1).

A   B

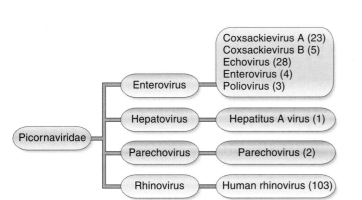

FIGURE 32-1 ▪ **Members of the Picornaviridae family.**
A. Four genera of picornaviruses cause human disease.
B. The members of each genus include a number of
known viral serotypes (indicated in parentheses).

Enteroviruses

Enteroviruses derive their name from their capacity to
replicate in the gastrointestinal tract. The most notorious
enteroviruses are the polioviruses, and more is known
about their molecular biology and pathogenesis than the
other members of this group (see Fig. 32-1). There are
three antigenic types, or serotypes, of polioviruses; most
epidemics were caused by **type 1.** Other enteroviruses
include **coxsackieviruses,** first isolated during a polio outbreak in Coxsackie, New York; and echoviruses (for "enteric cytopathic human orphan viruses"). Echoviruses
were so named because they were initially isolated from
the feces of individuals who had no symptoms, and the
viruses could not be linked to any human disease. More
recently discovered enteroviruses are simply assigned a
number, as in enterovirus 70.

 Hepatitis A virus was originally classified as enterovirus type 72. Information about the biology and
replication of this virus, and comparisons of the nucleotide and amino acid sequence of the viral genome
with that of other picornaviruses, led to reclassification
of hepatitis A virus into a separate genus, hepatovirus.

ENCOUNTER AND ENTRY

Like all enteroviruses, polioviruses are excreted in large
amounts in stool. In the outbreak of poliomyelitis at the
school in Connecticut, the likely source of contamination was a single individual who shed high amounts of
virus from the gastrointestinal tract. In countries with
temperate climates, outbreaks of enterovirus disease usually occur in the summer or early fall; in the tropics the
diseases caused by these viruses are endemic and occur

Case

Outbreak of Poliomyelitis

In October 1972, 11 of 130 students attending a private school
in Greenwich, Connecticut, were diagnosed with paralytic poliomyelitis. Three weeks elapsed between the first and the last
cases. Nine of the 11 cases were boys 12 to 17 years of age,
and all 9 were members either of the football or soccer team.
The clinical histories of those patients were similar: they reported "flulike" symptoms, fever up to 39°C, sore throat, and
muscle pains. Symptoms lasted on average 13 days. Two to
three days later they complained of stiff neck, increased muscle pain, and fever up to 41°C. Those symptoms were followed
by flaccid paralysis of the legs that varied in intensity from relatively minor to totally incapacitating. During the first 3 weeks
of October, 17 other students were seen at the school infirmary with nonspecific complaints that suggested an acute
viral syndrome.

 Poliomyelitis was diagnosed by serological studies that
demonstrated a rising titer of antibodies to type 1 poliovirus,
but not types 2 and 3. The diagnosis was confirmed by the
isolation of type 1 virus from the feces and throat washings of
patients with paralytic disease. More than 50% of the
school's students had not received oral polio vaccine because
of religious convictions. A small number of day students at
the school lived at home, where they interacted with friends
from surrounding towns in activities that included swimming
classes at the local YMCA. Paralytic disease did not occur
among youths who did not attend the private school. An immunization survey of the public schools revealed that more
than 95% of their students had been vaccinated.

 This case raises several questions:
1. What was the origin of the virus, and how did it spread
   among the students?
2. What caused the illness among the 17 students who
   complained of nonspecific signs and symptoms?
3. Why did the disease not spread to all the students or to
   the community outside the school?
4. How does poliovirus cause paralysis and other
   symptoms of disease?
5. What could have been done to halt further spread of
   poliovirus in the school?

 Poliomyelitis has been eradicated from the United States
and nearly eliminated from most countries. Paradoxically, its
dreaded consequences, paralysis and death, are more common in unvaccinated individuals living in countries with a high
standard of sanitation. Poliomyelitis remains an excellent
model for understanding the epidemiology and pathogenesis of
viral infections because of its well-understood and compara-
tively simple replication cycle and the relative ease with which
it can be studied in the laboratory. Several related viruses
(other enteroviruses) continue to cause important diseases in
the United States.

throughout the year. The major portal of entry is the mouth, and transmission is primarily from person-to-person via the fecal–oral route, through contaminated surfaces or drinking water.

SPREAD AND REPLICATION

After ingestion, poliovirus replicates in the oropharyngeal and intestinal mucosa, most likely in epithelial and lymphoid cells. Virus particles then traverse the basement membrane, invade the subepithelial tissues, and enter the bloodstream to establish a **viremia.** From the blood the virus can spread throughout the body (Fig. 32-2). In most infections virus replication does not progress beyond the mucosa or the initial stage of viremia. These infections may not be apparent (i.e., no symptoms are evident) or present as minor illnesses characterized by fever and headache. The incubation period for a minor illness is usually 1 to 3 days. Poliovirus can continue to replicate in the intestine and be shed in the stool for weeks to months after the symptoms subside. In the school outbreak, virus continued to circulate and infect new students for some time. The capacity to replicate weeks to months after infection explains the varying onsets of symptoms in students at the Connecticut school over a 3-week period.

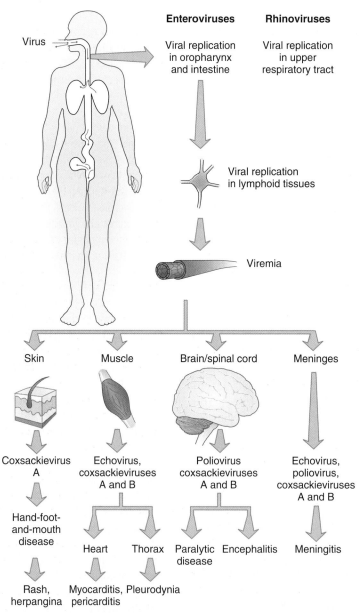

FIGURE 32-2 ▪ Pathogenesis of enteroviruses and rhinoviruses. Enterovirus infections begin in the alimentary tract; spread of virus through the blood to target organs is shown. The various clinical syndromes caused by some enteroviruses are listed. Rhinovirus infection initiates in the respiratory tract and is largely limited to epithelial cells of the upper respiratory tract.

FIGURE 32-3 ▪ **Picornavirus genome organization. A.** The poliovirus RNA genome has VPg protein covalently attached to the 5′ end. **B.** In the polyprotein precursor, viral polyprotein is cleaved by two virus-encoded proteases, 2A^pro and 3C^pro. Cleavage sites for each protease are indicated. The protease responsible for cleavage between VP4 and VP2 has not been identified.

In about 1% of infections, the viremia persists, leading to virus invasion of the brain and spinal cord. Virus can enter the central nervous system directly from the blood or by retrograde axonal transport in peripheral or cranial nerves. Paralysis usually occurs 4 to 10 days after infection.

Although the viremia allows virus access to all sites in the body, the organs infected by poliovirus are limited. The basis for this restricted **tropism,** defined as the organs where the virus replicates, is not known. The poliovirus receptor is necessary but not sufficient for poliovirus tropism. The protein is expressed by a broad range of animal tissues, some of which do not serve as sites for poliovirus replication. Thus, poliovirus tropism appears to be determined by a step following entry, such as translation or replication of the viral RNA.

The replication cycle of poliovirus is better understood than that of the other enteroviruses, in part because the virus multiplies rapidly and produces high virus yields in cell culture. Polioviruses are a prototype of **positive-sense RNA viruses,** which means that the **genomic RNA** can be translated and is therefore a messenger RNA (mRNA). The first step in the poliovirus replication cycle is attachment of the virus to a cellular receptor, which is a glycosylated membrane protein called **poliovirus receptor (PVR)** or **CD155.** The receptor binds to a cleft, called the canyon, on the surface of the viral capsid. It is thought that the interaction of CD155 with poliovirus at the cell surface leads to release of the genomic RNA into the cytoplasm, where replication and assembly take place. Poliovirus RNA is single stranded and, like most eukaryotic mRNAs, has a **poly(A) tract** at the 3′ end. The 5′ end of the genomic RNA is unusual in that it lacks the 5′-terminal-cap structure typical of many eukaryotic mRNAs (Fig. 32-3). Instead, the 5′ end of the genomic RNA is covalently linked to a viral protein called **VPg.** That protein is a primer for the viral RNA-dependent RNA polymerase.

Studies of the synthesis of poliovirus proteins have revealed several unexpected findings. The genomic RNA is translated by internal ribosome binding mediated by an **internal ribosome entry site (IRES)** within the 5′ untranslated region. The viral genome is translated in the cytoplasm by the cellular translation apparatus to produce a single polypeptide, called a **polyprotein** (see Fig. 32-3). The production of a polyprotein allows the synthesis of multiple proteins from a single RNA genome. The protein precursor is processed by two virus-encoded **proteases** to produce four **structural proteins** and 10 **nonstructural proteins.** The structural proteins, VP1, VP2, VP3, and VP4, are the constituents of the viral capsid. The nonstructural proteins include the viral proteases, an **RNA-dependent RNA polymerase,** VPg, and the other proteins involved in viral RNA synthesis.

The poliovirus RNA-dependent RNA polymerase, the enzyme that replicates the viral RNA genome, is an unusual enzyme not found in eukaryotic cells (which produce RNA from DNA templates). The viral enzyme copies the positive-sense RNA to form complementary negative-sense strands, which in turn serve as templates for the synthesis of additional positive-sense copies of the genome. The poliovirus RNA-dependent RNA polymerase uses the viral protein VPg linked to two U residues (VPg-U-U) as a primer for viral RNA synthesis. Late in the replication cycle, as the viral structural proteins accumulate, viral RNA is encapsidated into mature virions. The virus particles are released when the host cell lyses.

Under optimal conditions of cell culture, approximately 1,000 infectious virus particles are released per cell. A complete cycle of replication, from virus attachment to the release of progeny virions, is completed within 8 hours. The replication cycles of other enteroviruses are likely to proceed in a similar manner.

DAMAGE

Poliovirus is known as a **lytic** infection because virus replication leads to the destruction of infected host cells. The virus replicates in neurons of the gray matter of both the brain and spinal cord. The characteristic **flaccid paralysis** of limb muscles occurs when **anterior horn cells** of the spinal cord are destroyed. However, it is not known if those neurons are destroyed by viral lysis or by the immune response of the host. The most severe form of disease is **bulbar poliomyelitis,** the paralysis of the respiratory muscles resulting from involvement of the **medulla oblongata.** That type of poliomyelitis led to the development of "iron lungs," cumbersome predecessors of modern respirators that enabled patients to inhale and exhale by external changes in pressure. The mortality rate in paralytic cases of poliomyelitis is 23%.

In the outbreak of poliomyelitis at the Connecticut school, one strain of virus caused a spectrum of disease.

Why are poliovirus infections so frequently mild or asymptomatic? The answer is not known, but many factors are likely responsible. The size of the viral inoculum, the concentration of viruses in the blood, the virulence of individual virus strains, and levels of circulating antibodies all may determine whether an infection is symptomatic. Risk factors for poliomyelitis include physical exertion and trauma. Those factors may explain, in part, the observation that 9 of the 11 affected students were actively participating in football and soccer. Another predisposing factor for bulbar poliomyelitis is tonsillectomy, perhaps because the procedure leads to reduced levels of antibodies to poliovirus in the nasal secretions of immunized persons. Circulating antibodies play an important role in controlling enterovirus infections, emphasized by the fact that patients with hypogammaglobulinemias cannot readily resolve enterovirus infections.

Diseases Caused by Other Enteroviruses

The most frequent diseases caused by enteroviruses in the United States are caused by the coxsackieviruses (Table 32-1). These viruses produce a variety of illnesses, with some differences among the members of group A and group B. Viruses of both groups cause **aseptic meningitis,** a term used to describe nonbacterial meningitis. Group A

table 32-1 **Enterovirus Disease**

DISEASE	POLIOVIRUS	COXSACKIEVIRUS		ECHOVIRUS	ENTEROVIRUS 70	ENTEROVIRUS 71	PARECHOVIRUS
		TYPE A	TYPE B				
Asymptomatic infection	+	+	+	+	+	+	+
Paralytic disease	+	+	+	+	+	+	+
Encephalitis, meningitis	+	+	+	+	−	+	+
Myocarditis	−	+	+	+	−	−	−
Pleurodynia	−	−	+	−	−	−	−
Herpangina	−	+	−	−	−	−	−
Hand-foot-and-mouth disease	−	+	−	−	−	+	−
Acute hemorrhagic conjunctivitis	−	+	−	−	+	−	−
Respiratory tract disease	+	+	−	+	−	−	+
Gastrointestinal disease	−	−	−	+	−	−	+
Diabetes, pancreatitis	−	−	+	−	−	−	−
Orchitis	−	−	+	−	−	−	−

viruses cause **herpangina,** a fever of sudden onset with vesicles or ulcers on the tonsils and palate. Group B viruses also infect other organs, particularly the heart. In general, echoviruses produce similar diseases (see Table 32-1).

Most enterovirus infections are not sufficiently unique to allow diagnosis on clinical grounds alone. For example, the skin rashes (exanthems) caused by coxsackieviruses and echoviruses are indistinguishable. One important exception is **hand-foot-and-mouth disease,** a readily identifiable febrile illness that is associated with blisters on the palate, hands, and feet. This disease is usually caused by a specific type of coxsackievirus, **type A16,** and enterovirus 71 (see Table 32-1).

Most enterovirus infections are accompanied by viremia, allowing virus access to many organs. Nevertheless, the tropism of different enteroviruses is distinct (see Table 32-1). All enteroviruses replicate in the central nervous system, but some also replicate in the heart (**myocarditis**), the respiratory tract (**pleurodynia**), or the mucous membranes of the eye (**hemorrhagic conjunctivitis**). Infected newborns are at high risk for developing severe enterovirus disease unless they have acquired protective maternal antibodies. The neonatal immune system may not be sufficiently developed to curtail an enterovirus infection. Neonates can acquire coxsackievirus or echovirus by transplacental passage of the virus near term, from contact with maternal fecal material during birth, or from contact with an infected individual at or shortly after birth.

It has been suggested that **type 1 autoimmune diabetes mellitus** may be associated with enterovirus infection. Coxsackievirus B4 infection of certain strains of mice can lead to pancreatitis, and the virus has been isolated from rare cases of fatal human diabetes. In one hypothesis, an initial infection with coxsackievirus or echovirus of the pancreas may trigger autoimmune destruction of β cells in genetically susceptible individuals. Additional work is necessary to confirm or refute the role of enteroviruses as a possible cofactor in the etiology of diabetes.

DIAGNOSIS AND TREATMENT

Diagnosis of enterovirus disease is challenging because the symptoms of infection are generic. Further, during endemic months when enteroviruses circulate in a community, they can be readily isolated from throat washings or fecal specimens from symptomatic as well as asymptomatic people. Consequently, recovery of an enterovirus from the throat or feces of an ill person does not prove that the symptoms are the result of an enterovirus. However, certain epidemiological features of enterovirus infection may permit a presumptive diagnosis. For example, enterovirus infections are seasonal in temperate latitudes and tend to cause community outbreaks. There-

fore, cases of aseptic meningitis in the summer months are likely to be caused by an enterovirus.

Identification of enterovirus infection is done by inoculating a cell culture with a clinical sample, isolating the virus, and neutralizing by reference antisera. Typical specimens for isolating enteroviruses include stool samples, rectal swabs, throat swabs, and cerebrospinal fluid. Reverse transcription-polymerase chain reaction to detect viral genomic RNA is increasingly employed to diagnose enterovirus infections.

No drug therapy for enterovirus infections exists, although several antiviral compounds have been studied extensively in clinical trials. The administration of pooled immunoglobulin is effective in preventing central nervous system disease in immunocompromised persons with severe coxsackievirus or echovirus infections.

PREVENTION

Two excellent vaccines are available for preventing poliomyelitis. Both were made possible by the seminal finding of Enders, Weller, and Robbins in 1949 that poliovirus could be propagated in cultured nonneural cells. The formalin-inactivated, noninfectious **Salk vaccine** was introduced in the United States in 1955 and led to a precipitous decline in the incidence of poliomyelitis (Fig. 32-4). In 1961 the orally administered **live, attenuated Sabin vaccine** was introduced in the United States, and it soon replaced the Salk vaccine for routine use. Both vaccines have advantages and disadvantages (Table 32-2).

Both the Salk and Sabin vaccines induce serum antibody (Fig. 32-5). However, because the Sabin vaccine is administered orally, an infection of the intestine ensues that stimulates the formation of secretory antibodies. The immune response elicited by the live, attenuated vaccine therefore closely resembles the response brought about by natural poliovirus infection. In contrast, the Salk killed vaccine is administered by injection and produces immunity in the circulation but not in the intestine (see Fig. 32-5). A recipient of the killed vaccine is pro-

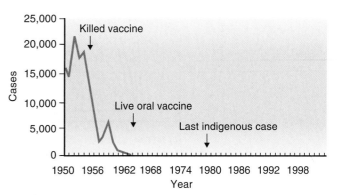

FIGURE 32-4 ■ **Impact of immunization on poliomyelitis cases in the United States, 1950–1998.**

table **32-2**	**Poliovirus Vaccines**	
	SABIN (LIVE, ATTENUATED)	**SALK (KILLED)**
Advantages	• Easy to administer • Produces intestinal immunity • Spreads to contacts (herd immunity) • Inexpensive	• When properly prepared does not cause disease • Safe for immunodeficient persons
Disadvantages	• May revert during intestinal replication (vaccine-associated poliomyelitis) • Not safe for immunodeficient persons	• Must be injected • Produces reduced intestinal immunity compared with natural infection • More costly than Sabin vaccine

tected from symptomatic disease, but poliovirus can still replicate in the intestine and spread to others. The Sabin vaccine is therefore highly effective at halting outbreaks of poliomyelitis because it interrupts the chain of virus transmission. Another advantage of the Sabin vaccine is that it can spread from immunized to unimmunized persons. That property is desirable because immunization rates in most countries do not approach 100%.

Compared with the killed vaccine, the live, attenuated vaccine has an important disadvantage. During replication of the Sabin strains in the human gut, the mutations that reduce the virulence of the vaccine strains can be lost. Consequently, vaccine recipients shed revertant viruses that can cause disease in either the recipients or their contacts. The risk of developing vaccine-associated poliomyelitis is one case of paralytic poliomyelitis per 1.4 million first doses of

vaccine. From 1980 to 1998, 144 cases of vaccine-associated paralytic poliomyelitis were reported in the United States. Of those cases, 59 occurred in vaccine recipients, 44 in healthy contacts of vaccine recipients, 30 in individuals with immune defects, and 7 in hosts with no known contact with recipients. From 1979 to 1999, all cases of poliomyelitis in the United States were consequences of the Sabin vaccine. The Advisory Committee for Immunization Practices thus recommended that the Salk vaccine be used exclusively in the United States beginning in 2000.

Because only three serotypes of poliovirus exist and humans are the only known reservoir for the virus, it is a candidate for eradication. Smallpox is the only virus that has been eradicated; the last case occurred in 1978, and the virus is known to exist only in secure freezers in the United States and Russia. In 1988 the World Health Organization

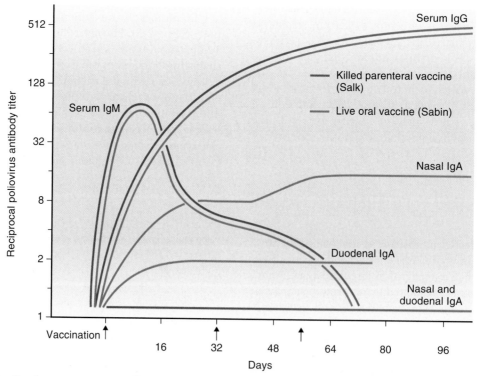

FIGURE 32-5 ▪ **Antibody responses to poliovirus vaccines.** Serum and secretory (IgA) antibody response at different times after immunization with Salk vaccine (black line) or Sabin vaccine (blue line). The y-axis is the reciprocal of the dilution of antiserum that causes 50% inhibition of poliovirus infectivity.

declared that poliovirus would be eradicated from the globe by 2000. Although that goal was missed, eradication is imminent. In 2003 only 748 cases of poliomyelitis were reported worldwide, down from more than 350,000 in 1988. Paradoxically, the eradication campaign is threatened by the use of the Sabin vaccine, which has been instrumental in the reduction of poliomyelitis worldwide. Vaccine revertants now circulate freely in global sewage and aquifers, capable of causing poliomyelitis in unimmunized recipients. That problem confounds the plan to cease poliovirus immunization, a step that is anticipated to occur within the next 5 to 10 years. Once vaccination against poliovirus stops, will circulating revertant poliovirus vaccine strains cause outbreaks of paralytic disease? That question remains unanswered but is a significant cause for concern.

Human Rhinoviruses

Human rhinoviruses are the viruses most frequently isolated from patients with mild upper respiratory infections (common cold) and are probably the most frequent causes of acute infectious human illness. Rhinoviruses are members of the Picornaviridae family, but they have been placed in a separate genus because they differ markedly from enteroviruses (see Fig. 32-1). Antigenic diversity is a striking characteristic of the rhinoviruses, with more than 100 serotypes recognized to date (any two rhinovirus isolates are considered to be of different serotypes if their infectivity is not neutralized by the same antiserum). Because incorporating such diversity into a rhinovirus vaccine is seemingly impossible, researchers have little enthusiasm for the task.

Case

Common Cold

Ms. C., a 28-year-old woman, realized she was getting a cold when she noticed a scratchy feeling in her throat, sneezing, nasal discharge, low-grade fever, and malaise. The symptoms worsened, reaching a peak after 48 hours. Her nasal discharge thickened and was slightly yellowish. It slowly subsided over the next several days. All her other symptoms resolved completely within about 7 days of onset. She thought that she had acquired the illness from her 7-year-old child, who had similar symptoms a few days earlier.

This case raises several questions:

1. What viruses can cause these symptoms?
2. How was the infection transmitted from the child to the mother?
3. Will this infection induce immune responses that protect against future infections of the same type?

The differences in the physical properties of rhinoviruses and enteroviruses partly explain why the two agents cause very different diseases. Enterovirus particles are highly resistant to gastric acidity (pH 3.0) and to bile; therefore, enteroviruses can initiate infection in the alimentary tract. Rhinoviruses are acid labile and are readily inactivated by gastric secretions. Rhinoviruses replicate best at 33°C, a temperature found within the upper respiratory tract. Those features of rhinoviruses may help explain why they infect the upper respiratory tract and not the gastrointestinal tract.

ENCOUNTER

Rhinovirus infections are very common. The average person experiences approximately one rhinovirus infection per year, and school-age children and their contacts may experience many more. Rhinovirus infections occur most commonly in the fall and spring. Multiple serotypes circulate simultaneously, but the prevalent serotypes change from year to year.

Infected humans, particularly children, are the only known reservoir for rhinoviruses. The mode of transmission has been the subject of intense experimental study. One series of experiments demonstrated that transmission occurs if individuals touch their nose or eyes after their hands become contaminated with rhinovirus (either from contaminated nasal secretions or environmental objects). In other experiments, susceptible volunteers played cards with persons who had symptomatic rhinovirus infection, and the volunteers became infected even if they were restrained from touching their faces. The finding indicates that rhinovirus infection can be transmitted by **aerosols** as well as by direct contact. Sneezing effectively produces and disperses aerosol droplets. Results of experimental infections demonstrate that a small inoculum of rhinovirus is sufficient to initiate an infection.

ENTRY, SPREAD, AND REPLICATION

Once rhinovirus has entered the respiratory tract, the first step in infection is the binding of the virus to specific receptors on respiratory epithelial cells. The cellular receptor for 91 rhinovirus serotypes, also known as the "major group," is **intercellular adhesion molecule 1 (ICAM-1),** a cellular adhesion protein that plays a role in the recruitment of inflammatory cells. The remaining rhinovirus serotypes, the "minor group," bind to the **very low density lipoprotein (VLDL) receptor.** The results of structural studies have revealed that ICAM-1 binds within a cleft or "canyon" on the capsid surface of the major group rhinoviruses in a manner similar to the binding of CD155 by poliovirus. In contrast, the VLDL receptor binds to a flat dome at one end of the capsid of minor group viruses. The replication of rhinovirus within the infected cell is similar to that described for poliovirus.

The primary site of rhinovirus infection is the epithelial surface of the nasal mucosa. The release of rhinovirus particles from infected cells is thought to facilitate spread through the respiratory epithelium. In experimental colds the **posterior nasopharynx** is the site of the most intense infection. The incubation period, from infection to onset of virus shedding, is 1 to 4 days. Virus shedding decreases after 2 to 3 days but may be detectable for up to 3 weeks, long after symptoms have subsided. Such prolonged asymptomatic virus shedding likely facilitates transmission.

DAMAGE

The nose of a patient with a cold becomes swollen and red (**hyperemic**), as a consequence of blood vessel dilation. The thin nasal discharge contains large amounts of serum proteins. As the cold progresses, the discharge becomes **mucopurulent** and contains many cells, especially **neutrophils.** Respiratory epithelial cells are also present, some of which contain rhinovirus antigens, indicating that they are infected by the virus. Biopsy of the mucosa early in the course of a cold reveals edema of subepithelial connective tissue with relatively small numbers of inflammatory cells. In contrast to other viral respiratory infections, particularly influenza, a cold causes only minimal histopathological changes, even in areas where viral antigens are present.

What produces the symptoms of the common cold? A clear correlation exists between the severity of the cold and the amount of rhinovirus recovered from the respiratory tract. However, even when high levels of virus particles are produced, tissue destruction does not occur. The clinical symptoms of a rhinovirus infection are probably not caused by virus-induced cytopathology but are **immunopathological,** a consequence of the immune response to the virus. Supporting that hypothesis is the finding that nasal secretions of persons with colds contain large amounts of the vasoactive substance **bradykinin** and **proinflammatory cytokines** that recruit inflammatory cells into the infected area. In addition, rhinovirus infection of a cell leads to increased expression of ICAM-1 on the cell surface. Because ICAM-1 is an important mediator of inflammatory cell recruitment, its upregulation is likely to play a role in airway inflammation. Understanding the immunopathology of rhinovirus infection might allow development of therapies to treat the symptoms of a common cold.

Most rhinovirus common colds are mild, although they may involve secondary complications such as **sinusitis** or **otitis media,** which are usually caused by bacterial infections that develop because the normal draining of the sinuses or the middle ear is blocked. Rhinoviruses also can cause **lower respiratory tract disease** and **asthma exacerbations.** Rhinoviruses are the second most frequently isolated virus from infants, children, older adults, and immunocompromised hosts with pneumonia and bronchiolitis. Infection with rhinovirus is associated with up to 50% of asthma attacks in children and adults, many of which require hospitalization. Understanding the physiological basis of airway inflammation that occurs during rhinovirus infection is clearly essential for developing therapies for virus-induced asthma exacerbations. Thus, the medical consequences of rhinovirus infections are likely to be much greater than previously thought.

PREVENTION AND TREATMENT

Following most rhinovirus infections, neutralizing antibodies develop in serum and nasal secretions. Unfortunately, those antibodies are only effective in preventing infection by the same rhinovirus serotype. Therefore, reinfection with a different serotype can readily occur. A vaccine to prevent rhinovirus infection does not appear feasible because it would have to comprise more than 100 serotypes. Nevertheless, several novel approaches to prophylaxis have been explored. One is the use of **recombinant interferon-α** administered by nasal spray. When given for 5 days before viral infection, interferon was 80% effective in preventing illness. However, when given for longer than 5 days, interferon led to nasal symptoms as bothersome as those of a cold (see Chapter 44). Interferon treatment of rhinovirus infection is no longer being pursued because it is not effective in clearing an established viral infection. Antiviral drugs that inhibit various stages of the viral life cycle have been developed. They include compounds that bind the viral capsid and block uncoating of the viral RNA and inhibitors of the viral proteases. Although some of the compounds have proven safe and effective in clinical trials, their effectiveness is reduced by the emergence of resistant viral strains. Further compromising the effectiveness of antiviral drugs is the short duration of virus shedding and illness.

Coronaviruses and SARS

Coronaviruses are a family of enveloped, positive-sense RNA viruses that have been known for more than 30 years to cause significant and economically important illnesses of many animal species, including dogs, cats, cattle, pigs, and chickens. Studies of human coronaviruses in the 1960s and 1970s demonstrated that the viruses cause up to 30% of common colds. However, the lack of severe human disease and the difficulty in growing human respiratory coronaviruses from clinical specimens posed impediments to studies of new coronaviruses and their potential to cause other diseases.

Research using model coronaviruses such as mouse hepatitis virus has revealed substantial information about the molecular biology and pathogenesis of this virus family. Importantly, the work has demonstrated in the laboratory and in animals the potential for coronaviruses to undergo rapid genetic change with alterations in clinical disease and trans-species movement to new animal hosts. Those laboratory observations were dramatically confirmed in nature during the spring and summer of 2003 with the recognition that a new human coronavirus was the cause of **severe acute respiratory syndrome (SARS)**. Within several months of its emergence in the Guangdong province of southeastern China, the SARS coronavirus demonstrated worldwide spread and the potential for high mortality as well as dramatic economic and social disruption.

Where did the SARS coronavirus come from? Why was it able to cause such severe disease in humans? Will it reemerge to cause new outbreaks of disease? What is the potential for new coronaviruses to enter the human population and cause disease? Those questions have no clear answers yet, but the known biology of the coronaviruses gives important clues. The coronaviruses contain positive-sense RNA genomes. The process of intracellular replication of coronaviruses requires synthesis of full-length negative-sense intermediate templates and new full-length positive-sense genome copies. Coronaviruses also synthesize a set of short mRNAs (subgenomic mRNAs) that are used as templates for translation of structural and other viral proteins. To accomplish those steps in RNA synthesis, coronaviruses use a viral RNA-dependent RNA polymerase in a mechanism that requires the polymerase to "jump" across a template or between two different templates, resulting in RNA–RNA recombination. In addition, the polymerase has a significant error rate, with the potential to introduce multiple nucleotide changes each time a template is copied. The combination of RNA recombination and polymerase error during virus replication leads to the generation of both recombinant viruses and viruses with mutations that might allow adaptation to new environments or hosts.

The SARS coronavirus has characteristics suggesting that it came from another animal species and was transmitted to humans from infected animals used for food. The SARS coronavirus genome is thought to be a recombinant between mammalian and avian coronaviruses. The genome sequences from SARS patient isolates show additional genetic mutations, suggesting further adaptations during the course of the epidemic. It appears that coronaviruses are undergoing continual change in nature and have the potential to cause severe disease in humans. However, the SARS outbreak also demonstrates that the biological potential for emergence of new human coronaviruses may be limited by natural barriers and is likely to be a rare event. Studies to identify the natural host for the SARS coronavirus, and to determine the capacity in nature for coinfection, recombination, and trans-species movement of coronaviruses, will lead to a greater understanding of the role of coronaviruses in human disease.

Conclusion

Enteroviruses commonly cause infections in humans. Although readily communicable, only rarely do they cause severe disease. Illnesses caused by enteroviruses may be highly tissue-specific (poliovirus) or can affect many organs (coxsackievirus and echovirus). These diseases are often difficult to distinguish clinically, and their presumptive diagnoses are often based on epidemiological features. The success in eradicating poliovirus with vaccination is providential, because no other way is known to control the disease.

Rhinoviruses cause half of all common colds. Although it is a benign illness, associated complications such as asthma and lower respiratory tract infection can be life threatening. It is therefore essential to develop effective means of controlling rhinovirus infections. Because conventional vaccine approaches do not appear feasible, current efforts are directed towards identifying effective antiviral compounds against rhinoviruses.

chapter **33**

Arthropod-borne Viruses

Diane E. Griffin

key **concepts**

Arthropod-borne viruses:

- Are transmitted by mosquitoes, ticks, and sandflies.

- Replicate in invertebrate and vertebrate hosts.

- Are maintained in natural cycles between insects and birds, wild animals, or humans.

- Belong primarily to the Flaviviridae, Togaviridae, and Bunyaviridae families of enveloped RNA viruses.

- Have seasonal transmission in restricted geographic regions.

- Cause encephalitis, rash, arthritis, or hemorrhagic fever.

- Are usually diagnosed by serology or reverse transcription-polymerase chain reaction.

- Cannot be treated, but vaccines exist for a few and are under development for others.

Arthropod-borne viruses (**arboviruses**) are transmitted by insects, usually mosquitoes, ticks, or blood-feeding flies. More than 100 arboviruses are known to infect humans. These viruses belong to several different virus families, the most important of which are the Togaviridae, Flaviviridae, and Bunyaviridae. Human infection is often asymptomatic, but when disease occurs it can be manifested by mild to severe febrile illness, rash, arthritis, meningitis, encephalitis, or hemorrhagic fever. Each virus causes a characteristic spectrum of illness, but the same virus can produce diseases of differing severity depending on the viral inoculum and host factors such as age, genetic background, and immunological status.

An arbovirus must replicate in its insect vector and spread to the arthropod's salivary glands before the virus can be transmitted. After an infected insect bites a human or reservoir host, the virus replicates locally, enters the blood, and then spreads to target cells and organs, such as the brain, liver, skin, or endothelium. Virus in the blood provides the means for infection of new insects that feed on the infected individual during that time. The transmission increases the number of infected mosquitoes, ticks, or flies and amplifies the infection in nature. The amount of virus in the blood determines the likelihood of the insect becoming infected during feeding. For many arboviruses humans are "dead-end" hosts because the viremia is of short duration and levels of virus in blood are low. For these viruses, amplifying infections occur in birds or small mammals (Fig. 33-1). However, for yellow fever and dengue viruses, humans are important vertebrate hosts for amplifying viral infection. The paradigm provides a fundamental understanding of infection by arthropods.

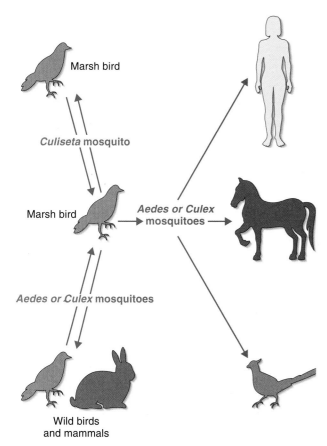

FIGURE 33-1 ▪ **Life cycles of mosquito-borne arboviruses with nonhuman reservoirs.** For eastern equine encephalitis virus, the natural cycle is maintained between birds in salt marshes and *Culiseta* mosquitoes. Transmission to other hosts requires infection of "bridge" mosquito species, such as *Aedes* and *Culex*, that feed on a variety of hosts, including humans. Other animals, such as humans and horses, are susceptible to these infections but are unimportant for maintaining these viruses in nature. Other arboviruses may use the same mosquito species for transmission to humans and other hosts.

Arboviruses

Case

West Nile Virus

Mrs. K., a 72-year-old, previously healthy woman, was admitted to a hospital in Illinois in early September with high fever and altered mental status. For several days she had experienced fever, headache, cognitive decline, and difficulty walking. Mrs. K.'s past medical history was unremarkable. She was active outdoors (president of the local garden club), had not traveled out of the area, and her husband was not ill.

On admission her temperature was 39.5°C, and her heart rate was 120 beats per minute. On physical exam she was disoriented, and her left leg was weak. Her white blood cell count was 6,500/mm^3; and cerebrospinal fluid (CSF) showed 150 cells/mm^3, with 75% mononuclear cells, glucose of 100 mg/dL, and protein of 90 mg/dL. Mrs. K. was given antibiotics for the fever but did not respond and became increasingly obtunded. No bacteria were isolated from blood or CSF.

Five days after admission Mrs. K. had two generalized seizures, became deeply comatose, and required mechanical ventilation. Muscle tone was flaccid, and deep tendon reflexes were absent. She showed no signs of improvement over the next 2 weeks and life support was withdrawn on day 19 of hospitalization. CSF and serum samples were positive for IgM antibody to West Nile virus, and RNA of the virus was detected by reverse transcription-polymerase chain reaction (RT-PCR). Serum collected just prior to death was positive for IgG antibody to West Nile virus.

This case raises several questions:

1. How and where did Mrs. K. become infected with West Nile virus?
2. What was her most important risk factor for severe disease?
3. How could this infection have been prevented?

West Nile virus is widespread throughout Africa, the Middle East, and southern Europe. It was not recognized as an important cause of neurologic disease in those regions until the mid-1990s, suggesting the recent emergence of a new, more virulent strain of the virus. In 1999 an outbreak of viral encephalomyelitis in Queens, a borough of New York City, was surprisingly found to be caused by West Nile virus, which was not previously known to exist in the Western Hemisphere. Whether it came across the Atlantic with an infected mosquito, bird, or human is not known. However, appropriate mosquito vectors and avian hosts were available in the new environment, and the virus spread throughout the Americas within a few years. In 2003 West Nile virus caused illness in approximately 10,000 people in the United States. Seventy percent of those people had only a febrile illness, and the rest had neurologic disease along with fever. The median age for those with any illness was 47 years, but for those with neurologic disease it was 77 years. Most deaths occurred in patients over age 60 (Fig 33-2).

Principles of Arthropod-borne Infection

Many of the infections described in this text are acquired by exposure to arthropods. Nearly any insect that feeds on humans can also be a vector for infection, including mosquitoes, ticks, sandflies, tsetse flies, black flies, reduviid bugs, fleas, and lice. Viruses, bacteria, rickettsia, protozoa, and helminths are among the infectious agents that can be transmitted by insects. A few general principles can be applied to the infections transmitted by various arthropods.

In most instances the infectious agent must develop and multiply within the vector before it can be transmitted. Agents that do not infect arthropods (e.g., HIV) are rarely, if ever, transmitted by passive contamination of a biting insect's mouth parts.

The geographical distribution of an arthropod-borne infection is determined by the habitat requirements of the vector. The temperature, humidity, altitude, and vegetation determine whether vector and host will survive in a specific location.

The feeding behavior of the vector often influences the epidemiology of an arthropod-borne infection. Human disease requires vectors that feed on humans. For example, despite the wide distribution of the virus, eastern equine encephalitis virus has a low incidence of disease because *Culiseta* mosquitoes prefer to feed on birds that maintain the natural cycle. Only when there is "spill over" into mosquito species that feed on mammals do equine and human cases occur (see Fig 33-1).

Human behaviors influence the likelihood of contact with arthropods. Diseases transmitted by fleas and lice are commonly associated with impoverished conditions or war. Mosquito-borne diseases tend to occur in locations where humans do not have the means to protect themselves from exposure, particularly at night.

Arthropods expose humans to agents that are otherwise restricted to animals or birds. For instance, mice are the reservoir for Lyme disease, and ticks transmit the agent to humans, as well as to mice.

FIGURE 33-2 ▪ Age-dependent mortality caused by infection with West Nile virus in the United States. A graph of the percentage of all fatalities that occurred in each age group shows the largest proportion in patients older than 60 years. (From data from the Centers for Disease Control and Prevention Web site, http://www.cdc.gov.)

Case

Yellow Fever Virus

Mr. W., a 20-year-old college student, was admitted to the hospital with high fever, jaundice, and renal failure. Two days before admission he had been seen in the emergency department for the abrupt onset of fever, chills, back pain, headache, nausea, and vomiting. At that time his face was flushed, temperature was 39°C, and his heart rate was 65 beats per minute. He was previously well and had recently returned from a 2-week trip to the Amazon basin where he collected plants for a summer research project. A malaria smear was negative. Gastroenteritis was considered the most likely diagnosis, and symptomatic treatment was prescribed. The next day he felt better. However, the day of admission his headache and back pain had returned, and he developed bloody diarrhea and was too weak to walk.

On admission he was jaundiced but alert and had a temperature of 38°C, heart rate of 60 beats per minute, and blood pressure of 110/70 mm Hg. His white blood cell count was 4100 /mm³, creatinine 6.9 mg/dL, and bilirubin 3.5 mg/dL. He had albuminuria, and over the next 2 days, urine output declined to less than 100 mL in 24 hours. Hemodialysis was initiated. On the third day his prothrombin time was very low, and he started to bleed from injection sites as well as mucosal surfaces. He was transfused, but died from massive gastrointestinal bleeding and hypovolemic shock 4 days after admission. RT-PCR on plasma taken at the time of admission was positive for yellow fever virus RNA.

This case raises several questions:

1. How and where did Mr. W. become infected with yellow fever virus?
2. What was the reason for his bleeding disorder?
3. What could have been done to prevent infection?

Yellow fever is a historically important arbovirus. It was first recognized as a clinical entity in the Yucatan in 1648, but the virus was probably introduced from Africa. Summertime epidemics occurred as far north as Boston and Halifax into the twentieth century. Demonstration by Walter Reed that the disease was transmitted by the ***Aedes aegypti* mosquito** led to massive vector control programs (see the box titled "Yellow Fever Board"), and in the 1930s *Aedes aegypti* was eradicated from much of its range in the Americas. However, mosquito control was not sustained; thus, *Aedes aegypti* has gradually repopulated its old habitats, and yellow fever is an emerging threat. Yellow fever virus can be maintained in a "jungle cycle" involving forest mosquitoes and monkeys. Humans that go into forested regions, as Mr. W. did for his summer project, can become infected. The disease typically has a biphasic course corresponding to the viremic and hepatic phases of infection and is fatal in 50% of cases. An effective live virus vaccine is available, which should be administered to individuals traveling to endemic regions.

EPIDEMIOLOGY

Arboviruses are a large group of viruses that share three characteristics: transmission by arthropod vectors, enveloped virions, and an RNA genome (Table 33-1). Many cause encephalitis, while others produce fever, rashes, arthritis, hepatitis, or hemorrhagic fever. Arboviruses are often named after the disease they cause or the place where they were first isolated (e.g., La Crosse, Rift Valley, Venezuelan equine encephalitis, Ross River, West Nile, etc.). Vectors include mosquitoes, ticks, and biting flies. The natural cycle for many arboviruses involves transmission between the insect vector and wild animals or birds. Humans are only accidentally infected and unimportant for maintaining the virus in nature (see Fig. 33-1). However, for dengue and yellow fever viruses, humans are important hosts for the natural cycle and, in concert with the urban mosquito *Aedes aegypti* as a vector, can lead to explosive outbreaks of human disease.

The natural life cycle of the viruses that cause West Nile and eastern equine encephalitis involves birds and mosquitoes, while the natural cycle of Venezuelan equine encephalitis involves small mammals and mosquitoes (see Fig 33-1). Transmission of yellow fever can involve monkeys or humans and mosquitoes. Several viruses in the tickborne encephalitis group of flaviviruses are transmitted between animals by ticks. The insect becomes infected by taking a blood meal from an infected vertebrate host with sufficient levels of virus in the blood to initiate infection. Several days must pass before an insect that has acquired a virus can transmit it because the virus must first replicate in midgut cells and spread through the hemolymph to replicate in the salivary glands. Insect vectors survive infection with these viruses and remain infectious for life. For some virus–arthropod pairs transmission occurs through germline cells to the next generation of insects constituting a true reservoir of infection.

VIRUS CHARACTERISTICS

Members of the Togaviridae and Flaviviridae families are enveloped viruses that contain a nonsegmented, single-stranded, positive-sense RNA genome. The RNA serves as messenger RNA and is translated directly into

Yellow Fever Board

Large outbreaks of yellow fever affected the U.S. Army in Cuba during the Spanish-American War and caused high mortality in workers attempting to build the Panama Canal. In 1881 a Cuban physician, Carlos Finlay, proposed that the disease was transmitted by mosquitoes, but he was unable to demonstrate this experimentally by feeding mosquitoes on an ill person and then on a healthy person. The Yellow Fever Board was established by the U.S. Army in 1900 and went to Cuba to help determine how the disease was spread. Walter Reed led the group.

The investigators demonstrated that a filterable agent in the blood of patients could transmit disease. They also showed transmission by *Aedes aegypti* mosquitoes after a incubation period of several days. Jesse Lazear, one of the four members of the Yellow Fever Board, died from yellow fever during the investigations. Yellow fever was the first virus ("filterable agent") shown to cause a human disease and the first virus for which insect transmission was identified.

table **33-1**   Important Human Arboviruses

GENUS AND EXAMPLE	MAIN DISEASE	PRIMARY VECTOR	DISTRIBUTION
Togaviridae family			
Eastern equine encephalitis	Encephalitis	Mosquito	Eastern United States
			Caribbean
Venezuelan equine encephalitis	Encephalitis	Mosquito	Central and South America
Ross River	Rash, arthritis	Mosquito	Australia
Many others	Fevers, arthritis, rash, encephalitis	Mosquito	Worldwide
Flaviviridae family			
West Nile	Encephalitis	Mosquito	Americas, Africa, Middle East, Europe
St. Louis encephalitis	Encephalitis	Mosquito	North America
Japanese encephalitis	Encephalitis	Mosquito	Asia, India, Australia
Dengue	Rash, hemorrhagic fever	Mosquito	Caribbean, South and Central America, Asia
Yellow fever	Hemorrhagic fever	Mosquito	Africa, South America
Tickborne encephalitis	Encephalitis	Tick	Russia, eastern and central Europe, Japan
Many others	Encephalitis	Mosquito, tick	Worldwide
Bunyaviridae family			
California	Encephalitis	Mosquito	North America
Rift Valley	Fever	Mosquito	Africa, Middle East
Sandfly fever	Fever	Sandfly	Mediterranean
Crimean-Congo hemorrhagic fever	Hemorrhagic fever	Tick, culicoid fly	Europe, Africa, Asia
Others	Fever	Mosquito	Worldwide

large polyproteins that are subsequently processed into the individual proteins necessary for replication and assembly of new virions. Members of the Bunyaviridae family are enveloped viruses that contain a segmented, single-stranded, negative-sense or ambisense RNA genome. The virion carries an RNA polymerase for production of messenger RNA. For all groups the lipid-containing envelope, acquired during budding from host cell membranes, contains surface glycoprotein spikes that are important for attachment and entry of the virion into new cells. These viruses are inactivated by detergents that disrupt the lipid envelope.

Togaviruses that are important causes of human disease include the encephalitic eastern, western, and Venezuelan equine encephalitis viruses (**EEE, WEE,** and **VEE**) in the Americas and **Ross River virus,** which causes rash and arthritis, in Australia. Flaviviruses that are important causes of human encephalitis include the mosquito-borne **West Nile virus (WNV), St. Louis encephalitis** virus, and **Japanese encephalitis** virus and the tickborne encephalitis viruses. **Dengue** virus usually causes a febrile rash disease, but it also can cause a severe hemorrhagic fever. Like dengue virus, **yellow fever virus**

(YFV) causes hemorrhagic fever. Bunyaviruses are the most varied and numerous of the arboviruses and include the mosquito-transmitted **La Crosse virus** in North America and **Rift Valley fever** virus in Africa, a group of viruses that cause **sandfly fever** around the Mediterranean, and tickborne **Crimean-Congo hemorrhagic fever** virus in Africa and Europe (see Table 33-1).

Some diseases that are not transmitted by an arthropod vector are caused by viruses in the same families as arboviruses. For example, the virus that causes rubella belongs to the Togaviridae family, the virus that causes hepatitis C belongs to the Flaviviridae family, and the virus that causes hantavirus pulmonary syndrome belongs to the Bunyaviridae family.

ENCOUNTER

Acquisition of arbovirus infection is seasonal because transmission depends on the presence of the insect vector. In temperate climates infections are most likely in the warm months; in tropical climates they can occur year-round or in conjunction with the rainy season. Arboviruses, and therefore the diseases caused by them, are geographically restricted by the availability of the vertebrate and invertebrate hosts necessary to maintain the virus in its natural cycle (see Table 33-1). Viruses with birds as natural hosts can be spread over wide ranges, while those with mammals as hosts are usually confined to smaller regions. With modern travel the opportunity for expansion of these historically confined ranges is great. That opportunity was dramatically demonstrated with the introduction of WNV into North America in 1999. This virus was previously found only in Africa and the Middle East. The virus can infect a wide variety of birds and mosquitoes, which aided its successful introduction into this new region. Interestingly, **corvid birds** in North America are very susceptible to infection, and the spread of the virus across North America has been heralded by the deaths of large numbers of crows and blue jays.

With the resurgence of *Aedes aegypti* and the spread of Asian stains of dengue virus, the incidence of dengue and **dengue hemorrhagic fever** is increasing significantly. An estimated 50 million to 100 million cases of dengue fever and 250,000 to 500,000 cases of dengue hemorrhagic fever occur annually worldwide. Multiple serotypes are now circulating in Latin America and Asia.

Entry, Spread, and Replication

Arboviruses gain access to humans through the bite of an infected arthropod. Saliva containing virus is introduced into the capillary bed, and the virus can initiate infection at that site or be carried by Langerhans cells from the skin to local lymphatic tissue, where replication occurs. As the virus replicates and is released into the blood from the primary site of infection, a viremia is established. In individuals without protective antibody, fever often appears at this time, and the virus can spread to new target organs such as the central nervous system, joints, liver, and skin. In many cases infection does not progress past the stage of local replication. It is not known how encephalitic arboviruses cross the blood-brain barrier or why that only occurs in some infected individuals.

Other modes of infection are possible. Many arboviruses can cross the placenta to cause fetal infection that can result in abortion, stillbirth, or congenital disease. Tickborne viruses can be transmitted orally through the milk of infected animals, and Rift Valley fever can be contracted through contact with infected livestock. A number of cases of WNV have been acquired through transfusion of blood to a susceptible recipient from an asymptomatic viremic donor.

Diseases Caused by Arboviruses

Encephalitis

In addition to WNV, several other arboviruses can cause encephalitis. In the Americas these viruses include two togaviruses: eastern and Venezuelan equine encephalitis viruses. Eastern equine encephalitis virus is endemic in a natural cycle involving marsh birds and *Culiseta* mosquitoes along the Atlantic and Gulf coasts and in the Great Lakes Region of the United States. Eastern encephalitis has a high mortality, with the most severe disease occurring in children. Neurologic sequelae, such as mental retardation and motor deficits, are common in patients who survive. Fortunately, cases are few because the mosquito that transmits the virus between marsh birds does not usually feed on humans. Only when mosquitoes that feed on mammals become infected are people and horses at risk (see Fig. 33-1). Western equine encephalitis virus has caused large outbreaks of equine and human encephalitis in the western United States. However, for reasons that are not known, no cases have been recognized since 1994.

St. Louis encephalitis virus is a flavivirus related to WNV that is endemic in the United States. It causes periodic outbreaks of encephalitis and shares with WNV the capacity to cause more severe disease in the elderly. Japanese encephalitis virus is another flavivirus related to WNV and is the most important cause of encephalitis worldwide. It is widely distributed throughout Asia and causes at least 10,000 deaths from encephalitis each year. Many of the fatalities are children, probably because older individuals living in the region have already acquired infection and are immune. Adult travelers to endemic regions are susceptible to fatal disease.

La Crosse virus is a member of the California encephalitis group of bunyaviruses and one of the most common causes of central nervous system infection in the group. The spectrum of illness caused by the California serogroup viruses ranges from mild febrile illness to aseptic meningitis and encephalitis. Neurologic disease occurs primarily in children under the age of 10 years living in the central United States. The case fatality rate is less than 1%.

Rash and Arthritis

Ockelbo and Ross River viruses are togaviruses that cause summertime outbreaks of rash and arthritis in northern Europe and Australia, respectively. These viruses can cause substantial morbidity, with prolonged and recurrent joint pain, but little if any mortality.

Hemorrhagic Fever

Dengue virus is transmitted by the *Aedes aegypti* mosquito, and humans are the primary vertebrate host. It is the most common arbovirus-induced disease and is found in tropical and subtropical regions of much of the world. There are four dengue virus serotypes. The first infection with dengue virus is rarely fatal and provides solid protection against reinfection with that serotype. Clinical manifestations include the sudden onset of fever, headache, and lumbosacral pain (**"breakbone fever"**), often followed by the appearance of a generalized rash. This infection does not provide protection against other serotypes, and the partially cross-reactive immunity can result in enhanced disease on infection with a second dengue virus serotype. The enhanced disease is associated with increased capillary permeability and can lead to dengue hemorrhagic fever or dengue shock syndrome. Multiple serotypes are circulating in most regions of the world, including much of South and Central America and the Caribbean. Dengue is frequently imported into the United States by returning travelers but has not spread widely, perhaps because, in contrast to WNV, dengue virus requires the natural cycle to infect humans, who can avoid mosquito contact.

DAMAGE

The clinical symptoms in Mrs. K.'s case of West Nile fever are consistent with damage to the brain and spinal cord, while Mr. W.'s symptoms from YFV are consistent with damage to the liver. For WNV and other arboviruses that cause encephalitis, neurons are the primary target cell for virus replication and can be irrevocably damaged by the virus. Particular subsets of neurons may be more vulnerable to infection than others. Infection of spinal cord motor neurons leads to flaccid paralysis observed with flavivirus-induced neurologic disease, as seen in Mrs. K. Infection of basal ganglia neurons leads to symptoms resembling Parkinson disease in many individuals with Japanese encephalitis. In cases of eastern equine encephalitis, vascular damage is also prominent with many small hemorrhages throughout the central nervous system.

In YFV infection, the liver is the major target organ, and hepatocellular damage is mediated directly by viral infection. Failure to metabolize bilirubin leads to jaundice (and the name yellow fever). Decreased synthesis of vitamin K-dependent coagulation factors is an important part of the hemorrhagic disorder. The virus also infects monocytes and macrophages with extensive cell death in lymphoid tissue.

In dengue virus infection, mononuclear cells are also major targets for infection. Those cells have Fc receptors on the surface, and infection can be increased by the presence of cross-reacting antibodies, as seen during infection with a second dengue virus serotype. Through mechanisms that may be related to increased virus replication and cytokine production, a second infection can lead to increased vascular permeability manifested by serous effusions, hypovolemia, and shock. Additional signs of a second infection are bleeding associated with thrombocytopenia and disseminated intravascular coagulation.

DIAGNOSIS

Diagnosis of diseases caused by any arbovirus on clinical grounds alone is difficult, except in outbreak situations, because of the paucity of specific findings on physical examination. A travel history can provide important clues to virus exposure. Definitive diagnosis is usually made by detection of virus-specific IgM by enzyme immunoassay, viral RNA by reverse transcription-polymerase chain reaction (RT-PCR), or seroconversion.

TREATMENT AND PREVENTION

There is no specific therapy for any of the arbovirus diseases. Community mosquito control programs and the use of insect repellents and window screens for personal protection against mosquitoes are important for prevention of infection. Widespread aerial spraying of insecticides can decrease adult populations of mosquitoes, and treatment of water to control larvae can inhibit emergence. Vaccines against yellow fever, Japanese encephalitis, and tickborne encephalitis are available and should be used by travelers going to regions where exposure to these viruses is likely. Vaccines against other arboviruses, particularly WNV and dengue, are in development.

Conclusion

The diverse group of arthropod-borne viruses are transmitted by arthropods, most commonly mosquitoes, and can cause diseases that include fever, encephalitis, hemorrhagic fever, rash, and arthritis. No specific treatment for any of these diseases is available, so prevention of infection is key to inhibiting arbovirus-induced morbidity and mortality.

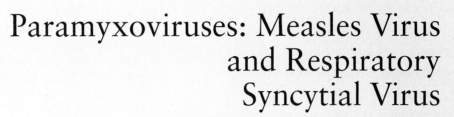

Paramyxoviruses: Measles Virus and Respiratory Syncytial Virus

John V. Williams and James E. Crowe, Jr.

key concepts

Paramyxoviruses:

- Have single-stranded, negative-sense RNA genomes.
- Have a lipid envelope derived from the host cell membrane.
- Contain membrane glycoproteins that are important functional and immunologic determinants of virulence.
- Are major causes of human diseases, including measles, mumps, and respiratory infections.
- Include some of the oldest pathogens known (measles) and some of the most recently discovered (human metapneumovirus).

The Paramyxoviridae family includes major causes of childhood diseases that have been recognized for centuries, such as measles and mumps (Table 34-1 and see History Box on Measles). This family also includes viruses that have recently emerged as causes of human disease, such as Hendra and Nipah viruses and human metapneumovirus (hMPV). Another member of the family, respiratory syncytial virus (RSV), is the most common cause of lower respiratory tract infection in infants and children worldwide and a significant cause of acute respiratory tract illness in the elderly. Parainfluenza viruses types 1, 2, and 3 are also major causes of acute respiratory diseases such as croup or laryngitis in children and adults. Thus, many of the paramyxoviruses are of major medical and socioeconomic importance, particularly for children. This chapter focuses on two paramyxoviruses that typify varying patterns of disease caused by members of this group of viruses: **measles virus** and **RSV**.

Common morphologic and genetic characteristics define the Paramyxoviridae. These viruses possess single-stranded, negative-sense RNA genomes (Fig. 34-1). Because humans do not possess RNA-dependent RNA polymerases, the virus particle must contain a polymerase.

A viral **RNA-dependent RNA polymerase (large** or **L protein)** is required to transcribe both mRNA and a positive-sense, full-length RNA copy of the genome used to make negative-sense RNA genomes for assembly of new infectious virus particles (Fig. 34-2). The viral polymerase transcribes individual mRNAs directly from the virus genome; the mRNAs are then translated by the host cell protein synthesis machinery. At some point during the viral life cycle, the polymerase switches to replicating only full-length genome for incorporation into progeny virions, which bud from the host cell membrane. The outer surface of the paramyxovirus is composed of a **lipid envelope** derived from the host cell plasma membrane. The envelope contains several integral membrane glycoproteins that are determinants of virulence and host cell tropism; those proteins also serve as targets for protective neutralizing antibodies (see Fig. 34-1). The surface glycoproteins also define antigenic subgroups of some paramyxoviruses, a characteristic with implications for vaccine development. In general, paramyxoviruses are spread by the respiratory route and cause respiratory infections, although the central nervous system is another target tissue for some viruses, notably measles, mumps, Hendra, and Nipah viruses.

Unlike influenza virus in the Orthomyxoviridae family, viruses with single-stranded, nonsegmented genomes cannot acquire genetic changes by mixing gene segments (reassortment). In addition, paramyxoviruses rarely undergo recombination. Therefore, genetic diversity of paramyxoviruses is achieved solely through the process of nucleotide point mutations arising from errors made by the error-prone viral RNA polymerase during virus replication.

table **34-1**	**Family Paramyxoviridae**
SUBFAMILY PARAMYXOVIRINAE	**SUBFAMILY PNEUMOVIRINAE**

Genus Respirovirus
  Parainfluenza virus 1, 3
	Genus Pneumovirus
	  Respiratory syncytial virus (RSV)

Genus Rubulavirus
  Mumps virus
  Parainfluenza virus 2, 4
	Genus Metapneumovirus
	  Avian pneumovirus (APV)
	  Human metapneumovirus (hMPV)

Genus Morbillivirus Measles virus	

Genus Henipavirus
  Hendra virus
  Nipah virus	

Case

Mr. B., a 19-year-old college student, returned from a trip to India. During his flight from New Delhi through Amsterdam and Detroit to Iowa, he developed a cough and conjunctivitis. On the day he arrived home, he had a rash. The rash began on his forehead and face and then spread to his trunk and extremities over the next several days. Initially, the rash consisted of discrete reddish macules (flat spots), which gradually coalesced and became brown. A physician reported the case to the local public health authorities. Subsequently, measles was confirmed serologically, and throat swab and urine specimens were collected for virus isolation. Because of religious objections, Mr. B. had not received measles vaccine.

This case raises several questions:
1. Why had this unvaccinated college student not acquired natural infection and immunity before the age of 19 years?
2. Is there a concern that he might transmit the infection to others?
3. How was this illness diagnosed as measles?

Mr. B. had traveled to India with a group of 28 other students from a college in Iowa. Many students from the college were also unvaccinated because of nonmedical reasons. Six students contracted measles while they were in India. The group had been scheduled to return to the United States, but to avoid potential spread, public health authorities recommended that the six students stay in India for at least 4 days after the onset of rash (i.e., the period of infectivity). Contacts of the infectious students who lacked immunity for measles were asked to stay in India for 18 days after the last possible exposure. Despite those recommendations, Mr. B. had returned to the United States early.

The Centers for Disease Control and Prevention issued a health advisory recommending that persons who had been on the plane with Mr. B., or had been in one of the airports at the same time as the student, be evaluated and receive measles vaccine or measles immune globulin if they were susceptible to measles virus infection. Measles vaccination clinics were held at the local departments of public health in Iowa and Michigan. Attempts were made to contact all passengers on flights with Mr. B. Public health measures were taken in other states in which exposed passengers resided to control the potential spread of measles.

Measles Virus

BIOLOGY

Measles virus contains an **RNA genome** that encodes eight proteins. The genome is complexed in a helical nucleocapsid with the **nucleocapsid protein** and the **phosphoprotein.** Alternate open reading frames within the

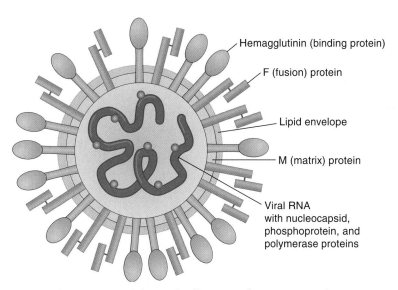

Hemagglutinin (binding protein)

F (fusion) protein

Lipid envelope

M (matrix) protein

Viral RNA
with nucleocapsid,
phosphoprotein, and
polymerase proteins

FIGURE 34-1 ▪ Schematic diagram of a paramyxovirus.

phosphoprotein gene encode two additional proteins designated **V** and **C**, which may have roles in virus replication and pathogenesis. **Matrix (M) protein** localizes at the inner face of the viral envelope and is necessary for virion assembly. Measles virus has two important membrane glycoproteins embedded in the viral envelope and displayed on the outer surface of virions. **Hemagglutinin (H)** serves as the attachment protein that binds to host cell receptors, and the **F protein** mediates fusion of the viral envelope with the host cell membrane to facilitate genome entry into the cell. The F protein also mediates cell-to-cell fusion of infected cells to adjacent uninfected cells,

History of Measles

Measles is one of the classical diseases of antiquity, first clearly described by the Baghdad physician Abu Bakr Muhammad ibn Zakariyya of Ray (latinized to Rhazes) in his AD 910 treatise on measles and smallpox. It is thought that measles virus became endemic within human populations when concentrated masses of people began living in urban areas. Humans are the only known host for measles virus, and infection leads to lifelong immunity. Therefore, the persistence of measles virus in a population requires a certain "size threshold" of susceptible humans being born or migrating into a population. That number has been estimated to be 250,000 at a minimum, and the first cities approaching that size developed in Sumer more than 5,000 years ago.

Measles has had a tremendous historical impact, perhaps surpassed only by smallpox and plague, because of its highly contagious nature and the significant morbidity and mortality associated with measles virus disease. The Italian physician Fracastorius appreciated the spread of measles from human to human in the sixteenth century, long before development of the germ theory.

Measles virus is one of the most contagious viruses known. In an outbreak between April and October 1846 in the Faro Islands near Iceland, more than 6,000 of the 7,782 inhabitants were infected. Because no measles outbreaks had occurred in this insular population for 65 years, Faro natives were almost universally susceptible. Crowding facilitates measles epidemics; for example, epidemics were common in armies and decimated many regiments of both the North and South during the American Civil War. The introduction of measles to the Fiji islands in 1875 led to more than 40,000 deaths, one fifth to one quarter of the population.

In 1857 the Scottish physician Francis Home provided the first demonstration of virus in blood (before the actual discovery of viruses) when he transmitted measles by injecting blood from infected patients into volunteers in an attempt to immunize the recipients. Growth of measles virus in tissue cell culture by John Enders and Thomas Peebles in 1954 paved the way for the study of measles virus and the development of a live, attenuated vaccine. Although measles is no longer endemic in the United States because of high levels of vaccine coverage (more than 90% by age 3 years), deaths from the disease exceed 750,000 annually worldwide, making measles a major vaccine-preventable disease.

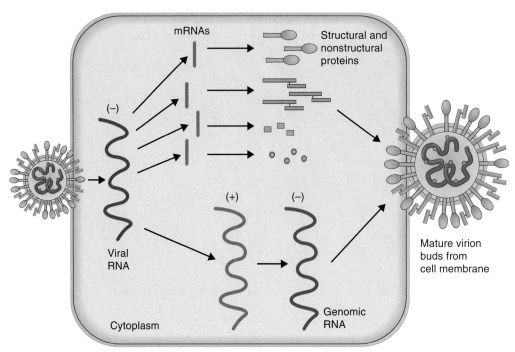

FIGURE 34-2 ■ Schematic representation of the transcription, translation, and genome replication of paramyxoviruses in the host cell cytoplasm.

forming **giant cells** or **syncytia,** a hallmark of measles virus cytopathic effect in tissue culture and in vivo (Fig. 34-3). Although mutations do occur in measles viruses that circulate in humans, only one measles virus serotype exists. Therefore, a single vaccine strain has proved effective at preventing disease caused by naturally circulating virus.

ENCOUNTER AND ENTRY

Persons infected with measles virus are most contagious 2 to 3 days before developing a rash, but they remain infectious until approximately 4 days after the rash appears. Thus, Mr. B. may have been infected by a contact

FIGURE 34-3 ■ **Formation of giant cells (syncytia) in measles pneumonia.** Notice the eosinophilic inclusions in both the cytoplasm and nuclei.

who had not yet become symptomatic. The virus is easily spread by **aerosolized droplets,** which can transmit infection during a brief encounter on an elevator, plane, or other public space. Careful history for potential exposures to infected or susceptible persons or for recent travel to endemic areas is important for raising suspicion of this diagnosis. Knowing whether a patient has received a vaccination or not is essential in determining that person's susceptibility to infection.

SPREAD AND REPLICATION

The route of infection is usually by inhalation or conjunctival inoculation, and virus initially replicates in respiratory epithelial tissues. Primary **viremia** spreads the virus to the lymph nodes, tonsils, lungs, gastrointestinal tract, and spleen. A few days later, a second wave of viremia coincides with the onset of major systemic symptoms and rash. This requirement for multiple cycles of replication and dissemination accounts for the 10- to 14-day incubation period for measles. Persons infected with measles virus are contagious prior to the onset of rash, so the potential for spread to susceptible individuals prior to diagnosis is high.

DAMAGE

Many of the clinical manifestations of measles virus infection can be attributed to damage of host epithelial and endothelial cells caused by measles virus cytotoxicity.

Infection of epithelial cells leads to the formation of giant cells, similar to that seen in tissue culture, while endothelial cell infection causes vascular dilation and increased vascular permeability. Although viral antigens are present in infected cells, histopathology of those lesions demonstrates intense inflammation and mononuclear cell infiltrates. Thus, the host immune response required to clear the infection also contributes to the disease. Epithelial giant cells are present in nasal secretions and conjunctivae, and the pathognomonic mucosal eruption (**enanthem**) of measles, **Koplik spots**, consists of epithelial giant cells with surrounding mononuclear cell infiltrates in the submucous glands. Measles virus infection is often accompanied by leukopenia. Organ-specific complications such as pneumonitis, diarrhea, and encephalitis can occur.

The host immune response is important for clearance of measles virus infection. The onset of rash coincides with the appearance of measles-specific antibodies in the normal host, initially of the IgM isotype. Over the next few weeks to months, IgG isotype antibodies appear and persist at low levels for life. Antibodies specific for measles virus are important for protection against disease and may play a role in clearance of acute infection. In a susceptible host exposed to measles, administration of measles virus–specific immune globulin ameliorates the course of disease. However, cellular immunity appears to be more important than humoral immunity for clearance of acute infection. Patients with primary antibody deficiencies (e.g., X-linked hypogammaglobulinemia) generally recover from measles virus infection, but patients with primary or acquired cellular immune deficiencies (e.g., severe combined immunodeficiency or AIDS) are prone to severe or fatal measles. Immunocompromised patients can develop giant cell pneumonia or chronic progressive encephalitis (measles inclusion body encephalitis), which is distinct from the encephalitis that can occur in normal hosts.

The most salient feature of the interaction of measles virus with the immune system is **immunosuppression** following measles virus infection. There is a very high rate of secondary infections following measles, particularly bacterial and viral pneumonias but also bacterial and protozoan intestinal infections. These infections are more frequent and associated with greater mortality in malnourished persons and those at the extremes of age. Historically, secondary infections were the greatest cause of death in measles outbreaks, and the availability of antibiotics and other public hygiene measures greatly decreased measles-associated mortality decades before the virus was identified or a vaccine developed. **Vitamin A deficiency** is particularly associated with poor outcome in measles virus infections in the developing world, and large studies have shown the benefit of vitamin A supplementation in that setting.

The exact mechanisms of immunosuppression following measles are not known, although several potential pathways exist. Two receptors for measles virus have been identified: **CD46** (membrane cofactor protein, expressed primarily on the apical surface of polarized epithelial cells) and **SLAM** (signaling lymphocyte activation molecule, expressed on B cells, T cells, and dendritic cells). Both molecules transduce powerful signals on binding their normal ligands, and interactions with measles virus might lead to attenuation of the immune response. In addition, measles virus nucleocapsid protein binds to an inhibitory immunoglobulin receptor on B cells (Fc-λ receptor II) to inhibit antibody production. It is likely that other mechanisms contribute to the immunosuppression observed following measles, which not only leads to secondary infections but also diminished responses to vaccines and tuberculin skin tests.

DIAGNOSIS

An experienced clinician can make a diagnosis of measles based on a patient's history and clinical presentation alone; almost all measles virus infections are symptomatic in susceptible persons. A 2- to 3-day prodrome of fever and the "three Cs" (cough, coryza, and conjunctivitis) followed by a rash are highly suggestive of the diagnosis. Koplik spots, which are small, bright-red spots with bluish centers that can be seen on the buccal mucosa during this period, are almost pathognomonic for measles (Fig. 34-4). The rash that follows the prodrome, with cephalocaudal progression and evolution from discrete maculopapules to confluence, is classic for the disease (Fig. 34-5). However, measles has become uncommon in many parts of the world, and many clinicians are no longer familiar with its presentation. Furthermore, manifestations may be altered in persons who were previously immunized and thus partially protected or those who are immunocompromised.

Definitive diagnosis of measles is made by virus isolation in culture. Virus can be recovered from respiratory or conjunctival secretions, peripheral blood mononuclear cells, or urine. However, measles virus culture is difficult,

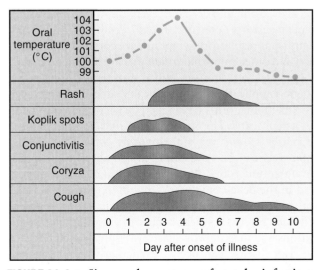

FIGURE 34-4 ▪ **Signs and symptoms of measles infection.**

FIGURE 34-5 ■ **A child with measles showing classic rash and runny nose.**

time consuming, and not widely available. Serology is now the laboratory method employed to diagnose measles. Ideally, acute and convalescent sera are obtained to document a fourfold rise in measles-specific serum IgG levels, but in a potential outbreak more rapid diagnosis is needed. Enzyme immunoassays to detect measles-specific IgM antibodies are available and can establish the diagnosis of measles using a single blood sample. Other methods that use immunofluorescent antibodies to detect measles virus proteins or reverse transcription polymerase chain reaction (RT-PCR) to detect measles virus genome are sensitive and specific but not widely available.

COMPLICATIONS

Immunologically normal, well-nourished people usually do not suffer major complications or long-term consequences from measles, but even for those individuals acute measles is not a mild disease. Profound malaise and significant respiratory symptoms are common. Malnutrition and other comorbid conditions are prevalent in most countries where measles still flourishes. The most frequent complications are respiratory superinfections such as pneumonia, otitis media, and laryngotracheobronchitis, usually caused by *Streptococcus pneumoniae, Staphylococcus aureus,* or *Haemophilus influenzae.* These infections can be devastating in the absence of appropriate antimicrobial therapy. Diarrhea also is common, and in the developing world that complication is a major cause of morbidity and mortality in young children. Vitamin A provides clear benefit for respiratory complications and may improve gastrointestinal outcomes.

Eye disease can occur, particularly in vitamin A–deficient children, and is an important cause of blindness

in measles-endemic areas of Africa and India. Cerebrospinal fluid pleocytosis is common in apparently uncomplicated measles and is usually asymptomatic. However, approximately 1 in 1,000 children with measles develop clinical signs of encephalitis, which appears to be caused by an inflammatory process known as **acute disseminated encephalomyelitis (ADEM).** The disease usually has an abrupt onset of fever and altered mental status within 2 weeks following the rash. ADEM appears to be an autoimmune-mediated demyelinating disease and can follow a variety of other infections besides measles. Most survivors of measles encephalitis have profound neurological sequelae such as deafness or mental retardation.

Although extremely rare (occurring in about 1 in 1,000,000 cases), a neurological complication of measles called **subacute sclerosing panencephalitis (SSPE)** can affect primarily immunocompetent children and young adults. The onset is insidious, 7 to 10 years after primary infection, with mental deterioration, personality changes, or myoclonus. The disease course is marked by relentlessly progressive neurological deterioration, with death occurring months to years after onset. The pathophysiology of SSPE is not completely understood. Measles virus particles with defects in the envelope-associated proteins have been isolated from the brains of affected patients, and measles-specific antibodies are present in the cerebrospinal fluid. The incidence of SSPE declined dramatically with the introduction of measles vaccine (Fig. 34-6).

PREVENTION

The cornerstone of reducing morbidity and mortality from measles is prevention through vaccination. There is no effective antiviral therapy for established measles virus infection, although measles immune globulin given soon after exposure can ameliorate disease. The World Health Organization recommends administration of vitamin A for children with measles in high-risk regions. Vitamin A is inexpensive and widely used, while immune globulin is expensive and primarily directed toward preventing severe measles in immunocompromised individuals.

Live, attenuated measles vaccine has greatly diminished the incidence of measles in every country in which it has been used. The vaccine strains were generated by manipulation of viruses in the laboratory. Wild-type measles virus strains were passaged in chick embryo fibroblast cell culture until they sustained mutations and became avirulent for primates. However, these attenuated strains can still induce protective humoral and cellular immune responses. A number of such strains have been developed and used since the 1960s. In the United States the current childhood vaccine employed for universal use is a combination measles-mumps-rubella (MMR) vaccine containing attenuated strains of all three viruses. A single dose, given intramuscularly at 12 to 15 months of age, induces measles-specific immunity in

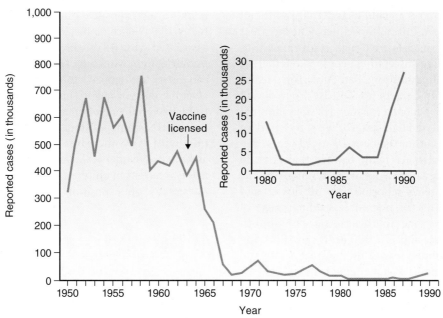

FIGURE 34-6 ▪ **Reported cases of measles in the United States, 1950–1990.** Immediately after the introduction of the vaccine, the incidence declined dramatically. A measles epidemic occurred between 1989 and 1991, with most cases affecting unvaccinated children younger than 5 years.

more than 95% of normal children. The recommended second dose at 4 to 6 years of age serves not as a booster of partial immunity but rather to seroconvert children who missed or did not respond to the first dose.

The presence of passively acquired maternal antibodies inhibits the response to measles vaccine, and this presents a problem in measles-endemic areas, where the risk of severe measles is greatest in infants and young children. If immunized at 12 months of age, most infants will seroconvert, but many infants with low maternal antibody levels will contract measles at ages younger than 12 months. Immunization at 6 months of age will protect some of these infants, but many others will fail to respond because of the presence of maternal antibodies and immunologic immaturity. These infants will require revaccination or will not be protected against later exposure.

Trials were conducted to evaluate the efficacy of a higher-titer, live, attenuated vaccine given to infants 4 to 6 months of age in an attempt to overcome the poor immunogenicity of the vaccine in young infants. The higher-titer vaccine induced higher rates of seroconversion, but female children in some trial sites had increased mortality as a result of all causes over the next few years of follow up. Although this observation has not been explained, the practice of immunizing 4- to 6-month-old infants has been discontinued. Current recommendations are for immunization at 9 months of age in endemic areas and 12 to 15 months in areas where measles is rare.

A formalin-inactivated vaccine used in the mid-1960s proved surprisingly ineffective. In fact, recipients of the inactivated vaccine developed **atypical measles** when they were subsequently infected with wild-type measles virus. The clinical features of this altered illness were high fever,

pneumonitis, and unusual rash consisting of vasculitic, hemorrhagic, or vesicular lesions with a centripetal spread differing from that of typical measles. Evidence points to the formalin inactivation steps used in vaccine preparation possibly altering the conformation of the F protein, thus inducing low-affinity antibodies that did not inhibit virus or protect recipients against infection. Instead, the antibodies may have reacted with wild-type measles virus to form immune complexes with resultant immune dysregulation. This episode illustrates the complexity of vaccine development for paramyxoviruses.

The currently licensed vaccine is safe and well tolerated, with occasional mild side effects similar to natural measles virus infection, such as rash or fever. However, in 1998 a group of researchers in Great Britain published a study of 12 children with autism and "enterocolitis," which the authors claimed was associated with measles vaccine based on histological stains of intestinal biopsies from the affected individuals. Methods of the study have been widely questioned, and no other investigators have been able to replicate the findings. Several epidemiologic studies involving hundreds of thousands of children in various countries subsequently failed to show any link between measles vaccine and autism. Nonetheless, immunization rates fell in Great Britain, and measles outbreaks occurred, resulting in the deaths of three children. In 2004, 10 of the original 13 authors of the 1998 report published a retraction of the article, and it was revealed that the senior author had received financial support from a law firm that was pursuing a suit against vaccine manufacturers.

Universal measles vaccination and the possible eradication of measles virus transmission face numerous obstacles. Sociopolitical upheaval and civil wars hamper the delivery of vaccine, and temperature instability of the live-virus vaccine requires a **"cold chain"** that is difficult and costly to maintain. Furthermore, many of the areas where measles virus persists have high birth rates, thus continually introducing susceptible people. Nonetheless, the World Health Organization, Pan American Health Organization, and the Centers for Disease Control and Prevention have set an agenda for measles virus elimination from the Western Hemisphere, with the goal of measles eradication within the next 10 to 20 years. Remarkable progress has been made toward that goal. In 2003 only 105 cases of measles were reported in the Americas, with outbreaks reported only in Mexico and the United States. Measles remains a leading cause of death in Africa, India, and Southeast Asia with an estimated 40 million cases and 777,000 deaths in 2000. Reduction of this continued loss of life, despite a safe and effective vaccine, remains a challenging task.

Respiratory Syncytial Virus

Respiratory syncytial virus (RSV) is a ubiquitous cause of respiratory tract disease in children worldwide. In both developed and developing nations, approximately 75% of

Case

In January, a mother brought her 2-month-old boy, N., to his pediatrician because the infant was coughing and breastfeeding poorly. The baby had rhinorrhea but no fever. His 2-year-old sibling was enrolled in a child care facility. On examination, the physician noted that N. was tachypneic, with subcostal retractions and diffuse expiratory wheezes on auscultation. Pulse oximetry showed his oxygen saturation to be low, and he was administered oxygen and an aerosolized form of the bronchodilator drug albuterol.

The treatment had little effect, and N. was admitted to the hospital for continuous oxygen therapy and intravenous hydration because he remained unable to nurse owing to tachypnea. A rapid antigen test performed on nasal secretions was positive for respiratory syncytial virus, and a chest radiograph revealed hyperinflation with peribronchial thickening. He was hospitalized for 3 days, during which time he improved, began nursing again, and was weaned from supplemental oxygen. He was discharged home in good condition but continued to cough for 2 more weeks.

This case raises several questions:

1. What was the role of N.'s sibling in this case?
2. What is the significance of hyperinflation with peribronchial thickening on the chest radiograph?
3. Why did N.'s cough persist for 2 weeks after hospitalization?

infants are seropositive for RSV by 1 year of age, and virtually all have been infected by age two. The classic illness associated with RSV is **bronchiolitis,** which is characterized by cough, wheezing, and dyspnea, although RSV also can cause laryngotracheobronchitis, or **croup,** and focal alveolar disease indistinguishable on chest radiographs from bacterial **pneumonia.** RSV is linked epidemiologically with asthma, although it is not clear whether infection with RSV increases a child's risk of developing asthma or whether RSV infection is more severe and thus more apparent in children who already have a genetic or physiologic predisposition for the illness.

BIOLOGY

RSV has **nucleocapsid, matrix, phosphoprotein,** and **polymerase** proteins, similar to measles virus, which serve analogous functions. RSV does not encode additional proteins within the phosphoprotein gene, but it encodes the **nonstructural** (NS) proteins **NS1** and **NS2,** which are involved in replication and modulation of the host immune response. RSV has an additional membrane glycoprotein, the small hydrophobic or **SH protein,** the function of which is not known. The major RSV surface glycoproteins are the highly glycosylated **G protein** and the **fusion** (F) **protein.** G protein mediates virus attachment to host cells, although a definitive receptor has not been identified. Diversity within G protein defines the two antigenic subgroups of RSV. F protein mediates fusion of the viral envelope and the host cell membrane and release of the viral genome into the cytoplasm to begin the virus replication cycle. F protein also promotes cell-to-cell fusion, another mechanism by which virus spread may occur. F protein is fairly well conserved between the two virus subgroups, and neutralizing antibodies to F protein generally protect against lower respiratory tract disease caused by viruses of either subgroup.

ENCOUNTER AND ENTRY

Humans are the only known host for RSV, and respiratory droplets and fomites readily transmit the virus. Reinfection occurs throughout life, with repeat infections generally milder than those in early childhood. In one study healthy adult volunteers were inoculated repeatedly with a single, wild-type strain of RSV and were reinfected successfully more than half the time. Many of these infections were symptomatic, causing rhinorrhea and cough. Thus, natural immunity to RSV protects against lower respiratory tract involvement but is not very effective at preventing disease of the upper respiratory tract. One of the features of RSV biology that has hindered successful vaccine development is the high rate of reinfection.

In temperate regions RSV infection is seasonal, occurring most frequently in the winter months. In the tropics infection occurs throughout the year but peaks in the rainy season. Almost all children are symptomatic with primary infection, and up to 40% of them have evidence of lower respiratory tract involvement. The risk of hospitalization is about 3% in normal, healthy infants, but the hospitalization rate is higher in children with underlying problems such as prematurity, cardiopulmonary disease, or immune deficiency. In the United States RSV is estimated to cause about 50,000 to 80,000 hospitalizations, at least 100 infant deaths, and 17,000 deaths in the elderly each year. Risk factors for acquisition of RSV include child care attendance and the presence of school-age siblings in the home. Risk factors for more severe disease include prematurity, male sex, secondhand exposure to tobacco smoke, and lack of breastfeeding.

SPREAD AND REPLICATION

In contrast to measles virus infection, RSV infection is limited to respiratory epithelial cells and does not involve distant body sites. Signs of upper respiratory infection occur before lower respiratory tract signs, although it is not known if infection spreads by cell-to-cell fusion or aspiration of respiratory droplets. Peak virus replication in the host precedes the peak of clinical illness; therefore, children are infectious for a few days before they become sick. The mean duration of virus shedding in immunocompetent children is 12 days; virus shedding is shorter in adults and much longer in immunocompromised persons.

DAMAGE

RSV is cytotoxic to respiratory epithelial cells, with resultant damage to ciliary function. Necrosis of RSV-infected cells with sloughing into the bronchiolar lumen is seen in autopsy specimens of fatal cases. However, as with measles, the host immune response plays an important role in the pathogenesis of RSV disease. The amount of virus present in nasal secretions peaks just before the development of severe illness. Often when infants are hospitalized, the amount of virus being shed is declining even as the illness worsens. Histopathology of fatal cases shows an intense inflammatory infiltrate in a peribronchiolar distribution, with edema of the airway contributing to the obstruction. Obstruction of small airways leads to the classic manifestations of bronchiolitis: wheezing, dyspnea, and air trapping, with hyperexpansion of the lung and decreased ventilation.

Immunopathologic components of RSV infection are not well understood. RSV infection of epithelial cells induces the production of certain cytokines such as interleukin 6 (IL-6), IL-8, tumor necrosis factor-α, and RANTES (regulated on activation, normally expressed and secreted by T cells). Animal models suggest that a skewed CD4 T-cell response, marked by Th2 cytokines, may play a role in immunopathogenesis. Severely immunocompromised persons, such as bone marrow transplant recipients, can develop fatal pneumonia with RSV that appears to be caused principally by cytotoxic viral damage.

PREVENTION

No highly effective antiviral therapy exists for RSV infection. The nucleoside analogue ribavirin has in vitro inhibitory activity, and it may have a role in severely immunocompromised patients. However, ribavirin is of no benefit to most hospitalized children with RSV. Supportive therapy with oxygen and intravenous fluids is of paramount importance. Bronchodilators have limited utility, underscoring the distinction between acute viral bronchiolitis and the reversible airway obstruction that occurs in asthma. Although the host immune response seems to be involved in disease production, immunomodulatory corticosteroids have shown no benefit in controlled trials. Currently, no licensed vaccine for RSV exists, although several promising vaccine candidates are under study in clinical trials. The history of RSV vaccine development provides another illustration of the complexity of designing strategies to prevent paramyxovirus disease.

A formalin-inactivated RSV vaccine candidate was tested in the late 1960s, but vaccine recipients developed altered immune responses and suffered more severe disease when infected subsequently with wild-type RSV, and several deaths occurred. Those events slowed RSV vaccine development for decades. Subsequent studies have suggested that, like the inactivated measles vaccine, RSV antigens did not retain a native conformation following formalin inactivation and induced a biased Th2 cytokine response with low-affinity antibodies that did not protect against wild-type RSV infection. Later, live, attenuated virus strains were developed using the techniques of serial viral passage in cell culture and chemical mutagenesis to generate stably attenuated viruses. Several of these vaccine candidates have been tested in clinical trials, and some are promising for infant vaccination.

One challenge to the development of a safe and effective RSV vaccine is the need to vaccinate very early in life to protect those at highest risk. The immunological immaturity of young infants hinders effective antibody responses to attenuated vaccines, but more immunogenic and less attenuated viruses can cause unacceptable side effects of respiratory infection. Thus, a perfect balance may be difficult to achieve between immunogenicity in the infant and suitable attenuation. Protein subunit vaccines have been found to be efficacious in older children, but in animal models these vaccines induce a biased Th2 cytokine response similar to that induced by the formalin-inactivated RSV vaccine.

The most effective preventive strategy currently available for high-risk infants is passive immunoprophylaxis. **Palivizumab** is a humanized monoclonal antibody specific for the F protein that has high neutralizing activity against most RSV strains. This licensed product was developed by cloning the antigen-binding domain from a murine monoclonal antibody into the framework of a human antibody gene, thus producing a recombinant antibody that is mostly human derived. Palivizumab reduces RSV-related hospitalizations in high-risk infants by about 50%. The antibody is expensive and must be given intramuscularly once a month during the RSV season for the first year of life. Palivizumab is one of the most successful and widely used monoclonal antibodies licensed for use thus far. Although RSV is not associated with the severe morbidity and mortality of measles, the high rates of hospitalization caused by this pathogen warrant continued efforts to develop a vaccine and prevent disease.

Newly Discovered Paramyxoviruses

Hendra and Nipah Viruses

In 1994 an outbreak of severe respiratory disease in Australia killed 14 horses and affected two humans, one of whom died. The causative agent was determined to be a paramyxovirus based on virion morphology and genetic analysis. The virus was named **Hendra virus** after the location of the outbreak. Evidence for a latent reservoir of virus in horses or humans was not found, and the virus has not reemerged.

In September 1998 an outbreak of febrile encephalitis eventually resulted in 283 human cases and 109 deaths in Malaysia and Singapore. Most of the affected individuals had direct contact with pigs on farms or in slaughterhouses; the pigs were found to have a mild respiratory illness. More than 1 million pigs were destroyed in an effort to stop the outbreak, which subsided in May 1999. Another novel paramyxovirus was found to be the cause of this outbreak and was called **Nipah virus** after the village where it was recovered.

Extensive epidemiological and environmental investigations identified a **fruit bat** species as the asymptomatic natural host for both Hendra virus and Nipah virus. It appeared that deforestation had encroached on the fruit bat's natural habitat, thus bringing the animals into closer contact with domesticated pigs and allowing interspecies transmission. Subsequently, Nipah virus was shown to infect dogs, cats, horses, and goats, thus exhibiting a remarkable ability to infect a variety of host species. In 2004 an outbreak of a "Nipah-like" virus occurred among people in Bangladesh involving more than 100 cases, including dozens of fatalities, and evidence for the same virus was found in fruit bats. The long-term relationship of these viruses with humans is not clear, but technological advances in modern molecular biology have allowed these new viruses to be rapidly identified and characterized.

Human Metapneumovirus

Investigators in the Netherlands in 2001 described a previously undetected paramyxovirus associated with severe acute respiratory tract infections in children and adults. Genetic analysis of the virus showed that it was similar to RSV but was also closely related to an important bird pathogen called avian pneumovirus. Thus, the new virus was designated human metapneumovirus (**hMPV**; see Table 34-1). The virus was difficult to grow and detect in culture, requiring special cells and conditions, likely accounting for the delay in its recognition. Further studies using molecular tests such as RT-PCR found evidence of the virus worldwide. A large prospective study in the United States found hMPV to be one of the most common viruses associated with lower respiratory infection in children, causing bronchiolitis, croup, and pneumonia. hMPV also is a common cause of upper respiratory infections, and reinfections can occur later in life, as with RSV. Phylogenetic analyses of different virus strains suggest that there are two antigenic subgroups. Serological studies of archived sera indicate that hMPV has been infecting humans for at least 50 years and probably longer.

Conclusion

Paramyxoviruses cause some of the most ancient as well as the newest diseases that plague humankind. Vaccines have dramatically diminished the incidence of diseases caused by some viruses in the Paramyxoviridae family, such as measles and mumps viruses. Others, like RSV and the parainfluenza viruses, are major causes of respiratory disease and so far have eluded the development of effective vaccines. Three paramyxoviruses—Hendra virus, Nipah virus, and hMPV—have emerged in the last decade. All paramyxoviruses share common structural and genetic features and cause either respiratory or neurological infections or both. All are important human pathogens deserving of continued studies into mechanisms of pathogenesis and immunity.

Rabies

Charles E. Rupprecht

key concepts

Rabies:

■ Is a zoonosis caused by a lyssavirus, such as rabies virus, transmitted to humans by the bite of an infected wild or domesticated animal.

■ Is mainly a disease of dogs in developing countries, and in developed countries is perpetuated by wildlife such as bats and mammalian carnivores (foxes, skunks, raccoons, coyotes, mongooses, and jackals, among others).

■ Spreads from the site of the bite in the peripheral nervous system via nerves to the central nervous system; then the virus travels back from the brain to peripheral sites.

■ Manifests after a variable incubation period of approximately 1 to 3 months, but the incubation period can range from a few weeks to more than 1 year.

■ Signs and symptoms include acute, progressive fever, headache, difficulty swallowing, paresthesia, increased muscle tone, hypersalivation, paralysis, and hydrophobia.

■ Lesions are minimal and nonspecific in the brain, but microscopic pathology may include intracytoplasmic inclusions in neurons (known as Negri bodies).

■ Can be diagnosed postmortem by fluorescent antibody demonstration of viral antigen in the brain, or antemortem by detection of viral antibody in patient serum or cerebrospinal fluid, viral antigen in a skin or brain biopsy, or viral nucleic acid or infectious virus in saliva.

■ Can be controlled by vaccination of domesticated and wild animals, stray animal removal, and local leash laws.

■ Has been prevented in humans with local wound treatment, passive administration of rabies immune globulin, and rabies vaccination.

Rabies is an acute, progressive, incurable encephalitis. It is a disease that has instilled terror in human society, and with good reason. Virtually all people who are bitten by a rabid animal and develop symptoms will die. Many of the symptoms are dramatic and frightening. In developed countries the disease in dogs has been controlled with veterinary vaccines, and consequently human rabies cases are rare. Surveillance in developed countries is still important, however, because the rabies virus is commonly found in a variety of wild animals (including bats, foxes, skunks, and raccoons). A limited number of places are considered "free" of the disease, mainly islands such as Hawaii and Japan and many of the small Caribbean islands. The disease is common in many developing countries, where canine rabies persists, and millions of people are vaccinated after being bitten by potentially rabid animals, mainly dogs.

This chapter discusses the distribution of rabies in various parts of the world and the animals involved, as well as the replication and spread of virus in those animals, the diagnosis of the disease, and prevention of persons exposed (including the crucial question of whether or not to use postexposure prophylaxis).

Rabies Virus
ETIOLOGY

Rabies virus can infect dozens of mammalian species, including humans. The reason for its unusually broad host range is not known. The agent that causes rabies

Case

A Dog Bite

As Mrs. X., a 38-year-old accountant, was jogging through her neighborhood in suburban Seattle, Washington, she was chased by an average-size black dog that bit her on the right ankle. The dog then ran away. Mrs. X. thought she recognized the animal as a Labrador-mix from a few streets away, but she was not sure. Mr. X. cleaned his wife's puncture wounds when she got home. Both Mr. and Mrs. X. were concerned about rabies and called the local health department. An official told them that no cases of rabies in dogs had been reported in Washington for decades. Only bats had been reported rabid in the last few years. The couple was told not to worry about rabies in the dog. The county animal control department was dispatched to search for the dog, found a likely suspect, and placed the animal in quarantine, where it remained healthy for the next 10 days before being claimed by its owner.

This case raises several questions:

1. Should Mrs. X. still be concerned about rabies exposure?
2. If the dog had not been found, would the treatment have been different?
3. If this incident occurred outside the United States, would the protocol have been the same?

Case

A Bat Bite

Mr. R., a 66-year-old retiree residing in Trinity County, California, was bitten on the right index finger by a bat while in his bed. He washed the wound, but he did not obtain medical care for the bite immediately following the injury. Five weeks later, he complained of headache, malaise, drowsiness, and pain and weakness in his right hand and went to the local emergency department. Based on his history of bat bite, he was admitted and treated with rabies vaccine, rabies immune globulin, ribavirin, and interferon-α.

Over the next few days, Mr. R. had steady neurological decline. He became febrile, confused, and disoriented. On the fourth day of hospitalization, Mr. R. was intubated for airway protection. His electroencephalogram exhibited diffuse slowing by the fifth day. Despite supportive therapy, Mr. R.'s condition continued to deteriorate, and he died 7 days after admission.

Mr. R.'s saliva was found to be positive for rabies virus nucleic acid by a nested polymerase chain reaction test. Based on genetic sequencing, the rabies virus variant was identified as identical to those viruses found in silver-haired bats. Because of possible contacts Mr. R. had with people, including family and medical personnel while sick, rabies postexposure prophylaxis was begun for six persons.

This case raises several questions:

1. Is this a "typical" case of rabies in the United States?
2. What prophylaxis would Mr. R. have received had he gone to the emergency department immediately after he was bitten?
3. What would have been the chances of success if Mr. R. had been provided with the appropriate prophylaxis against rabies?
4. On average, how many cases of human rabies occur in the United States each year?
5. Approximately how many persons are vaccinated against rabies in the United States each year?
6. Were Mr. R.'s symptoms characteristic of human rabies cases?

belongs to the Rhabdoviridae family, genus Lyssavirus. The best known member of that genus is rabies virus, but rabies-related viruses from the Old World can also cause the disease. Rabies and rabies-related viruses are rod or bullet shaped and contain an envelope. These viruses are fairly large compared with most other viruses (approximately 180 nm in length and 75 nm in width; Fig. 35-1). The rabies virus consists of only five genes that each encodes a single protein. The virus contains an **envelope glycoprotein (G protein)**, a **matrix (M) protein** underlying the envelope, and a **helical ribonucleoprotein (RNP) core,** or nucleocapsid, in which the **unsegmented single-stranded RNA** is tightly

FIGURE 35-1 ■ **Neuron of a dog inoculated with rabies virus.** This ultrathin section of a cell shows randomly spaced viral matrices (M) and virions (arrow) budding from endoplasmic reticulum membranes. (Original magnification, × 62,560.)

encased with the **nucleoprotein (N protein).** Because the genome of rabies virus is of **negative polarity,** the virions contain an **RNA-dependent RNA polymerase (L) protein.** A **phosphoprotein (P protein)** also is found in the RNP core. The replication cycle of rabies viruses takes place entirely in the cytoplasm of infected cells and results in the formation of numerous virus particles. Masses of nucleocapsids accumulate in the cytoplasm of neurons to form inclusions, called **Negri bodies,** which can be seen in specially stained preparations or by immunofluorescence (Fig. 35-2).

Resistance to rabies infection has long been correlated with the presence of neutralizing antiviral antibodies, and that relationship has been well established in a variety of experimental animal studies. Some of the

FIGURE 35-2 ■ **Negri bodies in a neuron of a rabid dog.** Hematoxylin–eosin stained section. (Original magnification, × 560.)

viruses in this group may elicit the formation of antibodies that cross-react against other members of the group.

EPIDEMIOLOGY

Typically, only one to three human rabies cases are reported in the United States each year. Those cases are either imported or associated with exposures to wild or unidentified animals. Tens of thousands of cases of animal rabies occur annually worldwide, most of which are in domestic animals. Consequently, humans from regions of endemic rabies are vaccinated after exposure to dogs and cats that are known to be rabid or have escaped examination and observation. In contrast, most rabies cases in the United States are found in wild, not domestic, animals.

Rabies epidemiology varies greatly from country to country. In almost all of Africa, Asia, and Latin America, rabies continues to be a disease of dogs that accounts for more than 90% of human rabies deaths. Where canine rabies persists, human rabies remains common, and millions of persons are vaccinated annually for exposures to rabid animals, mostly dogs. Worldwide, an estimated 50,000 to 100,000 persons die of rabies every year, and most of those cases occur in developing countries. In much of the developed world, where rabies in dogs has been controlled, the disease primarily affects a variety of wild animals and the animals that they bite. In western Europe, for instance, the red fox is the primary transmitter of rabies, and most cases are found in that species. In the United States and Canada, rabies is maintained by skunks, raccoons, foxes, and insectivorous bats.

It is crucial to monitor the exact location of rabid animals within each state through state health departments or federal health agencies, because that information will assist in deciding whether to recommend treatment for persons bitten by animals. If a given species has not been reported to be rabid in a certain area (e.g., terrestrial animals in the Pacific Northwest), treatment of persons exposed to that species in that area is usually unnecessary. However, a person bitten by a bat in a geographic area where rabid bats have been found will require treatment. Some animal species are almost never diagnosed as rabid, including rodents (mice, rats, hamsters) and lagomorphs (rabbits and hares). Approximately 25,000 to 40,000 persons are vaccinated against rabies each year in the United States. Only a small number of people who are vaccinated are known to have actually been bitten by rabid animals.

The bite of a rabid animal does not necessarily result in rabies. Contrary to popular beliefs, humans are somewhat refractory to the rabies virus. Historical records show that the average occurrence of disease after the bite of a known rabid dog is about 15%, although the percentage rises to more than 60% with severe bites on the face and head.

The problems of encounter with the rabies virus are very different from those with other viral diseases in which contact may be unknown, because the location and time of possible virus entry (by bite) are usually obvious in rabies. The following questions relate particularly to rabies:

- Did the bite result in a skin break?
- Has rabies been reported in the state or region where the bite occurred?
- Was the biting animal rabid? Is it available for laboratory diagnosis, or did it escape?
- Is the species known commonly to be infected with the virus?
- Is the biting animal a dog, cat, or ferret that can be observed? (If so, the period of shedding or potential virus transmission is usually concomitant with illness, or a few days before, up to a maximum of 10 days, which allows a generous safety margin. If a person has been bitten by a dog 11 days before the dog gets sick, no treatment is needed.)

SPREAD AND REPLICATION

After rabies virus enters the body through a bite, the **incubation period** is usually between 1 to 3 months but can last up to 12 months and, in rare cases, years. The length of the incubation period depends in part on the size of the viral inoculum, the length of the neural path from the wound to the brain, and the type of virus. Thus, a severe bite on the face or head typically results in a shorter incubation period.

Studies using experimental animals have shown that during the incubation period the rabies virus may move into the nervous system or remain at or close to the bite. It is not known exactly where the virus resides during that period or what factors stimulate the virus to advance to the peripheral and central nervous systems. When the virus eventually reaches the peripheral nerves, it quickly advances to the spinal ganglia, spinal cord, and brain. The virus moves passively within the **axoplasm of peripheral nerves** to the central nervous system in a retrograde fashion.

From the brain, the virus often returns to the periphery using the same axoplasmic route as used for centripetal movement. A favored peripheral site is the highly innervated **salivary glands,** but toward the end of the disease course, the virus may be found in many other tissues. In some cases the virus never reaches the salivary glands or any exit route, and the host can die from acute encephalitis. The levels of virus in the salivary gland tissue of rabid animals may be 1,000 or more times the level found in the brain, suggesting that the virus replicates at those sites as well. The location in the salivary glands helps explain the transmission of virus from one animal to another through infectious saliva.

DAMAGE

A surprisingly limited amount of histopathological change occurs in the central nervous system of animals or humans dying of rabies. Neurons of infected animals and humans contain typical intracytoplasmic inclusions, the **Negri bodies.** These inclusions are highly pathognomonic—that is, indicative of the specific disease. In the case of rabies, Negri bodies may be the only diagnostic sign, but they are not always detectable. In some cases perivascular cuffing and limited neuronal necrosis also occur. These limited histopathological changes are in striking contrast to the marked symptoms seen in human rabies.

Symptoms usually start with fever, headache, **difficulty in swallowing,** and **increased muscle tone. Hydrophobia** (contractions of the muscles involved in swallowing) is sometimes elicited by the mere sight or sound of water or other liquids. Eventually, patients develop signs of extensive damage to the central nervous system, progress to coma, and die. Rabies virus can be detected in and isolated from almost all tissues in the body of the deceased host.

DIAGNOSIS

For the first half of the twentieth century, rabies diagnosis in suspect animals was limited to the detection of Negri bodies in the Ammon horn and cerebellum (the inclusions were found in approximately 75% of positive cases) and intracerebral inoculation into mice of suspected brain specimens. Those tests resulted in immediate diagnosis of some positive cases but a delayed diagnosis of the remaining cases. Usually, a period of 24 days elapsed until the inoculated mice either died of rabies or survived.

In 1958 the **fluorescent antibody technique** was introduced. That test involves staining suspect brain impressions with a fluorescein-tagged antibody to rabies virus. Diagnosis also can be made in persons with encephalitis by fluorescent staining of skin biopsies of the nape of the neck where many hair follicles are found (the infected nerve network around hair follicles fluoresces) during the encephalitic period. The fluorescent antibody technique has become the diagnostic procedure of choice for use early in the disease. Neutralizing antibodies are found in the serum and cerebrospinal fluid later in infection, usually 8 to 10 days after the encephalitic symptoms appear. Virus can be isolated from saliva in cell culture, or viral nucleic acid can be amplified from infected tissues by the

History of Rabies

Disease associated with the bite of many kinds of animals has been recognized for thousands of years. For example, in the Mesopotamian Eshunna Code, dating from about 2300 BC, it is written: "If a dog is mad, and if the authorities have made its owner aware of this fact; if . . . it bites a man and causes his death, the owner must pay two thirds of a mina." That amounted to about 40 shekels of silver. Whether this account was an early recognition of rabies or merely outright death from a vicious dog is uncertain. Nevertheless, in the glory that was Greece and the grandeur that was Rome lurked the horror that was recognized by the great thinkers of the time, including Democritus, Aristotle, Celsus, and Galen.

Evidence that saliva was infective came in the early nineteenth century when Georg Gottfried Zinke, a German scientist, demonstrated that saliva from a rabid dog placed in contact with the wounds on the leg of an uninfected dachshund caused the disease. In 1881 Louis Pasteur delineated the role of the central nervous system in rabies when he injected rabbits intracerebrally (rather than intramuscularly) with a suspension of brain taken from a rabid cow and thus reproduced the disease. Pasteur produced the first rabies vaccines by passing infectious spinal cord material (he did not know it was a virus at the time) through a series of rabbits. The then infected spinal cords were partially inactivated by drying over potash for various periods. Pasteur's first rabies vaccination injection consisted of cords dried for 14 days. Subsequent injections used cords dried for shorter periods, until the last injection employed fully virulent cord suspensions.

Although Pasteur's early studies of vaccine were performed on dogs and other animals, the results from those studies led to the triumphant use of a spinal cord vaccine in a human in July 1885, when a 9-year-old boy, Joseph Meister, was successfully treated for severe wounds received from a rabid dog. Over the next few decades, the original vaccine underwent many changes, including chemical inactivation of the virus. Early vaccines were prepared from virus growing in nervous system tissue. Regrettably, those vaccines resulted in postvaccine demyelination and tissue destruction in approximately one third of vaccinated individuals.

Today safe and effective vaccines are produced from inactivated viruses grown in nonneural tissue culture. Recombinant rabies vaccines are also being tested and have been used to control rabies among wildlife in Europe and North America.

---

polymerase chain reaction test performed by a qualified reference diagnostic laboratory.

PREVENTION

Vaccination of Animals

Rabies is a zoonosis, a disease transmitted to humans by animals—in this case, by infected mammals. The best protection against the disease can be achieved by the elimination of rabies virus in dogs (and preventing exposure to cats) by requiring **vaccination of pets** by law, thereby creating a barrier to human exposure by the interruption of animal-to-animal transmission (either dog-to-dog or wild animal-to-dog). An additional approach is to vaccinate wild animals. Vaccination of red foxes has been performed successfully on a mass scale in Europe and Canada by dropping baited oral vaccines from airplanes. A similar strategy is being used to vaccinate raccoons, the major reservoir in the northeastern United States, and gray foxes and coyotes in Texas.

Prophylaxis of Humans

Because the incubation period of rabies is usually long, and because disease is preventable if neutralizing antibodies are present when the virus emerges in the central nervous system, rabies is one of the few infectious diseases for which there is highly effective prevention afforded by primary and secondary immunization after exposure to the infectious agent. Once the decision to provide postexposure prophylaxis has been made, treatment of humans consists of three steps: (1) **local wound treatment,** (2) **passive administration of antibody** (antiserum or rabies immunoglobulin), and (3) **vaccination.** Superficial wounds can be washed with soap and water. The passive antibody administered in developed countries is **human rabies immune globulin (HRIG)** collected from immunized persons and administered as soon as possible after rabies exposure at a dose of 20 IU/kg; as much as possible is infiltrated at the bite site, and the remainder is administered intramuscularly.

Vaccination with modern tissue culture vaccines consists of a series of five doses, all administered intramuscularly in the deltoid region, 1 mL each, over a 4-week period (days 0, 3, 7, 14, and 28). The most common vaccines are prepared with avian embryos or several kinds of human or monkey cells in culture from which the virus is purified and inactivated. All individuals given such treatment have developed the expected level of antibodies. When the combination of globulin and vaccine has been properly applied promptly, no treatment failures have been noted, and complications have been rare.

People in certain professions, such as veterinarians and animal handlers, are considered at higher risk of rabies exposure. These individuals may receive preexposure vaccination (usually three doses of vaccine on days 0, 7, and 21 or 28), and two booster vaccinations (on days 0 and 3) if they ever have a known exposure (such as an animal bite).

Conclusion

Rabies is a viral disease of mammals. The virus is neurotropic and shed in the saliva. Rabies is almost always caused by a bite. The disease may be prevented by avoiding exposure to animal bites. Rabies is fatal after the onset of illness. A large part of disease control encompasses measures to prevent an opportunity for rabid animals to bite people. In the developing world, the prime offenders are dogs, and canine vaccination is essential in those areas. In many parts of the developed world, wildlife is the source of exposure. All mammals may be susceptible, but only certain hosts maintain the disease. Common animals include bats and carnivores such as foxes, raccoons, skunks, mongooses, and coyotes.

Avoiding contact with strange-acting animals and wildlife can prevent exposure. Vaccinating pets and being a responsible owner by supervising pets are critical to avoiding rabies. Prompt first aid after a bite, and proper prophylaxis by immune globulin and vaccine, can prevent the disease. State and national public health officials can provide information on the current epidemiology of the disease and answer questions about the risk of acquisition from various exposure scenarios.

chapter **36**

Influenza and Its Viruses

Peter Palese

key concepts

Influenza:

- Is caused by influenza viruses infecting the respiratory tract.

- Occurs in epidemics and pandemics in the winter (seasonality).

- Causes clinical symptoms, including common cold, pharyngitis, tracheobronchitis, and bronchiolitis or croup in children.

- May be associated with complications such as viral pneumonia, secondary (bacterial) pneumonia, central nervous system syndromes, or Reye syndrome.

Influenza viruses:

- Contain a genome of segmented negative-sense RNAs.

- Belong to three types: A, B, and C.

- Can infect birds, horses, pigs, and other animals, including seals (type A); types B and C in general do not have an animal reservoir.

- Possess hemagglutinin and neuraminidase as major surface antigens.

Influenza can be a serious disease in humans and is characterized by repeated **epidemics** and **pandemics** (global epidemics). The cyclical nature of influenza reflects the characteristic of the virus to undergo **antigenic drift** (accumulating changes in the antigenic sites of the hemagglutinin and neuraminidase) or **antigenic shift** (capturing novel hemagglutinin or neuraminidase by exchange of genes with another virus, a process called **reassortment**). Despite the availability of vaccines and antiviral drugs, influenza ranks among the major public health problems in the United States, causing annually an average of about 20 million respiratory illnesses, 100,000 hospitalizations, and more than 20,000 deaths. Influenza virus types A and B (but not C) are mostly responsible for the disease in humans.

363

Influenza Viruses

CHARACTERISTICS

All influenza viruses possess a common structure (Fig. 36-1). Each RNA segment is encapsidated by the **viral nucleoprotein (NP)** and the three **virus-encoded polymerase proteins (PA, PB1, and PB2)**. The encapsidated RNAs are surrounded by the **matrix (M) protein.** This in turn is surrounded by the host-derived lipid membrane, into which the surface glycoproteins, hemagglutinin (**HA**) and neuraminidase (**NA**), are embedded. The RNA genome of influenza A viruses consists of eight segments coding for up to 11 proteins (Fig. 36-2). Antibodies made against the internal proteins of a single strain of influenza A virus cross-react with the proteins of all other type A strains but not with those of an influenza virus type B or C. Influenza virus types B and C have diverged sufficiently from type A influenza viruses (and from each other) that no cross-reactivity with antisera can be detected. Possibly because they have an **animal reservoir,** only influenza A viruses (not influenza B or C virus) occur as **subtypes;** there are currently 16 HA subtypes and 9 NA subtypes.

Case

A woman brought her 2-year-old son, P., to the family doctor early in January. The day before, her 6-year-old son, F., had developed high fever, sore throat, and muscle aches. When F. developed a runny nose, the boys' mother became concerned about P. He showed signs of crankiness, and his mother thought P. might have contracted the same disease as his older sibling.

The doctor did not order any laboratory work but wrote a prescription for an antipyretic and an antiviral drug active against influenza virus. In fact, he asked the mother to take that same drug as well. After the doctor found out that the other members of the household, the father and another boy (15 years of age), did not show any signs of illness, he suggested that they (but not the 6-year-old) also take that drug to prevent influenza.

This case raises several questions:

1. Why did the physician think P. would develop influenza, even though no laboratory tests supported the assumption?
2. What was the most likely drug the physician prescribed to the patient and other family members? Why did he not give the medication to the 6-year-old sibling?
3. What should the physician have asked regarding all family members, and what should he have recommended the family do next year?

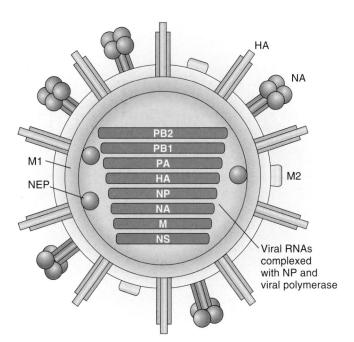

FIGURE 36-1 ▪ **Diagram of an influenza virus particle.** The hemagglutinin (HA) is found as a trimer, the neuraminidase (NA) as a tetramer, and the M2 ion channel as a tetramer. The matrix protein (M1) underlies the plasma membrane–derived lipid envelope. A nuclear export protein (NEP) is also associated with the virus. The viral RNA segments are coated with nucleoprotein (NP) and are bound by the polymerase complex (PA, PB1, and PB2).

FIGURE 36-2 ▪ **RNA segments of influenza A/Puerto Rico/8/34 and A/Hong Kong/8/68 viruses.** The viral RNAs are separated on a polyacrylamide gel. The proteins encoded by the RNAs are indicated. The PB1 gene codes for the polymerase protein PB1 and the proapoptotic PB1-F2. The M gene codes for the matrix protein (M1) and the ion channel protein (M2). The NS gene codes for the non-structural protein (NS1) and the nuclear export protein (NEP, formerly called NS2).

ENCOUNTER

Influenza viruses are transmitted from person to person by **airborne droplets** (1 to 5 μm in size). Coughing and sneezing are obvious ways in which the virus becomes airborne. The virus infects the mucosa of the respiratory tract, and initial infection of the lower respiratory tract also has been observed. Usually, the incubation period is 1 to 2 days, and virus shedding during uncomplicated influenza continues for 3 to 6 days. Influenza viremia or invasion of extrarespiratory tissues is documented extremely rarely.

EPIDEMIOLOGY

Three instances of antigenic shift occurred in the twentieth century. Figure 36-3 shows the circulation of influenza A viruses starting with the pandemic of 1918. During that well-documented event at the end of World War I, an estimated 50 million people died of what was called the **Spanish flu,** and countless millions had severe disease. Following the 1918 pandemic, influenza A viruses of the H1N1 subtype remained prevalent until 1957. During the next 11 years, from 1957 to 1968, H2N2 viruses (**Asian flu**) circulated, and since 1968 the **Hong Kong** subtype (H3N2) has predominated. Interestingly, H1N1 viruses reemerged in 1977 and have cocirculated with the H3N2 viruses since that time.

Predictions about the characteristics of novel pandemic strains cannot be made with certainty, but if the past is any guide to the future, we would expect the introduction of a novel HA (or a novel HA and another gene) into the backbone of a circulating human strain. For example, in 1968 a novel HA (H3) replaced the H2 HA, and the PB1 gene also changed. It is likely that the two genes were captured from an avian strain, and the

Antigenic shift

FIGURE 36-4 ▪ **Antigenic shift: reassortment of a human H2N2 and an animal (avian) influenza virus.** The H3N2 virus responsible for the pandemic in 1968 is postulated to have derived its PB1 and HA genes (red lines) from an animal strain and its remaining six RNAs from an H2N2 parent (blue lines).

remaining six genes were derived from the H2N2 virus circulating in humans during the previous subtype period (Fig. 36-4).

Antigenic drift occurs with both influenza A and B viruses. In general, drift over a period of 3 to 5 years is sufficient to allow a novel strain to cause disease. The antigenic sites in HA that undergo mutations (antigenic drift) have been defined (Fig. 36-5). Antigenic drift (as well as the occasional antigenic shift) is responsible for the need to change the vaccine formulations each year (see "Treatment and Prevention"). At the beginning of the twenty-first century, H3N2 and H1N1 influenza A viruses, as well as influenza B virus strains, are responsi-

FIGURE 36-3 ▪ **Epidemiology of influenza A and B viruses.** The appearance of new influenza A virus subtypes in 1918, 1957, and 1968 resulted in pandemics. The broken lines indicate the probable prevailing strains before isolation of the first human influenza viruses. Sequence analysis of viral RNA obtained from formalin-fixed and frozen tissue samples indicates that the 1918 pandemic strain was an H1N1 virus (solid square).

Receptor binding site

Antigenic sites

Fusion peptide

FIGURE 36-5 ▪ **Ribbon representation of the hemagglutinin monomer from the 1918 influenza virus based on X-ray diffraction analysis.** The five predicted antigenic sites surround the sialic acid receptor binding site. Viruses counter antibody reactivity by mutating these sites or by introducing new glycosylation sites (existing glycosylation sites are colored orange) through a process called antigenic drift. Towards the membrane proximal end (bottom) is the fusion peptide. (Contributed by James Stevens and Ian Wilson.)

ble for disease in humans. Thus, the current vaccine formulation must contain three different strains.

Infections from influenza virus types A and B usually appear in the Northern Hemisphere between October and April, with peaks between December and March. Influenza C virus infections are usually nonseasonal, and most occur in children between 1 and 4 years of age. In general, infections with influenza virus type C are less severe than those caused by influenza A and B viruses.

table **36-1**	**Characteristics of Influenza Virus Types A, B, and C**		
CHARACTERISTIC	**A**	**B**	**C**
Frequency of isolation	+++	++	+/−
Severity of disease	+++	++	+/−
Animal reservoir	Yes	No	No
RNA segments	8	8	7

+++ High; ++ Medium; ±Infrequent

Most adults and children over six years of age are seropositive for influenza C viruses (Table 36-1).

ENTRY

Influenza viruses infect the upper and lower respiratory tracts. The first cells to be infected are the nonciliated epithelial cells. The preferred receptor for the virus on those cells is a terminal sialic acid in a (2-6) linkage to galactose. Whether the virus "takes" depends mostly on the presence or absence of **neutralizing antibodies** in the host and on the capacity of the virus to overcome host **innate immune response.**

SPREAD AND REPLICATION

Infection of cells by influenza viruses is initiated by attachment of the HA to the viral receptor (sialic acid-containing glycoproteins or glycolipids on the cell surface) and subsequent uptake of the virus into an endocytic vesicle. Under the acidified conditions within the vesicle, the HA undergoes a structural change leading to fusion of the viral membrane with that of the endocytic vesicle. At the same time, the M2 protein of the virus, which has **ion channel activity,** allows the influx of H^+ ions from the vesicle into the interior of the virus, facilitating the uncoating of the virus and release of the viral gene segments (ribonucleoprotein) into the cytoplasm. The processes of viral uncoating and release are inhibited by the antiviral drugs **amantadine** and **rimantadine.** Subsequently, the viral ribonucleoprotein enters the nucleus, where viral mRNA is synthesized. Viral protein synthesis and amplification of the viral RNA allows the formation of viral ribonucleoproteins and the assembly and budding of new particles from the cytoplasmic membrane. The function of the neuraminidase is to remove the sialic acid receptors from the virus particles and from the cell surface; thus, the viruses do not self-aggregate and they do not remain glued to the surface of the infected cell. **Neuraminidase inhibitors** (**oseltamivir** and **zanamivir**) effectively prevent the removal of the sialic acid receptors, thereby inhibiting the spread of virus particles from infected cells to uninfected cells.

Paradigm **Box**

Influenza Pandemic of 1918: Lessons Learned

A **pandemic** occurs when a highly virulent and transmissible virus surfaces to which most people lack prior exposure and thus immunity. In the case of influenza, the virus can acquire a new surface antigen (e.g., HA) by exchanging its "old" HA for a "new" one. If a human influenza virus and an animal influenza virus happen to infect the same cell, a novel virus can form through **reassortment** of the genes of the two viruses (see Fig. 36-4). Influenza pandemics occurred in the twentieth century in 1918, 1957, and 1968. In each case it is likely that an antigenic shift occurred when the human strain acquired a new HA from an avian virus infecting the same cell. The estimated death toll from the 1918 pandemic exceeds 50 million people worldwide. Among the U.S. military approximately an equal number of men died from influenza as from direct military action in World War I.

Although no live 1918 virus is available, recent technological breakthroughs allow RNA sequences to be obtained from formaldehyde-treated lung samples (in paraffin blocks) by **reverse transcription polymerase chain reaction (RT-PCR)**. Based on its sequence, a gene can be reconstructed by using synthetic oligonucleotides. Virus containing genes from the 1918 strain can then be rescued (in a high-containment facility) from the DNA by a technique called **reverse genetics**. Study of such **recombinant viruses** in animal models has revealed that the virus was unusually virulent. In fact, the reconstructed extinct 1918 virus can kill mice in as few as 3 days, faster than any other human virus ever tested. However, currently available antivirals would be effective against the 1918 pandemic virus. Vaccines also have been shown (in mice) to be effective against the 1918 strain. Thus, we have learned valuable lessons from the 1918 pandemic virus. Not only have we gained an understanding of why the virus was so virulent, but also we know that we have developed effective countermeasures: antivirals and vaccines.

DAMAGE

In uncomplicated cases of influenza, respiratory epithelial cells are affected by the infection and edema, and mononuclear cell infiltrates in the lamina propria are observed. In more severe disease, gross pathologic findings include hemorrhagic and airless lungs, and necrotizing tracheobronchitis and bronchiolitis are found. Later in the infection, severe alveolar damage can occur, sometimes with extensive fibrosis. A direct cytopathic effect is most likely responsible for the pathologic changes observed following infection, and the direct involvement of the upper and lower respiratory tracts can account for most of the signs and symptoms of the disease (see the box titled "Clinical Manifestations of Influenza"). In addition, **complications** have been described including primary viral pneumonia and **secondary bacterial pneumonia**. Reye syndrome in children is associated with infections of influenza virus type B (and occasionally type A), leading to brain swelling and a fatty degeneration of the liver. Interestingly, the incidence of Reye syndrome has been lowered dramatically as a result of the decreased use of aspirin (acetylsalicylate), which had previously been identified as a cofactor of the disease.

DIAGNOSIS

The laboratory diagnosis of influenza in many cases still relies on virus isolation from clinical samples, including sputum and nose and throat washings or swabs. Embryonated chicken eggs or Madin-Darby canine kidney

Clinical Manifestations of Influenza

Symptoms and signs		Complications
Malaise	Respiratory symptoms	Pneumonia
Myalgia	Cough	Secondary bacterial pneumonia
Fever	Substernal burning	Otitis media
Chills	Gastrointestinal symptoms (rare)	Reye syndrome
Headache		Encephalitis (possibly Parkinson disease)

(MDCK) tissue culture cells are the preferred substrates for isolation of the virus. Viral antigens can be detected in clinical samples by a variety of immunoassays, and more recently RT-PCR has been used to detect viral RNA. Prior infections (as evidenced by the presence of anti-influenza virus antibodies) can be demonstrated by the classical **hemagglutination inhibition test.** Sera from patients are used to measure the inhibition of hemagglutination of chicken or human red blood cells by known influenza viruses. It should be noted, however, that the majority of clinical diagnoses do not involve the use of laboratory tests but are based on clinical symptoms, epidemiological evidence in the community, and knowledge concerning the seasonality of the virus.

TREATMENT AND PREVENTION

Influenza is frequently treated only symptomatically. However, there are now specific treatment modalities available (Table 36-2). Amantadine and rimantadine are effective only against influenza A viruses. That drawback—combined with known adverse reactions, including dizziness, central nervous system symptoms, and cases of drug resistance—make those antiviral approaches less desirable. Neuraminidase inhibitors such as oseltamivir and zanamivir not only are efficacious in the treatment of both influenza A and B viruses but also can be used prophylactically. Resistance during clinical use is rare, and mutant strains that are resistant to neuraminidase inhibitors may be less pathogenic than the wild-type virus. The successful development of these antiviral drugs has been helped by the availability of animal models, including mice and ferrets, which allow the study of influenza viruses in vivo. Clearly, in most cases of influenza the use of antibiotics is not indicated.

The most cost-effective treatment modality remains prophylactic vaccination (see the box titled "Influenza Virus Vaccines"). Currently, **inactivated vaccines** and **live, attenuated, cold-adapted vaccines** are available. The inactivated vaccines are formaldehyde-treated prepara-

table **36-2**	**Antiviral Drugs Active Against Influenza**	
GENERIC/(TRADE NAME)	**ANTIVIRAL ACTIVITY**	**ROUTE OF ADMINISTRATION**
Amantadine	Influenza A	Oral
Rimantadine (Flumadine)	Influenza A	Oral
Oseltamivir (Tamiflu)	Influenza A and B	Oral
Zanamivir (Relenza)	Influenza A and B	Inhalation

Influenza Virus Vaccines

Killed (inactivated) virus
Split or whole (formaldehyde treated)

Live (attenuated) virus
Cold adapted

Genetically engineered viruses
In development

tions of whole virus or disrupted split virus. They are injected intramuscularly, and their level of efficacy is generally in the range of 60 to 90% in healthy children and adults. The injection may cause local reactions, but the killed inactivated vaccine cannot cause influenzalike symptoms in the recipient. Immunization with the injectable vaccine does not result in mucosal immunity. On the other hand, the live, attenuated, cold-adapted influenza virus vaccine induces a **local mucosal response** because it is given as a nasal spray, resulting in low-level replication in respiratory epithelial cells. Immunization with the live, attenuated virus vaccine also may induce a response that is more cross-reactive against different viral variants and thus may offer longer-lasting immunity than that resulting from vaccination with the inactivated preparation. Adverse reactions associated with the live influenza virus vaccine in certain subpopulations are currently being evaluated.

Immunization against influenza not only is of paramount importance in curbing the disease itself but also may reduce the risk of myocardial infarction in patients with coronary disease and dramatically reduce the incidence of otitis media in young children. Thus, the use of influenza virus vaccines may not only be cost effective but also may bring added benefits to certain risk groups. Efforts are ongoing to improve existing vaccines (through development of genetically engineered strains) and to establish the safest and most effective regimens for special populations using the currently available vaccines.

Genetic Engineering of Influenza Viruses: Reverse Genetics

Influenza viruses are negative-sense RNA viruses whose RNA is not intrinsically infectious. Thus, viral RNA transfected into cells does not produce infectious virus.

Viral RNA expression plasmids

FIGURE 36-6 ■ **Plasmid-based rescue of infectious influenza virus.** Twelve plasmids are introduced into mammalian cells. Eight plasmids express precise copies of the eight viral RNA segments (PA, PB1, PB2, HA, NP, NA, M, and NS). Four plasmids lead to formation of the viral polymerase complex (formed by the PA, PB1, PB2, and NP proteins) required for replication of viral RNAs. The production of viral RNAs and proteins leads to the formation of infectious (recombinant) influenza viruses.

To introduce specific changes into the genome of influenza viruses (**genetic engineering**), cells are transfected with plasmids expressing the eight viral RNAs as well as helper plasmids that express the viral polymerase proteins. That system, called **reverse genetics**, results in the rescue of infectious virus from DNA and thus can be used to study genetic changes in the virus (Fig. 36-6). Reverse genetics also allows the generation of **attenuated viruses** for possible use as vaccines. Similar techniques have been developed to generate from cDNA other infectious negative-sense RNA viruses, including bunyavirus, Ebola virus, and measles virus.

Conclusion

Three types of influenza virus (A, B, and C) occur in nature. Antigenic drift (A and B) and antigenic shift (A only) define the epidemiology of this family of negative-sense RNA viruses. Pandemics such as the one in 1918 are characterized by high morbidity and mortality in the human population. Recent developments have resulted in improved antivirals and vaccines against influenza.

chapter **37**

Rotaviruses, Noroviruses, and Other Viral Agents of Gastroenteritis

Robert L. Atmar and Mary K. Estes

key **concepts**

Viral gastroenteritis:

■ Is caused by several viruses

■ Presents clinically in a manner that prevents distinguishing which virus is causing the disease.

■ Is transmitted primarily by person-to-person contact through the fecal–oral route.

■ Is not treatable by any specific therapy; rather, treatment is supportive to provide and maintain hydration.

Rotaviruses:

■ Are wheel-shaped, double-stranded RNA viruses.

■ Are the most common cause of viral gastroenteritis in young children.

■ Cause a disease with seasonal distribution in the United States, with peak incidence in the winter months.

■ Are transmitted by the fecal–oral route.

■ Cause changes in the small intestine mucosa that lead to diarrhea.

■ Induce long-term immunity.

Noroviruses:

■ Are small, single-stranded RNA viruses that currently cannot be cultivated.

■ Are the cause of almost all (more than 95%) of the outbreaks of nonbacterial gastroenteritis and are the most common cause of outbreaks of foodborne and waterborne viral gastroenteritis.

■ Are the leading cause of viral gastroenteritis in adults and the second leading cause of severe disease in children.

■ Are transmitted primarily by the fecal–oral route.

■ Are associated with disease in diverse settings, including schools and day care centers, nursing homes, vacation settings (e.g., camps and cruise ships), military ships and maneuvers, restaurants and catered meals, and hospitals.

■ Cause changes in the mucosa of the small intestine that may be related to diarrhea.

■ Are associated with susceptibility to infection and disease based on histoblood group antigen expression (e.g., blood type and secretor status).

Other enteric viruses that cause gastroenteritis:

■ Two serotypes of adenovirus, which cause diarrhea especially in children under the age of 2 years.

■ Sapoviruses, which cause institutional outbreaks of diarrhea.

■ Astroviruses, which cause enteric disease mainly in children.

■ Aichi viruses, which cause disease in children and adults.

cute gastroenteritis is one of the most common diseases in humans and continues to be a significant cause of morbidity and mortality. Worldwide, 2.5 million children die each year from the complications of **infectious gastroenteritis.** In the United States fewer than 500 children per year die from infectious diarrhea, but more than 200,000 children under age 5 are hospitalized for diarrhea-induced dehydration. Before the 1970s, although viral agents were suspected to cause diarrhea, the only etiologic agents for diarrhea that could be diagnosed were bacteria or protozoa. Viral agents of diarrhea were difficult to identify because they do not grow well in cultured cells.

In the 1970s electron microscopy allowed detection of viruses in stool specimens, and in 1972 Norwalk virus, a **norovirus** that is a type of **calicivirus,** was the first agent of viral diarrhea identified by electron microscopic analysis of stool. When a convalescent serum specimen was mixed with a diarrheal stool specimen, clumped virions were observed. Norwalk virus is now recognized as the most common cause of outbreaks of viral diarrhea in adults, and it is increasingly being identified as the second most important cause of diarrhea in children. In 1973 **rotavirus** was identified by electron microscopic examination of stool specimens. Rotavirus is now known to be the most commonly recognized agent of gastroenteritis in children. Four additional viral agents of gastroenteritis have been identified: **enteric adenoviruses, sapoviruses, astroviruses,** and **Aichi virus** (Table 37-1). It is likely that additional viral agents will be discovered as causes of gastroenteritis because 40 to 50% of diarrhea cases are still of uncertain etiology.

Case

M., a 7-month-old girl living in Washington, D.C., was recently switched from breastfeeding to bottle feeding. Usually a satisfied and happy child, M. became irritable on March 29, began to vomit, and had a low-grade fever. She also had mild upper respiratory symptoms, with cough, nasal discharge, and pharyngitis. After 2 days she was brought to the pediatrician, who diagnosed rotavirus gastroenteritis by detecting viral antigen in the stool with an enzyme-linked immunosorbent assay (see Chapter 58). Oral rehydration solution was given at home, and M. made an uneventful recovery by the sixth day.

This case raises several questions:

1. How did M. acquire the virus?
2. Is it significant that M.'s disease occurred in the spring?
3. Will M. ever have the same disease?
4. Why did the pediatrician suspect this etiological agent?

immunocompromised may experience mild illness. Parents of young children experiencing a primary rotavirus infection may have mild symptoms. Certain individuals known to be at increased risk for complications of dehydration due to viral gastroenteritis include malnourished children and adults, particularly in developing countries, and the elderly, who may experience waning immunity with age.

Rotavirus-induced disease has a **seasonal distribution** in the United States, peaking in the winter and becoming rare in the warmer months. In tropical countries endemic rotavirus infection occurs throughout the year. Other viruses, such as influenza virus and respiratory syncytial virus, also have characteristic seasonal appearances in temperate climates, but the reasons for the seasonality are not known. As with other viral illnesses, some children will develop rotavirus gastroenteritis without having had contact with symptomatic individuals. Acquisition may result from an encounter with an individual who is asymptomatically shedding virus. Such asymptomatic excretion of rotavirus can occur for weeks before the onset of diarrhea and for days following resolution of symptoms. Other children can shed rotavirus and never experience symptoms.

Rotavirus
ENCOUNTER

Essentially every child in the United States becomes infected with rotavirus. The peak incidence of rotavirus infection in the United States occurs between 6 months and 2 years of age. Most individuals have experienced infection and are immune to severe rotavirus disease by age 4. Seropositive older children or adults who are reexposed to a high inoculum of virus or who become

ENTRY

Endemic rotavirus disease is caused primarily by **person-to-person transmission.** The principal means of transmission is by the **fecal–oral route.** Rotavirus is excreted at levels that reach 10^{12} infectious particles per milliliter of stool. Transmission of as few as 10 infectious particles can result in infection. Outbreaks due to contamination of municipal water supplies and foodborne transmission have been reported but appear to be rare. Speculation

table 37-1 | Viral Causes of Gastroenteritis in Humans

ETIOLOGIC AGENT	VIRUS FAMILY	GENOME	SEASONALITY	MEDICAL SIGNIFICANCE
Rotavirus	*Reoviridae*			
Group A		Segmented dsRNA	Predominantly winter	Major cause of diarrhea in children 6–24 months
Groups B and C		Segmented dsRNA		Rare in United States
Norovirus	*Caliciviridae*	(+) ssRNA	Winter peak, year-round occurrence	Major cause of diarrhea outbreaks in children and adults
Sapovirus	*Caliciviridae*	(+) ssRNA	Year-round	Infects children and adults
Enteric adenovirus	*Adenoviridae*	Linear dsDNA	Year-round	Infects mainly children, 2–10 years old
Astrovirus	*Astroviridae*	(+) ssRNA	Year-round	Infects mainly children
Aichi virus	*Picornaviridae*	(+) ssRNA	Not known	Infects children and adults

(+), positive-sense polarity; ds, double-stranded; ss, single-stranded.

exists that rotavirus may spread by the **respiratory route** via infectious aerosol. That possibility is based on well-described epidemics in which fecal–oral transmission cannot be documented and on the observation that respiratory symptoms may precede the development of gastroenteritis by a day or two.

STRUCTURE AND REPLICATION

Rotaviruses are among the few human viruses with a **double-stranded RNA genome,** which resembles double-stranded DNA in structure. Another distinguishing property (shared by the orthomyxoviruses) is that the genome of rotaviruses is **segmented.** Rotavirus particles are shaped like wheels with short spokes and an outer rim (*rota* means "wheel" in Latin; Fig. 37-1). The particle possesses an icosahedral structure with inner and outer capsids. Infectivity requires an intact outer capsid layer that helps establish **acid stability,** a critical characteristic for microorganisms that gain entry through the gastrointestinal tract. Two outer-capsid proteins, a hemagglutinin (VP4) and a glycoprotein (VP7), induce development of neutralizing antibodies.

The capsid contains 11 segments of double-stranded RNA as well as a viral **RNA-dependent RNA polymerase (transcriptase)** for transcription of individual RNA segments into messenger RNA (mRNA). The enzyme is absent in animal cells and must be introduced with the virion during infection. Most rotavirus strains require treatment with a protease to become infective. Virus penetration into cells is enhanced by proteolysis of the VP4 outer-capsid protein. Virus replication proceeds in the cytoplasm, resulting in the formation of both positive- and negative-sense RNA (Fig. 37-2). The positive-sense RNA functions as a template for both

translation (like mRNA) and replication of negative-sense RNA. Production of negative-sense RNA using positive-sense RNA as a template results in the formation of progeny, double-stranded RNA gene segments. Virus particles are assembled in the cytoplasm and mature by budding through the endoplasmic reticulum. Mature virus particles are released into the extracellular environment with lysis of the infected cell.

Six groups of rotaviruses (A through F) have been identified based on antigenic characteristics. **Group A rotaviruses** share a common antigen and are the only rotaviruses recognized to cause frequent infections in the United States. **Group B rotaviruses** are best known as a cause of diarrhea in swine, but these viruses have caused outbreaks in children and adults in China. The other rotavirus groups are either infrequent or their role in human disease is not clear.

FIGURE 37-1 ■ Electron micrograph of negatively stained virus particles. **A.** Norwalk virus. **B.** Rotavirus.

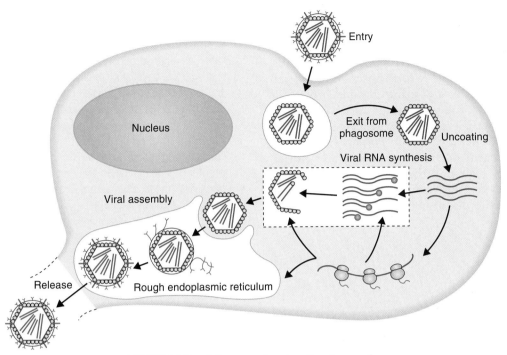

FIGURE 37-2 ■ **The rotavirus replication cycle.**

DAMAGE

Rotaviruses produce a spectrum of disease ranging from asymptomatic infection to severe diarrhea with potentially fatal dehydration. Severe gastroenteritis generally occurs in children between 6 and 24 months of age, as in the case of M. Rotavirus infections typically have a 2-day incubation period. Vomiting often precedes the onset of diarrhea by 2 or 3 days. Watery diarrhea can last 3 to 8 days in infants who become symptomatic. Fever and abdominal cramps are common. Red blood cells or leukocytes are generally not found in the stool of patients with rotavirus gastroenteritis.

Morphological changes have been identified from biopsies of the mucosa of the proximal small intestine of infants and children with rotavirus gastroenteritis. Among the changes are shortening and atrophy of the villi, denuded villi, and mononuclear cell infiltration of the lamina propria. Virus invasion of the epithelial cells of the small intestine causes destruction of the mature absorptive cells that are then replaced with young, virus-free cells. That process results in diarrhea for at least four reasons: First, immature replacement cells have a reduced ability to absorb salt and water. Second, immature cells have a reduced ability to produce disaccharidases, which results in malabsorption of carbohydrates. Third, the virus produces a protein that functions as an enterotoxin, is released from virus-infected cells, and stimulates chloride and water secretion in the gut. Fourth, the enteric nervous system is activated. The severity of rotavirus-induced diarrhea may not be proportional to the extent of mucosal damage in the small intestine because the enterotoxin can cause diarrhea in the absence of histological changes.

In infants younger than 6 months of age, rotavirus diarrhea is less common, except for premature neonates who may acquire the infection during outbreaks in newborn nurseries. Normal full-term infants often become infected but remain asymptomatic even while shedding rotavirus in the stool, for reasons not well understood. It may be that maternal antibodies transferred during the third trimester protect term infants, while premature infants born before they can acquire maternal antirotavirus antibodies are susceptible. In children older than 6 months of age, rotavirus is a major nosocomial pathogen and is frequently the cause of disease in child care settings.

Adults generally experience a mild or even asymptomatic infection from rotavirus because long-term immunity generally follows a primary infection. Symptoms become apparent when the inoculum size is large enough to overcome preexisting immunity. In some instances rotavirus causes travelers' diarrhea in children and adults, although it is a less common agent of that disease than are other pathogens.

Chronic diarrhea and prolonged shedding have been associated with rotavirus infection in children with T-**cell immunodeficiencies.** Patients undergoing immunosuppression for bone marrow transplantation are also at increased risk.

DIAGNOSIS

Because most of the viral agents that cause gastroenteritis grow poorly in cell culture, assays that detect viral antigen in stool specimens have become the most commonly employed diagnostic strategies. **Antigen detection** assays, as used in M.'s case, are widely available for rotavirus detection, but the commercially available assays detect only group A rotaviruses. Electron microscopy also is used, and group B and C rotavirus infections are often only suspected following use of that test. Electron microscopy also allows the identification of other enteric viruses. However, electron microscopy is not available in many clinical laboratories, and a relatively high viral titer must be present in the stool specimen for the virus to be detected by that method. Serologic diagnosis is possible but generally not useful.

Treatment and Prevention

At present no specific therapies for the management of viral gastroenteritis are available. Adherence to standard precautions for infection control, such as hand washing and barrier methods (e.g., gloves and gowns) are important for minimizing disease spread. Patient care is directed at supportive measures with particular attention to preventing dehydration by using intravenous hydration or oral rehydration therapy.

Oral immunization with a **live, attenuated rotavirus vaccine** is effective for preventing severe rotavirus disease. Live, attenuated vaccines induce a protective immune response without inducing disease. Rotaviruses of rhesus, bovine, or human origin have been evaluated as candidate vaccines. The first licensed rotavirus vaccine (derived from a rhesus rotavirus strain) was withdrawn from the market after one year owing to an unexpected, temporal association with **intussusception,** a telescoping of the intestine into itself. Another approach under evaluation involves the generation of recombinant rotaviruses that contain genes from both human and animal strains. Two important concerns include (1) the ability of high-risk neonates to mount an effective immune response against a vaccine strain and (2) ensuring that the attenuated vaccine virus cannot cause disease in susceptible contacts.

Norovirus

Encounter

Norwalk virus is the prototype strain of the noroviruses, which were previously called Norwalk-like viruses or small, round, structured viruses (SRSVs; see Fig. 37-1). Noroviruses are members of the **Caliciviridae** family and the genus *Norovirus*. Norovirus strains are named after

Case

Mr. S., a 25-year-old chef who had just returned from a vacation on a cruise ship, presented to his primary care physician with a 2-day history of diarrhea. He also had abdominal cramps, vomiting, and malaise but no fever. He was anxious to go back to his job at a restaurant. His wife had also been sick for 1 day, but she only had vomiting. Their two children, who did not go on the cruise, were in good health. Without ordering any diagnostic tests, Mr. S.'s physician sent him home with the recommendation to drink fluids and be careful to wash his hands and disinfect the bathroom to prevent spreading the illness to others. Although he was advised to return to work when his illness ended, Mr. S. was cautioned to continue using good hygiene practices and to be sure to wear gloves when handling food.

This case raises several questions:

1. How did Mr. S. acquire the virus?
2. Why did the physician not perform any diagnostic tests?
3. Why did the physician tell Mr. S. to use good hygiene practices at home and at work?
4. Will Mr. S. ever have the same disease again?

the geographic area where an outbreak occurs (e.g., Hawaii agent, Snow Mountain agent, and Montgomery agent) and are genetically very diverse. The viruses usually come to attention through the occurrence of **explosive outbreaks** of disease, with an incubation period of 1 to 2 days following a common source exposure. A seasonal peak of disease occurs in the winter, but infection can happen throughout the year. Noroviruses are highly stable in the environment and are transmitted by contaminated **food** or **water** and by person-to-person contact. Fecal–oral transmission is the usual route, but transmission by aerosol also can occur following vomiting.

Noroviruses can infect persons of any age, but they are most frequently diagnosed in adults and school-aged children who are involved in outbreaks. However, noroviruses increasingly are being recognized in ill preschool children and are now thought to be second to rotaviruses as a cause of diarrhea in children, including children hospitalized with gastroenteritis. Noroviruses cause outbreaks in nursing homes, on cruise ships, and in essentially any setting where individuals are confined in close contact. International common source outbreaks related to food and water also can occur. Asymptomatic infection is common, and virus shedding can occur for prolonged periods (2 to 3 weeks) after an individual recovers from illness. Transmission of virus from persons asymptomatically shedding virus is likely to be the source of many infections.

Host Factors Affect Infection

Early volunteer studies showed that some individuals are resistant to infection with noroviruses. Recent studies have found that genetic factors affecting histoblood group antigen expression; including secretor status and ABO blood group type, influence whether an individual becomes infected with Norwalk virus. Nonsecretors are resistant to infection, and individuals with a blood group type B are less likely to become infected or develop symptomatic infection. Resistance to other norovirus strains that are genetically distinct from Norwalk virus is not well understood. Norovirus infection induces short-term immunity (6 to 8 weeks) to reinfection and disease, but reinfection with the same strain 1 to 2 years later can again lead to gastroenteritis.

REPLICATION AND DAMAGE

The human noroviruses cannot be cultured in the laboratory, so knowledge about the pathogenesis of disease caused by these viruses has primarily come from volunteer studies. Norovirus gastroenteritis is generally considered to be mild and self-limiting, although illness can last from 24 to 48 hours and can be incapacitating during that time. A spectrum of clinical manifestations has been seen in adults infected with the same virus, with some adults having significant vomiting and diarrhea and others having only diarrhea or vomiting. Common symptoms (seen in more than 50% of patients) include nausea, abdominal cramps, diarrhea, vomiting, and malaise. Chills and fever occur less frequently. Bloody diarrhea does not occur. Small bowel biopsies of infected volunteers show villous blunting in the ileum and proximal jejunum, with the intestinal mucosa remaining intact. Gastric emptying is delayed, and malabsorption of fat, D-xylose, and lactose has been observed.

DIAGNOSIS

Currently, no commercial diagnostic assays for noroviruses are available in the United States, although there are new enzyme-linked immunosorbent assays available in Europe. The usual method for diagnosis of norovirus infection is by identification of the viral RNA in stools by using RT-PCR, assays. Electron microscopy, antigen detection in stool, and serologic diagnosis using paired sera also are used but are not available in most clinical laboratories.

TREATMENT AND PREVENTION

No specific treatments for norovirus-induced disease exist. Symptoms usually resolve without complications, and oral fluid and electrolyte replacement therapy is normally sufficient to manage fluid loss. If severe vomiting or diarrhea occurs, parenteral administration of fluids may be needed. Vaccines to prevent norovirus disease are being evaluated, but otherwise prevention relies on the same basic infection control measures described for rotavirus infections.

Other Enteric Viruses

Whereas rotaviruses and noroviruses are the most widely recognized causes of viral enteric infections, other agents are clearly important. **Adenoviruses** are best known as a cause of upper respiratory tract disease (see Chapter 39). However, two serotypes (40 and 41) are now recognized to cause diarrhea, especially in children who are less than 2 years of age. Outbreaks due to **sapoviruses**, another type of **calicivirus**, have been described, mainly in institutions. Based on the prevalence of specific antibodies, most individuals have been infected with those viruses by 12 years of age, but infections in adults are being recognized more frequently. **Astroviruses** are another group of viruses that cause enteric disease, primarily in children less than 5 years of age. **Aichi virus** is a **picornavirus** that causes disease in children and adults. Diagnostic assays for the adenoviruses, sapoviruses, astroviruses, and Aichi virus are not routinely available. Treatment for infections by those agents is supportive, similar to that described for the rotaviruses and noroviruses.

Conclusion

Rotaviruses and noroviruses are the most common causes of viral gastroenteritis worldwide. Rotavirus infections are almost universal in children; norovirus infections are associated with explosive outbreaks of disease. Both viruses are spread by the fecal–oral route. Rotaviruses and noroviruses contain RNA genomes and replicate in the cytoplasm of host cells. Virus replication leads to secretory diarrhea. Treatment of rotavirus and norovirus disease relies on fluid replacement. Vaccines are not currently available for rotaviruses and noroviruses. However, vaccine development is an active area of research.

chapter 38

Human Retroviruses: AIDS and Other Diseases

Robert T. Schooley

key concepts

Retroviruses:

- Are RNA viruses that contain the enzyme reverse transcriptase, which allows them to use RNA as a template to make DNA.

- Are capable of causing chronic disease long after initial infection because the viral DNA integrates with the host cell genome.

- Include HIV, the virus that causes AIDS; human T-cell lymphoma/leukemia virus 1 (HTLV-1), which is associated with leukemia and lymphoma; and HTLV-2.

HIV:

- Preferentially binds to the CD4 receptor found on helper T cells and monocytes; the destruction of these cells ultimately disables the immune system and makes the infected individual vulnerable to opportunistic infections.

- Is transmitted through sexual contact, injection drug use, and vertically (mother to child).

- Displays antigenic variation.

- Has a long latency period (average of 10 years).

- Can be suppressed by antiviral drugs but is otherwise nearly 100% fatal.

I n the decades since five previously healthy homosexual men were diagnosed with *Pneumocystis jiroveci* (formerly *P. carinii*) pneumonia in May 1981, AIDS has grown from an epidemiologically isolated medical condition to a worldwide epidemic of mammoth proportions. During the initial phase of the epidemic, it became apparent that the disease was likely caused by an infectious agent with a prolonged incubation period that could be transmitted sexually or parenterally (bloodborne). By 1983 initial reports linked the presence of a retrovirus (subsequently designated human immunodeficiency virus type 1, or HIV-1) to the syndrome, and the agent responsible for the illness had spread far beyond its initial epidemiological and geographic boundaries.

The number of AIDS cases in the United States and Europe rose steadily through the mid-1990s and then plateaued as the combined effects of antiretroviral chemotherapy and increasingly effective prevention efforts synergized to delay the onset of new cases and reduce transmission of the etiologic retrovirus. In contrast to the situation in the United States and Europe, the disease has continued to spread in resource-limited settings where it now exerts its most devastating medical and social effects. By the beginning of 2004 nearly 38 million people were living with HIV-1 (Fig. 38-1). The most cases are reported in sub-Saharan Africa, but the number of cases in Asia has been rising steadily.

Nearly 10% of people with HIV-1 succumb to the illness each year. Two attributes make AIDS unique among infectious diseases: it is uniformly fatal, and most of its devastating symptoms are not direct results of the causative agent. With suppression of the host immune response by HIV-1, opportunistic organisms cause a number of clinical syndromes. In fact, most symptoms seen in persons with AIDS result from secondary infections rather than the virus itself. The clinical manifestations of AIDS are described in Chapter 71.

Human Immunodeficiency Virus

Pathobiology

Structure

Retroviruses have a small, protein capsid surrounded by a lipid envelope (Fig. 38-2). The genome consists of a single-stranded, positive-sense RNA and is present in two identical copies in the virion. These molecules resemble eukaryotic messenger RNA (mRNA) because they contain a **cap structure** at the 5′ end and **poly A tail** at the 3′ end. Four viral genes are necessary for the replication of retroviruses (Fig. 38-3). The *gag* gene encodes several core (Gag) proteins. The *pro* gene encodes a protease necessary for cleaving the Gag and Pol polyproteins to their active forms. The *pol* gene encodes **reverse transcriptase** or **RNA-dependent DNA polymerase** (Pol), the enzyme responsible for making a DNA copy of the genome, as well as **integrase,** the enzyme necessary for integration of the DNA copy into the host cell genome. The *env* gene encodes the two **envelope glycoproteins.** Noncoding sequences include terminally redundant regions and unique regions near the ends of the genome.

Case

A baby boy, G., was born by cesarean section after a 36-week gestation to a 19-year-old commercial sex worker with AIDS. The mother had been diagnosed 4 years previously when she developed *Pneumocystis jiroveci* pneumonia, but she had not had regular medical care since that time. She came to the hospital in labor. The delivery staff did not immediately inquire about her past medical history because her labor was quite advanced; thus, her prior history of *P. jiroveci* pneumonia was not known until after the delivery.

IgG antibodies to HIV were detected in the infant by both an enzyme-linked immunosorbent assay and immunoblot (Western blot) analysis (see Chapter 58). By 4 months of age G. experienced poor weight gain, thrush (oral candidiasis), diffuse lymphadenopathy (enlargement of lymph nodes), and persistent diarrhea. HIV RNA and proviral DNA were detected in his peripheral blood, and a diagnosis of AIDS was made. Antiretroviral drugs were administered, and over several months G.'s symptoms disappeared and weight gain resumed.

This case raises several questions:

1. Was the presence of HIV antibodies in G.'s blood diagnostic for HIV infection?
2. What was the basis of the initial diagnosis?
3. How was the diagnosis confirmed?

Reverse transcriptase molecules are associated with the genome and are packaged in the virion.

In addition to the genes common to all retroviruses, *gag, pro, pol,* and *env,* the HIV genome contains at least six other genes (as discussed in the next section). These genes encode functions that are important in regulating the complex replication cycle of this virus, which may exist in a latent state in the infected cell and then undergo rapid replication at the appropriate time.

Life Cycle of the Virus

The replication cycle of HIV includes the following steps (Fig. 38-4):

- **Binding:** Once in close proximity to a **helper T lymphocyte,** HIV recognizes and binds to the **CD4 receptor** molecule via the gp120 portion of its envelope glycoprotein. Antibodies to either the viral envelope protein or the cell receptor block that interaction and prevent infection. The presence of the CD4 molecule on the cell surface, which plays an important role in immune function (see Chapter 7), determines the primary target cells for infection. After binding to the CD4 molecule, a secondary attachment event occurs in which the viral envelope binds to one of two coreceptor molecules (CCR5 or CXCR4). These molecules serve physiologically as receptors for chemokines, but

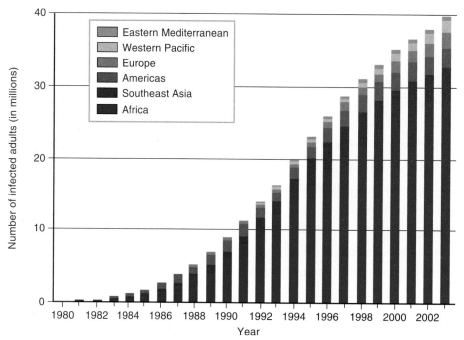

FIGURE 38-1 ▪ **Estimated number of individuals infected with HIV-1 by region, 1980–2003.** (From World Health Organization. The world health report 2004: changing history. Available at: http://www.who.int/whr/2004/en/ report04_en.pdf. Accessed October 28, 2005.)

in the case of HIV-1 infection, they facilitate tight binding of the virus to the cell membrane and induce a conformational change in the viral envelope glycoproteins bringing a hydrophobic domain of gp41 into approximation with the cell membrane.

- **Fusion:** Fusion of the viral envelope with the cell membrane is facilitated by a hydrophobic interaction between the viral envelope and the cell membrane. Following the fusion event, the virion loses its integrity and characteristic morphology. Genomic RNA within the virus core, which includes molecules of reverse transcriptase, is released into the cytoplasm.
- **Synthesis of DNA:** Reverse transcriptase synthesizes a complementary DNA molecule corresponding to the

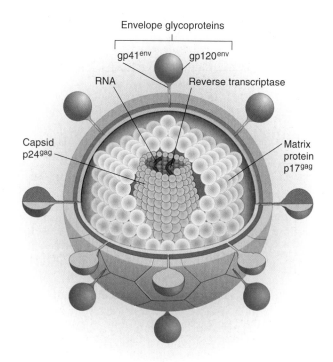

FIGURE 38-2 ▪ **Retrovirus structure.** A schematic drawing showing the virion proteins and other structures.

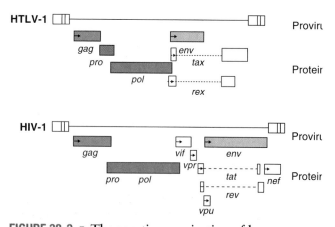

FIGURE 38-3 ▪ **The genetic organization of human retroviruses.** The top line in each group shows the provirus with control LTR sequences shown as boxes at the ends. The lower boxes indicate the location of the viral genes, with dotted boxes showing genes whose functions are uncertain. Notice that both of these viruses have genes in addition to those that encode viral proteins (*gag, pol,* and *env*).

CD4 receptor — Coreceptor

Penetration

Virus RNA

Reverse transcriptase

Double-stranded DNA

Host DNA — Integration into host DNA — Host DNA

Provirus

Transcription

Single-stranded RNA (viral messenger RNA and progeny RNA)

Translation

Viral proteins

Assembly

Nucleocapsid

Budding

Release

FIGURE 38-4 ▪ **The retrovirus replication cycle.**

viral RNA genome. The enzyme then synthesizes the second DNA strand (complementary to the first), generating a double-stranded DNA molecule. In the process of making the DNA, portions of the ends of the genomic RNA are copied twice, resulting in a structure at each end of the DNA called the **long terminal repeat (LTR).**

- **Integration:** The double-stranded DNA molecule is transported to the nucleus and integrated into the host cell genome. The virus-encoded enzyme integrase is responsible for that reaction, which involves joining the ends of each LTR to cellular DNA. The retrovirus inte-

gration process resembles the mechanism used by some transposable elements of bacteria (see Chapter 4). In the integrated state, viral genetic material is called the **provirus.** The provirus behaves like a cellular gene in that it is passed to daughter cells at cell division and contains signals that control its transcription into RNA.

- **Synthesis of progeny virus:** In the "productive phase," viral DNA is transcribed into messenger RNA by host cell DNA-dependent RNA polymerase. Signals that direct the host cell RNA synthetic machinery (promoters) are found in the LTR and resemble signals that the cell uses to make its own RNA. After transcription, some of these viral RNA molecules are used as mRNA for synthesis of viral proteins. Others become incorporated as genomes into progeny virus particles. Assembly of virions takes place at the cell surface. The structural proteins assemble with genomes and acquire their envelope by passage through the host cell membrane (Fig. 38-5). Following budding through the membrane, the viral protease cleaves the viral protein precursors (Gag and Gag-Pol), and morphological changes in the virion are observed.

- **Latency and transactivation:** In general, the replication cycle described so far is common to all retroviruses. HIV and some related viruses have additional features:
  - Infection can also involve a **latent** phase in which infected cells contain a provirus but do not express viral RNA or proteins.
  - Expression of HIV macromolecules is subject to regulation by viral gene products that operate as soluble elements (in "trans"). This phenomenon is known as **transactivation.** At least two HIV genes, called **tat** and **rev,** function as **transactivating factors,** which greatly increase the expression of viral RNAs and proteins. Tat enhances the production of RNA by host DNA-dependent RNA polymerase, and Rev affects the way that newly synthesized RNAs are processed and transported into the cytoplasm.
  - HIV proviruses contain promoters that can induce viral gene expression when HIV-infected cells are stimulated by antigen or infected by other viruses (such as herpesviruses). These features appear to be related in an important way: after infection of lymphocytes and integration of the provirus, the infection process may be halted and then reinitiated much later in an explosive way by unknown stimuli. The outcome is a high level of transactivation, resulting in a burst of virus production and rapid death of the cell. Although only a small fraction of infected cells enter the latent state, those cells can defeat attempts to eradicate infection by antiviral therapy, even when used for extended periods.
  - In addition to the regulatory effects of Tat and Rev, HIV-1 has other gene products that interact with host cell proteins to facilitate evasion of virus-specific immune responses and intracellular protective mechanisms that can limit virus replication. For example, the **Nef** protein downregulates the presence of major

FIGURE 38-5 ▪ **Electron micrographs showing successive stages in the assembly and budding of HTLV-1 (upper panels) and HIV-1 (lower panels).** Panels a, b, and c show sequential stages of the assembly and budding process. Notice the difference in the structure of the mature cores of the two types of viruses in panels c.

histocompatibility complex (MHC) class I molecules on the surface of cells responsible for presenting antigen to virus-specific cytotoxic T cells. Another protein (**Vif**) facilitates destruction of a cellular protein (APOBEC 3G) capable of blocking reverse transcription when packaged within the virus particle.

Antigenic Variation

A unique characteristic of infection by HIV is that the immune response of the host is unable to completely curtail virus replication (although it may be important in partially suppressing it during the latent phase of the disease). That characteristic is a paradox because for most other viral infections the presence of antibody indicates immunity, protection from infection, and a favorable prognosis. How is HIV able to survive despite the host immune response? Several mechanisms may be at work: viral gene products may be relatively invisible to the immune response; the virus may be able to mask or change its antigenic specificity; and the virus may primarily replicate in lymphoid follicles, locations within lymphoid tissues in which virus-directed immune cells do not migrate freely.

Which HIV gene products are important in directing the immune response of the host? A clue comes from studies of the genetic diversity of the viral genes. HIV genes that encode internal viral proteins (*gag* and *pol*) show relative stability from one isolate to the next, but the *env* gene displays frequent mutations that lead to variations in its products, the surface and transmembrane glycoproteins. Although antibodies to the Gag and Pol proteins are found in infected individuals, these antibodies do not

seem to be important in containing the infection. Some antibodies to the envelope proteins, on the other hand, can neutralize the virus. However, titers of these antibodies are very low compared with other viral infections. HIV envelope glycoproteins have two unusual features. First, they are extensively coated with polysaccharide side chains that, because they are added by host enzymes, are antigenically invisible to the host. Second, they contain **hypervariable regions** that permit the virus to present new antigenic configurations. In contrast, segments of the surface glycoprotein that are involved in interactions with cellular receptors must be conserved. Conserved segments may be hidden and protected from neutralizing antibodies by the carbohydrates and the hypervariable regions. As a result, HIV can constantly vary its surface antigenic composition, which may allow it to avoid inactivation. Thus, HIV resembles influenza viruses and trypanosomes of sleeping sickness in its capacity to withstand the immune response by changing major surface antigens. Such a mechanism hinders the development of an effective vaccine.

ENCOUNTER

The distribution of HIV infection in the population is consistent with an agent that is extremely labile and cannot readily enter through intact body surfaces. In that respect HIV resembles (but is much less contagious than) hepatitis B virus, which has a similar epidemiological pattern in the United States. HIV has been detected in a number of body fluids, including peripheral blood, semen,

History of Retroviruses

Understanding the role of retroviruses as the etiologic agent of AIDS requires a historical detour through the puzzling connection between viruses and cancer. This history includes a challenge to a traditional tenet of molecular biology that genetic information flows from DNA through RNA intermediates to protein. In the late 1960s researchers identified an unusual class of viruses that carried genetic information in molecules of RNA. Although RNA-containing viruses were not a novelty, the newly discovered viruses were unique because they contained the formerly unrecognized enzyme called reverse transcriptase. Using RNA as a template, the enzyme reverses the conventional flow of genetic information by synthesizing a copy of complementary DNA that ultimately integrates into the genome of the host cell. The DNA, called the provirus, serves as an intermediate stage in the replicative cycle.

Some of the newfound viruses (now called retroviruses in recognition of their reverse or "retro" mode of replication) are capable of causing tumors. A virus of this type was first isolated in 1911, when Peyton Rous reported that tumors in chickens could be caused by a virus (later known as Rous sarcoma virus, or RSV) readily transmissible by filtered extracts. Since then hundreds of retroviruses have been isolated from many groups of vertebrates. In the early 1960s a cancer-inducing virus was discovered in cats. Now called feline leukemia virus, the discovery proved to be important in understanding the biology of retroviruses for two reasons. First, the virus induces in cats an immunodeficiency similar to the one later observed in humans with AIDS. Second, feline leukemia virus is transmitted among cats in a household setting, providing a valuable model for epidemiological analysis of retrovirus infection.

Until the late 1960s, considerable skepticism surrounded the theory that a virus could mediate the transmission of cancer. Because cancer appeared to be a genetic alteration, it was difficult to conceive how an RNA-containing virus could interact with the DNA of the host cell to produce oncogenic changes. The discovery of reverse transcriptase suggested a mechanism for the induction of permanent genetic change.

Since 1980 two groups of retroviruses capable of causing disease in humans have been isolated and characterized (Table 38-1). For several years before 1980, researchers suspected that retroviruses might be agents of human disease, but the point could not be proved because these viruses did not grow in cultured cells. Several advances in cell culture technology overcame that obstacle. One of the most important was the discovery of interleukin 2 (IL-2), which stimulates the

table **38-1**	**Pathogenic Human Retroviruses**
HTLV Group	
HTLV-1	Causative agent of certain cutaneous T-cell lymphomas and HTLV-1 myelopathy (also called tropical spastic paraparesis)
HTLV-2	Not conclusively linked to a specific disease; found in cases of hairy cell leukemia
Lentiviruses	
HIV-1	Causative agent of AIDS
HIV-2	Related to but distinct from HIV-1; described as a cause of AIDS, particularly in West Africa

HTLV, human T-cell lymphoma/leukemia virus.

growth of T lymphocytes in vitro. These lymphocytes could then be used for the isolation of human T-cell lymphoma/leukemia viruses (HTLVs).

The first of these viruses, HTLV-1, was isolated from the cells of two patients with adult T-cell lymphoma. Subsequent HTLV-1 isolates from other patients with leukemia were shown to be closely related, as determined by serology and nucleic acid hybridization. Epidemiological studies suggested a causal relationship between a childhood infection with HTLV-1 and the development of lymphoma in a small percentage of infected individuals as many as 40 years later. A similar virus, HTLV-2, was later isolated from a patient with hairy cell leukemia, but its role in human disease is less clear. The malignant diseases caused by HTLV-1, adult T-cell leukemia and lymphoma, are uniformly fatal but are relatively rare (even in infected individuals) and have been limited to certain specific populations. HTLV-1 infection also has been associated with certain progressive spinal cord diseases, such as tropical spastic paraparesis and HTLV-1–associated myelopathy.

HTLV-1 attracted considerable attention, both because it was the first known human retrovirus and because of the novel features of its biology. Although the virus is uncommon in the United States, concerns about the spread of HTLV-1 through the blood supply have resulted in routine screening of donated blood for the presence of the virus. Fortuitously, studies of HTLV-1 provided the technology needed for the isolation of the AIDS agent several years later. Thus, AIDS was shown to be caused by a retrovirus within three years after the disease was first described in 1981. When first isolated, the virus had several names, but it is now known as human immunodeficiency virus, or HIV.

cervical secretions, breast milk, urine, cerebrospinal fluid, saliva, and tears (the last four of which do not represent important means of transmission). With few exceptions HIV transmission occurs by one of three routes: sexual contact, injection drug use, and vertical passage from infected mothers to offspring. In 1991 homosexual and bisexual men accounted for approximately 70% of AIDS cases in the United States (including 8% who were also injection drug users). Since that time men who have sex with men have represented a progressively smaller proportion of total cases, and injection drug use and heterosexual transmission have become more important, especially among people of color. Injection drug users have become the second-largest group with HIV infection in the United States, about 25% of total cases. Importantly, this group acts as a bridge for the spread of HIV infection to the heterosexual population. Transmission among drug users occurs by sharing contaminated needles and syringes that contain residues of blood (including infected white blood cells) from previous users.

HIV transmission by blood transfusion has been exceedingly rare since March 1985, when routine screening of blood products was instituted. Hemophiliacs have long been identified as a group at risk for bloodborne viruses such as hepatitis B and C viruses because they receive preparations of factor VIII and factor IX obtained from plasma pooled from thousands of donors. Since 1984 factor VIII concentrates have been unlikely to contain HIV because blood donors are screened for HIV antibodies. In addition, since 1984 plasma products have been treated with heat and chemicals to inactivate contaminating viruses. Approximately 80% of recipients of factor VIII before 1984 are now infected with HIV or deceased.

Vaginal intercourse can result in HIV transmission to partners of either gender, although the risk is somewhat higher for women. The lower rate of transmission of HIV from females to males versus males to females is not fully understood. Vaginal transmission from females to males may occur less frequently due to unfavorable factors for HIV survival in the vagina and because such transmission may require penile ulcerations or damage to the male urethral mucosa. Transmission rates to long-term heterosexual partners of AIDS patients vary widely, from less than 10% to 70%. In some instances transmission occurs after only one or two sexual contacts. However, the low transmission rate seen in spouses of HIV-infected hemophiliacs suggests that, in many instances, the virus is not easily transmitted even over a period of several years.

Variation in the rate of HIV transfer from infected to uninfected partners implies that genetic factors may influence susceptibility to infection. One such factor has been identified as the gene encoding CCR5, a chemokine receptor that serves as a coreceptor for HIV. The defective form of this gene is found in about 10% of individuals of European descent, but it is much less frequent in other populations. In the 1% of this group who are homozygous, it confers a very high (although not absolute) level of resistance to HIV infection. Heterozygous individuals are not protected from infection but seem to have a slower rate of progression to AIDS. Individuals with high levels of HIV in plasma—those with acute HIV infection and those in the later stages of illness in which viral titers generally rise—are more likely to transmit the virus to sexual partners.

Heterosexual transmission is now the most common mode of HIV spread in most countries other than the United States and northern Europe. For example, the overall ratio of male-to-female AIDS cases in sub-Saharan Africa is approximately 1:1 as opposed to 13:1 in the United States. Regardless of differences in rates of transmission in the various groups, the prevention of major heterosexual epidemics must focus on all young, sexually active individuals. In many areas of Africa, AIDS is now the leading cause of death among adult males.

Congenital transmission, as in the case of the baby boy G., is the most important route of transmission of pediatric AIDS. The Centers for Disease Control and Prevention estimates that between 1978 and 1993, 15,000 newborns in the United States acquired HIV infection by vertical transmission. Since the recognition that intervention with antiretroviral drugs can interrupt maternofetal transmission, new cases of pediatric AIDS have fallen sharply in the United States and Europe. In the absence of such intervention, between 25 and 33% of HIV-infected women transmit HIV-1 to their children. When infection of the mother is recognized and antiretroviral intervention is employed in the mother and child, the transmission rate falls to less than 1% of births.

Although HIV transmission among health care workers is an area of particular concern, extensive studies have confirmed that HIV transmission in medical settings is exceedingly rare. The risk of infection following accidental injury with needles used to draw blood from HIV-infected patients is less than 0.3%. The risk from exposure to mucous membranes or by contamination of intact skin is considerably less. With the general adoption of "universal precautions," which assume that blood or other fluids from all patients are potentially infectious, HIV spread to health care workers should remain rare. Its rate can be reduced still further by immediate postexposure treatment with a combination of antiviral drugs. The spread of HIV from health care workers to patients is even less frequent. Spread of HIV among nonsexual household contacts or coworkers is exceedingly rare. More than 12 studies involving over 700 family members or boarding school contacts of persons with AIDS failed to detect a single instance of transmission. Although arthropod vectors have been proposed as a route of transmission, no evidence supports that theory. If arthropods, such as mosquitoes or ticks, were important carriers of the virus, children in developing countries would be frequently infected, as they are often victims of bites. In fact, the occurrence of AIDS in children outside recognized risk groups is highly unusual, making vectors an unlikely mechanism of transmission.

ENTRY, SPREAD, AND REPLICATION

The mechanism by which HIV establishes an infection in the host is poorly understood because of the variable course of the disease and the scarcity of infected cells, especially during the long, latent phase of infection. HIV may enter the host as part of infected cells, such as macrophages, lymphocytes, or spermatozoa, or as free virus. Entrance to the body can be through microabrasions on the surface of mucous membranes, penetration of intact skin with a needle, or exposure to grossly intact mucosal surfaces.

The two major groups of cells in the body that serve as preferred targets for infection by HIV are helper T lymphocytes and monocytes. The surfaces of these cells contain CD4, which serves as the receptor necessary for virus entry, as well as appropriate coreceptors (Fig. 38-6). Most of our knowledge about HIV replication comes from studies using cells derived from human T-cell tumors, which can be grown in the laboratory.

DAMAGE

The molecular events that modulate lymphocyte damage in HIV-infected persons have not been fully elucidated.

However, on the basis of known abnormalities in humoral and cellular immunity, it is possible to outline a sequence of events that follow HIV infection.

Infection and Depletion of Helper T Cells

Because of its primary receptor, HIV preferentially infects helper T cells—that is lymphocytes that express the CD4 surface protein or monocytes that also express that receptor. During acute HIV-1 infection, the virus infects helper T cells within local mucosal surfaces and then rapidly establishes infection in local lymphoid tissues. The virus quickly disseminates, systemically infecting remote lymphoid tissues as well as the central nervous system in a brush fire of infection during which the virus exhibits some of its highest replication rates in the natural history of the disease. The virus quickly appears in genital secretions, and as in many other infectious diseases, the propensity to transmit the virus may be highest during this initial phase of infection. The infected individual may be asymptomatic at this stage or may manifest fever, headache, malaise, and an evanescent rash. These symptoms can be confused with acute infectious mononucleosis.

Within weeks of the initial infection, virus-specific cytotoxic T cells appear in the peripheral blood and lymphoid tissue, and shortly thereafter neutralizing antibodies may be detected in the plasma. During this period of rapid virus replication, the lifelong process of virus diversification is initiated. The host is confronted with the challenge of developing an adequate immune

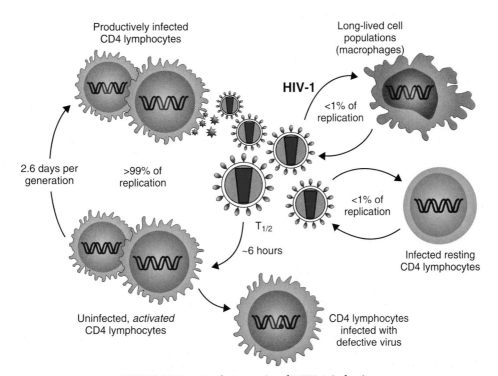

FIGURE 38-6 ■ Pathogenesis of HIV-1 infection.

response to a rapidly changing virus at the same time the virus is destroying the CD4 cell pool—especially virus-specific CD4 cells—that is required to drive and shape the immune response. Because HIV-1 reverse transcriptase has an error rate of about 1 in 10,000 bases copied, on average a new base is introduced into the virus with each replication cycle. Up to a billion virus replication cycles occur in each HIV-1 infected person each day, resulting in enormous implications for the emergence of viral variants at both the individual and population levels. For example, in the case of the viral envelope, virus diversity can occur at such a rate that 15 new amino acid changes become fixed within the host each year.

Infected cells can be killed directly by virus replication or indirectly by virus-specific immune effector mechanisms (primarily HIV-1-specific cytotoxic T cells or antibody dependent cellular cytotoxicity). After the first several months of infection, a balance is established among virus replication, immune effector mechanisms, and cells available for virus replication, and the infection enters its chronic phase during which the patient is generally asymptomatic. The so-called set point to which virus replication settles following acute infection is the most important determinant of the rate of disease progression within an infected individual. After the initial primary phase of HIV infection, virus replication is confined largely to the lymphoid organs, where activated CD4 lymphocytes are the primary target in which approximately 99% of virus replication is thought to occur (see Fig. 38.6). The remaining 1% of virus replication occurs in monocytes and resting CD4 cells, which are the cell populations responsible for virus latency.

Loss of the CD4 cell population results in progressive immunodeficiency that ultimately leads to severe opportunistic infections and malignancies. Although great variation exists between infected individuals, the duration of the symptom-free period before the appearance of AIDS-defining infections is approximately 10 years. During that interval, CD4 counts drop from the normal level of about 1,000 to less than 500 cells/μL^3. Patients with advanced HIV disease usually have CD4 counts of less than 200 cells/μL^3. The risk of opportunistic infections is greatest in late-stage AIDS, when the CD4 count drops to fewer than 50 cells/μL^3. Serial measurements of CD4 cell counts serve as indicators for the risk of such infections, as well as a guide for the management of antiretroviral therapy.

The rate of immunological and clinical progression is directly related to the extent of virus replication, and it varies considerably from individual to individual. Virus replication rates within the host are highly correlated with the number of copies of HIV-1 RNA in plasma as quantitated by polymerase chain reaction (PCR) technology. Individuals with high viral loads (10^5 copies/mL or more) are at greater risk for disease progression within a few years; infected individuals with lower loads (less than 10^4 copies/mL) may not progress to AIDS for 10 years or more.

Damage to and depletion of helper T cells during HIV replication results in a characteristic change in the ratio of helper/suppressor cytotoxic cells. Depletion of helper T cells results in a reduction in total circulating lymphocytes (lymphopenia) and a relative increase in the number of suppressor cytotoxic lymphocytes. In addition to quantitative T-cell deficits, HIV induces abnormalities in T-cell function. Normally, T cells modulate the function of other cells in the immune system, including B cells, monocytes, and natural killer cells. Although many patients with AIDS have elevated immunoglobulin levels in their sera, their ability to produce antibodies against specific antigens may be impaired. For example, children with HIV infection do not generate antibodies against the specific capsular polysaccharide antigens of *Streptococcus pneumoniae* and *Haemophilus influenzae* type B. This defect may be due to direct impairment of B lymphocytes as well as to the loss of helper T lymphocytes.

The specific CD4 marker characteristic of helper T lymphocytes is also expressed by other cell types, including circulating monocytes and macrophages, natural killer cells, certain B lymphocytes, and cells of the central nervous system, such as glial cells. These cells also may become infected and damaged by virus replication or may serve as a reservoir for virus latency. Defects in killing secondary invading microorganisms may be attributes of HIV infection of macrophages and monocytes, which are likely augmented by the loss of helper T cells. Furthermore, macrophage-related cells called Langerhans cells, which form part of epithelial surfaces, have been found to be highly sensitive to HIV and may be an important entry point for sexually transmitted infection.

Some Clinical Consequences

AIDS represents the terminal stage of infection by HIV. Clinical syndromes vary with different stages of infection. Primary HIV infection may be associated with a mononucleosis-like illness that develops a few weeks following exposure. The infected individual then usually becomes asymptomatic, but HIV-specific antibodies can be detected in serum, and virus replication continues during a period of clinical latency that is variable from person to person but averages 8 to 10 years. As virus replication proceeds and CD4 cells are depleted, the infected individual may remain completely asymptomatic or may develop persistent generalized lymphadenopathy. Lymphadenopathy may persist or resolve before progressing over months to years to pre-AIDS conditions characterized by diarrhea, oral candidiasis, weight loss, and fever.

HIV-infected individuals will eventually progress to AIDS with opportunistic infections or malignancies, such as Kaposi sarcoma or B-cell lymphomas. The specific distribution of AIDS-associated opportunistic infections that cause morbidity in a given population is highly dependent on the background prevalence of these pathogens in the population infected with HIV-1. For example, in the United States and Europe *Pneumocystis jiroveci* pneumonia is the most common initial clinical manifestation in patients not receiving prophylaxis for this agent; in Zimbabwe, *Mycobacterium tuberculosis* is the most common clinical manifestation. A significant fraction of adult AIDS patients also develop neurologic symptoms. Neurologic manifestations of AIDS may be due to virus replication in the central nervous system or secondary infection by opportunistic organisms such as the protozoan *Toxoplasma gondii* or the fungus *Cryptococcus neoformans*. Neurologic manifestations of AIDS also can be caused by development of malignancies in the central nervous system. It is not known whether damage to brain cells is caused by the release of toxic substances from monocytes or by direct damage to brain tissue by replicating virus.

The single most important factor in the development of AIDS in HIV-infected individuals is time. In the absence of antiretroviral chemotherapy, most if not all HIV-infected individuals will ultimately develop AIDS. More than 95% of HIV-infected persons progress to AIDS within 15 years of infection. The remaining small fraction of long-term nonprogressors have very low viral loads and may survive for very long periods, perhaps indefinitely. Several factors affect survival rates, including virulence determinants and host factors such as age, gender, and immune status. Effective antiretroviral chemotherapy (as assessed by the use of antiretroviral drugs that drive HIV-1 RNA levels in the plasma to levels below the current limits of detection [50 copies/mL]) may reverse immunologic progression and delay the onset of symptoms indefinitely.

Paradigm **Box**

New Epidemics of Infectious Diseases

How do new epidemics of infectious diseases arise? In some cases, such as influenza virus, the virus is already present in the human or animal population and undergoes antigenic change to produce new, more virulent strains. In other instances, the agent is present as a relatively innocuous commensal in animals, and by a genetic change it becomes virulent in humans.

In the case of the AIDS epidemic, considerable genetic evidence suggests that viruses related to HIV have existed in nonhuman primate populations for a long time. The prevailing evidence is that retroviruses similar to HIV-1 were present in primate (simian) species and that the strain most like HIV-1, termed SIV$_{cpz}$, was carried by chimpanzees. In that host the virus appears to be less pathogenic than in humans. Several transmissions of the virus from chimpanzees to humans are thought to have occurred in equatorial West Africa in the early part of the twentieth century, probably in association with the butchering of chimpanzees for food. The most important variable that has accounted for the rapid global spread of HIV-1 is increasing travel, which presented the virus an opportunity to become established in the human population and be transmitted widely by sexual intercourse and mother-to-infant spread.

Will the AIDS epidemic ever come to an end? The AIDS epidemic of today has a vivid historical parallel.

At the end of the fifteenth century, an apparently new disease, syphilis, swept through Europe in epidemic proportions. For the first 60 years of its history, syphilis was a very different illness from that we now know: instead of progressing (if untreated) to the chronic manifestations of the tertiary stage, syphilis at that time was an acute disease with a high mortality rate. We do not know what caused the abrupt change in the pathological picture of syphilis, but this is a likely scenario: For any disease that is spread directly among humans, an agent that causes death of the host eliminates infected contacts. As a result, transmission of the agent is greatly reduced. Eventually, the deadly strain of the agent will be supplanted by a milder one that causes a chronic illness and thus has a greater chance of being transmitted to new hosts.

The hypothesized course of syphilis just described may in fact have occurred for HIV or HIV-like viruses in monkeys and apes. AIDS in humans, on the other hand, is unlikely to result in such a balanced situation any time in the near future. An HIV-infected person can be the source of transmission of the virus over a long period. Thus, the biological basis for the abatement of the AIDS epidemic is not at all obvious. Interrupting the AIDS epidemic cannot depend on evolutionary changes in either the host or the virus, but it will require effective antiviral vaccination or chemotherapy.

DIAGNOSIS

Before the viral etiologic agent was identified, the diagnosis of AIDS was based solely on clinical findings. The presence of specific opportunistic infections or certain tumors such as Kaposi sarcoma in high-risk groups was necessary before the disease could be suspected. Patients in the early stages of infection could not be identified. In 1993 the Centers for Disease Control and Prevention issued revised criteria for a **case definition of AIDS** based on the presence or absence of laboratory evidence of HIV infection and either a CD4 lymphocyte count less than 200/μL; or the presence of an AIDS-defining opportunistic illness (see the box titled "AIDS-defining Opportunistic Infections in HIV-Infected Individuals Over 13 Years of Age"). Evidence of infection is generally based on the presence of antibodies to HIV. The presence of virus in blood or tissues can be documented by growth of the virus in cell culture or by molecular methods, such as PCR assays that detect viral genetic material. Serologic tests for HIV infection detect HIV-specific antibodies in serum. The ability to grow HIV in culture provided the antigens that made such tests possible. It is now clear that close to 100% of HIV-infected individuals have measurable antibodies in sera. The exceptions are a small group of individuals either in the earliest stages of the disease (before seroconversion) or even more rarely in the terminal stages (when B cells are unable to synthesize antibodies). On very rare occasions, certain individuals may "serorevert" (lose detectable antibodies while still carrying the virus). Therefore, in a limited number of circumstances the absence of antibodies does not completely exclude HIV infection. The persistence of detectable antibodies specific for HIV is generally accepted as an indication of infection and the ability to transmit the virus.

Initial tests for HIV serology generally are performed by using an enzyme-linked immunosorbent assay (ELISA). If the serum is found to be positive for HIV antibodies, the test is usually repeated and confirmed by a secondary antibody test such as an immunoblot (Western blot). See Chapter 58 for a full discussion of ELISA, immunoblots, and diagnostic principles.

The ELISA test has a false-positive rate of less than 0.1%. With confirmatory immunoblot tests, the joint false-positive rate approaches a remarkable 0.005%. Before the advent of effective antiretroviral therapy, it was necessary to carefully weigh whether low-risk individuals should be tested. The impact of a positive test result on a person's state of mind, social interactions, marriage, insurance eligibility, and employment opportunities is enormous. It is now recognized that the beneficial effects of initiating anti-HIV therapy before the onset of AIDS clearly justifies testing of individuals at risk for HIV infection.

AIDS-Defining Opportunistic Infections in HIV-Infected Individuals Over 13 Years of Age

- Candidiasis of the trachea, bronchi, or lungs
- Esophageal candidiasis
- Disseminated coccidioidomycosis
- Extrapulmonary cryptococcosis
- Chronic cryptosporidiosis, with diarrhea for more than 1 month
- Cytomegalovirus infection (other than liver, spleen, or nodes)
- Cytomegalovirus retinitis (with vision loss)
- HIV encephalopathy
- Herpes simplex: chronic ulcers for more than 1 month, or bronchitis, pneumonia, or esophagitis
- Disseminated or extrapulmonary histoplasmosis
- Isosporiasis, with diarrhea for more than 1 month
- Kaposi sarcoma
- Non-Hodgkin lymphoma of B cell or unknown phenotype, including Burkitt lymphoma
- Primary lymphoma of the brain
- Disseminated *Mycobacterium avium* complex or *M. kansasii*
- *Mycobacterium tuberculosis*, either pulmonary or extrapulmonary
- Other disseminated or extrapulmonary mycobacterial infections
- *Pneumocystis jiroveci* pneumonia
- Recurrent pneumonia
- Progressive multifocal leukoencephalopathy
- Recurrent *Salmonella* septicemia
- Toxoplasmosis of the brain
- Wasting syndrome owing to HIV
- Invasive cervical cancer

PREVENTION

Control of HIV transmission has proved to be difficult because a vaccine is not yet available. Effective control of the disease requires a reduction in sexual activities associated with virus transmission or cessation of the use of contaminated needles or syringes associated with injection drug use. Education is an important means of reducing the spread of AIDS at the present time. The most important measures include curtailing high-risk practices, such as multiple sexual contacts for both homosexual and heterosexual persons; awareness of the danger of anal intercourse; and the use of uncontaminated needles for injection drug users.

Evidence that education has an impact on sexual practices comes from experience in the gay community in San Francisco as well as in heterosexual persons in resource-limited countries where governments have openly dealt with the epidemic. Although not yet proven, effective integration of prevention and treatment programs will likely be even more successful in reducing spread of the virus. Making medical care available to those who need it acts as an incentive for individuals to submit to voluntary testing for HIV infection. Prevention messages targeted at the infected population can only be effective when those individuals are identified. Moreover, persons using effective antiretroviral therapy are less infectious, further slowing spread of the disease.

What problems are encountered in designing an AIDS vaccine? The capacity of HIV to change its antigenicity complicates conventional approaches to vaccine development and presents perhaps the most serious barrier to effective vaccine development. Since the initial introductions of HIV-1 into the human population 70 to 80 years ago, the virus has diversified widely into multiple types, subtypes, and recombinant viruses. Early results with viral envelope proteins prepared by genetic engineering techniques have failed to prevent virus transmission in phase 3 clinical trials in humans. Although it is clear that vigorous virus-specific immune responses develop during the course of infection, and that these immune responses are partially effective in controlling virus replication, it is not clear which (if any) of these immune responses are associated with reductions in acquisition of the virus. Furthermore, recent data indicating that superinfection with multiple strains of virus among highly exposed individuals occurs with a frequency approaching 50%, despite the presence of antiviral immune responses, should provide a sobering reminder that it is possible that an effective AIDS vaccine may not be developed for several decades, if at all.

Nonetheless, the challenge of AIDS vaccine development has been met with a number of innovative approaches for antigen presentation and has scientifically revitalized the field of vaccinology. These efforts must be vigorously supported, but enthusiasm for the development of an effective vaccine must not attenuate current efforts in prevention and treatment. If a vaccine is developed, modifying public health strategies to encourage vaccination will be much easier than to facing the long-term consequences of inadequate investments in these areas.

TREATMENT

Over the past 20 years major progress has been made in the development of antiretroviral therapy (see Chapter 44). Because the life cycle of retroviruses is intimately connected with the replication of mammalian cells, only a limited number of metabolic reactions can be singled out for inhibition by specific therapeutic agents. Reverse transcriptase is an attractive target because inhibition of this enzyme should have no effect on the host cell. Several FDA-approved anti-HIV drugs inhibit this unique virus function. Zidovudine (azidothymidine, or AZT) was the first of several dideoxynucleotides to be tested in clinical trials. Other approved drugs in this category include didanosine (ddI), emtricitabine (FTC), lamivudine (3TC), stavudine (d4T), tenofovir, and zalcitabine (ddC). These drugs inhibit reverse transcriptase after being phosphorylated intracellularly. Inhibition takes place by premature termination of growing strands of DNA into which the drugs have been incorporated. Mammalian DNA polymerases are more resistant to these drugs than viral reverse transcriptase.

A second class of reverse transcriptase inhibitors, the nonnucleoside reverse transcriptase inhibitors (NNRTIs), act by directly binding to the enzyme at a site away from the active site. That class includes the drugs delavirdine, efavirenz, and nevirapine.

A third class of antiviral drugs approved for use against HIV comprises inhibitors of the viral protease, such as amprenavir, indinavir, nelfinavir, ritonavir, saquinavir, and lopinavir/ritonavir. These drugs do not affect early stages of virus replication but rather prevent cleavage of viral proteins into their mature, active forms. Drugs in a fourth class of antivirals prevent viral envelope fusion with the host cell membrane. The first of these agents (enfuvirtide) has entered clinical practice.

The use of all antiviral agents is limited by the development of resistance. Any of the antivirals individually is capable of rapidly and effectively halting most or all virus replication in the body. However, in virtually all cases of monotherapy, virus replication rapidly rebounds and remains resistant to further treatment with the same or related compounds. Much more durable results, with strong suppression of virus replication combined with marked clinical improvement, can be achieved in most HIV-infected individuals by using combinations of three or four agents with diverse mechanisms of action. The use of such regimens, tailored for individual safety and adherence, can drive virus replication rates below the limit of detection, as assessed by currently available tests, and should be successful for many years. Additional improvement in the condition of many persons with AIDS has been achieved by therapy directed at preventing and treating opportunistic infections (see Chapter 71).

Conclusion

AIDS is a uniquely devastating disease: it kills all those who exhibit symptoms. It is a chronic illness, often manifested years after the virus is acquired and after the individual has had the opportunity to transmit it. In the United States the number of new AIDS cases has stabilized in recent years, and the number of AIDS deaths is declining because of the use of potent antiretroviral drug combinations.

By inactivating a central cellular component of the immune system, the helper T lymphocyte, HIV produces severe impairment of both humoral and cellular immunity. The disease is lethal because the defense mechanisms against opportunistic pathogens are eradicated. Diseases that were practically unseen before AIDS (e.g., encephalitis caused by *T. gondii*), or under reasonable control (e.g., mycobacterial infections), have become common and highly dangerous among persons with AIDS.

AIDS runs counter to the tenet that a successful parasite does not cause lethal injury to its host, suggesting that HIV may be a relative newcomer among human pathogens. The disease appeared suddenly in the United States, and its etiology was established with remarkable speed. Researchers have acquired a great deal of knowledge about HIV and other retroviruses, but many of the features of the disease are still inexplicable. The virus is particularly elusive to immunotherapeutic approaches because of variability in surface antigens and other features of its structure and replication.

Prolonging survival among those who have acquired the virus presents a major challenge. In the absence of an effective vaccine or curative treatment, prevention of HIV transmission among uninfected members of the population depends on education about the mechanisms of virus spread.

Adenoviruses

Gary Ketner

key concepts

Adenoviruses:

- Most often cause mild infections of the respiratory and gastrointestinal systems. More severe infections caused by adenoviruses include epidemic keratoconjunctivitis and an acute, severe form of pneumonia. Disseminated adenovirus infections can be fatal in immunocompromised individuals.

- Are large, nonenveloped, DNA-containing viruses with icosahedral symmetry.

- Express their genes following penetration into the host cell in three phases: immediate-early, early, and late.

- Employ both virally encoded and host proteins in the replication process.

- Can evade antiviral host defenses by multiple mechanisms, including preventing host cells from expressing major histocompatibility complex proteins, inducing resistance to tumor necrosis factor, and abrogating the interferon response.

- Have oncogenic potential owing to interactions between viral proteins and cellular tumor suppressor proteins.

Adenoviruses are among the most common causes of viral disease. They frequently cause acute respiratory diseases that range in severity from a sore throat to serious pneumonia and can cause diarrhea in children. Adenoviruses also are a common cause of eye infections. Adenoviruses comprise many serotypes associated with various disease manifestations (Table 39-1). A healthy person can harbor an adenovirus for a long period, and adenoviruses are often isolated from the tonsils, adenoids, and stool of asymptomatic individuals. People with persistent infections can shed adenoviruses over months or years.

Case

Over a period of 3 months, 83 patients who had visited an ophthalmologist's office in Erie, Pennsylvania, reported redness of the eyes, eyelid swelling with discharge, photophobia, and change in vision. Only two of those patients had fever or diarrhea. The patients ranged in age from 18 to 89 years, and all had visited the office between 3 and 29 days before the onset of symptoms. Eventually, all the patients recovered spontaneously. No further outbreaks were reported after ophthalmologist's office instituted preventive measures, including reducing the use of procedures that required instruments.

Epidemiologists from the Centers for Disease Control and Prevention in Atlanta studied the Erie outbreak of **epidemic keratoconjunctivitis** and documented the presence of adenovirus serotype 37 in 20 of the 22 patients from whom specimens were obtained. The procedures used were immunofluorescence microscopy of eye specimens and viral culture using human kidney cells. The virus also was found in the ophthalmologist's office. Virus was isolated from instruments used to measure visual acuity, work surfaces, eye drops, and the air-conditioning filter. Neither the ophthalmologist nor members of the staff tested positive for the virus or for specific antibodies.

This case raises several questions:

1. What was the source of the virus that caused the disease?
2. Why did the disease resolve spontaneously?
3. What measures helped prevent further spread of the disease?
4. Why were the medical personnel in the ophthalmologist's office not affected?

■ ■ ■ ■ ■

Adenoviruses most frequently cause **mild infections of the respiratory and digestive systems.** These infections resemble those caused by other agents and usually remain undiagnosed. Much of our knowledge of adenovirus infection stems from **outbreaks** such as the one

table 39-1	Association of Adenovirus Infections With Specific Phenotypes
DISEASE	**COMMON ADENOVIRUS SEROTYPES**
Respiratory infections	1, 2, 5, 6
Pharyngoconjunctivitis	3, 7, 14
Acute respiratory disease	4, 7, 21
Gastrointestinal infection	40, 41
Associated with celiac disease	12
Conjunctivitis	2, 3, 5, 7, 8, 19, 21
Epidemic keratoconjunctivitis	8, 19, 37

described in the case. Outbreaks of adenoviruses that lead to eye infections are frequently reported, indicating that transmission from a contaminated environment (instruments, surfaces, etc.) readily occurs. Other outbreaks of eye infections (**"pink eye"**) can be caused by contaminated swimming pools. The most serious outbreaks of adenoviral infections are seen among military recruits in the form of serious acute pneumonia. Crowding and physical stress appear to contribute to the occurrence of such outbreaks, which can be controlled by vaccination.

For all their disease importance, adenoviruses are common human commensals and relatively mild human pathogens. Although their pathogenic mechanisms are not well known, a great deal is known about their structure and mode of replication. Emphasis in this chapter is on basic aspects of the replicative strategy of adenoviruses, which serves as a well-studied example of replication among the large DNA viruses.

Adenoviruses
▪ Virus Structure

An adenovirus virion is a **nonenveloped icosahedral particle** (Fig. 39-1). The shell of the virion is made up of two kinds of capsomeres, **hexons** and **pentons.** Hexons have six neighbors, and pentons, located at the vertices of the icosahedron, have five neighbors. The **pentons** have projecting knobbed **fibers** that give the virions their characteristic appearance. Inside the virion, the viral DNA is associated with several basic proteins in a structure called the **core.** The predominant protein component of the viral core is an arginine-rich basic protein that presumably aids in the spatial organization of the viral DNA and neutralizes its negative charge. The core protein serves to package the adenoviral DNA in a manner similar to that of histones in the packaging of cellular chromatin.

The genome of the human adenoviruses is a **linear double-stranded DNA** molecule of 30,000 to 36,000 base pairs, depending on the serotype. The adenoviral genome has two unusual structural features. First, it possesses **inverted terminal repeats:** approximately 100 base pairs are repeated in an inverted orientation at each end of the genome. Second, each strand of the genome is covalently attached at its 5' end to a protein molecule (the **terminal protein,** or **TP**). Both the terminal repeats and the terminal protein play key roles in the replication of adenovirus DNA.

Adenovirus genes with related functions tend to be clustered on the genome and expressed from a common promoter. That arrangement, which is more characteristic of prokaryotes than eukaryotes, is also

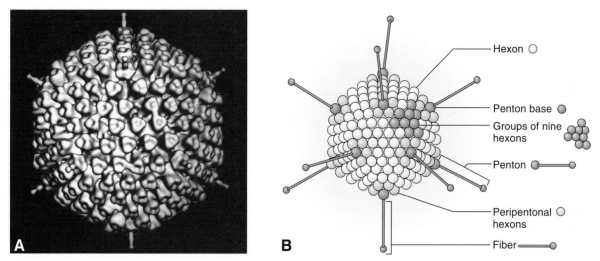

FIGURE 39-1 ▪ The adenovirus particle. A. Three-dimensional image of the adenovirus capsid reconstructed by computer from electron micrographs. **B.** Schematic view of the adenovirus particle with the locations of individual capsid proteins shown.

found among other DNA viruses, such as the papillomaviruses and polyomaviruses. Clustering provides an economical mechanism for coordinating expression of genes whose functions are required at similar times during infection. Examples of clustered adenoviral genes are those whose products (1) interact with the host immune system (the genes of early region 3 [E3]; see Figure 39-2); (2) participate in posttranscriptional events in gene expression (E1B, E4); (3) are essential for viral DNA replication (E2); and (4) are components of the virion or are involved in its assembly (L1 through L5).

ENTRY, SPREAD, AND REPLICATION

Attachment and Penetration

Adenoviruses attach to receptors on the host cell surface through the fiber protein. Different serotypes employ different receptors. For the commonly studied adenovirus serotypes 2 and 5, the receptor is a member of the immunoglobulin superfamily of proteins called

FIGURE 39-2 ▪ Temporal regulation of adenovirus transcription. The portions of the adenoviral genome transcribed during the immediate-early, early, and late phases of viral infection are indicated by arrows under a scale that shows position on the viral DNA molecule. The regions denoted by solid lines encode mRNAs that appear in the cytoplasm. The regions indicated by stippled lines are transcribed but are removed by splicing events from the RNA molecules that enter the cytoplasm. The early regions are numbered E1A through E4. The major late promoter (MLP) drives transcription of the late regions L1 through L5.

CAR (coxsackievirus and adenovirus receptor). CAR is present on most human cells and many other vertebrate cell types at up to 10^5 copies per cell. The normal function of CAR is not known. Following attachment, the virus–receptor complex migrates to **clathrin-coated pits,** which form endosomes that carry the virus particles into the cell. Internalization of adenovirus is dependent on the interaction of a second virion protein (penton base) with other cell surface proteins, members of the integrin family of membrane proteins. The pH of the endosome falls, inducing the virions to shed their penton capsid proteins and attached fibers. A conformational change in the virions causes the endosome to rupture and releases the partially disassembled virions into the cell cytoplasm. The particles migrate to the nucleus of the infected cell, probably along microtubules, and bind to proteins at the nuclear pore. The viral core then enters the nucleus, leaving behind most of its remaining capsid proteins. The stage is now set for viral gene expression.

Adenovirus Gene Expression

All DNA viruses display **temporal regulation** of gene expression. That is, viral gene expression takes place in two or more fairly distinct phases, each characterized by the synthesis of a specific set of viral proteins. Temporal regulation of gene expression presumably contributes to the efficiency of the viral life cycle. For example, in most cases synthesis of the proteins required for viral DNA replication occurs before the synthesis of proteins that form the virus particle. That sequence of events ensures that a large pool of viral DNA has accumulated before the packaging of viral DNA into capsids begins.

Temporal regulation of adenovirus gene expression is accomplished by a regulatory cascade in which each phase of gene expression depends on the expression of specific genes in the previous phase. In adenoviruses, gene expression occurs in three phases: immediate-early, early, and late (see Fig. 39-2). Most regulatory events in adenovirus gene expression occur at transcriptional or posttranscriptional steps in cytoplasmic messenger RNA (mRNA) production. Those events take place in the following order:

1. During the **immediate-early phase,** only the portion of the genome called **E1A** is transcribed. Because viral proteins have not yet been synthesized, transcription of the E1A genes depends entirely on host enzymes. The E1A transcript is spliced (as are essentially all adenoviral mRNAs) to yield two stable cytoplasmic E1A mRNAs. From those transcripts, two proteins are produced. Both proteins are **transcriptional regulators,** which induce transcription from five viral promoters that are inactive during the immediate-early phase. The E1A proteins also stimulate transcription of many cellular genes—generally, genes that are active in the DNA synthesis (S) phase of the cell cycle and are required by

the virus to provide the proper intracellular environment for viral DNA replication. The activation of those genes is responsible for transformation by adenoviruses. The E1A proteins stimulate transcription indirectly by increasing the activity of endogenous host cell transcriptional factors.

2. The E1A-dependent activation of the five viral promoters marks the beginning of the **early phase** of gene expression. During that phase, the newly activated viral promoters direct the transcription of four early regions (**E1B, E2, E3,** and **E4**) and one (questionably named) late region (**L1**). Most of the regions contain several genes and encode several proteins. The early RNA transcripts are spliced to yield the individual mRNAs. Protein products of at least six early genes participate in the events necessary for progression to the late phase of gene expression. Three encode the viral proteins necessary for viral DNA replication, and three are required for posttranscriptional events in mRNA synthesis during the late phase.

3. Viral DNA replication is catalyzed by three of the early proteins along with certain host proteins. Coincident with the onset of viral DNA synthesis is the transition from the early phase to the **late phase** of virus replication. The most dramatic events of the transition affect RNA synthesis, which is directed by the so-called **major late promoter.** Transcription from the major late promoter greatly increases until it makes up the majority of new RNA synthesized in the infected cell. The transcript is a large RNA molecule that, when spliced, produces about 20 distinct late viral mRNAs. Those mRNAs are then transported to the cytoplasm for translation. Early phase gene products are required for both the splicing and transport steps in late mRNA production. Because of the efficiency with which late RNA is transcribed and processed and because of the large number of viral genomes present in the infected cell (owing to DNA replication), late mRNAs and proteins are abundantly produced.

Viral DNA replication is a prerequisite for late gene expression. Why? We do not really know, although some evidence suggests that the physical act of replication is in some way necessary for an individual DNA molecule to serve as a template for late gene expression.

As the expression of the viral late genes increases during the early–late transition, the expression of cellular genes decreases. Adenovirus infection interferes with host gene expression in two ways. First, the accumulation of cellular mRNAs in the cytoplasm is prevented by **inhibition of the transport of host mRNAs** from the nucleus to the cytoplasm. Products of early regions E1B and E4 are responsible for the inhibition. Second, a virally encoded late protein **inhibits the translation of existing host mRNAs** in the cytoplasm. The consequence of those two actions is that during the late phase of infection, essentially all the proteins produced in the infected cell are viral products.

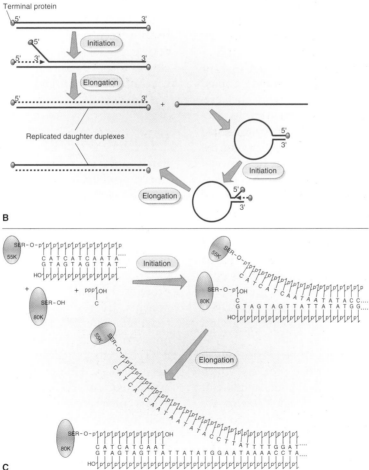

FIGURE 39-3 ▪ **Adenovirus DNA replication. A.** An electron micrograph of a DNA molecule of the type diagrammed in the second line of part B—that is, a duplex with one single-stranded branch. **B.** Schematic representation of the events in adenovirus replication. **C.** Details of the initiation of adenovirus DNA replication showing the priming of DNA synthesis by the preterminal protein (pTP is labeled 80K; TP is labeled 55K).

DNA Replication

DNA-containing animal viruses rely to various extents on host cell proteins for the replication of their genomes. The papillomaviruses (see Chapter 40) make a single viral protein that redirects host replication enzymes to replicate the viral genome, whereas herpesviruses (see Chapters 41 and 42) encode a large number of the enzymes involved in viral DNA replication. The adenoviruses fall between those extremes, employing both virally encoded and host proteins in replication.

Replication is initiated within the inverted repeats at one or the other end of the adenoviral DNA molecule (Fig. 39-3). The two ends of the DNA molecule have identical sequences, and initiation of DNA replication takes place at either end with about equal frequency. After initiation, DNA synthesis proceeds along the template DNA. One parental strand is copied and the other is displaced. Completion of the synthesis of the first daughter strand produces a duplex molecule consisting of one parental strand and one daughter strand, plus a displaced parental single strand. Because of the inverted terminal repeats, the displaced single strand assumes a **"panhandle"** configuration containing a short double-stranded region identical in sequence to the ends of the normal double-stranded genome. DNA synthesis is initiated on the panhandle, and the displaced single strand then serves as the template for the synthesis of the second daughter strand.

Synthesis of viral DNA differs from that of host DNA in three respects. First, a single DNA strand is copied at each virus replication fork, whereas in host cell replication, both strands are copied concurrently. Second, the synthesis of all new viral DNA is continuous; that is, it occurs by the uninterrupted elongation of the growing chain across the entire genome. In host cell DNA replication, one strand at each replication fork is produced continuously, but the other is synthesized discontinuously as short pieces (Okazaki fragments) that must be joined to produce the finished strand. Finally, host chromosomes replicate by a well-regulated process that occurs once in a division cycle, whereas virus replication is uncoordinated and takes place continuously over time. The latter strategy is presumably a response to the need to produce as many viral DNA molecules as possible over the short course of a viral infectious cycle.

Adenovirus DNA replication can be carried out in vitro in a system composed of purified proteins, which has led to a fairly detailed biochemical understanding of the events in viral DNA replication. Six proteins are required for optimal viral DNA replication in vitro (and presumably in vivo). Three of the proteins are virally encoded—a **DNA polymerase**, a **DNA-binding protein (DBP)**, and the **preterminal protein (pTP)**, which is the precursor of the terminal protein found in virions. All three proteins are products of the E2 region. The remaining three replication proteins are cellular products. Two are DNA-binding proteins that normally function in the transcription of cellular genes in uninfected cells; the third is a topoisomerase.

The initiation of DNA replication is carried out by the adenoviral DNA polymerase and pTP, which associate in the cytoplasm after their synthesis and migrate as a complex into the nucleus. The complex binds to about 18 nucleotides at the end of the genome, a process **stimulated by the binding of host transcription factors** to adjacent blocks of nucleotides in the terminal repeats. The end of the viral DNA molecule is unwound, exposing single-stranded DNA that serves as the template for the actual initiation event. That event is the formation of a phosphodiester link between deoxycytosine monophosphate (dCMP, the first residue at the 5′ end of the new DNA strand) and a serine residue in the pTP molecule. In that way, **pTP serves as the primer for adenoviral DNA replication** (see Fig. 39-3, Panel C). Protein priming of DNA replication is most unusual; in most systems, primers for DNA replication are actually short RNA molecules.

After formation of the initial pTP–dCMP linkage, elongation of the new daughter strand proceeds conventionally. Viral DNA polymerase sequentially adds nucleotides to the 3′ OH group of the pTP-bound growing chain. The viral DBP is essential for elongation and coats the displaced single strand, protecting it from nuclease attack. As DNA is packaged, proteolytic processing cleaves the pTP molecule bound to each DNA strand to generate the form found in mature virions.

Virion Assembly

Particle assembly begins when sufficient amounts of capsid proteins have accumulated. The first step is the assembly of free polypeptide chains into hexon and penton capsomeres. Pentons are assembled spontaneously, but hexon assembly requires the participation of a protein that does not appear in the mature particle. Such proteins that assist in assembly but that do not appear in virions are common and are referred to as **scaffold proteins.** Hexons, as well as several minor virion components, are next assembled into an intermediate structure that is later filled with DNA and core proteins. It is not clear how the DNA enters the empty shell, although it has been suggested that it may pass through one of the open vertices. Finally, the pentons and fibers become associated with the capsid, and a series of proteolytic events converts precursor proteins within the virion into their mature forms. After assembly, adenovirus particles remain associated with the dying cell and are slowly released as the cell lyses. A viral protease and the colorfully named adenovirus death protein (from E3) both participate in the destruction of the host cell and virus release.

Paradigm Box

DNA Virus Replication and Control of the Cell Cycle

The study of DNA viruses can teach us a great deal about the complicated workings of normal cells. Because DNA viruses either make use of host cell machinery (frequently modified by viral proteins) or employ general strategies similar to those of their host cells, understanding the events that occur in virus-infected cells often reveals much about the events that take place in uninfected cells. Adenoviruses have been particularly useful in that regard. For example, **mRNA splicing** was first discovered in studies of the synthesis of adenoviral late mRNAs, and only later was it shown that the process also occurs in normal eukaryotic cells. Similarly, in vitro eukaryotic DNA replication systems first developed for adenovirus and polyomavirus DNAs have been extremely useful in understanding the biochemistry of cellular DNA replication. Studies of adenoviruses, papillomaviruses, and polyomaviruses also have contributed to our understanding of mammalian cell cycle control that, for example, guarantees that cellular DNA replicates exactly once per cell division and that cells divide only on receipt of appropriate signals. Aberrations in cell cycle control are central to the growth abnormalities of cancer cells.

Most DNA viruses, including adenoviruses, exploit at least some elements of the cellular DNA replication machinery. That exploitation is economical for the virus, but it also creates a timing problem because the shared cellular factors are normally expressed only during the S phase of the cell cycle. For a virus it is not advantageous to wait for the cell to begin its division cycle, and many of the cells targeted by DNA viruses are differentiated and do not divide at all (e.g., superficial epithelial cells). To overcome that difficulty and maintain a continuous high level of replication and a large supply of the necessary host cell proteins, adenoviruses and most other DNA viruses force infected cells into the S phase of the division cycle.

Viral proteins force the S phase by interacting with key regulators of the normal cell cycle. In the case of adenoviruses, the products of the **E1A** region bind to and inactivate the cellular protein **pRb,** which normally maintains S-phase genes in a silent state. Inactivation of pRb is primarily responsible for continuous S-phase gene expression in adenovirus-infected cells. A second adenoviral protein, expressed from **E1B,** binds to and inactivates the cellular protein **p53,** which cooperates with pRb in preventing a cell from advancing into S phase and which also can induce **apoptosis** (programmed cell death) in cells that overexpress S-phase genes. Together, the viral proteins inactivate two key negative regulators of the S phase of the cell cycle and permit the cell both to overexpress factors necessary for DNA replication and to survive the cell death pathway that would be the normal consequence of overexpression.

Because of their effects on pRb and p53, adenoviruses possess **oncogenic potential.** Indeed, the cellular proteins are known as **tumor suppressors,** since mutations in their respective genes are associated with a wide range of human cancers. Adenoviruses are not alone in their effects on tumor suppressors: papillomaviruses, polyomaviruses, and some herpesviruses produce proteins that subvert the functions of pRb and p53, resulting in the induction of tumors. Of note, both pRb and p53 were originally identified on the basis of their interactions with DNA virus proteins.

Interactions with Host Defense Systems

Adenoviruses carry several genes whose functions seem to be to stop antiviral host defenses. The main immunological defense against viral infection, cell-mediated immunity, involves destruction of infected cells by cytotoxic T lymphocytes (CTLs). CTLs have receptors for specific complexes of viral peptides bound to a host protein found on the surface of almost all cells, the **major** histocompatibility complex (MHC) class I. Those receptors enable CTLs to recognize infected cells. Cells that do not possess MHC class I molecules on their surface do not become targets for destruction by CTLs. Adenoviruses evade cell-mediated immune response using two separate mechanisms that interfere with expression of MHC class I molecules. The first mechanism is mediated by an early viral protein that **blocks the production of MHC class I mRNA** in infected cells. The second mechanism is mediated by a glycoprotein from E3 that **prevents the transport of newly synthesized MHC class I protein** molecules to the cell surface. In an animal model system (cotton rats), infections of the lung with viral mutants that do not express the E3 protein induce a striking pulmonary infiltration of neutrophils, suggesting that this protein in fact influences the course of disease in vivo.

Another way by which adenoviruses protect themselves from cellular immunity is through resistance to signals from immune cells that would otherwise cause premature death of the infected cell. For example, both **tumor necrosis factor (TNF)**, produced by activated macrophages, and **Fas ligand,** found on the surface of many immune cells, can activate intracellular pathways that result in the death of many types of virally infected cells. Adenoviruses produce proteins that block those death pathways and render cells relatively resistant to both death stimuli. In addition, a cell surface receptor required for killing by Fas ligand is removed from the surface of infected cells by adenoviruses.

A third line of defense against viral infection is the antiviral state induced in cells by **interferon-α** and **interferon-β.** Among other effects, the interferons prevent protein synthesis in virus-infected cells by initiating a chain of events that culminates in the inactivation of the cellular translation machinery. Central to inhibition of translation is a host cell protein (PKR) that is activated by double-stranded RNA produced in most viral infections, including adenoviral infection. Adenoviruses break the interferon chain and prevent the inhibition of protein synthesis through the action of small RNA molecules (**VA RNAs**) encoded by viral genes. The VA RNAs fold into partially double-stranded structures that bind to and prevent activation of PKR, preserving the cellular translational apparatus for use by the virus. Obviously, adenoviruses do not completely blunt the immune response by those mechanisms, because most adenoviral infections eventually are cleared. However, it is likely that reductions or delays in the immune response caused by the viral proteins contribute to the success of adenoviruses as common human pathogens.

Oncogenicity and Cell Transformation

Adenovirus type 12 was the first DNA-containing virus shown to cause cancer in animals. That discovery sparked a massive search for evidence that adenoviruses (and other animal DNA viruses) were etiological agents of human cancer. Enormous efforts also have been spent to determine mechanisms of tumorigenesis by animal DNA viruses. Those studies have contributed significantly to knowledge about the molecular basis of carcinogenesis. It is now clear that some DNA viruses, including papillomaviruses (see Chapter 40), are important causes of human cancer, but generally studies have

revealed no convincing association between adenoviruses and cancer. All adenovirus serotypes tested induce phenotypic changes in cultured cells that resemble those that occur during natural carcinogenesis. That process is referred to as **transformation.** Because adenoviral infection of human cells results in production of progeny viruses and cell death, transformation is apparent only in cells, such as rodent cells, in which the virus does not grow productively, or in human or animal cells containing incomplete fragments of the viral genome. Transformation by adenoviruses requires the products of the E1A and E1B regions.

The adenovirus E1A and E1B proteins transform cells largely by interacting with the cellular tumor suppressor products pRb and p53 (see the paradigm). Both proteins play important roles in mechanisms that regulate the normal cell cycle: pRB acts as a negative regulator of S-phase gene expression; and p53 is responsible for the induction of programmed cell death (apoptosis) in response to a number of signals, including excessive S-phase gene expression. Adenoviruses induce S-phase gene expression in infected cells to enhance the capacity of the cell to synthesize viral DNA. That enhancement is accomplished by inactivation of pRB by the E1A proteins. Concomitantly, an E1B product inactivates p53, preventing programmed cell death that otherwise would be induced by the action of E1A and would prematurely abort the viral infection. Together, the disruptions of the cell cycle regulatory machinery are primarily responsible for transformation, although additional host cell genetic changes are needed for maintenance of the transformed phenotype. Importantly, tumorigenesis by adenoviruses is only an incidental consequence of the mechanisms that regulate viral gene expression.

DAMAGE

Adenovirus infections are widespread in human populations, accounting for 5 to 10% of all viral infections. Most infections occur in childhood; 75% occur before 14 years of age, and over half occur before 5 years of age. Most adenoviral infections affect either the **respiratory tract** or the **gastrointestinal tract,** in about equal numbers. Although most patients with adenoviral respiratory diseases recover, some mortality has been associated with pneumonia.

The usual symptoms of adenoviral respiratory infections resemble those of the **common cold,** including nasal congestion, inflammation of the upper respiratory tract, and cough. Systemic symptoms such as chills, headache, muscle aches, and fever are common, and **conjunctivitis** sometimes accompanies the other symptoms (**pharyngoconjunctival fever**). In severe cases **pneumonia** can develop. Different serotypes are associated with dif-

Adenoviruses as Vectors for Gene Delivery

Virus particles efficiently introduce foreign nucleic acid (the viral genome) into living cells. Interest has developed in using that viral property to introduce non-viral genes into animals or animal cells. Because adenoviruses have been studied extensively and much is known about their biology and genetics, adenoviruses are considered to be particularly promising vectors for foreign gene delivery.

The safe and effective vaccines developed to combat acute respiratory disease makes the use of recombinant adenoviruses to immunize against pathogens other than adenovirus itself an attractive idea. Several candidate **adenovirus-based vaccine strains** have been constructed. In those strains, a segment of DNA encoding an antigen derived from a pathogen, along with regulatory signals to direct expression of the antigen, replaces a segment of the adenoviral genome. Such genetically engineered adenoviruses direct the production of the foreign antigen in infected cells. Vaccines against pathogens including HIV, rabies virus, and the malaria parasite have been shown to induce strong cellular and humoral immune responses and to protect against the target pathogen in animal model systems.

A second potential application for adenovirus is as a vector for the introduction of an exogenous gene into an individual for therapeutic purposes. **Gene therapy** is usually envisioned as a therapeutic approach to inherited disease. For example, the blood-clotting disorder hemophilia A results from the inheritance of nonfunctional alleles of a particular gene (the factor VIII gene) from both parents. Administration of purified factor VIII to affected persons corrects the defect. Therefore, delivery of the normal factor VIII gene to appropriate cells in a patient might restore enough factor VIII function to relieve the symptoms of the disease. Accordingly, genetically engineered adenoviruses carrying the factor VIII gene in place of E1 (such viruses cannot conduct a lytic growth cycle in normal cells) have been constructed, and clinical improvement has been demonstrated in a murine hemophilia A model after the administration of recombinant adenovirus. Significant technical problems, such as short-lived expression of the exogenous genes, need to be overcome before gene therapy of the sort becomes practical. The tragic death of a human volunteer in an adenovirus gene therapy trial in 1999 points out the social and ethical problems that also accompany the development of gene therapy.

A final promising application for adenoviral vectors is in cancer treatment. Numerous clinical trials with recombinant adenoviruses designed specifically to kill cancer cells are under way. Cell death is variously accomplished by delivery of toxic genes, by delivery of genes that stimulate antitumor immunity, or by use of adenovirus mutants that grow selectively in cells with genetic abnormalities frequently found in cancer cells. As with vaccination and gene therapy by adenoviruses, much work remains before adenoviral anticancer therapy becomes clinically useful.

---

ferent disease manifestations. Serotypes 1, 2, 5, and 6 are endemic in most populations, and 80% of all young adults have neutralizing antibodies to those types. Other serotypes (4 and 7) are associated with outbreaks of a fairly severe febrile respiratory infection (**acute respiratory disease, or ARD**).

ARD affects primarily military recruits during basic training. As many as 80% of some groups of recruits are affected, with one fourth to one half requiring hospitalization in some outbreaks. Crowded conditions and fatigue presumably favor the spread of the disease and increase its severity. However, college freshmen, many of whom are similar in age to military recruits, do not suffer from ARD. ARD is a sufficiently severe problem that a live adenovirus vaccine was developed by the military in the 1960s. Given to newly inducted military personnel, it effectively eliminated ARD from the military for three decades. Recently, production of the vaccine was ended for economic reasons and ARD has reappeared, resulting in at least one fatality.

Vaccine manufacture is now being reestablished, and it is likely that the disease will again come under control. The military experience with ARD graphically illustrates the hazard to health created by eliminating costly vaccination programs when funds are short and the problem seems to have disappeared (because of the vaccine).

Adenoviruses are also an important cause of acute gastrointestinal disease in children and may be responsible for up to 15% of childhood intestinal infections. Many serotypes of adenoviruses are present, not only in the stool of patients, but in normal stool as well, in contrast to other serotypes that are only associated with disease. Adenovirus type 12 (Ad12) has been implicated in the development of celiac disease (gluten enteropathy). The development of that illness appears to depend on protein sequence homology between an Ad12 early protein and gliadin-α, a component of the cereal grains that activate the disease. It has been suggested that exposure to Ad12 induces an antibody response to gliadin-α, which predisposes to celiac disease in some persons.

Less common than respiratory and gastrointestinal disease is adenovirus-induced conjunctivitis without other symptoms. Mild **"swimming pool conjunctivitis"** is probably most often a result of adenoviral infection, as is the more serious, highly contagious **epidemic keratoconjunctivitis.**

Latent adenovirus infections are very common; adenoviruses can be recovered from as many as 80% of the tonsils or adenoids removed from children and young adults. The mechanism of persistence in those cases is not known. It has been reported that viral DNA can persist in tonsillar tissue free of infectious virus, but it is also possible that persistence may be caused by a low-level active infection imperfectly controlled by the immune system. In fact, the majority of healthy adults examined have very small numbers of peripheral lymphocytes apparently undergoing a typical adenoviral lytic cycle. Early gene products that interfere with host defense mechanisms may play a role in persistence.

Adenoviruses can be recovered from immunocompromised individuals. Numerous isolations from patients with immunodeficiency resulting from HIV infec-

tion have been reported, and infection has been associated in some cases with mortality. Disseminated adenovirus infections also are a significant cause of mortality among bone marrow transplant recipients.

Conclusion

Adenoviruses are commonly found among healthy persons but also cause many types of infections that range in severity. The eye, the upper and lower respiratory tracts, and the gastrointestinal tract are often involved. Adenoviruses are capable of cellular transformation in some circumstances, but convincing evidence linking adenoviruses to cancer in humans is lacking. Adenoviruses are double-stranded DNA viruses whose life cycle has served as a model for the study of eukaryotic DNA replication and gene expression. The expression of viral genes follows a defined program, some genes being expressed early, others late. Modified adenoviruses may be suitable candidates for recombinant vaccines to be used in immunizing against a variety of antigens, or for introducing genes into humans for correction of genetic diseases.

Human Papillomaviruses and Warts

Elliot J. Androphy

key concepts

Human papillomaviruses (HPVs):

■ Are a group of small, nonenveloped, nonlytic DNA viruses that replicate within squamous epithelial cells.

■ Cause local infections that may appear as warts (papillomas) at various sites, including the hands, feet, and genital region.

■ Are spread by direct skin-to-skin contact, sexual transmission, or through contact with contaminated inanimate objects.

■ Chronic infection with specific HPV types can lead to malignancy—most commonly, cancer of the cervix.

■ Infections are usually diagnosed by clinical signs and history; treatment includes surgical, chemical, or laser destruction of infected tissue.

Human papillomaviruses (HPVs) are a large group of genetically related nonenveloped viruses with a small, circular DNA genome. Clinical manifestations of warts can range from inapparent (subclinical) to large bulky growths. Warts usually appear as **slow-growing bumps** of the skin and mucous membranes. The majority of patients with warts seek medical attention because of physical discomfort or concern about the appearance of a new skin lesion. While most papillomavirus-induced warts are biologically benign, some warts may become cancers. Indeed, **cervical cancer** is one of the most common neoplasms of women and develops from lesions caused by specific types of HPVs.

Case

As a healthy 26-year-old, Mr. M. was almost in a panic. Four months ago he noticed a small bump on the shaft of his penis, but he decided to ignore it with the hope that it would go away on its own. When he found two new growths, he and his wife became worried that he had genital warts. The dermatologist he saw immediately confirmed that diagnosis without performing any tests and applied liquid nitrogen to destroy the warts. He told Mr. M. that genital warts are transmissible and that his wife needed to be examined. Mr. M. was anxious about spreading a virus that could cause his wife of two years to acquire cervical cancer. The doctor discussed HPV infection and reassured him that with routine gynecological care his wife should be fine.

This case raises several questions:

1. How and when did Mr. M. acquire the HPV infection?
2. Is Mrs. M. also infected, and what are the clinical implications?
3. What if any laboratory tests should be performed on Mr. and Mrs. M.?
4. If Mrs. M. has cervical warts, will they eventually result in cancer?
5. How can Mr. M. and his wife be treated for the HPV infection?

■ ■ ■ ■

Human Papillomaviruses

CHARACTERISTICS

Human papillomaviruses (HPVs) belong to the Papillomaviridae family. Particles of these viruses are formed by two tightly packed viral proteins and contain a single copy of the circular viral genome (Fig. 40-1). Virus particles are released as the infected epithelial cells are desquamated. Because the viruses do not bud from the cell, they do not have a lipid **envelope.** The absence of an envelope causes HPVs to be resistant to detergents, desiccation, and heat. Therefore, they can remain infectious in the environment for long periods. Because papillomavirus genomes are only about 8,000 base pairs, or one twentieth the size of herpesviruses, they encode only a few proteins. They do not encode a DNA polymerase to replicate their genome and thus must rely on host cell DNA replication proteins to reproduce. Nucleoside analogs directed against viral polymerases and used in the treatment of herpesvirus infections (or even HIV) are not effective against warts.

Papillomaviruses are pathogens of humans, monkeys, dogs, cattle, birds, fish, and most other species. The viruses are species specific, and only HPVs can cause warts in humans. HPVs are subclassified into types on

FIGURE 40-1 ■ Electron micrograph of purified wart viruses.

the basis of their **DNA sequences.** If the nucleotide sequence of a short, highly conserved region found in all papillomaviruses varies by more that 10% from all other known HPV sequences, the isolate is defined as a new type, or more accurately, a new **genotype.** According to that scheme, presently more than 100 HPV genotypes exist (Table 40-1). Minor variants that differ at only a few nucleotides have been described within several genotype groups, thus expanding the genetic and possibly the biologic diversity of HPVs.

HPV types 1 through 4 were the first to be discovered because they are found in the majority of **cutaneous warts.** The HPVs in **genital warts,** also called **condyloma,** are usually types 6, 11, 16, 18, 31, 33, and 35. Those HPV types cause warts of the penis, vulva, and anus and can infect the mucosal epithelium of the vagina, cervix, and oropharynx. The genital-associated HPV types were identified later because the amount of viral DNA present in genital lesions is very low. In general, each HPV type is associated with infection of a specific anatomic region or epithelial environment. For instance, HPV-1 is most frequently found in plantar warts. HPV-2 causes common cutaneous warts but has been isolated from genital warts, especially in children. HPV-6 and HPV-16 typically cause genital lesions but have been infrequently isolated from cutaneous warts.

ENTRY

HPV particles are present on the surface of warts and the associated keratotic scale. The particles are spread by direct skin-to-skin contact with other people or with

table 40-1 Lesions Associated With Human Papillomavirus (HPV) Types

LESIONS	
Plantar and palmar warts	HPV-1, 4
Common cutaneous warts	HPV-2, 4
Flat warts	HPV-3, 10
Anogenital warts, respiratory papillomatosis, cervical papillomas; "low risk" for becoming malignant	HPV- 6, 11, 40, 42, 43, 44, 54, 61, 70, 72, 81
Common warts in meat handlers	HPV-7
Epidermodysplasia verruciformis; immunosuppression	HPV-5, 8, 9, 12, 14, 15, 17, 19 to 29
Focal oral epithelial hyperplasia	HPV-13
Penile, vulvar, vaginal, and anal warts, Bowenoid papulosis; "high risk" for cervical and anal dysplasia and carcinoma	HPV- 16, 18, 26, 31, 33, 35, 39, 45, 51, 52, 53, 56, 58, 59, 66, 68, 73, 82

oneself—for example, a wart on the side of one finger touching the adjacent finger. However, normal skin is highly resistant to entry. HPVs are not highly contagious, and epidemics are rare, even within a family. Breaks in the skin barrier promote entry, and scratching a wart can spread the virus to uninvolved areas. Infection also takes place more readily when the virus comes in contact with mucous membranes or with macerated skin. Despite the low content of virus particles in genital warts, such contact is sufficient to propagate the infection, because transmission of the virus during sexual contact occurs with high efficiency. Being nonenveloped, papillomaviruses are quite stable and remain infectious after exfoliation. Therefore, it is likely that papillomaviruses present on inanimate objects can be a source of infection. Warts of the soles of the feet probably result from implantation of virus present on microabrasions of the feet caused by contact with rough surfaces, like the concrete surfaces of swimming pools.

ENCOUNTER

The location of a lesion is determined by the site of virus entry and may be influenced by the HPV genotype involved. The most frequent sites of warts are commonly traumatized skin surfaces such as the fingers, hands, soles, knees, and elbows. The numerous warts often seen on the hands and fingers of butchers are caused by the inoculation of virus into cuts sustained at those sites. Microabrasions that occur with vaginal, anal, or oral sex and the moist, mucosal epithelia promote efficient virus spread to the penis, anus, vulva, vagina, cervix, and less frequently, the oropharynx and larynx. Rarely, transmission from mother to child occurs during birth with aspiration of HPV. Infection by that route can cause the devastating disease **respiratory papillomatosis** in the infant. There is no evidence of hematogenous spread of papillomavirus.

Host immunity plays an important role in susceptibility and maintenance of HPV infection. Individuals with defective cell-mediated immunity (e.g., transplant recipients receiving immunosuppressive drugs) may have numerous warts that are highly resistant to treatment. Men and women with AIDS are at high risk for development of HPV-associated carcinomas. In the rare disease **epidermodysplasia verruciformis,** the individual is susceptible to specific HPV genotypes, presumably owing to an inability to mount an immune response to the virus. Widespread and longstanding warts may occur, and if infected with an oncogenic cutaneous HPV type such as type 5 or 8 (see Table 40-1), the individual may develop multiple invasive skin cancers.

Recent studies using polymerase chain reaction (PCR) suggest that trace levels of HPV DNA can be found on skin and in hair appendages from normal individuals. The low level of virus may represent the environmental reservoir for the more rare types of HPVs that are usually found in immunocompromised patients. Thus, HPVs may be maintained as subclinical infections in the normal population and arise in an individual when host immune surveillance is decreased.

EPIDEMIOLOGY

It is estimated that 20 million to 30 million persons are infected with HPV in the United States, with about 3 million new individuals infected each year. Genital warts are the single most common sexually transmitted infection that leads people to seek medical attention and are second only to chlamydial infections as the most common sexually transmitted disease. Worldwide an estimated 600,000 new cases of cervical cancer arise each year, leading to more than 230,000 deaths annually, 4,500 of which are in the United States.

Many people become infected with wart viruses during their lifetime without exhibiting symptoms.

Alterations in the epithelium may be so slight that the infection is not recognized. HPVs can lie dormant in the epithelial layers of the skin or mucosa. Compelling evidence of frequent asymptomatic infection derives from PCR studies of cervical and vaginal cells obtained from healthy women presenting for routine gynecological care. Prospective studies of college women found that 20 to 60% become HPV DNA positive, although the majority of their cervical cells showed normal histology. Many of those HPV DNA–positive women subsequently became negative on repeat examination several months later. Those findings provide evidence that most cervical HPV infections are transient.

HPV infections are of special concern because of the association with progression to cancer (see the paradigm). Virtually all cervical carcinomas contain a subset of so-called **high-risk** HPV genotypes (see Table 40-1). HPV 16 is the prototype of the group and is found in about 50% of all cervical cancers. Other HPVs found in genital and cervical lesions are rarely found in cancers and are therefore called **low-risk types.** The high-risk HPVs also have been identified in about 90% of anal cancers, 25 to 30% of penile and vulvar cancers, and a minority of epithelial malignancies of the larynx and oropharynx.

Although several other cancers have been reported to contain HPV DNA using highly sensitive PCR-based techniques, those findings often represent detection of much less than one copy of viral DNA per tumor cell. In malignancies caused by HPVs such as that of the cervix, all tumor cells contain HPV DNA and express the viral E6 and E7 genes.

The major risk factors for progression of HPV infection to malignancy are the HPV type, persistence of the viral DNA, and host immune status. Why some warts persist in the skin or cervix is not known.

Spread and Replication

HPVs have a genetic content that is minuscule compared with the human genome. Thus, like all viruses, papillomaviruses must use the host cell machinery to synthesize their macromolecules. To orchestrate those papillomavirus activities, proteins directly or indirectly coordinate the viral life cycle in concert with the cells that they infect. A papillomavirus protein called **E1** maintains the viral DNA as a covalently closed circular molecule or **episome** that does not integrate into the host cell genome. In that form the viral genome replicates to high numbers at the proper time, independent of cellular DNA. A second viral protein called **E2** binds to a specific DNA sequence within the viral genome. E2 also binds to the E1 protein, and that complex binds with high-affinity and specificity to the viral DNA. The E1 protein is a **helicase** that unwinds double-stranded DNA to initiate replication, and it also binds cellular DNA replication proteins and localizes those to the viral episome. The E2 protein is also a **transcription factor** that regulates expression of the viral genes by directing the assembly of cellular transcription factors and RNA polymerase.

Papillomaviruses probably establish infection in the **basal cell layer** of the epithelium. That layer represents the replicative compartment of the skin, where cells continuously divide to replenish the desquamating surface and to heal wounds. One or at most a few copies of viral DNA are maintained as **extrachromosomal episomes.** Papillomaviruses are not **lytic;** that is, they do not replicate to copy and kill the basal cell. Therefore, HPVs do not cause any immediate damage to the infected cells. The viral episome is initially duplicated in synchrony with cellular chromosomes; the replicated viral genome segregates into the daughter cell. As those cells mature and migrate toward the skin surface, the viral episome is transported to upper levels of the epithelium. There viral genes are expressed and viral genome amplification begins.

Virus reproduction occurs in concert with the normal differentiation program of **keratinocytes.** Those cells are destined to form a nonreplicating, physical barrier that preserves the integrity of the subcutaneous organs and protects the body from exogenous insults. As an epithelium differentiates, upper-level epithelial cells lose their nucleus and are filled with stable, insoluble, structural proteins. The flattened cells are shed as scales into the environment, with fresh cells continually replacing them from below. The papillomaviruses exploit that process for their replication and transmission. After passage to the outer skin layers, the virus somehow senses the differentiated status of the keratinocyte and directs transcription of the late mRNAs that encode its **capsid** proteins called **L1** and **L2.** Those proteins are transported into the nucleus of the keratinocyte. The newly replicated episomes are packaged into the capsids to form progeny **virions,** which are then shed from the surface of the epithelium.

Viruses such as herpes simplex virus and HIV-1 incorporate part of the cell membrane into their virus particles as they bud from infected cells. Because of the lipid bilayer, those virions are readily inactivated by heat, drying, or detergents. In contrast, papillomaviruses are **nonenveloped** because they do not bud from a cell membrane. Their stable protein **capsid** allows papillomaviruses to remain infectious after long periods in the environment.

Damage

Papillomavirus-induced alterations in the host epithelium develop slowly and are often clinically inapparent. Changes may not be visible for many months after infection has begun.

Warts look different at different sites. Common warts of the hands and other cutaneous surfaces are elevated, firm, fleshy lesions with a sharp border (Fig. 40-2). On the

Paradigm Box

Viral Oncogenesis

The recognized human oncogenic viruses include **papillomaviruses, Epstein-Barr virus** (associated with **Burkitt lymphoma** and **nasopharyngeal carcinoma**), **hepatitis B virus** (associated with primary **hepatocellular** carcinoma), and **human herpesvirus 8** (associated with **Kaposi sarcoma**). Most human cell lines in culture are derived from cancers, whereas normal human cells placed in culture do not continuously proliferate and thus are not "**immortal.**" The oncogenes derived from some oncogenic viruses can induce cell immortalization; that is, the cells do not undergo **senescence,** which is characteristic of normal diploid cells in culture. Establishment of the immortal phenotype is an early step in progression to cancer. Some oncogenic viruses can **transform** established cell lines. **Transformed cells** can be recognized by their altered morphology, loss of contact-inhibited growth, and decreased nutritional requirements. In many cases transformed cells are malignant; that is, they form tumors when injected into immunodeficient animals.

How and why do viruses transform cells? The paradox of papillomavirus replication is that it occurs in the upper epithelium, which is normally composed of nondividing, differentiated cells. Because papillomaviruses do not encode DNA replication enzymes, they must both prevent the exit from **cell cycle** and activate the cellular pathways that replicate DNA. Many different mechanisms of transformation are used by different viruses, but two recurring themes are inhibition of normal growth regulatory processes and stimulation of cell division.

A finite series of molecular events appears to be necessary for neoplastic progression. First, immortalization requires repeated entry into the cell cycle, which is restricted by the cellular **retinoblastoma (Rb)** protein; inactivation of that **tumor suppressor** pathway is found in many types of cancer. Second, the cellular tumor suppressor protein **p53** is disrupted; p53 normally induces **programmed cell death (apoptosis)** that would occur following Rb inactivation. Third, the ends of **chromosomes** must be protected from progressive erosion that normally occurs with each replicative cycle. The process is reversed by the expression of **telomerase,** which protects cells from senescence. Proliferative immortal cells subsequently acquire malignant characteristics by mutations in normal growth regulating genes or by infection with an oncogenic virus.

Tumor induction by high-risk HPVs exemplifies the molecular processes. Among the eight proteins encoded by high-risk HPVs, only two, **E6 and E7,** are always expressed in cervical cancer cells. Using in vitro cell culture assays, the E6 and E7 genes have been shown to immortalize human keratinocytes and to increase their growth rate. E6 and E7 also transform established mouse cell lines. Those findings demonstrate that the viral proteins target fundamental growth regulatory pathways.

The molecular details of how high-risk E6 and E7 proteins cause cellular changes are incomplete but are becoming clearer. E7 has amino acid similarities to other viral oncogenes—namely, adenovirus E1A and simian virus 40 (**SV40**) **large T** (tumor) antigen. Those viral proteins can form complexes with the **Rb** family member called **p105,** the name reflecting its size (105 kilodaltons). The development of retinoblastoma is associated with the absence of p105-Rb. Thus, the protein is considered to be a natural suppressor of cell proliferation. By complexing with p105-Rb, viral oncoproteins prevent Rb from exerting its normal check on cell proliferation. Binding to p105-Rb releases a **transcription factor** called **E2F,** which has been shown to activate expression of a series of genes necessary for DNA synthesis and entry into the cell cycle. E7, E1A, and SV40 large T also bind other Rb family proteins, which inactivate other E2F family members necessary for different stages of cell division. Unlike E1A and SV40 large T, high-risk E7 also induces Rb protein degradation.

The high-risk E6 proteins inactivate the p53 tumor suppressor pathway by taking advantage of normal cellular mechanisms to **degrade** unwanted proteins. High-risk E6 binds to a cellular factor called E6-AP, which is a component of the **ubiquitination proteolysis pathway. Ubiquitin** is a short peptide covalently attached to other proteins to mark them for proteolytic degradation. The E6/E6-AP complexes with p53 and induces its polyubiquitination and subsequent proteolysis. As a result, levels of p53 are very low, and its effects as a tumor suppressor are inhibited. Interestingly, E6 proteins from low-risk HPV types do not bind p53.

Although high-risk HPV E6 and E7 proteins block the functions of the p53 and Rb tumor suppressors, respectively, the viral proteins are known to interact with many other cellular factors. E6 stimulates expression of telomerase and can therefore efficiently induce cell immortalization. Furthermore, inactivation of p53 by E6 allows accumulation of genetic mutations that would normally be eliminated by apoptosis. Such a mutation in a critical regulatory gene would promote tumorigenesis. The requirement for cellular mutations along with expression of E6 and E7 explains why cervical cancers only develop after several years of persistent high-risk HPV infection.

FIGURE 40-2 ▪ Common warts.

face, knees, or arms, warts tend to be flat and are more likely to be clustered (Fig. 40-3). On the soles of the feet, they tend to be more deeply embedded and more keratotic than those on the hands. Anogenital warts (**condyloma**) may be either flat, slightly elevated, or pedunculated. Cauliflowerlike lesions may surround the anus, labia, or shaft of the penis (Fig. 40-4). Warts of the uterine cervix are usually flat and may be missed during visual speculum examinations.

Warts of the oropharynx occur in infants and adults. In some cases the warts lead to progressive impairment of laryngeal function and may compromise the airway. Hoarseness is the usual presenting symptom. Respiratory distress and secondary bacterial pneumonias occur in children and signify the presence of obstructing lesions in the bronchial tree. The virus types associated with **respiratory papillomatosis** are the same as those that cause anogenital warts and suggest transmission at birth. Oral–genital transmission may be responsible for that clinical syndrome in adults.

FIGURE 40-3 ▪ Multiple flat warts on knee.

FIGURE 40-4 ▪ Penile warts.

How does the host respond to papillomavirus infection? It is thought that cell-mediated immunity is necessary to restrict HPV. Persons who are deficient in cellular immunity (transplant recipients, or those with AIDS) are more likely to have multiple chronic warts.

DIAGNOSIS

The diagnosis of warts is made by morphologic appearance and clinical history. Warts often show plates of thin scale or rough keratotic debris that may form thin finger-like projections and hence "verrucous." As warts enlarge, dermal capillaries proliferate. When the capillaries become thrombosed, usually because of trauma, they create black dots or "seeds," which can be useful in diagnosing warts. Another diagnostic clue to the identification of HPV infection is the absence of normal skin lines.

Papillomaviruses are not easily cultivated in vitro, so a skin specimen cannot be tested by inoculating cultured cells. No routine clinical test exists for determining whether HPV is present in a lesion. Identification of HPV is possible in a research setting, where the tissue is reacted with HPV type-specific nucleic acid probes to specifically amplify viral DNA using PCR. Although exquisitely sensitive, the test is also fraught with the problems of sample contamination. Thus, it is currently limited to research laboratories.

Papanicolaou (Pap) smears of exfoliated cervical cells are routinely used to detect cytological abnormalities typical of HPV infection. Because the presence of a specific HPV type has implications for the level of risk of progression to cervical cancer, it may be important to confirm the presence and specific type of HPV in the specimens. A nucleic acid-based test is available that uses highly specific probes to test for the presence of specific HPV types.

TREATMENT

About 50% of cutaneous warts probably regress spontaneously within 2 years, although new warts also can appear during that time. Because it is not possible to predict which warts will regress and whether new warts will develop, treatment is not always necessary for cutaneous warts. Anogenital warts may be obstructive and raise the concern of sexual transmission and cervical infection. In the uncommon disease respiratory papillomatosis, significant and life-threatening impairment of laryngeal function can occur. Unfortunately, no specific treatments exist for warts. Nearly all modes of treatment are ablative, such as **liquid nitrogen cryotherapy, surgical excision,** destruction with **laser** beams, or application of **caustic, keratolytic, or cytotoxic chemicals.** Those approaches and others have been used with variable efficacy and long-term success. **Imiquimod** is thought to act by stimulating immune response to anogenital HPV infection. Treatment may have to be repeated several times. Not only does destruction of the host cell impair wart virus replication, it also may expose the virus to the immune system.

It is not known whether successful treatment of warts actually results in viral cure—that is, whether HPV DNA is completely gone. The risk of spread is likely reduced, since most patients who have complete remission do not develop new warts. Because the viruses can persist subclinically in apparently normal tissue, only molecular methods can prove whether low amounts of viral DNA persist. Destruction of the lesion may remove one focus of infection but may leave a residual inoculum nearby that later results in local recurrence.

PREVENTION

The intact skin is an effective barrier to wart virus transmission. Complete avoidance is not practical because papillomaviruses can be transmitted by inanimate objects. There is no evidence that condoms reduce the risk of transmission of HPV. Women with a history of genital warts should have regular examinations of the external genitalia, vagina, and cervix, including Pap tests. "Painting" the cervix or other suspected mucosal lesions with 3 to 5% acetic acid whitens them, making the papillomas easier to visualize with magnification (colposcopy). Biopsies of suspicious lesions can then be done to detect precancerous changes in time to permit effective treatment. HPVs are slow viruses, often clinically inapparent, and it is not possible to determine when infection occurred.

Laryngeal warts in the neonate may be prevented if an infected woman is aggressively treated before pregnancy. Some have suggested Cesarean sections for pregnant women with genital warts; however, the risks of surgery are probably greater than the likelihood of the baby developing respiratory papillomatosis.

An exciting development currently in clinical trials is a prophylactic vaccine to prevent HPV infection. Synthesis of the L1 protein at high levels in organisms such as yeast or *Escherichia coli* results in the spontaneous assembly of viruslike particles (VLPs) that exhibit the same epitopes as native virus. VLPs do not contain viral genomes and hence cannot cause warts. Injection of VLPs induces high-titer neutralizing antibodies to the specific HPV L1 type. An early report suggests that immunization with VLPs may protect against cervical HPV infection.

Conclusion

Warts are caused by a large group of related DNA viruses, the papillomaviruses. Papillomaviruses cause a wide variety of clinical manifestations ranging from common cutaneous warts to more serious, proliferative lesions. Fortunately, the benign manifestations are by far the most common. Wart viruses have been associated with various epithelial cancers, especially of the cervix.

chapter **41**

Alphaherpesviruses: Herpes Simplex Virus and Varicella-Zoster Virus

Patricia G. Spear and Stephen E. Straus

key **concepts**

Alphaherpesviruses:

- Include herpes simplex virus types 1 and 2 (oral and genital herpes) and varicella-zoster virus (chickenpox and shingles).

- Invariably establish latent infections following primary infection. Latency allows the virus to persist for the life of the infected individual and can lead to reactivation of virus replication and recurrent outbreaks of symptoms.

- Are ubiquitous in humans; for example, almost all individuals have been infected with herpes simplex virus type 1. Most infections, however, are asymptomatic.

- Are diagnosed in humans by clinical presentation or through virus isolation in cell culture.

- Can be treated with antiviral agents such as acyclovir. However, antiviral therapy cannot prevent recurrences. A varicella-zoster virus vaccine is available to prevent chickenpox.

The term *herpesvirus* refers to many human and animal viruses, the most widely known of which are the **herpes simplex viruses (HSV)**. These viruses are the causative agents of fever blisters and a sexually transmitted genital infection. Herpes simplex virus types 1 and 2 (**HSV-1** and **HSV-2**) are members of the alphaherpesvirus subfamily, which also includes **varicella-zoster virus (VZV)**, the causative agent of varicella (chickenpox) and zoster (shingles). Latent infections of neurons permit these viruses to persist for life. Reactivation of virus replication after recovery from primary infection can cause recurrence of disease symptoms. Rare manifestations of disease caused by HSV and VZV are life-threatening encephalitis and severe disseminated disease.

Despite recent public awareness, herpesviruses are not new causes of human disease. Ancient Greek medical texts described oral infections similar to those now recognized as associated with HSV. The infections are probably what Shakespeare had in mind when he wrote these lines in *Romeo and Juliet* (act 1, scene 4):

> *O'er ladies' lips, who straight on kisses dream*
> *Which oft the angry Mab with blisters plagues*

Case

Mr. H., a 26-year-old graduate student, returned home from his first real vacation in years. While on vacation, Mr. H. had engaged in both vaginal and oral sex with Ms. C., who was staying at the same resort. Several days after his last sexual contact with Ms. C., he noted painful, itchy sores on the shaft of his penis and a sore throat. During a difficult telephone call, Ms. C. acknowledged past episodes of genital herpes. "Could I have herpes?" Mr. H. wonders? He had heard about herpes infections and knew that there are several types and that some recur.

This case raises several questions:

1. What tests would be required to confirm Mr. H.'s suspicion that he has genital and oral herpes?
2. Is it likely that Ms. C. would have engaged in sex when she had active herpetic lesions? If she had no lesions, how could she have transmitted herpes to Mr. H.?
3. What are some of the more severe symptoms that can be associated with primary genital herpes?

Alphaherpesviruses

CHARACTERISTICS

Members of the herpesvirus family can be recognized by properties of the virion and by their mode of replication. All herpesviruses, including the alphaherpesviruses, have large, double-stranded DNA genomes encoding at least 100 proteins. As shown in Figure 41-1 the genome in the virus particle is packaged within an icosahedral protein shell called a nucleocapsid. The nucleocapsid is covered by a layer of proteins called the tegument, which in turn is enclosed within a lipid-containing membrane or envelope. The envelope contains about a dozen viral glycoproteins in addition to lipids. In their replication, herpesviruses make use of the cell nucleus for viral gene transcription, viral DNA replication, and assembly of progeny nucleocapsids. Viral proteins are made in the cytoplasm. Envelopment of the nucleocapsids occurs at the inner nuclear membrane, followed by elimination of that envelope at the outer nuclear membrane and acquisition of the final envelope at a cytoplasmic membrane.

The human and animal herpesviruses are classified into three subfamilies based on their evolutionary relationships and biological properties. The subjects of this chapter are the human alphaherpesviruses: HSV-1, HSV-2, and VZV. The betaherpesviruses (cytomegalovirus and human herpesviruses 6 and 7) and gammaherpesviruses (Epstein-Barr virus and human herpesvirus 8) are discussed in Chapter 42. Members of the various subfamilies can be distinguished by the types of cells in which the viruses can replicate and establish latency. The human alphaherpesviruses replicate in epithelial cells of skin or mucosa, causing vesicular, mucocutaneous lesions. They also can replicate in other cell types. The alphaherpesviruses establish latent infections in neurons.

ENCOUNTER

Infection with one or more herpesviruses is inevitable for virtually everyone. Most of us have probably spread HSV-1 by kissing or exchanging saliva. The virus is usually acquired during childhood or during sexual activity when, either through oral–oral or oral–genital contact. Nearly two thirds of adults have antibodies to HSV-1, indicating prior infection. HSV-2 also can be acquired by oral–oral and oral–genital contact, but it is primarily spread by genital–genital contact. Although uncommon before adolescence, HSV-2 infection rapidly becomes more prevalent with increased sexual activity. About one fifth of all adults are infected with HSV-2, depending on the nature and number of sexual encounters. VZV is usually acquired through the respiratory route, but infection by direct contact with vesicular fluid or secretions also can occur. Primary disease caused by VZV is

FIGURE 41-1 ■ Electron micrographs and schematic drawing of a herpesvirus.

Capsomeres

100 nm

Nucleocapsid

Bilayer membrane (envelope)

Tegument proteins

Nucleocapsid

Envelope glycoprotein

much more contagious than that caused by HSV-1 or HSV-2, in part because direct contact is not required for VZV infection.

Most infections with HSV-1 or HSV-2 are **asymptomatic.** Perhaps only one third of the individuals who harbor the virus recognize symptoms from it. However, asymptomatic infected persons can transmit the virus, because shedding from epithelial surfaces can occur even if lesions are not large enough to be noticeable. Clinically evident infection with HSV-2 is increasing. Rough estimates suggest about a tenfold increase occurred between 1965 and 1985. Primary infections with VZV are usually (but not always) symptomatic, resulting in chickenpox.

ENTRY

Herpesviruses are fragile and susceptible to drying and inactivation by heat, mild detergent, and solvents. Their susceptibility is imposed by their membrane envelope. Because the viruses do not survive well on environmental surfaces, infection with the herpesviruses usually requires direct inoculation of virus into areas where they can replicate. Mucous membranes of the mouth, eye, genitals, respiratory tract, and anus are the sites most readily infected by HSV-1 or HSV-2. The first line of defense against HSV is the skin, which under normal conditions is not readily penetrated or infected by the virus. It is likely that the thick keratin layer of the superficial epidermis prevents access of HSV to their receptors. Because the mucous membranes do not present such a formidable barrier, those surfaces are more readily infected. Inhalation of VZV contained in **aerosols** is the main way individuals contract chickenpox. However, direct inoculation is possible. Thus, the mucous membranes provide the primary portal of entry for these herpesviruses.

SPREAD AND REPLICATION

The life cycle of herpesviruses resembles that of other large DNA viruses that encode many of the enzymes required for virus replication. Although these viruses encode many enzymes, they are still dependent on cellular enzymes, energy, and metabolite resources. Infection begins with the attachment of virus particles to susceptible cells (Fig. 41-2). Virions interact with specific cell surface receptors through glycoproteins that project from the viral envelope. The alphaherpesviruses can bind to cells through the interaction of viral glycoproteins with heparan sulfate chains on cell surface proteoglycans. Although binding is not sufficient for virus entry into the cell, it serves to bring the virus into close proximity to other cell surface molecules that serve as entry receptors. In the case of HSV-1 or HSV-2, several kinds of entry receptors have been identified, any one of which can mediate virus entry. It seems likely that these viruses use different receptors to infect different cell types. The entry receptors used by VZV have not been identified.

Binding of one of the viral glycoproteins to an entry receptor triggers fusion of the virion envelope with a cell membrane, either the plasma membrane or the membrane of an endosome. That fusion causes release of the viral nucleocapsid into the cytoplasm. Following transport of the nucleocapsid to nuclear pores, the viral

FIGURE 41-2 ▪ **Schematic representation of events during productive infection of a cell by a herpesvirus.** The virions are not drawn to scale; in reality they are much smaller in proportion to the cell.

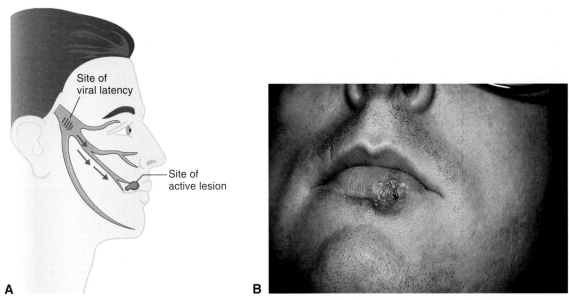

FIGURE 41-3 ▪ **A.** The sites of active and latent herpes simplex virus infections after perioral inoculation. **B.** Recurrent lower-lip lesion caused by HSV-1.

genome is released into the nucleus. If the cell is capable of supporting virus replication, as is true for mucosal epithelial cells, then the viral genes will be transcribed in a temporal fashion, leading to synthesis of viral proteins, replication of the viral genome, and assembly of progeny viruses. If the cell is latently infected, then the viral genome circularizes in the nucleus and persists as an episome with only minimal transcription of viral genes. In the case of HSV and perhaps VZV, virus gains access to nerve cell endings that extend toward the epidermis and is transported to the nerve cell bodies in peripheral ganglia, where latent infections are established (Fig. 41-3).

During productive infection (i.e., an infection in which virus replication occurs), **immediate-early genes** are transcribed with the assistance of an **activating protein** carried in the virion tegument, the space between the nucleocapsid surface and the envelope. Proteins encoded by the immediate-early genes activate expression of about a dozen **early genes** whose protein products are needed to replicate the viral DNA. Following DNA synthesis the viral **late genes** are expressed. Those genes encode proteins that assemble and comprise the progeny virions. Included among the late proteins are glycoproteins inserted into cell membranes. As the new viral nucleocapsids are assembled in the nucleus, they bud through the inner nuclear membrane to acquire a temporary envelope, which they then lose by fusing with the outer nuclear membrane. The final viral envelope is acquired by budding into cytoplasmic vacuoles derived from the Golgi apparatus. Within the final envelope is the full set of viral glycoproteins. The vacuoles containing mature virions then transport the virions to the cell surface for release by exocytosis.

Unlike many other viruses, newly formed herpesvirus particles are not efficiently released into the extracellular space. Rather, as they are released from the host cell, they immediately attach to and penetrate adjacent cells, a process reminiscent of that used by some bacteria, such as *Rickettsia* and *Shigella* . The process of cell-to-cell spread has several important implications for the pathogenesis of disease associated with each herpesvirus and the host responses to infection by this virus group. Diseases induced by HSV, for example, are characterized by local spread and progression of lesions. HSV infection at multiple distant sites is rare and probably requires the circulation of infected cells rather than free virus. HSV rarely causes systemic disease, except in newborn infants or severely immunocompromised individuals. VZV, on the other hand, causes systemic multiorgan disease—a feature that may be partly the result of its ability to infect and be transported by circulating leukocytes. Infected leukocytes can deliver virus to multiple organs and to skin by cell-to-cell contact.

HOST DEFENSES

The innate and adaptive immune responses to herpesvirus infections are multifaceted. Host defenses are usually adequate to limit the duration and severity of infection and, in some persons, are capable of preventing symptomatic primary disease or recurrences, at least in the case of HSV-1 and HSV-2. The host defenses do not prevent latent infections, however, and cannot eliminate latent virus, largely because the latently infected cells apparently do not trigger immune responses.

As is true for many viruses, infection with HSV-1, HSV-2, or VZV induces immediate innate responses, such as activation of neutrophils and natural killer cells and production of interferons and other cytokines. Within several days of infection, antibodies to some of the viral proteins appear in the circulation, and T lymphocytes responsive to viral antigens are amplified in number and activated.

It is thought that antiherpesvirus antibodies play a minor role in recovery from primary HSV or VZV disease. The development of antibodies may occur too late to modify the course of infection. In addition, antibodies probably have little impact on recurrent disease. In fact, persons who are unable to make antibodies have no particular problems with herpesviruses. The likely reason is that the viruses spread from cell to cell, and their mode of spread provides little opportunity for antibodies to come into contact with the viruses. However, antibodies can contribute to prevention of primary disease. Before a VZV vaccine was available, anti-VZV antibodies were administered to prevent infection in immunocompromised children at risk for severe disease. The efficacy of VZV vaccine partly stems from its capacity to induce antiviral antibodies.

Cell-mediated immune mechanisms are most important for recovery from disease caused by HSV or VZV and for prevention or control of recurrent disease. How do the **lymphocytes** involved in cell-mediated immunity control herpesvirus replication and spread? They do so by detecting the "foreign" viral antigens displayed on the surface of infected cells in the form of viral peptides presented by major histocompatibility complex (MHC) class I or class II proteins. T lymphocytes that are activated by interaction with peptide–MHC complexes can then directly kill infected cells or secrete cytokines and chemokines to attract macrophages that can be activated to attack cells infected by virus. No better proof of the primacy of lymphocyte-mediated responses in the control of herpesvirus infections can be found than in the response of severely immunocompromised persons to the infections. About two thirds of all bone marrow transplant recipients experience reactivation of HSV infections within the first month after transplantation. Some of those infections may be severe and destructive. Similarly, children with leukemia and persons with AIDS experience frequent and prolonged HSV infections.

The ability to mount an adequate cellular immune response to herpesviruses changes with age. The relevant immune effector cells gradually mature during the first month of an infant's life. Until maturation is complete, herpesvirus infections can be devastating. In fact, neonatal HSV infection is often fatal, in part because of immunological immaturity and perhaps because the cells of developing organs may have greater innate susceptibility to HSV infection. By 1 month of age, however, the infant tolerates the virus well. Some herpesviruses become problematic at the other end of the age spectrum. Reactivation of VZV leading to zoster occurs with increasing frequency as a function of age, perhaps because of senescence of antiviral immune responses. The likelihood of having zoster is about 10 times greater at age 80 years than at age 8 years.

Herpesviruses encode proteins that allow the virus to evade host immune defenses. For example, HSV-1, HSV-2, and VZV express envelope and cell surface glycoproteins that bind to the Fc domain of antibodies and to complement components to abrogate antiviral activities of those molecules. Certain HSV proteins can reverse the antiviral effects of interferons. Others can prevent the cell surface expression of peptide-loaded MHC proteins, thereby preventing recognition of infected cells by T lymphocytes. HSV and VZV can persist in latently infected neurons despite antiviral immune responses because the cells do not routinely express MHC antigens and they express few if any viral proteins.

DAMAGE

Both HSV and VZV are destructive of the epithelial cells in which they replicate in skin and mucous membranes (Fig. 41-4). As virus replication and spread are contained by immune responses, the epithelium fully regenerates. In other ways, HSV and VZV diseases differ in pathology.

FIGURE 41-4 ■ **Skin lesion biopsies. A.** Photomicrograph of a biopsy of a skin lesion from a patient with HSV infection. Numerous multinucleated cells containing eosinophilic intranuclear inclusions are apparent (red arrow). **B.** Biopsy of a skin lesion from a patient with chickenpox showing a fluid-filled vesicle in the skin (clear space) and giant cells (red arrows) and intranuclear inclusions (green arrow).

table **41-1**	**Usual Course of Herpes Simplex Virus Infection and Disease**
STAGE	**EVENTS**
Acute disease (facial or genital lesions, stomatitis, or keratitis); localized	• Exposure of skin, mucosa, or cornea to secretions containing virus.
	• Replication of virus in epithelial cells, causing vesicular mucocutaneous lesions, stomatitis, or keratitis.
	• Spread to peripheral sensory or autonomic nerve endings and ganglia.
Recovery	• Healing of lesions and establishment of latent infections in neurons.
Latency	• Maintenance of latent infections in neurons.
Recurrent disease (cold sores, fever blisters, keratitis, or genital lesions); localized	• Reactivation of latent virus and distal spread. • Recurrent lesions caused by virus replication in epithelial cells.

HSV lesions are usually localized, with spread of virus restricted to regional nerves. Some damage or inflammation of the nerves can occur during the acute phase of disease, causing symptoms of itching, tingling, burning, or pain. Similar sensations (prodrome) can indicate that recurrent lesions are about to develop. Certain factors trigger the reactivation of latent HSV, including sunburn, systemic infections, immune impairment, emotional stress, and menstruation. It is not yet known how seemingly unrelated factors induce viral reactivation. Reactivated HSV travels down the axonal processes to infect contiguous mucocutaneous epithelial cells. The usual course of events in HSV infections are summarized in Table 41-1.

HSV infection can result in a variety of diseases (Table 41-2). Corneal infections can cause immune responses that damage the cornea irreparably and cause blindness, necessitating corneal transplant for recovery of vision. Primary genital herpes, particularly that caused by HSV-2, can progress to meningitis. HSV-1 can pass from peripheral nerves to the central nervous system (CNS) to cause life-threatening encephalitis, characterized by an unusually progressive and destructive inflammation of a unilateral and focal nature. Persons with no known predisposing risk factors can have CNS involvement, but fortunately it occurs rarely. Newborn infants are especially susceptible to disseminated or neurological disease and, if they survive, might be developmentally impaired. Persons with inadequate cell-mediated immunity are at risk for developing severe disseminated HSV infections that can spread widely across the skin and to viscera, especially the lungs, esophagus, liver, and brain.

Chickenpox, caused by VZV, is a systemic febrile disease with mucocutaneous lesions. Cells of the lymphatic system are infected at the usual portal of entry in the respiratory tract. The spread of virus-infected leukocytes throughout the lymphatic system induces the types of cytokine responses that result in fever, malaise, and headache. During the course of secondary viremia, circulating leukocytes transmit virus to epithelial cells of the skin and mucosa, and the characteristic lesions of chickenpox occur. Latent infections are established in peripheral ganglia. Recovery can be uneventful with no further symptoms from the latent virus unless and until zoster develops years later. Complica-

table **41-2**	**Different Types of Disease Associated With Herpes Simplex Virus Infections**				
INFECTION	**PREDOMINANT VIRUS TYPE**	**FREQUENCY**	**AGE GROUP**	**USUAL OUTCOME**	**RECURRENCE**
Ocular herpes	1	Common	All	Resolution, visual impairment	Yes
Oral herpes	1 > 2	Very common	All	Resolution	Yes
Genital herpes	2 > 1	Common	Adolescents, adults	Resolution	Yes
Neonatal herpes	2 > 1	Very rare	0–4 weeks	Developmental impairment	No*
Meningoencephalitis	2	Uncommon	Adolescents, adults	Resolution	Yes
Encephalitis	1	Very rare	All	Severe neurologic impairment, death	No
Disseminated herpes (immunocompromised)	1 > 2	Rare	All	Resolution or death	No

* Skin lesions can recur; disseminated disease does not.

table 41-3	Usual Course of Varicella-Zoster Virus Infection and Disease
STAGE	**EVENTS**
Acute disease (chickenpox); asymptomatic incubation period followed by systemic disease with skin lesions	• Exposure of respiratory tract to aerosols containing virus. • Replication of virus in regional lymph nodes. • Primary viremia (cell-associated virus); replication in liver and spleen. • Secondary viremia; transport of virus in mononuclear cells to skin and mucous membranes. • Lesions of chicken pox, release of virus from lesions and from respiratory secretions, and spread of virus to dorsal root ganglia. • Spread of virus to sensory and autonomic ganglia.
Recovery	• Healing of lesions, recovery from systemic symptoms, and establishment of latent infections in neurons (also possibly in satellite cells).
Latency	• Maintenance of latent infections in neurons.
Reactivation disease (zoster or shingles); usually localized, but can spread over large areas of body surface	• Reactivation of latent virus and distal spread. • Vesicular lesions along dermatome of nerve harboring reactivated virus; pain.

tions of chickenpox include cerebellar ataxia in otherwise healthy children and encephalitis in immunocompromised persons.

Zoster lesions (shingles) are not unlike the lesions of chickenpox except that they appear on the body surface along the dermatome of the nerve from which VZV was reactivated. The neurological symptoms (pain) associated with zoster are much more severe than for HSV recurrences, probably because there is more viral damage to the affected nerves and supporting cells. The usual course of events in VZV primary disease (chickenpox) and reactivation disease (zoster) are summarized in Table 41-3. As with HSV, VZV can cause severe disseminated disease in immunocompromised individuals.

DIAGNOSIS

The astute clinician who understands the biology and pathophysiology of HSV and VZV infections will have little difficulty diagnosing oral or genital herpes, chickenpox, and zoster. The patient's clinical presentation, coupled with his or her history, is usually sufficient. To establish the diagnosis, the presence of virus or its components in active lesions can be demonstrated. Scrapings or a biopsy of lesions can be examined microscopically for multinucleated giant cells whose nuclei contain **eosinophilic inclusions** (see Fig. 41-4), the hallmark of herpesvirus replication in tissues. Scrapings also can be stained with specific fluorescein-labeled antisera that will bind to viral proteins and fluoresce when examined by a microscope with an ultraviolet light source. The definitive diagnostic tool is virus isolation in cell culture. HSV grows well in a wide variety of fibroblast and epithelial cell lines from animals or humans. Replicating viruses induce characteristic changes in cell shape and appearance (Fig. 41-5). The combination of

FIGURE 41-5 ■ **Human diploid fibroblasts. A.** 48 hours before inoculation with HSV-2. **B.** 48 hours after inoculation.

the appearance of cytopathic changes and immunofluorescence allows a definitive diagnosis of HSV. VZV is more difficult to propagate in cell culture and more fastidious about cell type, but similar methods can be used for definitive diagnosis.

PREVENTION

Herpesviruses are ubiquitous, and it is not practical to avoid contact with all individuals with herpesvirus infections. It is appropriate, however, to avoid sexual contact during active genital herpes infections. Unfortunately, safe and effective vaccines have not been developed for HSV. Even if an effective vaccine were available, it would probably not help people with existing infections. It is unlikely that a vaccine could induce a better immune response than natural infection, which does not suffice to prevent recurrence. Preventative measures for VZV infection are available. Severe chickenpox in immunodeficient children may be partially prevented by administration of specific human immune globulin promptly after exposure. A live, attenuated VZV vaccine prevents chickenpox in normal and some immunologically impaired (leukemic) children (see Chapter 45). Research continues to develop an HSV vaccine and to improve the VZV vaccine.

TREATMENT

Antiviral therapy is still an evolving science. Some of the first antiviral drugs developed were those for the treatment of HSV infections. Nucleoside analogs have been developed that are preferentially used by viral synthetic pathways (see Chapter 44). The most useful antiviral drug to be studied extensively in humans is **acyclovir.** An analog of guanosine, acyclovir can be phosphorylated by herpesvirus enzymes, but not cell enzymes, and then

Paradigm **Box**

Virus Persistence and Latency

Chronic and latent infections are strategies that some viruses use to maintain themselves in the host for long periods and enhance their spread to other hosts. Both types of infection require the viruses to deter or avoid host immune responses. In chronic infections the virus continues to replicate at a low level, whereas in latent infections viral genomes are maintained in specific cell types without virus replication. Periodically, latent viruses may shift to a state of virus replication, with production of infectious virus particles and possible clinical consequences.

Virus latency is an integral part of the life cycle of herpesviruses, papillomaviruses, and retroviruses. The processes involved in establishing and maintaining latency are only partially understood. However, it is apparent that different viruses use different mechanisms to achieve it. Two well-studied herpesviruses, Epstein-Barr virus (EBV) and herpes simplex virus (HSV), illustrate that diversity.

EBV establishes latent infections in B lymphocytes. After virus entry into the cell, the viral genomes circularize and are maintained in the nucleus as episomes. Maintenance of the viral genomes requires the expression of a limited set of viral proteins, some of which ensure that the viral genomes are tethered to cell chromosomes, replicated when cell DNA replicates, and partitioned equally to daughter cells during cell division. Interestingly, the minimal set of EBV proteins required to maintain latent infections fails to induce effective immune responses.

HSV establishes latent infections in neurons, cells that are postmitotic—that is, unable to undergo further cell division. The HSV genome also circularizes following its delivery to the neuronal cell nucleus. Apparently, the expression of viral proteins is not necessary for maintaining the viral genome in latently infected cells. However, a specific HSV transcript is produced (called the **latency-associated transcript,** or **LAT**), and introns are excised from the transcript. Those introns accumulate in the nuclei of latently infected cells. The roles of the LAT and LAT-derived introns have not been definitively established, but some evidence suggests that the RNAs influence the establishment of latent infection.

The factors that influence virus reactivation and recurrence of disease are not well understood for either EBV or HSV. Reactivation and shedding of virus may or may not have clinical consequences but certainly enhances the transmission of virus to uninfected individuals.

incorporated into viral DNA as a chain-terminating nucleotide. Thus, acyclovir is active principally in virus-infected cells and has little or no toxicity for uninfected cells.

Acyclovir, however, is not a cure because it does not prevent entry of virus into neurons and cannot eliminate latent viral genomes. Therefore, patients treated with acyclovir remain susceptible to later recurrences. Long-term treatment with acyclovir will suppress recurrent infections, and such a regimen can be prescribed for persons with frequent troubling recurrences. Varicella and zoster infections also can be ameliorated by acyclovir or a closely related nucleoside analog, **famciclovir.** Now that successful antiviral treatment has become routine, so has the emergence of drug-resistant viruses. Resistance is currently a concern only in selected patients with severe immune deficiencies.

Conclusion

Alphaherpesviruses display a wide range of biological properties and clinical manifestations. Key features of their biology and pathogenesis are the capacity to establish latent infections in neurons and to be activated from the latent state to cause new episodes of clinical disease. Latent infections account for the capacity of these viruses to persist for the lifetime of the host. High prevalence of HSV is partly a result of asymptomatic reactivation and shedding of virus, such that healthy people can inadvertently transmit infection. High prevalence of VZV in human populations is principally a result of contagion during primary disease (varicella or chickenpox). Infection of neurons and spread to the CNS account for some of the most life-threatening and rare forms of alphaherpesvirus disease.

chapter **42**

Betaherpesviruses and Gammaherpesviruses: Cytomegalovirus and Epstein-Barr Virus

William J. Britt

key **concepts**

Betaherpesviruses

- Include human cytomegalovirus, human herpesvirus 6, and human herpesvirus 7.

- Are ubiquitous in humans. Most individuals are infected with betaherpesviruses by young adulthood. Infections are characterized by lifelong persistence with intermittent virus shedding from mucosal surfaces.

Cytomegalovirus

- Is rarely associated with clinical symptoms in normal individuals but represents a common opportunistic pathogen in immunocompromised hosts, including the developing fetus, organ transplant recipients treated with immunosuppressive drugs, and persons with AIDS.

- Can be diagnosed by isolation of replicating virus from patient specimens, demonstration of viral nucleic acids by polymerase chain reaction, and detection of viral antigens in blood or biopsy specimens.

Gammaherpesviruses:

- Include lymphocryptoviruses (Epstein-Barr virus) and rhadinoviruses (human herpesvirus 8, or Kaposi sarcoma herpesvirus).

Epstein-Barr virus

- Establishes lifelong persistence in B cells with intermittent shedding from mucosal sites.

- Is associated with human cancers, including lymphomas and nasopharyngeal carcinoma.

- Causes infections in early childhood that are usually asymptomatic, but infection during adolescence can be associated with a mononucleosis syndrome. In contrast to normal individuals, immunocompromised persons infected with the Epstein-Barr virus are susceptible to acquiring lymphoproliferative syndromes (e.g., posttransplant lymphoproliferative disease, or PTLD) that in some cases progress to malignant lymphomas.

- Causes infection in immunocompetent persons that is usually diagnosed by detection of heterophile antibodies (monospot test) or specific Epstein-Barr virus serologies. In immunocompromised hosts the diagnosis is most often made by detection of Epstein-Barr virus nucleic acids.

The family of human herpesviruses is divided into subfamilies based on genetic attributes and biological properties. The **betaherpesviruses** and **gammaherpesviruses** exhibit remarkable differences in the organization of their genomes and, more importantly, their biological characteristics compared with the alphaherpesviruses (see Chapter 41). The prototype member of the betaherpesvirus subfamily is **human cytomegalovirus (CMV)**; the prototype member of the gammaherpesvirus subfamily is **Epstein-Barr virus (EBV)**. Both CMV and EBV are ubiquitous in humans, and infection with either or both agents by adulthood is nearly universal in the developing world. In the developed world, particularly in North America and Northern Europe, infections with CMV and EBV tend to occur later in life, and about 50 to 60% of adults are infected.

Fortunately, infection with CMV or EBV in immunocompetent individuals is self-limited and infrequently leads to clinically apparent disease. In contrast, infection with either virus in an immunocompromised person can result in serious illness and in some cases death. Persistent infection is a hallmark of all herpesvirus infections and, as with other herpesviruses, CMV and EBV persist for the life of the infected host. In the case of EBV, the virus establishes persistent infection in B lymphocytes, and a well-characterized sequence of viral gene expression events can lead from a state of latency to lytic, productive infection. In contrast, even though latent CMV infection has been described in hematopoietic cells, CMV appears to persist in the human host as a chronic productive infection in a variety of tissues. CMV persistence is not associated with overt evidence of organ dysfunction or clinical disease.

Intermittent excretion of either CMV or EBV in the absence of any clinical symptoms is common and likely responsible for spread of the viruses among humans. Diagnosis of CMV infection in the immunocompromised host is important because effective antiviral therapy is available. Currently, no effective antiviral agents are available to treat EBV infection. Efforts to develop vaccines are under way, but in neither case is a vaccine available.

Case: EBV

Immunocompetent Host

D., a 16-year-old high school student and a member of her school's dance team, recently began dating a 19-year-old student from a nearby college. About two months after they began dating, D. developed a sore throat with a white exudate on her tonsils, swollen but minimally tender lymph nodes in her neck, and a slight yellow tinge to her eyes. She scheduled an appointment with her doctor when her symptoms increased, her energy waned, and her appetite declined. Her new boyfriend had no symptoms. D.'s physician noted that she had exudative pharyngitis and icteric sclera. As part of her evaluation, he ordered a complete blood count and a chemistry panel. The laboratory studies revealed a lymphocytosis with atypical lymphocytes and elevation in the levels of hepatic transaminases.

This case raises several questions:

1. What is noteworthy about D.'s symptoms, and how are they related to her age and behavior?
2. How will the physician use the laboratory to confirm the diagnosis?
3. Should D. be given an antiviral drug?

Case: CMV

Immunocompromised Host

At the age of 20 years, Mr. J. received a kidney transplant for underlying end-stage renal disease. The donor was an unrelated accident victim who was 50 years old. The surgical procedure was uneventful, and Mr. J. tolerated the posttransplant immunosuppressive therapy. About 6 weeks after the transplantation, Mr. J. developed a fever, a drop in his white blood cell count, and decreased appetite. After an extensive medical evaluation, a diagnosis was made with the aid of the clinical pathology laboratory.

This case raises several questions:

1. What factors predispose Mr. J. to infection with either CMV or EBV?
2. Does the limited amount of information that has been included in the clinical history provide clues to the possible causes of his clinical illness?
3. What laboratory tests were used to make the diagnosis?
4. Is treatment with antiviral chemotherapy indicated?

Cytomegalovirus and Epstein-Barr Virus

PATHOBIOLOGY

Overview of Replication and Spread

Human CMV and EBV share many similarities in overall virus structure and replication strategies. Both CMV and EBV are **large, enveloped, double-stranded DNA viruses** that use virus-encoded enzymes to replicate their nucleic acids in the nucleus of infected cells. Both viruses follow a highly regulated and **orderly pattern of viral gene expression** during lytic replication leading to a program of sequential transcription of immediate-early, early, and late viral genes that are required for the production of progeny virus. Abortive infection can lead to incomplete expression of the program and, in the case of EBV, result in restricted expression of viral genes and latency in B cells. Activation of latent EBV infection leading to productive replication requires the expression of viral immediate-early genes that initiate the cascade of viral gene expression. Similar mechanisms have been proposed for CMV, but that virus apparently uses other strategies to persist, including evasion of host immune responses and chronic productive replication in epithelial cells.

Newly replicated viral DNA of both viruses is encapsidated in the nucleus, progeny virions are assembled in the cytoplasm of infected cells following the application of a second layer of protein (tegument layer), and

progeny virions become coated with a lipid-containing envelope of viral glycoproteins (Fig. 42-1). During assembly several host cell proteins also are incorporated, and some are thought to play important roles in the early stages of infection by newly assembled virions. The complexity of the assembly process of these viruses is illustrated by the finding that the CMV virion contains **more than 100 virus-encoded proteins**.

Acquisition of CMV and EBV infection in nonhospitalized persons usually occurs following exposure of mucosal surfaces, such as the oropharynx, to infectious virus. Both viruses can be isolated from secretions collected from the oropharynx and the genital tract. In addition, CMV is readily transmitted in breast milk, and ingestion of breast milk containing CMV is likely the most common mode of infection in infants. CMV infects a wide variety of cells in vivo, including epithelial and endothelial cells, blood mononuclear cells, and supporting cells of the CNS. EBV is more restricted in its cellular tropism and infects B lymphocytes and epithelial cells. Although both CMV and EBV can be transmitted to other hosts in the form of cell-free virus in mucosal secretions, both viruses likely traffic within the infected host as cell-associated virus and not as free virus particles.

Virus Entry, Genome Replication, and Virus Assembly

CMV and EBV attach to target cells through nonspecific interactions with glycosaminoglycans followed by specific interactions with high-affinity cell surface receptors.

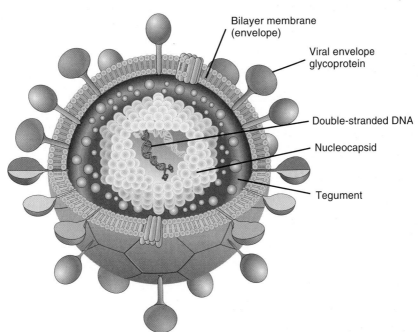

Bilayer membrane (envelope)

Viral envelope glycoprotein

Double-stranded DNA

Nucleocapsid

Tegument

FIGURE 42-1 ■ **Schematic of herpesvirus virion.** A virion is shown with double-stranded DNA in the center of the particle surrounded by an icosahedral nucleocapsid. Proteins in the tegument layer are shown located between the capsid and the lipid membrane, with viral envelope glycoproteins, inserted through the lipid membrane. Modified from a figure provided by Dr. Jay Nelson and Andrew Townsend (Oregon Health Sciences University; Portland, Oregon).

In the case of EBV, a major viral **envelope glycoprotein (gp350/220) attaches to cell surface receptor CD21** and initiates the entry process. Although several candidate proteins have been identified, the cell surface receptor for CMV is not known. However, binding of CMV glycoproteins to the cell surface initiates both virion entry as well as a complex host cell response that is characterized by altered expression of nearly 1,400 cellular genes. Following fusion and penetration of CMV or EBV, viral nucleocapsids containing infectious DNA are translocated to the nucleus by a pathway that appears to involve microtubular transport.

Once the virion DNA has entered the nucleus, the transcriptional program is initiated by cellular factors that activate expression of viral immediate-early genes in the absence of expression of viral proteins. Proteins contained within the virion tegument also enter the nucleus and serve to disarm intrinsic antiviral responses such as the production of interferons. In addition, specific virion proteins also function as transcriptional activators and facilitate expression of a restricted set of viral genes shortly after the viral genome enters the nucleus. Expression of the viral immediate-early genes leads to the sequential expression of the viral early genes, which are required for viral nucleic acid synthesis, including the viral DNA-dependent DNA polymerase, and the viral late genes, which encode virion structural proteins. Both CMV and EBV encode proteins that inhibit apoptosis and block induction of innate immune responses. Both functions ensure host cell survival for a period sufficient to allow production of progeny virus.

The assembly of CMV and EBV virions includes steps in capsid formation, viral DNA packaging, and envelopment that are likely shared by all herpesviruses. The pathway of virus assembly involves both nuclear and cytoplasmic steps. Within the nucleus, the viral capsid is formed around a scaffold provided by one of the virion protein components, resulting in formation of a **130-nm icosahedral nucleocapsid**. Viral DNA is synthesized as long chains of genome-length DNA (concatamers) that are cleaved into unit-length genomes during packaging and capsid maturation. Capsids are thought to exit the nucleus by sequential budding through the inner and outer leaflets of the nuclear membrane, acquire a protein layer (tegument), and eventually become enveloped in the cytoplasm. The size of the mature virus is about 200 to 300 nm. Release of infectious virus is thought to occur either by **exocytosis** or following death of host cells late in infection.

Persistence and Latent Virus Infection

The establishment and maintenance of persistent infection by CMV is poorly understood. Cell culture models suggest that the virus can persist in **hematopoietic progenitor cells** as well as in macrophages. The importance of that mode of persistence in vivo is unclear, and studies of CMV-infected humans suggest that persistence can be more readily explained by chronic productive infection in selected tissues. In contrast, latent infection with EBV is characterized by persistence of the viral genome in **memory B cells**. Reactivation of EBV from latency in vitro can be accomplished by treatment of cells with nonspecific activators of gene expression, such as phorbol esters. Reactivation in vivo is well documented, but the specific stimuli that lead to productive infection in vivo are less clear. **Latency-associated transcripts** have not been convincingly demonstrated in CMV latency. EBV encodes proteins during latent infection of B cells that are required for B cell proliferation and episomal replication of the EBV genome.

Host Responses

Host immune responses play a critical role in the pathobiology of CMV and EBV. The importance of host immunity is most readily illustrated by the finding that deficits in innate or adaptive immunity can lead to enhanced disease following infection with either virus. Patients with primary immunodeficiencies that affect natural killer (NK) cell or T-lymphocyte function, acquired immunodeficiencies such as HIV infection, and immunodeficiencies associated with antirejection therapy in allograft transplantation are at increased risk for development of severe disease following CMV or EBV infection.

NK cells and virus-specific cytotoxic T lymphocytes (CTLs) **control virus replication** during primary infection and **provide surveillance** during viral latency, which limits reactivation within the host. Loss of those responses can lead to reactivation and eventually virus dissemination. Antiviral antibodies also contribute to control of virus spread. Ongoing virus replication can result in end-organ damage and disease. Clinical trials using passive transfer of ex vivo–expanded CMV- or EBV-specific CTLs into allograft recipients have demonstrated the in vivo protective activity of the immune effector cells.

Perhaps one of the most intriguing aspects of the relationship of CMV and EBV with the host cell is the multitude of virus-encoded genes that function specifically in antagonism of host innate and adaptive immunity. In the case of CMV, some viral gene products mediate downregulation and degradation of major histocompatibility complex (MHC) class I and II proteins, and other viral gene products modulate NK-cell receptors and activation antigens. Mechanisms that limit the function of antiviral antibodies also have been documented. CMV encodes a number of functional cytokines, such as interleukin 8 (IL-8) and IL-10, and chemokine receptors that are thought to modulate the host inflammatory response to favor virus persistence in the host. Together, those properties contribute to virus persistence, ensuring the survival of virus-infected cells by limiting the activity of virus clearance mechanisms and preventing apoptosis of infected cells.

table 42-1   Herpesvirus Proteins That Block Host Antiviral Functions

HOST ANTIVIRAL RESPONSES	VIRUS AND VIRAL PROTEIN	FUNCTION
Intrinsic	HSV (alphaherpesvirus), ICP 34.5	Inhibits host cell antiviral response, blocks cell death
	CMV (betaherpesvirus), UL37	Inhibits caspase activity and prevents apoptosis
	EBV (gammaherpesvirus), BHRF1	Similar to cellular Bcl-2, prevents apoptosis
Innate	HSV, IE genes	Infection of NK cells leads to decreased activity
	CMV, UL83 (pp65), UL16	Inhibition of NK receptor activation
Adaptive	HSV, ICP47	Blocks TAP function resulting in decreased antigen presentation
	CMV, US2, US11	Degrades MHC class I and class II molecules with resultant decreased antigen presentation
	EBV gp 42	Blocks MHC class II molecule interactions with T-cell receptor

CMV, cytomegalovirus; EBV, Epstein-Barr virus; HSV, herpes simplex virus; MHC, major histocompatibility complex; NK, natural killer; TAP, transporter associated with antigen presentation.

EBV apparently uses similar strategies to antagonize host immune responses, such as the expression of anti-apoptotic functions, cytokines, and immunomodulatory molecules, including those that inhibit antigen presentation by MHC molecules. An additional novel mechanism of immune evasion used by EBV is the presence of glycine–alanine amino acid repeats within the major target antigen for EBV-specific CTLs. Those unique sequences restrict antigen processing and thus presentation of the antigen to CTLs. Many of the strategies used by CMV and EBV to antagonize host immune responses are conserved in other herpesviruses (Table 42-1) and in other DNA viruses, such as adenoviruses and poxviruses.

EPIDEMIOLOGY

CMV and EBV are ubiquitous in humans with near universal infection in most parts of the world. In developing countries more than 95% of adults are infected with CMV, whereas in the United States about 50 to 60% of adults are infected with the virus. CMV is acquired early in life following exposure to virus-infected breast milk or from exposure to virus-containing secretions from infected children or adults. An increase in the rate of virus acquisition occurs in adolescence and likely results from exposure during intimate and sexual contact. CMV is a sexually transmitted infection, and near universal rates of infection are observed in sexually active populations.

EBV infection follows a similar epidemiologic pattern. However, transmission through breast milk is not an important route of virus spread. As with CMV, almost all adults in the developing world are infected with EBV, whereas EBV infection in the United States and northern Europe is more variable. Infection with EBV is common in the urban poor and less frequent in individuals from middle and upper socioeconomic groups. In populations with limited exposure to EBV during childhood, infection in adolescence more frequently results in clinical symptoms (**infectious mononucleosis,** or **"kissing disease"**). Primary infection with either CMV or EBV rarely results in symptomatic disease, particularly in infants and children.

In addition to community exposure, specific hospital treatments put certain groups of patients at risk for CMV and EBV infections. Infection with either virus can follow **blood transfusion** or **transplantation of an allograft from an infected donor.** Infection following blood transfusion can result in symptomatic disease, which can be especially severe in immunocompromised patients. Similarly, transplantation of an allograft from an infected donor often results in infection of the recipient. Infection with either CMV or EBV in transplant recipients also can be associated with significant morbidity and mortality.

The developing fetus and newborn infant are also at high risk for severe CMV infection. CMV can readily cross the placenta and infect the developing fetus, resulting in a congenital (present at birth) CMV infection. **Congenital CMV** is the most common viral infection of the fetus in humans and can lead to severe disease and permanent neurological damage, including hearing loss and learning disabilities. A summary of modes acquisition and the spectrum of disease associated with CMV and EBV is provided in Table 42-2.

SIGNS AND SYMPTOMS

The vast majority of acute CMV and EBV infections are **clinically asymptomatic,** particularly in young children. Acute infection in young adults can be associated with a mononucleosis syndrome that consists of pharyngitis, cervical lymphadenopathy, low-grade fever, fatigue, and peripheral blood monocytosis that may include the presence of atypical lymphocytes. That presentation is classic for EBV infection, but CMV accounts for about 20% of patients presenting with those symptoms. The clinical

table 42-2 | CMV and EBV Infection: Acquisition and Clinical Syndromes Associated With Infection

HOST	MODE OF EXPOSURE	CLINICAL MANIFESTATIONS
Community Acquired		
Fetus and newborn infant	Intrauterine transmission to fetus (CMV); breast milk transmission (CMV); intrapartum (CMV)	Congenital CMV infection (cytomegalic inclusion disease) with CNS disease, hepatitis, thrombocytopenia. Asymptomatic infection with CNS sequelae (hearing loss). Asymptomatic infection with prolonged virus shedding.
Children	Saliva (CMV, EBV); urine (CMV)	Asymptomatic infection (CMV, EBV). Infrequent mononucleosis-like syndrome (CMV, EBV).
Adolescents and young adults	Saliva (CMV, EBV); sexual transmission from virus in genital tract (CMV)	Mononucleosis syndrome (pharyngitis, fever, lymphadenopathy, hepatitis, and lymphocytosis with atypical lymphocytes) (CMV, EBV). Asymptomatic infection (CMV, EBV).
Hospital acquired		
Patients receiving blood transfusions	CMV, EBV present in white blood cells (acute and latently infected)	Mononucleosis syndrome with more severe symptoms; fever; fatigue (CMV, EBV).
Organ transplantation patients	CMV and EBV present in allograft; blood transfusion	Mononucleosis syndrome, fever (CMV, EBV). Leukopenia, thrombocytopenia (CMV). Hepatitis (CMV, EBV). Lymphoproliferation (EBV). Chronic graft rejection (CMV).

CMV, cytomegalovirus; CNS, central nervous system; EBV, Epstein-Barr virus.

symptoms associated with acute CMV and EBV infections in immunocompetent persons resolve in almost all cases, and the preponderance of evidence suggests that antiviral therapy is of little value in treating the infections.

In contrast to the self-limited disease associated with CMV and EBV infections in immunologically normal individuals, infection with either virus in an immunocompromised person can result in organ dysfunction and in some cases death. Acute CMV infection in transplant recipients often presents as a mononucleosis-like syndrome that includes fever, hematologic abnormalities, and hepatitis. In many cases the infections are self-limited, but CMV infection in allograft recipients can progress to organ-specific and life-threatening disease, including hepatitis, colitis, and pneumonia.

Similarly, EBV infection is an important cause of disease in the immunocompromised host. Infection with the virus can lead to an acute mononucleosis-like syndrome with lymphoid proliferation. In some patients, uncontrolled virus replication secondary to immunosuppression can result in increased expression of viral genes associated with B-cell immortalization and transformation. In immunocompromised persons EBV infection can result in lymphoproliferation, yielding **posttransplant lymphoproliferative disease (PTLD)**. Some cases of PTLD progress to the development of lymphomas. Loss of immunological control of EBV gene expression may be involved in human hematopoietic malignancies linked to EBV infection, such as **Hodgkin disease** and **African Burkitt lymphoma.**

Before the introduction of effective antiretroviral therapy, CMV was a frequent cause of retinitis and colitis in persons with AIDS. As therapy for HIV has improved, the incidence of CMV disease has declined precipitously, providing further support for the hypothesis that acute disease with CMV requires significant immunosuppression.

Newborn infants infected in utero with CMV can develop serious illness secondary to CMV infection. The infant acquires the CMV infection following a maternal infection with CMV that is usually asymptomatic. The virus is transmitted from the pregnant mother to the developing fetus. Infected infants can exhibit significant multisystem disease secondary to unrestricted replication of the virus, presumably as a result of immunological immaturity. In contrast to other immunocompromised hosts, infants infected with CMV in utero often have central nervous system (CNS) involvement as well as hepatitis and hematologic abnormalities. CNS disease in infants can include **encephalomalacia, hydrocephalus, retinitis,** and **damage to the auditory system** (Fig. 42-2). The disease manifestations associated with liver and bone marrow involvement are self-limited, but structural damage in the CNS results in long-term sequelae. It is estimated that CMV infection results in more than 3,000 neurologically impaired infants in the United States each year, with sensorineural hearing loss being the most common long-term manifestation of the infection.

Persistent infections with CMV and EBV have been associated with chronic inflammatory diseases and

A

B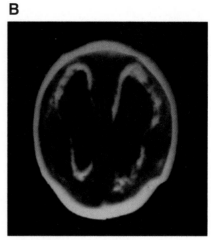

FIGURE 42-2 ▪ **Clinical appearance and radiologic findings of infants with congenital cytomegalovirus. A.** Infant with severe congenital CMV with stigmata of disease, including petechial rash, microcephaly, jaundice, and abnormal posture of upper extremities secondary to central nervous system (CNS) damage. **B.** Computerized tomographic image of an infant with CNS damage secondary to congenital CMV with severe periventricular calcifications (white signal lining the ventricles) and enlargement of the cerebral ventricles (ventriculomegaly).

cancer. Findings from studies of cardiac allograft recipients and epidemiological studies of patients with atherosclerotic vascular disease have linked CMV infection with coronary artery disease. However, the biological significance of the association is not clear. The persistence of CMV in allograft recipients is also thought to be a major contributor to chronic graft rejection. EBV infection has been epidemiologically linked to **African Burkitt lymphoma** and **nasopharyngeal carcinoma.** In addition, EBV nucleic acids can be detected in tissue from more than 40% of patients with Hodgkin lymphoma and in biopsy specimens from patients with breast cancer. Several latency-associated proteins of EBV have oncogenic potential and can transform cells in vitro.

DIAGNOSIS

The diagnosis of CMV and EBV infections can be established by the isolation of the virus in tissue culture, detection of viral antigens or viral nucleic acids in clinical specimens, or measurement of serological responses following infection. Isolation of CMV from urine, saliva, blood, and tissue specimens is readily accomplished. Although EBV can be isolated from clinical specimens, its recovery in tissue-culture systems is difficult and rarely undertaken.

Polymerase chain reaction (PCR)-based assays, both qualitative and quantitative, are commonly employed to identify CMV and EBV in clinical specimens. Application of quantitative (real-time) PCR provides additional precision in diagnosing invasive CMV infection in immunocompromised persons as well as in identifying

patients at risk for the development of EBV-associated PTLD. That approach also permits classification of infants at risk for hearing loss following congenital CMV infection. Techniques for the detection of CMV and EBV antigens in tissue specimens, including routine light microscopy, are useful for confirmation of infection with the viruses.

Histopathological detection of **large ("owl eye") inclusions** in tissue specimens is considered definitive pathological evidence of CMV infection (Fig. 42-3). A widely employed method for the diagnosis of CMV infection in immunocompromised patients is the antigenemia assay. That technique utilizes immunofluorescence to detect a highly expressed CMV antigen in circulating mononuclear and polymorphonuclear leukocytes (see Fig. 42-3). Detection of CMV antigen in peripheral blood leukocytes using the antigenemia assay is predictive of actively replicating CMV, and in transplant patients a positive test often predicts virus dissemination and end-organ disease. Results from the antigenemia assay are used to guide administration of antiviral chemotherapy in transplant patients.

Acquisition of serologic reactivity (seroconversion) is considered strong evidence for primary infection with CMV or EBV. In addition, detection of IgM antibodies specific for either CMV or EBV suggests a recently acquired infection. However, detection of IgG antibodies reactive with either CMV or EBV in a single serum specimen provides no information about the duration of the infection. EBV infection induces the production of a large number of antibodies during acute infection, including antibodies that recognize antigens found on red blood cells of heterologous species. That serologic reactivity forms the basis of the **heterophile antibody or**

FIGURE 42-3 ■ **Laboratory findings of cytomegalovirus infection. A.** Extensive cytopathic effect of human fibroblasts infected with CMV. Notice rounding of cells and large nuclei (arrow). **B.** Fluorescent antibody detection of CMV antigen in circulating polymorphonuclear leukocytes (antigenemia assay) from an allograft recipient. **C.** Nuclear inclusions and cytoplasmic inclusions (arrows) in infected alveolar epithelium of an infant with congenital CMV infection. **D.** Immunohistochemical staining of infected cells (arrow) in a renal biopsy specimen from a transplanted kidney in a patient with CMV infection.

"monospot" test, a simple and rapid agglutination test that is commonly employed in outpatient clinics for the diagnosis of acute EBV infection. Although far from ideal, serologic testing continues to be used in the diagnosis of CMV and EBV infections in immunocompetent persons. However, serology is of little value in the laboratory diagnosis of CMV or EBV infections in immunocompromised persons for several reasons, including the relatively high incidence of preexisting infection in these patients and, perhaps more importantly, because their underlying immune dysfunction often leads to inconsistent serologic responses.

TREATMENT AND PREVENTION

CMV and EBV infections in immunocompetent individuals are almost always self-limited and rarely if ever require treatment. In contrast, antiviral chemotherapy is indicated for treatment of disseminated CMV and EBV infections in immunocompromised patients. Two agents, **ganciclovir** and **foscarnet,** inhibit replication of CMV in cultured cells and in vivo, and both agents are routinely used in the prevention and treatment of invasive CMV infection. Ganciclovir is a nucleoside analog that is phosphorylated by the virus-encoded phosphotransferase UL97. The phosphorylated form of ganciclovir blocks virus replication by directly inhibiting the viral DNA-dependent DNA polymerase and by serving as a DNA chain terminator following incorporation into the newly synthesized viral DNA. Foscarnet also inhibits the viral DNA polymerase. Both agents exhibit dose-related toxicity, and resistance to both agents can develop during therapy.

In contrast to CMV therapy, treatment of EBV infection in the immunocompromised host is problematic. Ganciclovir and the related nucleoside analog **acyclovir** have activity against EBV, and treatment with both drugs can limit virus replication. However, use of ganciclovir and acyclovir to treat PTLD in EBV-infected transplant recipients is of uncertain value, possibly because the viral genes thought to be responsible for lymphoproliferation can be expressed in the absence of viral DNA replication. Alternative approaches have included passive infusion of cytotoxic antibodies specific for EBV-transformed B lymphocytes or ex vivo-expanded CTLs directed against EBV-infected cells. Epithelial malignancies associated with EBV do not respond to treatment with currently available antiviral agents.

Prophylaxis of CMV and EBV infections includes either **prophylactic or preemptive antiviral chemotherapy** to limit disease manifestations. Prophylaxis with antiviral chemotherapy is standard in many transplant centers and is based on the observations that CMV and EBV infections occur during the initial period of intense immunosuppression, and that reduction of virus replication and therefore virus burden limits virus dissemination and disease. Preemptive therapy relies on monitoring the virologic status of the patient and instituting therapy when there is laboratory evidence of increasing virus burden. Both approaches reduce disease caused by CMV in immunocompromised transplant recipients. The effectiveness of the approaches for EBV infection in transplant recipients has not been defined.

Immunoprophylaxis of CMV and EBV disease in transplant recipients has been used for decades. Passive transfer of antiviral antibodies in the form of intravenous immunoglobulin attenuates disease in CMV-infected kidney and liver transplant recipients, and although extraordinarily costly, it is used routinely in some centers. The efficacy of that approach in the hematopoietic transplant recipient is not clearly established. Transfer of ex vivo–expanded, virus-specific T lymphocytes protects hematopoietic allograft recipients from severe CMV infections, which is definitive evidence of the role of T lymphocytes in resistance to CMV disease. Similarly, transfer of EBV-specific T lymphocytes lessens disease associated with EBV infection in hematopoietic and solid-organ allograft recipients. Although a number of candidate vaccines designed to limit virus infection and modify disease associated with CMV and EBV infections are under development, none is currently available.

Conclusion

Betaherpesviruses and gammaherpesviruses have limited intrinsic pathogenicity and restricted tropism in cell culture and in vivo. Compared with alphaherpesviruses, members of both the beta and gamma subfamilies of herpesviruses exhibit more delayed replication cycles but establish similar lifelong persistence in the host. As with all herpesviruses, CMV and EBV enter the host through epithelium and eventually target reservoirs of persistence, hematopoietic and epithelial cells. The replication and assembly of CMV and EBV are similar to that of other herpesviruses. Mechanisms of host-derived resistance to CMV and EBV infections and associated disease include NK cells, CTLs, antiviral antibodies, and soluble effectors such as interferons. Those components of host defense control virus replication, but there is little evidence that they can prevent infection. CMV and EBV express a complex array of virus functions that antagonize various components of host defense, including viral gene products that block apoptosis of infected cells and inhibit recognition of infected cells by immune effector cells.

Although clinically apparent disease following infection with either virus is rare in immunocompetent individuals, a variety of clinical diseases can develop in immunocompromised hosts. In some cases CMV and EBV infections can have significant morbidity with organ-specific and life-threatening manifestations. Effective antiviral therapy is available for CMV infection, but the value of antiviral agents in immunocompromised patients with EBV infection has not been established. Vaccines to prevent infection with either virus are not available.

Viral Hepatitis

Donald E. Ganem

key concepts

Viral Hepatitis
- Is a clinical syndrome characterized by fever and signs and symptoms of liver injury.

- Can be caused by several viruses (known as hepatitis viruses A through E) that are antigenically and genetically unrelated to each other. However, all the agents of hepatitis demonstrate marked tropism for liver cells.

- Shows clinical signs that are initially variable and are indistinguishable among initial infections caused by all of the hepatitis viruses.

- Can be identified by testing for the presence of specific viral proteins, specific antibodies against those proteins, or viral nucleic acid associated with the causative agent.

- Can produce only a transient infection followed by resolution (hepatitis A and E viruses).

- Can produce lifelong persistent infections, with ongoing virus replication in the liver and persistent viremia (hepatitis B, C, and delta viruses).

Many viruses can infect the liver and cause disease. These viruses include adenovirus, cytomegalovirus, Epstein-Barr virus, herpes simplex virus, Lassa virus, varicella-zoster virus, and yellow fever virus. However, all of those viruses also cause diseases affecting organs or tissues in addition to the liver. In contrast, the viruses discussed in this chapter can be thought of as "professional" hepatitis viruses: they have a strong tropism for the liver and preferentially replicate in the **hepatocyte,** the predominant cell type of that organ. As a result, the viruses discussed here are associated primarily with liver disease and only rarely produce disease outside that organ.

The professional hepatitis viruses are a diverse group that includes members from five taxonomic families (Table 43-1). **Hepatitis B virus** (HBV) is the best understood of the group and is therefore the focus of this chapter.

table 43-1 Properties of Human Hepatitis Viruses

AGENT	SIZE (NM)	NUCLEIC ACID COMPOSITION	VIRUS FAMILY
Hepatitis A	27	Linear (+) single-stranded RNA	Picornaviridae
Hepatitis B	45	Nicked, circular, mostly double-stranded DNA	Hepadnaviridae
Hepatitis C	?	Linear (+) single-stranded RNA	Flaviviridae
Hepatitis delta		Circular (−) single-stranded RNA	Deltaviridae
Hepatitis E	27	Linear (+) single-stranded RNA	Caliciviridae

(−), negative-sense polarity; (+), positive-sense polarity.

Virus Replication in the Liver

As the largest organ of the body, the liver represents a potentially major site for virus replication. Approximately 85% of liver cells are **hepatocytes,** the principal epithelial cell in the liver and the target cell type for most hepatitis viruses. However, the liver is also armed with potent immune defenses. It is extensively wired with circulatory and lymphatic networks that provide excellent access to the immune system, including its innate components (e.g., interferons) and its adaptive responses (e.g., antibodies and cytotoxic T cells). Liver-specific macrophages, known as Kupffer cells, undergo inflammatory responses (e.g., cytokine release) that also can aid in the clearance of virus from the liver, either directly or by evoking the influx of additional inflammatory cells from the circulation. The liver is home to many distinctive populations of T cells, some of which—natural killer T (NKT) cells, for instance—are strikingly overrepresented there. NKT cells belong to the innate immune system and are known for dramatic cytokine production when activated. The immunology of the liver is a complex and understudied area, and much remains to be learned about how viruses are eradicated from liver tissue and how (in the case of hepatitis B and C viruses) they often can escape such eradication.

Infection Strategies Used by Hepatitis Viruses

Despite their differing genetic makeups, the hepatitis viruses display two broad patterns of infection in human hosts (Table 43-2). The simplest is exemplified by **hepatitis A virus (HAV)** and **hepatitis E virus (HEV),** which are acquired from the environment by the fecal–oral route. Following uptake in the intestine, the viruses home in on the liver, where replication takes place. Virus is shed into the bile ducts and returned to the intestine, where it can pass out with the feces to contaminate food or drink. Importantly, infected hosts mount an effective immune response that clears virus from the liver and blood and generates lasting immunity to reinfection. Thus, infection by HAV or HEV produces only a transient, self-limited infection. Although the infection can be severe, fatalities are uncommon and resolution is generally the rule.

In contrast, **HBV, hepatitis C virus (HCV),** and **hepatitis delta virus (HDV)** are capable of either transient or persistent infection. They first initiate an acute infection that may or may not result in disease symptoms but always leads to extensive replication of the virus. The immune response that follows, however, is not invariably effective in clearing the infection. The net result is that, although some infected persons do clear the acute infection, many do not and develop a persistent infection that frequently is lifelong. Persistent infection is characterized by continued virus replication in the liver and release of infectious particles into the bloodstream (Table 43-3).

For HBV and HCV, the weight of evidence is that virus replication in hepatocytes is not directly injurious to the cell. How then does the liver damage of hepatitis result? Current evidence favors the theory that liver damage is caused not by viral replication but by **the host**

table 43-2 Transmission of Hepatitis Viruses

	A	B	C	D	E
Fecal–oral	Yes	No	No	No	Yes
Sexual	Yes[a]	Yes	Yes	Yes	Yes[a]
Vertical	No	Yes	Yes	Yes	No
Parenteral	Yes[b]	Yes	Yes	Yes	Yes[b]

[a] From the combined practices of anal and oral sex.
[b] A brief window of viremia exists in which parenteral transmission can occur.

table **43-3**	Clinical Comparison of Disease Associated With Hepatitis Viruses				
	HEPATITIS VIRUS TYPE				
CHARACTERISTIC	**A**	**B**	**C**	**D**	**E**
Incubation period (days)	15–40	60–180	60–120	60–180	21–42
Asymptomatic infection	Often	Often	Often	Can occur	Often
Chronicity	No	Yes (5%)	Yes (80%)	Yes	No
Long-term sequelae	No	Yes[a]	Yes[a]	Exacerbation of HBV infection	No

[a] Includes cirrhosis and hepatocellular carcinoma.
HBV, hepatitis B virus.

immune response to it. That response generates cytotoxic T cells (CTLs) directed against viral antigens displayed on MHC class I proteins on the hepatocyte surface. When antiviral CTLs recognize the antigens, the hepatocytes are killed. In addition, cytokines are released from the T cells that promote further inflammation and tissue injury. When the immune system kills or injures infected hepatocytes, enzymes that normally exist only within those cells, such as aminotransferases (also known as transaminases) are liberated into the bloodstream. If hepatocyte death is extensive and liver function impaired, bilirubin—an intermediate of heme metabolism that is normally detoxified in the liver—accumulates in the blood, causing the patient's skin and eyes to become yellow, which is known as **jaundice.** In fact, clinicians use the magnitude of elevations in serum aminotransferases and bilirubin to gauge the severity of liver injury.

Therefore, the immune response to hepatitis viruses is a double-edged sword: on the plus side, it kills infected cells and clears the infection; on the minus side, it causes liver injury and results in disease symptoms. If the response is sufficiently robust, the primary infection is resolved, as in HAV or HEV infection. The host immune response clears about 95% of adult HBV infections but only 15 to 20% of primary HCV infections. In the remaining cases the immune response is inadequate to clear the virus and persistent infection results. However, the inadequate response continues to injure infected hepatocytes, generating a syndrome of sustained liver damage called **chronic hepatitis.**

The liver responds to sustained damage in a stereotyped way, with regeneration and, in some cases, with scarring (fibrosis). If those two processes are extensive, the resulting disease is **cirrhosis,** in which nodules of regenerating hepatocytes are accompanied by large bands

of connective tissue. Cirrhosis usually indicates extensive loss of functioning liver cells (not made up for by the amount of regeneration), and many such patients go on to liver failure, a condition that is fatal without liver transplantation. In addition, decades of hepatocyte death and regeneration may lead to liver cancer, possibly in connection with viral factors. Chronic infections by HBV and HCV account for more than half the cases of **hepatocellular carcinoma (HCC)** worldwide.

Hepatitis B Virus

Case

Mr. L., a 23-year-old grocery clerk, came to the emergency department because of jaundice. For several days he had felt increasingly weak, nauseated, and feverish and had pain on the right side of his abdomen and joints. He had no appetite. Mr. L. thought that he had picked up a bad case of the "stomach flu" until, while shaving, he noted that his eyes were yellow. He reported that he had experimented with a variety of oral and injectable drugs, but he denied being addicted. He had a stable job and a girlfriend with whom he was sexually active.

The emergency physician suspected that Mr. L. had contracted HBV infection. The laboratory reported increased levels of serum aminotransferases, bilirubin, and alkaline phosphatase, all indicative of liver injury. Antibodies to hepatitis A and C viruses were absent. A surface antigen associated with HBV, called HBsAg, was detected in his serum, although antibodies directed against that antigen were not found. The findings confirmed the diagnosis of HBV infection. The medical personnel who had been exposed to Mr. L. or his blood samples were not particularly concerned about becoming infected because all had received the hepatitis B vaccine.

This case raises several questions:

1. By what route or routes might Mr. L. have become infected?
2. What caused Mr. L.'s symptoms?
3. What was the significance of finding viral surface antigen but not antisurface antibodies?
4. What follow-up tests will be needed to determine his long-term prognosis?
5. What treatment could be instituted?
6. What advice can Mr. L. be given to avoid further transmission?

HBV belongs to the **hepadnavirus** family, a group of viruses with unusual properties, including a partially double-stranded circular DNA and replication via **reverse transcription.** In addition, HBV exhibits a marked tropism for human liver cells (**hepatocytes**) and cannot be grown in cells in culture. One reason for the tropism is that hepadnaviruses only infect cells that express liver-specific transcription factors. Many standard, immortalized cell lines that have been established in the laboratory do not express such proteins and thus cannot transcribe the viral genome. Some cell lines derived from liver tumors do express liver-specific transcription factors, and those cells can produce HBV virions if they are transfected with viral DNA using special laboratory procedures. However, tumor-derived cells cannot be infected by authentic HBV virions, leading scientists to conclude that they lack another factor, most probably a surface receptor that allows binding and internalization of the virus. The lack of infectable cell lines has greatly hampered research on HBV replication. Much of the information about HBV comes from studies of animals infected by other hepadnaviruses.

GENOME AND VIRION STRUCTURE

A map of the HBV genome is shown in Figure 43-1. With less than 3,200 nucleotides, HBV has the smallest genome of any human virus (the HDV genome is smaller but, as discussed later, it is not a traditional virus). HBV uses its genome economically by encoding different proteins within the same region of DNA in different reading frames. About half the nucleotides in the genome are used to code simultaneously for two different proteins, and all of the nucleotides encode at least one protein. The regulatory signals of HBV are not contained in separate regions as in most genomes; instead, they overlap with coding sequences. The cis-acting signals are needed for transcription (promoters and enhancers), polyadenylation, and replication (packaging and reverse transcription). Such unprecedented genome compression limits the degree to which the virus can naturally mutate, because mutations in one base can affect multiple viral proteins.

The structure of HBV DNA is unique: it is a partly double-stranded circular molecule. The minus strand (i.e., noncoding) is nicked and a polymerase molecule is attached to its 5′ end. The plus strand contains a short RNA oligonucleotide at its 5′ end and is shortened at its 3′ end. Thus, the circular DNA genome has a single-stranded gap (see Figure 43-1).

The infectious HBV virions are surrounded by an **envelope** and contain only five proteins. The names of the proteins include the letters *HB* and *Ag* as well as various other letters. The **envelope** layer contains three surface antigens, **HBsAg-S, HBsAg-M,** and **HBsAg-L** (the *S, M,* and *L,* are for "small," "middle," and "large"), embedded in a lipid bilayer. Each protein is translated from a different initiator methionine codon on its messenger RNA (mRNA), but the proteins share much of their carboxy-terminal sequence. HBsAg-S is the main constituent of the envelope and is important for virion assembly. HBsAg-L, which contains all of HBsAg-S plus additional amino acid sequences at its N terminus, is involved in receptor binding and is essential for infection. The function of HbsAg-M is unknown.

The HBV capsid is icosahedral and composed entirely of **core proteins** (**HBcAg**) that surround the viral DNA and the reverse transcriptase, which is also known as the **Pol** protein. A processed form of the core protein, called **e antigen** (**HBeAg**), is made when translation of the precore message begins upstream from the usual start site. The HBeAg is secreted from infected cells and found free in the blood (i.e., not within virions). Although it has the same primary sequence as a portion of the core protein, HBeAg adopts a unique conformation that exposes different epitopes, which makes it a useful marker of HBV infection.

The HBV **reverse transcriptase** has some properties in common with those of the retroviruses. Both kinds of enzymes can copy RNA into DNA and DNA into RNA. Furthermore, both enzymes have RNase H domains that digest the RNA template soon after it is copied. However, the HBV *pol* gene has a unique amino terminal region, called the **terminal domain,** that is covalently attached to virion DNA. The significance of the covalent linkage is explained in the next section.

In addition to infectious virions, the blood of HBV-infected individuals contains many particles with empty envelopes (i.e., lacking the core and genome). The titer of these HBsAy **particles** in the blood can reach

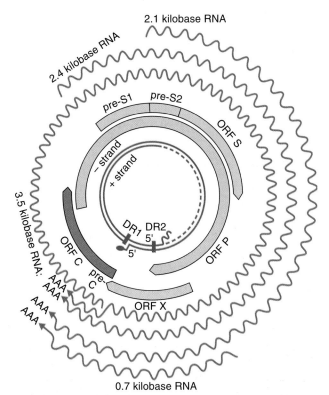

FIGURE 43-1 ■ **Hepatitis B virus genome structure and mRNA transcripts.**

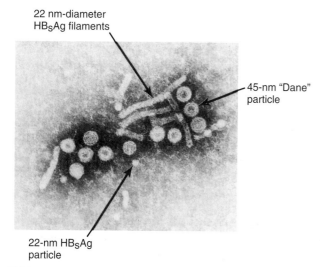

22 nm-diameter HBₛAg filaments

45-nm "Dane" particle

22-nm HBₛAg particle

FIGURE 43-2 ■ **Electron micrograph of hepatitis B virus.** The image includes 22-nm small, spherical aggregates of hepatitis B surface antigen (HBsAg) particles, 22-nm-wide filamentous aggregates of the antigen, and 42- to 45-nm hepatitis B virus ("Dane") particles.

10^{13}/mL. Most of the empty particles are spherical and composed mainly of HBsAg-S. Filaments enriched for HBsAg-L are found in smaller amounts (Fig. 43-2). The role of the empty particles in virus replication and disease is uncertain.

REPLICATION

The HBV replication cycle involves several steps:

1. Following its introduction into the bloodstream, HBV travels to the liver and attaches to the surface of hepatocytes. Attachment involves the interaction of the large surface antigen with unidentified receptors.
2. After uptake and uncoating, the viral genome is delivered to the nucleus, where the partially double-stranded nicked viral DNA is converted into a fully double-stranded, covalently closed, circular species (**cccDNA**). In that process the RNA on the plus strand and the Pol protein on the minus strand are removed, the gapped single-stranded region is filled in, and the resulting termini are ligated.
3. The cccDNA serves as the template for transcription of viral RNA, which is synthesized by a **host RNA polymerase.**
4. The single viral RNA that is to be used for reverse transcription is packaged into an immature viral capsid, along with the viral Pol protein.
5. Viral RNA is used as a template for reverse transcription, resulting in the formation of viral DNA.
6. The virus particles are assembled, and progeny virions are released from infected cells.

Several steps have characteristics exclusive to HBV. For example, HBV transcription has properties that help explain its tropism for liver cells. HBV encodes two enhancer elements that have binding sites for host transcription factors uniquely enriched in liver cells. In addition to expressing five mRNA molecules (for making HBsAg-S, HBsAg-M, HBsAg-L, HBe antigen, and a protein called **X**), HBV makes a sixth, longer transcript called the **pregenomic RNA** (pgRNA). Following its synthesis, pgRNA is transported to the cytoplasm, where it performs two functions: it serves as mRNA for translation of the remaining viral proteins (core and pol) and as a template for viral genome synthesis.

Reverse transcription in HBV replication is a complex process consisting of the following steps:

1. The polymerase binds to a unique stem-loop structure located at the 5′ end of pgRNA (Fig. 43-3, step 1). No other viral or host RNA is known to have such a structure at its 5′ end. This step ensures that only the appropriate RNA is reverse transcribed.
2. Reverse transcription begins, using a mechanism unique to hepadnaviruses. Instead of using a host transfer RNA (tRNA) molecule to prime synthesis (as is done by retroviruses), the hepadnaviral polymerase uses one of its own amino acids for that purpose. As a result, the first deoxynucleotide synthesized is covalently joined to a specific tyrosine residue within the terminal domain of the polymerase.
3. Reverse transcriptase makes a short stretch of three to four deoxynucleotides covalently bound to the polymerase, using as a template a single-stranded bulge region within the RNA (see Fig. 43-3, step 2a).
4. The polymerase translocates to a direct repeat on the 3′ end (DR1) that includes nucleotides complementary to those attached to the polymerase. The deoxynucleotides base pair with DR1, and the polymerase elongates to make a DNA copy (see Fig. 43-3, step 3). As the front end of the polymerase copies RNA into DNA, its trailing portion concomitantly destroys the portion of the template that has already been copied (see Fig. 43-3, step 4). When the polymerase reaches the 5′ end of the pregenomic RNA, minus-strand synthesis is complete, and a short RNA oligonucleotide at the 5′ end remains undigested.
5. The RNA oligonucleotide that remains after minus-strand synthesis is used as a primer to initiate plus-strand synthesis. After a complex series of synthetic events that include two additional strand translocations (see Fig. 43-3, steps 5 and 6), DNA synthesis stops. For reasons that are not understood, the polymerase pauses before completing the plus strand, and a single-stranded gap remains in the final product.

Following reverse transcription, most of the "mature" cores become enveloped by insertion into surface antigen particles that bud from the endoplasmic reticulum. Those particles are transported to the Golgi apparatus, where

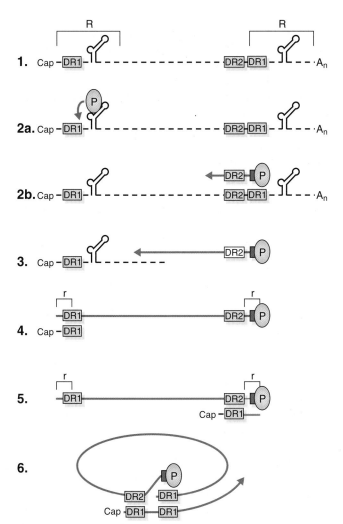

FIGURE 43-3 ▪ **Hepatitis B virus genome replication. 1.** Reverse transcription begins with the polymerase binding to a unique stem-loop structure, located at the 5′ end of pregenomic RNA. **2.** The polymerase (P) uses one of its own amino acids to prime synthesis and copies three or four nucleotides derived from a bulged region of the stem-loop structure (2a). The polymerase then translocates to the 3′ copy of direct repeat 1 (DR1), which includes nucleotides that are complementary to those attached to the polymerase (2b). **3.** Reverse transcription is extended from that point. As the leading front of the polymerase copies RNA into DNA, its trailing portion destroys the template that has already been copied. **4.** When the polymerase reaches the 5′ end of the pregenomic RNA, minus-strand synthesis is complete. The short pregenomic RNA oligonucleotide that remains undigested is then used to prime plus-strand DNA synthesis. That RNA includes the 5′ copy of DR1 and is translocated to a new and complementary region near the 5′ end of the minus DNA strand termed direct repeat 2 (DR2). **5.** Once the second translocation has occurred, plus-strand synthesis begins. During plus-strand synthesis, when the polymerase reaches the end of the minus-strand template, a third and final translocation event occurs. The minus DNA strand has two small terminal redundancies, termed "r". **6.** The 5′ copy of r is dissociated from the plus DNA strand and replaced with the 3′ copy. That dissociation results in the circularization of the DNA molecule and enables further extension of the plus strand cap, 5′-terminal cap; A_n, poly(A) tract.

their envelope proteins become glycosylated. They are secreted from the cell as infectious virus. However, a small percentage of mature core particles are not enveloped. Those particles travel to the nucleus, and following gap repair, replenish the pool of cccDNA.

Readers who find hepadnaviral replication complex and puzzling are not alone. Researchers who have spent much of their scientific careers studying these mechanisms continue to be amazed. The molecular gymnastics that occur during HBV replication are even more remarkable considering that the acrobatic polymerase is conducting its maneuvers within the restrictive confines of the capsid, all the while tethered to the 5′ end of the minus DNA strand.

ENCOUNTER AND ENTRY

HBV is one of the most clinically important viral pathogens of humans. It is estimated that nearly one third of the world's population has been exposed to HBV, and more than 300 million people are chronically infected. Because most of those individuals will continue to produce infectious virus for many years to come, they represent an enormous viral reservoir.

Patterns of HBV infection are not uniform throughout the world. In the United States, Canada, and northern Europe, HBV infections are common only within high-risk groups such as intravenous drug users. In most of Asia, parts of southern Europe, Africa, and South America, HBV infection is far more prevalent in the general population; from 5 to 15% of all human beings in those parts of the world are chronically infected. HBV transmission occurs through the exchange of body fluids such as blood, semen, and vaginal secretions. Before effective screening for HBV in donated blood supplies, transfusions were a common route of transmission. Today that route continues to be a problem only in countries that lack the resources necessary for proper blood screening. Another form of HBV transmission is vertically from mother to infant, probably as a consequence of the child's exposure to maternal blood during birth.

CLINICAL OUTCOMES

The clinical pattern of HBV infection is complex and can follow several paths. The events can be monitored by determining the presence of viral products and specific antibodies in the patient's blood. The serologic events accompanying primary infection are depicted in Figure 43-4. Following infection is an incubation period in which viral infection becomes established but symptoms of liver injury have yet to begin. If the liver injury is very mild (reflecting a mild CTL response), some patients remain asymptomatic and learn only later from serological testing that they had a prior HBV infection. Those with more robust CTL responses, however, develop signs and symptoms of liver injury, which at that stage is called **acute hepatitis.**

From that point, two outcomes are possible. In about 95% of otherwise healthy adults, the immune response is sufficient to clear the infection. In those cases viral gene products in the blood decline precipitously, and anti-HBs IgG antibodies appear (see Fig. 43-4). Those antibodies probably play a role in virus clearance and provide protective immunity against reinfection. In contrast, about 5% of patients progress to chronic infection. Those individuals usually have little or no freely circulating anti-HBs IgG. However, viral products such as HBsAg and HBV virions may be found in the blood for decades (Fig. 43-5). The persistence of HBsAg in the blood for 6 months or more confirms the diagnosis of chronic HBV infection. Results of serologic assays for HBV at various stages of the infection are summarized in Table 43-4.

We know little about why immune responses of some persons can clear the infection while those of others cannot. Before infection most chronic carriers display "normal" immune function and have no prior evidence of an

table **43-4**	Interpretation of Serologic Assays for Hepatitis B Virus				
HBsAg	**ANTI-HBs**	**ANTI-HBc**	**ANTI-HBe**	**HBeAg**	**INTERPRETATION**
Neg	Neg	Neg	Neg	Neg	No prior exposure
Neg	Pos	Neg	Neg	Neg	Prior vaccination
Neg	Pos	Pos	Pos	Neg	Prior acute infection, resolved
Pos	Neg	Pos	Neg	Pos	Acute or chronic infection
Pos	Neg	Pos	Pos	Neg	Later stage in chronic infection

Neg, negative; Pos, positive.

immune deficiency. Clearly, however, they must have a subtle defect in the way they respond to HBV-specific antigens, though what that represents remains a mystery. Likewise, it is not known if host genetic factors have an impact on the outcome of infection. As might be expected, chronicity rates are much higher for individuals whose immune responses are immature or suppressed, like newborn infants or persons with advanced HIV infection. For instance, the rate of progression to chronic infection among exposed newborns (whose T-cell responses are still developing postnatally) is about 85 to 90% compared with 5% among normal adults.

Once a chronic infection is established, the patient is likely to suffer from sporadic episodes of active

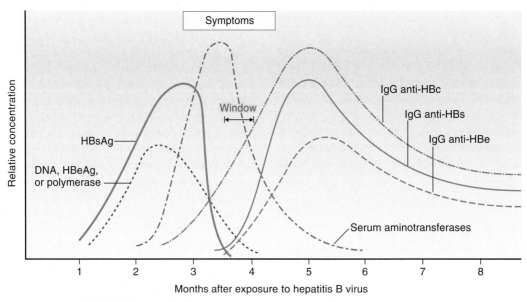

FIGURE 43-4 ■ Typical course of acute hepatitis B virus infection.

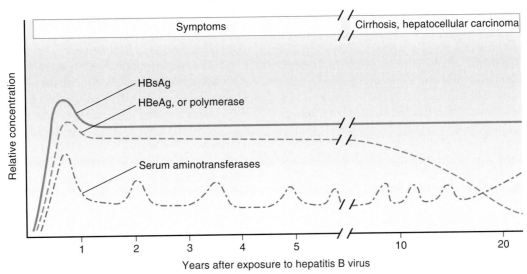

FIGURE 43-5 ▪ **Typical course of chronic hepatitis B virus infection.** After years of undulating symptoms and aminotransferase levels, circulating HBsAg, as well as viral DNA, HBeAg, and polymerase, may decline or even disappear. However, cirrhosis and hepatocellular carcinoma may still develop.

hepatitis associated with liver cell death, which is readily demonstrated by high serum aminotransferase levels (see Fig. 43-5). After many years of persistent infection and associated scarring of the liver, some patients progress to cirrhosis, a potentially fatal condition. In addition, after two to four decades of chronic infection, the risk of developing HCC is increased 100-fold. Several diverse factors participate in the induction of liver cancer during a chronic infection. In persons with chronic hepatitis B, hepatocytes are constantly dying and being replenished as the immune system attempts to clear the infection. The net result of chronic HBV infection is a large increase in the total number of cell divisions in the liver. Because each cell division introduces the chance for mutations that can lead to cancer, perhaps the enhanced rate of liver cell turnover accounts for HBV-induced tumorigenesis. Compounding that effect is the production of peroxides and other mutagenic free radicals that accompanies immune-mediated necrosis.

In addition to mechanisms related to the immune response, viral factors might directly contribute to tumorigenesis. The product of the HBV X gene is able to transactivate promoters not only from the virus but also from the host. Thus, the HBV X protein can potentially induce overexpression of host factors involved in cell cycle progression. In some animal model systems, the HBV X protein induces tumors when expressed at high levels. Integration of HBV DNA into the host genome also might contribute to tumorigenesis. Hepadnaviruses, unlike retroviruses, have no obligatory integration step in their life cycle. The hepadnavirus analog to the retroviral provirus is the cccDNA, which exists as an episomal **plasmid**. Despite the existence of the plasmid, following many years of chronic infection, portions of the HBV

genome can be found integrated at apparently random sites in the host genome. Integration near important growth regulatory genes might deregulate their expression and predispose the host to cancer. That mechanism has been shown to be important in some animal hepadnavirus-induced forms of HCC, but its relevance to human HCC is unclear.

PREVENTION AND TREATMENT

An effective vaccine against HBV is now available. It consists of HBsAg particles obtained from yeast engineered to express an HBsAg-encoding DNA. The HBV vaccine was the first recombinant vaccine approved for use in humans. Currently, HBV vaccination is recommended for all infants in the United States and many other countries. In addition, infants of HBV-seropositive mothers should receive both the vaccine and anti-HBs IgG. Although vaccination programs have reduced the rate of HBV transmission, the virus is far from eradicated. The vaccine requires multiple boosters and is expensive to produce, which has limited its use in some resource-poor countries. However, many countries in Africa and Asia are aggressively vaccinating their populations, and where that has happened, rates of HBV infection and liver cancer are rapidly declining. Nonetheless, since the vaccine is of no benefit to the world's 300 million chronic carriers, much remains to be done before HBV-related diseases disappear.

Treatment options for chronic carriers of HBV are expanding rapidly. For many years injections of interferon-α, a natural antiviral cytokine, were the main-stay of therapy. However, that treatment is expensive, toxic, and of limited efficacy. For approximately 70% of HBV-infected persons, the benefit of interferon-α treatment is transient, and viral levels rebound following cessation of therapy. The discovery that HBV replication involves reverse transcription has led to the development of a number of nucleoside analogs that selectively inhibit the viral enzyme. Some of these, like adefovir, lamivudine, and tenofovir, were initially developed for use against HIV. Those drugs were subsequently noted to have activity against the HBV Pol protein. (Interestingly, adefovir is much more active against HBV than HIV and is not approved by the Food and Drug Administration for treatment of HIV.) Others, including several drugs still in clinical trials, were developed specifically for HBV and are more specific for that virus.

Hepatitis Delta Virus

HDV is not a true virus but rather a subviral agent incapable of disseminating without help from HBV. The RNA genome of HDV encodes a single protein, hepatitis delta antigen (HDAg), which binds to the viral RNA and is important in viral replication and assembly. HDV does not encode any envelope proteins. Instead, it requires the presence of HBV to provide the envelope proteins (HbsAg-L, -M, and -S) necessary for HDV envelopment. As a result of this requirement, HDV only infects persons who are simultaneously infected with HBV (coinfection) or who are already HBV chronic carriers (superinfection). The requirement for a helper virus is a rare property among human viruses. Only one

other helper-dependent infectious agent of humans is known (the adeno-associated virus, a parvovirus that requires adenovirus as a helper).

HDV is associated with an increased risk of fulminant hepatitis during the acute phase of hepatitis and increases hepatitis severity during the chronic phase (Fig. 43-6). Not surprisingly, HDV is acquired by the same routes as HBV, but HDV is not found at equal rates in all parts of the world where HBV is endemic. Furthermore, since the HDV envelope contains HBsAg, the HBV vaccine also protects against HDV infection. The presence of antibodies directed against HDAg in HBV carriers is diagnostic of HDV infection. As yet, there are no effective treatments specific for the HDV component of concurrent HBV and HDV infections.

Hepatitis C Virus

HCV is responsible for the most cases of non-A, non-B hepatitis. The number of persons chronically infected with HCV worldwide is an estimated 200 million. In the United States roughly 15 of every 1,000 persons have chronic HCV infection. HCV, like HBV, is spread by the exchange of body fluids. Before the elimination of HCV from donated blood supplies, transfusions were a common route of infection. HCV is frequently associated with intravenous or percutaneous drug use and is efficiently transmitted by that route. Sexual spread of HCV occurs, although HCV is much less efficiently transmitted by sexual contact than is HBV. HCV-infected mothers also can transmit the virus to their newborn infants. HCV infections are diagnosed by the appearance of antibodies directed against viral proteins and by the

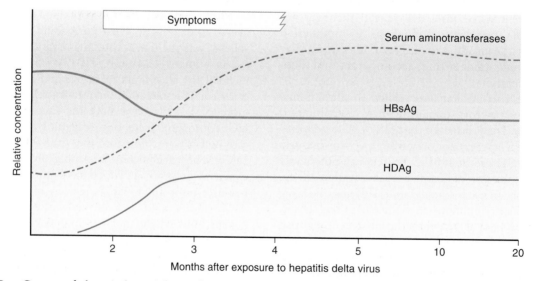

FIGURE 43-6 ▪ **Course of chronic hepatitis B infection exacerbated by infection with hepatitis delta virus.** The levels of aminotransferases may increase, and the liver histology may shift from that of chronic persistent to chronic active hepatitis.

detection of viral RNA in blood using a variation of the polymerase chain reaction.

The liver diseases caused by HCV are similar to those caused by HBV, although they are often somewhat milder, especially in the early stages of infection. However, the long-term consequences of chronic infection with HCV can be as devastating as those caused by HBV. That fact is particularly ominous because the rate at which acute infections progress to chronicity in otherwise healthy adults is much higher for HCV than for HBV (80% compared with 5%). Following several decades of chronic HCV infection, the incidence of liver cirrhosis and HCC is substantial. HCV infection is also associated with extrahepatic diseases, the most notable of which is **mixed cryoglobulinemia,** an immune complex disorder of the kidneys and other sites. In that disease antiviral antibodies complexed to virions are deposited in affected tissues, triggering inflammatory responses that result in tissue damage.

HCV is an enveloped, single-stranded, positive-sense RNA virus in the Flaviviridae family (see Chapter 33). Like HBV, HCV cannot be routinely grown in cultured cells. The only susceptible laboratory animal is the chimpanzee. What little is known about HCV replication has been inferred from its sequence and homology to other viruses, from the expression and analysis of recombinant viral proteins, and from the study of viral RNA synthesis in cell cultures transfected with cloned viral RNA.

Like other single-stranded, positive-sense RNA viruses, the HCV RNA genome is translated on entry into the cell. HCV RNA is not capped, yet most ribosomes usually first recognize the presence of a cap structure at the 5′ end of an RNA molecule before initiating translation. HCV has circumvented the cap requirement by using an **internal ribosome entry site (IRES)** at its 5′ end as a ribosomal binding sequence that directs internal initiation of RNA translation. The product of translation is a single large polyprotein. Within that polyprotein are two protease domains capable of cleaving the polyprotein into a number of functional subunits. The x-ray crystallographic structure of one of those proteases has been determined, giving information that is likely to be useful for the design of specific antiviral protease inhibitors. Once the HCV polyprotein is processed, viral nonstructural proteins participate in genome replication. One of those, the viral RNA-dependent RNA polymerase, first copies the positive-sense RNA into negative-sense RNA and then copies the negative-sense RNA into more positive-sense RNA.

Currently, no vaccine is available to prevent HCV infection. Vaccine development has been hampered by at least two properties of HCV. First, the virus has many genotypes, each with numerous subtypes. Second, during HCV replication, hypervariable regions within the envelope genes are constantly undergoing mutation. Thus, an infected individual carries not one unique virus but a whole population of related viruses, termed a **quasi species** (reminiscent of HIV).

Few treatment options exist for HCV infection. Current therapy with interferon-α (together with ribavirin, an antiviral agent of uncertain mechanism) results in lasting responses in 40 to 50% of infected individuals. Although the responses result in sustained clinical benefit, the regimen is expensive and difficult to tolerate. Clearly, more selective antiviral agents are needed, and that is an active area of research.

Hepatitis A Virus

HAV is responsible for most cases of **infectious hepatitis.** HAV is a nonenveloped, single-stranded, positive-sense virus in the Picornavirus family (see Chapter 32). It is fairly closely related to other picornaviruses, such as poliovirus, and is thought to replicate similarly. Unlike other hepatitis viruses, HAV can replicate in primates, such as marmosets, as well as in liver cells cultured from those animals. The capacity to replicate in cell cultures has facilitated HAV research and vaccine development.

HAV is spread primarily through the ingestion of fecally contaminated food or water. Once HAV reaches the intestine, it is thought to be absorbed into the bloodstream and to reach the liver through the portal system. The virus initiates a rapid acute infection before the development of an immune response (Fig. 43-7). Newly synthesized virus particles are shed into the bile ducts and from there are eventually excreted in the feces. To a lesser extent, virus is also released into the bloodstream, causing a transient viremia and a brief period in which HAV can be transmitted parentally or by blood transfusion.

Symptoms usually appear coincident with the initiation of an immune response, as gauged by the appearance of IgM antibodies specific for the structural proteins of the virus. The extent of illness varies among individuals, but generally symptoms are more severe in adults than in children. In highly endemic regions where sanitation is generally poor, nearly all children become infected in the first few years of life, although most remain asymptomatic. In contrast, adults from nonendemic regions who become infected are more likely to display symptoms, though death associated with fulminant HAV infection is rare. Following development of an immune response, the virus is rapidly cleared, and patients are left with lasting immunity to reinfection. **HAV does not cause chronic or persistent infections.**

An inactivated HAV vaccine has proven to be safe and highly effective. Vaccination is recommended for members of high-risk groups such as military personnel, frequent travelers to developing countries, and the staff of child care facilities and institutions for the severely mentally handicapped. Also, persons exposed to HAV (for example, those who have been served food by an HAV-infected food handler) can be offered administration of serum γ globulin (pooled antibody from normal

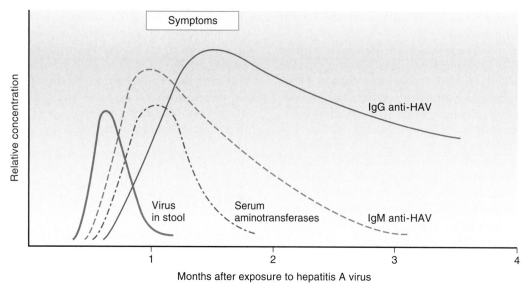

FIGURE 43-7 ▪ Typical course of acute hepatitis A virus infection.

blood donors), which generally has high titers of anti-HAV antibodies. If given soon after HAV exposure, serum γ globulin can prevent HAV infection or reduce its extent and severity.

Hepatitis E Virus

HEV is another cause of foodborne and waterborne hepatitis, especially in the developing world. It resembles HAV in its routes of transmission and associated diseases. Therefore, HEV and HAV infections can only be distinguished serologically. Symptoms associated with acute HEV infections may be more severe than those induced by HAV. That is particularly true for pregnant women, for whom HEV infection can be life threatening. Like HAV, HEV is a nonenveloped, single-stranded, positive-sense RNA virus that causes only acute disease. Efforts to develop an HEV vaccine are currently under way.

Conclusion

The hepatitis viruses are a diverse group of viruses that replicate by a variety of mechanisms. The one attribute shared by hepatitis viruses is a common tissue tropism:

each targets the hepatocyte as its focal point for infection. From the standpoint of disease, the hepatitis viruses can be grouped into two categories. Hepatitis A and E are "hit and run" viruses that are transmitted by the fecal–oral route and replicate prior to the development of an immune response. Ultimately, HAV and HEV are cleared from the liver and thus only cause acute infections. In contrast, hepatitis B, C, and delta viruses are transmitted through body fluids and are capable of persisting in the liver even in the presence of an immune response. After one or more decades, the resulting chronic infection can have profound consequences, including the induction of liver cirrhosis and HCC. Effective vaccines exist only to prevent the spread of HAV and HBV.

During the acute phase of infection, the symptoms induced by all hepatitis viruses are fairly similar and arise as a consequence of damage to the liver. Elevated serum levels of liver enzymes such as aminotransferases and alkaline phosphatase as well as bilirubin (resulting in jaundice) are indicators of liver damage. Determination of the particular virus responsible for the associated disease depends on the use of serological and molecular methods that assay for the presence of specific viral proteins, antibodies directed against those proteins, or viral nucleic acid. Obtaining such a diagnosis is critical for determining the long-term prognosis of the infected individual. Treatment options for chronic HBV and HCV infection are improving, but much work remains to be done in the prevention and treatment of both disorders.

Antiviral Treatment Strategies

Richard T. D'Aquila

key **concepts**

- Antiviral drugs must block a specific step in virus replication.

- Virus replication relies on, and is intertwined with, essential cellular processes in diverse ways.

- Toxicity of antiviral drugs is often related to drug effects on host cell processes.

- Antiviral drug discovery exploits structural, functional, and genomic information to maximize specific inhibition of virus replication and minimize inhibition of cellular processes that might cause toxicity.

- Replication of hepatitis B and C viruses, herpesviruses, HIV, and influenza viruses are targeted by current drugs.

- Resistance to antiviral drugs mandates diagnostic testing and ongoing development of new drugs.

- Other advances in antiviral therapy may come from learning how to better detect and minimize virus resistance and how to better exploit cellular mechanisms with specificity for aiding virus replication or evading drug effectiveness.

The key to successful antiviral chemotherapy is specificity against virus replication. An effective antiviral agent must impair the capacity of a virus to replicate while sparing host cells from potentially toxic effects. This chapter describes some of the chemotherapeutic strategies that have proven successful for combating viral infections in humans. Although interferons, which work in part by augmenting innate immune responses, are mentioned here, the chapter focuses on antiviral drugs used to treat viral infections. Approaches used to induce immunity through vaccination, a highly effective and important means of preventing viral infections, are described in Chapter 45.

Antiviral drugs have been sought since the early days of animal virology. Hundreds of thousands of compounds have been screened against viruses in many taxonomic groups. Many substances inhibit virus replication but are also toxic to host cells. **A strategy for virus inhibition that uses adverse effects on the host cell to interrupt virus**

replication is doomed to fail because of drug toxicity. Because virus growth is tightly linked to host cell processes, one of the first steps following discovery of an agent that can inhibit virus replication is to attempt to select for drug-resistant virus strains. Selection of a resistant strain is an indication that the agent alters a virus-specific process rather than simply causing host cell toxicity. Resistance caused by a mutation in the viral genome will not be selected if virus replication is only indirectly inhibited because of the effects of the virus on the host cell.

Studies of virus–host interactions are increasingly revealing potential points where the Gordian knots that link viruses and their host might be severed. Researchers have elucidated biochemical targets at which replication of certain viruses may be impaired, including viral polymerases and proteases. Many drugs have been found to be safe and effective against some viruses—in particular, hepatitis B and C viruses, herpesviruses, HIV, and influenza viruses. **No truly "broad spectrum" antiviral drugs** yet exist, as they do for bacteria. The diversity of strategies that viruses use to replicate in host cells suggests that development of such agents may not be possible, even as the number of antiviral agents continues to

increase. This chapter summarizes the major strategies to inhibit virus replication that have been successfully deployed in the treatment of human viral diseases.

Approaches to Antiviral Drug Discovery

Each step and biochemical reaction involved in virus replication is conceivably a target for chemotherapeutic intervention. However, inhibition of viral processes that depend on host metabolic pools, host energy sources, and host cell enzymes is likely to result in unacceptable cell toxicity. Fortunately, **some steps in virus replication differ sufficiently from cellular processes in that they can be inhibited with little or no impact on the host cell.** Examples of such specific processes include virus penetration, uncoating, nucleic acid synthesis, protein processing by virally encoded enzymes, assembly of virus particles, and release of the virus from the infected cell. The steps in an idealized virus growth cycle that various agents inhibit are shown in Figure 44-1. Current drugs and agents in development that affect the virus-specific steps in replication are described here. Drugs also have been identified and developed based on a more empiric approach to

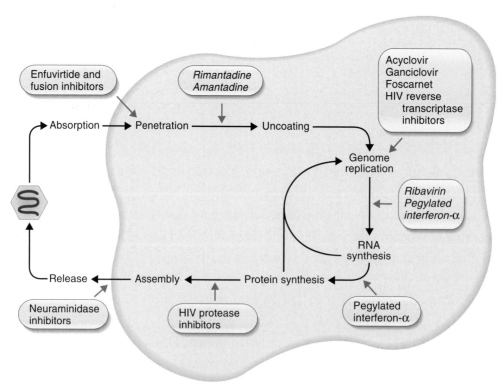

FIGURE 44-1 ▪ **Viral life cycle.** Schematic drawing showing the steps at which replication can be inhibited by antiviral drugs (in italics) or classes of drugs (in regular typeface). The light blue area is the intracellular space.

screening for inhibitors of virus replication without targeting a particular mechanism or virus process.

Although empiricism (along with luck) remains important in antiviral drug discovery and accounts for some of our current therapeutic armamentarium, the acceleration of advances in antiviral discovery in recent years has come from leveraging knowledge of the structure and function of specific viral target proteins and viral genomics. Following early exploitation of herpesvirus polymerase inhibition based on biochemistry (e.g., acyclovir), many advances occurred in the search for HIV inhibitors. Those advances included additional applications of polymerase biochemistry for inhibitor development (e.g., HIV reverse transcriptase inhibitors). The first design of specific inhibitors based on viral protein structure also quickly followed the first determination of crystal structures of the HIV reverse transcriptase (e.g., nevirapine) and the HIV protease (e.g., indinavir, nelfinavir, ritonavir, saquinavir, and subsequent HIV protease inhibitors). The design of inhibitors active against specific drug-resistant mutants (e.g., lopinavir) and other viral targets (enfuvirtide, directed against the HIV gp41 membrane fusion apparatus) have emphasized the power of structure-based drug design.

Agents Developed by an Empiric Approach

Interferon and ribavirin represent two empirically derived agents that are now used to treat hepatitis C virus (HCV) infection. Indeed, HCV infection is one of the next frontiers for advances in antiviral therapy, because drugs developed to specifically target viral enzymes are finally in development. However, the empirically derived agents represent currently used examples of successes of the earlier approach to antiviral drug development.

Interferons

Interferons were the first extensively studied antiviral substances. They are not synthetic drugs but rather natural proteins made by the body. The discovery of interferons by Alick Isaacs and Jean Lindenmann in 1957 involved a brilliant and fortuitous observation, somewhat analogous to Alexander Fleming's recognition of penicillin in moldy cultures. Isaacs was interested in the process of **viral interference,** a poorly understood phenomenon in which infection by one virus renders a cell resistant to subsequent infection with a different virus. Interference of virus-infected cells allowed, for example, the first laboratory detection of rubella virus; although that virus does not produce visible damage to cells in culture, it does render them refractory to secondary infection with other viruses that can produce cytopathic damage.

In studying viral interference, Isaacs and Lindenmann noted that resistance to viral infection could be transferred to uninfected cultures by the addition of media from infected cell cultures. The cell-free factors that mediated the transferable resistance to virus infection were found to be proteins, which they termed interferons. Two properties of interferons were quickly appreciated. First, interferons released from cells in response to infection by one virus provide resistance to infection by many other viruses; thus, interferons are not virus specific. Second, interferons are present in extremely small amounts, indicating that they are very potent molecules. It was reasoned that if interferons could be purified in sufficient quantities, they might be potent therapeutic agents with a broad spectrum of activity. As natural substances, they were likely to be relatively nontoxic, although one might wonder why large amounts are not mobilized spontaneously during infections.

Today we know that many of the early assumptions about interferons were naive and only partially correct. Large amounts of interferons can now be generated by sophisticated purification methods or by recombinant DNA technology, and their mechanisms of action, biological properties, and therapeutic potencies are relatively well defined. In both animals and humans, the effect of treatment with interferons is more complex than in cell cultures because the compounds not only inhibit virus replication but also modulate host immune responses to infection. Numerous clinical trials have shown that interferons in therapeutic doses, despite their natural origin, cause fatigue, fever, myalgias, bone marrow suppression, and neuropsychiatric problems. In fact, it is now thought that many of the constitutional complaints that accompany common viral infections may result from host responses mediated by interferon.

Although interferon treatment ameliorates some severe herpesvirus infections, that action is not sufficiently efficacious to make it the treatment of choice. Nucleoside analogs are much more effective (as discussed in the next section). Similarly, nucleoside analogs such as adefovir and lamivudine are now preferred over interferon for hepatitis B virus (HBV) infection. However, HCV infection responds to recombinant interferon, and effective alternatives are not yet available (see Chapter 43). Interferon therapy in persons with HCV infection results in significant improvements in hepatic function. Longer-lived forms of interferon (e.g., pegylated interferon), used in combination with ribavirin, have yielded sustained virus clearance in some patients.

Why do interferons not show more dramatic clinical activity for all viruses? Inadequate dosage cannot explain their limitations, because circulating levels of the newer recombinant interferon preparations can exceed those observed in untreated infections. There are two possible explanations for the failure of interferons to provide broad-spectrum antiviral activity. First, the production of an interferon may be different in response to different viruses. For a given infection, the antiviral activity achieved may depend on the relative amount of each interferon expressed at a particular site. That effect may not be precisely duplicated by exogenous administration. Second, interferons exhibit the most potent activity against RNA viruses, many of which do not cause serious human disease. Interferons are not very active against DNA viruses and retroviruses.

Ribavirin

Ribavirin is a purine nucleoside analog with a relatively broad antiviral spectrum in cell culture. It inhibits some DNA viruses and many RNA viruses, including influenza A and B viruses, measles virus, parainfluenza virus, respiratory syncytial virus, and several arenaviruses. Ribavirin appears to inhibit virus replication by several different mechanisms, perhaps explaining its range of activity. The triphosphate form of ribavirin inhibits virus-encoded, DNA-dependent DNA polymerases and possibly RNA-dependent RNA polymerases as well. Ribavirin monophosphate inhibits inosine monophosphate dehydrogenase, leading to an overall reduction in cellular pools of GTP. That in turn restricts viral (as well as cellular) nucleic acid synthesis. In addition, ribavirin impairs capping of virus-specific messenger RNA (the addition of methylated guanine nucleotides to the 5′ end of RNA molecules).

The relatively broad spectrum of ribavirin is accompanied by a concomitant lack of potency at nontoxic doses, probably because the mechanisms by which it inhibits viruses are nonspecific and also inhibit cellular enzymes. Lack of specificity translates into poor clinical activity for most viral infections. Oral and intravenous ribavirin appears useful in the treatment of hemorrhagic fevers caused by Lassa virus. It also has been administered through aerosols for severe respiratory syncytial virus infections in children; however, that is no longer standard treatment. Ribavirin remains useful as an adjunct to pegylated interferon for the treatment of HCV infections.

Steps in Virus Replication Targeted by Current Drugs and Agents in Development

Virus entry into cells, virus genome replication, virus protein processing, and virus release from infected cells are each targets of currently available antiviral drugs and new virus-specific inhibitors now in development.

Virus Entry

Entry of virions into host cells can be subdivided into attachment of virions to host cell receptors, cell membrane penetration, and virion uncoating (or disassembly) following successful internalization. Those processes differ for different viruses. HIV, for example, binds to target cells such as T lymphocytes through adsorption of its envelope glycoprotein, **gp120,** to CD4 molecules on the cell surface (Fig. 44-2). That binding event leads to conformational changes in gp120 that facilitate additional interactions with one or more coreceptors. Several chemokine receptors serve as **coreceptors** for HIV, the most common of which are **CCR5** and **CXCR4.** After gp120 engages its coreceptor, further conformational changes trigger the HIV transmembrane protein gp41 to refold to allow fusion of virus and cell membranes. **Membrane fusion leads to entry of virion contents into the cytoplasm,** where the internalized particle undergoes further uncoating before the initiation of genome replication. Additional cellular proteins, including the TRIM family of proteins, can modulate the cytoplasmic virion uncoating process. Mechanisms by which viral proteins interact with cellular proteins to mediate uncoating are just beginning to be defined for HIV. Agents currently in development block the binding of gp120 to CD4 or one of the coreceptors. A currently available drug, enfuvirtide (previously called T-20), specifically interferes with HIV penetration into cells.

Enfuvirtide

Enfuvirtide is a peptide that acts extracellularly to bind the specific domain in HIV gp41 that folds back onto itself to draw the membranes of both virus and cell into proximity to mediate membrane fusion (see Fig. 44-2). By occupying that very specific site, the peptide inhibitor prevents gp41 from undergoing the conformational changes required for membrane fusion, thus inhibiting the penetration step of HIV entry. Given the highly conserved nature of the target motif in gp41, the peptide is effective against a broad range of HIV isolates. It has no known activity against other viruses or cellular proteins. Specific substitutions in the gp41 motif to which enfuvirtide binds mediate antiviral resistance. Because its mechanism of action differs from other currently available anti-HIV drugs (protease and reverse transcriptase inhibitors), enfuvirtide has been used primarily to treat patients with extensive prior antiretroviral drug treatment and concomitant multidrug-resistant HIV. It also differs from other antiretroviral drugs in requiring subcutaneous injection because it is a peptide. It is likely to be further developed for use at earlier stages of HIV treatment.

Amantadine and Rimantadine

The anti-influenza drugs amantadine and rimantadine target the entry of influenza viruses into host cells. The drugs were identified through more empiric means but are now

FIGURE 44-2 ▪ **The process of HIV entry into target cells. A.** Initial attachment of the HIV gp120 envelope protein to the CD4 molecule. **B.** Secondary interaction of HIV gp120 with a chemokine receptor such as CCR5 or CXCR4, which is facilitated by initial CD4 binding. **C.** Stepwise interaction of the HIV gp41 transmembrane protein with the cell membrane, which requires interactions between domains of gp41 that bring membranes of both virus and cell into close proximity for fusion. **D.** Fusion inhibitors, such as enfuvirtide, interact with gp41 intermediates and prevent membrane fusion mediated by gp41 refolding.

known to specifically target the late stages of the entry process of influenza viruses. Amantadine (Fig. 44-3) and rimantadine (not pictured) are primary symmetrical amines chemical structures that provide no clues about how they inhibit influenza A virus replication (see Chapter 36). The primary mechanism of action of the drugs involves disrupting virus entry by preventing virion disassembly.

The influenza A virion contains a transmembrane protein, **M2,** that is well-conserved among human and avian strains (Fig. 44-4). The M2 protein functions as a hydrogen ion channel. Influenza virus enters cells through endosomes, and the M2 protein allows hydrogen ions to move from endosomes into the virion interior during the entry process. The flux of hydrogen ions decreases pH in the virion, which is necessary for conformational changes in the influenza virus nucleocapsid protein that allow movement of the viral ribonucleoproteins (containing the viral genome segments) into the cell nucleus to establish infection. Amantadine and rimantadine **inhibit the ion channel function of M2,** presumably by their large structures blocking the channel through which the ions flow. That effect impedes influenza **virion disassembly** after

internalization into endosomes. Resistance to amantadine and rimantadine occurs with single amino acid substitutions at particular points in the transmembrane region of M2 that prevent drug binding within the channel. Up to 30% of treated patients may shed resistant virus, although illness usually persists only in those who are immunocompromised. Resistant influenza virus strains are genetically stable, but they remain susceptible to neuraminidase inhibitors (as discussed later in the chapter).

The anti-influenza activity of amantadine was first reported in 1961, but enthusiasm for its clinical activity was low. Controlled studies of laboratory-induced or naturally occurring influenza A virus infections demonstrate that the drug should be used when the encounter with influenza A virus can be predicted, such as during epidemics. When treatment is initiated before exposure to the virus, amantadine and rimantadine prevent clinical disease in more than 75% of cases. For patients who begin treatment shortly after the first signs of influenza appear (within 2 days of symptom onset), the reduction in severity of symptoms drops to about 50%. If an index case is found, an entire household or exposed group

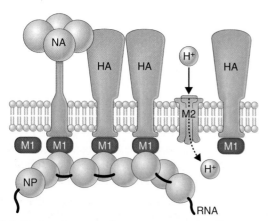

FIGURE 44-3 ■ **Structures of some clinically useful antiviral chemotherapeutic agents.** The structure of the physiologic nucleotide deoxyguanosine (highlighted blue) is shown for comparison to its analogs.

should be treated simultaneously to minimize the spread of resistant virus. It is uncertain whether treatment reduces complications in high-risk patients.

Both amantadine and rimantadine are fairly well tolerated at the therapeutic dose level. About 3 to 5% of amantadine recipients (but fewer rimantadine recipients) report mild central nervous system reactions, including anxiety, insomnia, and difficulty concentrating. The main use has been for prophylaxis in individuals who are at increased risk of severe infection during suspected influenza A virus epidemics. People at high risk include the

elderly and patients with chronic cardiopulmonary disease. It is also recommended that treatment be initiated in those groups at the first sign of influenza in the community. A major limitation of amantadine and rimantadine is that the drugs are not active against influenza B strains; drug disruption of M2 function is specific for influenza A strains.

Virus Genome Replication

Following entry and uncoating, viruses replicate their genomes using virus-specific polymerases. The processes vary among virus families depending on the nature of the genome (DNA or RNA) and the type of enzyme that catalyzes genome synthesis. However, several drugs specifically inhibit viral polymerases. Acyclovir was the first selective inhibitor of a viral polymerase to be developed, and it remains a model for antiviral drug specificity. Many other compounds are now available that target the HIV reverse transcriptase and the HBV polymerase.

Acyclovir

Acyclovir is the prototype antiviral agent and standard against which all other antiviral drugs are compared. It was the first antiviral drug approved for clinical use that resulted from a rational and directed search for antiviral compounds (see Fig. 44-3). It also illustrates how antiviral drugs can be modified to yield increased activity and

FIGURE 44-4 ■ **Structural components of influenza virus relevant to the action of amantadine, rimantadine, oseltamivir, and zanamivir.**

FIGURE 44-5 ▪ Phosphorylation of acyclovir by viral and host *kinases.*

table **44-1**	**Typical Concentrations of Acyclovir Required for 50% Inhibition of Herpesvirus Replication in Cell Culture**
VIRUS	**μg/mL**
Herpes simplex virus 1	0.1
Herpes simplex virus 2	0.3
Varicella-zoster virus	3
Epstein-Barr virus	3
Cytomegalovirus	>40

better pharmacologic properties, such as longer half-life or better gastrointestinal absorption.

Acyclovir is an inhibitor of the DNA polymerases of several herpesviruses. When its activity against cellular and viral polymerases is compared, acyclovir exhibits a therapeutic ratio (i.e., the ratio of specific therapeutic effects relative to nonspecific toxic effects) that substantially exceeds—by about a thousandfold—that of earlier empirically discovered herpesvirus DNA polymerase inhibitors (e.g., vidarabine). The reason is interesting: For acyclovir to inhibit any DNA polymerase, it must be phosphorylated (Fig. 44-5). Herpes simplex virus (HSV) encodes a **thymidine kinase** that has the unique property of phosphorylating acyclovir far more efficiently than does the thymidine kinase of the host cell. The resulting monophosphate is then further phosphorylated by cellular enzymes to generate acyclovir triphosphate. This moiety inhibits herpesvirus DNA polymerase because its incorporation into nascent strands of DNA **blocks further elongation.** Viral DNA polymerase is incapable of attaching bases beyond the point of addition of acyclovir, because the drug lacks the 3′ carbon of the sugar ring at which phosphodiester bonds link nucleosides together.

How do the biochemical mechanisms of acyclovir translate into the in vitro potency of the drug for each herpesvirus? HSV types 1 and 2 are effectively inhibited with submicrogram concentrations of acyclovir (Table 44-1). Epstein-Barr virus (EBV) and varicella-zoster virus are less sensitive to the drug because their kinases phosphorylate it less well, and cytomegalovirus (CMV) is even less well inhibited.

The clinical response to acyclovir therapy in humans is similar to the in vitro activity of the drug. The most significant benefits are observed in patients with HSV infections. Clinical responses to acyclovir therapy also are seen in patients with varicella and zoster, but higher doses are required to treat those infections. Acyclovir has not reproducibly helped alleviate CMV infections or EBV infections.

The greatest benefit from acyclovir comes in the treatment of prolonged or severe mucocutaneous HSV infections, including primary herpes infections of immunocompetent persons or any infection of immunocompromised hosts. Topical, oral, and intravenous formulations of acyclovir speed the clearing of virus, hasten the resolution of symptoms, and shorten the healing time (Fig. 44-6). HSV infections in immunocompetent individuals, which are inherently milder, are not helped by topical acyclovir, and the infections do not warrant intravenous therapy. A modest reduction in the severity of the milder forms of HSV infections can be achieved with prompt administration of oral acyclovir.

Acyclovir does not prevent or terminate herpesvirus latency. Therefore, the infection is as likely to recur whether or not acyclovir treatment is instituted. Nevertheless, there is an effective way of circumventing that limitation. Long-term treatment with oral acyclovir suppresses most expected herpetic recurrences (Fig. 44-7). The suppressive effect of the drug is limited to the period of treatment. Even after years of continuous treatment, recurrences can develop after its termination. That

FIGURE 44-6 ▪ Comparison of intravenous acyclovir and placebo for inhibition of virus shedding in immunocompetent individuals with first episode of genital herpes.

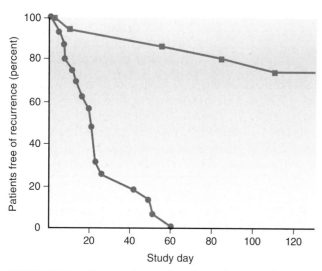

FIGURE 44-7 ■ **Comparison of oral acyclovir (red) and placebo (black) for suppression of recurrent genital herpes.** The likelihood of remaining free of recurrence is shown by study day.

scenario leads to a dilemma for practitioners. Should patients take prolonged treatment for a nonprogressive illness like recurrent herpes? An additional source of concern is that the virus may develop resistance to the drug, although that is rare in immunocompetent persons (as discussed later in the chapter). Most practitioners reserve long-term acyclovir therapy for patients with frequent, painful recurrences of oral or genital herpes.

Ganciclovir

The most serious gap in the antiviral spectrum of acyclovir is its lack of activity against CMV. As a major cause of morbidity and mortality in transplant recipients and persons with HIV infection, CMV has long been a target for antiviral chemotherapy.

In studying modifications of the acyclovir molecule, one compound, ganciclovir, was found to have greatly improved activity against CMV (see Fig. 44-3). Its mechanism of action is similar to that of acyclovir, with preferential phosphorylation by viral enzymes and inhibition of the viral DNA polymerase. The CMV-encoded kinase that phosphorylates ganciclovir is much more efficient in that activity than the enzymes of other herpesviruses that phosphorylate acyclovir. However, it is more toxic than acyclovir, possibly because some cellular polymerases can utilize ganciclovir triphosphate better than acyclovir triphosphate.

Ganciclovir was the first agent shown to reduce the amount of CMV in an infected person. CMV-induced retinitis and gastroenteritis in AIDS patients are stabilized by the drug, but reactivation and progressive infections are seen in many patients once treatment is stopped. Therefore, therapy must be continued for the duration of immunosuppression and possibly for life. In some AIDS patients with CMV disease, treatment has to be changed

because of the bone marrow toxicity of ganciclovir or the emergence of drug-resistant strains.

Organ and bone marrow transplant recipients are also at risk for serious CMV infections, especially pneumonia. Ganciclovir treatment is less effective in those cases because the disease often causes significant lung injury before it can be correctly diagnosed. A good strategy is to observe transplant recipients closely, taking frequent blood cultures or nonculture diagnostics for CMV (e.g., polymerase chain reaction or specific CMV protein detection). When ganciclovir is initiated as soon as an evolving CMV infection is evident from laboratory tests and before any clinical symptoms appear, the likelihood that pneumonia will develop is greatly diminished. That strategy is referred to as **preemptive therapy.**

New Antiviral Drugs Similar to Acyclovir

Acyclovir and ganciclovir have become established as the standards of therapy for a spectrum of herpesvirus infections ranging from simple and recurrent to rare and life threatening. However, the two drugs have important limitations, which have led to focused efforts to improve drug potency and availability. Acyclovir is not very soluble and thus is poorly absorbed from the gastrointestinal tract. Therefore, the maximum serum levels that can be achieved with oral acyclovir are relatively low. **Valacyclovir** is an acyclovir analog that is very well absorbed. It has a valine side chain that is enzymatically removed as the drug traverses the liver, yielding higher, and clinically more effective, acyclovir blood levels. Valacyclovir is considered a "prodrug" that is converted to an active antiviral compound. A similar modification of ganciclovir to **valganciclovir** has improved the **oral bioavailability** of that drug as well. Using the modified drug, immunocompromised patients with persistent CMV infection can be treated with oral rather than intravenous therapy.

Another limitation of acyclovir is its relatively short half-life. After oral or intravenous administration, acyclovir disappears so quickly from the blood that it must be given 5 times per day to be most effective. Of the many new antiherpesvirus synthetic compounds, penciclovir, which is similar in activity to acyclovir but with a much longer half-life, was chosen for clinical development. Unfortunately, penciclovir is also poorly absorbed. Therefore, a penciclovir prodrug was designed by adding two acetyl groups that are removed after it is delivered into the bloodstream. The prodrug, called famciclovir, is effective when given orally 2 to 3 times daily.

Foscarnet

The antiherpesvirus drugs discussed previously are nucleoside analogs that must be phosphorylated before they can inhibit herpesvirus DNA polymerase. Another antiherpesvirus drug, foscarnet, is a phosphonate rather than a nucleoside (see Fig. 44-3). It directly inhibits the enzymatic activity of herpesvirus DNA polymerases.

Foscarnet requires intravenous administration and is moderately toxic.

Drug-resistant herpesvirus strains have been recovered from patients. The good news is that, in the immunocompetent host, resistance has not proven to be especially troublesome. There are two major reasons for that observation:

- Most herpesvirus infections (and infections by many other viruses) resolve spontaneously as a result of cellular immune defenses. The goal of antiviral therapy in most instances is to speed resolution. Emergence of drug resistance may lead to delay in virus clearing, but in general the resistant viruses present a problem mainly for individuals with impaired immune defenses.
- Development of drug resistance may actually reduce the inherent virulence of some viruses. Most acyclovir-resistant strains of HSV have mutations in the gene encoding thymidine kinase. However, thymidine kinase deficiency renders those strains less virulent in animals and less likely to establish latent infection in sensory neurons. In fact, patients with strains resistant to acyclovir often do not suffer severe infections. Moreover, recurrences are associated with reactivation of the original drug-sensitive strains that remain unaltered in sensory ganglia.

Unfortunately, antiviral resistance is a problem for severely immunocompromised persons. The best-studied examples are acyclovir- and ganciclovir-resistant herpesvirus infections in AIDS patients. Foscarnet, with its completely distinct mechanism of action, is currently recommended for the treatment of those resistant infections.

Nucleoside Inhibitors of the HIV Reverse Transcriptase and the HBV Polymerase

The strategy of polymerase inhibition that led to the development of effective antiherpesvirus agents has now been widely exploited, particularly in the urgent search for agents that inhibit HIV reverse transcriptase. Screening compounds expected to inhibit the enzymatic activity of HIV reverse transcriptase, such as nucleoside reverse transcriptase inhibitors (NRTIs), identified many candidates for clinical testing. The NRTIs act as DNA chain terminators after they are converted to the triphosphate form intracellularly. Each lacks a 3′ hydroxyl required for chain elongation and therefore stops chain growth after incorporation by reverse transcriptase. Some NRTIs are too toxic because they also block cellular polymerases, but several nucleoside analogs have become mainstays of HIV therapy. However, long-term toxicity of even the best available anti-HIV drugs (including those in the other classes discussed later in the chapter) has led most experts to recommend initiation of lifelong therapy only when a certain degree of immune impairment has been reached.

Zidovudine (ZDV or AZT) was the first anti-HIV drug to be used clinically (see Fig. 44-3). It inhibits HIV replication at concentrations of 0.1 to 0.5 μg/mL, which are readily achieved following oral or parenteral administration and fall below the cytotoxic level. A series of related nucleosides were developed after AZT that comprise an "alphabet soup" of drug options for HIV-infected persons: abacavir (ABC), didanosine (ddI; see Fig. 44-3), lamivudine (3TC), stavudine (d4T), tenofovir (TDF), and zalcitabine (ddC). Although it is not important at this point to know them all (and the list continues to grow), it is valuable to appreciate their merits and limitations as a group. Each has its own toxicity profile, dose schedule, and evolving role in HIV therapy. They are well absorbed after oral administration, as is required for virtually lifelong, daily therapy. Current practice is to combine two or three of the HIV-targeted nucleoside analogs with at least one agent from a different class, either a nonnucleoside reverse transcriptase inhibitor (NNRTI) or an HIV protease inhibitor. Certain combinations within the nucleoside class are inappropriate because of additive toxicity (e.g., ddI and d4T) or antagonism based on intracellular metabolism (e.g., ZDV and d4T).

It is noteworthy that HIV variants resistant to NRTIs can be selected by using various mechanisms. Some substitutions in the reverse transcriptase impair binding of the NRTI triphosphate. Other substitutions increase the capacity of the reverse transcriptase to excise the chain terminator and gain a "second chance" to incorporate the natural analog. New analogs in development are more active against viruses resistant to current NRTIs.

Some nucleoside analogs also are effective against the HBV polymerase, which in some ways acts like the HIV reverse transcriptase. Adefovir and lamivudine are active at lower doses in vivo against HBV than they are against HIV. Other nucleoside inhibitors of HBV are under development. Adefovir produces renal toxicity when used at the higher doses required to treat HIV but not at the lower doses required to treat HBV. Adefovir is related to tenofovir, which also has in vitro activity against HBV. Although interferons were formerly used to treat HBV infections, the use of nucleoside analogs has supplanted those agents. Other nucleoside analogs with activity only against the HBV polymerase are in advanced stages of development.

Nonnucleoside Inhibitors of the HIV Reverse Transcriptase

Like the NRTIs, the NNRTIs, including delavirdine, efavirenz, and nevirapine, inhibit HIV reverse transcriptase, but they do so by a different mechanism. NNRTIs do not block chain elongation. Instead, they inhibit the catalytic step in reverse transcription by binding to a site of the reverse transcriptase that differs from that bound by natural nucleoside analogs (and NRTIs). Structural studies have shown how the nonnucleoside inhibitors act and have elucidated mechanisms of drug resistance. Those mechanisms are now being used to guide the development of new NNRTI derivatives active against variants resistant to the first-generation compounds. Some second-generation NNRTIs are now in clinical trials. Of note, first-generation NNRTIs are active only against HIV-1 and do not inhibit the closely related lentiviruses HIV-2 and simian immunodeficiency virus (SIV). It turns out that the reverse transcriptases of HIV-2 and SIV naturally contain the residues that are selected when HIV-1 develops resistance to the first-generation drugs.

Virus Protein Processing

Following genome replication, production of virus proteins is an essential part of the replication cycle of all viruses. For many viruses, new virus proteins require cleavage by virus-specific proteases to become fully functional. The HIV protease cleaves a long Gag-Pol precursor polypeptide to yield the shorter, mature HIV proteins. The cleavage events are triggered when the newly formed virion begins to bud from an infected cell. If the mature HIV proteins are not formed by multiple, ordered cleavages, the virion is not infectious. An understanding of the structure of the HIV protease and modeling of its natural peptide substrates led to development of **peptidomimetic inhibitors** of the protease. Those pseudosubstrates bind to the protease but are not cleaved, thus preventing cleavage of the natural substrates. HIV protease inhibitors introduced into an infected cell before virion budding begins block polyprotein cleavage and act to maintain virions in a noninfectious state. Many such compounds are now in clinical use, including amprenavir (and the better-absorbed prodrug fos-amprenavir), indinavir, nelfinavir, ritonavir, and saquinavir (see Fig. 44-3).

Some HIV protease inhibitors have unexpected pharmacologic activities that have improved their utility. For example, ritonavir is a very potent inhibitor of **cytochrome P450 3A4,** the enzyme responsible for metabolism of most protease inhibitors. Combining low doses of ritonavir with other protease inhibitors leads to pharmacologic "boosting" of the blood level of the codosed protease inhibitor, increasing drug effect and half-life. The need for higher blood levels of protease inhibitors, as well as the structure-based design of new agents based on resistance to first-generation protease inhibitors, led to the development of newer coformulations of lopinavir and ritonavir. Specific inhibitors of other essential virus proteases are also being developed, including those required for replication of CMV and HCV.

Since the late 1990s the standard for anti-HIV chemotherapy has been to use at least three drugs in combination to increase potency and minimize the emergence of drug resistance. This advance is called highly active antiretroviral therapy (HAART). Unfortunately, the earlier use of single agents and combinations of two drugs has left a legacy of persons in the United States and Europe who harbor multiple drug-resistant viruses. Intense, multinational efforts to determine which combination of several drugs with distinct actions would be

best have to date been stymied by that legacy and other factors. Treatment decisions are now guided, in part, by drug resistance testing to determine which resistant mutants are present in an individual patient. Consensus guidelines about HIV therapy are updated frequently. Contemporary anti-HIV regimens appear to be less likely to select resistant variants when they fail, but the hope that resistance will be less with the use of only potent combinations is being carefully monitored as treatment expands globally into resource-poor countries.

Virus Release

Inhibitors of the influenza virus neuraminidase (NA) are the first example of antiviral drugs that inhibit virus release from infected cells. The influenza virus NA is a virion surface protein that cleaves terminal sialic acid residues (see Fig. 44-4). Another influenza virus protein, hemagglutinin (HA), is used to attach the virion to sialic acid, which serves as the cellular receptor. Cleavage of terminal sialic acid residues abrogates binding of HA to the cell surface. Removal of sialic acid is essential for release of virus from infected cells and effective spread of virus through the respiratory tract. In the absence of NA cleavage of terminal sialic acid, newly produced influenza virus aggregates as it is released and cannot spread efficiently from cell to cell. Animal studies indicate that NA activity at the time of virion release is essential for virulence of both influenza A and B virus strains.

Oseltamivir and zanamivir each potently inhibit influenza virus NA; they do not inhibit NAs from cells or other pathogens except at much higher concentrations. Clinical studies have shown prophylactic activity, including activity against influenza viruses resistant to either amantadine or rimantadine. If used within 2 days of symptom onset, signs, symptoms, and virus shedding caused by established infection are also diminished. There is hope that oseltamivir and zanamivir will be effective against pandemic influenza virus strains expected in the future.

Conclusion

Antiviral drugs that target virus-specific processes have been successful in the treatment of viral infections without producing undue cellular toxicity. Successful antiviral therapy targets viral enzymes, such as polymerases and proteases, and virus entry mechanisms. Viral enzymes essential for virion release from the infected cell also have been targeted. New advances in antiviral therapy may come from learning how to better detect and minimize virus resistance and from developing strategies to exploit cellular mechanisms that specifically aid virus replication or evade drug effectiveness.

Vaccines and Antisera for the Prevention and Treatment of Infectious Diseases

Kathryn M. Edwards and Natasha B. Halasa

key concepts

- Either active immunization (the administration of all or part of an infectious agent to induce antibodies or other immune responses) or passive immunization (the administration of exogenously produced antibodies) can be effective in the prevention or therapy of infectious diseases.

- Vaccines can be live, attenuated microorganisms; killed microorganisms; components of microorganisms; or toxoids made from microbial products. In general, live vaccines provide longer immunity than those composed of killed organisms, components of organisms, or toxoids.

- In response to some vaccines, B-cell type–specific protective antibody responses are generated; for other vaccines, T-cell type–specific protective responses are seen.

- Some vaccines induce secretory immunity at critical sites of microorganism replication or penetration; examples include live, attenuated vaccines against polio, rubella, and cholera.

- Vaccines should be administered to infants, the elderly, and persons at risk for contracting diseases that for them can be particularly severe.

The dramatic decrease in the incidence of infectious diseases since the middle of the nineteenth century is due largely to two factors: improved sanitation and the development of vaccines. The availability of potable water supplies and sewage disposal, along with improvements in housing, have reduced the incidence of diseases transmitted by food and water and those associated with close living quarters, such as typhoid fever, cholera, tuberculosis, typhus, and plague. Administration of vaccines directed against a number of human pathogens also has remarkably reduced the morbidity and mortality associated with infectious diseases. Examples include the use of vaccinia virus to eradicate smallpox; live, attenuated vaccines to decrease the incidence of polio, measles, rubella (German measles), mumps, and varicella; and toxoid vaccines that have caused an extraordinary decline in cases of diphtheria, tetanus, and pertussis in the United States and abroad. Nevertheless, infectious diseases still cause havoc in developing countries because of inadequate sanitation or the unavailability of vaccines. Roadblocks to controlling infectious diseases often represent failures of economics and politics rather than deficiencies in scientific knowledge or public health awareness.

Even in industrialized countries, despite advances in sanitation and the use of vaccines, infectious diseases continue to cause serious morbidity and mortality. Vaccines have not been developed for many pathogens, and institutional public health control measures have proven difficult for others. Unconquered infections include many viral diseases, particularly those affecting the respiratory and gastrointestinal tracts; sexually transmitted diseases (syphilis, gonorrhea, and chlamydia); and HIV. While rejoicing in the triumphs over many infectious diseases, the health care community should not be complacent about the tremendous tasks ahead in dealing with microbes that continue to attack the human population.

Approaches to Immunization

Vaccinations to prevent infectious diseases have been enormously successful. The benefits of vaccination include partial or complete protection against infections both for the vaccinated person and for society as a whole. Benefits for the individual include protection from symptomatic disease, improved quality of life and productivity, and even prevention of untimely death. Benefits to society include establishment and preservation of herd immunity against communicable diseases, prevention of disease outbreaks, and decrease in health care–related costs. However, no vaccine is completely safe or effective. The risks or side effects of vaccination range from common, minor, and local adverse effects to rare, severe, and even life-threatening conditions. Therefore, recommendations for immunization practices must weigh the scientific evidence of the benefits for each person and for society against the potential costs and risks of the vaccination program.

Several immunization strategies are available to prevent or to treat infectious diseases; the choice depends on the type of microorganism, the age of the host, and the time frame of contact between the host and the pathogen. **Active immunization** with vaccines or toxoids leads to prolonged immunity and is generally preferred to **passive immunization** (administering immune globulins) for prevention of infection (see the box titled "Terminology" for more complete definitions of these and other terms used in this chapter). Vaccines currently licensed for use in the United States are listed in Table 45-1.

Vaccination alone may not ensure protection from disease. As a rule, antibody responses to killed vaccines or toxoids can take several weeks to develop and often require two or three doses at 3- to 4-week intervals for the development of an adequate and persisting immune response. In contrast, **most individuals will develop protective immunity within 2 weeks after administration of a live vaccine.** However, this is not always the case. A small population (less than 5%) will not respond to one dose of MMR vaccine and require a second dose. Likewise, for varicella vaccine, for which approximately 20% of persons 13 years of age or older will not respond to the first dose of vaccine, but close to 99% of persons will seroconvert after two doses. To maintain protective antibody concentrations, many vaccines must be repeated as booster doses. For example, booster doses of tetanus and diphtheria toxoids should be given every 10 years.

Terminology

Active immunization: Involves the administration of all or part of a microorganism or a modified product of that microorganism to evoke an immunologic response mimicking that of natural infection but that presents little or no risk to the recipient.

Vaccine: An immunizing agent derived from microorganisms (or parasites), consisting of the following:

- Live, attenuated microorganisms (e.g., Sabin polio vaccine and measles, mumps, rubella [MMR] vaccine).
- Killed microorganisms or components of microorganisms.
- Killed whole agents (e.g., Salk polio vaccine).
- Extracts of microorganisms, such as soluble capsular polysaccharide (e.g., pneumococcal vaccine) or immunologically active subunits (e.g., hepatitis B vaccine).

Toxoid: An inactivated bacterial toxin that has lost its damaging ("toxic") properties but is capable of inducing protective antibody; diphtheria and tetanus toxins are inactivated and adsorbed with aluminum salts to produce their respective toxoids.

Passive immunization: Administration of exogenously produced or preformed antibodies for the amelioration or prevention of infectious diseases.

Immune globulin: A mixture of antibodies produced by fractionating large pools of blood plasma.

Specific immune globulin: Antibody produced by fractionating donor blood pools selected for high antibody titer to a specific microorganism.

Attenuate: To reduce the severity, virulence, or vitality.

table **45-1**	Vaccines Licensed for Use in Humans in the U.S.		
PATHOGEN		**TYPE OF VACCINE**	
	LIVE	**KILLED**	**SUBUNITS**
Virus	Measles	Hepatitis A	Hepatitis B (recombinant viral surface glycoprotein)
	Mumps	Influenza (whole virus)	Influenza ("split" vaccine)
	Polio (Sabin)	Polio (Salk)	
	Rubella	Rabies (human diploid)	
	Varicella	Japanese encephalitis	
	Yellow fever		
	Vaccinia (smallpox)		
	Influenza (cold-adapted)		
Bacteria	BCG (tuberculosis)	Cholera	Diphtheria (toxoid)
	Typhoid (oral)	Pertussis (whole cell)	*Haemophilus influenzae* B polysaccharide conjugate vaccines
		Plague	Meningococcal (polysaccharide)
		Typhoid	Pertussis (acellular)
			Pneumococcal (polysaccharide-23 valent and polysaccharide conjugated to protein)
			Tetanus (toxoid)
			Typhoid (Vi capsular polysaccharide)

Because most infectious diseases have a short incubation period, usually less than 2 weeks, it is often ineffective to use active immunization for postexposure control. If available, passive immunization with specific globulins or antitoxins can be used after contact (Table 45-2). Passive immunization can be achieved with several types of products. Their use depends on the type of antibody desired, route of administration, and interval after exposure, among other factors. These products can be categorized as immune globulin (IG) and specific (hyperimmune) IG administered intramuscularly, IG administered intravenously (IVIG) and specific (hyperimmune) IG administered intravenously, human plasma, and antibodies from animal origin. Pooled IVIG is used to treat a variety of infectious diseases, immunodeficiencies, and inflammatory conditions—for example, primary immunodeficiencies, Kawasaki syndrome, chronic B-cell lymphocytic leukemia, bone marrow transplantation in adults, immune-mediated thrombocytopenia, and chronic inflammatory demyelinating polyneuropathy. Importantly, antibody-containing products can inhibit the immune response elicited by live vaccines. Therefore, the administration of live vaccines (e.g., MMR and varicella) should be delayed until passive antibody has degraded.

For diseases that have long incubation periods (e.g., the incubation period for hepatitis B is 6 to 24 weeks) or variable incubation periods (e.g., rabies and tetanus), both active and passive immunization are used for postexposure control.

table **45-2**	Specific Immune Globulins and Antitoxins	
HUMAN IMMUNE GLOBULINS	**EQUINE ANTITOXINS**
Cytomegalovirus	Botulism (types A, B, E)
Hepatitis B	Diphtheria
Rabies	
Respiratory syncytial virus (as both an intravenous and an intramuscular monoclonal antibody preparation)	
Tetanus (antitoxin)	
Vaccinia (smallpox)	
Varicella-zoster	

Live Versus Killed Vaccines

Vaccines are made with live, attenuated microorganisms; killed microorganisms; or microbial extracts or purified components. Influenza, polio, and typhoid vaccines are available in live or killed versions. Killed vaccines have traditionally been used because they are easier to manufacture and pose no risk of vaccine-associated infection. The advantages and disadvantages of the two types of polio vaccines are discussed in Chapter 32 and are listed in Table 32-2.

Vaccines are generally designed to stimulate antibody or cell-mediated immune responses directed against critical virulence factors of the organism. Examples include the capsular polysaccharides of the pneumococcus organism, the surface glycoprotein of hepatitis B virus, and the hemagglutinin and neuraminidase proteins of the "split" inactivated influenza virus. In general, **immunity generated by a killed vaccine is not as effective or long lasting as immunity stimulated by a live, attenuated vaccine,** which more closely mimics the natural disease. Additionally, live vaccines often elicit both cell-mediated immunity and neutralizing antibodies, which provide prolonged, and often lifelong, immunity.

The recent approval of the live, attenuated, intranasal, cold-adapted influenza vaccine (sometimes called, more simply, the live, attenuated influenza vaccine) offers another live vaccine alternative. Containing a weakened form of live influenza virus instead of killed virus, the vaccine is administered by nasal spray instead of injection. The term *cold-adapted* indicates that the virus can grow in the nose and throat but not in the lower respiratory tract where the temperature is higher.

Attenuation of a virulent pathogen to an avirulent vaccine strain can be technically difficult to accomplish. Even when successful, a small but finite danger exists that the attenuated vaccine strain will revert to a more virulent strain in a susceptible host. For example, **vaccine-acquired paralytic poliomyelitis (VAPP)** occurs after approximately 1 in every 1 million to 3 million doses of live polio vaccine administered. Because wild-type poliovirus transmission was eliminated in the United States in 1979, and the only cases of paralytic disease since that time have been due to VAPP, exclusive use of inactivated polio vaccine was recommended in 1999. However, in other countries where wild-type poliovirus still exists, live, attenuated polio vaccine is the primary vaccine used because of its excellent ability to produce intestinal immunity and induce **herd immunity.** Unfortunately, localized outbreaks of paralytic polio have been reported in several countries including the United States where the attenuated vaccine strain has reverted to virulence and spread among previously unimmunized persons. Therefore, immunization rates must be kept high to prevent outbreaks.

Another example of adverse events associated with vaccines is the previously licensed rotavirus vaccine. After licensure of a live, attenuated rotavirus vaccine, it was found to be associated with an increased rate of intussusception. As a result, its use was discontinued. Live viral vaccines remain excellent immunogens, but their potential for adverse events must be carefully considered.

Type of Immune Response and Correlation of Protection

The type of immune response elicited by a vaccine is dependent on which vaccine is administered. For example, active immunization with a live, attenuated organism (e.g., poliovirus) induces B cells, $CD8^+$ T cells, and $CD4^+$ T cells, whereas active immunization with inactivated organisms (e.g., rabies, inactivated polio), protein antigens (e.g., diphtheria, tetanus, pertussis), and capsular polysaccharide plus a protein carrier (e.g., *Haemophilus influenzae* type B polysaccharide linked to a bacterial toxoid) induces B cells and $CD4^+$ T cells. Immunization with capsular polysaccharides (e.g., pneumococcal capsular polysaccharide) induces B cells only.

Immunizing agents can produce immunity through B-cell proliferation leading to antibody production, with or without helper T cells. Both pneumococcal capsular polysaccharides (see Chapter 13) and the polysaccharide of *H. influenzae* type B (HIB) induce B-cell production of antibody without a contribution of helper T cells. These **T cell–independent antigens** are characterized by low antibody titers, particularly in children less than 18 months of age, and little memory response. By covalently coupling (conjugating) the *H. influenzae* polysaccharide known as polyribosylribitol phosphate (PRP) to a protein antigen such as diphtheria toxoid or the outer membrane protein of *Neisseria*, the conjugated HIB vaccine produces a T cell–dependent antibody response. The conjugate HIB vaccine induces high antibody levels in young infants and primes for strong booster responses with revaccination. Since widespread use of the conjugated HIB vaccines, the incidence of invasive HIB disease has fallen dramatically (more than 99%) compared with the prevaccine era.

The conjugation of pneumococcal capsular polysaccharides to protein antigens also has been used to generate a 7-valent conjugated pneumococcal vaccine. The vaccine, which also produces a T cell–dependent response, was licensed in 2000. Since licensure, the pneumococcal conjugate has decreased invasive pneumococcal disease in vaccinated children ages 2 months to 59 months and in unimmunized individuals of all age groups, suggesting that herd immunity has been achieved.

Secretory IgA antibodies produced at the mucosal surface offer protection against some mucosal pathogens such as influenza virus, poliovirus, respiratory syncytial virus, rotavirus, rubella virus, *Neisseria gonorrhoeae*, and *Vibrio cholerae*. Live, attenuated vaccines delivered to mucosal sites can induce secretory immunity at the site of initial pathogen contact. Several such vaccines have been produced, including live, attenuated adenovirus, influenza virus, and poliovirus vaccines. Oral typhoid vaccines also induce local immune responses.

The favored approach in vaccine development is to define the **"correlates of protection,"** or the host immune responses associated with disease prevention. Vaccines that protect solely or principally by induction of serum antibodies include hepatitis A, polio, rabies, yellow fever, diphtheria, Lyme disease, pertussis, tetanus, and extracellular encapsulated bacteria. Both antibody levels and their function are important correlates of protection for mumps, rubella, meningococcal, and pneumococcal vaccines. Secretory antibodies play a role in protection against infections caused by agents that must first replicate on mucosal surfaces such as influenza virus, poliovirus, and rotavirus. Lastly, vaccines for which T-cell responses are essential include measles, varicella, and tuberculosis. Induction of T-cell immunity is an important goal of current efforts to develop an HIV vaccine.

Age of Immunization

Because they receive a supply of serum IgG antibody from their mothers, newborns have transient protection against diseases to which their mothers were immune. Breast milk also contains secretory IgA antibodies that provide protection against intestinal and respiratory tract infections to which the mother has developed immunity. Although the humoral immune system is not fully functional at birth and generates poor responses to certain polysaccharide antigens, it generally responds well to protein antigens like those seen in the diphtheria, pertussis, and tetanus vaccines when given at 2 months of age. When given at birth, hepatitis B vaccine is also immunogenic. Some vaccines, particularly those that contain live, attenuated viruses, like MMR, are given after the first year of life because of the potential interference of maternally derived antibodies with the ability to generate an adequate immune response.

As with infants, the elderly have a reduced antibody response to vaccines and an increased susceptibility to certain infections such as those caused by influenza virus and pneumococcus.

Selection of Antigens

Although infecting pathogens contain an enormous quantity of various types of antigens, immune responses are often targeted to surface components that the pathogen encounters when it invades. In some instances, a vaccine confers protection against all strains of the infecting organism. In contrast, other infectious agents, such as the pneumococcus, have several distinct capsular polysaccharide types, and immunity to one polysaccharide type does not confer immunity to the others. Thus, the pneumococcal vaccine is a mixture of antigens comprising the most common serotypes causing invasive pneumococcal disease.

Another complicated problem with antigen selection is seen with the influenza virus. The vaccine is formulated annually to protect against the strains expected to circulate during the following year. Minor antigenic changes in influenza virus, called antigenic drift, occur annually, whereas major antigenic changes, known as antigenic shift, occur approximately every 10 years. Vaccines must therefore be modified to accommodate antigenic drift and shift (see Chapter 36).

Immunization of Special Populations

Certain individuals are at higher risk for vaccine-preventable diseases and should be targeted for immunization. Examples include persons with underlying heart or lung disease or those more than 65 years of age who are at greater risk for morbidity and mortality from influenza (Table 45-3). Some individuals also are at greater risk for disease because specific immune system defects reduce their ability to generate adequate immune responses.

Because of functional asplenia, persons with sickle cell disease are at risk for infections with encapsulated organisms, particularly pneumococci. Those individuals should be vaccinated with pneumococcal vaccine, which may not be totally effective but nevertheless will provide some protection. Similarly, a person who is either born without a spleen or has had the spleen surgically removed also is at high risk for overwhelming infections with encapsulated organisms, such as pneumococci, meningococci, and *H. influenzae* and should receive the appropriate vaccine. Other special groups that should be targeted for vaccination are the elderly, for influenza and pneumococcal vaccines; health care workers, who may be exposed to hepatitis B and rubella; and travelers, depending on local health conditions at their destinations.

Live, attenuated vaccines generally should be avoided in immunocompromised persons because the attenuated organism may be sufficiently pathogenic to cause disease in those individuals. If the safety of administering a live, attenuated vaccine in an immunocompromised patient is in question, the clinician should consult vaccine experts.

DTaP (Diphtheria, Tetanus, Acellular Pertussis) Vaccine

DTaP vaccine is the oldest and most successful combination vaccine used in children. It consists of a combination of two toxoids (**diphtheria** and **tetanus**) and purified components of *Bordetella pertussis*. The pertussis vaccines

table 45-3	Immunization of Special Populations	
POPULATION	**IMMUNIZATION**	**COMMENT**
People with sickle cell disease; splenectomized patients	Pneumococcal, meningococcal, and *Haemophilus influenzae* vaccines	Infections are often fatal
Elderly	Influenza vaccine; 23-valent pneumococcal polysaccharide vaccine; diphtheria, pertussis, tetanus vaccine	High risk (immunity has waned)
Children with immunodeficiency (including HIV)	Varicella-zoster immune globulin (postexposure)	Chickenpox causes severe, often fatal disease in this population
Health care workers	Hepatitis B vaccine; measles, mumps, rubella vaccine; influenza vaccine	If not immune
Travelers	Hepatitis A and B, yellow fever, rabies, Japanese encephalitis, measles, meningococcal, polio vaccines	Depends on local conditions
Pregnant women	Hepatitis B vaccine, tetanus toxoid, influenza vaccine	Prenatal screening for HbsAg; newborns of carriers receive HBIG and vaccine;[a] particularly in developing countries to prevent neonatal tetanus;[b] higher risk for morbidity due to influenza, especially in third trimester[c]

[a] Hepatitis B vaccine
[b] Tetanus toxoid
[c] Influenza vaccine

consist of inactivated bacterial components. All pertussis vaccines include pertussis toxin, and many contain differing amounts of filamentous hemagglutinin, pertactin, and fimbriae. Clinical trials have shown high protection rates and fewer side effects with acellular pertussis vaccines than the previously used whole-cell preparations. The preferred schedule for DTaP vaccination is 2, 4, and 6 months of age, followed by booster doses of vaccine at 15 to 18 months and 4 to 6 years. Thereafter, a booster of tetanus toxoid (full dose) and diphtheria toxoid (reduced dose) is given every 10 years. In 2005, two new vaccines comprised of tetanus toxoid, reduced-dose diphtheria toxoid, and pertussis components (Tdap) have been licensed in response to the increased incidence of pertussis in adolescents and adults. The American Academy of Pediatrics currently recommends universal vaccination with Tdap for adolescents at 11 to 12 years of age, as well as a catch-up vaccination of older adolescents, to boost protection against pertussis.

Conclusion

The use of vaccines has had a major impact on the health and well-being of many millions of persons throughout the world. The success stories of vaccines are exemplified by the eradication of smallpox and the dramatic decrease in the prevalence of many other infectious diseases. With success comes controversy: issues of the safety and side effects associated with vaccines have become a major focus of attention. Those issues pose challenges for the introduction of new vaccines required to prevent infectious diseases that remain important causes of morbidity and mortality in humans.

chapter **46**

Introduction to the Fungi and Mycoses

Carol A. Kauffman

key concepts

Fungi:

■ Are eukaryotes and constitute a separate kingdom called Fungi.

■ Can be multicellular and comprise filamentous structures (molds) or unicellular forms (yeasts). Some species are dimorphic; that is, they exist in either form depending on environmental conditions.

■ Cause superficial, cutaneous, subcutaneous, and systemic infections.

■ Are typically free living in nature and acquired from environmental sources; some are part of normal human flora.

■ Cause disease by eliciting an inflammatory response or through direct invasion or destruction of tissues.

Fungal infections, or **mycoses,** are usually classified by the area of the body primarily affected and the type of infection induced, rather than by taxonomic criteria that are not very meaningful clinically.
- **Endemic mycoses** are infections caused by pathogens that are restricted geographically and are true pathogens because they have the ability to cause serious systemic infection in healthy individuals.
- **Opportunistic mycoses** are caused by fungi that not true pathogens because they cause life-threatening systemic disease only in immunosuppressed patients.
- **Subcutaneous mycoses** are a group of fungal diseases that involve the skin, subcutaneous tissue, and lymphatics.
- **Superficial and cutaneous mycoses** are common fungal infections limited to the skin and skin structures.

Types of Pathogenic Fungi

Fungi belong to a discrete kingdom, the Fungi, and are classified on the basis of their mode of sexual and asexual reproduction, morphology, life cycles, and to some extent physiology. The kingdom Fungi comprises at least 100,000 species found all over the globe. Most exist only in the environment, and far less than 1% cause disease in humans. A crucial role for fungi is to degrade organic waste in the environment. They also cause widespread damage to food and fabrics. Fungi are used

FIGURE 46-1 ▪ **Yeast cell reproducing by budding.** The buds are called blastoconidia.

A

B

FIGURE 46-3 ▪ **Hyphae. A.** In a hypha from a mold that is nonseptate, the protoplasm is continuous and multinucleated. **B.** In a hypha from a mold that is septated, the protoplasm is interrupted by cross walls.

commercially in many fermentation processes producing steroid hormone derivatives and antibiotics.

Fungi are **eukaryotes,** with a defined nucleus enclosed by a nuclear membrane, a cell membrane that contains lipids, glycoproteins, and sterols; mitochondria; Golgi apparatus; ribosomes bound to endoplasmic reticulum; and a cytoskeleton with microtubules and microfilaments. The sterols comprising the cell membrane largely consist of **ergosterol,** whereas mammalian cell membranes are primarily cholesterol. More importantly, fungi have **cell walls** predominantly made of chitin, mannan, and glucan; mammalian cells do not have cell walls, and the cell walls of bacteria and plants differ markedly from those of fungi.

In nature most fungi derive their nutrients from decaying matter. They require an exogenous source of organic carbon for growth. Unlike plants, fungi do not have chlorophyll and do not undergo photosynthesis. Almost all fungi are strict aerobes. Although environmental fungi can tolerate extremes of temperatures, fungi that cause disease in humans favor 35°C to 37°C.

The fungi that cause disease in humans have two forms: a **unicellular** form called **yeast** and a multicellular **filamentous** form called **mold.** Yeasts are single cells that are ovoid or spherical. Most yeasts divide by budding (asexually), and the bud is called a blastoconidia (Fig. 46-1). On agar, yeasts form moist colonies that appear similar to, but larger than, those of bacteria (Fig. 46-2).

Molds grow as microscopic, branching, threadlike filaments. The filaments are called **hyphae** and are collectively referred to as the **mycelium.** Hyphae are either

septate (divided by partitions or cross walls perpendicular to the length of the hyphae) or nonseptate (multinucleate without cross walls; Fig. 46-3). On agar, part of the mycelium grows into the agar to provide nutrients to the aerial hyphae that form a "fuzzy" outgrowth or mold above the surface of the agar (Fig. 46-4). Aerial hyphae provide support for the reproductive structures of molds.

Many pathogenic fungi display both growth forms and can exist as either molds or yeasts. This phenomenon is called **dimorphism,** and the shift frequently occurs when a free-living organism infects a living host. With most fungi that cause systemic infections, the yeast is the parasitic form, and the mold form is found in the environment. In a few unusual instances that rule is reversed and the mycelial form is found in host tissues.

Fungi reproduce by either an asexual or sexual process. Asexual reproductive structures are termed **conidia.** The appearance of conidia varies enormously and is used for identification of fungi (Fig. 46-5). The conidia can be formed at the tips of the growing hyphae on a specialized structure called a conidiophore, directly off the hyphae, or within the hyphae themselves. Sexual reproductive structures are termed spores and often are formed into complex structures. Many of the sexual stages of fungi, especially those causing disease in humans, have yet to be described.

FIGURE 46-2 ▪ **Colonies of *Candida albicans,*** a typical yeast, growing on blood agar.

FIGURE 46-4 ▪ **Growth of a mold on an agar plate.** Notice the "fuzzy" growth (aerial hyphae) above the surface of the plate.

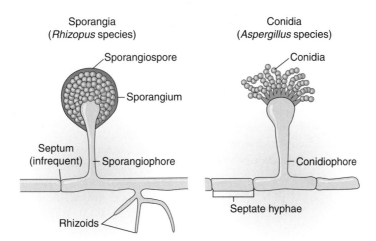

FIGURE 46-5 ▪ **Mold morphology.** Molds can assume various forms, starting with the basic hyphal structure that can then differentiate into various reproductive structures (conidia and spores).

ENCOUNTER

The human host encounters infection-causing fungi through two main mechanisms. Most fungi live freely in the environment, and people encounter them incidentally in the course of everyday living. Several important human pathogens are geographically restricted so that only people who enter that habitat are at risk for infection. Others are ubiquitous in the environment, and healthy hosts are continually exposed with no dire consequences. However, markedly immunosuppressed hosts can develop progressive fatal infection after exposure to seemingly innocuous fungi dispersed throughout the environment.

The other source for pathogenic fungi is the normal human flora. Mere colonizers in healthy hosts, these organisms, mostly yeasts, can become pathogenic and cause serious disseminated infection in the immunocompromised host.

ENTRY

The level of innate immunity to pathogenic fungi is high in most humans, as witnessed by the fact that most fungal infections are mild and self-limiting. The intact skin and mucosal surfaces are the primary barriers to infection. Desiccation, epithelial cell turnover, fatty acids, and the low pH of the skin are believed to be important factors in host resistance. In addition, the bacterial flora of the skin and mucous membranes compete with fungi and hinder their unrestricted growth. Alterations in the balance of the normal flora by the use of antibiotics or changes in nutrition allow fungi such as *Candida albicans* to proliferate, thus increasing the likelihood of entry and subsequent infection. Violation of the natural barriers by trauma or foreign bodies allows entry of fungi into sterile areas of the body.

SPREAD AND MULTIPLICATION

Tissue reaction to the presence of fungi varies with the species, the site of proliferation, and the duration of infection. Some mycoses are characterized by a low-grade inflammatory response that does not eliminate the fungi; for the most part, however, the organisms are not very virulent and serious disease does not result. In general, nonspecific inflammatory reactions are critically important in eliminating fungi. **Neutrophil phagocytosis and killing** are the primary mechanisms that prevent the establishment of many fungal infections. The extent of disease caused by opportunists like *Candida* and *Aspergillus* is greater in patients with low numbers of neutrophils or with disorders of neutrophil function, such as chronic granulomatous disease or myeloperoxidase deficiency.

Fungi that are too large to be ingested can, nevertheless, be killed. Instead of "ingesting" and "digesting" filamentous fungi, phagocytic cells line up along the surface of the hyphal structure and secrete lysosomal enzymes that damage the organisms. Antibodies play a role in the elimination of fungi from the body by participating in the extracellular killing of some filamentous fungi and yeasts by phagocytic cells, but overall the role of antibodies in host defense is minor.

The most important host defense in the elimination of many fungi is **T cell–mediated immunity.** Several important human pathogens persist within macrophages without being killed until specific T cell–mediated immunity develops. The clinical observation that AIDS patients with low CD4 lymphocyte numbers are especially prone to invasive and serious systemic fungal disease corroborates the importance of cell-mediated immunity.

DAMAGE

As in all infections, the **outcome is determined by the virulence of the infecting organism, the size of the inoculum, and the adequacy of the host defenses.** Tissue damage varies with each organism and the organ involved but typically results from the direct invasion of the organism, with the associated displacement or destruction of vital structures, and from the toxic effects of the inflammatory response. Fungi that cause invasive disease are not known to secrete toxins that harm the host. In subsequent chapters, specific clinical syndromes related to each organism are discussed.

DIAGNOSIS

Fungal infections are diagnosed in the laboratory by **direct microscopy, histopathology, culture, serology, and antigen detection.** Some fungi are large enough to be identified by **direct examination** of body fluids or purulent material. For direct examination, 10% potassium hydroxide is used to dissolve tissue debris so that the fungi, whose cell walls remain intact, can be observed, or a fluorescent dye, such as calcofluor white, that binds to chitin, is used to highlight the fungal cells. On **histopathological examination,** special stains are usually needed to detect fungi; morphological characteristics are distinctive enough in some fungi to aid in their identification. That is particularly useful in the diagnosis of serious systemic infections, providing an immediate and reasonably reliable identification of the causative agent.

Pathogenic fungi may be recovered from infected tissues using **culture** procedures. In general, growth of a fungus from a normally sterile body site always implies infection. Culturing clinical specimens does not always result in growth of the organism, and some medically important fungi take weeks to grow. Thus, in a severely ill patient, cultures are used to confirm a diagnosis but cannot be relied on to establish the diagnosis, and therapy cannot be withheld while awaiting culture results. On the other hand, some pathogenic fungi are ubiquitous in the environment or are part of the normal flora of humans; for those fungi, growth in the laboratory does not always establish a diagnosis of infection but may reflect merely contamination or colonization. The laboratory uses the morphological characteristics of fungi to identify fungi that have grown in culture.

The detection in the serum of **antibodies** to fungal antigens is helpful in the diagnosis of several of the endemic mycoses but rarely helpful in the diagnosis of opportunistic fungal infections. The detection of fungal **antigens** in body fluids, urine, and serum has proved both sensitive and specific for the diagnosis of several fungal infections. Polymerase chain reaction techniques will likely prove useful in the future.

TREATMENT

Not all fungal infections require treatment. For those that do require systemic antifungal agents, toxicity is a problem because fungi share with mammalian cells many pathways and structures targeted by antifungal agents. Compared with antibacterial agents, the number of effective antifungal agents is quite small. Antifungal agents are discussed in Chapter 50.

Conclusion

Fungi constitute a separate kingdom composed of at least 100,000 species. They are eukaryotes, which means that they share some metabolic pathways and structural components with mammalian cells. Although most human encounters with fungi do not lead to infection, if the fungal inoculum is large or the human host is immunocompromised, serious and even life-threatening infection can ensue. A variety of diagnostic tests are available to determine if a fungal infection is present.

Endemic Mycoses

Carol A. Kauffman

key concepts

Histoplasmosis:

- Is caused by *Histoplasma capsulatum*, a mold that grows in soil enriched with bird and bat excreta and transforms into a yeast after being inhaled into the alveoli.

- Occurs throughout the Mississippi and Ohio River valleys.

- Immunity depends on T cells and activated macrophages.

- Occurs in both acute and chronic forms of pulmonary and disseminated disease.

- Is treated with amphotericin B for severe disease and with itraconazole for mild-to-moderate disease.

Blastomycosis:

- Is caused by *Blastomyces dermatitidis*, a soil mold that transforms into a yeast after inhalation into the alveoli.

- Occurs in the Mississippi River Valley and southeastern and north-central states.

- Triggers immunity that depends on both polymorphonuclear leukocytes (PMNs) and T cells and macrophages.

- Causes characteristic skin lesions, pulmonary disease, and disseminated infection.

- Is treated with amphotericin B for severe disease and with itraconazole for mild-to-moderate disease.

Coccidioidomycosis:

- Is caused by *Coccidioides immitis*, a mold that grows in the desert of the southwest United States and converts to a large endospore-containing spherule in the body.

- Triggers immunity that depends on both PMNs and T cells or macrophages.

- Causes a wide spectrum of pulmonary disease, skin and osteoarticular lesions, abscesses, and meningitis.

- Is treated with amphotericin B for severe disease and with itraconazole or fluconazole for mild-to-moderate disease; meningitis is treated for life with fluconazole.

The endemic mycoses result from fungi that are geographically restricted to certain environmental areas and are true pathogens in that they have the ability to infect healthy people, not only those who are immunosuppressed. The diseases that occur in the United States include histoplasmosis, blastomycosis, and coccidioidomycosis. A fourth endemic mycosis, paracoccidioidomycosis, occurs in South America and is not discussed here. All the fungi that cause endemic mycoses are dimorphic, existing in the environment as molds and in hosts as either yeasts or spherules.

Histoplasmosis

Case

An infectious diseases specialist who practiced in the endemic area for histoplasmosis reflected on the varied manifestations of pulmonary histoplasmosis she had seen in the previous week. One patient was a 14-year-old boy from New York City who was spending the summer on his uncle's farm. Approximately 2 weeks after helping his uncle clean out some chicken coops, he developed fever, cough, chest tightness, and malaise. An oral macrolide for a week had provided no benefit, and his cough was worsening. The physical examination was normal; the chest radiograph showed hilar lymphadenopathy and a patchy lower lobe infiltrate (Fig. 47-1). Although the differential diagnosis was broad, she thought that acute pulmonary histoplasmosis was the most likely

FIGURE 47-1 ■ Patchy pneumonitis and hilar lymphadenopathy typical of acute pulmonary histoplasmosis in an immunocompetent host.

FIGURE 47-2 ■ Kidney transplant recipient with diffuse pulmonary infiltrates that proved to be caused by *Histoplasma capsulatum*.

possibility and ordered acute and convalescent antibody titers to help establish the diagnosis. She did not think that antifungal therapy was warranted and counseled the boy and his uncle that the illness was a self-limited one and would resolve in another few weeks.

The following day, she was consulted on a 58-year-old woman who was in the intensive care unit and had received a kidney transplant 18 months before. She was on prednisone, mycophenolate, and cyclosporine to prevent rejection. She had developed the acute onset of fever, chills, dyspnea, and cough. The Po$_2$ was 65 mm Hg, white blood cell count was 4,600/mm^3, and creatinine was 1.8 mg/dL. The chest radiograph showed diffuse bilateral infiltrates (Fig. 47-2). A bronchoscopic lung biopsy showed tiny oval, budding, intracellular yeasts in alveolar macrophages, and a diagnosis of pulmonary histoplasmosis was made. Therapy with amphotericin B was begun immediately.

Later that week a 66-year-old man who had a long history of chronic obstructive pulmonary disease (COPD) returned to her office for a follow-up visit. She had initially seen the man 6 months earlier when he came into the hospital with increasing fatigue, dyspnea, fevers, night sweats, anorexia, 20-pound weight loss, and cough productive of yellow sputum mixed with blood. A chest radiograph taken in the hospital had shown extensive upper-lobe cavitary infiltrates (Fig. 47-3). Sputum cultures had grown *Histoplasma capsulatum* after 5 weeks incubation, antibody titers were positive for that organism, and a diagnosis of chronic cavitary pulmonary

FIGURE 47-3 ▪ Chronic cavitary pulmonary histoplasmosis with bilateral cavitary upper-lobe infiltrates and lower-lobe scarring.

histoplasmosis had been made. Treatment with itraconazole was begun, and after one month he had noticed improvement in cough and sputum production. Fevers and night sweats had disappeared, and he began to gain weight by the second month of therapy. The plan was to treat him for 12 to 18 months with itraconazole. At 6 months he appeared to be responding well to treatment.

These cases raise several questions:

1. What is the main reason that the manifestations of pulmonary histoplasmosis were so different in the three patients?
2. What was the source of *H. capsulatum* that infected each patient? Can a discrete point source be found for most patients?
3. Why was therapy unique for each patient? Do most patients with histoplasmosis require treatment with an antifungal agent?

CHARACTERISTICS OF THE ORGANISM

Histoplasma capsulatum is a **dimorphic** fungus that in the environment exists as a mold that produces macro (tuberculate) conidia and microconidia, the infectious

FIGURE 47-4 ▪ Temperature dimorphism of *H. capsulatum*. **A.** The environmental form is a mold with small microconidia that are inhaled and cause infection and distinctive macroconidia with tuberculate projections on the surface. **B.** The tissue form is a yeast, shown here within macrophages.

form. In the body at 37°C, *H. capsulatum* assumes a yeast-like form (Fig. 47-4).

ENCOUNTER

Histoplasmosis occurs primarily in the Mississippi and Ohio River valleys, in Central America, and in some areas of South America (Fig. 47-5). In addition, microfoci occur in caves and other focal areas in several eastern states. In the endemic area in the United States, as much as 90% of the population has been infected.

H. capsulatum is a soil fungus whose growth is enhanced by the high nitrogenous content of earth that has been fertilized by bird or bat guano, as might occur under blackbird roosts, around chicken coops, and in caves and old buildings. Clusters of infection occur with spelunking, demolition of old buildings, and construction work

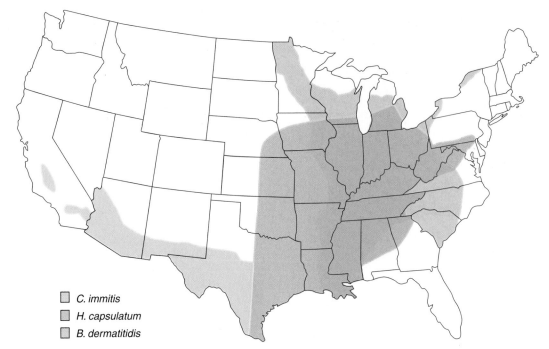

FIGURE 47-5 ▪ Geographic distribution of the major endemic mycoses, *Histoplasma capsulatum*, *Blastomyces dermatitidis*, and *Coccidioides immitis*, in the United States.

that disrupts soil. The largest outbreak reported involved more than 100,000 people infected after the demolition of an old amusement park in Indianapolis.

ENTRY

When *H. capsulatum* enters the lungs, the organism transforms into the yeast phase. That process is complex and not fully understood but clearly is essential for pathogenicity. The yeasts are phagocytosed by macrophages and neutrophils, but killing is problematic.

SPREAD AND MULTIPLICATION

Histoplasmosis should be viewed as an **infection of the reticuloendothelial system.** The organisms remain viable within macrophages by modulating the phagolysosomal pH and capturing essential growth factors from the cell. More than for other fungal organisms, immunity to *H. capsulatum* is mediated through the **cell-mediated immune system of CD4 T lymphocytes and activated macrophages;** antibody appears to play no role in resolution of infection. Only after T-cell sensitization, leading to the release of interleukin-2 and interferon-γ, are macrophages able to kill the intracellular yeasts. That generally takes several weeks, and until

then the organism spreads locally through the lymphatics to the hilar and mediastinal lymph nodes and then hematogenously within macrophages throughout the reticuloendothelial system.

When cell-mediated immunity to *H. capsulatum* is established, the infection is curtailed and resolves. Immunity is lifelong, but reinfection has been noted with exposure to a huge inoculum of *H. capsulatum.* The cell-mediated immune response is reflected in the development of **granulomas** with caseous necrosis and a positive skin test to *Histoplasma* antigens. Ultimately, the granulomas calcify. However, yeast cells can remain viable within granulomas for years and are a source for **reactivation infection** should cell-mediated immunity wane.

DAMAGE

The extent of infection and clinical disease manifestations are dependent on both the numbers of conidia inhaled and the cell-mediated immune response. The majority of infected persons have no clinical disease or mild pulmonary and systemic symptoms often ascribed to a viral-like illness. A small proportion of patients will have fever, chills, anorexia, fatigue, and dry cough; **patchy pneumonitis** and **hilar or mediastinal lymphadenopathy** are noted on chest radiograph. With extensive exposure, even in healthy hosts, severe pneumonia can occur, causing bilateral diffuse nodular infiltrates and hypoxemia. Patients who have underlying chronic obstructive pulmonary disease are at risk for developing **chronic cavitary pulmonary histoplasmosis,** a progressive and eventually fatal infection that mimics reactivation pulmonary tuberculosis.

Although dissemination occurs in virtually everyone infected with *H. capsulatum*, symptomatic disease is uncommon and clearly more likely to occur in people with cell-mediated immune deficiencies, such as AIDS, and those treated with immunosuppressive agents. **Acute disseminated histoplasmosis** is characterized by fever, chills, fatigue, mucous membrane ulcers, hepatosplenomegaly, and pancytopenia; in some cases adrenal insufficiency, sepsis syndrome, and disseminated intravascular coagulation occurs. **Chronic progressive disseminated histoplasmosis** is seen in older adults who have no obvious immune deficiency but for some reason are unable to contain *H. capsulatum*. If not treated, patients with the chronic disease die from progressive infection of the liver, spleen, bone marrow, adrenals, and other organs.

DIAGNOSIS

Histoplasmosis can be diagnosed by growing the organism from sputum, blood, tissues, or body fluids. Although definitive, growth in vitro can take up to 6 weeks and is not successful in many laboratories. Histopathological demonstration of the small intracellular yeasts in samples from bone marrow, liver, lung, or lymph nodes using special stains is rapid and highly suggestive of histoplasmosis. Polysaccharide antigen from the cell wall of *H. capsulatum* can be detected by enzyme immunoassay in urine or serum in most patients with disseminated infection and some with primary pulmonary histoplasmosis, but very few with localized and chronic forms of the disease. The demonstration of antibody to *H. capsulatum* is helpful in the diagnosis of acute and chronic pulmonary and disseminated forms of the disease but not in immunocompromised hosts who cannot mount an antibody response.

TREATMENT AND PREVENTION

Mild-to-moderate pulmonary or disseminated histoplasmosis is treated with **itraconazole,** usually for 3 to 12 months depending on the extent of disease. Patients who have severe infection, generally those with dissemination, should receive **amphotericin B** initially and then can be switched to itraconazole after their condition has stabilized.

Guidelines for prevention of histoplasmosis in the workplace have been issued by the Centers for Disease Control and Prevention. Use of respirators when tearing down old barns and chicken coops or other areas that have housed birds and bats is highly recommended. Immunosuppressed persons should not take part in those activities.

Blastomycosis
CHARACTERISTICS OF THE ORGANISM

Blastomyces dermatitidis is a **dimorphic** fungus that in the environment exists as a mold and in the body at 37°C, assumes the yeast form. The yeast is large and thick-walled and produces a single broad-based bud (Fig. 47-6).

ENCOUNTER

Blastomycosis occurs primarily in the Mississippi River Valley and the southeastern states and extends northward into central Canada and the St. Lawrence River Valley (see Fig. 47-5). The ecology of *B. dermatitidis* is less well known that than of *H. capsulatum*, but soil and decaying wood are presumed sources. Small outbreaks have been described, but most cases appear sporadically.

ENTRY

The conidia of *B. dermatitidis* are inhaled into the lungs, where the organism transforms to the yeast phase. The yeast is phagocytosed by macrophages and neutrophils.

FIGURE 47-6 ■ Yeast form of *B. dermatitidis* demonstrating the thick cell wall and distinctive broad-based budding of the daughter cell.

Spread and Multiplication

B. dermatitidis multiplies initially in the lungs and causes pneumonia. However, the hallmark of blastomycosis is the development of skin lesions, which arise as the result of hematogenous dissemination. Cell-mediated immunity is clearly important in eradication of infection, but it appears that neutrophils also play a role in containing the organism. The histopathological picture reflects the **mixed granulomatous and pyogenic response.** As with histoplasmosis, it appears that yeast cells can remain viable within granulomas for years and can be a source for later reactivation.

Damage

Most infected persons have only mild pulmonary infection, and many present only with skin or osteoarticular lesions following a silent pulmonary infection. Those who have more extensive pulmonary disease have fever, chills, anorexia, fatigue, dry cough, and patchy pneumonitis on chest radiograph. With extensive exposure, even in healthy hosts, bilateral diffuse nodular infiltrates, hypoxemia, and acute respiratory distress syndrome can occur. The **cutaneous lesions** may be single or multiple, have **heaped-up borders,** and have **small central microabscesses** (Fig. 47-7). Other organs can be involved with disseminated infection.

Diagnosis

Blastomycosis is diagnosed by growing the organism from sputum, skin, or other tissues. Unfortunately,

FIGURE 47-7 ▪ **Skin lesions that had been present for several months in a patient with blastomycosis.**

growth in vitro may take weeks. Histopathological demonstration in tissues of **large, thick-walled yeasts with single broad-based buds** is highly suggestive of blastomycosis. Serological tests for *B. dermatitidis* are not helpful.

Treatment and Prevention

Mild to moderate pulmonary or cutaneous blastomycosis is treated with **itraconazole,** usually for 6 to 12 months depending on the extent of disease. Patients who have severe pulmonary or disseminated infection should receive **amphotericin B** initially and can be switched to itraconazole after their condition has stabilized. Preventative measures have not been established.

Coccidioidomycosis
Characteristics of the Organism

Coccidioides immitis is another dimorphic fungus, but its dimorphism is not temperature dependent. In the environment it is a mold that forms **arthroconidia,** the infectious form. In tissues it forms a huge structure called a **spherule,** which is 50 to 100 μm in size. Inside each spherule are hundreds of **endospores** that, when released, propagate the infection (Fig. 47-8).

Encounter

C. immitis exists only in a distinctive ecosystem termed the **lower Sonoran life zone.** In the United States the zone includes Arizona, southern California, several of the arid interior valleys in California, and parts of New Mexico and Texas (see Fig. 47-5). A semiarid environment fosters the growth of *C. immitis*, most likely in the burrows of desert animals. When conditions of rainfall, heat, and wind are correct, huge "blooms" of the organism occur, and outbreaks among humans often follow. In highly endemic areas as much as 80% of the population have evidence of prior infection with *C. immitis*.

Entry

The arthroconidia of *C. immitis* are highly infectious and easily inhaled into the alveoli. In the lung the arthro-

FIGURE 47-8 ▪ **Tissue dimorphism of C. immitis. A.** Segmented barrel-shaped arthroconidia are found in the environment. **B.** The tissue form, called a spherule, contains hundreds of endospores.

conidia transform into distinctive large spherules that fill with endospores. Although arthroconidia can be phagocytosed and killed by neutrophils, the spherules resist phagocytosis.

SPREAD AND MULTIPLICATION

The primary target organ for infection with *C. immitis* is the lung, but in many hosts the organism spreads hematogenously and infects many different organs. The **host response to C. immitis is a mixture of neutrophils and T lymphocytes and activated macrophages.** Ultimate control of the infection requires development of cell-mediated immunity that allows eradication of the spherules. In hosts with deficient CD4 function, such as AIDS patients, severe disseminated infection is frequent. As with the other endemic mycoses, reactivation of an old focus of infection is possible years later.

DAMAGE

Most people with coccidioidomycosis have no symptoms or a mild viral-like illness. Symptomatic **acute pulmonary infection** occurs a few weeks after exposure and is usually manifested by fever, anorexia, fatigue, dry cough, and chest pain. Arthralgias and skin nodules (erythema nodosum) can develop during the illness and reflect the host response to the organism. The syndrome is often called **desert rheumatism** or **valley fever.** For most patients it is a self-limited illness. However, in a small number of people disease progresses to **chronic pulmonary infection** that often cavitates and requires antifungal therapy.

  Disseminated coccidioidomycosis occurs more often in dark-skinned individuals, pregnant women, and people with cell-mediated immune deficiencies. Cutaneous, subcutaneous, and osteoarticular infection are common (Fig. 47-9), but any organ can be involved. **Chronic meningitis** is the **most feared complication** because it is fatal if not treated, and those who do respond to antifungal therapy will relapse if therapy is ever stopped.

DIAGNOSIS

The diagnosis of coccidioidomycosis is made by growing the organism from involved tissues or body fluids. *C. immitis* will grow on most media in several days. The laboratory must always be warned that coccidioidomycosis is a possibility, because the mold form is highly infectious and has led to numerous outbreaks among laboratory workers. Histopathological demonstration of spherules in tissues is also diagnostic. Various assays for antibodies against *C. immitis* are quite helpful diagnostically when performed by a laboratory experienced with the assays.

FIGURE 47-9 ▪ **Patient with coccidioidomycosis and a cutaneous lesion on the face.**

TREATMENT AND PREVENTION

Of all the endemic mycoses, coccidioidomycosis is the most difficult to treat. Some patients will have recurrent and relapsing disease throughout their lives. Mild-to-moderate coccidioidomycosis is treated with **itraconazole** or **fluconazole,** usually for 12 to 24 months depending on the extent of disease. Patients who have severe infection should receive **amphotericin B** initially and then can be switched to an azole after their condition has stabilized. Coccidioidal meningitis can usually be treated successfully with fluconazole, but therapy must be life-long. Prevention is difficult in the endemic area because the organism is so readily dispersed. Avoiding dust storms may be helpful.

Conclusion

The endemic mycoses are common infections that exist within restricted geographical areas. Most persons who are infected are asymptomatic or have only mild self-limited symptoms. Cell-mediated immunity is essential for successful resolution of histoplasmosis and probably coccidioidomycosis and contributes to immunity to blastomycosis. Clinical manifestations are unique to each organism, but the lung is prominently involved with all three. Symptomatic disseminated histoplasmosis and coccidioidomycosis are most common in people with deficient cellular immunity. Azoles have revolutionized the treatment of the endemic mycoses; amphotericin B is required only for patients with severe infection.

chapter 48

Opportunistic Fungal Infections

Carol A. Kauffman

key concepts

Candidiasis (primarily *C. albicans*):

- Caused by yeasts that are part of the normal human flora.

- Disease is associated with overgrowth of other normal flora and when the host immune response, (especially neutrophil function) is diminished.

- Mucous membranes and skin commonly affected (thrush, vaginitis, and diaper rash); disseminated infection and sepsis syndrome less common.

- Topical antifungals treat superficial disease; systemic antifungals are required for dissemination

Cryptococcosis (caused by *Cryptococcus neoformans*):

- Caused by encapsulated, environmental yeast; acquired by inhalation.

- Because of neurotropism, disease is usually chronic lymphocytic meningitis.

- Treated with amphotericin B plus flucytosine, followed by fluconazole.

Aspergillosis (usually *Aspergillus fumigatus* and *Aspergillus flavus*):

- Due to common environmental molds; not normal human flora.

- In profoundly immunocompromised patients, these angioinvasive molds cause hemorrhage and tissue infarction (usually nodular disease in the lungs).

- Treated with expanded-spectrum azoles, echinocandins, or amphotericin B.

Zygomycosis (members of the genera *Rhizopus*, *Mucor*, and others):

- Ubiquitous, environmental molds that are angioinvasive in tissues.

- Invasive disease (pulmonary and rhinocerebral) occurs in neutropenic patients and in diabetics with ketoacidosis.

- Treated with amphotericin B and aggressive surgical debridement of all involved tissue.

Pneumocystosis (*Pneumocystis jiroveci*):

- Occurs in AIDS patients with low CD4 lymphocytes.

- Causes pneumonia with hypoxemia as alveoli fill with proteinaceous fluid.

- The agent cannot be grown in vitro; treated with trimethoprim-sulfamethoxazole.

Opportunistic fungi are **not considered true pathogens** because they cause disease only when host defenses are decreased. The group of opportunistic fungi encompasses a variety of disparate organisms. The three most commonly encountered genera are *Candida,* yeasts that are part of the normal flora of humans; *Cryptococcus,* yeasts found in the environment; and *Aspergillus,* molds that are ubiquitous in the environment. This chapter focuses on organisms in those three classes and briefly discusses the Zygomycetes, a class of environmental molds, and *Pneumocystis jiroveci,* an organism formerly named *Pneumocystis carinii* and classified with the protozoa but recently renamed and reclassified as a fungus.

Patients at high risk for opportunistic fungal infections include individuals who are immunosuppressed because of hematological malignancies, solid organ or hematopoietic stem cell transplantation, neutropenia, HIV infection, or corticosteroids or other immunosuppressive drugs. Other patients at risk for opportunistic fungal infections include those who have major burn wounds, trauma, or illnesses that require long-term use of central intravenous catheters, have received broad-spectrum antibiotics, are receiving parenteral nutrition, are diabetic, or have renal insufficiency requiring dialysis. Neonates with very low birth weights are also at risk for infection from opportunistic fungi.

Candidiasis

CHARACTERISTICS OF THE ORGANISM

Candida species are round or oval **yeasts** that reproduce by forming buds or blastoconidia (Fig. 48-1). They have the potential to form **hyphae** in vivo, and that form is seen in invasive infection with some, but not all, species of *Candida.* The most important member of the genus is *Candida albicans,* which is the predominant species colonizing humans and is responsible for most infections. Other species of increasing importance are *Candida glabrata,* which is resistant to some antifungal agents, and *Candida parapsilosis,* which is a common cause of catheter-related infections.

Case

Mrs. D., a 60-year-old woman who had a perforated colon, had been in the intensive care unit for 3 weeks after surgery. She had renal failure and required intermittent hemodialysis. Mrs. D. also had an **ileus** (a nonfunctioning intestinal tract) and was obtaining parenteral nutrition through a central intravenous catheter. She was on a ventilator and had congestive heart failure. A prior pneumonia had been documented on day 12, and she was treated with piperacillin-tazobactam for that complication. On day 20 in intensive care, Mrs. D. became febrile to 39.3°C, her blood pressure fell to 90/50 mm Hg, and she became less responsive. Cultures of blood, urine, and sputum were obtained, and she was started on meropenem and vancomycin. The catheter was removed, and the tip was cultured. One day later the laboratory called to report that the blood culture was growing a yeast; the next day, the culture of the catheter tip also showed yeast, and the organism from the blood was noted to be **germ-tube** positive and identified as *Candida albicans.*

This case raises several questions:

1. What factors put Mrs. D. at risk for developing candidemia?
2. Where did the *C. albicans* come from?
3. What does the term "germ-tube positive" mean to the clinician?

ENCOUNTER

Candida species normally colonize the gastrointestinal tract from the mouth to the rectum, the vagina, and the skin. Most infections are **endogenous**—that is, derived from the host's normal flora. In addition to immunosuppressed patients, especially those with neutropenia,

FIGURE 48-1 ■ Budding yeasts typical of *Candida* species.

a major group at risk for developing candidiasis comprises patients in intensive care units. Risk factors include broad-spectrum antibiotics, renal failure requiring dialysis, central intravenous catheters, and parenteral nutrition.

ENTRY

Candida species do not cause infection unless the ecology of the normal flora is disrupted. The simplest reasons for disruption of normal flora are use of broad-spectrum antimicrobial agents, which allow *Candida* to proliferate on the mucosa, and macerations of the skin, which open that site to proliferation of the organism. **Decreased T-cell immunity** also increases *Candida* proliferation on mucosal surfaces. Circumstances that allow the escape of *Candida* from the gut into the bloodstream include **neutropenia** and use of chemotherapeutic agents that destroy the mucosal barrier of the gut. *Candida* species also gain access into the bloodstream through **central intravenous catheters.**

SPREAD AND MULTIPLICATION

The main host defense that holds *Candida* in check on mucosal surfaces is **T cell–mediated immunity.** Patients with advanced HIV infection and low CD4 lymphocyte numbers frequently have oropharyngeal and vaginal candidiasis. Despite extensive proliferation of *Candida*, no invasion through the mucosa occurs.

Neutrophils are the main host defense against invasion through the mucosa and subsequent dissemination. Monocytes and macrophages play a less important role in phagocytosis and killing of *Candida*. Antibodies do not appear to play a role in host defense. In neutropenic patients *Candida* spread hematogenously to many organs but especially to the eyes, kidneys, heart, brain, liver, and spleen.

DAMAGE

Mucosal candidiasis is characterized by thick, white, adherent plaques on the oropharyngeal and vaginal mucosa (Fig. 48-2). The lesions, often termed **thrush,** are not painful. Proliferation of *Candida* in warm moist areas of the skin, especially in the groin and under pendulous breasts, is termed **intertriginous candidiasis** and in babies, **diaper rash.** In all circumstances, underlying tissues are not damaged, and after the infection resolves patients suffer no long-term consequences.

FIGURE 48-2 ▪ **Extensive thrush on the palate of a patient with AIDS.**

Disseminated infection can present as unexplained fever, sepsis, or organ dysfunction. **Candidemia** is sometimes the only manifestation of dissemination; when visceral involvement is documented, the usual histopathologic picture is one of multiple **microabscesses** in many organs. The clinical manifestations vary according to the end organ involved. **Meningitis, chorioretinitis** with subsequent **endophthalmitis, hepatosplenic abscesses,** and **vertebral osteomyelitis** are common complications of disseminated candidiasis. **Endocarditis** occurs mostly on prosthetic valves.

DIAGNOSIS

The diagnosis of mucosal candidiasis is simple. Scrapings of the lesions show budding yeasts and often pseudohyphae (elongated buds attached one to another), and cultures readily yield *Candida*. **Invasive candidiasis is more difficult to document.** Growth of *Candida* from normally colonized sites is not helpful in the documentation of invasive disease. Culture of blood is the simplest technique to document disseminated infection, but it is not very sensitive. Biopsy of involved tissues will show invasion with a mixture of budding yeast and hyphae that is quite characteristic of candidiasis (Fig. 48-3), and culture of involved tissues should yield the organism.

Candida species readily grow in a few days on blood agar or Sabouraud's agar. *C. albicans* can be

FIGURE 48-3 ▪ Biopsy of the esophagus in a leukemic patient who had pain with swallowing, showing tissue invasion with yeast and hyphal forms of *Candida albicans.*

differentiated from other species in a few hours by the development of **germ tubes** (elongated buds from the yeast) when the yeast is exposed to calf serum. Identification of other species of *Candida* by utilization of sugars takes several more days.

TREATMENT AND PREVENTION

Mucosal candidiasis and intertriginous candidiasis are treated with local application of antifungal agents; however, extensive mucosal involvement may require treatment with a systemic antifungal agent. Invasive infection should always be treated with systemic antifungal agents. The most commonly used agent is **fluconazole,** but there are an increasing number of *Candida* species, especially *C. glabrata,* that are resistant to this agent. Other options include the expanded-spectrum azole, **voriconazole,** an echinocandin such as **caspofungin,** or the polyene **amphotericin B.** Candidemia with no obvious end-organ involvement is usually treated for a minimum of 2 weeks; depending on the organ involved, invasive candidiasis may need to be treated for many months.

Mucosal infection in AIDS patients can be prevented by prophylaxis with antifungal agents, but resistance develops when those agents are used for many months. Patients at high risk for disseminated infection, such as those who are neutropenic or have undergone stem cell transplantation, are usually treated with prophylactic fluconazole during the period of highest risk. Careful attention to hand cleansing and care of devices used in the

intensive care unit can help prevent candidemia; prophylaxis is generally not used in that setting.

Cryptococcosis
CHARACTERISTICS OF THE ORGANISM

The etiologic agent of cryptococcosis is an environmental yeast, *Cryptococcus neoformans,* which reproduces by budding. In tissues, but not in the environment, the organism is surrounded by a huge polysaccharide capsule. Other species of *Cryptococcus* are generally not pathogenic.

ENCOUNTER

C. neoformans is **found worldwide in soil** contaminated with bird excreta and in a variety of other environmental niches. Patients most at risk for cryptococcosis are those who have **AIDS** or a **hematologic malignancy,** have received an organ or bone marrow **transplant,** or have been treated with **corticosteroids** or other immunosuppressive drugs. In contrast to the situation with other opportunistic fungi, **about 20% of patients who have cryptococcosis appear to be immunocompetent.**

ENTRY

The yeast is inhaled into the alveoli and begins to produce the polysaccharide capsule, a major virulence factor.

SPREAD AND MULTIPLICATION

The host defense against *C. neoformans* is complex. Neutrophils and macrophages are important in initial phagocytosis and killing of the yeast, but as **capsule** production increases, phagocytosis is inhibited. If phagocytosis does occur, the capsule appears to forestall intracellular killing. The capsule also appears to downregulate the development of Th1 mediators. T-cell immunity is crucial to control of infection with *C. neoformans.* A measure of the importance of T-cell immunity is the observation that prior to effective therapy for HIV infection, 5 to 10% of AIDS patients in the United States developed cryptococcosis. The production of the pigment **melanin** by *C. neoformans* also appears to enhance virulence, possibly by providing a kind of "armor" in the fungal cell wall that resists enzyme degradation and free radicals.

A striking aspect of infection with *C. neoformans* is its **neurotropism.** No explanation currently exists for why the organism preferentially infects the central nervous system. Another unique aspect of infection with *C. neoformans* in some, but not all, patients is the lack of inflammatory response. Although pulmonary lesions may be granulomatous, the inflammatory response in the central nervous system is minimal.

DAMAGE

Pulmonary infection is usually asymptomatic, and patients most often present with **meningitis,** which is subacute to chronic in nature. Symptoms include headache that worsens over days to weeks, fever, cranial nerve palsies, and mental status changes. Signs of **increased intracranial pressure** are often present. Dissemination is common in AIDS patients, who can present with meningitis associated with diffuse pulmonary infiltrates, skin lesions, and widespread visceral infection.

DIAGNOSIS

The diagnosis of cryptococcal meningitis is made by performing a lumbar puncture and examining cerebrospinal fluid for **encapsulated budding yeast** cells that can be highlighted by adding a drop of India ink to the slide (Fig. 48-4). The fluid classically shows a predominance

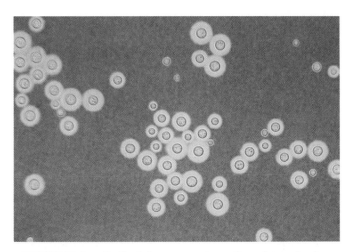

FIGURE 48-4 ▪ **India ink preparation of cerebrospinal fluid that shows many encapsulated yeast cells, some of which are budding, that are diagnostic of *Cryptococcus neoformans* meningitis.**

Case

Mr. S., a 35-year-old man with myelocytic leukemia, had received initial induction treatment with a combination of chemotherapeutic agents that caused severe and prolonged neutropenia and thrombocytopenia. On day 10 of neutropenia, when his absolute neutrophil count was 50/mm^3, Mr. S. had bacteremia with *Klebsiella pneumoniae* documented, for which he received broad-spectrum antibiotics. On day 21 of neutropenia, while still on antibiotics, Mr. S. developed fever to 39.7°C, complained of pleuritic right-sided chest pain, and developed a cough, hemoptysis, and shortness of breath. A computed tomography (CT) scan showed a nodular lesion in the right lower lobe (Fig. 48-5). A sample obtained by bronchoalveolar lavage revealed acutely branching septate hyphae, and cultures showed a mold that was identified as *Aspergillus fumigatus*.

This case raises several questions:

1. Why was Mr. S. at risk for an opportunistic fungal infection?
2. Why did Mr. S. have pleuritic chest pain and hemoptysis?
3. How useful is a bronchoalveolar lavage showing septate hyphae?

of lymphocytes, a high protein, and a decreased glucose concentration. A **latex agglutination test for the capsular polysaccharide antigen** is both sensitive and specific and should be performed on both cerebrospinal fluid and serum. *C. neoformans* grows on many types of agar media in a few days and is easily identified by clinical laboratories.

TREATMENT AND PREVENTION

The initial treatment of cryptococcal meningitis is the combination of **amphotericin B** and **flucytosine** for several weeks followed by consolidation therapy with **fluconazole** for at least several months. Some patients with T-cell defects require lifelong fluconazole suppression to prevent relapse of infection. Other forms of cryptococcosis, such as pulmonary infection, can often be treated with fluconazole as primary therapy.

With the advent of effective therapy for HIV, cryptococcal meningitis has become uncommon as an AIDS-associated infection in the United States. No prophylactic regimens are currently suggested for AIDS patients or other at-risk populations, such as transplant recipients.

FIGURE 48-5 ▪ Chest computerized tomography scan showing a right lower-lobe nodule surrounded by a halo, indicating hemorrhage.

Aspergillus

CHARACTERISTICS OF THE ORGANISM

Aspergillus species are filamentous fungi that form a mycelium of **septate hyphae** and reproduce by forming **conidia** on aerial **conidiophores.** The major pathogenic species are *A. fumigatus* and *A. flavus* (Fig. 48-6), but hundreds of species exist in the environment. Species are differentiated by the arrangement of conidia on the conidiophore (Fig. 48-7). *Aspergillus* species are not part of the normal flora of humans.

FIGURE 48-6 ▪ Colony of *Aspergillus fumigatus.*

FIGURE 48-7 ▪ Distinctive conidia on a conidiophore of *Aspergillus terreus,* an uncommon pathogenic species.

ENCOUNTER

Aspergillus species are **ubiquitous** in soil, manure, and decomposing vegetation throughout the world and can be cultured from air and water. Outbreaks in hospitals have occurred during construction, which widely disperses the conidia. The usual hosts are those who are **neutropenic,** are on **corticosteroids** or other immunosuppressive drugs, or are **transplant recipients.**

ENTRY

The **conidia are inhaled** into the upper and lower respiratory tracts. Invasive infection does not occur in the absence of profound immunosuppression. The initial event after entry is **germination of the conidia into hyphae,** which then invade into tissues.

SPREAD AND MULTIPLICATION

Neutrophils and macrophages are the main host defense against infection with *Aspergillus.* Pulmonary macrophages phagocytose and kill conidia that reach the alveoli but are unable to kill the hyphal forms. Neutrophils cannot phagocytose hyphae but instead line up along their surfaces and secrete reactive oxygen intermediates that kill the organism. Antibodies and T lymphocytes do not appear to be play a role in host defense against these filamentous fungi. *Aspergillus* is an **angioinvasive fungus;** the hyphae invade through blood vessel walls, causing **tissue infarction, hemorrhage,** and **necrosis.**

DAMAGE

Aspergillosis almost always presents initially as pulmonary or sinus infection. The usual histopathologic picture is one of hemorrhagic infarction and necrosis;

FIGURE 48-8 ▪ Invasion of tissue by *Aspergillus* species showing acutely branching septate hyphae.

with special stains, acutely branching septate hyphae are seen invading through tissues. The clinical manifestations of **invasive pulmonary aspergillosis** include fever, pleuritic chest pain, cough, hemoptysis, and dyspnea. Chest radiograph and CT scan show multiple pulmonary nodules, hemorrhage around the nodules, and cavitation (necrosis). Acute facial pain is a herald of **sinus invasion.** Dissemination is common because of the propensity of the organism to invade the blood vessels. However, *Aspergillus* species are rarely found in blood cultures. Common clinical manifestations of disseminated aspergillosis include **necrotic skin lesions** and **brain abscess** presenting as stroke, seizures, or mental status changes. Multiple areas of hemorrhagic infarction and abscesses are found in many organs.

DIAGNOSIS

Aspergillus species readily grow on Sabouraud's agar in a few days. The major issue for the clinician is to differentiate contamination from infection as these ubiquitous fungi are frequent laboratory contaminants. Tissue biopsy is important to document tissue invasion (Fig. 48-8), but is not specific for *Aspergillus* because other angioinvasive fungi also demonstrate septate hyphae in tissue biopsies.

TREATMENT AND PREVENTION

Aspergillosis is treated with the expanded-spectrum azole, **voriconazole, amphotericin B**, or the echinocandin **caspofungin.** Because the mortality is very high unless therapy is started before extensive tissue invasion

has occurred, empiric treatment is often initiated based on clinical manifestations and CT scan results in a high-risk patient.

Prevention of aspergillosis in high-risk patients is aimed at decreasing exposure by providing filtered air in high-risk units, such as transplant units; decreasing exposure to construction dust; and discouraging patients from activities likely to lead to exposure to these environmental molds. Prophylaxis with antifungal agents has shown variable success, and no standard regimen has been accepted at all centers.

Other Filamentous Fungal Opportunists

Severely immunocompromised hosts are at risk for infections caused by a large number of opportunistic fungi. Several fungal genera look very much like and behave in a similar fashion to *Aspergillus* species. The **Zygomycetes** are a class of molds that differ from *Aspergillus*-like organisms in that their hyphae are broader and have **no septae** (Fig. 48-9), but they are similar to *Aspergillus* in their **angioinvasive** properties. The major pathogens in this group are the genera *Rhizopus* and *Mucor*. The patients at risk are those who have **hematologic malignancies, are neutropenic, or are on corticosteroids;** in addition, **patients with diabetes mellitus who have ketoacidosis** are a major risk group. The reason diabetics are at risk probably relates to the adverse effects of acidosis on neutrophil chemotaxis and phagocytosis.

The presentation in diabetics is usually **rhinocerebral zygomycosis,** in which the fungi spread from the nares and sinuses into the palate, orbit, and soft tissues of the face and then invade the cavernous sinus and brain

FIGURE 48-9 ■ Biopsy of lung showing invasion of tissues by large, nonseptate hyphae characteristic of the Zygomycetes.

FIGURE 48-11 ■ Lung biopsy stained with hematoxylin and eosin from an immunosuppressed patient with pneumonia caused by *Pneumocystis jiroveci*. Notice the proteinaceous material filling the alveoli.

(Fig. 48-10). Pulmonary and disseminated zygomycosis also occurs and mimics aspergillosis. The treatment of zygomycosis is **amphotericin B** and aggressive **surgical debridement** of all infected and necrotic tissue.

Pneumocystosis

The organism that causes pneumocystosis previously was thought to be a protozoan. The fact that the organism has **never been grown in vitro** has contributed to the confusion about its nature. It is now clear, on the basis of sequence analysis of genes coding for ribosomal RNA and proteins made by the organism, that the organism is a fungus. The name has recently been changed from *Pneumocystis carinii* to *Pneumocystis jiroveci*. It is presumably inhaled from the environment, but its ecological niche has not been found. Most people likely have been infected early in life, but disease only occurs when immunosuppression intervenes. The most common risk factor is **T-cell deficiency**, as demonstrated by the fact that pneumocystic pneumonia (PCP) was the most common opportunistic infection in AIDS patients prior to the advent of effective antiviral therapy for HIV.

FIGURE 48-10 ■ Rhinocerebral zygomycosis in a diabetic with ketoacidosis.

FIGURE 48-12 ■ Diffuse bilateral pulmonary infiltrates in an AIDS patient with PCP.

FIGURE 48-13 ▪ Silver stain of lung biopsy showing organisms typical of *Pneumocystis jiroveci* in the alveolus.

The organism only very rarely is found outside the lungs. Histopathologically, the alveoli are filled with **foamy proteinaceous material**, desquamated alveolar cells, and organisms (Fig. 48-11). Patients present with dyspnea, dry cough, fatigue, and mild or absent fever. A chest radiograph shows bilateral **diffuse infiltrates** (Fig. 48-12); hypoxemia, which can be severe, is almost always present. The diagnosis of PCP is made by demonstration of the organism by silver stain (Fig. 48-13), direct fluorescent antibody techniques, or polymerase chain reaction on material obtained by bronchoalveolar lavage or biopsy. The treatment of choice is **trimethoprim-sulfamethoxazole**, which is also a highly effective prophylactic regimen in high-risk populations.

Conclusion

Advances in the fields of transplantation of organs and stem cells, treatment of hematologic malignancies and autoimmune disorders, and critical care medicine have resulted in an ever-increasing number of patients at risk for opportunistic fungal infections. Invasive infections caused by *Candida* species occur in patients who are neutropenic and also in those in intensive care. Cryptococcosis and pneumocystosis occur primarily in patients who have defects in T-cell immunity; before effective antiviral therapy for HIV became available, they were prominent opportunistic infections seen in AIDS patients.

Aspergillus species cause invasive infection almost entirely in severely immunosuppressed hosts. The Zygomycetes target diabetics as well as the profoundly immunosuppressed population. A large number of molds that occur in the environment and that have not been discussed here have been reported to cause life-threatening infection in patients who are immunosuppressed. Infections with opportunistic fungi constitute a major diagnostic and therapeutic challenge for infectious disease specialists.

chapter **49**

Subcutaneous, Cutaneous, and Superficial Mycoses

Carol A. Kauffman

key **concepts**

Sporotrichosis:

- Is caused by *Sporothrix schenckii*, a dimorphic fungus.

- Classically begins with inoculation of the organism from soil, moss, or decaying vegetation.

- Presents as an isolated cutaneous ulceration or a series of ulcerated nodules along the lymphatic distribution of the initial lesion.

- Is best diagnosed by culture of material from a lesion.

- Is treated with itraconazole.

Mycetoma and chromoblastomycosis:

- Are seen mostly in the tropics.

- Are caused by inoculation of environmental fungi into subcutaneous tissues.

- Usually require surgical extirpation.

Dermatophyte infections:

- Are caused by the genera *Trichophyton*, *Microsporum*, and *Epidermophyton*.

- Infect the stratum corneum, hair shafts, and nails.

- Cause tinea, meaning wormlike infections of various skin structures (tinea corporis, tinea pedis, etc.).

- Are treated with local antifungal creams and lotions, except for onychomycosis, which must be treated with systemic antifungal agents.

Superficial mycoses:

- Are caused by *Malassezia* species, normal colonizers of human stratum corneum.

- Cause tinea versicolor and seborrheic dermatitis, both of which are treated with antifungal creams or shampoos.

The most common fungal infections of humans are those affecting skin, skin appendages, and subcutaneous tissue. These infections almost always remain localized and, although annoying, are rarely severe. The dermatophytes are responsible for most superficial skin infections and nail infections. They are adapted to live in the keratinized tissues of hair and nails and the stratum corneum. Inoculation of a variety of different fungi that live in the soil or on plants leads to chronic, often disfiguring, subcutaneous infections. Sporotrichosis, the subcutaneous mycosis most commonly seen in the United States, spreads regionally through the lymphatics draining the inoculation site. In markedly immunocompromised persons, several of the environmentally acquired fungi that cause sporotrichosis can disseminate and cause serious, even life-threatening disease.

FIGURE 49-1 ▪ Multiple ulcerated nodules on the forearm in the distribution of the lymphatic drainage from an initial lesion that occurred on the back of the hand.

Case

Mr. J., a 53-year old dairy farmer who also raised Christmas trees for a living and whose hobby was raising tropical fish, noticed the appearance of a small nodule on his left hand. The growth enlarged over the next week to about the size of a quarter and then spontaneously opened and began to drain cloudy yellow material. The lesion was not painful or itchy. Mr. J. treated the open sore with an over-the-counter antibiotic ointment. Three weeks later he noticed two new nodules going up his arm in a line. Those lesions subsequently ulcerated, and several new ones developed proximal to them (Fig. 49-1). At that point Mr. J. decided to visit his physician.

The physician noted a total of seven nodules along the lymphatic distribution of the original lesion. She saw that the original lesion and several others were ulcerated; the rest were small subcutaneous nodules that were not tender. After taking biopsies of several of the ulcerated lesions for culture and histopathologic examination, Mr. J.'s doctor elected to wait for the results before starting therapy, because the lesions could have been manifestations of infection with several different pathogens. The biopsy was read as granulomatous inflammation with no organisms seen, but the culture was reported after 8 days as showing growth of a mold, which was later identified as *Sporothrix schenckii*. Therapy with itraconazole was begun and continued for 4 months until all the lesions had resolved.

This case raises several questions:

1. Where did Mr. J. acquire the organism? Was it related to his dairy farming, raising Christmas trees, or keeping tropical fish?
2. What other infections, besides sporotrichosis, were in the physician's differential diagnosis?
3. Why was Mr. J. treated with itraconazole, which costs approximately 10 times more than the treatment long used for this infection, potassium iodide?

Sporotrichosis
CHARACTERISTICS OF THE ORGANISM

Sporothrix schenckii is a **dimorphic fungus,** similar to fungi that cause endemic mycoses. In the environment *S. schenckii* exists as a mold whose hyphae produce small conidia that are the infectious form. At body temperature *S. schenckii* assumes the yeast form.

ENCOUNTER

S. schenckii is found in soil, sphagnum moss, and decaying wood and vegetation throughout the world. Most cases occur in those who have **outdoor vocations or avocations,** such as farming, landscaping, and gardening, that expose them to the fungus and are associated with a risk of penetrating trauma.

ENTRY

The organism is inoculated into the dermis or subcutaneous tissues by thorns, splinters, or other sharp vegetation. Entry can also occur through animal scratches. Most infections are seen on the upper extremities or face. On rare occasions the organism is aerosolized and inhaled, resulting in pulmonary sporotrichosis.

SPREAD AND MULTIPLICATION

The initial site of inoculation evolves over several weeks into a nonpainful or mildly painful nodular lesion that subsequently ulcerates. In some patients one cutaneous lesion is the only manifestation of infection (**cutaneous sporotrichosis**), and further spread does not occur. In others, like Mr. J., multiple nodules appear in the distribution of the lymphatics draining the area (**lymphocutaneous sporotrichosis**).

DAMAGE

Sporotrichosis is generally a localized infection with few systemic symptoms. Local tissue necrosis is uncommon, and lesions generally resolve with little scarring following antifungal treatment. However, in **immunosuppressed hosts**, especially those with AIDS, **widespread cutaneous and/or life-threatening visceral infection can occur**. Osteoarticular and pulmonary sporotrichosis, often seen in alcoholics, result in significant residual tissue damage.

DIAGNOSIS

Several bacterial infections, especially those caused by *Nocardia* and atypical mycobacteria, mimic lymphocutaneous sporotrichosis. Biopsy of a skin lesion or subcutaneous nodule should be performed for culture and histopathology. The characteristic picture is one of **granulomatous inflammation**. The small, cigar-shaped yeasts are rarely seen on histopathological examination, and **culture is the most reliable diagnostic test.**

TREATMENT

Sporotrichosis rarely resolves without antifungal therapy. The treatment of choice is **itraconazole.** It has been known for a century that potassium iodide is effective for cutaneous and lymphocutaneous sporotrichosis, but the mechanism of action is still unknown. However, potassium iodide is poorly tolerated, and most clinicians and patients prefer itraconazole. Treatment should be continued until the lesions have resolved completely, usually 3 to 6 months. For the uncommon case of osteoarticular, pulmonary, or disseminated infection, initial therapy with amphotericin B may be required, and itraconazole is subsequently given for 1 to 2 years.

Other Subcutaneous Mycoses

Most subcutaneous mycoses occur in tropical areas of the world. **Mycetoma** is a chronic infection characterized by nodules, sinus tracts, and discharge of visible grains composed of fungal colonies. **Chromoblastomycosis** is characterized by nodular, verrucous lesions and the presence of thick-walled, pigmented, sclerotic bodies seen on histopathological examination of involved tissues. Both conditions occur mostly on the lower extremities in persons who go barefoot. Many soil fungi can cause the infections, and treatment is problematic. Itraconazole can be tried, but often **surgical debridement or amputation** is necessary.

Dermatophytes

Infections caused by dermatophytes are the most common fungal infections of humans. They are among the most common skin disorders in children under the age of 12 and the second most common skin disorders in older adults. Infection of the skin is often called **ringworm,** which is a confusing term for patients because there is no connection with worms. A better term is **tinea,** the Latin word for worm. Both words denote the serpentine nature of the lesions that characterize dermatophyte infections on skin. The term *tinea* is used in conjunction with the Latin word for the part of the body affected—for example, **tinea capitis** (head), **tinea pedis** (feet), **tinea corporis** (body), **tinea cruris** (crotch), and **tinea unguium** or **onychomycosis** (nails). Other familiar terms often used to describe these diseases include **athlete's foot, jock itch,** and **jungle rot.**

CHARACTERISTICS OF THE ORGANISM

Three genera of dermatophytes, *Microsporum*, *Trichophyton,* and *Epidermophyton,* cause infection in humans. These molds take days to weeks to grow at 25°C in the laboratory.

ENCOUNTER

Different species of dermatophytes have different ecological niches. Dermatophytes are not members of the normal skin flora. Some organisms grow in soil, while others are found in association with animals, especially dogs and cats, and still others are found almost exclusively in association with humans. Close contact is usually required for transmission to occur among humans and between animals and humans. The ability of dermatophytes to survive on wet surfaces, like locker room showers, likely contributes to transmission.

ENTRY

For disease to occur, the person must not only be exposed to the fungus but also have breaks in the skin so that the relatively avirulent organisms can gain access. Maceration of tissue, especially common in the feet and groin, contributes to the development of infection. **Genetic and hormonal factors** also are important in the ability of the organism to gain entry and cause infection. For example, the incidence of dermatophyte infections is higher in males than in females, with ratios of 3:1 for tinea capitis and 6:1 for tinea pedis. Tinea cruris, common in males, is rare in females.

SPREAD AND MULTIPLICATION

The dermatophytes spread through the stratum corneum but rarely invade the dermis. The ring shape characteristic of dermatophyte lesions is the result of the organism growing outward in a centrifugal pattern. The area of the lesion that yields viable fungal elements is located at the margin. The central area generally has few or no viable fungi. Fungal invasion of nails occurs through the lateral or superficial nail plates and then spreads throughout the nail. When hair shafts are invaded, the organisms can be seen either within the shaft or surrounding it. Keratinases and mannans present in dermatophytes may play a role in invasion of keratinized tissues.

DAMAGE

Tinea infections manifest at various anatomic sites, depending on the age of the host. Tinea capitis is most common in children, with the highest incidence in 3- to 7-year-olds; after puberty the disease is much less common. Tinea pedis, tinea cruris, and onychomycosis rarely occur in childhood but are common in adults, especially men.

Many of the clinical features of tinea infections are related to the **inflammatory response** in the epidermis and dermis to fungal antigens that diffuse from the site of fungal invasion. Children with **tinea capitis** present with well-demarcated scaly patches where hair shafts have broken off right above the skin. **Tinea corporis** is manifested by well-demarcated, pruritic (itchy), scaly lesions that un-

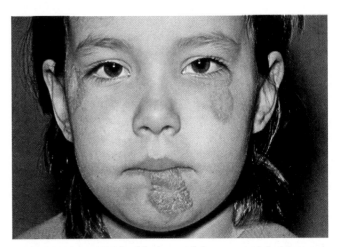

FIGURE 49-2 ■ **Typical lesions of tinea corporis (ringworm) in a child.** Notice the discrete borders with scaling and central clearing.

dergo central clearing as the lesion expands (Fig. 49-2). Often one or several small lesions are present, but in rare cases extensive involvement over much of the trunk occurs (Fig. 49-3). **Tinea cruris** presents as a pruritic, erythematous rash with a scaly border in the groin area. **Tinea pedis** causes fissures between the toes and a scaly pruritic rash along the lateral and plantar surfaces of the feet. Nails infected with dermatophytes become thickened, discolored, and lifted off the nail bed (onycholysis).

DIAGNOSIS

Scrapings should be taken of the involved area (at the border of skin lesions) and observed under the micro-

FIGURE 49-3 ■ **Extensive tinea corporis in a man who had no underlying medical illness.** Notice the well-demarcated border typical of dermatophyte infections. It is not clear why this patient had such extensive lesions; he required systemic azole therapy to cure the infection.

scope after treatment with potassium hydroxide. The presence of hyphae confirms the diagnosis of a dermatophyte infection, but culture is required to identify the specific organism.

TREATMENT

Tinea infections usually respond to treatment with topical antifungal creams and lotions, including tolnaftate, allylamines, and azoles. The exception is **onychomycosis,** which **always requires systemic antifungal agents** to achieve an effective response in the nail. Either terbinafine, which is an allylamine, or itraconazole can be used. For onychomycosis, therapy must be given for a minimum of 3 to 4 months. Relapses are the rule with tinea pedis and tinea cruris. Early institution of topical antifungal agents at the first signs of relapse generally keeps the infection in check.

Superficial Mycoses

Virtually all adults have colonization of the stratum corneum with the yeast *Malassezia* (formerly called *Pity-* *rosporum*). Usually no symptoms are associated with the colonization. However, the fungi can cause **seborrheic dermatitis,** which is characterized by pruritic, erythematous patches with greasy scales in the eyebrows, mustache, and scalp. They also cause **tinea versicolor,** which usually appears on the chest or neck as hypopigmented or hyperpigmented patches with slight scaling. Superficial mycoses are treated with topical antifungal creams or shampoos.

Conclusion

The superficial, cutaneous, and subcutaneous mycoses are the most common fungal infections of humans. They rarely lead to serious disease and in many cases are infections with which patients will live for years. Superficial and dermatophyte infections of the skin are treated with antifungal creams, lotions, or shampoos; infection of the nails must be treated with systemic antifungal agents. Subcutaneous infections require therapy with systemic antifungal agents, and some can be treated only with surgical debridement or amputation.

Antifungal Agents

Carol A. Kauffman

key concepts

- Polyenes interfere with ergosterol synthesis in the fungal cell membrane and have broad antifungal activity, but their use is limited by the high rate of adverse events.

- Allylamines interfere with ergosterol synthesis in the fungal cell membrane but are useful only for superficial fungal infections.

- Azoles target ergosterol in the fungal cell membrane and are relatively safe drugs. Each agent has a unique spectrum of activity and drug interaction profile.

- Echinocandins target the fungal cell wall and have very few side effects; however, they have a limited spectrum of activity.

- Pyrimidine inhibition is the target of flucytosine, an agent with limited use and a high rate of toxicity.

Compared with the number of antibacterial treatments, the drugs available for treating fungal infections seem woefully inadequate (Table 50-1). A major deterrent to the development of antifungal agents has been the shared metabolic and physiologic pathways of eukaryotic fungal and mammalian cells. Given that many antifungal agents have nonselective effects on mammalian cells, toxicity has consistently limited their usefulness. Introduction of the azole class of antifungal agents allowed many patients to be treated with drugs that were far safer than the polyene amphotericin B, which had been the standard antifungal agent for 30 years. With the development of the echinocandins, selective inhibition of fungal growth with minimal adverse effects has been achieved.

The majority of fungal infections are dealt with solely by the normal immune response without recourse to any antifungal treatment. However, the immune response, even in a normal host, can be overwhelmed by exposure to a large fungal inoculum; in such cases antifungal agents can be lifesaving. Many patients who require antifungal agents for systemic fungal infections are immunosuppressed and unable to eradicate the organism themselves.

table 50-1 | Major Classes of Antifungal Agents

CLASS	MECHANISM OF ACTION	AGENTS	FORMULATION	PATHOGEN OR INFECTION AFFECTED
Polyenes	Bind to ergosterol causing disruption of cell membrane	Amphotericin B	Intravenous	*Candida, Cryptococcus, Aspergillus,* Zygomycetes, endemic mycoses, other molds
		Nystatin	Topical	*Candida* (mucous membrane and skin)
Allylamines	Block ergosterol synthesis in cell membrane	Terbinafine	Topical Oral	Dermatophytes
Azoles	Block ergosterol synthesis in cell membrane	Ketoconazole	Oral	Endemic mycoses, dermatophytes
		Itraconazole	Intravenous, oral	Endemic mycoses, *Aspergillus,* dermatophytes
		Fluconazole	Intravenous, oral	*Candida, Cryptococcus*
		Voriconazole	Intravenous, oral	*Aspergillus,* other molds, *Candida*
Echinocandins	Inhibit cell wall synthesis	Caspofungin	Intravenous	*Candida Aspergillus*
Pyrimidine inhibitor	Inhibits DNA and protein synthesis	Flucytosine	Oral	*Cryptococcus, Candida*

Polyenes

The polyenes act by **binding to ergosterol,** a major component of the cell membrane in fungi. Binding leads to altered membrane permeability, leakage of cell constituents, and cell death. The polyenes also bind, although less avidly, to cholesterol in mammalian cell membranes, thus accounting for their toxicity. Two polyene agents are currently available. **Nystatin** is quite toxic and used only as a topical agent. **Amphotericin B**, introduced in the 1950s, has been the standard of therapy for serious fungal infections until recently.

Amphotericin B is available only as an **intravenous formulation** and is prepared as a colloidal dispersion with sodium deoxycholate because of its insolubility in water. The drug is highly protein bound to serum lipoproteins and penetrates poorly into cerebrospinal and other body fluids. The half-life is very long (terminal half-life is 15 days or more), and activity can be recovered from urine for several months after discontinuation. Amphotericin B has a **very wide spectrum of activity.** It has excellent in vitro activity against yeasts, including *Candida* species and *Cryptococcus neoformans*; molds, including *Aspergillus* species and the Zygomycetes; all the endemic mycoses; and most organisms causing subcutaneous and skin infections.

The major drawback to the use of amphotericin B is its **inherent toxicity.** Some degree of nephrotoxicity occurs in almost every patient receiving the agent, anemia is expected with prolonged therapy, and infusion reactions (chills, fever, nausea, myalgias) are common and can be severe. Because of its serious adverse event profile, new formulations have been introduced that mask much of the toxicity by wrapping the active drug in lipid layers or within liposomes. The introduction of three **lipid formulations of amphotericin B** has ameliorated, but not eliminated, the toxicity of the agent.

Although used less now than it was just a few years ago, amphotericin B remains the drug of choice for infection with the Zygomycetes and is the most appropriate initial therapy for cryptococcal meningitis, severe histoplasmosis, blastomycosis, coccidioidomycosis, and some forms of candidiasis. The introduction of new classes of antifungal agents has markedly diminished the need for amphotericin B.

Allylamines

Terbinafine, the major allylamine agent, **inhibits squalene epoxidase activity,** blocking ergosterol synthesis in the fungal cell membrane. This agent has activity against dermatophytes that cause skin and nail infections, and it has some activity against *Candida albicans*. It is available in both tablet and topical formulations.

The drug is extensively metabolized by cytochrome P450 enzymes in the liver and **concentrates in the stratum corneum, hair follicles, and nails.** Terbinafine is indicated for the treatment of **dermatophyte infections** of the skin that have not responded to application of creams and for fungal nail infections. It is not indicated for any systemic fungal infection.

Terbinafine is usually well tolerated. Changes in taste perception can occur and can interfere with appetite. Hepatic dysfunction and rarely liver failure have been reported in connection with the use of terbinafine.

Azoles

Three first-generation systemic azole antifungal agents, **ketoconazole, itraconazole, and fluconazole,** and one second-generation azole, **voriconazole,** are currently available. In addition, many topical azole agents are used for localized yeast infections. The second-generation azoles have a broader spectrum of activity compared with the first-generation agents. All azoles inhibit fungal growth through the same mechanism, inhibition of cytochrome P450-dependent 14α-lanosterol demethylation, a vital step in **cell membrane ergosterol synthesis.** Differences in selectivity for fungal cell membranes compared with mammalian cell membranes predict toxicity of the azoles.

Ketoconazole, the first oral azole, had a significant number of side effects and drug interactions and has largely been supplanted by **itraconazole,** with its greater intrinsic activity against many fungi and improved safety profile. Itraconazole is active against *Candida* species, *Cryptococcus, Aspergillus*, the endemic fungi, and dermatophytes. It is available as both oral and intravenous formulations. Absorption of itraconazole is problematic in that both food and gastric acid are required for maximum absorption. Itraconazole has become the drug of choice for the endemic mycoses and for dermatophyte infections of the skin and nails.

The antifungal spectrum of **fluconazole** is narrower than that of other azoles. It has activity against most *Candida* species but not *C. glabrata* or *C. krusei* and is not active against most molds. Fluconazole is water soluble and available in both intravenous and oral formulations. It undergoes less cytochrome P450-mediated metabolism, and renal excretion occurs. Fluconazole is widely used for treatment of *Candida* and *Cryptococcus* infections and for prophylaxis against fungal infections in immunosuppressed patients.

Voriconazole is the first second-generation azole available for use. In addition to activity against yeasts, such as *Candida*, the second-generation azoles have enhanced activity against molds, including *Aspergillus*, a characteristic that sets them apart from the first-generation agents. Voriconazole is available as both intravenous and oral formulations and is extensively metabolized by several cytochrome P450 enzymes.

Overall, the azoles are safe antifungal agents. The two most problematic issues are hepatitis, which is an uncommon side effect seen with all azoles, and drug interactions, which differ for each agent and must be monitored carefully to avoid serious and sometimes life-threatening reactions.

Echinocandins

The echinocandins are the newest class of antifungal agents. They have a **unique target, the synthesis of β-(1,3)-D-glucan,** an essential component of the fungal cell wall. Because mammalian cells do not have cell walls, the echinocandins are more selective than the agents discussed earlier that target the synthesis of cell membrane components. β-(1,3)-D-glucan is an important component of the cell walls of all *Candida* and *Aspergillus* species but is not present or occurs only in small amounts in other fungi. Thus, the spectrum of activity of the echinocandins is rel-

atively narrow (*Candida* and *Aspergillus*) compared with amphotericin B and the second-generation azoles.

Caspofungin was the first echinocandin to be made available. Micafungin has recently been approved and anidulafungin will soon be approved. All are available only as intravenous formulations. Hydrolyzed and then acetylated to inactive metabolites, the echinocandins are neither metabolized by nor inhibitors of the cytochrome P450 system.

Given their selective fungal cell wall target, the echinocandins have **minimal toxicity.** Infusion-related reactions (flushing, fever, chills) occur in less than 1% of patients. Rash, headache, nausea, and vomiting have been reported but are uncommon.

Pyrimidine Inhibition

The only agent in this class, **flucytosine** (5-fluorocytosine), is an oral fluorinated pyrimidine that is converted to 5-fluorouracil by fungal cells. It **interferes with fungal protein and DNA synthesis.** Flucytosine is active against *C. neoformans* and *Candida* species. Because resistance develops quickly, flucytosine is never used alone but must be paired with another antifungal agent. Another major drawback to using this agent is dose-related **bone marrow suppression** and hepatotoxicity. It is used almost entirely only for the initial treatment of cryptococcal meningitis.

Other Agents

Griseofulvin is an oral agent used only for treatment of superficial dermatophyte infections. The mechanism of action is unique in that it interferes with microtubule function. The use of griseofulvin has largely been supplanted by terbinafine and itraconazole. **Tolnaftate** is another agent used only for superficial dermatophyte infections. The mechanism of action is not known. It is available only in topical formulations.

Potassium iodide has been used for more than a century against cutaneous sporotrichosis, but the mechanism of action remains unknown. It is available as an oral solution. Side effects (metallic taste, thyroid dysfunction, rash, salivary gland swelling) are common.

Conclusion

The three major classes of antifungal drugs—polyenes, azoles, and echinocandins—are able to eradicate many previously fatal fungal infections. All have side effects, but the newer agents are markedly safer than the first antifungal drug, amphotericin B. The host immune response remains the most important determinant of the outcome of infection, even with the new antifungal drugs recently made available.

chapter 51

Introduction to Parasitology

Cary Engleberg

key **concepts**

- Knowledge of parasitic life cycles is essential to understanding the rationale for preventive interventions.

- Local ecology (e.g., climate, arthropods) and socioeconomic factors (e.g., sanitation, housing) govern the geographic distribution of disease by determining whether a particular parasite can complete its life cycle.

- Parasites that have evolved within human hosts usually cause asymptomatic infections; thus the host response does not usually hinder the completion of the parasitic life cycle. Symptoms typically result from a high parasite burden or prolonged duration of infection. Among the few notable exceptions to that generalization is malaria.

- Many parasites survive in the human host by evading or subverting the immune response. Damage induced by those pathogens is usually a direct consequence of host hypersensitivity.

- For many parasitic infections, the capacity to occupy certain tissues (tropism) is an essential feature of the life cycle.

- Diagnosis often depends on direct identification of parasitic forms in human samples. Therefore, knowledge of tissue tropisms and modes of transmission determines which samples should be collected and examined.

Parasitic infections are among the most prevalent infectious diseases worldwide (Table 51-1). Some diseases—malaria, schistosomiasis, and hookworm, for example—cause morbidity and mortality on a massive scale in many tropical countries. In most developed countries, where "tropical diseases" have no potential for transmission, parasites are regarded as strange and exotic. That perception may be misleading, however, because developed countries have their own complement of common parasitic diseases, albeit ones with less morbidity and sociomedical impact (Table 51-2). In either geographical context, common parasitic infections often cause no clinical symptoms at all. Yet the AIDS epidemic and more advanced immunosuppression for organ transplantation or following cancer treatment have given certain parasitic diseases new clinical significance.

table **51-1**	Estimated Worldwide Prevalence of Parasitic Infections
INFECTION	**PREVALENCE**
Toxoplasmosis	1–2 billion
Ascariasis	1 billion
Hookworm disease	800–900 million
Amebiasis	200–400 million
Schistosomiasis	200–300 million
Malaria	200–300 million
Filariasis	250 million
Giardiasis	200 million
Pinworm infection	60–100 million
Strongyloidiasis	50–80 million
Guinea worm infection	20–40 million
Trypanosomiasis	15–20 million
Leishmaniasis	1–2 million

Infection Versus Disease

As with other agents, parasitic infection must be distinguished from parasitic disease. For example, a large number of adults in the United States are infected with the protozoan *Toxoplasma gondii*, as demonstrated by the prevalence of antitoxoplasma antibodies in the population. However, few people become ill from the infection. Another example is hookworm infection. Hookworms consume small amounts of blood to survive, mate, and release eggs in the human intestine. Because the amount of blood consumed by each worm is small (0.03 to 0.15 mL/day), infections with only a few worms are clinically insignificant. However, infections with large numbers of hookworms can produce a life-threatening anemia.

Like other infectious agents described in this textbook, parasites have evolved to exploit their hosts in order to grow and procreate. Because they depend on the host for their survival and to complete their life cycle, killing or disabling the host is not to the parasites' advantage. Consequently, disease associated with many parasites is often the consequence of **prolonged, repeated, or unusually burdensome infection.** Parasitic diseases are usually **subacute or chronic** and, even if untreated, are rarely fatal over short periods. There are, however, important exceptions, such as malaria caused by *Plasmodium falciparum*, which may be rapidly fatal (within 3 to 5 days). Moreover, parasites that normally produce quiescent, asymptomatic infections in immuno-

competent hosts can cause disseminated and potentially lethal diseases in immunocompromised persons (e.g., toxoplasmosis).

Parasitic Infections as Zoonoses

Several parasitic infections of humans are **zoonoses;** that is, they are caused by agents that infect animals such as birds, reptiles, and other mammals (see Chapter 73 and the Chapter 33 paradigm). Many human parasites require both human and nonhuman hosts to complete their life cycles. For example, people can carry an adult beef tapeworm in the intestinal lumen, but an infected person cannot transmit the parasite to another person. To complete its life cycle, the parasite must undergo larval development in the muscles of cattle (cysticercosis). Humans can become infected with the tapeworm by eating undercooked beef. Both stages (adult and larval) and both hosts (cattle and humans) are required to complete the life cycle of the tapeworm. Other animal parasites do not require a developmental stage in humans but can nevertheless infect humans and cause disease. In those cases humans are **dead-end hosts.** For example, the blood fluke (schistosome) of birds alternates between birds and snails. Although humans can sometimes "substitute" for birds as vertebrate hosts, the life cycle of the parasite is not completed in humans. The infecting larvae cannot penetrate beyond the skin but die there, causing an irritating dermatitis called "swimmer's itch" that resolves spontaneously.

Types of Parasites and Modes of Transmission

Protozoa

Protozoa are one-celled eukaryotes. Protozoal parasites of medical importance include *Plasmodium* species (the agents of malaria) as well as species of *Giardia, Cryptosporidium, Leishmania,* and trypanosomes. Infections with any of those pathogens can be initiated by relatively small inocula. Disease is generally a consequence of the replication of the parasites in large numbers within the host. Replication may be intracellular (e.g., plasmodia, which grow within red blood cells, and *Leishmania* species, which grow within macrophages), or it may occur extracellularly, such as in the lumen of the gastrointestinal tract (e.g., amebas and *Giardia* species).

As unicellular organisms bounded by only a cell membrane, many protozoa are unable to withstand desiccation

table 51-2 Geographic Context of Parasitic Infection

CURRENTLY OR HISTORICALLY INDIGENOUS TO THE U.S. MAINLAND	IMPORTED
Intestinal Helminths	
Ascaris lumbricoides (roundworm)	*Ancylostoma braziliensis* (hookworm)
Enterobius vermicularis (pinworm)	*Schistosoma mansoni* (schistosomiasis)
Trichuris trichiura (whipworm)	*Schistosoma hematobium*
Strongyloides stercoralis (threadworm)	*Schistosoma japonicum*
Necator americanus (hookworm)	
Taenia saginata (beef tapeworm)	
Taenia solium (pork tapeworm)	
Diphyllobothrium latum (fish tapeworm)	
Hymenolepis nana (dwarf tapeworm)	
Toxocara canis, T. cati (visceral larva migrans)	
Trichinella spiralis (trichinosis)	
Echinococcus	
Echinococcus granulosus (cystic hydatid disease)	*Echinococcus multilocularis* (cystic hydatid disease)
Filaria	
Dirofilaria immitis (canine filariasis)	*Wuchereria bancrofti*
	Brugia malayi
	Onchocerca volvulus
	Loa loa
	Dracunculus medinensis
Flukes	
	Paragonimus westermani (lung fluke)
	Clonorchis sinensis (liver fluke)
Protozoa	
Entamoeba histolytica (amebiasis)	*Plasmodium vivax, falciparum, ovale, malariae*
Giardia lamblia (giardiasis)	*Leishmania donovani, L. tropica, L. mexicana, L. braziliensis*
Toxoplasma gondii (toxoplasmosis)	*Balantidium coli* (balantidiasis)
Babesia microti (babesiosis)	*Trypanosoma cruzi* (Chagas disease)
Pneumocystis carinii (pneumocystosis)	*Trypanosoma brucei* (African sleeping sickness)
Trichomonas vaginalis (trichomoniasis)	*Isospora belli* (isosporiasis)
Free-living amebas (meningoencephalitis, skin and eye infections)	
Cryptosporidium parvum (cryptosporidiosis)	
Cyclospora cayetanensis (cyclosporiasis)	

(drying) in the external environment. Consequently, their life cycles usually do not include free environmental stages, and their transmission from one host to another depends on **arthropod vectors**. For example, plasmodia are transmitted by mosquitoes. An alternative strategy used by some protozoa is to alternate between two distinct forms: an active **trophozoite** form that grows and replicates by binary fission with the host, and a dormant, non-replicating **cyst** form that is adapted for survival in various environmental extremes as it transits between hosts. Protozoal cysts are relatively impermeable because of their double membranes and thus can resist desiccation in the external environment. Protozoa that infect the gastrointestinal tract employ this strategy, and they are transmitted between hosts by the fecal–oral route.

Protozoal pathogens can be classified based on their life cycles and **locomotion** (Fig. 51-1):

- **Amebas** (or Sarcodina): formless cells that move purposefully by extending **pseudopods** toward an attractive stimulus and then **streaming** their cytoplasm in the desired direction. Amebas are intestinal parasites that alternate between trophozoite and cyst forms.

- **Flagellates:** intestinal and blood protozoa that use one or more flagellae for locomotion. Like the amebas, flagellates that infect the gastrointestinal tract form environmentally resistant cysts. Flagellates that infect the tissues or blood are transmitted by arthropods.

- **Ciliates:** protozoa covered with tiny cilia that provide locomotion. Pathogenic ciliates are extremely unusual and are not covered in this textbook.

- **Apicomplexans** (or **sporozoa**): very important pathogens that include the agents of malaria, toxoplasmosis, and several common intestinal parasites. Apicomplexans share the feature of intracellular replication. Based on observations of *T. gondii*, it is thought to move using a "tractor-tread" mechanism of **gliding motility**, and the same mechanism permits its forced entry into host cells (see Fig. 51-1).

Helminths

Helminths (worms) are **multicellular animals** (metazoa) and are considerably larger than protozoa. Because they **reproduce sexually**, productive infections require both

Ameboid movement

Flagellae

Gliding motility (Apicomplexa)

FIGURE 51-1 ■ **Mechanisms of protozoal locomotion.**

male and female worms. However, some tapeworms are **hermaphroditic,** having both male and female reproductive organs. Helminths of medical importance include the following:

- **Roundworms:** circular in cross section. Adult worms of various roundworm species range in size from a few millimeters to 20 centimeters. One human intestinal roundworm *(Ascaris lumbricoides)* bears a remarkable resemblance to an earthworm; however, unlike annelids (e.g., earthworms), roundworms have **no visible body segmentation.**
- **Flatworms:** asymmetric in cross section. They comprise two main types:
  - **Flukes** (e.g., *Schistosoma, Fasciola*): relatively short flatworms with nonsegmented bodies.
  - **Tapeworms:** segmented worms that vary in size from millimeters to several meters in length. A tapeworm can be thought of more as a colony than as an integrated multicellular organism. The segments are generated from a germinal worm head that contributes to a growing chain of flat segments, each with its own nutritional and reproductive organs.

Because of their large size, helminths are typically extracellular. However, the larvae of some helminths, such as the roundworm that causes trichinosis (*Trichinella spiralis*) and most tapeworms, develop into dormant cysts. Protected by an impermeable **cuticle,** helminths often have complex life cycles involving environmental or animal reservoirs. With rare exceptions, no helminthic parasite completes its life cycle within a single human host. Therefore, disease is not normally a consequence of helminths growing in number within the host, as it is with protozoa. Instead, the parasitic burden (and the likelihood of pathologic consequences) is directly related to the number of helminthic parasites that the host acquires from the environment.

Vectors

Vectors are living transmitters of disease. Most vectors are **arthropods.** Perhaps the best-known example of a vector is the female *Anopheles* mosquito, which transmits malaria. Other important vectors include tsetse flies, which transmit sleeping sickness; black flies, which transmit the tissue roundworm infection called river blindness; reduviid ("kissing") bugs, which transmit Chagas disease; and ticks, which transmit babesiosis. Arthropods can transmit not only parasites but also bacteria (e.g., the agents of Lyme disease and Rocky Mountain spotted fever) and viruses (e.g., yellow fever, dengue, and encephalitis viruses).

Arthropods are not simply passive agents that transfer parasites from one mammalian host to another. They also are involved in essential steps of the parasitic life cycle. To a large extent the prevalence of a parasitic disease in a given geographical location may depend on whether the local conditions are favorable to arthropod breeding—for example, stagnant water for mosquito breeding, or foliage, moisture, and suitable animal hosts for the propagation of ticks. Because of the obligatory role that arthropods play in the development of some protozoal and helminthic pathogens, their elimination from the environment can theoretically eradicate the respective diseases they cause in humans.

Reservoirs

Reservoirs are sources of parasites in the environment that do not participate directly in transmission to humans. Reservoirs of human parasites include other humans (e.g., for malaria parasites and amebas), other animals (e.g., pigs for trichinosis and pork tapeworm, cattle for beef tapeworm and cryptosporidiosis) and the environment (e.g., soil contaminated with parasitized human feces).

Parasitic Infections and Disease

ENTRY

One intriguing aspect of human parasites is the number of strategies they have evolved to enter the host (Table 51-3). Infections can be transmitted by the fecal–oral route (e.g., amebiasis, ascariasis), by the direct penetration of unbroken skin infection (e.g., hookworm, schistosomiasis), or by the bites of arthropod vectors (e.g., malaria, filariasis).

With the first two routes of transmission, acquisition usually results from ingestion of **contaminated food or water** or from **inadequate control of human wastes** in soil or water. Although many of the parasites using those routes of transmission live in the gastrointestinal tract, several invade and infect the internal organs or skin, and a few cause disease in both the intestine and deeper tissues.

Most arthropod-borne infections are transmitted to humans through bite wounds. Transmission through arthropods can be extraordinarily efficient. In fact, malaria can be acquired from the bite of a single infected mosquito during a stop at an airport in an endemic area. In addition, some arthropod-borne infections can be transmitted by the transfusion of blood from asymptomatic infected humans.

SPREAD AND MULTIPLICATION

Inoculum Size

The effective inoculum size has been determined for a few parasites by experimental infections in human volunteers and animals, usually in conjunction with quantitative epidemiologic studies. For example, large inocula are required to cause amebiasis in humans, whereas symptomatic cryptosporidiosis can be produced by the ingestion of relatively few cysts. In most helminthic infections the severity of the infection is proportional to the inoculum size (or the cumulative inoculum if exposure continues over time).

Parasite Survival Mechanisms in Immunologically Normal Hosts

Like other microorganisms, parasites elicit both antibody and cell-mediated responses (see the box titled "Parasitic Mechanisms for Evading the Host Immune Response"). However, they are adept at circumventing those host defenses. For example, adult schistosomes (blood flukes) coat themselves with host plasma proteins and are thus not recognized as foreign by the host's immune system. As a result, they are able to persist within the bloodstream for decades without immune-mediated destruction. Trypanosomes elude their hosts' immune systems by varying their surface antigens. In contrast, intracellular parasites are protected by special adaptations. For example, *Leishmania* species, which live in the phagolysosomes of macrophages, secrete a superoxide dismutase that protects them from the toxic superoxide produced in the phagolysosome. Like other protozoal parasites, *Leishmania* species also directly influence the host immune response to their advantage, directing lymphocyte proliferation into the Th2 rather than Th1 pathway.

Parasitic Mechanisms for Evading the Host Immune Response

- **Antigenic variation:** trypanosomes, *Plasmodium* species, *Giardia* species
- **Intracellular infection:** plasmodia, *Toxoplasma* species
- **encystation:** amebas, cestodes
- **Camouflage:** schistosomes
- **Cleavage of antibodies or complement components:** amebas, *Leishmania* species
- **Suppression or redirection of the cellular immune response:** plasmodia, *Leishmania* species, schistosomes

---

Species and Tissue Tropisms

The life cycles of parasites are determined by species and tissue **tropisms,** which define the hosts that parasites can infect and the organs and tissues in which they can survive. As yet, very little is known about the biologic basis of tissue tropisms. Thus, it is not clear why the larvae of *Strongyloides* species invade the intestinal wall, whereas those of hookworms remain in the intestinal lumen. Nor is it clear why the pork tapeworm can cause cysticercosis (infection of the deep tissues) in humans but the beef tapeworm cannot. Recent studies have shown that some tropisms depend on specific receptors. For example, the presence of the Duffy factor antigen on the surface of the red blood cell is necessary for the entry of *Plasmodium vivax* malaria parasites (merozoites) into human red blood cells. Thus, subjects whose red blood cells lack the Duffy factor (black Africans) are resistant to *P. vivax* infection.

Temperature also plays an important role in the ability of parasites to infect humans and cause disease. For example, *Leishmania donovani* replicates well at 37°C and causes visceral leishmaniasis (kala-azar), a disease of the bone marrow, liver, and spleen. (Note that the temperature of those tissues is, of course, 37°C). In contrast, *L. tropica* grows well at 25°C to 30°C but poorly at 37°C and causes infections of the skin (where temperatures are 25°C to 30°C). Temperature changes also induce stage-specific transitions in many parasites. For example, *Leishmania* species change from the promastigote form to the amastigote form when they move from a cooler insect vector to a warmer human host (from 25°C to 37°C). They also synthesize heat-shock protein.

DAMAGE

As with other infectious agents, the clinical manifestations of parasitic disease may reflect tissue damage by the parasite, the effects of the host immune response, or both. The pathogenic amebas are examples of pathogens that cause most of their tissue damage by a direct cytolytic effect. For example, amebic liver abscesses are produced by direct destruction of host cells, with the host contributing an ineffective acute inflammatory response. In contrast, many other parasitic infections that involve deep tissues elicit an inflammatory response that may be exclusively responsible for the histopathology. **Chronic inflammation** is the hallmark of diseases such as schistosomiasis and cutaneous filariasis. In these helminthic infections, the adult parasites are innocuous, but their progeny (i.e., microfilaria and eggs of *Schistosoma* species) induce intense inflammatory responses when they degenerate in host tissues. In some parasitic diseases (e.g., trichinosis) the **host inflammatory response may cause persistent disease** even after the parasites have died. In cysticercosis the infected individual may remain asymptomatic for a long period until the parasite dies. Then the leakage of parasite antigens into the tissues may trigger a hypersensitivity reaction and produce symptoms in the host.

Eosinophilia

Eosinophils are leukocytes that participate in neutralizing infections with parasitic worms. In helminthic infections, eosinophils may appear in the blood in large numbers. This eosinophilia occurs in response to the parasites' surface glycoproteins and polysaccharides, particularly when the parasites invade or migrate through tissues. Eosinophilia is typically accompanied by increased levels of IgE and is driven by **elevated levels of interleukin-5.** Together, eosinophils and IgE play a critical role in killing multicellular parasites. Because eosinophilia and increased levels of IgE occur with helminthic infections and are most striking with helminths that invade the deep tissues, they are useful in diagnosis. In contrast, the responses are not a feature of most protozoal infections.

Timing of Clinical Complications

The most important complications of many parasitic diseases occur years after the initial infection. For instance, persons with schistosomiasis typically have bleeding from either the gastrointestinal tract (*Schistosoma mansoni*) or the urinary tract (*S. haematobium*), which continues for years. Decades later people with heavy, chronic infections may develop complications such as portal hypertension with esophageal varices (*S. mansoni*), or obstructions or cancer of the urinary tract (*S. haematobium*).

Important complications also can occur at distant sites. For example, intestinal pork tapeworm (*Taenia solium*) infections are asymptomatic. However, late complications result if tapeworm eggs are ingested and larval forms of the parasite hatch in the intestine, cross the mucosa, enter the bloodstream, and encyst in the deep tissues as **cysticerci.** The cysts are small (0.5 to 1.5 cm) and produce no signs or symptoms if they lodge in skeletal muscle or the central nervous system. However, when they infect the central nervous system, the cysts may eventually leak their contents into tissue, causing seizures or hydrocephalus (by blocking the flow of cerebrospinal fluid).

A chronic protozoal infection called Chagas disease (American trypanosomiasis) typically produces a relatively trivial skin lesion at the time of the initial infection. Although in rare cases among young children the initial infection progresses rapidly to death, it is usually asymptomatic or minimally symptomatic. Years later, older persons with chronic infection can develop heart block from damage to the cardiac conducting system, or impaired swallowing or defecation from damage to the nerves responsible for the motility of the esophagus or colon. Although late complications are rare, there are no predictors to identify the people at greatest risk of developing them.

Environmental Constraints on Transmission

Examination of the parasitic life cycle often explains why a given parasitic disease is found in one area of the world and not another (see Table 51-2). For example, the transmission of schistosomiasis depends on an intermediate snail host that is not present in North America or Europe. Thus, viable eggs in the stool or urine of infected persons cannot produce the forms infective for humans (**cercariae**) because there are no intermediate snail hosts in which the parasite can mature. For that reason, schistosomiasis is not endemic in the United States and will not be, unless an intermediate snail host becomes established. It does not matter how many persons infected with schistosomiasis enter the United States and contaminate the environment with infective eggs. In contrast, *Anopheles* mosquitoes capable of transmitting malaria are found in the United States. Therefore, recent immigrants or travelers who acquired malaria in endemic areas may infect the indigenous mosquito pool. Local transmission of malaria by that mechanism occurs a few times each year in the United States (recent cases have occurred in California, New Jersey, and Michigan). Those rare events are diagnostic puzzles because infected individuals typically have no histories of foreign travel. Ongoing malaria surveillance is therefore particularly important when large numbers of people from malaria-endemic areas enter the United States and settle in parts of the country where substantial numbers of *Anopheles* mosquitoes are present.

DIAGNOSIS

Most parasitic infections are diagnosed by identifying the parasites or their characteristic progeny (cysts, eggs, or larvae) in clinical specimens. To pursue the most effective diagnostic strategies, it is important to understand the parasite's life cycle (Fig. 51-2). For instance, in the life cycle of hookworms, the adult female lives in the lumen of

the human intestine, suggesting that she will release her eggs into the stool. Consequently, examination of the stool for hookworm eggs is an effective and sensitive method for the diagnosis of hookworm infection. In contrast, in the life cycle of *Strongyloides* species, the adult female invades the intestinal wall to release her eggs. Intact eggs are rarely seen in the stool. However, the larvae that emerge from eggs in the intestinal wall can be found in the stool of a person with *Strongyloides* infection, and their presence is diagnostic for that infection.

One species of filarial helminths, *Wuchereria bancrofti*, is transmitted to humans by mosquitos that bite primarily at night. To maximize their transmission to mosquitos, the parasites release their microfilaria into the human bloodstream during the late-evening hours. Thus, to examine blood for *W. bancrofti,* samples are typically drawn at midnight!

Traditionally, parasitic infections are diagnosed by visualizing the parasite or its progeny (eggs, cysts, or microfilaria) in clinical specimens. In recent years, immunologic and DNA-based detection of the organisms has assumed new importance because the techniques are both highly sensitive and better adapted for rapid testing of large numbers of samples.

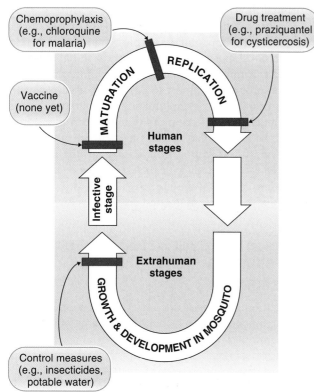

FIGURE 51-2 ▪ **Idealized (model) parasite life cycle and points of intervention.** The human stages of the life cycle are located in the top half of the diagram. The extrahuman stages (in animate or inanimate reservoirs) are in the lower half. When the parasite reaches the infective stage, it invades the human host, matures, replicates, and ultimately completes the life cycle by producing infective forms. The infective forms are taken up by a vector or released into the environment. Control measures interfere with the replication or survival of the extrahuman stages of the parasite. They reduce the incidence of infection by reducing the number of infective stages to which humans are exposed. Immunization (vaccination) prevents symptomatic infection by inhibiting or killing the parasite as it enters (or replicates within) the human host. Chemoprophylaxis is used to inhibit parasite replication and thus prevent symptomatic infection. Neither immunization nor chemoprophylaxis prevents the initial entry of the parasite. Drug treatment is used to prevent death or severe morbidity in persons with established infections.

TREATMENT AND PREVENTION

Antiparasite strategies fall into three general categories: drugs for prevention (chemoprophylaxis) and treatment, immunization, and control measures in the field. Eradication programs have generally been effective only when at least two strategies were used simultaneously.

An understanding of the parasitic life cycle is helpful in selecting antiparasitic drugs. For example, different drugs are necessary for the different stages (intestinal and tissue) of the pork tapeworm (*T. solium*): niclosamide is effective against intestinal infection (taeniasis), and praziquantel is used to treat the tissue stage of the infection (cysticercosis).

The parasite life cycle also provides important clues for treatment and control strategies (see Fig. 51-2 and Table 51-3). For example, hookworm larvae from eggs in human stool mature to the filariform stage in the environment; they then cause infection by penetrating unprotected human skin. Therefore, sanitation (appropriate disposal of human waste) and wearing shoes can reduce the transmission of hookworms and thus decrease the number of people infected. Hookworm infection and disease were very common in the southern United States until those preventive measures were instituted on a large scale by the Rockefeller Commission in the 1930s. Sanitation is particularly effective in reducing rates of parasitic infections transmitted through contaminated stool or urine, such as ascariasis, strongyloidiasis,

table 51-3 Modes of Spread of Some Parasitic Diseases

MODE OF EXIT	MODE OF ENTRY	HUMAN-TO-HUMAN	ANIMAL-TO-HUMAN
Feces	Mouth	Cryptosporidiosis	Cryptosporidiosis
		Amebiasis	Toxoplasmosis
		Giardiasis	Visceral larva migrans
		Strongyloidiasis[a]	Echinococcosis
		Ascariasis[b]	
		Trichuris infection[b]	
		Pork tapeworm	
Feces	Skin	Strongyloidiasis	Creeping eruption (dog or cat hookworm)
		Hookworm	Schistosomiasis [c]
Arthropod bite	Arthropod bite	Lymphatic filariasis	Trypanosomiasis (sleeping sickness, Chagas disease)
		Leishmaniasis	Leishmaniasis
		Malaria	
		Onchocerciasis	
None (parasite encysts in muscle)	Ingestion (inadequately cooked meat)		Trichinosis
			Toxoplasmosis
			Beef tapeworm
			Pork tapeworm
			Fish tapeworm

[a] Usually transmitted by fecal–cutaneous contact but may also be transmitted by the fecal–oral route.
[b] May require a period outside the human host to be infectious.
[c] Mode of exit may also be urine; development in an intermediate host is obligatory.

and hookworm infection. Paradoxically, according to the so-called "hygiene hypothesis," extremely hygienic environments that help prevent infections with minor intestinal helminth infections among children may also contribute to the development of allergies.

Drugs

Chemoprophylaxis

Drugs used for chemoprophylaxis must meet more stringent requirements than do drugs used only for treatment. Minor drug side effects acceptable for short periods in sick persons (e.g., headache, nausea, or gastrointestinal disturbances) are unacceptable for prolonged periods in persons who are healthy.

One example of successful chemoprophylaxis is the use of chloroquine to prevent malaria. Chloroquine is effective against all four species of *Plasmodium* that cause malaria in humans. Oral administration once a week produces effective plasma levels of the drug because chloroquine is well absorbed and has a plasma half-life greater than 4 days. The main disadvantage of chloroquine is that strains of *P. falciparum* in most

malarious areas of the world have become resistant to it. The development of resistance is always a concern when relatively lower doses of drugs are used for chemoprophylaxis.

Treatment

When does treatment influence the transmission of parasites? Mass treatment may be an effective control strategy for diseases that depend on humans as a reservoir. In contrast, treatment of people with zoonotic and dead-end infections will not influence the occurrence of those diseases. In general, treatment of symptomatic infections is usually an inefficient strategy for controlling transmission because a long delay often occurs between the initial infection and the onset of symptoms (e.g., 10 to 20 years or more for schistosomiasis). During the long asymptomatic interval, infected humans are able to transmit the infection. If treatment is to be effective in reducing transmission, it must be given to all infectious persons, both symptomatic and asymptomatic.

The goal of many treatment regimens for parasitic infection has been to prevent the long-term complications of infection (such as portal hypertension in schistosomiasis or seizures in cysticercosis). In the last 10 years, several new drugs have appeared that represent significant advances in the treatment of parasitic diseases, such as albendazole for cysticercosis, praziquantel for schistosomiasis, ivermectin for onchocerciasis, and difluoromethylornithine (DFMO) for African sleeping sickness. The drugs previously available to treat those diseases were toxic and often ineffective. Prior to praziquantel, no medical treatment existed for cysticercosis (the tissue-invasive form of pork tapeworm infection). Now researchers expect widespread use of the available drugs to significantly decrease seizures and hydrocephalus from cysticercosis, cirrhosis from schistosomiasis, and blindness from onchocerciasis.

Immunity and Immunization

Major Problem in Designing Vaccines: Evasion of the Host Immune Response

Many important parasites survive to produce disease because they can avoid the effects of the host immune response. Schistosomes masquerade as the "self" (host) by covering themselves with host antigens. Because of that protection, circulating antibodies against schistosomal antigens (produced spontaneously or by immunization) are unlikely to bind to the relevant schistosomal antigens and are thus unlikely to be effective against the parasites. Trypanosomes use another strategy to evade the host immune response: they alter their surface antigens (see Chapter 52 and the Chapter 14 paradigm). When the host develops an effective immune response to one antigen, clones of the trypanosomes emerge that express different antigens on their surfaces, leading to successive bouts of high-grade parasitemia. An effective vaccine against all antigenic types seems extremely unlikely.

Other Problems in Designing Vaccines: Stage-Specific Antigens

Parasites typically have different proteins or polysaccharides on their surfaces at different stages of their life cycles. Many of those surface components are antigenic, imparting different immunological characteristics to each stage of the parasite life cycle. For example, the form of the malaria parasite that is injected into humans by the mosquito is antigenically distinct from the form that infects red blood cells. Consequently, a person immunized with the mosquito stage (the sporozoite) is susceptible to infection by the red blood cell stage of the parasite (the merozoite). An effective malaria vaccine will likely need to contain major antigens derived from each of the several different stages of the parasite's life cycle. Efforts to develop vaccines are under way for several important parasitic diseases in addition to malaria, including schistosomiasis, onchocerciasis, lymphatic filariasis, and toxoplasmosis.

Control Measures

Effective control measures are potentially available for all parasitic diseases. The best measures are based on the mode of transmission defined by the parasite's life cycle (see Fig. 51-2). For example, mosquitoes that transmit malaria often bite at night while most people are sleeping. Because many of the mosquitoes rest under the eaves of houses after biting humans, insecticides such as dichlorodiphenyltrichloroethane (DDT) have reduced malaria transmission substantially when sprayed at those sites. Unfortunately, that strategy is limited because many mosquitoes have developed resistance to DDT and the strategy selects for mosquitoes that bite outside the house during daylight hours.

In developed areas like North America and Europe, transmission of parasitic disease is typically low because sanitation interrupts the parasite's life cycle. However, in developing countries, where the major parasitic diseases are endemic, even simple sanitary methods of interrupting transmission are difficult to implement. Potable water, for example, is unavailable or too expensive in many parts of the world. During the dry season, the transmission of infection by waterborne and fecal–oral routes increases in those regions because the small amounts of water available are used for both washing and drinking.

Conclusion

The most striking differences between parasites and other infectious agents are the variety of hosts, vectors, and stages in parasitic life cycles. The life cycles of parasites provide important clues to understanding parasitic diseases and help in diagnosis and in the development of public health strategies. In most cases the biological basis for the ability of different stages of parasites to invade different hosts and different types of tissues is still unknown.

Although parasitic diseases are more prevalent in areas with inadequate sanitation, they are also found in regions with apparently high sanitary standards, such as Europe and North America. The presence of parasitic diseases in developed countries is frequently related to the susceptibility of immunocompromised patients to the infections. For example, toxoplasmosis is quite prevalent in developed countries but does not produce severe disease in immunologically normal individuals. In immunocompromised patients, some parasites can escape their usual constraints and multiply to high and dangerous numbers.

Blood and Tissue Protozoa

Cary Engleberg

key **concepts**

- Most tissue invasive protozoa have intracellular stages in their life cycles.

- Fever is a cardinal symptom of disseminated protozoal infections. Some species become dormant in tissues and cause prolonged, asymptomatic infection.

- Malaria is transmitted among humans by *Anopheles* mosquitoes. Its propagation depends on the presence of a reservoir of partially immune, asymptomatic human carriers. Nonimmune persons (e.g., young children in endemic areas and adult travelers from nonendemic areas) may experience severe, or even fatal illness. Because it is more virulent and more likely to be resistant to antimalarial drugs, *Plasmodium falciparum* must be distinguished from other plasmodia and treated promptly.

- Like malaria, babesiosis is a protozoal infection of erythrocytes, but it is more geographically localized and less prevalent, partly because it is transmitted by ticks rather than mosquitoes.

- Cats are the definitive (intestinal) host for *Toxoplasma gondii*; all other animals develop dormant toxoplasmic cysts in their muscles and viscera. Humans acquire infection by ingesting oocysts from cat feces or muscle cysts in undercooked meat. Manifestations in humans include a mononucleosis-like primary infection, chorioretinitis, congenital infection, or mass lesions in the brain (in person with AIDS).

- Virulence attributes of various *Leishmania* species determine whether infection results in a chronic skin ulcer at the site of the sand fly bite or a disseminated chronic febrile illness involving the liver, spleen, and lymph nodes.

- Longstanding infection with the agent of Chagas disease, *Trypanosoma cruzi*, may result in immunopathologic damage to the heart and the gastrointestinal tract.

- The agent of African sleeping sickness, *Trypanosoma brucei*, evades the host immune response by a genetically determined mechanism of antigenic variation.

Protozoa that produce bloodstream infections typically cause anemia by effecting the destruction of red blood cells. Malaria and babesiosis are examples of protozoal bloodstream infections. Protozoa that infect tissues can cause significant damage to the eyes, brain, or heart (toxoplasmosis); to the brain (African sleeping sickness); or to the heart and gastrointestinal tract (Chagas disease). The major blood and tissue protozoa are presented in Table 52-1.

table **52-1**	**Comparison of Major Blood and Tissue Protozoa**		
ORGANISM	**RESERVOIR**	**MODE OF TRANSMISSION**	**CLINICAL MANIFESTATIONS**
Blood protozoa			
Plasmodium species (malaria)	Infected humans	Vectorborne by the female *Anopheles* mosquito	Fever and chills with red blood cell lysis
Babesia species (babesiosis)	Rodents (voles), deer, mice	Vectorborne by the hard-bodied *Ixodes* tick	Fever and chills with red blood cell lysis
Tissue protozoa			
Toxoplasma gondii (toxoplasmosis)	Sheep, pigs, cattle, cats	Foodborne by the ingestion of inadequately cooked beef or lamb	Intrauterine (congenital) infection can cause severe retardation in the neonate
			Mononucleosis-like illness most common
		Fecal–oral by the ingestion of infectious oocysts in cat feces	
			Infection of the brain (encephalitis) or heart (myocarditis) in severely immunocompromised patients
Leishmania species (leishmaniasis)	Infected humans, dogs, jackals, foxes, rats, ground squirrels, gerbils	Vectorborne by infected *Phlebotomus* sand flies	Trivial or mild (self-healing) skin lesions
			Disfiguring mucocutaneous lesions
			Systemic illness with involvement of liver, spleen, and bone marrow
Trypanosoma cruzi (Chagas disease, American trypanosomiasis)	Wildlife, domestic animals (zoonosis)	Vectorborne by reduviid bugs followed by rubbing infected feces in the bite wound	Gastrointestinal tract dysfunction from autonomic nerve damage (megacolon, megaesophagus)
			Cardiac dysfunction from damage to the conducting system (right bundle branch block)
Trypanosoma brucei gambiense or *T. brucei rhodesiense* (West and East African trypanosomiasis, respectively sleeping sickness)	Infected humans, wildlife, cattle	Vectorborne by the tsetse fly	Systemic illness with fever, headache, muscle, and joint pains
			Progresses to central nervous system involvement with altered speech, gait, and reflexes (encephalitis)

Parasites of Red Blood Cells

Plasmodium Species

Malaria is the most important of all protozoal diseases and is said to have caused "the greatest harm to the greatest number" of all infectious diseases. It occurs in many tropical and semitropical regions of the world, with approximately 200 million to 300 million cases annually (see Table 51-1). An estimated 2 million to 3 million people die of malaria each year, especially malnourished African children. Malaria in humans is caused by four species of the *Plasmodium* protozoa: *P. falciparum, P. vivax, P. ovale,* and *P. malariae.* Infected humans are the only reservoir for the plasmodia that infect humans; transmission occurs through the bite of infected female anopheline mosquitoes.

ENCOUNTER AND ENTRY

Malaria is transmitted to humans by the mosquito vector 9 to 17 days after a female *Anopheles* mosquito ingests blood from a person infected with a species of *Plasmodium* that infects humans. Infected persons typically develop malaria symptoms 8 to 30 days later. Most cases of malaria that occur in Europe and North America are acquired in endemic areas and then imported into

Case

Ms. M. is a 54-year-old businesswoman from Liverpool who traveled to East Africa (Kenya and Tanzania) on a business trip and then went on a photographic safari. After 1 week in Nairobi, she embarked on a 10-day trip through the wildlife preserves of Serengeti and Ngorogoro, with a final visit to Mombassa on the Indian Ocean. During her flight home, 9 days after leaving the game parks, Ms. M. developed a "flu-like" syndrome, with headache, muscle aches, and a temperature of 38°C. After she returned to Liverpool she saw a physician, who diagnosed influenza. She had returned to England in February during an outbreak of influenza A.

Ms. M. was given acetaminophen, which initially reduced her fever and muscle aches. However, she felt worse the next day. She suddenly developed an intense chill that lasted for about 30 minutes, followed by a fever to 40.2°C that lasted for 6 hours. As the fever abated, Ms. M. became drenched in sweat and felt exhausted and drained. Her symptoms continued to worsen, and she was brought to the hospital unconscious 2 days later. On examination, she had edema of the lungs. She showed no signs of endocarditis, and a lumbar puncture was negative for bacterial meningitis.

The attending physician, drawing on his experience while serving in the armed services abroad, recognized that Ms. M.'s clinical manifestations were typical of a **malarial paroxysm.** The recent history of travel to endemic areas gave credence to his suspicion of the disease, and the diagnosis was confirmed when a Giemsa-stained smear of Ms. M.'s blood revealed large numbers of parasites within red blood cells. The parasites were identified as *Plasmodium falciparum* by their characteristic ring shape. Ms. M.'s hematocrit (packed red cell volume) was 18% (normal is 40 to 45%). Urinalysis revealed dark urine, suggesting extensive hemolysis. Her serum creatinine (a measure of renal function) was 5.4 mg per 100 mL (normal is 1 mg or less per 100 mL).

Because Ms. M. had traveled in Kenya, a country in which drug-resistant malaria is endemic, treatment was begun with intravenous quinidine, which is effective against *P. falciparum* strains resistant to other antimalarial drugs. Ms. M. was also given intravenous glucose as a precaution against hypoglycemia (which can produce coma in patients with severe *P. falciparum* malaria). Hypoglycemia can result both from consumption of glucose by large numbers of parasites and from the direct release of insulin from the pancreas caused by quinidine or quinine. For her pulmonary edema Ms. M. required artificial ventilation with a respirator. She was given multiple transfusions for her anemia and was put on a dialysis machine because of her kidney failure. She recovered and was discharged after spending 10 days in the intensive care unit.

This case raises several questions:

1. Why did Ms. M.'s fevers occur in paroxysms (episodes) of shaking chills followed by fever and then drenching sweats?
2. Why did she have dark urine?
3. Why did she develop edema of the lungs and an elevation of the serum creatinine?

the nonendemic areas during the incubation period (**imported malaria**). However, mosquitoes that can serve as vectors (*Anopheles*) exist in the United States. Although malaria can no longer take hold in temperate, industrialized countries like the United States, in rare cases persons who have never traveled abroad have contracted the disease. It is assumed that such cases occur when potential vector mosquitoes feed on blood from a malaria carrier (i.e., an immigrant or traveler from an endemic country) and then survive long enough to become infectious and bite again. Introductions of malaria have occurred when a large number of infected soldiers have returned from war and when a region has received a large number of immigrants at one time. Malaria also can be transmitted by blood transfusion or by the sharing of needles among intravenous drug users (**induced malaria**).

SPREAD AND MULTIPLICATION

The life cycle of the malaria parasite is complex and rich in morphological detail (Fig. 52-1). In the infected mosquito, plasmodia inhabit the salivary glands as **sporozoites,** a stage of the parasite that is infectious for humans. The organisms are injected into the human bloodstream when infected mosquitoes bite and feed. The sporozoites travel through the bloodstream and enter liver cells within 30 minutes of injection. Over the next 8 to 14 days the sporozoites multiply and mature inside liver cells to very large numbers. At the end of that period (**the hepatocellular cycle**) they are released once again into the bloodstream in a form that can invade red blood cells (**merozoites**). Once inside red blood cells, the organisms divide and mature. After 2 or 3 days the cells burst, liberating a new generation of infective merozoites that infect previously unparasitized red blood cells (the **erythrocytic cycle**).

In the liver and red blood cells the parasites multiply asexually (i.e., by fission). A minority of the merozoites in the blood develop into forms capable of sexual reproduction, called **gametocytes.** Male and female gametocytes are taken up by biting mosquitoes. In the mosquito gut the haploid male and female gametes fuse to form a diploid zygote. That event represents the sexual part of the malaria life cycle. After the zygote is formed the parasite undergoes further changes in the mosquito gut and then divides by meiosis to generate sporozoites. Sporozoites migrate to the salivary glands and once again become infective for humans. All the subsequent asexual stages in the human, up to and including the gametes, are haploid. In each of those stages the plasmodial cells are morphologically distinguishable (see Fig. 52-1).

The four species of plasmodia that cause human malaria vary in their virulence. One reason for the variation is that different plasmodial species prefer red blood cells of different ages: *P. falciparum* invades erythrocytes of all ages, producing the highest parasitemias and the

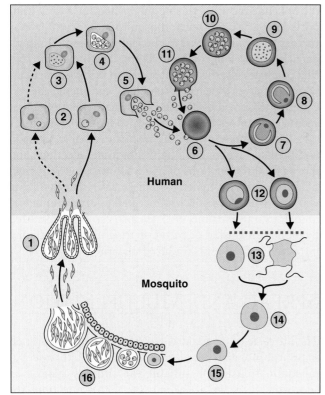

FIGURE 52-1 ▪ **Life cycle of *Plasmodium* species.** Sporozoites released from the salivary gland of the female *Anopheles* mosquito are injected under a person's skin when the mosquito bites (1). They then travel through the bloodstream and enter the liver (2). Within liver cells, the parasites mature to tissue schizonts (3–4). They are then released into the bloodstream as merozoites (5) and produce symptomatic infection as they invade and destroy red blood cells (RBCs). However, some parasites remain dormant in the liver as hypnozoites (see the dashed lines from stages 1 to 3). Those parasites (in *P. vivax* and *P. ovale*) cause relapsing malaria. Once within the bloodstream, merozoites (5) invade RBCs (6), and mature to the ring (7–8), trophozoite (9), and schizont (10) asexual stages. Schizonts lyse their host RBCs as they complete their maturation and release the next generation of merozoites (11), which invades previously uninfected RBCs. Within RBCs, some parasites differentiate to sexual forms, male and female gametocytes (12). When gametocytes are taken up by a female *Anopheles* mosquito, the male gametocyte loses its flagellum, producing male gametes. The male gametes fertilize the female gamete (13) to produce a zygote (14). The zygote invades the gut of the mosquito (15) and develops into an oocyst (16). Mature oocysts produce sporozoites, which migrate to the salivary gland of the mosquito (1) and repeat the cycle. The dashed line between stages 12 and 13 indicates that absence of the mosquito vector precludes natural transmission through this cycle. Note that infection by the injection of infected blood bypasses that constraint and permits transmission of malaria among intravenous drug addicts and to persons who receive blood transfusions from infected donors.

greatest risk of mortality. *P. vivax* prefers reticulocytes and young red blood cells, while *P. malariae* favors older red blood cells. Both *P. vivax* and *P. malariae* infect only 1 to 2% or less of red blood cells, thus producing less severe disease. The fourth species, *P. ovale*, is virtually identical to *P. vivax* clinically and morphologically. *P. vivax* and *P. ovale* are also notable for the fact that some infected hepatocytes may harbor parasites for a long period before they are released into the bloodstream. Thus, infection with either species can cause a series of relapses to occur months or even years after the initial episode. Recurrent malaria is prevented by treatment with an antimalarial agent that targets the dormant parasites (**hypnozoites**) within liver cells.

The intracellular location of the malaria parasite within the red blood cell has two important consequences:

- The presence of plasmodia within red blood cells makes the cells less deformable. The spleen recognizes and removes older and less deformable red blood cells from the circulation, thus removing parasitized red blood cells from the circulation. Not surprisingly, malaria may cause enlargement of the spleen (**splenomegaly**), and splenectomized people have higher degrees of parasitemia and more-severe infections.

- A red blood cell infected with *P. falciparum* develops special "knoblike" structures on its surface that contain the parasite-derived protein **pfEMP-1**. The protein binds the infected red blood cell to receptors on the endothelial cells of venules and capillaries, such as **intercellular adhesion molecule 1 (ICAM-1)** and CD36. When multiple parasitized red blood cells adhere and accumulate on the endothelium, blood flow through the deep vascular beds is impeded. Thus, *P. falciparum*–infected cells are prevented from circulating to the spleen and being removed from the circulation. However, the obstruction of blood flow in the microcirculation may have dire pathological consequences for the host.

DAMAGE

The main manifestations of malaria are fever, chills, and anemia. The typical malarial paroxysm (as in Ms. M.'s case) coincides with the lysis of many red blood cells and the release of large numbers of merozoites. In the process parasite molecules, such as membrane molecules, are also released, and some of those molecules, such as membrane **glycophosphatidylinositol (GPI)**, stimulate the production of tumor necrosis factor and interleukin-1 in macrophages. The surge in those cytokines is the stimulus for the sudden chill and fever characteristic of a malaria paroxysm.

Parasite replication can become synchronized so that all infected red blood cells lyse at the same time. As a result, a regular, periodic fever pattern may develop, depending on the length of the intracellular replication cycle: every 2 days with *P. vivax* or *P. ovale*, every 3 days with *P. malariae*. In contrast, the fever pattern is often irregular with *P. falciparum*. Other frequent clinical presentations include a syndrome similar to influenza (fever, muscle aches, and malaise) and gastroenteritis (nausea, diarrhea, and vomiting). Patients with those signs and symptoms are often misdiagnosed, especially if the physician is not acquainted with malaria or fails to obtain a history of recent travel to an endemic area.

The anemia that occurs in malaria is usually more severe than can be accounted for by the degree of para-sitemia. Thus, uninfected red blood cells may also be destroyed prematurely, presumably by an immunologically mediated mechanism.

Diagnosis

Malaria is diagnosed in the laboratory by microscopic examination of a Giemsa-stained smear of peripheral blood using the oil immersion objective (Fig. 52-3). Wright's stain, which is used more often in the clinical

Human Genetics and Malaria

Genetic polymorphism of several human genes affects the entry, multiplication, and survival of malarial parasites. Genes are also important in determining the outcome of the infection. For example, parasite invasion of red blood cells depends on the presence of specific surface molecules. For *P. falciparum* and *P. vivax*, the surface molecules are glycophorin A and the Duffy blood group antigen, respectively. The variable susceptibility of African Americans to *P. vivax* infection is consistent with the distribution of Duffy antigen. Black Africans are Duffy-negative and are thus resistant to *P. vivax* infection.

Because *P. falciparum* malaria is such a devastating disease, it has probably been a powerful selective force in human evolution. Many epidemiological studies have shown that sickle cell disease—a recessive genetic disorder that causes red blood cells to become sickle shaped—is common in areas of Africa with a high incidence of *P. falciparum*. A defective form of hemoglobin, called sickle cell hemoglobin (HbS), causes the disease. Malaria is seldom found in heterozygous carriers of HbS (sickle cell trait), which suggests that the genetic determinant imparts a selective advantage to people living in areas where the parasite is common. Furthermore, in vitro studies have shown that at oxygen tensions similar to those in tissue, the parasites grow poorly in red blood cells from persons with sickle cell disease or the sickle cell trait (Fig. 52-2). Thus, in the black African population, a trade-off exists between the risk of a fatal disease—sickle cell disease in those who are homozygous for HbS—and the protection of a larger group of the population, the heterozygous HbS carriers. That is an example of a balanced genetic polymorphism.

How does the sickle cell trait protect from malaria? *P. falciparum*–infected red blood cells adhere to the walls of blood vessels using knobs that form as the parasites mature. Adherence to the peripheral microcircu-

FIGURE 52-2 ▪ **Effect of hypoxia on parasite growth in sickle hemoglobin red blood cells.** In 18% oxygen (left panel), *Plasmodium falciparum* grows as well in sickle hemoglobin (SS) red blood cells (black circles) as in either heterozygous (SA) red blood cells (red-black circles) or normal (AA) RBCs (red circles). In contrast, at 3% oxygen, *P. falciparum* parasites grow less well in SS and SA cells than in AA cells (right panel).

lation sequesters the parasitized red blood cells in an area of reduced oxygen tension, which facilitates sickling, potassium loss, and the killing of the parasites.

Other genetic abnormalities that restrict the growth of malarial parasites within red blood cells are glucose-6-phosphate dehydrogenase deficiency (G6PD) and thalassemia. In the case of G6PD, the reduced ability of the red blood cells to produce NADPH via the pentose phosphate shunt is thought to cause an oxidative stress that inhibits parasite growth.

FIGURE 52-3 ▪ **Malarial parasites in blood cells.** This schematic drawing illustrates the most prominent morphological features that distinguish human malarial species in blood smears. The nuclear chromatid bodies of all of the malarial parasites are shaded in dark blue–gray in this diagram but actually appear red in Giemsa-stained preparations. *P. falciparum* usually appears as small, fine, ring forms, sometimes more than one per red blood cell. More-mature forms of the species are not usually seen in the peripheral blood. The gametocyte is characteristically banana shaped. *P. vivax* and *P. ovale* are distinguished by details not illustrated here. Infected cells and ring forms are larger than those of *P. falciparum*. At the trophozoite stage, red Schüffner dots are seen. The schizont contains more than a dozen merozoites before it ruptures. *P. malariae* infects smaller, senescent cells. Schüffner dots are not present. At the schizont stage, 8 to 12 merozoites are arranged peripherally around the central malarial pigment.

hematology laboratory, stains the parasites less well. If the degree of parasitemia is low, a "thick smear" can be used to increase sensitivity. Because red blood cells are lysed in the preparation of thick smears, this procedure provides no information about the size of the infected red blood cells or about the intracellular location of the parasite within the red blood cells (central or peripheral). Morphological characteristics that can be seen on a "thin smear" of blood can be used to differentiate among the Plasmodium species.

In acutely ill patients the malarial species is usually either *P. falciparum* or *P. vivax*. In contrast, *P. malariae* most often causes subacute or chronic infections (but can produce acute infections in nonimmune people). *P. ovale* malaria is clinically so similar to *P. vivax* malaria that the distinction of the two species is usually of no practical importance. *P. vivax* can be differentiated from *P. falciparum* on the basis of morphological characteristics. For example, *P. vivax* causes infected red blood cells to progressively enlarge as the parasite matures and produces eosinophilic "stippling" in the red blood cells (**Schüffner dots**). Neither red cell enlargement nor Schüffner dots occur with *P. falciparum*. That distinction is important because *P. falciparum* infection poses a greater risk of death and may be

resistant to treatment with chloroquine, whereas *P. vivax* may cause posttreatment relapses caused by slow-growing or dormant parasites in the liver.

Serologic testing is of little value for the diagnosis of malaria in the acutely ill patient. The reason is that treatment must begin within 1 to 2 days of the onset of symptoms, and patients do not develop species-specific antibodies to the parasites for 3 to 5 weeks. Diagnosis using polymerase chain reaction (PCR) is more accurate than microscopy, but it is expensive and requires special equipment and technical expertise (see Chapter 58). Rapid antigen detection tests also have been developed and are being evaluated for general use in the field.

PREVENTION AND TREATMENT

Natural immunity to malaria is imperfect. Persons who have lived in malarious areas all their lives and who have evidence of humoral and cellular responses to parasite antigens are nevertheless infected on a regular basis. However, their infections tend to be less severe than those of nonimmune persons, suggesting that the immune response plays a significant role in controlling infection. Some researchers have shown that antibodies directed against sporozoites, the form introduced by the insect (see Fig. 52-1), are not sufficient to protect against infection. Unfortunately, the major surface protein of the merozoite stage (**MSP-1**) is capable of undergoing antigenic variation (see Chapter 14 paradigm), an immune evasion mechanism that often thwarts both natural immunity and vaccine production. Protective immunity may involve cell-mediated cytotoxicity of infected liver cells or antibodies against certain surface proteins of the merozoite stage. Consequently, effective future vaccines will probably stimulate cell-mediated immunity and include conserved antigens derived from merozoites and possibly from the other stages of the parasite in humans as well.

Chloroquine was once the most widely used drug for antimalarial chemoprophylaxis and treatment. Chloroquine, and other quinine-based drugs, enter the parasite's food vacuole, where RBC hemoglobin is degraded for the nutrition of the parasite. Normally, toxic heme released by this degradation is detoxified and converted to harmless malarial pigment. Chloroquine blocks heme detoxification and kills the parasite. Chloroquine resistance occurs by mutation of a vacuolar membrane protein that causes chloroquine to be pumped out of the food vacuole and permits heme detoxification to resume. Unfortunately, chloroquine-resistant *P. falciparum* is now widespread in most of Southeast Asia, South America, and Africa, complicating the prophylaxis and treatment of malaria acquired in those geographic areas. Thus, Ms. M. might well have acquired *P. falciparum* infection in East Africa, even if she had been on chloroquine chemoprophylaxis. In contrast, she would have been protected in Haiti, where there is no chloroquine resistance.

Patients infected with chloroquine-resistant *P. falciparum* can be treated with other agents, such as Malarone (a fixed combination of atovaquone and proguanil), mefloquine, quinine, quinidine, halofantrine, or artesunate. At present, *P. falciparum* cases acquired in areas where drug resistance is prevalent are usually treated in the United States with a combination of doxycycline and quinine, Malarone, or quinidine. Mefloquine, a quinine derivative, is also active against chloroquine-resistant strains but is often toxic at treatment doses. However, it is a mainstay for chemoprophylaxis in travelers to most areas with chloroquine-resistant malaria. Unfortunately, resistance to mefloquine has also been detected in parts of Southeast Asia, and travelers to that area are now being advised to take daily doxycycline to prevent infection.

Although all of the antimalarials mentioned are effective in controlling acute infection caused by *P. vivax* or *P. ovale*, none is effective against the liver (hypnozoite) stages of those species. **Primaquine**, a derivative of **quinine**, is effective against the hypnozoite stages. It is used with chloroquine to prevent late relapses associated with maturation of the hypnozoite to the tissue schizont stage and the subsequent release of infectious merozoites. However, primaquine is more toxic than chloroquine and causes nausea, vomiting, and diarrhea. In patients with G6PD deficiency, primaquine induces hemolysis. Primaquine is not indicated for either *P. falciparum* or *P. malariae* infections because those parasites do not produce a dormant (hypnozoite) stage in the liver.

Mosquito control with insecticides and drainage of aquatic breeding sites have been used to control malaria in many countries, resulting in a dramatic decline in the incidence of the disease. Unfortunately, those control measures have some drawbacks: they are expensive and not always effective because mosquitoes can become resistant to some insecticides. In endemic areas individuals should protect themselves with mosquito netting, house screening, and insect repellents. The best hope for controlling malaria is the development of improved antimalarials and/or an effective vaccine.

Babesia Species

Like the plasmodia of malaria, *Babesia* species are protozoal parasites that cause illness by infecting red blood cells and generating fever on release. Unlike malaria, babesiosis is endemic in the United States. *Babesia microti* is the most recognized cause of human babesiosis in the United States. Interestingly, it is concentrated geographically in the same area as endemic Lyme disease because *B. microti* and *Borrelia burgdorferi* (the bacterial cause of Lyme disease) infect the same animal reservoir—the white-footed mouse—and are transmitted to humans by the same deer tick, *Ixodes scapularis* (see Chapter 25). Cases of babesiosis outside that geographic area (e.g., from the Midwest to the Pacific Coast) appear to be caused by other *Babesia* species more closely related to the principal European species, *B. divergens*, than to *B. microti*.

CLINICAL AND PARASITOLOGICAL FEATURES

Babesiosis is difficult to recognize clinically because the illness it causes is nonspecific. Infected persons experience a flulike illness, with fever, chills, sweats, muscle aches, and fatigue. Because the illness usually occurs in the summer months, when ticks are feeding, babesiosis has been likened to a "summer flu." Illness is usually mild, but as in malaria, more severe disease occurs in splenectomized patients. In a person with an intact spleen, the proportion of infected red blood cells is usually 0.2% or less, but it can rise to more than 10% in a splenectomized patient. In fact, the disease was first detected in postmortem studies

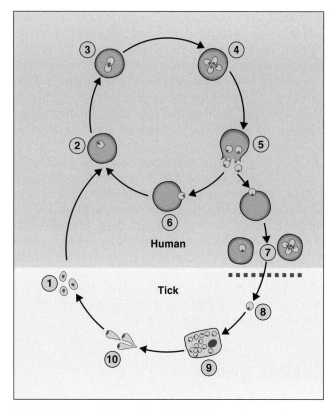

Human

Tick

FIGURE 52-4 ▪ **Life cycle of *Babesia* species.** Infectious merozoites are injected under the skin by the hard-bodied tick (*Ixodes*) vector (1) and they invade red blood cells directly (2). Unlike malaria, babesiosis has no intermediate liver stage. Once within the red blood cells, parasites replicate asexually by binary fission (3). *Babesia* species characteristically form tetrads (4), lyse their host red blood cells as they mature (5), and complete the cycle when parasitized red blood cells are ingested by the tick vector (6). The dashed line between stages 7 and 8 indicates that natural transmission does not occur in areas lacking the hard-bodied tick.

of splenectomized patients. As in malaria, the spleen is thought to remove the less deformable *Babesia*-infected red blood cells from the circulation.

The life cycle of *Babesia* species is shown in Figure 52-4. The epidemiology of the disease is restricted by the presence of a suitable tick vector and wildlife reservoir, as well as by human contact with them. Humans are infected accidentally in endemic areas and are not thought to contribute to the maintenance of the parasite's life cycle.

DIAGNOSIS AND TREATMENT

The laboratory diagnosis of babesiosis depends on finding the parasites in Giemsa-stained blood films using the oil immersion objective. The parasites are seen as

small rings, often in tetrads. That is the only form of the parasite found in peripheral blood and may be easily missed when parasitemia is low. The ring shape makes the parasites easy to confuse with a similar form of *P. falciparum*. The distinction between the two parasites is important because *Babesia* infections are treated with different chemotherapeutic agents than malaria: clindamycin plus quinine for babesiosis versus a variety of drugs for malaria (as discussed earlier).

Antibodies to *Babesia* species can be detected in most infected persons. However, they often appear too late (3 to 4 weeks after the onset of infection) to be helpful in the diagnosis and treatment of acute babesiosis. PCR-based diagnosis is available in specialized laboratories and is highly accurate.

Tissue Protozoa

Toxoplasma gondii

Infection with the agent of toxoplasmosis, *Toxoplasma gondii*, is common in humans. However, less

Case

Mr. H., who is 22 years old, had mild fever, malaise, muscle aches, and headache for 2 weeks. On several occasions he took his temperature orally and found that it ranged from 37°C to 38°C. On physical examination his physician detected no stiff neck or pharyngitis; however, Mr. H. had several enlarged cervical lymph nodes bilaterally. The liver and spleen were not enlarged on palpation, and the remainder of the examination was normal, including funduscopic examination of the retinas. Routine laboratory tests were similarly unremarkable and included a normal white cell count and normal liver function tests.

Additional history revealed that Mr. H. had no significant contact with animals and no pets at home. He was of Middle Eastern descent and lived with his first-generation immigrant parents. The family occasionally dined on kibbeh, a Middle Eastern dish made with lamb (sometimes raw), bulgur wheat, and spices.

Antibody tests for mononucleosis and cytomegalovirus were negative. However, IgM and IgG serologies for *Toxoplasma gondii* were positive. Mr. H. was advised to rest and to treat fever and muscle aches with acetaminophen. He was given no specific antimicrobial therapy. After 3 weeks, his symptoms were gone and the lymphadenopathy had receded. A repeat IgG serology for *T. gondii* showed an eightfold increase in titer from the first test.

This case raises several questions:

1. How did Mr. H. acquire the infection?
2. What was the purpose of the second serology?
3. Why was the patient given no treatment?

than 1% of those infected are ever diagnosed with toxoplasmosis. In the few persons with signs and symptoms of active infection, the clinical presentation of the disease varies. Toxoplasmosis is particularly damaging for immunocompromised patients, such as those with AIDS, and for the developing fetus. *T. gondii* can cause three distinct syndromes:

- A mononucleosis-like syndrome in which tests for the common viral agents of mononucleosis—Epstein-Barr virus and cytomegalovirus—are negative.
- A congenital infection that may have severe consequences if acquired in the first trimester of pregnancy (for more detail on the effects of *T. gondii* on the developing fetus, see Chapter 72).
- Infections in immunocompromised hosts (especially people with AIDS), often involving the brain or the heart.

ENCOUNTER

People acquire *Toxoplasma* infections by eating inadequately cooked meat or by ingesting the infectious oocysts found in the feces of cats (Fig. 52-5). The most common mode of transmission appears to be through the ingestion of inadequately cooked meat (lamb, mutton, and possibly beef) that contains parasitic tissue cysts produced by asexual reproduction (Fig. 52-6). Less frequently, humans become infected by accidentally ingesting minute amounts of cat feces containing fertile cysts called **oocysts**. The frequency with which that type of transmission occurs is in

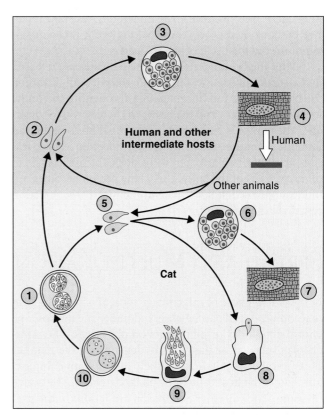

FIGURE 52-6 ▪ Life cycle of *Toxoplasma gondii*. Humans and other mammals become infected with *T. gondii* by ingesting inadequately cooked meat containing tissue cysts or by ingesting infectious oocysts excreted in the feces of infected cats (1). Once in the human host, the oocysts mature to tachyzoites (2). Tachyzoites enter the bloodstream and disseminate throughout the body (3). After the initial acute infection, most people mount a successful immune response that eliminates the active infectious (tachyzoite) form of the parasite and leaves only tissue cysts with dormant organisms (4). A similar progression is observed within the cat (1–4), where the parasite also invades intestinal epithelial cells (6). In addition, the organism establishes a sexual cycle (8–9) in the cat, in which infectious oocysts are formed (10) and released (11). The solid line below stage 4 in the upper half of the diagram indicates that human tissue infection is a dead end. Unless an animal or human consumes infected human flesh, human tissue cysts disintegrate after the death of the host.

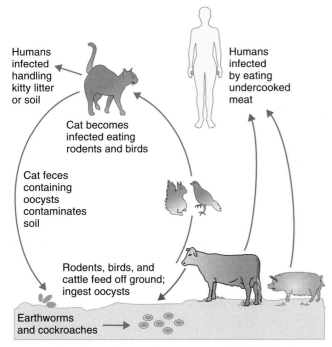

FIGURE 52-5 ▪ **Transmission and spread of *Toxoplasma gondii*.**

dispute and is difficult to determine for two reasons: only a small percentage of *T. gondii*–infected cats excrete oocysts in their stools, and how frequently humans accidentally ingest cat feces is not known.

The evidence that cats are important in transmitting *T. gondii* to humans comes from the observation that toxoplasmosis is absent from areas that do not have cats, such as isolated Pacific atolls. Once cats are introduced into an area, humans become infected. Cats harbor the sexual cycle of the organisms (analogous to the mosquito in malaria) and produce environmentally resistant infective cysts in their stool, thus making them necessary to maintain the life cycle of the parasite.

After the host ingests them, the parasites are released in the small intestine and penetrate the gut wall, invading the bloodstream and disseminating throughout the body, including the brain and the heart. In the first 4 to 6 weeks after the parasites enter the body, normal hosts mount an immune response that controls the infection. The parasites are not eliminated but form dormant tissue cysts in different parts of the body. Unless the person becomes immunosuppressed at some time in the future, the infection remains inactive.

SPREAD AND MULTIPLICATION

In the active phase of infection, *T. gondii* is found within macrophages and can be observed under the microscope with the high-dry or oil immersion objectives. The intracellular survival of the parasite depends on the manner of its uptake. *T. gondii*, and likely all other apicomplexans, enters the host cell not by phagocytosis but by active invasion. The secretory and motility functions of the parasite are used to contact the host cell membrane and force the parasite into a membrane-bound vesicle that is devoid of the cellular membrane proteins normally associated with the endocytic pathway. Altering the membrane in that manner has dramatic consequences. Namely, the **parasitophorous vesicle** becomes "invisible" to the host cell and cannot be appropriately targeted to a lysosome by the normal intracellular pathways. In contrast to a resting macrophage or monocyte, activated macrophages can actively phagocytose *T. gondii*. When the macrophage initiates and controls the uptake, the parasite can be appropriately dealt with and killed.

DIAGNOSIS AND TREATMENT

In the immunologically competent host, the diagnosis of acute toxoplasmosis is made by an elevated antibody titer, especially of IgM antibodies. Most previously healthy persons do not need treatment for self-limited, acute toxoplasmosis. Serologic diagnosis is often insensitive in the immunocompromised patient, such as a person with AIDS, who may be unable to produce a diagnostic rise in antibody titer. Other methods must be used to diagnose toxoplasmosis in immunocompromised patients. The appearance of new neurologic symptoms and the presence of multiple ring-enhancing lesions on a computerized tomography scan or magnetic resonance imaging of the brain should raise suspicion of nervous system toxoplasmosis. On biopsy the trophozoites associated with acute infection may be difficult to detect morphologically. Staining brain biopsy material with fluorescent or peroxidase-labeled antitoxoplasma antibodies increases the sensitivity of detection. In the absence of an adequate immune response, *T. gondii* causes local inflammation that can result in severe necrosis, tissue damage, and death. Because biopsy of the brain is a complicated and potentially hazardous procedure, most AIDS patients with a suggestive history, positive brain scan, and serological evidence of prior toxoplasmic exposure (e.g., specific IgG antibody) are treated presumptively for cerebral toxoplasmosis. Lifesaving treatment is usually initiated with pyrimethamine plus either sulfadiazine or clindamycin.

T. gondii may be transmitted to a developing fetus if the mother acquires infection during pregnancy. Because most of the potential damage occurs in utero, treatment for congenital infections after the baby is born is usually too late. Therefore, most physicians screen women for antitoxoplasma antibody when they get married or when pregnancy is first detected. Women with preexisting antibodies at the time of pregnancy (indicating prior infection) have virtually no risk of producing a congenitally infected child. Women who are seronegative can be given preventative advice, and those who seroconvert during pregnancy can be counseled, offered therapeutic abortion (if early in pregnancy), or given treatment with experimental drugs, such as spiramycin. The risk of severe complications in the fetus is greatest for women who seroconvert in the first trimester of pregnancy. The frequency of congenital infection is greatest in the third trimester, but most of the children infected late in gestation have no detectable disease at the time of birth. **Chorioretinitis**, which many infants develop early or many years after birth, is sometimes the only manifestation of congenital infection. Unfortunately, various developmental problems may also be seen among initially "asymptomatic" children later in childhood.

Leishmania Species

Leishmania species produce a spectrum of clinical syndromes, from superficial ulcers to severe lesions of the

Case

Ms. Q., a 26-year-old graduate student in anthropology, returned from a 6-month expedition to Peru with a nonhealing 2 × 5–cm lesion on her right shin. A smear taken from the edge of the lesion stained with Giemsa revealed *Leishmania*-containing macrophages. Ms. Q. was given the antimony-containing, antiprotozoal drug pentostam for 4 weeks. The lesion began to heal slowly, and she eventually recovered completely.

This case raises two questions:

1. How did Ms. Q. acquire the infection?
2. How would this case have evolved if Ms. Q. had not received treatment?

liver, spleen, and bone marrow accompanied by systemic signs such as fever, weight loss, and anemia. Several species are pathogenic for humans. The reason for the wide diversity in clinical disease is not well understood, but it is probably owing in part to the temperature preferences of the various species. Superficial lesions are produced by *Leishmania* species that grow better at lower temperatures (25°C to 30°C), whereas those that invade the viscera grow better at 37°C.

ENCOUNTER

Leishmania species are small protozoa that belong to the flagellates because they possess a prominent flagellum during part of their life cycle. The flagellum is connected to an organelle called the **kinetoplast**, which, like the mitochondria, has its own DNA. The protozoa are transmitted by the bite of sand flies—small, short-lived insects that feed on many mammals. The **phlebotomine sand flies** that transmit leishmaniasis are generally found in tropical or subtropical parts of the world, which explains why the disease is rare in North America and Europe. However, phlebotomine sand flies are occasionally found in more temperate regions, and indigenous cases have been reported in the United States. Like malaria, leishmaniasis in the United States is seen mainly among travelers returning from tropical countries and has been observed in military personnel who participated in the 1991 Gulf War. Reservoirs of *Leishmania* parasites include rodents, dogs, other animals, and infected humans.

PATHOGENESIS, DIAGNOSIS, AND TREATMENT

The genus *Leishmania* comprises several species, each with unique tissue tropisms and clinical manifestations. The diseases they cause include localized skin ulcers, mucocutaneous lesions (espundia), disseminated cutaneous leishmaniasis, and disseminated visceral leishmaniasis (kala azar). Ms. Q. had a form of cutaneous leishmaniasis that usually heals poorly and requires treatment.

The life cycle of *Leishmania* species is shown in Figure 52-7. A protein on the parasites' surface binds to one of the complement receptors on macrophages. Phagocytosis then takes place with a minimal degree of oxidative burst. *Leishmania* species also produce superoxide dismutase, which protects them from superoxide produced by the macrophages. After they are taken up into phagosomes, the parasites differentiate into a nonflagellate form, called the **amastigote**. Although the parasite-containing phagosomes fuse with lysosomes, the amastigotes are resistant to killing by lysosomal enzymes. In ad-

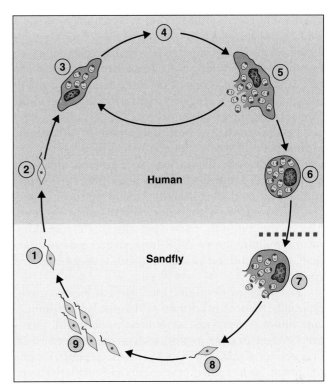

FIGURE 52-7 ▪ **Life cycle of *Leishmania* species.** The flagellated (promastigote) insect form of the parasite (1) is injected under the skin by the sand fly (*Phlebotomus*) vector (2). Once within the human host, the parasite transforms into a nonflagellated (amastigote) form that is more capable of evading the host immune response than the promastigote form (it stimulates less release of H_2O_2 from mononuclear cells than the promastigote and produces its own superoxide dismutase). The parasite then invades lymphoreticular cells (3), replicates (4), lyses the cells (5), and repeats the same sequence in other reticuloendothelial cells (6). In endemic areas, the cycle is completed when previously uninfected sand flies acquire infectious leishmanial amastigotes by biting infected humans (7). The amastigotes then transform into flagellated promastigotes (8) and replicate in the gastrointestinal tract of the sand fly (9). Infective promastigotes are injected under the skin of another human when the parasitized sand fly takes a blood meal (1–2). The dashed line between stages 6 and 7 indicates that transmission is blocked at this point in nonendemic areas such as the United States because the sand fly vector is not present.

dition, the amastigotes depend on the low pH of the phagolysosomes for the uptake of nutrients such as glucose and proline.

Immunity against leishmaniasis involves cell-mediated mechanisms and the induction of interferon-γ (a Th1 response; see Chapter 7). It is thought that the parasite may facilitate its own survival by possessing immunodominant antigens that preferentially induce a Th2 response, which is not protective. Patients with AIDS, who lack coordinated cell-mediated immunity altogether, may develop severe *Leishmania* infections. In fact, leishmaniasis is one of the most common causes of unexplained fevers in persons with AIDS who live in the Mediterranean region.

Leishmaniasis is best diagnosed by histologic examination of biopsy material using the high-dry objective. However, the various species look alike and cannot be distinguished morphologically. *Leishmania* species can be distinguished by culturing them in special media and then analyzing patterns of isoenzymes. That is done in only a few specialized reference laboratories. Alternatively, PCR has become a more practical and rapid technique for both diagnosis and speciation.

A variety of drugs are used to treat leishmaniasis, especially the invasive forms of the disease. Antimony-containing compounds are modestly successful. However, disease of deep organs, such as the bone marrow, may produce fatal anemia and granulocytopenia, despite treatment. Some forms of cutaneous leishmaniasis can be treated with allopurinol or ketoconazole.

Trypanosoma cruzi

Chagas disease, caused by *Trypanosoma cruzi*, occurs throughout Latin America. Overt disease is much less common than infection, but the reasons for the difference are poorly understood.

Case

Senhor R., a 58-year-old Brazilian businessman, was admitted to a hospital in Sao Paulo for the evaluation of chronic constipation. Radiologic examination of his gastrointestinal tract revealed a large, dilated colon (megacolon) and a somewhat less dilated esophagus (megaesophagus). A blood sample revealed antibodies to *Trypanosoma cruzi*. Because no drugs are effective after the onset of complications, Senhor R. was not given antiparasitic treatment. His chronic constipation was treated symptomatically with a high-fiber diet. A few years later, Senhor R. was hospitalized for treatment of cardiomyopathy with congestive heart failure. Although that complication was adequately compensated with medical therapy, Senhor R. expired suddenly at home 1 year later.

This case raises two questions:

1. What does the case reveal about Senhor R.'s past?
2. Why were antiparasitic drugs not given?

PATHOGENESIS

The life cycle of *T. cruzi* is shown in Figure 52-8. In the endemic areas of South and Central America, most persons are infected by *T. cruzi* in childhood by the bite of an infected **reduviid bug** (or "kissing bug"). A chancre or tissue and lymph node swelling may develop at the bite site. Although some persons develop serious (even fatal) illness, most develop a relatively mild disease with fever, recover spontaneously, and remain asymptomatic. A small proportion of individuals infected with *T. cruzi* develop complications 10 to 20 years later. The complications of Chagas disease result from damage to nerves in the gastrointestinal tract (**megaesophagus, megacolon**), the conducting tissue in the heart (**right bundle branch**

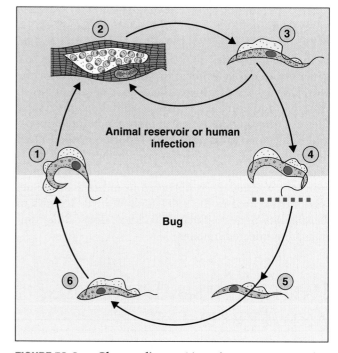

FIGURE 52-8 ■ **Chagas disease (American trypanosomiasis).** The reduviid bug vector deposits feces containing infectious trypomastigotes on the skin (1). The human host rubs the itching bite wound, allowing the parasites to enter the bloodstream. In the human host, the trypomastigote transforms into an amastigote (analogous to the leishmanial amastigote) as it invades tissue such as muscle (2). Cells containing large numbers of amastigotes often rupture, liberating large numbers of trypomastigotes (3). Trypomastigotes invade other host cells (arrow from 3 back to 2) or may be taken up by the vector to complete the cycle (4). In the vector the parasite replicates as an epimastigote (5) and produces additional infectious trypomastigotes (6). The dashed line below stage 4 indicates that natural transmission does not occur in areas lacking the reduviid bug vector. Although reduviid bugs are present in the southern United States, indigenous cases are rare.

block), or the heart muscle (**cardiomyopathy**). Sudden death from cardiac arrhythmia is common. Infected reduviid bugs are present in the southern United States and are presumably responsible for the sporadic cases of Chagas disease observed among lifelong residents of Florida, Louisiana, Mississippi, and California.

It is not clear why infection with *T. cruzi* produces autonomic nerve damage in the gastrointestinal tract or why it damages the cardiac conduction system. Usually, few organisms and a number of lymphocytes are seen in damaged tissue. **Fibrosis** is the hallmark of the pathology. Consequently, several investigators have postulated that autoimmune mechanisms may play a significant role in the pathogenesis of those complications.

DIAGNOSIS AND TREATMENT

The diagnosis of early infection is usually based on the appearance of the patient. Organisms often are found in the blood if it is cultured in an appropriate medium. Early infection can also be diagnosed by detecting infection in reduviid bugs that have purposely been allowed to feed on the patient. Antibodies appear in acutely ill patients within several weeks. Antibody titers usually remain positive for years. The diagnosis of chronic infection with complications is based on a positive antibody titer or history of exposure plus a known complication.

Patients with early acute Chagas disease may respond to treatment with either **nifurtimox** or **benznidazole**. However, no effective treatment is available for patients with late complications, perhaps because the critical damage has already occurred and is no longer reversible.

Trypanosoma brucei

African sleeping sickness is caused by *Trypanosoma brucei* (Fig. 52-9). The disease is endemic in Africa and transmitted by the bite of infected tsetse flies. *T. brucei* was one of the first microorganisms found to undergo **antigenic variation** of its immunodominant surface antigen, a process now known to occur in several parasitic pathogens.

T. brucei and its vectors differ in several biological characteristics from *T. cruzi* (the agent of Chagas disease) and its vectors. For example, *T. brucei* resides in the salivary glands of tsetse flies and is transmitted directly by bites. *T. cruzi*, on the other hand, grows in the intestine of reduviid bugs and is transmitted when feces deposited by the biting insect are introduced into the bite by scratching.

PATHOGENESIS AND DIAGNOSIS

The spread of African trypanosomiasis is restricted by the distribution of its tsetse fly vector (*Glossina*) and of

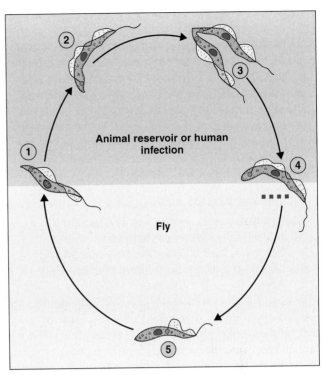

FIGURE 52-9 ▪ Sleeping sickness (African trypanosomiasis). The tsetse fly vector inoculates infectious trypomastigotes under the skin (1) when it bites humans or other mammals. Once inside the new host (2), the parasite replicates in the bloodstream by binary fission as a trypomastigote (3). Unlike *Leishmania* species and the trypanosome that causes Chagas disease, the trypanosomes that cause African sleeping sickness do not have promastigote or amastigote forms. The rate of movement of trypomastigotes from the bloodstream and lymph nodes to the central nervous system defines the point at which the illness changes from a systemic (hemolymphatic) infection to an encephalitis. Circulating trypomastigotes (4) taken up anew by tsetse flies complete the cycle. Within the tsetse fly the parasites replicate in the gastrointestinal tract and transform into epimastigotes (5). The dashed line below stage 4 indicates that natural transmission does not occur in countries such as the United States where the tsetse fly vector is not present.

its animal reservoirs. In East Africa the main reservoirs are wild game animals (such as impalas); West African reservoirs are infected humans and domestic animals, such as cattle. Several weeks to months after the initial infection, a patient develops a systemic illness with fever and swollen lymph nodes, and trypanosomes are present in the bloodstream. After several months (in the East African form) or years (in the West African form) the parasites invade the central nervous system and infect the brain and spinal fluid.

During months or years of chronic bloodstream infection, patients undergo bouts of parasitemia (Fig. 52-10). During each bout the parasite changes its dominant sur-

Case

Mr. B., a 32-year-old student from Senegal living in Canada, had fevers to 38°C and swollen lymph nodes at the back of his neck for 8 months. Two weeks ago, he developed a severe headache, stiff neck, and an aversion to light (photophobia). Trypanosomes were seen on Giemsa-stained specimens of blood and cerebrospinal fluid under the oil immersion objective. Mr. B. was treated with **eflornithine** for both the hemolymphatic and central nervous system infection. He recovered after 6 weeks of treatment.

This case raises two questions:

1. How did a parasite survive in Mr. B.'s blood for 8 months? Is he immunocompromised?
2. How would Mr. B.'s illness have been different if he had immigrated from South Africa rather than West Africa?

Case

E., a healthy 6-year-old girl living in rural Virginia, swam in a lake in the month of August. Two days later she developed a severe headache, neck stiffness, and eye pain on exposure to light (photophobia). Spinal fluid obtained a day later had 300 mononucleated cells/mm^3 and a few neutrophils. Many of those cells were actively motile in a wet mount, suggesting that they were not leukocytes but amebas. Despite treatment with antimicrobial drugs, E. died 3 days later.

This case raises one question:

1. How did amebas get into E.'s central nervous system?

face antigen (**variable surface glycoprotein**), thus avoiding immune destruction by the host. As with bacterial pathogens that undergo similar antigenic variation, the basis for variability is **genetic rearrangement**. Each parasite expresses only one glycoprotein gene from an "expression locus," but it also carries a repertoire of numerous alternative versions of the gene that are not expressed. When one of those "silent copies" recombines into the expression locus, the parasite expresses an immunologically distinct surface glycoprotein. For a full discussion of antigenic variation, see the Chapter 14 paradigm.

TREATMENT

In addition to eflornithine, several drugs (e.g., pentamidine and suramin) are useful in the systemic stage of the infection. However, treatment is much more difficult after the central nervous system becomes involved.

FIGURE 52-10 ▪ **Periodic fluctuation in the number of *Trypanosoma brucei* in the blood of a patient with African trypanosomiasis.**

Free-Living Amebas

In this section we discuss only the amebas that do not have human or animal reservoirs. Amebas with human or animal reservoirs, such as *Entamoeba histolytica*, are discussed in Chapter 53. A number of protozoa, principally *Naegleria*, *Acanthamoeba*, and *Hartmannella*, have no known animal reservoirs but may cause rare but serious systemic diseases.

There are two types of amebic meningoencephalitis. The first is a usually fatal disease caused by *Naegleria fowleri* that, as in E.'s case, typically occurs in young, previously healthy people. That form of amebic meningoencephalitis is associated with exposure to warm, freshwater lakes that harbor the amebas. The second form is a disease caused by *Acanthamoeba* or *Hartmannella* and is typically seen in older patients who are immunocompromised (such as those with lymphoma or diabetes). Both types of disease, once clinically apparent, tend to progress despite treatment. Although recovery using multiple drugs (amphotericin B, miconazole, and rifampin) has been reported, the regimens have not proven to be reproducibly effective.

In the meningoencephalitis caused by *N. fowleri*, the parasite is thought to enter the central nervous system through the cribriform plate along the olfactory nerve tracts. That site is the area in which the nervous system is in nearest proximity to the exterior; it can thus serve as a unique portal of entry into the central nervous system. *Acanthamoeba* or *Hartmannella*, on the other hand, are thought to spread to the central nervous system through the bloodstream, as suggested by the postmortem finding of foci of infection at distant sites, such as the lung.

Infection of the cornea (keratitis) is produced by *Acanthamoeba* and is an increasingly important (often undiagnosed) cause of visual loss among contact lens wearers or persons with other ocular trauma. It is important to recognize this infection (by morphologic examination of Giemsa-stained material using the high-dry or oil immersion objectives), because treatment with topical or systemic **imidazoles** can save the patient's sight. *Acanthamoeba* can gain access to the eye from contaminated fluids used to clean contact lenses.

Conclusion

The global morbidity and mortality associated with tissue-invasive protozoal infections is staggering. Malaria is a leading cause of death in young children in endemic regions. Toxoplasmosis is estimated to affect more than one billion people and is cosmopolitan in its distribution. Although public health measures to control vectors, mass treatment programs, and chemoprophylaxis (for malaria and toxoplasmosis) have dramatically reduced the impact of some diseases in countries that can economically support such measures, the best hope for worldwide eradication rests on the development of effective vaccines.

chapter 53

Intestinal and Vaginal Protozoa

Cary Engleberg

key **concepts**

- Intestinal protozoa are acquired by ingestion of cysts by the fecal–oral route of transmission, usually involving contaminated food or water.

- *Entamoeba histolytica* lyses cells in the colon and feeds on their contents, resulting in colonic ulcerations and dysentery (diarrhea with blood and mucus). Asymptomatic human carriers are the reservoir of infection; occasionally, the parasite enters the portal circulation and produces abscesses in the liver or other distant organs.

- *Giardia lamblia* and species of *Cryptosporidium, Cyclospora,* and Microsporidia are zoonotic and therefore cannot be prevented by control of human sanitation alone. They infect the small intestine and cause noninflammatory, watery diarrhea that can last for days or weeks.

- A chronic inflammatory response to persistent giardiasis may result in the loss of intestinal villi, malabsorption syndrome, and weight loss.

- Patients with AIDS and other immunodeficiencies may experience intractable diarrhea caused by these agents.

- Trichomoniasis is a common form of sexually transmitted vaginitis and urethritis that requires treatment of all contacts to ensure that reinfection will not occur.

The protozoa are classified according to their motility and their replicative cycles. The intestinal and vaginal organisms discussed in this chapter are a varied group: an **ameba** (*Entamoeba histolytica*), two **flagellates** (*Giardia lamblia* and *Trichomonas vaginalis*), three **apicomplexans** (genera *Cryptosporidium, Cyclospora,* and *Isospora*), and Microsporidia (a group of organisms that are difficult to classify because they possess features of both protozoa and bacteria; Table 53-1). The sporozoans (also known as apicomplexans) are intracellular parasites that reproduce by alternating sexual and asexual cycles (as do *Toxoplasma gondii* and malaria parasites; see Chapter 52).

Between 5 and 10% of all people in developing countries harbor the ameba *E. histolytica* in their stool. In the United States the figure is less than 1%. *Giardia* and

table **53-1**	Comparison of Major Intestinal and Vaginal Protozoa		
ORGANISM	**RESERVOIR**	**MODES OF TRANSMISSION**	**CLINICAL MANIFESTATIONS**
Entamoeba histolytica (amebiasis)	Infected humans	Fecal–oral transmission by the ingestion of feces containing infectious cysts	Bloody diarrhea (dysentery), distant abscesses (especially liver), asymptomatic intestinal infection
Giardia lamblia (giardiasis)	Infected humans, and other mammals	Fecal–oral transmission by ingestion of feces containing infectious cysts	Watery diarrhea; may also cause steatorrhea and malabsorption
Cryptosporidium parvum (cryptosporidiosis)	Infected humans and a wide variety of other animal hosts (zoonosis)	Fecal–oral transmission by the ingestion of feces containing infectious cysts	Watery diarrhea; intractable diarrhea in people with AIDS
Cyclospora cayetanensis	Unknown	Foodborne and waterborne; person-to-person spread unlikely	Watery diarrhea
Isospora belli	Infected humans	Foodborne and waterborne	Watery diarrhea; intractable diarrhea in people with AIDS
Microsporidia	Unknown	Unknown	Watery diarrhea, biliary tract infection, etc.

Cryptosporidium species are more frequent in the United States. Both have caused large waterborne outbreaks, but their prevalence varies considerably among U.S. regions. The *Cyclospora* genus was recognized as a human pathogen only recently, when it was implicated in a series of foodborne outbreaks. The genera *Isospora* and the Microsporidia are most serious when they affect persons with AIDS. Other protozoa that live in nonintestinal tissues include *Trichomonas vaginalis*, a common agent of vaginitis that is usually transmitted sexually.

Entamoeba Histolytica

Entamoeba histolytica causes a disease called **amebiasis.** As its species name indicates, *E. histolytica* may cause destruction of host tissue, especially in the colon. The lesions start as small ulcerations of the intestinal epithelium. Amebas within the lesions spread laterally as they encounter the deeper layers of the colon, sometimes producing **flask-shaped ulcers** that undermine the mucosal epithelium. Organisms may also spread through the portal circulation to produce abscesses in the liver and less commonly in the lung, brain, or other organs. Despite their pathogenic potential, organisms in the intestinal tract often cause few or no symptoms. In addition, many humans carry nonpathogenic amebas that are morphologically indistinguishable from *E. histolytica*. The species name *Entamoeba dispar* is used to designate the avirulent strains, which can be identified only by biochemical or nucleic acid–based techniques.

Case

Two years ago 26-year-old Mr. A. was discharged from the U.S. Army after 6 years of service. He was stationed abroad for 3 years, on tours of duty in Korea, Panama, and Germany. During the last 2 years he developed intermittent diarrhea, with blood and mucus visible in the stool (i.e., dysentery). Sigmoidoscopy (endoscopic examination of the colon) and a radiographic study of the intestine following a barium enema revealed pseudopolyps consistent with inflammatory bowel disease. He was diagnosed with ulcerative colitis, an inflammatory bowel disease of unknown cause, and was treated with steroids.

At the time of admission to the hospital, 4 months after beginning steroid therapy, Mr. A. reported a weight loss of about 24 lb (down to 147 lb) and a recent increase in bloody stools and abdominal pain. He had no fever (probably because he was medicated with large doses of steroids). Examination of his stool under the microscope showed many white and red blood cells but no amebas. However, a serological test for *Entamoeba histolytica* antibodies in serum (indirect hemagglutination) revealed a high titer (1:2,000). A computerized tomography scan showed an 8-cm abscess in the right lobe of the liver.

He had a stormy hospital stay with several episodes of bacteremia (secondary to disruption of the intestinal mucosa by the parasite). He finally recovered after the steroids were tapered and he was treated with the antiamebic agent metronidazole.

This case raises two questions:
1. Why were no amebas seen in Mr. A.'s stool?
2. What was the role of steroids in this case?

ENCOUNTER

E. histolytica is transmitted from person to person through the fecal–oral route. The protozoan has a simple life cycle with two forms: the actively growing, vegetative **trophozoite** and the dormant but highly resistant **cyst** (Fig. 53-1). The critical factors responsible for the transformation from trophozoites to cysts and vice versa are not understood. The transmission of *Entamoeba* and *Giardia* has a paradoxical aspect. Patients with diarrhea pose only a minor threat of transmission because they excrete the actively growing yet labile trophozoites; this form of the parasite is easily destroyed by drying in the environment and, if ingested, by acid in the stomach. Conversely, asymptomatic carriers excrete the durable cyst form of the parasite, which survives well in the environment and remains intact through the stomach. Asymptomatic carriers thus represent the greatest danger of transmission. That paradox illustrates the biological principle that successful parasites generally do not harm the host. When amebas are in balance with their host, they do not cause symptoms but are excreted as cysts, thus ensuring their transmissibility.

Because the parasite is infectious in the cyst stage and does not require a period of maturation in the environment, transmission of amebiasis is not restricted to warm climates. In fact, *E. histolytica* can even be transmitted in polar regions. The only requirement for transmission is that contaminated feces of the carrier be ingested with food or water. Sexual transmission (anal–oral or oral–genital) is also important, particularly among homosexual men.

SPREAD, MULTIPLICATION, AND DAMAGE

E. histolytica are frequently found in the human colon in persons without symptoms of disease. The amebas must adhere using a critical surface protein (or **lectin**) to specific receptors on host cells containing digalactose residues (i.e., Gal-galNAc). In experimental models, attachment to cells is inhibited by adding galactose. Attachment is also inhibited by intestinal mucus, which suggests that disruption of the mucus layer may be a critical event in the pathogenesis of amebiasis.

Damage to host cells requires intimate cell-to-cell contact and takes place in three steps: (1) receptor-mediated attachment to the mammalian target cell via the Gal-galNAc binding lectin; (2) contact-dependent killing, probably by insertion of pore-forming proteins (**amebapores**) into the host cell membrane; and (3) ingestion of the killed host cell by the ameba. Although certain strains of *E. histolytica* produce an enterotoxin, it is not yet clear whether enterotoxin production correlates with virulence.

Phagocytic cells do not control amebic infection in nonimmune hosts: pathogenic strains of amebas actually kill neutrophils and nonactivated macrophages (notice the reversal of the usual "phagocyte ingests invader" theme). The situation is different in immune hosts, in whom the most important line of defense appears to be cell-mediated immunity (which was suggested by the finding that amebas can be killed in vitro by activated macrophages). Furthermore, persons given steroids (which suppress cell-mediated immunity) tend to have disseminated infection despite high titers of antibodies, as was the case with Mr. A. Thus, circulating antibodies may not play a critical role in protection against amebic infection. Amebas are known to produce a **cysteine proteinase** that digests secretory IgA, IgG, and other proteins involved in the humoral immune response.

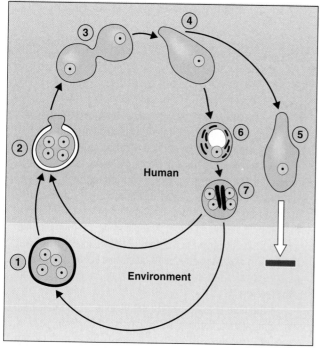

FIGURE 53-1 ■ Life cycle of *Entamoeba histolytica*. Humans acquire amebic infection by oral ingestion of the cyst form of the parasite (1). Viable cysts may be ingested from the external environment (where they remain stable and infectious for prolonged periods after excretion), from the stool of other infected persons, or from the stools of the patients themselves (the arrow from 7 to 2). In the upper gastrointestinal tract, the parasite excysts after passing through the stomach (2), replicates asexually by binary fission (3), and transforms to the potentially pathogenic trophozoite form (4), which is typically found in the large intestine. Trophozoites die rapidly when they are shed into the external environment (5; solid line represents dead end). When conditions in the gastrointestinal tract are unfavorable, trophozoites transform into cysts (6–7), which can remain dormant for long periods of time in the host and the environment.

DIAGNOSIS

The traditional method of diagnosis involves the microscopic identification of trophozoites in freshly passed dysenteric stool or in scrapings from colonic ulcers obtained through a sigmoidoscope. On a warm microscopic slide, organisms demonstrate ameboid movement. *E. histolytica* may contain ingested red blood cells. However, *E. histolytica* trophozoites without internalized red blood cells and cysts are indistinguishable from the nonpathogenic ameba *E. dispar*. Consequently, microscopic examination of stool from a patient without characteristic clinical features and colonic ulcers may be misleading. In that case alternative diagnostic methods may be helpful. In particular, a **stool immunoassay for E. histolytica antigen** may be more sensitive than microscopic examination and, in some formats, capable of distinguishing *E. histolytica* from *E. dispar*. Alternatively, serological diagnosis may be useful. Ameba serology is positive in 10 to 15% of asymptomatic carriers, in more than 80% of people with invasion of the intestinal mucosa, and in 96 to 100% of persons with metastatic infection (e.g., liver abscess). However, since antiameba antibodies persist for several years after infection, serology does not distinguish current from past infection and is therefore not useful in countries where amebiasis is endemic. However, in the United States, where less than 1% of the general population has antibodies to *E. histolytica*, a positive serology can be taken as evidence of active infection.

TREATMENT

The drug of choice for active amebic infection is **metronidazole**, the same antimicrobial used to treat infections caused by anaerobic bacteria. Pathogenic amebas carry out anaerobic metabolism and convert metronidazole to its active form in the same way as do species of *Bacteroides* (see Chapters 3 and 15). The drug is particularly effective for invasive infections because it penetrates well into most tissues, including the brain. Because metronidazole is less efficient at killing amebas within the intestinal lumen, a second drug is given to eradicate the luminal forms. Drugs such as diloxanide, paromomycin, and diiodohydroxyquin are used for that purpose and can also be used to treat asymptomatic carriers of pathogenic strains.

Giardia Lamblia

Giardia lamblia (also known as *Giardia intestinalis*) is the intestinal protozoan that causes **giardiasis**. *G. lamblia* is distributed all over the world. Giardiasis is a

Case

Thirty-six-year-old Ms. P. visited Colorado for 10 days of backpacking 2 months before seeing her physician. One week after returning she developed abdominal bloating, belching, and diarrhea with 3 to 5 watery stools per day. The stool contained no pus or blood, and she had no fever or chills. A stool examination was positive for *Giardia lamblia*. Ms. P. was treated with metronidazole and improved markedly over a 7-day period. Subsequently, symptoms recurred and the organisms were again found in her stool.

This case raises two questions:
1. How did Ms. P. acquire *Giardia* infection?
2. What prompted the physician to check for a parasite rather than to culture for agents of bacterial gastroenteritis?

zoonosis, an animal disease that affects humans only accidentally. It is commonly acquired by ingestion of water contaminated by feces from animal carriers. Because *Giardia* cysts are resistant to chlorine, waterborne outbreaks associated with municipal water systems have occurred in the United States and around the world. In the United States giardiasis is commonly found in areas of poor sanitation such as in day care centers, where there is frequent opportunity for direct fecal–oral transmission. Giardiasis is also an important infection among homosexual males. *Giardia* infection typically produces a mild but persistent diarrheal disease, with organisms often localized to the duodenum and jejunum. Occasionally, chronic infection causes intestinal malabsorption.

ENTRY, SPREAD, MULTIPLICATION, AND DAMAGE

As with *E. histolytica* infection, giardiasis is acquired by ingestion of the cyst form of the parasite (Fig. 53-2). *Giardia* cysts are highly resistant in the environment and are found in ostensibly "pure" mountain streams contaminated by the feces of infected animals or humans. When asked, Ms. P. admitted drinking water drawn directly from a mountain stream. Like pathogenic amebas, *G. lamblia* can be transmitted in cold as well as in warm climates.

Stomach acid does not kill *Giardia* cysts. In fact, stomach acid actually stimulates the cysts to transform into the vegetative trophozoite form in the duodenum. *Giardia* trophozoites attach to the epithelium of the duodenum and jejunum using a ventral sucking disk. The vegetative forms have the characteristic appearance of a face adorned with mustachelike flagella (see Fig. 53-2).

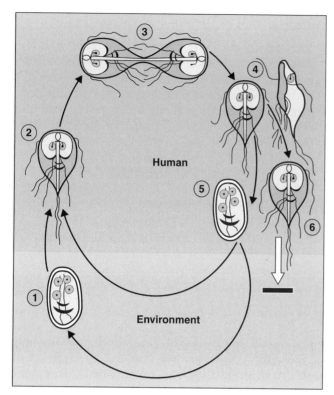

FIGURE 53-2 ▪ **Life cycle of *Giardia lamblia*.** Humans acquire giardiasis by ingesting the cyst form of the parasite (1). After contact with the gastric contents, the parasite excysts and transforms to a trophozoite in the upper gastrointestinal tract (2), where it replicates asexually by binary fission (3). Trophozoites cause disease by attaching to the epithelium of the small intestine via a ventral sucking disk (4). As indicated by the solid line and open arrow below stage 6, tropho-zoites are not infectious for others because they are readily killed by drying in the external environment. As in amebiasis, humans acquire infection by ingesting cysts from the external environment (1), from the stools of other patients, or from their own stool (arrow from stages 5 to 2).

FIGURE 53-3 ▪ **Scanning electron micrograph of *Giardia lamblia*. A.** *G. lamblia* adhering to the gastrointestinal epithelium using its ventral sucking disk. Patients with giardiasis may have a significant reduction in the amount of absorptive surface available because of the large num-ber of adhering parasites. **B.** On detaching from the in-testinal epithelium, the organisms often leave a clear impression on the microvillous surface (upper circles).

Signs of malnutrition resulting from malabsorption may occur as a result of extensive, prolonged infection. In those cases the organisms literally cover the mucosal surface of the small intestine (Fig. 53-3). Unlike *E. his-tolytica*, *G. lamblia* is not invasive and does not pro-duce bloody diarrhea or metastatic infection. However, the host responds to *Giardia* infection with a submu-cosal infiltrate of chronic inflammatory cells (mostly lymphocytes) and an effacement of the normal intesti-nal villi. With the loss of villi, the total absorptive area of the intestine is significantly diminished. In particular, malabsorption of fats can lead to greasy, foul-smelling stools; diarrhea associated with unabsorbed fatty acids in the lumen; deficiencies of fat-soluble vitamins (i.e., A, K, D, and E); and weight loss.

DIAGNOSIS AND TREATMENT

The classic approach to diagnosis of giardiasis is direct identification of parasites in stool or in duodenal aspi-rates. Trophozoites are actively motile in fresh specimens by virtue of their multiple flagellae. Cysts are small, ovoid, nonmotile bodies with four nuclei. Trophozoites are rarely seen in direct stool examinations, and it may take three or more stool examinations to find cysts in an infected patient or carrier. Fortunately, an antigen detec-tion assay for giardiasis is now available. This test is more sensitive than a single microscopic stool examina-tion in diagnosing giardiasis.

In the United States giardiasis can be treated with metronidazole, but relapses can occur. Alternative antimicrobial agents with a similar mechanism of action include **tinidazole** and **nitazoxanide.** Hikers and campers can prevent unpleasant episodes of diarrhea by boiling or filtering their drinking water or by treating it with adequate amounts of iodine or chlorine.

Cryptosporidium

Cryptosporidia cause a zoonosis first discovered among veterinary students and animal handlers who acquired it from calves they were treating for diarrhea. It is now clear that cryptosporidiosis is an important diarrheal disease in both developed and developing countries.

ENCOUNTER

Cryptosporidiosis is often acquired in rural areas because of greater contact with animals. However, it can also spread from person to person in crowded urban environments such as day care centers. It is now recognized as a frequent cause of diarrhea in Great Britain and the United States, and it has been identified as a potential cause of diarrhea in travelers to developing countries. Cryptosporidiosis is particularly troublesome in patients with advanced AIDS who lack the immune mechanisms necessary to resolve the infection.

Case

Mr. W., a 40-year-old homosexual with HIV infection, lives on a farm in rural Michigan. Despite a low CD4 count and periodic episodes of oral candidiasis, he had been well and had refused treatment. Six weeks ago he began to have watery stools 3 to 8 times a day. He denied fever or chills, and no blood or pus appeared in the stools. A microscopic examination of his stool after an acid-fast stain revealed the presence of acid-fast spherical organisms that were slightly smaller than erythrocytes. Although Mr. W. was treated with oral rehydration and a synthetic hormone that reduces intestinal secretion, he continued to have persistent watery diarrhea. He eventually agreed to treatment with a four-drug combination of antiretroviral agents and noted improvement in the frequency of diarrhea over the subsequent months.

This case raises several questions:

1. How did Mr. W. acquire cryptosporidiosis?
2. What other significant pathogens might be seen on an acid-fast stain of the stool?
3. Why was antiretroviral therapy given to control the diarrhea instead of an antiparasitic agent?

Recent attention has focused on outbreaks associated with public water systems. Cryptosporidium oocysts can be found in most surface waters in this country, and most public utilities draw on these sources to provide public water service. Several outbreaks of cryptosporidiosis have involved drinking water or swimming pools. The largest single waterborne outbreak of *Cryptosporidium* infection in the history of the United States occurred in Milwaukee, Wisconsin, in 1993. More than 400,000 persons were affected, and more than 4,000 people were hospitalized after contamination of the municipal water supply. More recently, outbreaks at swim clubs have followed fecal accidents in swimming pools by infected children. Cryptosporidia oocysts are highly resistant to chlorine, and the infectious particles are expelled in huge numbers in watery stool. Thus, even standard chlorination methods and massive dilution of the fecal organisms in the entire pool volume do not prevent transmission to swimmers who inadvertently swallow pool water. Currently, the only recourse in that situation is to close and drain the contaminated pool.

SPREAD AND MULTIPLICATION

Cryptosporidium parasites resembles *Toxoplasma* species in that infectious oocyst forms are produced in the intestine and spread to other animals. However, unlike *Toxoplasma* species, cryptosporidia do not invade the intestinal epithelial cells, nor do they disseminate to produce systemic infection. They carry out their entire life cycle among the microvilli of the small intestine (Fig. 53-4). In immunocompetent individuals the life cycle takes place only once or twice, resulting in a single episode of diarrhea that usually lasts 2 weeks or less. In immunocompromised patients (e.g., persons with AIDS) the life cycle of the organism is repeated many times and is associated with persistent and often intractable watery diarrhea.

DIAGNOSIS AND TREATMENT

The diagnosis of cryptosporidiosis can be made by identifying characteristic acid-fast cysts in the stool. A commonly used alternative is a stool antigen detection assay for cryptosporidia, which is less labor intensive than making stained smears of stool.

Nitazoxanide appears to have activity against cryptosporidia in immunocompetent hosts, but treatment with that agent has not resolved the problem of persistent diarrhea in AIDS. Supportive therapy with rehydration and antimotility agents is the mainstay in that setting. In addition, successful treatment with antiretroviral therapy

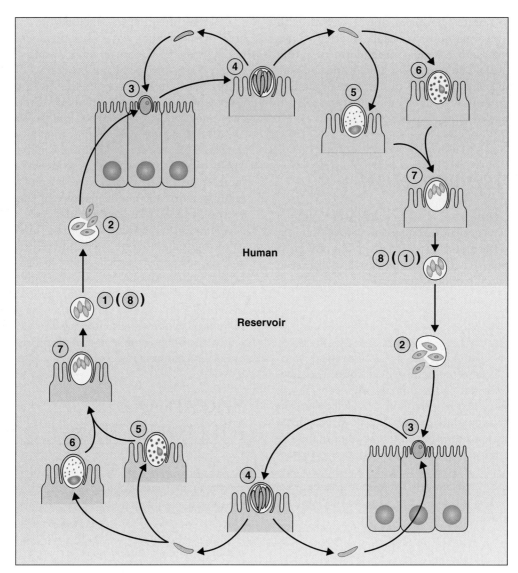

FIGURE 53-4 ■ **Life cycle of *Cryptosporidium* species.** Humans acquire infection by ingesting infectious oocysts (1) after direct contact with infected animals or humans, or by ingesting water or food contaminated with human or animal feces. Autoinfection can also occur. Once inside the human host (2), sporozoites are released from the oocyst, enter the epithelial cells of the gastrointestinal tract and develop into trophozoites (3). Trophozoites develop into structures containing individual merozoites (4). The trophozoites can either recapitulate the asexual cycle (3) or evolve into one of two sexual gametes (5–6). The gametes join and form oocysts (7). When mature and released, oocysts are the infectious form of the parasite that is excreted in the feces (8). Identical events take place in the reservoir.

and restoration of cell-mediated immunity can result in significant improvement of symptoms.

Cyclospora cayetanensis

Cyclospora cayetanensis is a protozoal parasite that resembles *Cryptosporidium* species in producing acid-fast cysts in stools, although the *Cyclospora* cysts are roughly twice the size of those caused by cryptosporidia (Fig. 53-5). In the late 1980s and early 1990s, *C. cayetanensis* was increasingly recognized as a cause of epidemic diarrhea in the United States and chronic diarrhea in developing countries around the world. In 1996 more than 40 outbreaks of cyclosporiasis occurred in several states. Most of those outbreaks were linked to ingestion of raspberries imported from Central America. In Lima, Peru, species of *Cyclospora* were found in the stools of 6 to 18% of young children, often associated with diarrhea. The species *C. cayetanensis* is named for the Peruvian University (Cayetano Heredia) where those observations were made.

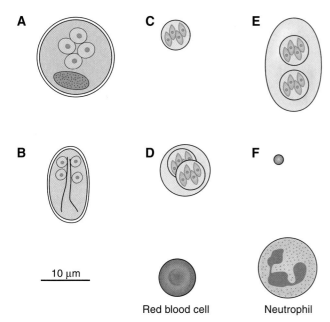

FIGURE 53-5 ▪ **Schematic representation and relative sizes of protozoal cysts and oocysts found in human feces. A.** Round *Entamoeba histolytica* cyst with four nuclei. **B.** Oval *Giardia lamblia* cyst with four nuclei and a central axostyle (encysted flagellae). **C.** *Cryptosporidium parvum* oocyst with four internal sporozoites. **D.** *Cyclospora cayetanensis* oocyst with two sporocysts, each containing four sporozoites. **E.** Oval *Isospora belli* oocyst containing two sporocysts. **F.** A tiny microsporidian organism with few distinguishing features by light microscopy.

SPREAD, MULTIPLICATION, AND DAMAGE

Unlike *Entamoeba* and *Giardia* cysts, *Cyclospora* oocysts are not infectious when excreted in human feces. The parasites become infectious (sporulate) only after days to weeks of incubation in environmental sites with warm temperatures and high humidity. Therefore, most new infections are acquired by ingestion of contaminated food or water. Person-to-person spread, if it occurs at all, is probably very rare.

Infection with *C. cayetanensis* causes watery diarrhea that may be associated with loss of appetite, bloating, cramps, nausea and vomiting, fatigue, muscle aches, and low-grade fever. The illness may last for only a few days, or it may persist for a month or longer. Relapses are common.

DIAGNOSIS AND TREATMENT

Diagnosis depends on the identification of the large acidfast oocyst in the stool. Treatment with trimethoprim-sulfamethoxazole relieves symptoms and shortens the course of infection.

Other Intestinal Parasites

Isospora belli

Isospora belli is a protozoan that causes transient watery diarrhea in healthy individuals. *Isospora* infection tends to occur more frequently in tropical areas. Cases recognized in the United States occur mostly in AIDS patients, in whom *I. belli* can cause a persistent watery diarrhea, like that associated with *Cryptosporidium* species.

The diagnosis is made by examination of stool for characteristic oocysts. Fortunately, trimethoprim-sulfamethoxazole appears to be effective in controlling infection in immunocompromised patients.

Microsporidia

Microsporidia belong to a phylum containing almost 1,000 species found ubiquitous among vertebrate and invertebrate animals and in the environment. They have been studied for decades as causes of insect and fish diseases; only recently have they been associated with human disease. The obligate intracellular parasites are very small relative to the other pathogens discussed in this chapter (see Fig. 53-5). They lack mitochondria and possess small ribosomal RNA, suggesting a prokaryotic origin. Those features distinguish them from other protozoa and have caused taxonomists to place the parasites into their own phylum, Microsporidia.

A few Microsporidia species have been associated with human diseases, particularly but not exclusively in immunocompromised patients. Various species have been associated with infections of the gastrointestinal tract, respiratory tract, urinary tract, liver, brain, or eye. The modes of transmission have not been clearly elucidated. Symptomatic intestinal infection is primarily associated with the species *Enterocytozoon bieneusi*.

E. bieneusi is believed to cause transient diarrhea in healthy hosts but a protracted watery diarrhea in AIDS patients. The organism infects the mucosal epithelial cells and, in AIDS patients, can also disseminate to distant sites. Thus, *E. bieneusi* may ascend into the biliary tree and cause symptoms of cholangitis. The diagnosis can be made by microscopic examination of stool or intestinal biopsy material after special staining procedures. Optimal treatment has not yet been found; common antibacterial and antiprotozoal drugs are not very effective. Oddly, the antihelminthic drug **albendazole** and a compound isolated from the fungus *Aspergillus fumigatus*, **fumagillin,** have been used with some success.

Trichomonas Vaginalis

Trichomonas vaginalis is a common inhabitant of the vagina and is found in 15% or more of women, in whom it occasionally causes vaginitis. Less common and less pathogenic species of *Trichomonas* are found in the gastrointestinal tract (*T. hominis*) or the mouth (*T. tenax*).

SPREAD, MULTIPLICATION, AND DIAGNOSIS

T. vaginalis infection is transmitted by sexual intercourse. Vaginitis is typically associated with a frothy creamy discharge. Most male partners of symptomatic women become infected; however, the majority of infections in men are asymptomatic. Symptoms sometimes seen among men include mild urethritis, epididymitis, or prostatitis.

DIAGNOSIS AND TREATMENT

It is usually possible to see these flagellates moving vigorously in wet preparations of vaginal secretions from infected women. Infection of male partners can be assumed. Single-dose metronidazole or tinidazole treatment is recommended by most investigators. In pregnant women (in whom there is particular concern about the potential carcinogenic effects of metronidazole), douching with vinegar can suppress symptomatic infection by lowering vaginal pH. Male sexual partners must also be treated to prevent "ping-pong" relapses, a common feature of many sexually transmitted diseases.

Conclusion

Most intestinal protozoa produce self-limited illness with watery diarrhea, abdominal cramps, and characteristic protozoal forms in the stool. Amebiasis is unique among these diseases because it involves direct destruction of tissues and occasionally disseminates to vital organs. Accordingly, the clinical features of amebiasis may include bloody stools (dysentery), fever, or abscess formation in the liver and elsewhere. Amebiasis is also distinct from the other protozoa in that the transmission depends on a reservoir of asymptomatic human carriers, rather than nonhuman sources. Thus, infection always results from a failure to dispose of human feces safely, in contrast to giardiasis and other intestinal protozoal infections, which may result from contamination of food and water at its source. Understanding the pathophysiologic differences among these parasites aids in the diagnosis of diarrheal illness, and an appreciation for their epidemiology may direct attention to the circumstances and source of infection.

Intestinal Helminths

Cary Engleberg

key concepts

- The common intestinal helminthic infections are caused by nematodes (roundworms) and cestodes (tapeworms). The life cycles of helminths require indiscriminate handling of human wastes leading to fecal helminth eggs contaminating soil, foodstuffs, animal feeds, and other materials.

- Nematode infections are acquired by ingestion of eggs (e.g., *Ascaris, Trichuris, Enterobius*) or by direct penetration of soil larvae through the skin (e.g., *Strongyloides*, hookworm). These infections are often asymptomatic unless the worm burden is very large. Pathologic features include intestinal obstruction (*Ascaris*), rectal prolapse (*Trichuris*), anal itching (*Enterobius*), and iron-deficiency anemia (hookworm).

- Sustained autoinfection is a unique feature of strongyloidiasis. Immunosuppressed individuals may develop a syndrome of *Strongyloides* hyperinfection with diarrhea, pneumonitis, rash, and eosinophilia.

- Three species of tapeworm can cause infections when people ingest encysted worm larvae in under-cooked tissues of beef, pork, or fish. Fish tapeworms may successfully compete for vitamin B_{12} and cause anemia in the host. The presence of beef or pork tapeworms in the intestines rarely produces systemic signs or symptoms.

- Diagnosis of intestinal helminths relies on identifying the characteristic eggs, larvae, or adult worms (or segments) in feces.

The helminths, or worms, are multicellular animals. They include many free-living, harmless species as well as some pathogenic species that infect a high proportion of all people on earth (see Table 51-1). Helminthic diseases are sometimes mistakenly considered a problem only for people living in the tropics. In fact, some infections are common in temperate zones; others are relatively rare but have major consequences when they go unrecognized, especially in immunocompromised persons.

Helminths are the largest parasites that affect humans, ranging in size from 10-yard-long tapeworms to barely visible pinworms. The three groups of helminths are **roundworms** (nematodes), **tapeworms** (cestodes), and **flukes** (trematodes). Each group is generally distinguished by its shape. Examples of each type of worm are

table **54-1**	Pathophysiologic Mechanisms in Helminthic Diseases

MECHANISM	EXAMPLE
Mechanical obstruction or mass effect	
Intestinal obstruction	*Ascaris* ("worm ball")
Lymphatic obstruction	Lymphatic filariasis (elephantiasis)
Displacement of normal tissue	Echinococcosis (cystic hydatid disease), cysticercosis
Facilitating bacterial invasion into normally sterile spaces	Strongyloidiasis
Anemia	
From consumption of blood	Hookworm
From vitamin B_{12} depletion	Fish tapeworm
Chronic inflammation	Schistosomiasis, onchocerciasis

intestinal helminths and the **tissue and blood helminths** (see Chapter 55). The generalities about helminths mentioned here apply to both intestinal and tissue-invasive helminths.

In small numbers, helminths often cause chronic infections that are well tolerated by their human host. Helminths reproduce sexually. Therefore, humans must harbor both a male and female worm for the infection to produce fertilized eggs or larvae. A few species (tapeworms) are hermaphroditic, enabling a single parasite to produce eggs. In massive numbers, intestinal parasites can cause disease by contributing to the malnutrition of their host, occluding the intestinal lumen, or triggering a symptomatic immune response (Tables 54-1 and 54-2). Tissue-invasive helminths in large numbers cause disease by immunopathologic mechanisms or by creating an obstructing mass in vessels or organs (see Table 54-1).

The developmental stages of some helminths (e.g., hookworms) take place outside the human body, sometimes involving insect vectors and/or animal reservoirs. In these complex life cycles, the hosts that harbor the

discussed in this and the next chapter. However, the number and range of all helminthic parasites is beyond the scope of this text, and specialized parasitology textbooks should be consulted for details. From the point of view of human disease, helminths can be divided into the

table **54-2**	Main Intestinal Helminths	
EXAMPLE	**RESERVOIR**	**CLINICAL MANIFESTATIONS**
Acquired by passage through the skin		
Roundworms		
Strongyloides stercoralis	Infected humans	Gastrointestinal manifestations that can mimic peptic ulcer or gallbladder disease; disseminated infection (hyperinfection syndrome)
Hookworms (*Necator americanus, Ancylostoma duodenale*)	Infected humans	Iron deficiency anemia from chronic gastrointestinal blood loss
Acquired by ingestion		
Roundworms		
Ascaris lumbricoides	Infected humans	Often asymptomatic except for passage of 25- to 30-cm worms; may produce biliary obstruction or peritonitis from intestinal perforation
Enterobius vermicularis (pinworm)	Infected humans, especially children	Itching of the perianal or genital region
Trichuris trichiura (whipworm)	Infected humans	Often asymptomatic. Damage to intestinal mucosa; malnutrition and anemia if severe
Tapeworms		
Taenia solium	Pigs	Intestinal infection (taeniasis) is typically asymptomatic; for cysticercosis, see Table 55.1
Taenia saginata	Cattle	Intestinal infection (taeniasis) is typically asymptomatic
Diphyllobothrium latum	Fish	Intestinal infection is typically asymptomatic but may lead to vitamin B_{12} deficiency

adult, sexual form of the parasites are called **definitive hosts,** and the animal hosts that harbor the developmental stages are called **intermediate hosts.** Because multiple steps are required for infectivity, direct transmission from human to human does not occur with these species. In some cases (e.g., *Enterobius* infections) an infected patient may pass feces containing eggs or larvae that are immediately infectious for other humans. Person-to-person transmission, or **autoinfection,** is then possible. In all these species, however, the total number of parasites does not increase during the course of infection because the life cycle cannot be completed entirely within the human body. As a result, the intensity of infection, called the **worm burden,** is determined by the size of single or repeated inocula (i.e., the number of eggs or larvae acquired from the external environment).

A few helminthic species (e.g., *Strongyloides*) can carry out their entire life cycle within the human body. A continuous reinfection cycle prolongs the duration of the infection long beyond the life span of a single worm. In infections of these species, the host immune system may provide a check on the continuous propagation of worms, but an immunocompromised individual may experience uncontrolled growth of the worm burden.

In general, established adult worm infections are not eliminated by the host immune response. Most helminth infections resolve spontaneously when the adult parasites reach senescence (after a few months or years, they die of old age). Longevity differs by species. In some infections immunity to progressive stages of the parasite may develop to keep continuous acquisition in check. Unfortunately, in most helminthic infections, the major contribution of the host immune response is to cause the pathophysiologic features of the disease. Most of the pathologic features of these infections do not result from the direct action of the parasite on tissues but rather on the host's response to the products of parasites (eggs, larvae, and soluble antigens).

Eosinophilia is often regarded as a characteristic host response to parasitic infection. Indeed, specific antibodies together with eosinophils can adversely affect some parasites. However, a significant systemic eosinophilia occurs only when parasites are invading or migrating through host tissues. Although some intestinal parasites have stages of migration through the tissues and lungs that may provoke eosinophilia, worm infections confined to the intestinal lumen do not cause that systemic response.

Intestinal Nematodes (Roundworms)

The comparative life cycles of intestinal roundworms (phylum Nematoda) are summarized in Figure 54-1. Some of these parasites enter the body through the mouth when eggs are ingested. Others develop into larvae that penetrate through intact skin. The species discussed here infect large numbers of people and cause infections that range from asymptomatic to severe.

Nematode Infections Acquired by Ingestion: Ascaris

Ascaris is one of the largest of the human parasites, up to 30 cm in length, and one of the most frequently encountered worldwide. It affects perhaps one quarter of the human population, including a substantial number of people in the southern United States. A few *Ascaris* are generally well tolerated, but a large worm load can cause serious illness.

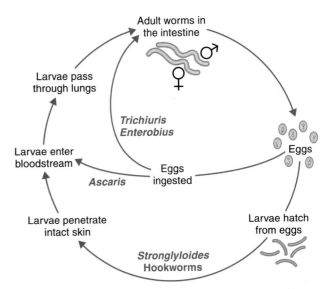

FIGURE 54-1 ▪ **Comparative life cycles of intestinal nematodes.**

Case

T., a 4-year-old-boy living in Georgia, had been well until 3 weeks before a visit to the doctor, although he had always been small for his age (height and weight at the tenth percentile). His parents reported that he passed "earthworms" with his stool. For the previous 2 to 3 weeks he had vague abdominal pain with nausea. His appetite had been poor, his abdomen was distended, and he had not had a bowel movement for 5 days. Radiographs of his abdomen were consistent with intestinal obstruction. Stool examination revealed large numbers of *Ascaris* eggs. He was given mebendazole and placed on intravenous fluids. One day after beginning treatment, he passed large numbers of *Ascaris*. Three days later, his abdomen was no longer distended, he was able to eat and drink, and he had a normal bowel movement.

This case raises two questions:

1. How did T. acquire the worms?
2. Is T.'s case typical of *Ascaris* infections?

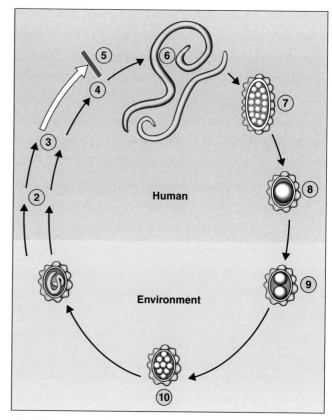

FIGURE 54-2 ▪ **Life cycle of *Ascaris lumbricoides* (human roundworm) and dog or cat roundworm (visceral larva migrans).** Humans acquire these infections by ingesting embryonated roundworm eggs from the environment (1). After ingestion the parasites hatch in the upper intestine (2), cross the bowel wall (3), and enter the bloodstream. The human *Ascaris* (innermost set of arrows in the top half of the diagram) enters the lung by crossing into the alveolus (4). It then travels up the trachea, is swallowed, and reenters the gastrointestinal tract to develop to a mature adult (6). The open arrow and solid line on the diagram indicate that neither dog nor cat *Ascaris* worms are able to enter the lung from the bloodstream. As a result, the parasites wander aimlessly through deep tissues and cannot return to the gastrointestinal tract (5). Stool examinations are therefore negative in patients with visceral larva migrans and positive in patients with human *Ascaris* infection (7). In the environment fertilized *Ascaris* eggs (8) germinate and divide (9) and produce embryonated eggs (10) that are infectious on oral ingestion. That process takes several weeks and requires a warm, moist climate. In visceral larva migrans the infectious eggs are shed by infected dogs or cats rather than humans.

ENCOUNTER AND PATHOBIOLOGY

After excretion in the stool, *Ascaris* eggs require several weeks in a warm environment to mature to the infective stage (Fig. 54-2). For that reason, ascariasis, like hookworm disease, is restricted to warm climates and to areas where the soil is contaminated by untreated human feces. The eggs must be ingested to complete the cycle. Ingestion occurs by placing soiled hands in the mouth or by eating food contaminated with soil-containing eggs. Fruits and vegetables growing near to the ground become contaminated by direct contact with fecally contaminated soil, either inadvertently or deliberately (as when human feces are used as fertilizer).

Once ingested, the eggs hatch in the small intestine and release larvae, which penetrate the mucosa and submucosa and enter venules or lymphatics. The parasites travel to the lung and migrate up the trachea to the pharynx, where they are swallowed to access the gastrointestinal tract. The worms mature in the intestinal lumen, and the females release their eggs into the stool.

Large numbers of larvae (from many ingested eggs) can produce a transient pneumonia as they cross from the bloodstream into the lungs. That reaction may be particularly severe if the patient has been sensitized by a previous *Ascaris* infection. Later, if adult worms are present in large numbers in the intestine, they may form a large mass (worm ball) and produce intestinal obstruction, as in T.'s case. Occasionally, individual worms produce biliary obstruction (by migrating up the bile duct and occluding it) or peritonitis (by perforating the

intestinal wall). Moderate intestinal worm burdens, on the other hand, can be totally asymptomatic.

Humans can also be infected by ingesting ascarid worms native to dogs, cats, or raccoons. Transmission is also by the fecal–oral route. The resulting infection is known as **visceral larva migrans.** Animals are the definitive hosts for these worms, which are unable to complete their cycle in humans. After leaving the intestine, dog or cat ascarid worms wander randomly through the tissues rather than crossing the lung to the trachea. Enlargement of the liver and spleen (hepatosplenomegaly) may result from the inflammatory response to the worms. **Eosinophilia** is usually marked because the worms invade the deep tissues. Because the worms cannot complete their life cycle in humans, they are considered **dead-end hosts** for the animal infections. The aborted nature of human infection by parasites of other primary hosts (dog or cat *Ascaris* in visceral larva migrans; dog or cat hookworms in creeping eruption) is a vivid reminder of the specificity of host–parasite interactions.

DIAGNOSIS AND TREATMENT

Usually, ascariasis is readily diagnosed by stool examination using low-power ($\times 100$) magnification, because each adult female worm releases approximately 200,000 eggs per day into the intestinal lumen. The number of eggs in the stool can be used to estimate of the number of worms present.

Mebendazole, albendazole, ivermectin, nitazoxanide, and several other drugs are effective in treating *Ascaris* infection of the gastrointestinal tract. Medical treatment with the anthelminthics typically relieves intestinal obstruction without surgical intervention.

Nematode Infections Acquired by Ingestion: *Enterobius* (Pinworm)

Pinworm infection is common in both temperate and tropical regions, affecting at least 200 million people worldwide. It is most prevalent among small children, who typically infect their siblings and parents, and among institutionalized persons. Pinworms seldom produce serious disease but may cause considerable discomfort.

Case

D., a healthy 3-year-old girl, was brought to the pediatrician because she had developed what the mother considers "unacceptable behavior"—she frequently scratched herself in the anal and vulval areas.

This case raises two questions:
1. What caused D.'s anal itching?
2. Should her mother be concerned that D. may become reinfected after being treated?

ENCOUNTER AND PATHOBIOLOGY

Pinworm eggs do not require a period of maturation outside the body; therefore, the infection can be transmitted readily by fecal–oral contamination (Fig. 54-3). The eggs also resist drying and may be transmitted from an infected person to other members of a household from bed clothes or dust. After oral ingestion, the eggs hatch in the duodenum and jejunum. The larvae mature in the ileum and large intestine. Gravid females migrate out of the rectum to the perianal skin to lay eggs. The most typical symptom of pinworm infection is perianal itching, which may be caused by dermal sensitivity to parasite egg antigens. Scratching facilitates the spread of the infection because infective eggs can be spread to the same person (autoinfection) or to others by putting contaminated fingers into the mouth. Other moist areas, such as the vagina, may also be affected. Occasionally, the parasite is found in the lumen of the appendix, although it rarely produces appendicitis.

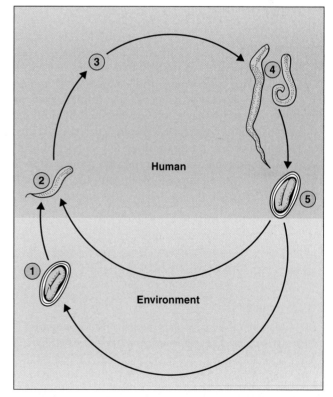

FIGURE 54-3 ■ **Life cycle of the pinworm (*Enterobius vermicularis*).** Humans acquire pinworm infection by the ingestion of embryonated eggs (1). After ingestion the eggs hatch in the small intestine (2), mature to adults in the large intestine (3–4), and produce eggs (5). Because the gravid female lays her eggs in the perianal area, the eggs may be shed into the environment (lower half of diagram) or inadvertently ingested by patients or their close contacts when fingers used to scratch the perianal area are licked or used to prepare food.

DIAGNOSIS AND TREATMENT

Pinworm infection is easy to diagnose using the microscope. The buttocks are gently separated, and a microscope slide covered with Scotch tape (adhesive side out) or its commercially prepared paddle version is placed between them before the patient arises in the morning. Pinworm eggs are large enough to be identified under the microscope using low-power ($\times$ 100) magnification.

Several anthelminthics, including albendazole, mebendazole, and pyrantel pamoate, are effective in the treatment of pinworm infection. Because one untreated person can easily infect others, the entire family must be treated (including relatives who live with or visit the infected child, baby sitters, and other children at the day care center).

Intestinal Nematodes That Penetrate the Skin: Hookworms and *Strongyloides*

Hookworms

Hookworm disease is caused by two species of roundworms: *Necator americanus* and *Ancylostoma duodenale*. Human hookworms penetrate human skin as **filariform larvae** (perhaps best remembered by thinking of them as "filing" their way through the skin). Thus, transmission of the parasites does not require the ingestion of contaminated feces; typically, transmission is through the fecal–cutaneous route, not the fecal–oral route.

Case

Hookworm Infection

V., a 4-year-old boy, underwent a routine medical examination and immunizations after immigrating to the United States from a rural town in a central African country. The physical examination revealed pallor of the conjunctivae, and the examining physician ordered a blood count, which showed a hematocrit of 28%. On a peripheral smear, V.'s erythrocytes were hypochromic and microcytic, suggesting iron deficiency. The astute physician also ordered a stool examination for ova and parasites, which was positive for eggs of *Ancylostoma duodenale,* a hookworm. Treatment of the hookworm infection with mebendazole and the iron supplementation resulted in a return of the hematocrit to 45% at a 3-month follow-up visit.

Case

Strongyloides Infection

Ms. C., a 57-year-old-woman, was hospitalized for her fourth episode of unexplained Gram-negative bacteremia. The only other pertinent medical history was that the patient had recently begun treatment with corticosteroids for asthmatic bronchitis. Paradoxically, her cough worsened with that therapy, and she began to experience abdominal pain and diarrhea. Likewise, the other episodes of bacteremia followed the initiation of steroid therapy.

A resident of Michigan, Ms. C. had lived in rural eastern Kentucky as a child and teenager. She was treated with antibiotics for the organism causing her bacteremia. Because a computerized tomography scan of Ms. C.'s abdomen showed a thickened intestinal wall, she underwent a small intestinal biopsy that revealed the presence of helminthic parasites attached to the mucosa. Subsequently, examination of the patient's stool revealed numerous immature larvae of *Strongyloides stercoralis*. More-developed larvae were identified in the patient's sputum.

These two cases raise several questions:

1. How did these patients acquire adult helminths in their intestinal tracts?
2. Why did V. have anemia while Ms. C. presented with recurrent Gram-negative sepsis?
3. Can these patients transmit their infections to other people?

ENCOUNTER AND ENTRY

People become infected with hookworms by contact with soil contaminated by human stool and subsequently filled with mature filariform larvae. As they penetrate the skin at the time of initial infection, hookworm larvae may cause local manifestations of itching and irritation ("**ground itch**"). In human hookworm infections, dermal manifestations are brief and resolve when the larvae enter the bloodstream and lymphatics. However, people can also become infected with cat and dog hookworm larvae, a condition known as "**creeping eruption**" (or **cutaneous larva migrans**). Unlike those of the human hookworm, the filariform larvae of dog or cat hookworms cannot find their way from the skin into the circulation and instead migrate randomly in the skin until they die. This process can produce an intensely itchy, red, serpentine track around the site of penetration that can persist for weeks.

Human hookworm larvae enter the circulation through the bloodstream or lymphatics, traverse the right side of the heart, and become trapped in the lungs. In the lungs the larvae break through the alveolar wall into the alveolar lumen, are coughed up, and are then swallowed into the gastrointestinal tract where they continue their life cycle (Fig. 54-4), primarily in the duodenum and jejunum. Female worms shed eggs into the stool. If the eggs hatch in a warm environment (usually soil in warmer climates), they yield larvae that mature by molting into the infective filariform larvae. That process requires a significant period of incubation outside the human host. Consequently, transmission of hookworms requires contamination of the soil with untreated human feces and subsequent exposure of unprotected human skin to the larvae that develop from the infected feces. Hookworm infection can be prevented by improved sanitation (using indoor or outdoor toilets or treating feces used for fertilizer) or by wearing shoes. Hookworm infection was common in some areas of the southern United States, where poor sanitary conditions were common until the early part of the last century.

DAMAGE

Hookworms produce chronic anemia by hanging onto the intestinal mucosa with their teeth, secreting an anticoagulant, and sucking the host's blood. That mode of attachment results in a slow, steady blood loss (0.03 mL per worm per day for *Necator americanus*, and 0.15 mL for *Ancylostoma duodenale*). Hookworms affect some 800 million to 900 million people throughout the globe; it has been estimated that the total loss of human blood to hookworms is at least 1 million liters daily. The severity of the anemia is proportional to the worm burden. Severe infections in children can produce chronic anemia, which may lead to developmental retardation.

DIAGNOSIS AND TREATMENT

The adult female hookworm releases 10,000 to 20,000 eggs per day into the bowel lumen, which makes it easy to diagnose significant hookworm infections by stool examination using low-power (× 100) magnification. In fact, it is possible to estimate the number of worms present and the average daily blood loss by quantitating the number of eggs in the stool.

Albendazole, mebendazole, and pyrantel pamoate can be effectively used to treat hookworm infection. Emergency treatment is not required because hookworms produce chronic but not acute or invasive disease. Patients with hookworm disease may require dietary supplementation with iron and folic acid to produce sufficient numbers of red blood cells to correct their anemia.

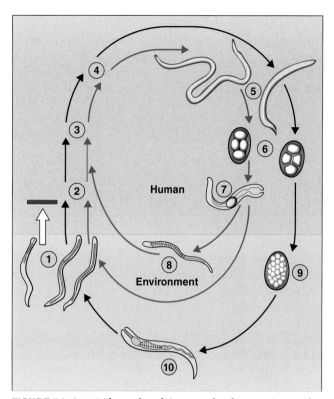

FIGURE 54-4 ▪ Life cycle of *Strongyloides* species and human hookworm. The invasive filariform larvae of these parasites penetrate unbroken human skin (1). Once inside the host, *Strongyloides* and human hookworm larvae migrate through the subcutaneous tissues to the bloodstream (2), enter the lung by crossing into the alveoli (3), travel up the trachea, and are coughed up and swallowed into the gastrointestinal tract (4). In contrast to *Strongyloides* and hookworm, the filariform larvae that cause creeping eruption (the larvae of dog or cat hookworms) are unable to enter the bloodstream and migrate to the lung. Instead, they wander through the subcutaneous tissues causing cutaneous larva migrans. The solid line and open arrow (above and to the left of stage 1) indicate that the larvae of the parasite are unable to complete their normal life cycle in a human host. The larvae of *Strongyloides* and the hookworm mature (5) within the upper gastrointestinal tract. As shown on the right side of the diagram, female hookworm larvae remain within the lumen of the gastrointestinal tract, releasing their eggs into the stool (6), which then pass into the environment (9). Because the female *Strongyloides* larvae enter the bowel wall, their eggs do not appear in the stool (left side of stage 6), and only the larvae (7) are normally found in the stool. Occasionally, the larvae mature to the filariform stage in the gastrointestinal tract (8) to produce endogenous reinfection (autoinfection). Because hookworm larvae require maturation in the environment to become infectious (9,10,1), autoinfection cannot occur in this disease.

Strongyloides stercoralis

Strongyloidiasis is prevalent in tropical areas of the globe but may also be found elsewhere. In large numbers, *Strongyloides stercoralis* worms may cause intestinal malfunction. They can perforate the intestinal wall, resulting in serious bacterial septicemias. In addition, they can reinfect the same host, especially one who is immunocompromised, to produce a lethal systemic disease.

ENCOUNTER AND ENTRY

The life cycle of *Strongyloides* species does not require an external soil phase (see Fig. 54-4). Consequently, in areas of poor sanitation, the worm may be transmitted directly through human feces and regardless of climate and soil temperature. Thus, outbreaks of strongyloidiasis have been reported from institutions for the mentally retarded in temperate zones, from Eskimo settlements north of the Arctic Circle, and from the tropics. In past decades strongyloidiasis was a common infection in the Appalachian region of the United States. Like hookworms, *Strongyloides* infects humans by direct penetration through intact skin. Their route of migration to the intestines is identical to that of hookworms (see Figure 54-4).

DAMAGE

After accessing the general circulation, *S. stercoralis* passes through the lungs, where it can elicit a transient response characterized by coughing, wheezing, and fever. Many people infected with *S. stercoralis* carry only a small number of the worms in the intestine, and few of those people have any clinical manifestations. However, if the worm burden is large, the infection may cause pain, vomiting, and diarrhea when the number of worms becomes large. Those symptoms occur because, unlike the other intestinal roundworms, the female *S. stercoralis* can invade the bowel wall to lay its eggs. That invasion may cause severe disease, because the early **rhabditiform larvae** that hatch from the eggs can cross the intestinal wall into the peritoneum and cause intestinal perforations, permitting intestinal bacteria to follow and producing peritonitis. As a result, strongyloidiasis can produce acute clinical syndromes (such as peritonitis) or mimic chronic abdominal problems such as peptic ulcer or gallbladder disease.

Because the female *S. stercoralis* lays her eggs in the bowel wall instead of the intestinal lumen, the larvae hatch and mature while still in the body. Reinfection may then occur from larval invasion of the perianal skin, even if the patient has not been exposed to new external sources of infection. *Strongyloides* **autoinfection** produces a characteristic snakelike (serpiginous) urticarial rash (**larva currens**), typically located near the anus.

Strongyloides infections may become chronic and produce symptoms for several decades. Persistent infections lasting more than 40 years have been described among former prisoners of war (from World War II). Those individuals often have chronic syndromes that are misdiagnosed as peptic ulcer or gallbladder disease and fail to respond to medical or surgical treatments for those conditions. Patients in whom autoinfection has been controlled can develop urticarial skin lesions from the migration of larvae at the surface of the skin.

In immunocompromised patients, the process of endogenous reinfection may produce a **hyperinfection syndrome** that is sometimes fatal. Ms. C. may have acquired the infection as a youth in rural Kentucky. She apparently maintained an asymptomatic *Strongyloides* infection by the mechanism of autoinfection. With the administration of corticosteroids later in life, the infection was no longer controlled, and she experienced respiratory and abdominal symptoms.

IMMUNOSUPPRESSION AND STRONGYLOIDIASIS

Patients immunosuppressed by malnutrition or drugs have a much greater risk of dissemination and progression to hyperinfection syndrome. In fact, strongyloidiasis is a major cause of death in kidney transplant recipients in the tropics. Presumably, those patients could control the infection before transplantation. However, they become unable to control the infection when their cell-mediated immunity is compromised by the immunosuppressive drugs used to prevent rejection of the transplanted kidney.

Because the hyperinfection syndrome is often seen in patients with impaired cell-mediated immunity, it seems likely that this kind of immunity is the critical factor in the control of strongyloidiasis. The relative role of mononuclear cells and eosinophils is not yet known.

DIAGNOSIS AND TREATMENT

Strongyloidiasis is often difficult to diagnose. Because the worms lay their eggs in the bowel wall, the eggs (which closely resemble hookworm eggs) are rarely found in the stool. It is more typical to diagnose strongyloides by identifying rhabditiform larvae in the stool.

Patients with strongyloidiasis typically have a marked eosinophilia (10 to 20% of white blood cells, more than 10,000 to 20,000 eosinophils per microliter of blood). However, lack of eosinophilia does not exclude the disease. The magnitude of the eosinophilia in persons with the hyperinfection syndrome may be limited by the basic T-cell defects predisposing to the syndrome, the outpouring of neutrophils resulting from secondary bacterial infection, and corticosteroid therapy. Patients thought to have strongyloidiasis should be studied first by stool examination. Even if three or more stool examinations reveal no larvae, examination of the duodenal contents or duodenal biopsy could be positive.

Albendazole and ivermectin are the drugs of choice for strongyloidiasis. Albendazole is thought to act by binding to β-tubulin of the parasite. Ivermectin paralyzes the worms by blocking γ-aminobutyric acid (GABA)–mediated neuromuscular transmission. The drug is nontoxic for humans because GABA-mediated synaptic transmission in mammals is found only in the central nervous system, and ivermectin does not cross the blood-brain barrier.

Intestinal Tapeworms

As the name suggests, tapeworms are long and ribbonlike and are composed of chains of rectangular segments. An individual tapeworm is actually an animal colony, because each segment (known as a **proglottid**) is a self-contained unit capable of reproduction, metabolism, and food uptake (a tapeworm has no common gut). A tapeworm attaches to the intestinal wall by a head (**scolex**) that has sucking discs or grooves (Fig. 54-5). In their intermediate animal host, tapeworms penetrate deep tissues and develop into infective, cystic larval forms.

Case

Mrs. N., the wife of a high-ranking government official, accompanied her husband on a trip to the Near East. During a diplomatic reception they were served steak tartare (highly seasoned raw beef), a traditional dish in that region. Three months later she noticed thin, white, rectangular segments in her stool (approximately 1 × 2 × 0.2 cm). She experienced nausea, apparently brought about by seeing the worms in her stool. Laboratory studies revealed that the segments were proglottids of *Taenia saginata*. The stool also contained eggs of the worm.

Mrs. N.'s physician assured her that the infection was unlikely to have clinical consequences in a healthy person. On the other hand, he could understand her revulsion at seeing the worm segments in her stool and visualizing the rest of the worm inside her. The physician prescribed niclosamide, which eliminated the rest of the tapeworm.

This case raises two questions:

1. How could this infection have been prevented?
2. What would have happened to Mrs. N. had she been given no treatment?

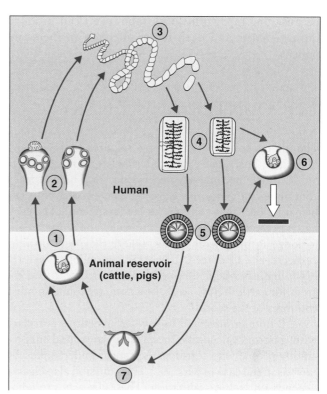

FIGURE 54-5 ▪ Life cycle of intestinal tapeworms *Taenia solium* (pork tapeworm) and *Taenia saginata* (beef tapeworm). Humans acquire intestinal tapeworm infections by ingesting the tissue stage of the parasite (cysticercus) in inadequately cooked meat (1). The parasite then hatches in the intestine (2) and matures to an intestinal tapeworm (3). The pork tapeworm (outside diagram) has a crown of spines on its head and fewer pairs of lateral uterine branches in its proglottids (segments) than the beef tapeworm (4). The eggs of both tapeworm parasites are identical morphologically (5). As shown in the diagram, only the pork tapeworm (*T. solium*) produces human cysticercosis (6). When human feces containing viable eggs are ingested by either pigs or cattle, the eggs hatch (7) and produce the tissue (cysticercal) stage of the infection in those animals (1) to complete the cycle.

The most common human tapeworms are acquired by eating uncooked or inadequately cooked beef (*Taenia saginata*), pork (*Taenia solium*), or fish (*Diphyllobothrium latum*). Tapeworms cause two types of disease:

▪ Intestinal infection (**taeniasis**) is caused by ingestion of larval cysts in undercooked pork, beef, or fish. The clinical picture of intestinal infection is generally mild and is essentially the same for all tapeworms.
▪ Deep tissue infection is caused by ingestion of eggs from the pork tapeworm (cysticercosis) or the canine tapeworm (echinococcosis or cystic hydatid disease). Tissue-invasive infections are discussed in detail in Chapter 55.

The two types of disease are very different and must be distinguished. Unfortunately, confusion is possible because one tapeworm (pork tapeworm) can produce both taeniasis and deep tissue infection in the same patient.

ENCOUNTER AND ENTRY

The life cycle of beef tapeworm requires both humans (definitive host) and cattle (intermediate host) (see Fig. 54-5). Cattle become infected by ingesting human feces containing the parasite's eggs; humans become infected by eating beef that contains larvae (**cysticerci**). The eggs hatch in the intestine of cattle and enter the bloodstream to lodge in peripheral tissues, where they develop into cysticerci (see Chapter 55). Beef tapeworm infection only exists in areas where infected humans defecate in grazing areas for cattle. Those areas, however, are found in most countries of the world.

All human intestinal tapeworm infections correlate with gastronomic preferences: they are found mainly among people who consume their meat undercooked or raw (as in the case of Mrs. N.). Transmission also clearly depends on lack of sanitation. These diseases are common in many parts of the world but are infrequent in western Europe and the United States. Cooking effectively destroys the larvae, but cooks have been known to become infected by tasting raw food during preparation. For example, fish tapeworm infection is said to be an occupational hazard of Jewish or Scandinavian women in the north-central United States who make gefilte fish or lutefisk.

DAMAGE

The infectious tissue larvae from the intermediate host (beef, pork, fish) hatch in the human small intestine and mature into adult tapeworms. The worms can live in the human intestine for several decades and attain lengths of up to 10 meters, which has given rise to the popular but mistaken notion that they increase a person's appetite by consuming a significant amount of their food intake.

Most patients are asymptomatic, but some have nausea, diarrhea, and weight loss. The infection is usually noted only because of the presence of proglottids in the stool. Almost half the people infected with fish tapeworm have **low levels of vitamin B_{12}**, leading to serious megaloblastic anemia. The B_{12} deficiency appears to be the result of competition between the host and the parasite for that vitamin in the diet. The intestinal disease caused by tapeworm is very different from the tissue disease (see Chapter 55).

DIAGNOSIS AND TREATMENT

Most tapeworm infections are readily diagnosed by stool examination. The proglottids are macroscopic and can be seen by the naked eye. The eggs are large enough (31 to 43 μm in diameter) to be seen using low-power ($\times$ 100) magnification. Although the eggs of pork and beef tapeworms are identical, their proglottids can be distinguished by the experienced observer (those of T. *solium* have uteri with fewer pairs of lateral branches).

Most patients (more than 90%) with intestinal tapeworms are cured with a single dose of **niclosamide**. Those who are not cured often have nausea or vomiting with their first treatment and typically respond to a second treatment with the drug. Patients with cysticercosis require a different approach to therapy (see Chapter 55).

Conclusion

Intestinal helminthic infections are usually benign but can cause significant illness if the worm burden is very large. With the exception of *Strongyloides*, helminthic parasites have no capacity to increase their numbers in the infected host. Therefore, the worm burden in infections other than those caused by *Strongyloides* is directly related to the size of the ingested inoculum (or the accumulation of repeated inocula). Because *Strongyloides* infection can be asymptomatic and sustained, the hyperinfection syndrome can occur during immunosuppression decades after the initial exposure.

Tissue and Blood Helminths

Cary Engleberg

key concepts

- Tissue-invasive helminths enter humans by ingestion (*Trichinella spiralis*, or invasive cestodes), penetration through the skin (schistosomes), or arthropod bites (various filariae).

- Trichinosis is maintained by a "cycle of carnivorism" in which predators and scavengers feed on each other and acquire larvae encysted in muscles. Humans usually acquire infection from undercooked meat from pigs or carnivorous game animals. Fever, severe muscle pain, and intense eosinophilia occur when larvae disseminate to human skeletal muscles.

- Invasive cestode infections occur when humans ingest tapeworm eggs (*Taenia solium*, or pork tapeworm, eggs from human feces or *Echinococcus granulosum* eggs from canine feces). Larvae that emerge from ingested eggs migrate to and encyst within the brain (*T. solium*) or in the liver or lungs (*E. granulosum*). Symptoms develop after prolonged infection because of pressure effects of the enlarging cysts or hypersensitivity to released parasite antigens.

- Schistosomiasis is prevalent in geographic areas where (1) fresh surface waters are used for bathing or washing, (2) waters are contaminated with human feces or urine, and (3) certain types of snails are present to host the intermediate stages of the parasite. In humans, adult worms localize to the mesenteric or pelvic veins. The manifestations of disease are caused by the granulomatous reaction to helminth eggs that are trapped in tissues (e.g., intestine, bladder, liver).

- Lymphatic filariasis results from chronic obstruction of lymph channels by adult worms and progressive swelling of extremities or genitals (e.g., elephantiasis). Adult worms are often inapparent in cutaneous filariasis, but their microfilaria (larvae) disseminate subcutaneously and produce chronic hypersensitivity reactions, which can lead to chronic dermatitis or blindness (e.g., onchocerciasis, or "river blindness").

Helminths cause a variety of diseases by establishing residence in deep tissues. As with the intestinal helminths, some are acquired by ingestion and others by penetration of the skin, either by direct entry of the parasites or by insect bites. The diseases they produce almost invariably involve chronic inflammation and thus are caused in part by the host immune response to the parasite. As with the intestinal helminths, when the worm burden is low, infections are rarely symptomatic. Because many worms are long lived in humans, they may gradually accumulate in large numbers as the consequence of repeated encounters. When present in sensitive target organs, helminths can produce severe disease and even death. Helminths that cause deep tissue infections include members of all three helminth groups: roundworms, tapeworms, and flukes (Table 55-1).

table 55-1 Main Tissue and Blood Helminths

EXAMPLES	RESERVOIR	MODE OF TRANSMISSION	CLINICAL MANIFESTATIONS
Acquired by ingestion			
Tapeworms			
Cystic hydatid disease (*Echinococcus granulosus*)	Sheep, cattle, horses	Fecal–oral (eggs)	Tissue-displacing and invasive lesions, most common in liver but seen in lung, CNS, and elsewhere
Cysticercosis (*Taenia solium*)	Pigs	Foodborne	Tissue-displacing lesions, most critical in CNS
Roundworms			
Visceral larva migrans (*Toxocara canis and T. catis*)	Dogs and cats (respectively)	Fecal–oral (eggs)	Systemic illness with malaise, eosinophilia, often enlarged liver and spleen
Trichinosis (*Trichinella spiralis*)	Pigs (and other carnivores)	Ingesting contaminated food	Mild infection produces malaise, mild diarrhea, and periorbital edema; severe infection may be life threatening, with CNS and heart involvement
Guinea worm (*Dracunculus medinensis*)	Infected humans (larvae)	Ingesting contaminated water	Malaise, fever, other systemic symptoms when the adult worm emerges 1 year after initial infection
Flukes			
Lung fluke (*Paragonimus westermani*)	Animals, possibly humans	Ingesting contaminated food (metacercariae in crabs)	Cysts rupture in lung, leading to secondary bacterial infection, chronic bronchitis, and tuberculosis-like picture
Liver fluke (*Clonorchis sinensis*)	Fish, animals, humans	Ingesting contaminated food (metacercariae in freshwater fish)	Often asymptomatic; if worm load is high, can lead to biliary stones, chronic inflammation, and liver cancer
Acquired by passage through the skin			
Blood flukes			
Schistosomes (*Schistosoma mansoni, S. haematobium, S. japonicum, S. mekongi*)	Infected humans	Skin contact with contaminated water (cercariae)	Symptoms vary with the intensity of infection, from asymptomatic to hematuria and bladder cancer (*S. haematobium*), to blood in stool and portal hypertension (*S. mansoni* and *S. japonicum*)
Roundworms			
Cutaneous larva migrans (hookworms of dogs, cats, and other animals)	Dogs, cats	Skin contact with contaminated feces (filariform larvae)	Superficial skin lesions progressing at a rate of 2 cm/day
Filaria			
Lymphatic filariasis (*Wuchereria bancrofti, Brugia malayi*)	Infected humans (larvae)	Mosquito bite	Vary from asymptomatic to massive enlargement of the legs, scrotum, and breasts with recurrent filarial fevers
Onchocerciasis ("river blindness") (*Onchocerca volvulus*)	Infected humans (larvae)	Black fly bite	Subcutaneous nodules (adults), itching (microfilariae); blindness from reaction to microfilariae in the anterior chamber of the eye

CNS, central nervous system.

Tissue Helminths Acquired by Ingestion

The main helminths that invade tissue and are acquired by ingestion are the roundworm *Trichinella spiralis* and the deep tissue–invading tapeworms.

Trichinella spiralis

The presence of *Trichinella spiralis* larvae in the heart, skeletal muscle, brain, or gastrointestinal tract causes trichinosis. Most infected people are asymptomatic and are not seriously ill. Only a few hundred clinically significant cases occur in the United States each year.

Case

Mr. Y., a 45-year-old immigrant from Laos living in Iowa, had been well until a few days after a family celebration that featured a highly seasoned but undercooked pork dish. Two days after the celebration, he developed diarrhea and abdominal pain. About a week after the onset of diarrhea, he developed severe muscle pain, swelling around the eyes, and headache. Physical examination revealed "splinter" hemorrhages in his fingernails. Laboratory studies demonstrated a marked eosinophilia ($12,000/mm^3$). Biopsies of Mr. Y.'s tender muscles and of the splinter hemorrhages revealed *Trichinella spiralis* larvae.

This case raises several questions:

1. How was did Mr. Y. acquire this illness?
2. What caused Mr. Y.'s diarrhea and abdominal pain?
3. Why was his eosinophil count elevated?
4. How could the illness have been prevented?

■ ■ ■ ■

ENCOUNTER AND PATHOBIOLOGY

The life cycle of *T. spiralis* is illustrated in Figure 55-1. After the ingestion of meat containing viable encysted *T. spiralis* (usually undercooked pork), the infective larvae hatch and mature in the small intestine of pigs or humans. After a few days the adult worms release larvae that cross the mucosa to enter the intestinal lymphatics and the bloodstream (producing diarrhea and pain in the process). The larvae are then carried to all parts of the body through the bloodstream. The larvae encyst in striated and cardiac muscle fibers and produce a marked initial inflammatory response. The cysts usually calcify, although the worms can remain viable for up to 30 years. The life cycle of the parasite is completed in nonhuman vertebrates when their muscle (meat) containing viable larvae is eaten by another carnivore. Thus, the propagation of *T. spiralis* infection depends on a "cycle of carnivorism" (Fig. 55-2).

Recently, the incidence of trichinosis has diminished, as judged by the prevalence of *T. spiralis* cysts at autopsy. The figure has decreased from 16% to less than 1% over the last 30 to 40 years, partly because of legislation prohibiting the use of uncooked garbage for feeding pigs, and partly because of increased public awareness about the danger of eating undercooked pork. *T. spiralis* is also found in other carnivorous animals such as wild pigs and bears, including polar bears, and has caused several outbreaks among hunters and in Eskimo communities.

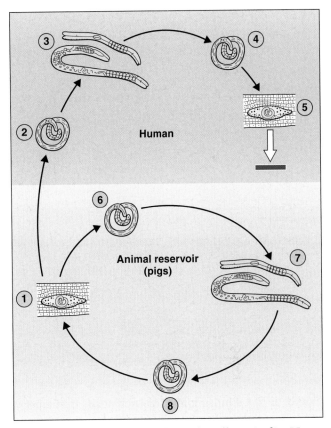

FIGURE 55-1 ■ **Life cycle of *Trichinella spiralis*.** Humans acquire trichinosis by eating undercooked pork containing viable encysted *T. spiralis* larvae (1). After ingestion, the larvae hatch in the intestine (2), mature to adults (3), and release larvae that invade the intestinal wall and enter the bloodstream (4). The larvae then encyst in striated or cardiac muscle (5). As indicated by the open arrow and solid line below stage 5 on the diagram, human infection is normally a dead end in the natural transmission of trichinosis. Similar phenomena are observed in the pig reservoir and in other carnivores that harbor *T. spiralis* larvae (6–8).

The manifestations of trichinosis correlate with the load of worms in tissues and range from asymptomatic to fatal. Several studies suggest that larger inocula (ingestion of many viable larvae) result in more severe disease with a shorter incubation period (2 to 3 days versus 10 days or more). Patients with 1,000 to 5,000 larvae per gram of tissue may die from involvement of the heart or central nervous system. Studies in experimental animals suggest that cell-mediated immunity is important in the control of *T. spiralis* infection.

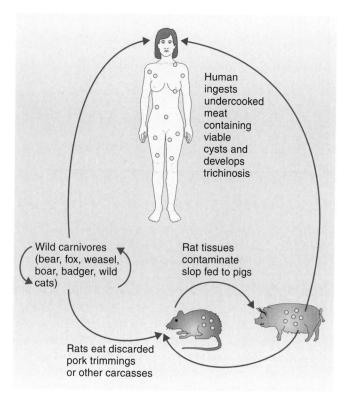

FIGURE 55-2 ■ Epidemiology of trichinosis. In temperate climates the infection is maintained in the food chain of wild carnivores by a "cycle of carnivorism." Carnivorous rodents contaminate garbage that is fed to domestic pigs, and humans become infected by eating undercooked pork or game meats. In arctic climates, indigenous peoples commonly become infected by eating undercooked bear, walrus, or seal meat. In the tropics, bush pigs and warthogs are potential sources.

Diagnosis and Treatment

A rise in antibody titer is diagnostic. However, the increase typically occurs 3 to 4 weeks or more after the initial infection and is thus useless for the management of severely ill patients (in whom the incubation period may be as short as 2 or 3 days). In severely ill patients like Mr. Y., muscle biopsy often reveals *T. spiralis* larvae under low-power (× 100) magnification and permits a definitive diagnosis long before serologic testing.

Treatment of trichinosis is problematic. In the early stages of infection, antihelminthic drugs (albendazole, mebendazole) are useful because they kill adult parasites in the intestine and may prevent ongoing production of invasive larvae. In contrast, antihelminthic agents are of little therapeutic value against the encysted larval forms and may actually provoke symptoms. Bed rest and anti-inflammatory agents (such as aspirin) are most useful for controlling symptoms. Corticosteroids have been used for their anti-inflammatory effects in severely ill patients with myocarditis and/or encephalitis.

Cases

Cysticercosis

Ms. F., a 33-year-old nurse, had been a Peace Corps volunteer in Thailand 10 years earlier. While in Thailand she had occasionally passed tapeworm segments (proglottids) in her stool, but she was never treated. Eight years after her return to the United States, Ms. F. developed multiple subcutaneous nodules across her chest and arms and began having headaches. After two generalized seizures, she was brought to the emergency room. A computerized tomography (CT) scan of her brain revealed numerous lesions consistent with cysticerci (tapeworm larvae). After treatment with praziquantel, Ms. F.'s headaches worsened. She then received corticosteroids to reduce brain swelling and antiepileptic drugs to control her seizures, and she was able to complete the praziquantel treatment. One year later Ms. F. was withdrawn from the antiepileptics and had no additional seizures.

Echinococcosis

A 39-year-old Navajo sheep farmer living in Arizona, Ms. K. was examined for abdominal pain. Two years previously she had first noticed a sensation of fullness in the right upper quadrant of her abdomen. Since then the sensation has increased, and she now has an obvious swelling (8 × 10 cm) in the area of the liver. Stool examination revealed no tapeworm eggs. A CT scan of the liver revealed a large (12-cm diameter) encapsulated lesion consistent with a hydatid cyst. Serologic testing revealed antibodies against *Echinococcus granulosus*. Because of the size of the liver lesion, the mass was removed surgically, using liquid nitrogen to freeze it and prevent its contents from spilling into the peritoneum.

These two cases raise several questions:

1. How did the two patients acquire their infections?
2. Why did Ms. F. have an intestinal tapeworm at some point but Ms. K. did not?
3. Can these patients be treated and cured?

Infections by Tissue Forms of Tapeworms

The larvae of a few species of tapeworms infect deep tissues of humans and cause diseases that may have severe manifestations. Illness caused by the tissue form of the pork tapeworm is known as **cysticercosis**; that illness caused by tapeworms of canines is known as **echinococcosis**. The life cycle of *Echinococcus* species is illustrated in Figure 55-3.

Encounter

Human **cysticercosis** is acquired by ingesting *Taenia solium* eggs from the feces of humans who harbor an

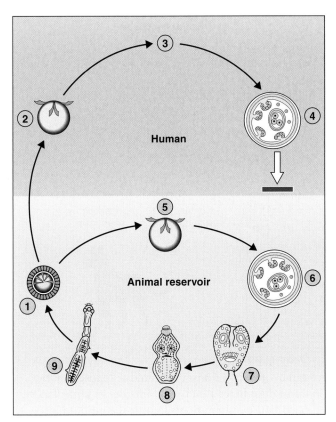

FIGURE 55-3 ▪ Life cycle of *Echinococcus* species.
Humans acquire infection by ingesting eggs in the feces of infected carnivores, such as dogs or wolves (1). After ingestion, the eggs hatch in the intestine (2). The larvae cross from the gastrointestinal tract to the tissues (3), where they develop into cysts containing daughter cysts and scolices (heads) from which tapeworms can develop under the appropriate circumstance (4). As indicated by the open arrow and solid line below step 4, this infection is a dead end in humans. However, domestic animals (e.g., sheep and goats) may acquire infection by grazing in fecally contaminated pastures (see Figure 55-4). The tissue cysts that develop in the animals are identical to those in humans (5–6), but when the animals eventually die in the pasture (often from unrelated causes), dogs or wolves may eat their remains and ingest the tissue cysts. In the canine intestine, the ingested heads (scolices) may develop into adult tapeworms (7–9), which eventually produce eggs (1) to complete the cycle.

adult tapeworm. The egg hatches into an invasive larva after passing through the acidic stomach. Occasionally, cysticercosis develops endogenously in a person who carries a tapeworm (by autoinfection with their own feces or by regurgitation of intestinal tapeworm eggs into the stomach). Endogenous infection may have been what happened to Ms. F.

The life cycle of *T. solium* requires that pigs become infected by ingesting the eggs of the parasite and that hu-

mans eat inadequately cooked pork (analogous to the beef tapeworm life cycle; Fig. 55-4). Conditions permitting this cycle to occur exist in many areas of the developing world. In Mexico as many as 15% of persons hospitalized for neurologic problems show evidence of central nervous system cysticercosis at autopsy.

Echinococcosis, or **cystic hydatid disease,** is found in most areas of the world, including the United States. *Echinococcus* infections are acquired by ingesting infectious eggs, rather than tissue cysticerci. The usual source of *Echinococcus granulosus* is the feces of dogs or other carnivores (e.g., wolves, coyotes). Thus, transmission is by the fecal–oral route, not by eating contaminated meat. The eggs hatch in the small intestine but do not reside there. Rather, they penetrate the intestinal wall and form so-called **hydatid cysts** in many organs.

The life cycle of *Echinococcus* species is maintained between sheep and sheep-herding dogs in the southwestern United States (see Fig. 55-4). Native Americans who keep sheep in that region are sometimes victims of the *E. granulosus* infection. A "sylvatic" cycle is also present in the northern United States and Alaska, with wolves as the carnivores and elk and other large game as the herbivores. *Echinococcus multilocularis* is an analogous parasite in colder climates, for which foxes and cats are the carnivore hosts and mice and voles are the herbivores.

PATHOBIOLOGY

The sequence of events in echinococcosis and cysticercosis is generally similar. The parasites lodge under the skin or within internal organs, such as the brain or liver, and develop a cyst wall surrounded by a fibrous capsule of host origin. In echinococcosis the hydatid cysts are lined internally by a germinal membrane that generates numerous embryonic tapeworm heads (each of which has the potential to develop into a tapeworm in the canine intestine). Most hydatid cysts occur in the liver or the lung. They usually produce few symptoms until they reach 8 to 10 cm or more in diameter, which may take years or even decades. The growing mass may produce symptoms by compression of vital structures, or the cysts may leak or rupture and pose a significant risk of death from anaphylactic reactions.

Tapeworm larvae (cysticerci) each contain only one potential tapeworm head. The cysts are generally more numerous than hydatid cysts but rarely grow larger than 1 or 2 cm. When a cyst dies, its contents leak into the surrounding tissues and induce a host inflammatory response. Cysts outside the central nervous system rarely produce symptoms. However, even small cysticerci in the brain can cause cerebral dysfunction, including seizures, increased intracranial pressure, and blindness. Cysticerci thus provide a good example of the correlation between the location and the severity of a disease. Cysticerci may

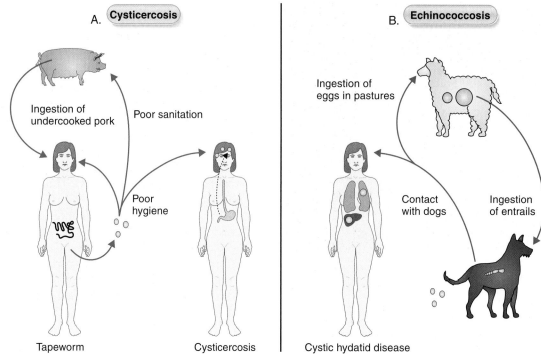

A. Cysticercosis

Ingestion of
undercooked pork

Poor sanitation

Poor
hygiene

Tapeworm   Cysticercosis

B. Echinococcosis

Ingestion of
eggs in pastures

Contact
with dogs

Ingestion
of entrails

Cystic hydatid disease

FIGURE 55-4 ▪ **Comparative epidemiology of two tissue-invasive tapeworm infections: cysticercosis (caused by the pork tapeworm _Taenia solium_) and echinococcosis, or cystic hydatid disease (caused by _Echinococcus granulosus_). A.** In pork tapeworm, the definitive host is the human, not the pig, because only humans harbor the adult tapeworms. Pigs are an intermediate host, since they develop only the tissue invasive form of infection (cysticercosis) after ingestion of eggs from feces of infected humans. Humans also develop the tissue-invasive stage of infection after ingesting eggs from human feces. Although tapeworm carriers can infect themselves with eggs from their own feces, many humans acquire cysticercosis directly by ingestion of fecally contaminated food and never actually harbor tapeworms themselves. **B.** The definitive host for the tapeworm that causes echinococcosis is the canine (dog, wolf, or fox). Intermediate hosts that harbor the tissue-invasive forms become infected by ingesting eggs from canine feces. In humans tissue-invasive disease with either tapeworm is considered a dead-end infection, since humans are rarely cannibalized (to complete the _Taenia_ life cycle), and human remains are buried or incinerated in most cultures (making completion of the echinococcal life cycle improbable).

cause symptoms when the parasites die and displacement of normal tissue is magnified by the host inflammatory response. That typically occurs 5 to 10 years after infection, but symptoms may not become apparent until as much as 50 years after the initial infection.

DIAGNOSIS AND TREATMENT

Because cysticerci can be present in patients without evidence of intestinal infection, _T. solium_ cysticercosis is usually diagnosed by its deep tissue manifestations (including lesions visible by CT scan or by a "soft" radiographic technique in the long axes of skeletal muscles). A positive serologic test for antibodies to _T. solium_ is helpful, especially among persons who live in Europe, the United States, or other areas of low incidence. The test is typically negative in persons with intestinal _T. solium_ infection only.

Praziquantel and albendazole are both effective in the treatment of cysticercosis. Drug treatment kills the organism and decreases the size of the lesions. The fluid-filled cysts collapse, and the parasite is ultimately resorbed by the host or calcified. During treatment, central nervous system symptoms may transiently worsen because of the inflammatory response to dying cysticerci. As with Ms. F., the concomitant use of steroids typically alleviates the headaches and seizures that the treatment can cause.

The antihelminthic drug albendazole administered over a period of weeks can kill growing echinococcal cysts as well. Alternatively, surgical removal of a large cyst can cure the infection, although great care must be taken to avoid spillage and dissemination of the infection. For the same reason, it is unwise to attempt blind needle aspiration of a cystic structure that may be a hydatid cyst. Nevertheless, and despite the potential hazard of needle puncture, procedures for aspiration of cysts have been developed that are safe and effective. Quite often patients with echinococ-

FIGURE 55-5 ▪ **Abdominal computerized tomography scan of an asymptomatic 55-year-old Lebanese woman.** The patient was scheduled to have surgery for an unrelated problem. A routine, preoperative chest radiograph showed a large calcified mass. The CT scan shows two large calcified structures in the liver that represent dead hydatid cysts (arrow).

cosis are discovered after their cysts have died. In those cases the cysts appear calcified in radiographs or CT scans, and no treatment is needed (Fig. 55-5).

Tissue Helminths That Penetrate Through the Skin

Two types of helminths enter the host through the skin: worms that can cross the skin directly (the schistosomes, or blood flukes), and those that penetrate via insect bites (the filariae, which are members of the roundworms).

Schistosomes

Case

Schistosoma mansoni Infection

Ms. U., a 48-year-old woman from Egypt, had noticed for many years that she had dark stools. During the past year she had two episodes of vomiting blood. Examination of her esophagus and stomach with a fiberoptic gastroscope revealed dilated veins in the esophagus that were oozing large amounts of blood. Because viable eggs of *Schistosoma mansoni* were found in her stool, she was treated with praziquantel.

Case

Schistosoma hematobium Infection

Born and raised in Europe, Mr. G., 38 years old, had worked in West Africa for 10 years on a rice-growing irrigation scheme. During the past year he noticed blood in his urine. Under the microscope his urine showed the presence of *Schistosoma hematobium* eggs. At cystoscopy his bladder had a cobblestone pattern, consistent with the granulomatous changes seen in schistosomiasis. Typical eggs were seen in the bladder biopsies taken during cystoscopy. He was treated with a single dose of praziquantel.

These cases raise two questions:

1. What caused the granulomatous changes associated with these infections?
2. Why was infection with *S. mansoni* associated with bleeding from the stomach whereas *S. hematobium* was associated with blood in the urine?

Schistosomiasis is an important and common disease in tropical regions. It is estimated that about 200 million to 300 million people are infected worldwide. Schistosomiasis produces a variety of clinical syndromes, depending on the anatomic location of the adult worms and the eggs they release. The three main pathogenic species of the genus *Schistosoma*—*S. haematobium*, *S. mansoni*, and *S. japonicum*—are mostly found in warm climates. However, each species has a unique geographic distribution that depends on the presence of the snail intermediate host (Fig. 55-6). The schistosomal life cycle is illustrated in Figure 55-7.

ENCOUNTER AND PATHOBIOLOGY

The life cycle of schistosomes requires development in certain species of freshwater snails, which are their intermediate hosts. The infective stage of the parasite emerges from the snails and swims in water until it finds a suitable host. Because these snails are not present in the United States, schistosomiasis cannot be transmitted in the United States, despite the migration of infected persons from Africa and the Middle East. Suitable snails are present in parts of the Caribbean.

The infective forms released from the snails are called cercariae. They are capable of burrowing through the skin of people standing, swimming, or walking in infected water, like the rice paddies in which Mr. G. worked. In the human body the cercariae lose their tails and change into forms called schistosomulae, which can enter the bloodstream. The parasites then pass through the pulmonary circulation to the portal venous system, where they mature. After several weeks,

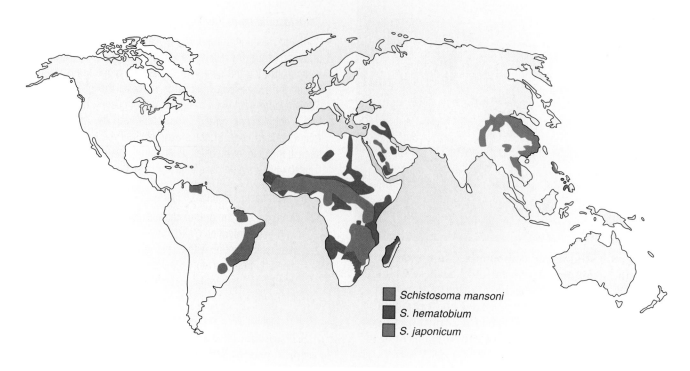

FIGURE 55-6 ▪ Geographical distribution of human schistosomiasis.

pairs of male and female adults move to the venous plexuses of the large intestine (*S. mansoni*), small intestine (*S. japonicum*), or bladder (*S. hematobium*). The mating worms remain locked together, copulating in the venous system for 10 years or more. The eggs they release may be excreted via the stool (*S. mansoni, S. japonicum*) or the urine (*S. hematobium*). The life cycle is completed when the eggs are released into fresh water, where they hatch and penetrate the appropriate snail intermediate host.

S. *mansoni* and *S. japonicum* adult worms reside in the venous plexuses of the intestine. There they release eggs that migrate to the intestine and the liver. Eggs trapped in host tissues induce the formation of granulomas (Fig. 55-8A). The granulomas eventually undergo fibrosis. Over many years of infection, that process results in the pathological changes of schistosomiasis, such as periportal fibrosis in the liver (Fig. 55-8B), which can lead to portal hypertension and thus to dilated collateral veins in the esophagus (esophageal varices, as in the case of Ms. U.). *S. hematobium* adults live in the venous plexus of the urinary bladder and produce blood in the urine (hematuria), granulomatous inflammatory changes in the bladder, and sometimes bladder carcinoma. Fibrotic changes in the bladder and ureters can cause ureterovesical obstruction and recurrent secondary bacterial infections of the bladder, leading occasionally to Gram-negative septicemia.

As in other helminthic infections that invade the tissues, eosinophilia and elevated IgE levels are common in

persons with schistosomiasis. Two important anomalous host–parasite interactions are central to the pathogenesis of schistosomiasis:

▪ Profound fibrotic reactions to schistosome eggs, probably mediated by cytokines, account for the important pathology of the disease and its long-term complications.

▪ Lack of an effective immune response to the male and female adult worms, which can reside in the vascular system for decades without being eliminated by the host. Studies have shown that adult worms adsorb host proteins (including serum albumin and HLA antigens) on their surfaces. Essentially, the parasite camouflages itself with those host proteins to evade the host immune response.

Cercariae often produce itching as they penetrate the skin. The cercariae of nonhuman schistosomes (of birds and fish) also cause itching as they penetrate the skin (swimmers' itch, clam diggers' itch), but do not enter the bloodstream or mature within the human body.

DIAGNOSIS AND TREATMENT

Most schistosome infections are diagnosed readily by microscopic examination of stool (*S. mansoni, S. japonicum*) or urine (*S. hematobium*) or by biopsy of a rectal

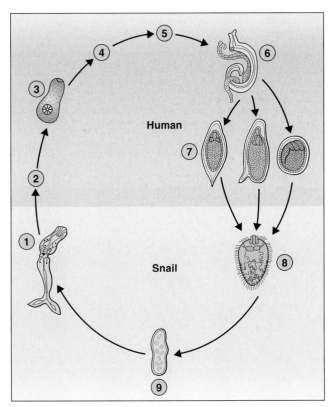

FIGURE 55-7 ▪ **Life cycle of *Schistosoma* species.** Humans acquire schistosomiasis by exposure of unprotected skin to water containing infectious cercariae (1). The cercariae penetrate unbroken skin (2), lose their tails, and become schistosomulae (3). They then travel throughout the bloodstream, cross the lungs (4), and mature (5) in the venous system of the liver to adult worms (6). After a period of 6 to 8 weeks, pairs of adult worms travel to the venous plexuses of the bladder (*S. haematobium*), the large intestine (*S. mansoni*), or the small intestine (*S. japonicum*), where they remain for decades releasing their characteristic eggs (7, left to right: *S. hematobium*, *S. mansoni*, and *S. japonicum*). Eggs released into fresh water hatch to miracidia (8), which invade the snail intermediate host where they mature to sporocysts (9). They then release cercariae (1) to complete the cycle.

valve (*S. mansoni*). Schistosome eggs are large enough (90 to 210 μm) to be identified easily under the microscope with low-power (× 100) magnification. Unfortunately, it can be difficult to find schistosome eggs in the stool or urine of patients who are chronically infected and at risk of developing long-term complications. In such patients, serologic testing for antischistosomal antibodies may be valuable. However, a positive serologic test does not distinguish between recent and old or mild and severe infections. Serologic testing is most useful in people who have had single, defined exposures in

FIGURE 55-8 ▪ **Liver sections from patients infected with *Schistosoma* species. A.** *S. japonicum* infection shows egg granulomas in two portal areas. **B.** "Pipe stem" fibrosis of the portal tracts characteristic of schistosomiasis.

endemic areas. It is of little use for lifelong residents of endemic areas because most are seropositive but not all experience complications.

Praziquantel is the treatment of choice for schistosomiasis. The drug exerts its lethal action by increasing the calcium permeability of the parasite. Drug treatment eliminates the production of eggs by killing the adult worms, but the fibrosis associated with chronic infection is not reversible. Disrupting any point in the parasitic life cycle can prevent schistosomiasis. Potentially effective public health measures and their rationales are shown in Table 55-2.

table 55-2	Control of Human Schistosomiasis
RATIONALE	**METHOD OF CONTROL**
Reduce carriers	Mass treatment program
Eliminate snail hosts	Molluscicides Destroy snail habitats Snail-eating fish
Prevent contamination of water	Provide latrines, sewage systems Public health education
Prevent human exposure	Provide clean water systems for washing, bathing, drinking, and recreation

Case

Onchocerciasis

Mr. L. is 32 years old and lives in a small Nigerian village near a rapidly running stream where men fish and hunt. Like many of his neighbors, Mr. L. began to lose his vision in his late twenties. He was prompted to go to a hospital in a nearby town for an evaluation because he had three nodules (2 × 3 × 2 cm) on his trunk. Skin snips revealed microfilariae of *Onchocerca volvulus*. He was treated with a single oral dose of ivermectin.

■ ■ ■ ■

Filaria

The main filarial infections in humans are onchocerciasis ("river blindness") and lymphatic filariasis (elephantiasis). In onchocerciasis the adult filarial worms live in subcutaneous tissue; in lymphatic filariasis the adult larvae live in lymphatic tissue. Their offspring, known as microfilariae, travel through the subcutaneous tissue or circulate in the blood. Some 50 million persons in Africa, Asia, and tropical Latin America have onchocerciasis. Unless they are treated, about 10% of those infected will become blind from the disease, and approximately 30% will have visual impairments. In some West African villages most people become blind from onchocerciasis by the time they reach adulthood. Lymphatic filariasis affects approximately 200 million people in tropical regions, especially in Asia. The disease leads to tissue swelling, sometimes to elephantine proportions (hence the name elephantiasis). Neither disease is endemic in the United States. The life cycle of filariae is illustrated in Figure 55-9.

Case

Lymphatic Filariasis

Mr. J., a 48-year-old native of a Philippine island, lived in a village where many men and women had elephantiasis. He first noticed swelling of his right leg when he was 20 years old. Subsequently, he had intermittent fevers as high as 39.0°C and red streaks from his groin to the foot on each leg. By the time Mr. J. went to a hospital for examination, both feet and his scrotum were chronically swollen. Typical microfilariae consistent with *Wuchereria bancrofti* were seen in a Giemsa-stained blood smear taken at 2:00 AM. His recurrent episodes of lymphangitis were treated with an antimicrobial effective against streptococci. The antifilarial drug diethylcarbamazine was given but discontinued when it produced shock and hypotension.

These cases raise two questions:

1. Why did Mr. L. became blind while Mr. J. developed swelling?
2. How did these patients acquire the infections?

■ ■ ■ ■

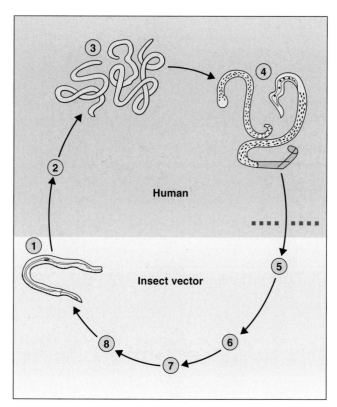

FIGURE 55-9 ■ **Life cycle of filariae (*Onchocerciasis*, lymphatic filariasis).** Humans acquire infection with the filariae that cause onchocerciasis or elephantiasis from the bite of black flies or mosquitos, respectively. After third-stage larvae (1) are injected under the skin by the vector, the larvae mature (2) to adult worms (3) that release microfilariae in the subcutaneous tissue (onchocerciasis) or in lymphatics (lymphatic filariasis; 4). Microfilariae ingested by the insect vector during feeding mature through a series of stages (5–8) to infectious third-stage larvae (1) within approximately 2 weeks.

ENCOUNTER AND PATHOBIOLOGY

The regional distribution of the vectors and infected human reservoirs limits the geographic distribution of filarial diseases. Onchocerciasis is transmitted by *Simulium* black flies, and lymphatic filariasis is transmitted by mosquitoes. Neither infection is transmitted within the United States; no reservoir of infected humans serves as a source of infection for susceptible insect vectors, and in the case of onchocerciasis, no *Simulium* flies exist to become infected. With both diseases filarial larvae enter the host during a bite by an infected insect.

The typical manifestations of lymphatic filariasis are low-grade fever and inflammation of lymphatics and lymph nodes induced by the adult worms (usually in the inguinal or pelvic nodes). With repeated episodes the lymphatics become occluded and fluids leak into tissues, producing severe swelling. After many years the lower limbs and the scrotum may swell to gigantic size. The diurnal cycle observed in lymphatic filariasis facilitates transmission because the microfilariae are more prevalent in the bloodstream at night, when mosquitoes bite more frequently.

In contrast, the microfilariae of onchocerciasis and other skin-dwelling filariae invade the subcutaneous tissues, where a biting fly can acquire them to continue the life cycle. The adult *Onchocerca* worms congregate in a subcutaneous nodule and, like adult schistosomes, are invisible to the host immune system. Females released by the adult female worms are disseminated under the skin in all directions from a mature nodule. The pathology of the disease is caused by a type III hypersensitivity reaction to antigens released from dying microfilariae (see Chapter 7). Thus, the clinical manifestations include chronic dermatitis and loss of eyesight (caused by nodules on the head with migration of microfilariae into the anterior chamber of the eye).

DIAGNOSIS AND TREATMENT

Infections that release microfilariae into the bloodstream (lymphatic filariasis) are diagnosed by examining smears of peripheral blood. The microfilariae may be scarce and difficult to find. The sensitivity of the method can be increased by lysing red blood cells and concentrating the remainder of the specimen and by sampling blood at night for microfilariae with nocturnal periodicity (e.g., with *Wuchereria bancrofti*). Onchocerciasis is diagnosed by examining for microfilariae in a superficial "skin snip." In all these specimens, microfilariae are identified with Giemsa stain under the high-dry or oil immersion objectives. Recent studies suggest that antigen detection using antifilarial antibodies may be a more sensitive and convenient method.

The treatment for lymphatic filariasis is less than ideal. The drugs diethylcarbamazine and ivermectin reduce the number of circulating microfilariae but do not eliminate the adult worms. In any form of filariasis, diethylcarbamazine can produce systemic reactions, presumably resulting from the sudden release of filaria antigens from damaged microfilariae (as in Mr. J.'s case). In heavy infections with *Onchocerca*, diethylcarbamazine

can cause severe reactions, including sudden blindness, vascular collapse, or even death. Ivermectin is less likely to produce those effects and is the preferred treatment for severe disease. This drug has been used in preemptive mass treatment campaigns in parts of the world where there is significant morbidity and blindness. Surgical resection of subcutaneous nodules in onchocerciasis removes the source of microfilariae and may thus decrease the risk of blindness. However, it is impossible to be sure that all nodules have been removed because they are often in deep tissue and not palpable.

A recent observation that *W. bancrofti* adult worms require colonization by a natural symbiont, *Wolbachia*, to maintain normal health and fertility has raised the possibility of treating the parasite infection by eradicating the symbiont. The *Wolbachia* bacteria are similar to rickettsiae and are susceptible to tetracycline. Initial trials treating *W. bancrofti* infection with tetracycline have shown promising results. It is still too early to say whether this approach will be useful for other treatment-resistant parasites.

Prevention of filarial diseases relies mainly on vector control. Unfortunately, the flies that transmit onchocerciasis breed in clean, fast-running streams and rivers. Although they can be controlled readily with insecticides, effective spraying may be difficult in those areas.

Conclusion

Tissue-invasive helminths are a diverse group of pathogens with distinct and complex life cycles. To diagnose and treat infections of these parasites, it is essential to know where they reside within the human host and which tissues, body fluids, or excreta harbor the characteristic eggs or larvae. Antihelminthic drugs are active against the parasites; however, infections of long duration with high worm burdens can produce chronic, fibrotic changes that are irreversible with treatment. To control infections in endemic regions, it is necessary to understand the parasitic life cycles and to know what environmental conditions, vectors, or intermediate hosts enable the tissue-invasive parasites to deliver their progeny from one human to the next.

chapter **56**

Prion Diseases

C. Alan Anderson and Kenneth L. Tyler

key **concepts**

Prion diseases:

■ Are transmitted by a pathologic isoform of a protein that causes a conformational change in the related normal host protein. The process occurs primarily in the central nervous system.

■ Usually present with dementia, abnormal movements, ataxia, and neuropsychiatric features.

■ Occur as sporadic, iatrogenic, hereditary, and transmissible diseases.

■ Are diagnosed by clinical features and neuropathological findings.

■ Are uniformly fatal.

Prion diseases are rare, fatal, rapidly progressive neurodegenerative diseases that occur in humans and other animal species. In all species they share common and recognizable neuropathologic features, namely the presence of small vacuoles within the neuropil, which produces a **spongiform** appearance, neuronal loss, and glial cell proliferation, which occur in the absence of an inflammatory response. These features were first recognized in a fatal neurodegenerative disease of sheep, called **scrapie.** As the prototype for prion diseases, scrapie was shown to be a transmissible disorder in the 1930s when the disease was successfully passed from a sheep to a goat. Because of the very long incubation period, measured in months or years, researchers originally thought that prion diseases were caused by "slow virus" infection.

Subsequently, a human disorder with similar neuropathology was observed among the Fore people of Papua New Guinea. Known as **kuru,** the disorder was thought to be transmitted by a form of ritual cannibalism that involved eating the brains of deceased relatives. Consistent with the notion that the ingestion of human neural tissue transmitted the disease, kuru has disappeared now that the cannibalistic rituals have been discontinued. However, the spongiform histopathologic changes seen in brains of kuru victims resemble another established neurodegenerative disease that occurs worldwide, Creutzfeldt-Jakob disease (CJD). Since the 1930s CJD has occurred both sporadically and in familial clusters. However, cases of iatrogenic transmission among humans through contaminated neurosurgical instruments, surgical grafts of dura mater, injections of human pituitary extracts, or even corneal transplantation also have been documented. In the late 1960s both kuru and CJD were transmitted from humans to chimpanzees, confirming that both are associated with a transmissible agent. The most puzzling aspect of the disorders is the absence of any appreciable nucleic acid in the material capable of transmitting the diseases.

Prion diseases are now known to be associated with the accumulation in the central nervous system of an abnormal form of a host protein called the prion protein (PrP). The "infectious agent" is not a virus but rather an abnormally folded, degradation-resistant form of the PrP protein. Several prion diseases have been identified in animal species (Table 56-1). In addition, five human prion diseases are currently recognized (see the box titled "Human Prion Diseases"). Although all are theoretically transmissible under appropriate circumstances, only kuru and variant CJD among the human diseases are thought to be predominantly acquired exogenously—that is, by ingestion of or contact with the prion protein from another human (kuru) or animal (CJD) source.

Prions

The term *prion*, (pronounced "pree-on" and derived from "proteinaceous infectious particle") refers to a

Human Prion Diseases

Kuru
Creutzfeldt-Jakob disease (CJD)
Variant Creutzfeldt-Jakob disease (variant CJD)
Gerstmann-Straussler-Scheinker syndrome (GSS)
Fatal familial insomnia (FFI)

small infectious agent that consists of protein but lacks nucleic acid. A host protein, PrP, appears to be the sole constituent of prions. The gene encoding PrP is found in the genomes of all humans and animals. It is expressed in most human tissues, with the highest levels in the central nervous system. Recent studies suggest that PrP is a copper-binding protein that may be involved in the cellular response to oxidative stress. It also might play a role in long-term memory. The pathological protease-resistant form of PrP isolated from the brains of animals with scrapie has been designated PrP^{Sc} (PrP^{Sc} also refers to the conformationally altered isoform of PrP in other prion diseases besides scrapie). Transgenic mice that cannot make PrP cannot develop prion disease, indicating that host PrP must be present for the development of illness.

Prion diseases appear to result from the **accumulation of abnormal isoforms of PrP**, which relies on the conversion of normal PrP into PrP^{Sc}. That conversion is not a chemical modification but a **conformational change in PrP** from a predominantly α-helical form to one that contains predominantly β-sheet. In the sporadic forms of prion disease (e.g., most cases of Creutzfeldt-Jakob disease), the first molecule of PrP^{Sc} seems to appear spontaneously, triggering the conversion of other PrP molecules to PrP^{Sc}, resulting in the assembly of long strands of polymerized proteins, or **amyloid** fibrils (Fig. 56-1). That process may be analogous to crystallization in solution in which a single seed crystal serves as a nidus for the continued growth of the crystal. A conformational change in PrP appears to be the necessary pathogenic first step in all forms of illness.

A common polymorphism (valine or methionine) at codon 129 in PrP appears to play an important role in determining susceptibility to acquiring prion disease. Most patients with sporadic and iatrogenic CJD, and all patients reported to date with variant CJD, are homozygous for methionine at codon 129. This polymorphism may influence other features of prion disease, including incubation time and clinical features of the illness. Other polymorphisms or inherited mutations in PrP explain how prion diseases may be sporadic (by spontaneous PrP to PrP^{Sc} conversion), heritable (by enhanced conversion because of an unfavorable, inherited PrP allele), or transmissible (by exogenous acquisition of PrP^{Sc}).

table 56-1   Animal Prion Diseases

DISEASE	ANIMALS AFFECTED
Bovine spongiform encephalopathy	Cattle
Scrapie	Sheep and goats
Chronic wasting disease	Deer and elk
Transmissible mink encephalopathy	Farmed mink
Feline spongiform encephalopathy	Zoological and domestic cats
Transmissible spongiform encephalopathy	Zoological ruminants and nonhuman primates

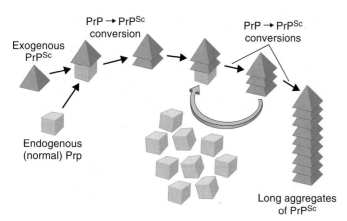

FIGURE 56-1 ■ One possible model for the conversion of normal PrP to PrP^{Sc} with subsequent polymerization and accumulation of amyloid.

Creutzfeldt-Jakob Disease

Sporadic and Iatrogenic CJD

EPIDEMIOLOGY AND ENCOUNTER

Prion diseases are rare, but CJD is the most common human prion disease, with an incidence of roughly one case per 1 million population worldwide each year. Its occurrence is mostly sporadic (90 to 95%), but familial clusters of CJD have been described. Men and women are at equal risk. The age at onset of disease is usually between 55 and 65 years, although rare cases of patients under 30 and over 80 years of age have been described. In the 1990s the appearance in Great Britain of numerous patients in their twenties led physicians to conclude that a variant of CJD was emerging.

ENTRY

In sporadic prion disease, spontaneous conversion of PrP to PrP^{Sc} is assumed to set in motion a continuous refolding and polymerization of normal PrP. Thus, no "entry" actually occurs. However, rare cases of iatrogenic CJD are associated with inoculation of PrP^{Sc} directly into the central nervous system. That may occur with corneal transplants, liver transplants, cadaveric human pituitary hormone, dural graft transplants, and the use of contaminated neurosurgical instruments or stereotactic depth electrodes.

Case

Mr. I., a 22-year-old native of England who had lived in Florida for 10 years, sought medical attention in November 2001 for depression and memory loss that was interfering with his work performance. He was referred to a psychologist for his complaints. However, in December he developed involuntary muscle movement, difficultly walking and dressing, and incontinence. In January 2002 he went to a local emergency room where a computerized tomography scan of the brain was found to be normal, and he was treated for an anxiety attack.

Later that month, at his mother's urging, Mr. I. returned to the family home in England. By then his symptoms had worsened: he experienced falls and could not shower or dress himself, recall his home phone number, or do simple arithmetic. An evaluation for variant Creutzfeldt-Jakob disease (CJD) was conducted: an electroencephalogram was normal, and magnetic resonance imaging of the brain showed high signal intensity in the pulvinar and thalamus bilaterally. Subsequently, a tonsil biopsy was performed. Tonsillar tissue was examined by immunoblotting and immunohistochemical staining for the protease-resistant form of prion protein (PrP^{Sc}). Both were positive and consistent with variant CJD. Sequencing of the patient's PrP genes showed homozygosity for methionine at position 129 but no mutations. Mr. I. had no history of transfusions, transplants, or major surgery.

In spite of an attempt at experimental therapy with quinacrine, the patient's decline continued. By September 2002 he was bedridden and unable to eat or communicate. (Adapted from Centers for Disease Control and Prevention. Probable variant Creutzfeldt-Jakob disease in a U.S. resident—Florida, 2002. Morb Mortal Wkly Rep. 2002; 51(41):927–929.)

This case raises several questions:

1. What features of Mr. I.'s case are characteristic of variant CJD?
2. How and when did he acquire the disease?
3. Should he be isolated to prevent transmission of the disease to others?
4. What are his chances for recovery?

A discussion of the circumstance and expression of Mr. I.'s case of variant CJD requires an understanding of how the sporadic form of Creutzfeldt-Jakob disease arises.

SPREAD, MULTIPLICATION, AND DAMAGE

The incubation period for sporadic CJD is unknown. In the case of iatrogenic disease, a better estimate is possible based on the timing of the inciting event (e.g., dural graft placement or initiation of hormonal therapy). One study of human growth hormone recipients with CJD found that most developed illness 8 to 12 years following exposure. The time to presentation is much shorter with transmission through contaminated neurosurgical instruments. In that case the mean incubation time is approximately 18 months.

The cardinal clinical manifestations of CJD are rapidly progressive dementia and myoclonus. The clinical features correlate with the distribution of PrP^{Sc} in the brain, and it is assumed that the abnormal accumulations of those proteins contribute to the focal neurologic features. Thus, most cases present with visual, cerebellar, thalamic, or striatal signs and symptoms, reflecting the distribution of PrP^{Sc} in those sites.

Attentional problems, memory loss, and judgment difficulties are frequent early signs. Cognitive disturbances involving language, visuospatial function, and other aspects of executive function emerge during the course of illness. Apathy and depression are common; less often euphoria, emotional lability, and anxiety can occur. As the disease progresses, dementia becomes prominent in most patients and advances rapidly. Death usually occurs within 1 year after the onset of symptoms.

Myoclonus (sudden involuntary jerking movements), especially provoked by loud noise or sudden movement, eventually occurs in more than 90% of patients, although in some cases presentation is late in the disease course. CJD should be considered in the differential diagnosis of a patient showing myoclonus and rapidly progressive dementia. Extrapyramidal signs, such as hypokinesia (reduced or slow movement) and cerebellar signs (nystagmus and ataxia), occur in most patients. The motor system also may be involved, with patients displaying weakness and, on examination, hyperreflexia, extensor plantar responses (Babinski sign), or spasticity.

Cranial nerve abnormalities, sensory abnormalities, and peripheral nervous system involvement, although occasionally present in CJD, should raise the suspicion of an alternative diagnosis, especially if those findings are a prominent part of the presentation. Sensory abnormalities are common in variant CJD but rare in other human prion diseases (as discussed later in the chapter).

DIAGNOSIS

No definitive diagnostic test for CJD is available, other than brain biopsy, but supportive evidence for the diagnosis is usually obtainable. Routine laboratory tests are generally normal, and the cerebrospinal fluid (CSF) contains no cells and has normal concentrations of glucose and protein. Recent studies have suggested that elevations of certain normally occurring central nervous sys-

tem proteins may serve as a marker of CJD. For example, an elevated CSF level of the **14-3-3 protein** has been suggested as a potential diagnostic test for the disease, although the protein may be a marker of brain cell death in general rather than of CJD in particular. Importantly, a negative test does not exclude the diagnosis of CJD, especially in persons with possible familial or variant CJD, and a positive test can occur in a variety of nonprion diseases, such as herpes simplex virus encephalitis, cerebral metastases, hypoxic encephalopathy, and metabolic encephalopathies, to name a few. Thus, the CSF level of the 14-3-3 protein should be considered an adjunctive rather than a definitive test for CJD.

The **electroencephalogram (EEG)** finding of periodic synchronous biphasic or triphasic sharp wave complexes is present in more than two thirds of patients with sporadic CJD at some point during the course of the illness. Although helpful in making the diagnosis, that EEG pattern is also not specific for CJD, and the finding can be masked by some neuroactive drugs and may not be seen in the initial or terminal stages of the disease.

As with the EEG, neuroimaging findings are not specific for CJD but can support the diagnosis. The **computerized tomography (CT)** scan is generally normal and serves mainly to exclude other diagnoses. **Magnetic resonance imaging (MRI)** is more informative. The most common MRI finding is increased T2 signal intensity in the putamen and head of the caudate (Fig. 56-2A). Less often, T2 hyperintensity is seen in the hemispheric white matter, globus pallidus, thalamus, cerebral cortex, and cerebellar cortex (Fig. 56-2B).

The typical neuropathological changes of CJD are spongiform vacuolation, neuronal degeneration, and glial proliferation (Fig. 56-3). The definitive test for diagnosis is the presence of PrP^{Sc} as determined by immunohistochemical testing of brain tissue.

FIGURE 56-2 ■ Magnetic resonance imaging of a patient with Creutzfeldt-Jacob disease. A. Increased signal intensity in the putamen and head of the caudate (arrows). **B.** Bilateral parieto-occipital cortical hyperintensity (arrows).

FIGURE 56-3 ■ Pathologic specimen from a patient with CJD demonstrating spongiform changes and neuronal loss.

TREATMENT AND PREVENTION

Currently, there is no specific treatment that alters the course of CJD. The disease remains inexorably progressive and invariably fatal. As with all prion diseases, care for CJD patients is supportive. Various antiviral, antibacterial, and immunomodulatory agents have been tested but were found ineffective. Despite the ability of chlorpromazine and quinacrine to inhibit PrPSc formation in tissue culture, human trials of the drugs have not been encouraging thus far.

Although there is no strategy to prevent the spontaneous development of CJD, the rare cases of iatrogenic transmission can be prevented. Fortunately, no evidence exists that CJD has been transmitted by blood transfusion. The majority of iatrogenic CJD cases followed either dural graft transplants or use of cadaveric pituitary hormones. Those iatrogenic routes of transmission have been dramatically reduced by changes in the process employed to prepare dural grafts and the use of recombinant-derived pituitary hormones.

One of the characteristic features of prions is their resistance to routine sterilization and decontaminating procedures. Therefore, special care and handling techniques are required for neuropathological specimens from patients with suspected prion disease. Similarly, neurosurgical instruments may be contaminated and require quarantine (pending a pathological diagnosis) and special decontamination protocols or must be discarded if the patient is determined to have a prion disease. PrPSc is resistant to processes affecting nucleic acids, such as hydrolysis or shearing. However, agents that digest, denature, or modify proteins do have activity against prions. PrPSc can be inactivated by prolonged autoclaving (at 121°C and 15 psi for 4.5 hours) or immersion in 1N NaOH (for 30 minutes, repeat three times) or in concentrated solutions of guanidine thiocyanate (more than 3M). However, certain cautions prevail; it appears that inadequate autoclaving can establish heat resistant subpopulations that fail to diminish with a further cycle of autoclaving. Stainless steel instruments also may retain infectivity even after treatment with 10% formaldehyde.

Variant CJD

Considerable evidence supports the hypothesis that variant CJD represents bovine-to-human transmission of **bovine spongiform encephalopathy (BSE)**, known popularly as **"mad cow disease."** For example, PrPs derived from different prion diseases and species differ in their glycosylation patterns and electrophoretic mobility. Evidence in favor of an association of variant CJD with BSE includes a pattern of glycosylation and electrophoretic mobility that has not been seen in other prion diseases. In addition, inoculating bovine PrPSc into transgenic mice expressing the human PrP gene can reproduce a disease resembling variant CJD.

Because of the unusual source of transmission of variant CJD, the initial reports in 1996 of cases of the disease focused intense interest on human prion diseases. Unique epidemiologic, clinical, and neuropathologic features of the illness led to the early recognition that the disease was indeed a "new variant," distinct from sporadic CJD.

EPIDEMIOLOGY AND ENCOUNTER

The variant form of CJD appeared in the late 1990s following an epizootic of BSE in Great Britain in the early 1990s (Fig. 56-4). Changes in the rendering process for bovine byproducts and the subsequent use of the products in cattle feed (a form of forced cannibalism) may have amplified the epidemic in animals. Variant CJD was initially reported in a 16-year-old girl from Great Britain in 1995. As of December 2, 2005, 153 cases of variant CJD have been reported worldwide, with 143 from Great Britain, six from France, and one each from Canada, Ireland, Italy, and the United States.

The average age at onset for variant CJD is about 30 years (ranging from 16 to 48 years) compared with 65 years for sporadic CJD. The variant form has a slower progression than sporadic CJD, with a mean survival of 14 months for variant CJD compared with 5 months for the sporadic form.

ENTRY

Although considerable experimental evidence links BSE and variant CJD, scant epidemiological evidence links

FIGURE 56-4 ■ Annual frequency of bovine spongiform encephalopathy (BSE) and variant CJD (vCJD) in Great Britain, 1988–2003.

variant CJD with the consumption of beef or any particular beef products. The assumption is that the PrP^{Sc} is ingested, but the exact circumstances of exposure are not known. A single case of variant CJD potentially related to a blood transfusion from an affected donor has been reported.

Humans have consumed an estimated 50,000 BSE-infected cattle. The majority of BSE cases have occurred in Great Britain, with spread to Europe, Asia, and the Middle East. A small number of infected animals have been identified in Canada, and two infected animals (one from a Canadian herd and the other from a native herd) have been identified in the United States. Fortunately, considering the number of persons exposed to BSE, the incidence of human cases has remained relatively low. Possible reasons include the following:

- Low levels of PrP^{Sc} in milk and meat, the main bovine products consumed by humans
- Inefficient transfer of PrP^{Sc} to the nervous system from ingested food
- Biologic barriers to transmission of disease between species
- Low incidence (about 30%) of homozygosity at PrP codon 129 in the human population

SPREAD, MULTIPLICATION, AND DAMAGE

As with sporadic CJD, the progression and specific manifestations of variant CJD depend on the locations of PrP^{Sc} accumulation in the nervous system. All forms of

CJD are uniformly fatal; however, in variant CJD the interval between the onset of symptoms and death is much longer than in sporadic CJD. In addition, the distribution of high-intensity signals by MRI scanning is different, accounting for the differences in clinical presentation.

Unlike patients with sporadic CJD, those with variant CJD commonly have prominent sensory disturbances (dysesthesias and paresthesias of the face, limbs, and torso) and psychiatric symptoms. Many cases of variant CJD in Great Britain presented with psychiatric symptoms, with depression being the most common. For example, Mr. I.'s first symptoms were diagnosed and treated as a psychiatric disorder. Apathy, anxiety, intermittent delusions, and psychosis also have been described. Once neurologic signs (typically ataxia) appear, the progression of the illness accelerates. Cognitive impairment, involuntary movements, immobility, paresis of upward gaze, unresponsiveness, and mutism are common signs as the disease advances. Abnormalities of gaze are noted in 50% of patients with variant CJD but are uncommon in other forms of CJD.

DIAGNOSIS

Laboratory and imaging studies are usually not helpful in the diagnosis of variant CJD. Typically, CSF has no cells, and levels of CSF protein are only mildly elevated. CSF 14-3-3 protein levels are usually not elevated in patients with variant CJD.

An EEG is usually abnormal due to excess slowing. However, the pattern is nonspecific, and periodic dis-

FIGURE 56-5 ▪ **Magnetic resonance imaging of a patient with variant CJD. A.** Increased signal intensity in the pulvinar ("pulvinar sign"). **B.** Increased signal intensity in the pulvinar and dorsomedial thalamus ("hockey stick sign").

charges like those seen in sporadic CJD do not occur. While an MRI can be normal in a patient with variant CJD, recent studies indicate that many patients have signal **hyperintensity in the pulvinar** (Fig. 56-5A) or in the pulvinar combined with the dorsomedial thalamus ("hockey stick sign") (Fig. 56-5B). As with sporadic CJD, an abnormal scan supports the diagnosis of variant CJD, but a normal MRI does not exclude the diagnosis. PrP mutations are not present in variant CJD, but like Mr. I., all patients tested to date are homozygous for a methionine at codon 129 in PrP, suggesting that host factors play a role in determining susceptibility to the disease.

The neuropathology of variant CJD also differs from that of sporadic CJD. The most striking difference is the presence of plaques, which stain intensely for PrPSc, throughout the cerebrum and cerebellum and to a lesser degree the basal ganglia and thalamus. The plaques have an eosinophilic center and a pale periphery and are surrounded by spongiform changes. The cerebellum is commonly involved in variant CJD but only occasionally affected in sporadic CJD.

PrP^{Sc} has also been identified in tonsil biopsy tissue from patients with variant CJD. That approach, which was used in Mr. I.'s case, may provide a less invasive way than brain biopsy than to make a pathological diagnosis of variant CJD. Of note, variant CJD is the only prion disease in which detection of PrP^{Sc} in nonneural tissue is currently useful for diagnosis.

In summary, variant CJD differs from typical sporadic CJD in the following ways:

- Younger age at presentation
- Slower progression of disease
- Different signs and symptoms at presentation
- Different neuropathology
- Detectable accumulation of PrP^{Sc} in nonneural tissue

TREATMENT AND PREVENTION

As with sporadic CJD, no specific therapy is available for variant CJD. The prohibition on ruminant-derived proteins in feeds for all animals and poultry in Great Britain and the ban in 1996 on consumption of animals over the age of 30 months have reduced the risk of human exposure to BSE and caused a dramatic decline in new cases of the disease.

Other Human Prion Diseases

Gerstmann-Straussler-Scheinker syndrome (GSS) is a rare human prion disease with an autosomal dominant pattern of inheritance and essentially complete penetrance. The incidence of GSS is 1 to 10 cases per 100 million population each year. GSS presents with progressive cerebellar degeneration accompanied by various degrees of dementia in patients entering midlife (mean age 45 years). The illness gradually progresses with a mean survival of 5 years after symptoms develop. Because the majority of cases are familial, all patients with definite GSS have been found to have PrP mutations.

Fatal familial insomnia (FFI) is a rapidly fatal midlife disease with a mean survival of 13 months following onset of symptoms. The disease presents with progressive insomnia, often associated with a dreamlike confusional state during waking hours. Inattention, memory loss, confusion, and hallucinations occur, but overt dementia is rare. Myoclonus, ataxia, and spasticity can occur late in the disease. FFI is the only prion disease to produce dysautonomia (hyperhidrosis, hyperthermia, tachycardia, and hypertension) and endocrine disturbances (decreased adrenocorticotropic hormone secretion, increased cortisol secretion, and disturbances in growth hormone, melatonin, and prolactin secretion).

Conclusion

Prion diseases are a unique group of illnesses resulting from a conformational change in a normal human protein. Occurring as sporadic, iatrogenic, hereditary, and transmissible forms of disease, they are relentlessly progressive and uniformly fatal. Ongoing concern about animal-to-human transmission has focused both popular and scientific attention on prions. Prion research may yield new insights into cellular physiology as well as treatments and methods of prevention for these unusual diseases.

Biological Agents of Warfare and Terrorism

Sandro K. Cinti and Philip C. Hanna

General concepts about bioterrorism:

- Biological agents provide a convenient and inexpensive way for rogue nations or organizations to foment terror.

- The National Institutes of Health and the Centers for Disease Control and Prevention have identified probable agents of bioterrorism and have grouped them into three categories for priority research.

- It is speculated that terrorists would attempt to disperse the most infectious agents in aerosol form.

Features of select agents:

- Anthrax causes a deadly hemorrhagic mediastinitis, septicemia, and meningitis when *Bacillus anthracis* spores are inhaled; however, the most common naturally acquired form of the disease in humans is an ulcerative skin lesion. It is not transmitted from person to person.

- Plague is a zoonosis naturally acquired from infected fleabites and causes suppurative lymphadenitis. However, *Yersinia pestis* can spread to the lungs to cause a pneumonia that can be transmitted among humans by droplets.

- Tularemia is a zoonosis usually acquired from contact with or ingestion of an infected animal. The typical infection involves skin and regional lymph nodes, but *Francisella tularensis* can also cause a serious pneumonia when inhaled.

- Smallpox (variola virus) is acquired by droplets spread from an infected individual. It causes a scarring, vesicular rash with high fever. Vaccination is an effective means of prevention but has not been widely used since the disease was declared eradicated.

- Hemorrhagic fever viruses (e.g., Ebola virus, Lassa fever, Marburg virus, and yellow fever) spread among humans mostly by contact. Features of the diseases vary but generally include fever, disseminated intravascular coagulation, and hemorrhagic manifestations.

- *Clostridium botulinum* toxin interferes with the release of acetylcholine at the neuromuscular junction and results in flaccid muscular paralysis without fever or changes in mental status.

Bioterrorism is the malevolent use of bacteria, viruses, or toxins against humans, animals, or plants in an attempt to cause harm and to create fear. Although concern about bioterrorism has always existed (see the box titled "Bioterrorism in History"), the 2001 anthrax attack in the United States that killed five people and prompted preemptive treatment of more than 10,000 others has

Bioterrorism in History

The use of biological agents for warfare has a centuries-long history, predating even the concept of germ theory. The first documented case was in 1346 when the Tartars, frustrated after years of laying siege to the Black Sea city of Kaffa, catapulted plague victims over the unassailable city walls. The Black Death epidemic that followed and eventually spread from Kaffa wiped out almost half of Europe. In 1763 Sir Jeffrey Amherst, the commander of British troops in America, sanctioned the use of smallpox-infected blankets as germ warfare implements against the American Indians who were highly susceptible to the deadly virus.

During World War I the Germans infected cattle destined for consumption by Allied forces with anthrax and glanders. That act resulted in the 1925 Geneva Protocol, which prohibited the use of biological weapons. In spite of that agreement and the 1972 Biological and Chemical Weapons Convention, sev-

eral nations continued to produce biological weapons. Biopreparat, the Russian biological weapons program, was the largest in the world, with 10,000 scientists working in 50 production facilities. In 1979 an accidental release of weaponized anthrax from a production plant in Sverdlovsk resulted in 66 deaths downwind of the facility. The program was dismantled in 1992 after Boris Yeltsin finally admitted that it existed.

Aum Shinrikyo, a Japanese cult, attempted several unsuccessful biological attacks with anthrax and botulinum toxin before releasing sarin gas in the Tokyo subway in 1995. The most successful biological attack in the United States was perpetrated by a religious cult, the Rajneeshees. In 1984, in an attempt to affect elections in a small Oregon town, the cult poisoned 10 restaurant salad bars with *Salmonella typhimurium* and sickened more than 700 people.

focused attention on bioterrorism as an imminent threat to national security. An understanding of the concern requires familiarity with the pathogens that are most likely to be used in any future attack and awareness of the available methods for detecting and responding to such an event. Consider how the following case—the first fatal case in the 2001 attack—came to light.

Case

On October 2, 2001, Mr. O., a 63-year-old photo editor at a Florida newspaper, awoke early with nausea, vomiting, and confusion. He was taken to a local emergency room for evaluation. Mr. O. had experienced malaise, fatigue, fever, chills, anorexia, and sweats beginning on September 27 during a trip to North Carolina. He denied headache, cough, chest pain, myalgias, dyspnea, abdominal pain, diarrhea, or skin rash. Medical history included hypertension, cardiovascular disease, and gout. He did not smoke.

On physical examination Mr. O. was alert and interactive but spoke nonsensically. His temperature was 39.2°C, his heart rate was 109 beats per minute, and his blood pressure and respiratory rate were normal. Initial pulmonary, heart, and abdominal examinations were normal, and his neck was not stiff. Mr. O. was not oriented to person, place, or time.

Laboratory testing included a normal total white blood cell (WBC) count, but the platelet count was low. A chest ra-

diograph showed prominence of the superior mediastinum and a possible small left pleural effusion (Fig. 57-1). A spinal tap was performed, and the cerebrospinal fluid (CSF) showed a WBC count of 4,750/mm^3 with 81% neutrophils, red blood cell count of 1,375/mm^3, glucose of 57 mg/dL (simultaneous serum glucose was 174 mg/dL), and protein of 666 mg/dL. Microscopy examination of the CSF showed many Gram-positive bacilli (Fig. 57-2). Anthrax was suspected. After only

FIGURE 57-1 ▪ Chest radiograph (anterior-posterior view) of patient infected with *Bacillus anthracis.*

FIGURE 57-2 ▪ Gram stain of cerebrospinal fluid obtained from patient infected with *Bacillus anthracis*.

7 hours of incubation of the CSF culture, *Bacillus anthracis* was isolated, and blood cultures were positive within 24 hours of incubation.

Mr. O. received a single dose of cefotaxime and was admitted to the hospital with a diagnosis of meningitis. Shortly after admission he had generalized seizures; an endotracheal tube was placed for airway protection. Initially he received multiple different intravenous antibiotics, but by day 2 Mr. O.'s ongoing therapy consisted of penicillin G, levofloxacin, and clindamycin. In spite of that combination therapy, he remained febrile and became unresponsive to deep stimuli. His condition progressively deteriorated, with hypotension and worsening renal function. Mr. O. died on October 5. A postmortem examination revealed hemorrhagic inflammation of the mediastinal lymph nodes, and immunohistochemical staining showed disseminated *B. anthracis* in multiple organs. (Adapted from Jernigan JA et al. Bioterrorism-related inhalation anthrax: the first 10 cases reported in the United States. Emerg Infect Dis 2001;7(6):933–944.)

This case raises several questions:

1. Why was anthrax considered early as a probable diagnosis in this case?
2. Why was bioterrorism suspected?
3. Why did antibiotic therapy fail to save Mr. O.'s life?

▪ ▪ ▪ ▪

Biological weapons, unlike other weapons of mass destruction, are inexpensive to make. Nuclear and chemical weapons programs are 800 and 600 times more costly to develop, respectively, than a comparable biological weapons program. The pathogens are relatively available, and the materials and equipment for producing biological weapons are the same as those used for peaceful purposes. For example, the organism that causes anthrax is present in the soil in many countries and can be grown in standard laboratory culture medium. The *Salmonella* species used in the Oregon attack described in the box titled "Bioterrorism in History" was easily obtained by a member of the Rajneeshee cult. The necessary culture media, incubators, and milling equipment are available for purchase, and information on cultivating the organisms and on generating antibiotic-resistant strains is available in the scientific literature and from the Internet.

Biological weapons produce fear and panic, as was apparent in the 2001 anthrax attack. The weapon can be released covertly, and its effects only become apparent days later when the terrorist is gone. Unlike that of chemical and nuclear events, the point of release of a biological agent may not be apparent. If it is a contagious agent, the uncertainty about who has been exposed could lead to widespread panic. Finally, the lethality of a biological attack could exceed that of other weapons of mass destruction. By one governmental estimate, 50 kg of powdered anthrax similar to that used in the 2001 attack released over a city of 500,000 people would cause death in 95,000 and incapacity in 125,000.

Epidemiology of a Bioterrorist Attack

A bioterrorist attack will have features that are similar to any naturally occurring epidemic of the involved disease. However, **certain epidemiologic features should increase suspicion that a biological agent has been released deliberately** and prompt further investigation (Table 57-1). For example, *B. anthracis* is found in soils around the world; however, naturally occurring anthrax in humans is uncommon. It is now so rare in the United States that any case, regardless of its clinical manifestations, should be investigated as a bioterrorist act. Thus, in the case of Mr. O., a deliberate biological attack was an early consideration.

Encounter With Biological Weapons

Biological weapons can be released by aerosolization, contamination of food, contamination of water, person-to-person transmission of a contagious agent, or release of infected insect vectors. **Aerosolization,** the dispersion of organisms into the environment, is the most feared and potentially lethal method of releasing biological agents. As mentioned earlier, a very small amount of weaponized anthrax (50 kg) could result in very high casualties (95,000). The Russian bioweapons program spent considerable resources developing effective methods of aerosolizing biological agents, especially anthrax, tularemia, and

table 57-1   Clues That Raise Suspicion for a Deliberate Release of a Bioterrorism Agent

CLUE	POTENTIAL SOURCE OR CIRCUMSTANCE
A large number of ill persons presenting at the same time with a similar disease, especially the following syndromes:	
Flaccid paralysis	Botulinum toxin
Hemorrhagic fevers	Ebola virus, Lassa fever
Vesicular/pustular rash with considerable mortality	Smallpox
Flulike illness associated with a widened mediastinum on chest radiograph and/or meningitis	Anthrax
Pneumonia with painful lymphadenopathy	Plague
Illness in animals and humans concurrently	Anthrax, encephalitis
A large number of unexplained deaths, especially in young healthy adults	Various agents
A single case of an uncommon organism	Smallpox, pulmonary anthrax, Ebola virus
Multiple disease entities presenting in one patient	Multiple agents released
An unusual disease presentation	Pneumonic instead of bubonic plague
An unusual geographic distribution	Ebola virus in the United States
An unusual seasonal pattern	Influenza in the summer
An illness that fails to respond to usual antimicrobials or vaccines	Engineered antibiotic- or vaccine-resistant anthrax
Clusters of a similar illness in noncontiguous areas, domestic or foreign	Various agents

smallpox. Both the 1979 Sverdlovsk outbreak of anthrax and the 2001 anthrax attack in the United States involved the release of finely powdered anthrax into the environment. Means of aerosolizing an agent include spraying devices (crop dusters), air-handling systems in buildings, incendiary devices (bombs), and the postal system (infected mail). However, aerosolization of a biological agent is not easy. Infectious particles **must be precisely the right size (0.5 to 5 μm) to enter and infect the lungs.** Furthermore, radiation from sunlight, shear forces from sprayers, or explosions from incendiary devices would likely destroy most of the released organism.

Contamination of the food or water supply with biological agents is another method of dissemination. The *Salmonella typhimurium* contamination of salad bars in Oregon restaurants is an example of a successful attack (see the box titled "Bioterrorism in History"). The most likely agents to be disseminated in this fashion include botulinum toxin, anthrax, and diarrheal agents including *S. typhimurium*. However, contamination of food and water would be difficult given inspection criteria, water purification, and filtering systems and increased security at water reservoirs and food distribution centers.

Dissemination through **person-to-person transmission** is a likely means of dispersing a contagious agent such as smallpox. As few as 100 smallpox-infected people could start an epidemic in a nonimmune population. The fear, panic, and quarantine measures that would result from such an epidemic could rapidly overwhelm health care resources and destabilize affected countries.

Zoonotic delivery, or the use of **insect vectors** to disperse a biological agent, is an unlikely method of bioterrorism because it is inefficient and unpredictable. The most likely agent to be delivered by zoonosis would be *Yersinia pestis* (plague) or viral hemorrhagic fevers (Ebola virus, Lassa fever).

The characteristics of an ideal agent for bioterrorism include **accessibility, durability, infectiousness, and communicability.** Although hundreds of agents and toxins may qualify, the Centers for Disease Control and Prevention (CDC) has developed **categories (A, B, and C) based on the perceived threat.** The characteristics of the pathogens in the CDC categories are listed in the box titled "Characteristics of Priority Biological Agents in Categories A, B, and C." Category A agents pose the greatest threat, and these agents are discussed individually in this chapter. A complete list of the pathogens listed in categories A, B, and C is included in the electronic supplement to this chapter.

Category A Agents

Anthrax

Anthrax, a disease most associated with grazing herbivores, has been reported throughout human history. It is believed to have been one of the Egyptian plagues at the time of Moses, and was described in detail by the ancient

Characteristics of Priority Biological Agents in Categories A, B, and C

CATEGORY A (E.G., ANTHRAX, SMALLPOX)

The most dangerous agents with the highest research priority for the following reasons:

- Can be easily disseminated or transmitted from person to person.
- Result in high mortality rates and have the potential for major public health impact.
- Might cause public panic and social disruption.
- Require special action for public health preparedness.

CATEGORY B (E.G., SALMONELLA SPECIES, VIRAL ENCEPHALITIS)

Represent a secondary priority for the following reasons:

- Are moderately easy to disseminate.

- Result in moderate morbidity rates and low mortality rates.
- Require specific enhancements of the CDC's diagnostic capacity and enhanced disease surveillance.

CATEGORY C (E.G., MULTIDRUG-RESISTANT TUBERCULOSIS, INFLUENZA)

Represent emerging pathogens that pose less of an immediate threat but may be genetically engineered in the future to produce more lethal disease or disease resistant to current antibiotics and/or vaccines for the following reasons:

- Are readily available.
- Can easily be produced and disseminated.
- Have a potential for high morbidity and mortality rates and major health impact.

Roman poet Virgil. Anthrax bacilli were used by Robert Koch to prove his theory that "germs" cause disease, and Louis Pasteur's celebrated public demonstration of the first attenuated vaccine showed protection of farm animals against anthrax.

Bacillus anthracis is a Gram-positive bacterium that forms stable endospores when nutrients are limited. These spores are extremely robust and capable of remaining dormant in the soil for decades or longer. **The spore is the infectious particle.** The natural stability of anthrax spores, their longevity and resistance to destruction, and their ability to cause lethal infections are likely reasons they were chosen as weapons. The **"weaponization"** of anthrax spores by drying and milling generates a unit spore size capable of reaching the recesses of the lung. In addition, spores prepared in this manner are easier to disperse in aerosols and remain airborne longer. Anthrax is **not known to spread from person to person.**

The virulence of *B. anthracis* depends on the presence of its **two large plasmids.** Plasmid pXO2 encodes the synthesis genes for an **antiphagocytic poly-D-glutamic acid capsule.** Plasmid pXO1 encodes for **two binary exotoxins** that act as potent enzymes in the cytoplasm of host cells. **Edema toxin** contains **edema factor, a calmodulin-dependent adenylate cyclase** that increases cellular cyclic adenosine monophosphate and upsets cellular water balance. Edema toxin probably contributes to the massive edema seen in anthrax infection. **Lethal toxin** contains **lethal factor,** a **zinc-metalloprotease** that cleaves a variety of cytoplasmic substrates and inactivates the signal-transducing enzyme MAPKK. Inoculation of purified lethal toxin kills test animals.

In addition to edema factor and lethal factor, each toxin has a second, shared subunit called **protective antigen.** Protective antigen is the binding subunit that mediates entry into host cells. Neither toxin is active without it, and the protective antigen subunit is the main ingredient of the anthrax subunit vaccine, underscoring the importance of exotoxins in the production of disease manifestations.

The **three main clinical forms** of anthrax are classified by the route of entry of the spores into the body: cutaneous, gastrointestinal, and inhalation (Table 57-2). **Cutaneous anthrax is by far the most common** and mildest form. Naturally acquired cases of cutaneous anthrax occur after contact with infected animals or their byproducts. However, during the postal attacks of 2001, half the people infected had the cutaneous form of disease. In cutaneous infections, spores enter the skin through minor cuts or abrasions, germinate to form growing bacilli, and cause local ulceration of the skin. The primary skin lesion is usually a painless itchy papule that appears 3 to 5 days after contact. In 24 to 36 hours, the lesion forms a vesicle that undergoes central necrosis and drying, leaving a typical smooth-edged, painless black crust, or **eschar,** surrounded by edema and a number of **purplish vesicles.** Cutaneous anthrax can be self-limiting, but antibiotic treatment is recommended to prevent any dissemination into the bloodstream. When treated, cutaneous anthrax heals completely and usually without scarring.

Gastrointestinal anthrax is extremely rare in developed countries. Symptoms appear 2 to 5 days after ingestion of spore-contaminated meat from diseased animals.

table 57-2 Disease Manifestations of Category A Agents

PRIMARY CLINICAL FEATURE	PATHOGEN	MODE OF ENTRY	COMMUNICABLE AMONG HUMANS?
Pneumonia	*Yersinia pestis*, *Francisella tularensis*	Inhalation Inhalation	Yes No
Single skin ulcer	*Bacillus anthracis* *F. tularensis*	Abrasion of skin Arthropod bite or abrasion of skin	No No

Lymphadenitis
  Mediastinal
  Regional
	B. anthracis
	Y. pestis (bubo)
	F. tularensis
		Inhalation
		Arthropod bite
		Arthropod bite or abrasion of skin
			No
			No
			No

Eye infection with lymphadenitis	*F. tularensis*	Direct inoculation of conjunctiva	No
Meningitis	*B. anthracis*	Inhalation, dissemination	No
Necrotizing intestinal infection	*B. anthracis* *F. tularensis*	Ingestion of spores Ingestion of bacteria	No No
Multiple skin vesicles	Smallpox	Respiratory droplet	Yes
Fever with hemorrhaging	*Y. pestis* Hemorrhagic fever viruses	Dissemination from skin or lung Arthropods, penetration through abraded skin, unknown inhalation	Yes Yes (some agents)
Paralysis	*Clostridium botulinum* toxin	Ingestion, inhalation	No

Gray highlighting indicates potential bioterrorist scenario.

They include fever and diffuse **abdominal pain and tenderness,** and patients often report either **constipation or diarrhea** and **black or bloody stools or vomitus.** Ulceration and inflammation of the gastrointestinal tract is typically accompanied by massive **edema, mucosal necrosis, and spread to the mesenteric lymph nodes.** Mortality from gastrointestinal anthrax is very high and is associated with blood loss and shock, intestinal perforation, or spread of the organism into the bloodstream.

Inhalation anthrax occurs after aerosolized spores are inhaled and thus represents the greatest concern as a bioweapon. Though extremely rare, naturally occurring disease has been reported in persons working with spore-contaminated furs or wools (thus the name **"wool-sorter's disease"**). Although the airways are the initial site of contact, inhalation anthrax is **not a true pneumonia** and in most cases no bacteria are found in the lungs. Rather, spores reaching the alveoli are engulfed by phagocytes and **transported to the mediastinal and peribronchial lymph nodes,** germinating en route. Illness may begin 1 to 6 days after exposure or after several weeks because of smaller inocula or delays in spore internalization by alveolar phagocytes.

Early symptoms of inhalation anthrax are "flulike" and include **fever, myalgia,** and **malaise.** As the bacilli multiply, **hemorrhagic mediastinitis** and **widening of the mediastinum** become visible on chest radiograph or computerized tomography scan (see Fig. 57-1). Symptoms of **shortness of breath, strident cough,** and **chills** develop at that point and are followed quickly by **massive pleural effusions, sepsis, shock,** and **death** as bacilli spread throughout the body in high numbers. Anthrax **meningitis** occurs

in up to 50% of inhalation cases and is almost always fatal in spite of intensive antibiotic therapy. Meningitis resulting from anthrax causes **extensive hemorrhage of the leptomeninges,** giving them a dark red appearance on autopsy, sardonically described as **"cardinal's cap."**

Anthrax can be successfully treated with antibiotics if they are administered prophylactically after spore exposure or early in the course of infection. During the anthrax outbreak of 2001, 6 of the 11 victims of inhalation anthrax survived with aggressive hospital care and multiple intravenous antibiotics. *B. anthracis* is naturally susceptible to **fluoroquinolones, tetracyclines,** and most other **antibiotics.** There is also an **anthrax vaccine** that is currently administered to military personnel, researchers, and some animal and human health care providers; however, it is not clear how well the current vaccine protects humans against inhalation anthrax.

Physicians will face many challenges during an anthrax outbreak. It is a disease with a rapid progression to death but manifesting vague early symptoms that are flulike and delay patients from seeking medical attention. Once the disease progresses and high numbers of organisms are disseminated to the blood, organs, and tissues, anthrax is difficult to treat and often requires intensive care with mechanical assistance for breathing.

Plague

Plague has been the cause of several pandemics, the most famous of which, the Black Death, began in 1346 and killed 30 million people in Europe. Although pandemics of plague have ceased with the advent of antibiotics and improved rodent control, outbreaks around the world continue to account for 1,700 cases per year, including a few each year in the southwestern United States. The bacterium that causes plague, *Yersinia pestis*, has several advantages as a biological weapon:

- It is relatively stable in the environment and can survive up to 1 hour in aerosolized form.
- The pneumonic form is contagious.
- Mortality from pneumonic plague is 100% without treatment.
- The mention of plague elicits considerable panic.
- Plague is highly infective, requiring only 100 to 500 organisms to cause infection.

The most feared method of disseminating plague is through aerosolization. Although the Japanese attempted to infect the Chinese by dropping plague-infected fleas during World War II, that method of delivering plague is inefficient and unpredictable. The Russian bioweapons program, Biopreparat, produced an aerosolized form of plague, 50 kg of which could have infected up to 100,000 persons and caused 36,000 deaths.

Y. pestis is a **Gram-negative coccobacillus.** The virulence of the organism depends on several factors:

- An **envelope antigen F1** is antiphagocytic.
- A **plasminogen activator** degrades fibrin and facilitates spread of the organism.
- **V and W antigens** are antiphagocytic and allow the organism to survive and reproduce in host cells.
- **Yops proteins** are antiphagocytic and prevent an effective inflammatory response.

In addition, *Y. pestis* produces a **lipopolysaccharide (LPS) endotoxin,** which causes most of the clinical manifestations of plague.

Plague is a **zoonotic infection of rodents.** In urban areas the animal reservoir is usually the rat, whereas in sylvatic areas squirrels, mice, or prairie dogs can carry the disease. In any case infection is transmitted among rodents by the bites of their fleas (Fig. 57-3). Natural transmission to humans occurs when an infected rodent flea attempts to feed on a human (see Table 57-2). After biting the host the inoculated bacteria migrate to lymph nodes, where they associate with mononuclear cells and multiply. An incubation period of 2 to 8 days results in the bite victim developing fever, chills, and a swollen tender lymph node, or **bubo,** the cardinal feature of **bubonic plague** (Fig. 57-4). Buboes are usually found in the groin, axilla, or cervical region and are often so tender that the affected individual cannot move the affected limb. If left untreated, bubonic plague can spread to the lungs (**pneumonic plague**) or disseminate in the bloodstream (**septicemic plague**). A biological attack with aerosolized *Y. pestis* would most likely present as primary pneumonic plague without buboes.

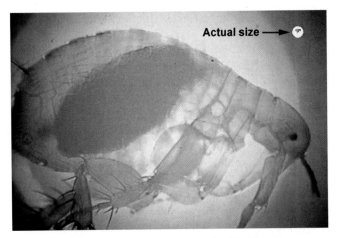

FIGURE 57-3 ▪ Flea engorged with blood.

Pneumonic plague can be primary or secondary. Secondary pneumonic plague results from the hematogenous spread of *Y. pestis* in untreated bubonic or septicemic plague. Primary pneumonic plague results from direct inhalation of plague bacilli from other humans or animals, particularly cats, with pneumonic plague. Clinically, patients have signs of pneumonia including fevers, chills, shortness of breath, and hemoptysis (coughing of blood).

Septicemic plague is characterized by **disseminated intravascular coagulation (DIC)**, necrosis of small vessels, and hemorrhages in the skin causing large purple or black lesions (**purpura and ecchymoses**). The skin lesions and necrosis of the fingers and toes that occurred in terminally ill persons during the fourteenth century plague pandemic are the features that inspired the name Black Death. The mortality rate of septicemic plague approaches 100% without treatment.

The diagnosis of plague from a biological attack would be difficult because most cases would present as primary pneumonic plague without the characteristic bubo present in naturally occurring plague. A chest radiograph would show a **bronchopneumonia,** and labo-

FIGURE 57-4 ▪ Bubo of the neck of a young woman with bubonic plague.

ratory data would be nonspecific and consistent with a systemic inflammatory response. Sputum Gram stain (and possibly blood smear) might show Gram-negative bacilli with **characteristic bipolar staining**. Although *Y. pestis* would eventually grow on culture, identification could take 6 days.

Treatment of pneumonic plague must be started within 24 hours of onset of symptoms, or mortality approaches 100%. Naturally occurring *Y. pestis* is sensitive to aminoglycosides, such as streptomycin and gentamicin; doxycycline; and fluoroquinolones. Because pneumonic plague can spread from person to person by droplet transmission, patients with this form of disease must be treated in respiratory isolation. In addition, persons in close contact with the affected individuals should receive prophylactic antimicrobial therapy.

Tularemia

Tularemia, the disease caused by the Gram-negative bacterium *Francisella tularensis*, occurs naturally throughout North America and Eurasia. Animal reservoirs of infection include rabbits, hares, voles, and squirrels. As with plague, transmission of the infection among those animals occurs through the **bites of ticks, flies, and mosquitoes**. Human infection is acquired by arthropod bites, handling infectious animal tissue, ingestion of contaminated food or water, and inhalation of aerosols.

F. tularensis is an intracellular pathogen that infects macrophages, hepatocytes, and epithelioid cells. Virulence factors include an **antiphagocytic capsule** and the enzyme **citrulline ureidase**. Although *F. tularensis* does produce an LPS endotoxin, the activity of the LPS is a thousandfold less than that of *Escherichia coli*. **Cell-mediated immunity** is the major host response to infection and results in a characteristic **granulomatous infiltrate** of the lymph nodes, liver, lung, spleen, and bone marrow. Tularemia can be misdiagnosed as tuberculosis if granulomas are caseating.

Tularemia also has a history as an agent of bioterrorism. The Japanese studied the disease in their bioweapons program in Manchuria (1932–1945) and the Russian Biopreparat program developed aerosolized forms of *F. tularensis* that were engineered to be resistant to antibiotics and vaccines.

In humans, **tularemia can present in various ways depending on the route of transmission and the site of entry into the body** (see Table 57-2). A bioterrorism attack would most likely involve aerosolized *F. tularensis*, with the predominant manifestations being pneumonic, typhoidal, septicemic, and possibly oropharyngeal. It has been estimated that one or two organisms are enough to produce infection. The mortality rate of untreated pneumonic or septic tularemia is as high as 60%. With treatment the case fatality rate is less than 2%. Isolation is not recommended for tularemia patients, given the lack of human-to-human transmission.

The diagnosis of a bioterrorist attack with tularemia would be difficult given the nonspecific presentation. Lymphadenopathy, the hallmark of naturally occurring tularemia, may not be present, and standard microbiological testing of sputum could miss *F. tularensis* or delay it by days to weeks.

The treatment of choice for pneumonic, septic, or typhoidal tularemia is an aminoglycoside antibiotic. Ciprofloxacin and doxycycline are also effective and would be preferred in a mass casualty setting. A live, attenuated *F. tularensis* vaccine is available for laboratory workers exposed to tularemia; however, in volunteer studies the vaccine did not protect all subjects from an aerosolized challenge.

Smallpox

The last naturally occurring case of **smallpox** was diagnosed in 1977 in Somalia. In 1980, 13 years after initiating an eradication program, the World Health Organization (WHO) certified the world free of smallpox and recommended discontinuation of the smallpox vaccine. Only two official repositories maintained the deadly **variola** (smallpox) virus, the Institute of Virus Preparations in Moscow and the CDC in Atlanta, Georgia. Thus, a case of smallpox anywhere in the world today could only arise as a result of a clandestine laboratory accident or a bioterrorist attack. Russia's now-dismantled Biopreparat program produced large amounts of smallpox as a biological weapon, and there is concern that some of those stocks may have fallen into the hands of rogue nations. A bioterrorist could initiate a smallpox epidemic by aerosol release or by sending intentionally infected individuals into an unsuspecting population. In a world that is no longer immune to the disease, the infection would spread rapidly from person to person. In its most pathogenic form, variola causes **disfiguring skin eruptions, fever, and a mortality rate of 30% or more** in unvaccinated persons.

Variola virus belongs to a group of large **DNA viruses** called the **orthopoxviruses**. Natural infection occurs when virus from respiratory droplets or skin lesions comes into contact with the oropharyngeal or respiratory mucosa. The infectious dose is thought to be very small, but historical outbreaks suggest that close contact is usually required to spread the disease. After migration to regional lymph nodes, an **asymptomatic viremia** transmits virus throughout the body. A nonspecific **prodrome** of **fever, malaise, and prostration with headache and backache** follows an **incubation period that averages 12 to 14 days** (ranging from 7 to 17 days). Abdominal pain and delirium also can occur. During the initial febrile prodrome, the patient is not contagious; therefore, monitoring for fevers is an excellent way of identifying exposed individuals who need to be isolated.

FIGURE 57-5 ■ **Progression of smallpox lesions.** Note early involvement of the face, hands (including the palms), and feet (including the soles).

Within 2 to 4 days of fever onset the patient develops a maculopapular rash on the mucosa of the mouth, pharynx, face, and arms that spreads to the trunk and legs. The patient is highly contagious at that point. Over the next several days the **rash becomes vesicular then pustular** as it covers the whole body (Fig. 57-5). If the patient survives, **lesions form crusts after 2 weeks** and leave **disfiguring scars.** The patient is most contagious during the first week of rash, but transmission continues to occur until all scabs have fallen off (about 3 weeks). Mortality is usually associated with **toxemia,** probably the result of **circulating immune complexes and soluble variola antigens** or, less often, to encephalitis or secondary bacterial pneumonia.

Differentiating smallpox (variola) from the more common chickenpox (varicella) can be challenging, but several discriminating features make accurate diagnoses possible (Table 57-3). Because laboratory testing for smallpox requires high-level containment facilities, suspected samples of vesicular or pustular fluid or scabs must be sent to the CDC for testing and cultivation. The large, brick-shaped virions of orthopoxviruses can be easily identified by electron microscopic examination (Fig. 57-6). Two other orthopoxviruses, cowpox and vaccinia, can be ruled out from the patient's history or the appearance of the lesions.

No antiviral therapy has been established for smallpox. One antiviral drug, **cidofovir,** has some activity against poxviruses, but it is toxic to the bone marrow and kidneys. **Vaccination with live vaccinia virus** has been the best way to prevent smallpox disease since the late 1700s, and mass vaccination would most likely occur in a widespread outbreak.

During an outbreak, infection control measures would be of paramount importance in preventing the

table **57-3**	**Features That Distinguish the Rash of Smallpox (Variola) and Chickenpox (Varicella)**

Smallpox   Chickenpox

	Smallpox	Chickenpox
Fever	Occurs 2–4 days before rash onset	Occurs at the time of rash, if at all
Rash		
• Distribution	More lesions on the face and extremities; lesions on palms and soles	More lesions on the body; no lesions on palms and soles
• Appearance	Large, deep-seated vesicles or pustules in the same stage of development	Small, shallow vesicles in various stages of development
• Course	Lesions resolve over 14-21 days	Lesions resolved within 7–10 days
Mortality	10–30%	Very uncommon

FIGURE 57-6 ▪ Electron micrograph of a variola virion.

spread of smallpox. All health care workers caring for smallpox patients would be vaccinated as soon as possible, and patients with suspected infection would be placed in high-level isolation. Public health officials would immediately begin contact tracing to identify other potential cases and candidates for vaccination.

Viral Hemorrhagic Fevers

In nature, humans are infected with hemorrhagic fever (HF) viruses from the bite of an infected arthropod (mosquito), from aerosols of rodent excreta, or from direct contact with an infected animal. Person-to-person spread of **Ebola virus** has been the cause of several devastating outbreaks in Africa. **Marburg virus** and possibly **Lassa fever** also spread through person-to-person contact, although aerosol spread was implicated in an outbreak of Lassa fever in Nigeria in 1969.

Several distinct groups of RNA viruses can produce a **viral hemorrhagic fever syndrome.** The pathogenesis of the syndrome is poorly understood. After an incubation period of 2 to 21 days, infected persons **develop fever, myalgias, headache, retro-orbital pain, and prostration.** A maculopapular rash and/or conjunctivitis may be present with Lassa fever and yellow fever. **Jaundice** is a hallmark of yellow fever and Rift Valley fever. In its most severe form viral hemorrhagic fever syndrome manifests as **hemorrhagic complications,** including diffuse bleeding in the skin and gastrointestinal tract. DIC and shock may be present. The mortality rate varies from less than 1% for Rift Valley fever to more than 70% from Ebola or Marburg virus.

The HF viruses—Ebola, Marburg, Lassa, Junin, and Machupo—were developed as aerosolized biological weapons in Russia until 1992. The United States developed Rift Valley fever and yellow fever viruses as

biological weapons before the U.S. program was dismantled in 1969. The most likely route of dissemination in a bioterrorist attack would be aerosolization.

Rapid diagnosis of HF viruses is problematic at present. Tests for a specific HF virus, including antigen detection by antigen-capture enzyme-linked immunosorbent assay (ELISA), IgM antibody detection by antibody-capture ELISA, and reverse transcription polymerase chain reaction are done in specialized laboratories. Viral culture should be attempted only at the CDC or the U.S. Army Medical Research Institute of Infectious Diseases.

Because of the potential for person-to-person transmission of some HF viruses (e.g., Ebola virus), infected individuals must be cared for in isolation rooms. Although the U.S. Food and Drug Administration has not approved any drug for viral hemorrhagic fever syndrome, **ribavirin**, a nucleoside analog, has reduced mortality from Lassa fever in some small trials. Ribavirin has no activity against Ebola virus, Marburg virus, or yellow fever. Except for yellow fever, there is no vaccine for any of the HF viruses.

Botulinum Toxin

Botulinum toxin, produced by the spore-forming anaerobe *Clostridium botulinum*, is the most potent toxin known to humans. It has already been used as a biological weapon by the Japanese cult Aum Shinrikyo, which attempted aerosol dispersions on U.S. military installations in Japan on three occasions between 1990 and 1995. Large amounts of weaponized botulinum toxin were also produced in the former Soviet Union and in Iraq. Methods of dispersion include aerosolization and poisoning of the food supply. Contamination of the water supply with botulinum toxin is impractical given that large amounts of toxin would be required, and standard water purification methods (e.g., chlorination) rapidly inactivate the toxin.

C. botulinum is ubiquitous in the soil and can be easily isolated in culture. Botulinum toxin exists in **seven distinct antigenic forms** (A through G) that make convenient epidemiologic markers in an outbreak. Most natural foodborne outbreaks of botulism occur with toxins A, B, and E. The lethal dose of botulinum toxin for a 70-kg human is 0.09 to 0.15 μg intravenously, 0.70 to 0.90 μg inhaled, and 70 μg orally. Therapeutic BoTox contains only 0.3% of the lethal inhalational dose and 0.005% of the lethal oral dose. Botulinum toxin does not permeate intact skin.

Botulinum toxin acts at the neuromuscular junction to prevent release of acetylcholine, a neurotransmitter that stimulates muscle contraction (Fig. 57-7). The clinical symptoms that result are manifestations of impaired muscle contraction. Symptoms typically appear 12 to 72 hours after ingestion of toxin, but inhalation botulism is likely to present within hours. The classic triad of botulism is (1) descending flaccid paralysis with prominent

A **Normal neurotransmission at the neuromuscular junction**

B **Inhibitory effect of botulinum toxin**

FIGURE 57-7 ■ **Mechanism of action of botulinum toxins. A. The** assembly of the SNARE mechanism that mediates fusion of acetylcholine-containing vesicles with the cell membrane and release of acetylcholine into the neuromuscular junction after normal excitatory stimuli. **B.** The actions of botulinum toxins: proteolytic cleavage of either synaptobrevin, syntaxin, or SNAP-25 (the main components of the SNARE complex).

bulbar signs, (2) normal body temperature, and (3) normal mental status. The patient remains lucid because the toxin does not penetrate the brain. The bulbar signs include the "4 Ds": **diplopia** (double vision), **dysarthria** (difficulty forming words), **dysphonia** (difficulty intoning words), and **dysphagia** (difficulty swallowing). Paralysis may progress to involve the muscle of respiration, in which case death results from asphyxiation or secondary infection (aspiration pneumonia).

In addition to foodborne botulism (see Chapter 76), the toxin can also be released from *C. botulinum* growing in wounds (**wound botulism**) or in the intestinal tracts of infants (**infant botulism**), particularly those fed honey.

Treatment of botulism consists of supportive care (e.g., **mechanical ventilation** is required in 20% of foodborne cases) and the administration of **equine antitoxin.** Antitoxin must be administered early because it will not reverse existing paralysis.

Conclusion

Several virulent bacterial and viral pathogens are potential agents for a bioterrorist attack. Some have already been used for that purpose. Certain terrorist groups or rogue nations may favor using these agents over nuclear or chemical weapons of mass destruction because they are relatively easy to obtain, cheap to produce in large quantities, and highly effective in creating human morbidity and panic. The category A agents are considered the most dangerous. A major release of these pathogens in a terrorist attack would likely involve large quantities of the agent release in aerosol form. Physicians of the future must be familiar with the clinical diseases caused by these pathogens, even though they are rarely seen today in clinical practice. In addition, physicians must be aware of the clues that signal that a terrorist attack may be under way.

part 3

Pathophysiology of Infectious Diseases

Diagnostic Principles

Cary Engleberg

The role of the clinical microbiology laboratory is to determine whether potential pathogens are present in tissues, body fluids, or secretions of patients and if present, to identify them. This service is indispensable to the modern clinician because information about a pathogen's identity is of critical importance in predicting the course of an infection and in guiding the selection of appropriate therapy. This information can be generated in four ways:

1. Microscopic examination of patient samples.
2. Cultivation and identification of microorganisms from patient samples.
3. Measurement of a pathogen-specific immune response in the patient.
4. Detection of pathogen-specific macromolecules in patient samples.

The extent and reliability of the information that the laboratory can provide varies depending on the nature of the pathogen. Some pathogens (e.g., *Staphylococcus aureus*) are easily detected, cultivated, identified, and characterized; others (e.g., *Toxoplasma gondii*) require extraordinary measures merely to establish their presence. However, thanks to technological advances in molecular biology, the capabilities of the modern clinical microbiology laboratory are expanding and improving rapidly. New diagnostic procedures are being introduced into clinical practice at an ever-increasing pace. Clinicians need to understand the principles underlying both the new and old methods to make an informed and critical assessment of their value and reliability and to use them wisely.

Assessing the Performance of Laboratory Tests

No laboratory test is perfect. Therefore, to interpret the results of tests, clinicians must have a sense of how reliable they are. When a microbiologic test correctly predicts the presence of a pathogen, the result is called **true-positive**. Similarly, a negative test obtained in the absence of the pathogen is **true-negative**. Inaccuracies occur either because the laboratory test is negative in the presence of the pathogen (**false-negative**) or positive in the absence of the pathogen (**false-positive**).

Test results

	Positive	Negative
Organism present	true-positives	false-negatives
Organism absent	false-positives	true-negatives

$$\text{Sensitivity} = \frac{\text{true-positives}}{\text{true-positives} + \text{false-negatives}} \times 100\%$$

$$\text{Specificity} = \frac{\text{true-negatives}}{\text{true-negatives} + \text{false-positives}} \times 100\%$$

$$\text{Positive Predictive Value} = \frac{\text{true-positives}}{\text{true-positives} + \text{false-positives}} \times 100\%$$

$$\text{Negative Predictive Value} = \frac{\text{true-negatives}}{\text{true-negatives} + \text{false-negatives}} \times 100\%$$

FIGURE 58-1 ■ **Definitions of terms used in evaluating diagnostic tests.**

The terms *sensitivity* and *specificity*, defined in Figure 58-1, are commonly used to describe the performance and value of all diagnostic tests. The **sensitivity** of the test is the likelihood that it will be positive when the pathogen is present. The **specificity** of the test measures the likelihood that it will be negative if the pathogen is not present.

In clinical practice, diagnostic tests with 100% sensitivity and 100% specificity do not exist. If available, a combination of tests often yield a higher level of diagnostic certainty. In addition, clinicians can use less-than-perfect tests to their advantage. Thus, a test that is very sensitive but not particularly specific can be useful in screening for the presence of an infection. For example, the so-called rapid plasma reagin (RPR) test or the Venereal Diseases Reference Laboratory Test (VDRL) are commonly used to screen patients for syphilis, even though several other infectious and noninfectious conditions can cause those tests to be false-positive. However, nearly all patients who have syphilis have positive RPR tests or VDRLs after the primary (chancre) stage. Therefore, either test has few false-negatives and is useful to "rule out" the diagnosis of syphilis. If the RPR test or VDRL is positive, then a second, confirmatory test must be employed to determine whether syphilis is actually present. In contrast to a screening test, a confirmatory test used to "rule in" a suspected diagnosis must be highly specific. Consider the example of a patient found to have a positive enzyme-linked immunosorbent assay (ELISA) screening test for HIV after a blood donation. A more specific (and costly) confirmatory test, the Western blot assay, is used to determine whether the patient actually has HIV infection or whether the screening test result was false-positive.

The predictive value of a diagnostic test is influenced by the frequency of the infection in the population being tested. Because the specificity of the ELISA for HIV is 99.8%, it will register as false-positive in one of every 500 negative individuals tested. If less than one person in 500 in a given population is infected with HIV, then there will be more false-positive tests than true-positive tests, and the positive predictive value will be poor (see Fig. 58-1). For example, HIV infection is extremely rare among elderly women with no apparent risk factors, and a positive result in such a patient is most likely to be false-positive. In contrast, in populations with a high prevalence of HIV infection—among intravenous drug users, for instance—the proportion of true-positive tests will be higher. The lesson is this: the interpretation of a laboratory test result depends not only on the technical accuracy of the method used but also on the prevalence of the infection in the population to which the patient belongs.

Diagnosing Infections by Microscopy

Because they possess characteristic morphologic features, staining properties, or movement, some pathogens can be accurately identified by direct microscopic examination of clinical material. For certain infections, microscopic diagnosis is highly sensitive and specific. It is also a rapid technique that permits the physician to initiate treatment without waiting for the results of a culture.

Most helminthic and protozoal infections are routinely diagnosed by microscopy. Many fungal pathogens also have characteristic morphologic features. Notably, *Cryptococcus neoformans* meningitis is diagnosed rapidly by finding encapsulated yeast in cerebrospinal fluid (CSF). By staining the CSF background with India ink, the transparent capsule of the yeast is visualized (see Fig. 48-4). In contrast, the morphology of most bacteria is too simple to permit microscopic identification; however, a few exceptions exist. Syphilis can easily be diagnosed by observing the characteristic helical form and bending motions of spirochetes from fresh scrapings of primary or secondary lesions. Although viruses cannot be seen in the light microscope, virus-induced changes in host cell morphology may be diagnostic. Examples include the multinucleated giant cells in scrapings from herpes simplex or varicella-zoster virus lesions (the Tzanck smear) and the specific intracellular inclusion bodies in tissues that are actively infected with cytomegalovirus.

Stains

Although a species identification is rarely possible, bacterial pathogens may be visualized and assigned to morphologic and functional groups using special stains. The basic principles of the **Gram stain** and the **acid-fast stains** were described in Chapter 3. The Gram stain is both rapid and simple to perform and can be carried out on virtually any body fluid or tissue sample. It can yield clinically useful information of three kinds:

1. The presence of bacteria in a normally sterile body fluid (e.g., CSF, pleural fluid, urine).
2. Staining properties and morphology of the organisms in a sample or culture that can direct further efforts at species identification and the empirical selection of antibiotics for the patient.
3. For certain clinical specimens, a diagnosis. For example, the presence of Gram-negative diplococci inside the leukocytes of urethral pus is highly specific for gonococci. The same morphologic type seen in samples of CSF is nearly always the meningococcus.

The Gram stain is much less useful when a sample is obtained from a nonsterile body site and thus contains normal flora. Considerable experience and skill are required to interpret Gram stains of coughed sputum specimens because they are typically contaminated with oropharyngeal bacteria that are indistinguishable from respiratory pathogens. In contrast, acid-fast bacteria (i.e., mycobacteria) are not normally found in the respiratory tract, and seeing them in a coughed sputum suggests pulmonary tuberculosis. In general, acid-fast bacteria in smears of sputum or normally sterile tissues are assumed to be *Mycobacterium tuberculosis* until proven otherwise.

A variety of other stains are used to visualize pathogens. Among the most commonly used stains are the **Giemsa stain** for systemic protozoal infections (e.g., malaria), iodine stains for intestinal helminths, and silver stains for systemic fungal pathogens. Special stains can be used to visualize the characteristic cysts of *Pneumocystis jiroveci* in a sample of bronchial fluid from an AIDS patient.

Antibody-Based Identification

The accuracy of microscopic identification of bacterial and viral pathogens is enhanced when **specific antibodies** are used in conjunction with direct microscopy. These procedures generally involve the attachment (or conjugation) of a detectable substance to antibody molecules so that the microscopist can actually see where the antibodies bind. For example, in a **direct fluorescent antibody (DFA) test** for *Cryptosporidium* protozoa, a monoclonal antibody has been conjugated to a fluorescent compound. To diagnose the infection, stool is fixed to a slide and then treated with the conjugated antibodies. After washing, the slide is examined using a **fluorescence microscope.** *Cryptosporidium* cysts appear as bright yellow–green, glowing spheres when illuminated with light of the appropriate wavelength. Because the organisms are so distinct against the dark background, they are easy to pick out when scanning the slide. The DFA technique can be used to identify any pathogen to which specific antibodies can be produced.

Clearly, the specificity of antibody-based identification of pathogens depends on the specificity of the antibodies used. Most antisera are polyclonal mixtures of antibodies that bind to different domains of different antigenic molecules (Fig. 58-2). Therefore, when polyclonal antiserum is used in a diagnostic test, the likelihood is high that unwanted cross-reactions with other

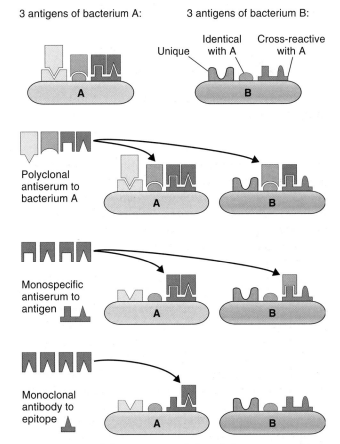

FIGURE 58-2 ■ **The cross-reactivity of three types of immunoglobulin preparations.** Antibodies raised to react with bacterium A may cross-react with bacterium B. Polyclonal antisera are cross-reactive because bacteria A and B have protein antigens in common. Additionally, monospecific antiserum raised against a single antigen of bacterium A is also cross-reactive, because one of the antibody-binding sites (epitopes) on this antigen is shared by an antigen of bacterium B. However, a monoclonal antibody against an epitope on this antigen was found to be unique to bacterium A and to have no cross-reactivity.

microorganisms will occur. The specificity of the test may be enhanced with the use of monoclonal (monospecific) antibodies, as suggested in Figure 58-2. The principles illustrated in the figure apply to all antibody-based methods of diagnosis, including the serologic antigen detection tests described in the next few sections of this chapter.

Diagnosing Infections by Culture

Culturing is usually the most specific way to establish the presence of a particular pathogen in a patient sample. However, in many situations culturing may not be sensitive or clinically practical. Culture is routine for most bacterial and fungal infections but is rarely performed for helminthic and protozoal pathogens. Some microorganisms cannot be cultured at all in clinical microbiology laboratories (e.g., hepatitis viruses, *Treponema pallidum*, *Mycobacterium leprae*, and *P. jiroveci*), either because the necessary conditions for their cultivation in vitro are not yet known or because the available culture systems are inefficient and impractical. Because chlamydiae and viruses are obligate intracellular pathogens, they can be propagated and identified only in appropriate cell cultures. Cultivation of other pathogens, such as rickettsiae, is shunned by most clinical laboratories because of the hazards involved in handling the microorganisms.

General Principles

In general, the choices of culture method and medium are tailored to the nature and source of the specimen and the question that the culture is meant to address. For example, when a specimen of pus from a brain abscess is cultured, the implied question is, What microorganisms are present in the abscess? The assumption is that any organisms present are causative and that chemotherapy directed against them will be beneficial. To look for the etiologic agents, the sample is cultured on a variety of agar-based media and in a broth medium under both aerobic and anaerobic conditions. The culture strategy is to recover all microorganisms that might inhabit a brain abscess.

In contrast to that open-ended approach, other cultures are performed primarily to determine whether a particular pathogen is present or not. An example is the throat culture for *Streptococcus pyogenes* in cases of exudative pharyngitis, because that is the only culturable bacterial agent for which treatment is indicated. Throat swab specimens are inoculated only onto nutrient sheep's blood agar plates, which not only support the growth of streptococci but also show the characteristic β-hemolysis of *S. pyogenes*.

Cultures from nonsterile body sites present yet another problem: the inhibition or obscuring of the pathogen's growth by an abundant normal flora. Thus, **selective media** are needed for those cultures. An example of a selective medium is Thayer-Martin medium, used to culture gonococci. Thayer-Martin is a chocolate agar (made with boiled blood, not chocolate) containing antibiotics that inhibit the growth of members of the normal flora in the genitourinary tract but not gonococci. Selective and semiselective media are also used to cultivate enteric pathogens from the bacteria-rich stool specimens or respiratory pathogens from sputum. One disadvantage of selective media is that they can inhibit the growth of some strains of the pathogen of interest. Therefore, selective media should be used only for specimens that are likely to contain contaminating normal organisms.

As with all diagnostic methods, culture results require interpretation by the physician. In some situations (e.g., meningitis, urinary tract infection), a negative culture is quite reassuring that the etiology of the patient's problem is not a bacterial or fungal infection. In other situations the sensitivity of culture diagnosis is relatively poor. For example, a negative culture for pneumococci does not rule out the agent as the cause of a bacterial pneumonia, because the sensitivity of sputum culture for this fastidious pathogen may be 50% or lower in some clinical settings.

Positive cultures always raise the question of whether the isolate is the actual cause of the patient's illness. In cultures from nonsterile body sites, the problem is whether the isolate represents normal flora (colonization) or an etiologic agent (infection). In cultures from normally sterile body sites, contamination can occur when patient samples are obtained using faulty sterile technique. Typically, specimens obtained by needle puncture are contaminated with normal skin flora (e.g., *Staphylococcus epidermidis*, diphtheroids, streptococci). Because these bacteria can occasionally cause true infections, the physician must consider the clinical circumstances of the individual patient to judge whether the isolate is a contaminant. In many cases it is necessary to reisolate the same organism by repeated cultures to be convinced of its significance. As another example, almost all voided urine collections have some degree of contamination; true infection is associated with a relatively high concentration of bacteria in the specimen. However, a urine sample that sits for hours becomes grossly contaminated as the microorganisms in the specimen start growing.

Blood Culture

The simplest blood culture involves the direct inoculation of a blood sample into nutrient broth, followed by incubation at 37°C and periodic checks for an indication of microbial growth. In the past, turbidity was used as an indicator of microbial growth. However, the development of visible turbidity can take days. Modern automated blood culture systems periodically assay culture bottles for a byproduct of microbial growth (e.g., CO_2). Using such sensitive techniques, growth of organisms can be detected long before visible turbidity develops. Once growth is detected, microorganisms from cultures are transferred to agar plates, or **subcultured,** to permit species identification.

Another method that works well for fungi, mycobacteria, and certain fastidious pathogens is the **lysis–centrifugation technique.** In this method, blood is collected directly into a tube containing a solution that lyses blood cells. The remaining dense material, which includes any microorganism, is pelleted by centrifugation to the bottom of the tube, where it is removed and inoculated directly onto an appropriate agar-based medium. In addition to its increased sensitivity for some pathogens, this technique has the advantage of bypassing the usual subculture step, because the isolates grow directly as colonies on agar plates.

Culture Identification

Classically, bacteria cultured from clinical specimens are identified by determining **phenotypic properties,** such as motility; utilization of various nutrient substrates; and production of enzymes, toxins, or byproducts of metabolism. Because regrowth is required for many of the tests on bacteria, definitive identification typically requires an extra day or more.

Microorganisms in culture are sometimes identified more rapidly using **antibody-based techniques,** which are discussed in more detail in the next section. Viruses are frequently identified in culture by their reaction with specific antiviral antibodies or by the ability of a specific antiserum to neutralize them when inoculated into fresh tissue culture.

Antimicrobial Sensitivity Testing

Perhaps the most important advantage of culturing is that the isolate can be tested for susceptibility to antimicrobial agents, often the most important piece of therapeutically related information to be obtained. Antibiotic sensitivity testing of bacteria is discussed in Chapter 30. Fungal and viral pathogens can also be tested for drug susceptibility, but those tests are beyond the capabilities of most clinical microbiology laboratories.

Measuring the Antibody Response to Infection

Serologic tests measure the patient's humoral immune response to an infection. Because human serum contains many antibodies, serologic tests are designed to measure only those directed at specific microbial antigens. Some of the common formats for **serology** of infectious diseases (i.e., agglutination, complement fixation, neutralization, and indirect fluorescent antibody tests) are discussed in the electronic supplement to this chapter. In those tests and others, the amount of specific antibody present in the patient's serum is quantified by testing dilutions of the patient's serum. The highest dilution of the patient's serum that still can exert the measured function, or **endpoint,** is the positive **titer** for that assay.

Later generations of serologic tests do not measure the activity of specific antibody but measure their presence directly. Most of these tests are **solid-phase assays,** which use either the pathogen or antigens from the pathogen fixed to a solid support, such as the wells of a microtiter plate, porous membrane, or inert beads. Patient serum is added to the system, and specific antibodies are bound and immobilized to the fixed antigen. All nonreacting an-

1. Patient serum incubated with antigen on solid support.

2. Unbound antibodies washed away.

3. Enzyme-labeled anti-immunglobulin binds to patient antibodies bound to the antigen on the solid support.

4. Amount of bound enzyme activity is measured.

Solid support

FIGURE 58-3 ▪ **Direct ELISA serology for the detection of specific antibodies in patient serum.**

tibodies and serum components are washed away. The presence of the bound specific antibody is typically detected by adding a labeled antibody directed against human immunoglobulin molecules (raised in animals by immunization with human antibodies). A popular format for these tests is the **ELISA** (Fig. 58-3). In an ELISA the "second antibody" is conjugated to an enzyme, such as peroxidase or alkaline phosphatase, which catalyzes the production of visibly colored compounds from colorless precursors and makes the detection far more sensitive. In addition, the second (conjugated) antibody may be made specific for IgG, IgM, or other immunoglobulins, permitting the ELISA to measure only antibodies of a certain class.

The specificity of a serologic test is determined largely by the character and purity of the antigen used to capture the patient's antibodies. An **immunoblot** (or **Western blot**) is one of the most specific serologic methods available because the antigens to which the patient's serum reacts are specified. In this test the antigenic molecules from a pathogen are first separated according to their size using electrophoresis. The whole series of antigens is then "blotted" onto a solid support and incubated with the patient's serum (Fig. 58-4). It is then possible to determine whether the patient's antibodies are directed against pathogen-specific or cross-reactive antigens. That additional level of analysis allows the discrimination of specific and nonspecific reactions. Western blotting has become a mainstay for confirming the diagnosis of HIV infection first detected by ELISAs.

Serological tests for particular infectious diseases can be both sensitive and specific, but their utility in clinical management is often limited. Because the tests depend on the immune response to infection, they have limited use in the early diagnosis of acute infections, be-fore the patient develops specific antibodies. Serology is typically more useful in determining whether infection with a particular pathogen has occurred in the past. The physician must decide whether the positive serology is the result of the patient's current illness or an infection that took place months or years earlier. There are two ways to make this determination. First, the patient's specific antibody titer can be measured at two points in time, usually several weeks apart (**acute and convalescent titers**). A significant increase in the amount of antibody indicates a recent or ongoing infection with the pathogen. The second way to diagnose a recent infection serologically is to measure specific **IgM antibodies** against the pathogen. In the course of most infections, IgM antibodies appear first and tend to disappear a few months after onset.

Diagnosing Infection by Detecting Microbial Macromolecules

In the investigation of a crime, a detective looks for traces left by the perpetrator. Similarly, the microbial culprit associated with an infection can often be identified by recognizing its products or parts, provided those parts are as specific for the pathogen as fingerprints are for a criminal. In microbiology identifications are made either by detecting an **antigen** or a **nucleic acid sequence** that is specific for a pathogen. As you know from recent, celebrated criminal cases, prosecutors also use laboratory methods when traces of blood or body fluids are the

1. Soluble proteins extracted from the pathogen are separated by size using gel electrophoresis.

2. Protein bands are transferred electrophoretically to a paper-like membrane support.

3. Direct enzyme immunoassay with patient serum; only those antigens to which the patient has antibodies are visualized.

Specific antigen
Cross-reactive antigen
Specific antigen

FIGURE 58-4 ■ **Western blot.** By noting the antigens ("bands") with which the patient serum reacts, it is possible to determine whether the reactivity is owing to specific or cross-reactive antibodies.

available clues.

Macromolecular detection tests have inherent disadvantages and advantages compared with standard culture diagnoses. Among the disadvantages are the imperfect specificity, the inability to further study the infecting pathogen (e.g., for antimicrobial sensitivity, strain typing), and the need to perform separate tests for each suspected pathogen. Advantages include the capacity to diagnose the infection within hours rather than days and greater sensitivity in certain settings (e.g., the detection of a pathogen after treatment with antimicrobials has rendered the culture negative).

Detecting Microbial Antigens

Antigen detection tests are like serologic tests in reverse; instead of using the microbial antigen to capture antibodies from patient serum, specific antibodies are used to capture microbial antigens from a patient sample. In most of these assays, the "capture" antibody is bound to a solid support. Certain antigens, such as capsular polysaccharides, can be detected by a simple agglutination assay (Fig. 58-5). Several widely performed tests use antibody-coated latex beads (**latex agglutination tests**) to detect capsular material from *C. neoformans*, meningococcus, pneumococcus, *Haemophilus influenzae*, and others.

For many antigens the presence of the "captured" molecule is detected using a second antibody (e.g., in the **enzyme immunoassay**; Fig. 58-6A); this test is analogous to the ELISA for antibody detection. The sample is incubated with an antibody-coated solid support, and the unbound material in the sample is washed away. An enzyme-labeled second antibody, which is also directed against the microbial antigen, is then added, forming a "**sandwich**" of the antigen between two layers of antibody. Another format for this test is the **competitive**

assay (Fig. 58-6B). In these systems the sample is coincubated with an enzyme-labeled antigen that competes with an unlabeled antigen in the sample for binding to a fixed amount of specific antibody. A positive test is one that fails to develop a enzymatic color reaction. These basic formats have been adapted to simple kits to test for several pathogens in office practice (e.g., influenza) or at home (e.g., pregnancy tests detecting human chorionic gonadotropin).

Nucleic Acid–Based Diagnosis of Infection

DNA is composed of two separate strands held together by hydrogen bonding between complementary bases. Because they are bound by relatively weak hydrogen bonds, the two strands of DNA can be separated into single strands by heating. When the temperature is again lowered, the complementary strands reconnect (or **hybridize**), reforming double-stranded DNA. Hybridization occurs only when the two strands are a genuine **complementary pair**. A short, single-stranded DNA sequence (or **probe**) can be chosen so that it hybridizes *only* to a perfectly complementary "**target**" sequence. The precision of this interaction accounts for the high degree of specificity of nucleic acid–based tests.

The **DNA probe test** was the first nucleic acid-based test to be used. Typically, a single-stranded DNA probe is labeled with a radioisotope, enzyme, or other detectable label, and the patient's sample is treated so that microorganisms are disrupted and DNA and RNA are released and then heat denatured (i.e., converted to single strands). The mixture of labeled probe and sample is incubated, and the amount of probe hybridized to nucleic acids is measured. The bound and unbound probes are distinguished, commonly by using probes attached to

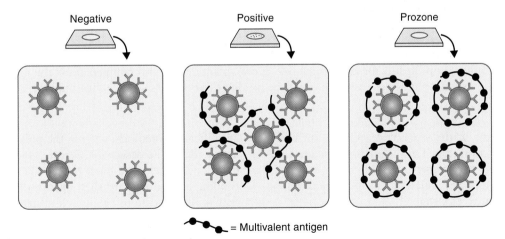

FIGURE 58-5 ■ **Detection of a polyvalent antigen by particle agglutination.** Particles are coated with specific antibodies. If a multivalent antigen is present in the patient sample, bridges form between the particles, causing clumping. When there is much more antigen than antibody in the mixture, a false-negative, or prozone phenomenon, may occur because no bridges between beads can form. Paradoxically, a serum sample that is negative because of a prozone reaction becomes positive when it is diluted.

A. ELISA for antigen detection
(direct "sandwich" assay)

1. Add patient sample.

2. Any antigen present in sample "captured" by immobilized antibodies.

3. Wash.

4. Enzyme-conjugated specific antibody added; binds to antigen, forming a "sandwich."

5. Wash; add enzyme substrate and measure color change.

Solid support

B. Enzymeimmunoassay for antigen detection
(competitive assay)

Sample containing *no* antigen

Pure radiolabeled antigen

Solid support

Wash | Count

Maximal binding of isotope to the solid support indicates no antigen present in the sample.

Sample containing antigen

Pure radiolabeled antigen

Solid support

Wash | Count

Reduced isotope binding to the solid support indicates antigen present in the sample.

FIGURE 58-6 ▪ **Enzyme immunoassays for microbial antigen detection. A.** In the "sandwich" assay format of the test, "capture" antibody bound to a solid support binds antigen from the patient sample. Nonspecific contents of the sample are washed away. The presence of the captured antigen is detected using a second, specific antibody conjugated to an enzyme. Lastly, the activity of the enzyme bound to the solid support is measured using a color-producing substrate; color production signals the presence of the antigen, which is sandwiched between the two antibodies. **B.** In the competitive assay format, the patient sample is coincubated with a measured, small amount of purified, enzyme-labeled antigen over the same captured antibody solid support. If the patient sample contains no antigen, all the labeled antigen will complex with the antibody, and all the added enzyme-labeled antigen will be bound in immune complexes. If the patient sample contains antigen, it will compete with the labeled antigen for binding to the available antibody, and there will be minimal enzyme associated with immune complexes.

a solid support, as in the separation steps in antibody and antigen detection tests. On the microscopic level, **in situ hybridization** may be performed on tissue sections. More detail about these formats can be found in the electronic supplement to this chapter.

Nucleic Acid Amplification

In many instances the amount of specific nucleic acid in a sample is insufficient for direct detection with a DNA probe. In such cases it may be possible to use **nucleic acid**

amplification methods, such as the **polymerase chain reaction (PCR).** To design a PCR test, a specific sequence of microbial nucleic acid must be known. Two short DNA probes, or **primers,** are then chemically synthesized so they will hybridize to the opposite strands of the target DNA sequence at a given distance (Fig. 58-7). In the assay, three components are added to DNA extracted from the patient's specimen: the two primers, deoxyribonucleotides (deoxynucleotide triphosphates, or dNTPs), and a heat-stable DNA polymerase. The reactants are subjected to repeated cycles of temperature shifts that result in denaturation of DNA (heating), hybridization of

FIGURE 58-7 ▪ **Nucleic acid amplification: the polymerase chain reaction (PCR).** The patient sample is mixed with specific primers, deoxynucleotide triphosphates (dNTPs), and a thermostable DNA polymerase enzyme. The reaction involves three steps repeated in sequence: (1) heat denaturation, which permits complementary strands of the target DNA to separate; (2) annealing, as the primers hybridize to opposite strands of the targeted sequence when the temperature is lowered; and (3) synthesis, as the polymerase incorporates the dNTPS into a new complementary strand of DNA, in a sequential and unidirectional manner, beginning at each hybridized primer. Note that synthesis from either primer generates a new site to which the opposite primer can hybridize in the next cycle. Each time this cycle is repeated, the number of double-stranded target DNA sequences available to bind the two primers doubles. One target DNA molecule subjected to 30 repetitions of the PCR would result in 2^{30} copies of the target sequence. The products of the reaction are detected by gel electrophoresis or by a gene probe specific for the sequences between the two primers.

the primers (cooling), and DNA synthesis. In each cycle of the reaction, the DNA spanned by the two primers is duplicated. With the synthesis of each new strand of DNA, new primer-binding sites are generated. Consequently, each new strand becomes a new template for subsequent rounds of primer-initiated synthesis.

With every cycle of the PCR the number of copies of the DNA segment between the primers doubles, thus doubling the templates for further synthesis. This "chain reaction" results in the geometric increase in the amounts of target DNA. In this respect, PCR is analogous to the biological process of DNA replication that occurs in populations of dividing cells; however, in PCR the exponential synthesis is limited to the DNA segment bounded by the two synthetic primers. The amplified sequences of a PCR (or **amplicons**) can then be analyzed by gel electrophoresis as fragments of a predicted size or "captured" and detected by conventional DNA probe hybridization. PCR assays to detect and confirm the presence of *M. tuberculosis* in a sputum sample, herpes simplex virus or enterovirus in CSF, or *Chlamydia trachomatis* in a urine specimen or cervical swab have been commercialized and are routinely available at many institutions.

Gel electrophoresis, while suitable for the research laboratory, is a cumbersome process for a clinical laboratory. Therefore, several strategies to detect and confirm the identity of amplicons have been proposed. To date the most efficient and practical strategy has been **real-time PCR**. Using this technique, the accumulating

amplicons in a PCR are quantified as they are generated using a fluorescent label. One commonly used method is illustrated in Figure 58-8A. The typical result of this method and others is that the intensity of the fluorescence in the reaction vessel increases as more amplicons are generated. Thus, real-time PCR adds two important features to the process: First, it combines the steps of amplification and amplicon analysis into a single process, simplifying the analysis of the amplicons. Second, it offers the possibility of quantifying the target nucleic acid sequence in the original sample by measuring the number of cycles required to reach a threshold of fluorescence detection (Fig. 58-8B). Quantitative PCR is now routinely used to detect and measure viruses in human fluid samples (e.g., HIV, cytomegalovirus, Epstein-Barr virus, hepatitis viruses).

The great power of PCR is its sensitivity. Theoretically, the chain reaction can be initiated by a single copy of the target sequence. However, the procedure's exquisite sensitivity is also its major drawback as a clinical diagnostic tool. A serious potential for cross-contamination (microcontamination) exists in laboratories that process many similar samples every day. The prevention of false-positive PCR results is a matter of great concern to physicians and lawyers because no equally sensitive, alternate method may be available to verify a positive PCR result. The most celebrated example of that pitfall occurred in the murder trial of O. J. Simpson, in which questions about mishandling of specimens and cross-contamination

A

1. Two primers and the detection probe are denatured and hybridized

2. DNA is synthesized with displacement of the detection probe

3. Detection probe cleaves by 5'-exonuclease activity of polymerase

4. Physically separated from the quencher, the fluorescent label becomes active

B

Fluorescence intensity

10^6 10^5 10^4 10^3

Threshold of fluorescence detection

Number of PCR cycles

FIGURE 58-8 ▪ **Real-time PCR. A.** In the TaqMan (Applied Biosystems) procedure for confirming and quantifying PCR products, the PCR vessel contains target DNA (pink and lavender), primers (dark purple), and a DNA detection probe that hybridizes specifically to the amplified sequence (blue). Conjugated to this detection probe is a fluorescent dye and a fluorescence quencher in close proximity to one another, such that the fluorescence from the dye is quenched and is undetectable. As DNA synthesis proceeds, the 5'-exonuclease activity of the polymerase digests the detection probe, releasing the fluorescent dye and the quencher. As they separate from one another, the fluorescent dye becomes active and emits a signal. With each round of PCR, more detection probes hybridize and are cleaved, increasing the fluorescent signal geometrically until all of the primers and probes are exhausted. **B.** Fluorescent signals obtained with real-time PCRs beginning with decreasing quantities of target DNA. As the number of copies of target DNA decrease, the fluorescence curve shifts to the right. For quantitative PCR a standard curve can be generated by determining how many cycles of PCR are required to exceed a predetermined threshold for fluorescence detection (purple horizontal line). By reference to these standards, the number of target nucleic acid molecules in a patient sample can be determined.

of evidence may have influenced the verdict. To avoid cross-contamination in clinical diagnostic laboratories, specimen preparation and amplification are performed in separate areas. Another strategy is to incorporate modified nucleotides in the PCR so as to render the products (amplicons) susceptible to enzymatic degradation should they contaminate a patient sample.

Microarrays

A disadvantage of nucleic acid–based tests and antigen detection assays is that they can tell the physician only

whether a particular pathogen is present in a sample. As a diagnostic tool, bacterial culture has an advantage over those methods because it does not require the physician to guess which pathogens may be present and to test for each individually. One culture can detect an enormous variety of pathogenic organisms by a single method. Advances in microchip technology have created the possibility of using nonculture diagnostics in a similar manner. A microchip can be printed to contain hundreds of oligonucleotide probes bound in an array no bigger than a microscopic slide.

Since bacteria have many conserved sequences (e.g.,

FIGURE 58-9 ▪ **Oligonucleotide microarray analysis to identify specific products of a nonspecific PCR amplification.** In this theoretical assay, PCR is conducted using primers that bind to all bacterial chromosomes but amplify intervening sequences that are different in each species. During the amplification process the amplicons are labeled with a fluorescent dye–conjugated primer. Finally, the amplicons are hybridized to a microarray that has bound oligonucleotides representing the inventing sequences from hundreds of bacterial species. In this case the amplicons bind to the sequences characteristic of *Escherichia coli*, identifying *E. coli* as the bacteria in the original sample.

16S ribosomal RNA) with intervening, nonconserved regions, it is theoretically possible to design PCR primers that will amplify a product from any bacterial species, albeit with different amplified sequences between the primers. Imagine that DNA extracted from a patient sample is incubated with these primers in a PCR. The products of such a reaction could then be hybridized with a microarray containing the known intervening sequences from hundreds of bacterial species. It would then be possible to determine which one (or ones) are present in the patient sample (Fig. 58-9). Tests of that kind are not currently available commercially but may represent the vanguard of new diagnostic development in the near future.

Conclusion

Many techniques are available to establish the presence of a pathogenic microorganism in an ill patient. All methods have the potential for inaccuracy, either in failing to detect a pathogen or immune response when present or in signaling their presence when the pathogen or the immune response is absent. Some tests are more sensitive or more specific than others, and those measures of performance determine how and when they are used. However, even when a test accurately analyzes a given sample, the simple presence of a microorganism in the specimen or of antibodies against a pathogen in patient serum does not always indicate active infection, nor does it necessarily establish the cause of illness. Therefore, interpretation is always necessary with any microbiologic test, regardless of its technical performance characteristics. In the final analysis there is no substitute for the interpretive skills of the clinician in placing microbiologic test results into the context of the patient's illness.

Principles of Epidemiology

David R. Snydman

Epidemiology is the study of the determinants of disease in a population. Epidemiologists deal with both infectious and noninfectious etiologies. When infectious agents are involved, the aim is to understand their mode of transmission and what predisposes a population to a particular agent. The practical purpose of epidemiology is to control the spread of disease in a population, either by limiting microbial transmission or by altering the susceptibility of a population. Common control measures include removing the source of the agent, controlling its transmission, and immunizing the population.

This chapter considers epidemiological concepts and methods through the examination of an epidemiological "case," the investigation of a new disease. Following the case discussion, the chapter considers general epidemiological issues.

Epidemiological Methodology

The Connecticut epidemiologists undertook what is known as an **epidemic investigation,** the study of the extent, characteristics, mode of transmission, and etiology of a cluster of cases. It is perhaps the most self-evident method used in epidemiology, but it is by no means the only one. Others, including **case-control studies, cohort studies,** and **epidemiological interventions,** are discussed in this chapter.

An epidemic investigation is undertaken when the number of cases of a disease increases over what is considered to be the norm or standard. In the Connecticut study it was necessary to determine first if the arthritis cases did indeed represent an epidemic. The determination of an epidemic depends solely on the background incidence of the disease in the population and not on an absolute cutoff point. For example, before the advent of the polio vaccine in the 1950s, about 50,000 cases of the disease occurred in the United States annually. After the vaccine was put into widespread use, the number of cases dropped dramatically to about 10 per year. Therefore, one or two cases of polio after widespread vaccination might be considered an epidemic.

In addition to epidemics, epidemiologists study **endemic** and **pandemic** diseases. An endemic infectious disease is one that is consistently found in the population, such as dental caries, gonorrhea, or athlete's foot. A pandemic is a worldwide epidemic; examples are the current AIDS pandemic and the Spanish flu pandemic of 1918.

Case

In October 1975 the Department of Health of Connecticut received separate calls from two mothers living on rural roads in the towns of Lyme and Old Lyme. They reported that several children in their households and their neighborhoods had what appeared to be arthritis. They had voiced their concern to local physicians and were not deterred by being told that arthritis is "not infectious."

This case raises several questions:

1. Were the cases reported in the two towns related?
2. Did any other people in either town have similar symptoms?
3. Did the children have an infectious form of arthritis?
4. What forms of arthritis are infectious?
5. What steps should epidemiologists take and what principles should they apply to studying the reported cases, after discussions with the parents and local physicians?

FIGURE 59-1 ▪ Clustering of cases of Lyme disease in three towns in Connecticut (Lyme, Old Lyme, and East Haddam) between 1972 and 1975.

Case Definition

The investigators of the cases of arthritis in Connecticut began by asking whether other individuals had the same disease. They first had to establish a set of clinical criteria known as the **case definition.** After all, many people have arthritis. From the mothers, physicians, and school nurses in the area, they obtained a list of other individuals who may have had the same symptoms. After examining those people and taking careful histories, the epidemiologists included, as fitting the case definition, individuals with the following clinical picture: a sudden onset of swelling and pain in a knee or other large joint lasting a week to several months, several attacks that recurred several times at intervals over a few months, and/or fever and fatigue.

Time, Place, and Personal Characteristics of Patients

Armed with a usable case definition, the investigators found other cases in Old Lyme and two adjacent towns. The best sources of additional cases were the two determined mothers who had made the original phone calls. From current and past episodes, the investigators collected 51 cases that conformed to the case definition. They could now proceed to determine what epidemiologists call the time, place, and personal characteristics of the cases. The **time characteristics** include the **time of onset** of the disease and its **duration.** As shown in Figure 59-1, many of the Connecticut cases clustered in the summer and early fall. The duration of each bout of the disease varied from a week to a few months, and 69% of the patients had recurrences of the symptoms. Not

knowing at the time the etiology of the disease, the investigators could not determine another important time characteristic, the **incubation period,** or the interval from exposure to the first onset of symptoms.

Place characteristics are primarily the site of residence and the area in which the patients lived. For occupation-related illnesses, the workplace is another location to consider. The Connecticut cases were concentrated in three adjacent towns on the eastern side of the Connecticut River. Most of the patients lived in wooded areas near streams and lakes. **Personal characteristics** include the age and sex of the patients and any possible genetic predisposition to the disease. Of the 51 Connecticut cases, 39 were children, nearly evenly divided by gender. No familial pattern was discerned.

Using the information they gathered on time, place, and personal characteristics, the epidemiologists listed the cases by times of onset and constructed what is called an **epidemic curve.** They dubbed the outbreak Lyme arthritis, although that name was later modified to Lyme disease.

The epidemiologists now posed other questions. Was the outbreak a surveillance artifact resulting from the many questions about arthritis that were being asked by outsiders? The simplest way to assess that possibility was to go elsewhere and ask the same questions. By surveying towns on the other side of the Connecticut River, the investigators determined that increased interest did not result in an increase in the number of cases of arthritis reported. In their early investigation, the epidemiologists wondered how common Lyme disease might be. Assessing the **attack rate** of an epidemic disease requires knowing the total number of cases (the numerator) and the total number of people who are "at risk" (the denominator). In the context of many confined outbreaks, it is possible to make that calculation. For example, if 25 of 125 guests who attended a wedding later developed staphylococcal food poisoning from eating the potato salad, the attack rate is 20% (i.e., 25 divided by 125).

In the first Lyme disease investigation, neither the total number of cases nor the number of at-risk persons was known. However, surveillance for the infection in subsequent years has yielded case reports from each state that can be used to calculate the local risk of Lyme disease in the United States. Those data can be reported as an **incidence** (the number of cases during a defined period divided by the population of the state during that time) or as a **prevalence** (the number of cases at any given time). For example, we now know that the annual incidence of Lyme disease in Connecticut (from 1992 to 1998) was 68 per 100,000 population, whereas in neighboring Massachusetts the annual incidence was only 5 per 100,000 population, an almost twelvefold lower risk.

Is Lyme Disease Communicable?

The investigating team then asked, Is this an infectious disease? The most common arthritic conditions of childhood, such as juvenile rheumatoid arthritis, are collagen vascular problems and are not known to be infectious. Nonetheless, the clustering of cases, with most cases beginning in the summer or early fall and most patients living in wooded areas along lakes or streams, suggested an arthropod-transmitted disease, possibly viral. If so, the investigators wondered, is the disease new? Many infectious diseases, like measles, polio, and tuberculosis, are **communicable.** Others, like a ruptured appendix, urinary tract infections, or osteomyelitis, are not. Was Lyme disease communicable, or did it merely affect susceptible individuals? To answer that question, the investigators attempted to trace contacts; but even in families with several affected members, the onset of illness had usually taken place in different years. When they tried to identify a common exposure, they could not find any. However, an intriguing clue surfaced. About one quarter of the patients had reported that the symptoms of arthritis were preceded by an unusual skin rash. The rash had started as a red spot that spread to form a 6-inch ring. What was the connection? An astute dermatology consultant remembered that similar rashes had been described in 1910 in Sweden and had been attributed to tick bites. The rash went by the impressive name of erythema chronicum migrans.

The investigators undertook a **case-control study** in 1977, in which the cases are matched with a similar group of control or unaffected persons. Note that case-control studies are always **retrospective;** that is, they begin by defining groups of ill or well subjects and then look to the past for potential exposures or **risk factors** that were more common among the ill than the well subjects. After matching for age, sex, and any other relevant factors, the epidemiologists found that those affected by Lyme disease were more likely to live in households with pets and thus were more likely to come in contact with the ticks that dogs and cats picked up in the woods of that region. In a roundabout way, that clue became more credible when the investigators remembered the suggestive clinical finding of the Swedish researchers.

So far, the connection between the rash and Lyme disease depended on **retrospective evidence.** To make the connection stronger, it became appropriate to ask if patients with the signs of erythema chronicum migrans progressed to develop Lyme disease. In 1977 the team set up a **prospective study,** looking for patients with the rash and observing them for some time. That type of study is referred to as a **cohort study.** In contrast to the case-control approach, a cohort study defines subjects by a clinical characteristic or suspected exposure and then follows the subjects to determine who becomes ill and who remains well. In the Connecticut study 19 of 32 new cases of erythema chronicum migrans progressed to Lyme disease.

Meanwhile, the "tick connection" became even more plausible after a thorough entomological survey. After collecting insects and ticks from Lyme and the surrounding areas, the investigators found that adult ticks were 16 times more abundant on the east side of the Connecticut River than on the west side. That finding corresponded roughly to the incidence of cases of Lyme disease in the two areas. In addition, many more tick bites were reported by the arthritis patients than by their neighbors without the disease. Thus, the tick–rash–arthritis connection seemed more and more plausible. The final proof of the investigators' scheme awaited the discovery of the etiological agent and the direct demonstration of its transmission by ticks.

At the same time, a **surveillance network** had been set up in Connecticut and parts of the adjacent states to gather information about other cases. A careful study revealed that, contrary to the early reports, the disease was more frequent in adults than in children. It was easier to recognize arthritis as an unusual occurrence in children. Many arthritis patients had serious manifestations, such as neurological dysfunction and myocarditis. Thus, the disease turned out to be considerably more complex than described by the original case definition. That illustrates an important epidemiological point: an early case definition is, by necessity, tentative and may be modified when the full spectrum of the disease becomes known. As an example of a complex case definition, consider the one developed for AIDS (see Table 38-4).

Search for the Etiological Agent

So far, the investigators could conclude with assurance that Lyme disease was an infection, most likely transmitted by ticks. It appeared to be a new clinical entity. However, the search for the etiological agent had proved unproductive. Despite many attempts, no laboratory had succeeded in isolating a virus, which at the time seemed to be a good candidate for being the agent of the disease. On the other hand, the investigators collected anecdotal evidence that tetracycline, erythromycin, and penicillin were clinically effective. With time, more physicians reported the beneficial effects of antibiotics, making a bacterial etiology more likely. At about that time, in 1979 and 1980, entomologists and microbiologists at the Rocky Mountain Public Health Laboratory in Montana, who were experts in tickborne diseases, examined ticks sent from the affected area and found that the gut of many specimens contained unusual spirochetes. Were those the agents of Lyme disease?

Using a culture medium that supports the growth of tickborne or louseborne spirochetes, the microbiologists succeeded in growing a newly recognized spirochete. Soon thereafter they isolated the spirochete from human cases, and the immune responses of patients were linked to that organism. The spirochete was classified in the *Borrelia* genus, a group that includes the agent of another tickborne disease also found in the United States, relapsing fever. The agent of Lyme disease was given the name *B. burgdorferi*, in honor of the entomologist who discovered the organism in the ticks.

With a simple diagnostic test at hand, investigators in many parts of the world could carry out serological surveys, or **serosurveys,** to determine the proportion of persons with antibodies to *B. burgdorferi*. In general, serosurveys enable investigators to recognize a wide range of clinical manifestations, from asymptomatic cases to full-blown disease. That recognition is important because in most infectious diseases there are many more asymptomatic than clinically overt cases. The use of serosurveys has led to diagnoses of Lyme disease in other parts of the United States, especially on both coasts, as well as in Canada, Europe, Asia, and Australia. It is considered a serious disease, mainly because of its important and chronic neurological manifestations.

Prevention Strategies

Once the agent was confirmed, investigators set about attempting to develop a vaccine against disease. That process was complicated and required knowledge of the immunology of infection and the role of the outer membrane proteins of *B. burgdorferi* and the establishment of animal models of infection with demonstrated protection. As with many infectious agents, a vaccine would be one way to prevent future cases of Lyme disease. In fact, a vaccine against the disease was developed and was shown to be effective, but manufacturers have stopped development because of concern about the potential risk of arthritis resulting from vaccine administration. Liability issues led to the vaccine becoming unavailable. Alternative prevention strategies, such as public health awareness of exposure, examination for tick bites or tick attachment, and use of a short course of antibiotics after exposure, have been shown to be effective in diminishing the risk of infection. Reducing the overabundant deer population through authorized deer hunting has been a controversial means of indirectly controlling *B. burgdorferi* transmission.

The puzzle of "Lyme arthritis" had been solved. A few years after the original phone calls, a new disease was described, its agent and mode of transmission were identified, and preventive and therapeutic measures had been instituted. Note that it took the joint efforts of epidemiologists, clinicians, entomologists, microbiologists, and alert and determined members of the public.

Routes of Transmission

Humans as Reservoirs

We now turn from a specific example to a more general consideration of epidemiological principles. These principles include the routes of transmission, incubation periods, communicability, and individual susceptibility. The first is the mode of transmission (Table 59-1). **Transmission from human to human** may take place from parent to offspring or between mature individuals. **Vertical transmission** refers to the passage of an agent from an infected mother to her fetus or infant. The most intimate mode is via the **transplacental route.** Examples of such congenitally acquired diseases are syphilis and rubella. A newborn can also pick up chlamydiae, gonococci, cytomegalovirus, or hepatitis B virus during passage through the birth canal. Other organisms are transmitted through breast milk.

Horizontal transmission can be among individuals in close proximity or living far away and includes intimate modes, such as sexual intercourse, or more casual contacts, such as touching another person or breathing aerosols. The actual path of an organism from one person to another depends on the way the agent exits the body of the donor. Thus, bacteria or viruses that infect the respiratory tract are often expelled as aerosols during coughing and even talking, and may be inhaled by bystanders. If the organism is resistant to drying, as is the case with the tubercle bacillus, the danger of inhalation can persist for a long time. Intestinal pathogens often cause diarrhea, which increases their distribution in the environment and, under conditions of poor sanitation, results in contaminated drinking water and foodstuffs.

table 59-1	**Modes of Transmission**		
MODE	**EXAMPLE**	**FACTOR**	**ROUTE OF ENTRY**
Direct contact			
Respiratory aerosol	Influenza Tuberculosis	Crowding? Household	Lung Lung
Nasal secretions	Respiratory syncytial virus	Household, nosocomial	Upper respiratory tract
Droplets	*Meningococcus*	Crowding	Nasopharynx
Skin	*Streptococcus* (impetigo)	Crowding	Skin
Semen	AIDS	Sexual contact	Mucous membrane
Transplacental	Hepatitis B	Carrier	Mother
Indirect contact			
Blood	Hepatitis B AIDS	Transfusion, needlestick Transfusion	Blood Blood
Stool	Hepatitis A	Ingestion	Gastrointestinal tract
Animal	*Salmonella* infection	Ingestion	Gastrointestinal tract
Inanimate	*Legionella* infection	Water contamination	Respiratory tract
Arthropod vector			
Tick	Lyme disease	Bite	Skin, blood
Mosquito	Malaria	Bite	Blood

Some diseases are acquired by breaching the skin or mucous membranes by trauma, insect bites, blood transfusions, or contaminated hypodermic needles. Agents transmitted in this fashion include the AIDS or hepatitis B viruses. Many of the agents that are transmitted by insect **vectors** have different life cycles in the vector and in the host. Note that some of these organisms may be transmitted by more than one of these routes. Thus, HIV infection can be transmitted transplacentally, by sexual intercourse, or by the use of needles.

Nonhuman Reservoirs

Other diseases are acquired from **nonhuman reservoirs.** These include the **zoonoses** (Chapter 73), in which the reservoir is an animal. Transmission from the animal may be direct, as in the bite from a rabid dog, or through insect vectors, as in the plague or the viral encephalitides. Lyme disease is another zoonosis; its natural reservoir is mice, and the infection is transmitted to humans by a tick that feeds on mice, deer, and a variety of other mammalian hosts. Indirect transmission can result from contact with a contaminated environment, such as with rodent excreta in the newly described hantavirus outbreak in the southwestern United States.

In other diseases the reservoir is the **inanimate environment** and the organisms live freely in nature. For example, the clostridia of gas gangrene are commonly found in soil. However, humans or animals can contribute to the frequency with which the agents are found in nature. Thus, cholera bacilli grow naturally in warm estuaries, probably on the surface of shellfish, but contamination from human feces can help the organisms become established in a previously unaffected area.

Incubation Periods and Communicability

The length of the **incubation period** differs considerably among infectious diseases, from a few hours to months and years (Table 59-2). Many factors influence the incubation period. For example, a large infective dose can shorten it, and a small one can lengthen it. To epidemiologists, the incubation period is particularly important because some diseases can be transmitted from asymptomatic patients during that time. Control of transmission may therefore rely on special surveillance methods that include infected but asymptomatic persons. The periods of incubation and of communicability are not always the same. For example, the incubation period in hepatitis A usually ranges from 2 to 6 weeks. However, individuals can communicate the virus for only 1 or 2 weeks before the onset of the disease.

The period of communicability may extend long after the disease symptoms abate, as in the case of a **chronic carrier.** For example, hepatitis B carriers can usually transmit the virus for the length of time they carry it. Many of the

table 59-2	Incubation Periods
DISEASE	**RANGE OF PERIOD**
Staphylococcal food poisoning	1–6 hours
Clostridial food poisoning	12–24 hours
Hepatitis A	14–42 days
Hepatitis B	30–180 days
Gonorrhea	2–9 days
Salmonellosis	0.5–3 days
Epstein-Barr virus infection	21–49 days
Mycoplasma pneumoniae infection	8–21 days
Varicella-zoster virus	10–21 days
AIDS	21 days to 5 years or more
Leprosy	7 months to 5 years

preceding chapters have discussed the carrier state at some length (see Chapters 14, 17, 27, 38, 41, and 42).

Individual Susceptibility

Humans differ in their susceptibility to infectious diseases. For instance, some individuals seem more prone to respiratory or intestinal infections than are most people. Often the reason for this variability is unknown. A person might have subtle deficiencies in certain defense mechanisms. When those deficiencies become severe and the risks more evident, the cause is often easier to ascertain.

Epidemiologists must be aware of the various susceptibilities of members of the population. Age, sex, nutritional status, previous exposure, and immune competence all influence susceptibility to a particular infectious disease. For instance, children and older persons frequently are more likely to contract bacterial pneumonia or intestinal infections. The incidence of the carrier state of hepatitis B is greater in males than in females. It is also more frequent among individuals with Down syndrome or those receiving hemodialysis.

Genetic factors are also known to play a role in susceptibility, although the specific genes or gene products that contribute to susceptibility are not yet known. Why do some colonized patients develop overwhelming meningococcal disease, for instance, and others do not? The importance of genetic factors is often difficult to differentiate from a myriad of socioeconomic factors that might contribute to the state of health and nutrition. Nonetheless, the role of genetic factors has been well established in certain diseases. It has been shown, for example, that among identical twins living apart, when one twin contracted tuberculosis, the other had a greater chance than average of getting the disease. Nonidentical twins did not show that pattern. One of the most intensively studied genetic effects is the decreased susceptibility to malaria of persons with the sickle cell trait (see Chapter 52). It is also well established that non-Caucasians are more prone to the disseminated form of coccidioidomycosis than are Caucasians.

Practical Aspects of Epidemiology

In a civilized society epidemiology is everyone's business. The practicing physician and all members of the health care team must be aware of the public health implications of a given patient's infectious disease. To safeguard both the public interest and individual rights to privacy, a considerable body of local and national laws has been developed in most countries of the world. For instance, in the United States **certain communicable diseases are notifiable;** that is, physicians are obliged to report cases to the U.S. Public Health Service. The information collected is published in a readily available pamphlet, the *Morbidity and Mortality Weekly Report (MMWR)*, which lists all routine information and calls attention to unusual occurrences. In addition, each state has its own surveillance mechanism and reporting requirements for the study of communicable diseases within its borders. Each has a **state board of health** and a **reference laboratory** equipped to carry out special diagnostic tests that are often outside the scope of hospital laboratories.

Conclusion

Epidemiology may appear to be a remote discipline practiced mainly by public health officials. In fact, it pervades all forms of medical practice and furnishes important clues to the diagnosis of infectious diseases. Thus, inquiry into time and place characteristics should be part of the usual process of taking a clinical history. Epidemiological information reveals how people encounter disease agents and helps reduce the exposure and spread of infectious diseases.

Digestive System Infections

David Acheson and James Nataro

The digestive system is a microbiologist's paradise. In health or disease the digestive tract is a microbial garden of unsurpassed variety and complexity. It varies in the level of colonization from the "buggiest" parts of the body at both ends to the nearly sterile environment of the mid–small intestine (Fig. 60-1). The alimentary tract is studded with various ecosystems occupied by site-specific microbial populations. The normal stomach is an effective sterilization chamber that limits the entry of microorganisms to the small bowel and beyond, thus providing nonspecific protection against many enteric pathogens.

A community of well over 400 distinct species of bacteria, in addition to a few fungi and protozoa, form the resident flora of the normal gastrointestinal (GI) tract. Bacteria in the colon are present at approximately one tenth the theoretical limit of packing cells into a defined space (about 10^{12} bacteria/g) and amazingly produce no intestinal dysfunction. On the contrary, the normal flora enters into a **symbiotic relationship** with the host (see Chapter 2). Although we furnish this microbial population with room and board, it provides a number of essential services for us: accessory digestive functions such as converting unabsorbable carbohydrates to absorbable organic acids, energy for colonic epithelial cells in the form of butyrate, vitamin K needed for synthesis of blood clotting factors, and assistance in the reabsorption and conservation of estrogens and androgens excreted in the bile. In addition, the mere presence of the bacterial flora helps us resist colonization by invading pathogens. The intestinal havoc and diarrhea that is sometime seen following the use of antibiotics is indicative of how the intestinal bacterial flora helps keep the intestine in good working order.

The frequency of infections of the digestive system varies from the most prevalent human infectious disease, dental caries, to fairly common diarrhea and food poisoning, to unusual opportunistic infections of immunocompromised patients. Diarrheal diseases are a far greater cause of morbidity and mortality worldwide than are the more familiar diseases of the industrialized nations (heart disease, cancer, and strokes). Unfortunately, infants and small children are disproportionately affected, especially in developing countries with poor nutrition and environmental sanitation.

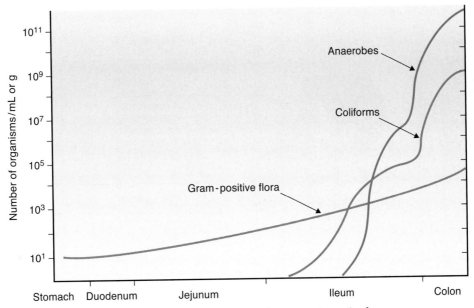

FIGURE 60-1 ▪ **Typical numbers of bacteria at the main sites in the gastrointestinal tract.**

Although diarrheal diseases do not usually cause fatalities in the United States, diarrhea remains among the most common complaints of people seen in general medical practice. Of the estimated 76 million cases of foodborne disease in the United States each year, much of the burden of illness is caused by gastroenteritis.

Intestinal infections range in severity from asymptomatic (e.g., enteroviruses) to mild diarrhea (e.g., most rotavirus infections) to life-threatening loss of fluid and electrolytes (e.g., cholera) and severe mucosal ulceration complicated by intestinal perforation (e.g., bacillary dysentery). This variation in clinical manifestations is not surprising when one considers the striking local differentiation in the alimentary tract and the variation in virulence genes among the pathogens (Fig. 60-2).

ENTRY

Barriers to Infection

Each portion of the alimentary tract has special anatomical, physiological, and biochemical barriers to infection (see Fig. 60-2). The most general impediment to infective agents is an **unbroken mucosal epithelium** covering all parts of the alimentary system. Its importance is evident in people receiving ionizing radiation or cytotoxic cancer chemotherapy, which interferes with the normal replacement of sloughed epithelial cells. Nausea, vomiting, and mucositis (superficial ulcerations of the mucosa of the entire GI tract) are some of the earliest manifestations of

damage. Members of the normal flora can reach deep tissues through these ulcerations and can even disseminate through the bloodstream to other organs, causing to life-threatening bacteremias.

Some defense mechanisms, such as **mucus formation** and **gut motility**, hinder the adhesion of microorganisms to the epithelial wall. In the intestine, the **mucus layer functions as a mechanical obstacle to protect the epithelium**; it also coats bacteria, which makes it easier to pass them along by peristalsis. Glycocalyx, the glycoprotein and polysaccharide layer that covers the surface of cells, has "decoy" binding sites that entrap certain invading organisms and facilitate their excretion in feces. However, in some instances mucus promotes virulence by triggering the synthesis of virulence factors. **Bile** plays an important role in selecting the bacteria and viruses able to colonize the intestine. Organisms that survive in the intestinal lumen, both normal flora and pathogens, are often resistant to the detergent action of bile salts. Most enteric viruses—hepatitis A virus and poliovirus, for example—lack a lipid-containing envelope that would make them sensitive to bile. Certain bacteria, including the Gram-negative typhoid bacillus and Gram-positive enterococci, are so highly resistant to bile that they can even grow in the gallbladder.

The defensive functions of several cellular and soluble factors are not as well understood. For instance, **secretory IgA immunoglobulins** and the protein **lactoferrin** in breast milk can help prevent colonization of the infant by certain bacteria. While it is likely that IgA has a similar function in older children and adults, it has been difficult to prove its role as a host defense mechanism, in part because some individuals with IgA deficiency (the most common immunoglobulin defect) have no evidence of an increase in susceptibility to infections. The intestinal tract is also the major disposal site for senescent

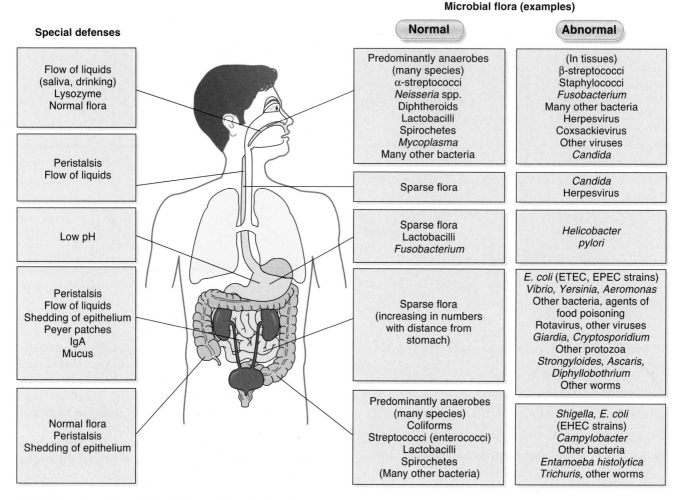

FIGURE 60-2 ▪ Microbiological overview of the digestive system.

white blood cells, especially neutrophils. It is likely, but not proven, that movement of those cells through the mucosa into the lumen of the gut plays a role in controlling pathogens or in maintaining balance with the normal flora. This putative role may explain the frequency of gut-based systemic infections in granulocytopenic patients, especially infections caused by bacteria in the Enterobacteriaceae family.

Establishment of Infectious Disease in the Digestive System

Several circumstances predispose to the establishment of infectious disease in the alimentary tract either by pathogens or members of the normal flora:

- **Anatomic alterations:** Obstructions to the flow of secretions remove one of the most powerful defensive mechanisms of the hollow organs. Thus, stones in the gallbladder or the common bile duct that impede the flow of bile predispose the biliary tree to infections. **Surgery may create intestinal "blind loops"** that are

isolated from the moving stream of the intestinal contents. Bacterial overgrowth can occur in the blind loop and result in malabsorption.

- **Changes in stomach acidity:** Alteration of the acid barrier of the stomach by disease, surgery, or drugs increases the survival of some but not all pathogens in this organ, allowing some ingested organisms greater access to the lower gastrointestinal tract. Thus, in persons with impaired gastric acidity, bacterial infection in the lower intestinal tract can occur after ingestion of smaller numbers of pathogens. This scenario is seen particularly in infections of acid-sensitive bacteria like *Vibrio cholerae* or *Salmonella* species but not in infections of *Escherichia coli* O157:H7 or *Shigella* species, which are naturally resistant to acid.

- **Alterations to the normal flora:** In the regions of the digestive tract that are most heavily colonized, the mouth and the colon, changes in the density or composition of the flora may permit pathogens to become established. The most frequent cause of such an alteration is the use of **broad-spectrum antibiotics.**

- **Encounter with specific pathogenic agents:** Certain viruses, bacteria, protozoa, and helminths cause disease even in the absence of predisposing host factors. At each site pathogens must be able to resist the specific local defenses. Because microorganisms face different survival problems in the mouth, stomach, small intestine, and colon, they must possess different attributes to live in each site.

DAMAGE

The signs and symptoms of infections related to the digestive system are caused by several general mechanisms:

- **Pharmacologic action:** Some bacteria produce toxins that alter normal intestinal function without causing lasting damage to their target cells. Typical examples are the **enterotoxins** made by *V. cholerae* or by some strains of *E. coli* (such as enterotoxigenic *E. coli*), which provoke copious watery diarrhea. Because the small bowel is primarily responsible for absorbing most of the 9 to 10 liters of fluid that pass through the gut each day, even small reductions in its absorptive capacity cause large amounts of fluid to enter the colon, overwhelming its relatively modest absorptive function. The excess unabsorbed fluid results in diarrhea, which can rapidly lead to profound dehydration, electrolyte loss, depletion of the intravascular volume, and shock, as seen in cholera.

- **Local inflammation:** In certain areas of the alimentary tract, an inflammatory reaction can occur as a consequence of microbial invasion. Often the invasion is limited to the epithelial layer, but it can spread to contiguous tissue and beyond. In the mouth, usually the gums, infections with anaerobic bacteria cause inflammation in the gingival pocket (periodontitis). In the large intestine, inflammation due to *Shigella* infection of the lamina propria can result in bloody diarrhea or dysentery.

- **Deep tissue invasion:** Some organisms are able to invade deeper and enter the circulation. Examples are the protozoan *Entamoeba histolytica* and the worm *Strongyloides*, which are capable of burrowing through the intestinal wall, and *Salmonella*, which penetrates the lamina propria and eventually reaches the bloodstream. Interestingly, *Strongyloides* itself is often colonized by gut bacteria; as a result, invasion by the worm can cause in polymicrobial septicemia.

- **Perforation:** When the mucosal wall is necrotic or perforated, the normal flora can spill into the usually sterile peritoneal cavity and invade the bloodstream, often with serious consequences. Thus, rupture of an inflamed appendix can lead to peritonitis, and traumatic perforation of the esophagus results in mediastinitis.

The variety of infectious agents and the intestinal diseases that they can cause is daunting. This chapter is organized by the principal sites of infection: the mouth, stomach, biliary tree, and intestine.

Infections of the Mouth

Virtually all the pathogens of the alimentary tract enter through the mouth. Because most of these pathogens come from the stools of infected persons, their route is known as **fecal–oral transmission.** The organisms reach the mouth by hitching a ride aboard food, fluids, or fingers.

The specific defenses of the mouth include the following:

- **Nonpathogenic resident flora:** Among the normal flora of the mouth are bacteria, fungi (e.g., *Candida*), and protozoa (e.g., the ameba *Entamoeba gingivalis*). These organisms resist the establishment of newcomers by occupying suitable sites and repelling other organisms, presumably by the production of acids and other metabolic inhibitors.

- **Mechanical actions of saliva and the tongue:** We produce more than a liter of saliva per day. With assistance from the tongue, saliva mechanically dislodges and flushes microorganisms from mucosal surfaces. If salivary flow is reduced, as with dehydration or during fasting, the bacterial content of saliva increases markedly.

- **Antimicrobial constituents of saliva, notably secreted antibodies and lysozyme:** Secretory IgA selectively inhibits the adherence of certain bacteria to mucosal cells or to tooth surfaces. Lysozyme is effective mainly against Gram-positive bacteria.

Several properties allow bacteria to evade host defenses. Some are able to stick to teeth or mucosal surfaces. Attachment to teeth is not direct; rather, bacteria adhere to a coating of sticky macromolecules, mainly proteins, called the **dental pellicle.** The bacteria themselves produce polysaccharides that help them adhere. For example, *Streptococcus mutans* transforms sucrose into polysaccharides that are particularly sticky. They are layered on the pellicle to form a matrix that allows adherence of other organisms. The result is **dental plaque,** one of the densest collections of bacteria in the body. Microbial metabolism in plaque transforms dietary sugar into acids, mainly lactic acid, which are responsible for dental caries (cavities). Other bacteria, especially strict anaerobes, reside in the gingival crevices between the tooth and gum, where they evade the washing effects of saliva and normal toothbrushing.

The bacteria of the indigenous oral flora are not highly virulent, but when a break occurs in the mucosal barrier, such as with advanced gingivitis (periodontal disease), they may invade surrounding healthy tissue. The mouth is also the likely portal of entry of α-hemolytic streptococci that cause subacute bacterial endocarditis in persons with rheumatic heart disease. A synergistic cooperation between several types of bacteria, both aerobic and strictly anaerobic, also can lead to a severe and rapidly advancing mixed infection of the soft tissues surrounding the oral cavity. **Ludwig angina**, a polymicrobial infection of the sublingual and submandibular spaces that arises from a tooth (often the second and third mandibular molars), is a cellulitis—an inflammation of submucosal or subcutaneous connective tissue—that can progress rapidly, press against the airway, and compromise respiratory airflow and threaten the affected individual with asphyxiation.

Candidiasis

Case

C., a 7-month-old girl, was treated by her pediatrician for a middle ear infection. She was prescribed a 10-day course of amoxicillin, which cleared the infection within 4 days. On the sixth day of antibiotic therapy, her mother noticed that the child was irritable and feeding poorly. During a follow-up visit, her pediatrician noted several creamy white, curdlike patches on the tongue and buccal mucosa. When scraped, they were clearly painful and left a raw, bleeding surface. Microscopic examination of the exudate scraped from the affected areas revealed yeast. Thrush, or oral **candidiasis**, was diagnosed. Antibiotics were stopped, a topical antifungal solution was administered, and the patches disappeared within 2 days.

This case raises several questions:

1. What aspects of normal physiology prevent the development of thrush?
2. Should C. be evaluated for an immune deficiency?

Pathobiology

In the case of C., the white patches adhering to the oral mucosa consisted of "pseudomembranes" made up of the yeast *Candida* mixed with desquamated epithelial cells, leukocytes, oral bacteria, necrotic tissue, and food debris. *Candida albicans* and related species are yeasts found in the environment that establish themselves in the alimentary tract early in life (see Chapter 48). The adult vagina is commonly colonized with these organisms, and they may be acquired by infants during delivery. Small numbers of *Candida* live harmlessly in the alimentary tract until the balance between indigenous bacterial flora and host defenses is upset. C.'s antibiotic therapy killed many of the normal oral bacteria and allowed *Candida* to proliferate.

Candida exploits changes in the normal host flora to multiply locally. If the number or function of neutrophils is decreased, or if defects in cellular immunity are present, they may invade beyond the mucosal surface.

Predisposing conditions for oral and other forms of candidiasis include diabetes, malnutrition, malignancy, immunosuppressive drugs, genetic abnormalities of the immune system, and HIV infection. Normally healthy individuals also are frequently affected. *Candida* vaginitis is commonly encountered in postpubertal women who are taking broad-spectrum antibiotics, often for a urinary tract infection. The prolonged use of inhaled steroids for asthma also can predispose to candidal overgrowth in the mouth. In more severe forms of immunodeficiency the organism can disseminate through the bloodstream and infect virtually any organ system but most commonly the liver, lung, and kidney.

Candida can invade the esophagus, an organ that is rarely prone to infection. Candidal esophagitis is seen in patients with specific T-cell abnormalities, such as chronic mucocutaneous candidiasis or AIDS. The differential diagnosis of esophagitis in immunocompromised patients includes infection by cytomegalovirus (CMV) and herpes simplex virus type 1 (HSV-1). Those infections can cause particularly troublesome mucosal ulcerations, with severe pain and difficulty swallowing.

Diagnosis

Thrush is characteristic in appearance, and the diagnosis is usually suspected on oral inspection. It is confirmed by examination of the exudate under a microscope and detection of characteristic yeast forms. Culture is not necessary and often misleading, because *Candida* is a commensal and can be cultured from the mouths of some healthy persons.

Prevention and Treatment

Because candidal colonization of the GI tract is frequent, prevention and treatment consist primarily of correcting the reversible predisposing factors and avoiding the unnecessary use of antibiotics. Candidiasis of the mouth is usually superficial and responds to oral antifungal agents such as nystatin. If the infection extends more deeply than the mucosa, it may be necessary to use an absorbed oral antifungal agent, such as fluconazole, or intravenous amphotericin B.

Stomach Infections

Until recently, the stomach received little attention as a locus of infections of the alimentary tract because it was considered insusceptible to infection. Rather, research focused on the important role the stomach plays in

table 60-1	Comparison of the Intestinal Flora of Human Adults			
BACTERIA SPECIES	**BACTERIA CONCENTRATION (Log₁₀/mL OR g)**			
	STOMACH	**JEJUNUM**	**ILEUM**	**COLON**
Total viable count	$0-10^3$	$0-10^5$	10^2-10^7	$10^{10}-10^{12}$
Aerobes or facultative anaerobes				
Enterobacteria	$0-10^2$	$0-10^3$	10^2-10^7	10^4-10^{10}
Streptococci	$0-10^2$	$0-10^4$	10^2-10^6	10^4-10^9
Staphylococci	$0-10^2$	$0-10^3$	10^2-10^5	10^4-10^{10}
Lactobacilli	$0-10^3$	$0-10^4$	10^2-10^5	10^4-10^{10}
Fungi	$0-10^2$	$0-10^2$	10^2-10^4	10^4-10^6
Anaerobes				
Bacteroides species	Rare	$0-10^3$	10^3-10^7	$10^{10}-10^{12}$
Bifidobacteria	Rare	$0-10^4$	10^3-10^9	10^8-10^{12}
Streptococci	Rare	$0-10^3$	10^2-10^6	$10^{10}-10^{12}$
Clostridia	Rare	Rare	10^2-10^6	10^6-10^{11}
Eubacteria	Rare	Rare	Rare	10^9-10^{12}

protecting the gut from infection further downstream by its secretion of acid. The majority of oral or foodborne bacteria, washed with saliva into the stomach, are destroyed by acid secreted by the stomach.

In some individuals, the stomach is indeed sterile, and in most others, the concentration of bacteria is very low, generally less than 10^3/mL (Table 60-1). The predominant bacteria found in the stomach are acid-resistant Gram-positives, like *Lactobacillus, Peptostreptococcus, Staphylococcus,* and *Streptococcus.* The normal stomach contains very few enteric Gram-negative rods, *Bacteroides,* or *Clostridium,* organisms that are usually associated with the lower GI tract.

It is now known that gastric infections do occur and much more frequently than was previously thought. In particular, *Helicobacter pylori* is able to colonize regions of the stomach and is involved in the pathogenesis of gastritis and peptic ulcers. Human and experimental animal studies have established that *H. pylori* is a pathogen of major clinical significance (see Chapter 22). Thus, gastric ulcers have now entered the ever-expanding ranks of infectious diseases.

Some bacteria, including pathogens, if introduced into the stomach with food, will survive and enter the small intestine alive. Survival depends largely on the buffering effects of food, especially in patients who do not produce normal amounts of gastric hydrochloric acid because of disease, partial or total gastrectomy, drug therapy (e.g., histamine-2 receptor [H2] or proton pump blockers), or antacid consumption. The infective dose of cholera bacilli or salmonellae in human volunteers, for example, is 10,000 times lower when the organisms are administered with 2 g of sodium bicarbonate.

Low or absent acid production, known as hypochlorhydria or achlorhydria, often leads to colonization of the stomach and upper small intestine by enteric Gram-negative rods. That colonization can have two important consequences: (1) development of a disease called the bacterial overgrowth syndrome (discussed later in the chapter) and (2) regurgitation of the abnormal gastric flora, which becomes a source of nosocomial (hospital-acquired) aspiration Gram-negative pneumonia (see Chapter 62).

Infections of the Biliary Tree and Liver

Infections of the gallbladder (**cholecystitis**) are a frequent complication of obstruction to the flow of bile caused, for example, by gallstones migrating into the cystic duct or common bile duct. The clinical presentation is often sudden and dramatic, with the obstruction leading to increased pressure and distention. Mechanical, chemical, and bacterial inflammation caused by enterococci, *E. coli, Klebsiella pneumoniae, Staphylococcus aureus,* or *Clostridium perfringens* can result. The hallmark of cholecystitis is **pain in the right upper quadrant of the abdomen,** which may build to a crescendo and then subside, only to recur rapidly. That pattern is called **biliary colic.** Nausea and vomiting usually accompany the pain and may be intractable. The majority of patients with common duct obstruction have shaking chills, high spiking fever, jaundice, and tenderness over the gallbladder. Biliary colic, jaundice, and chills and spiking fever, known as **Charcot triad**, are characteristic of acute cholecystitis.

Inflammation and infection can cause ischemia of the gallbladder wall, sometimes progressing to gangrene and perforation. Gangrene and perforation can lead to contamination of the peritoneal cavity with bacteria and abscess formation. The spread of infection from the biliary ducts to the liver, known as **ascending cholangitis**, is common. With complete obstruction, the combination of pus and increased pressure leads to abscess formation, bacteremia, and symptoms of septic shock.

Primary bacterial infections of the **liver parenchyma** are not common, partly because of the defensive capacity of the phagocytic Kupffer cells. Liver abscesses can develop from portal vein bacteremia from an infected intra-abdominal site, from systemic bacteremia via the hepatic artery, from ascending cholangitis, and from contiguous infections. Intracellular pathogens that survive in macrophages can cause granulomatous infections. Examples are the agents of typhoid fever, Q fever, brucellosis, and tuberculosis.

Infectious diseases of the liver are not discussed in detail here. The most important diseases stem from hepatitis viruses (see Chapter 43). The liver is also the site of several parasitic infections, including leishmaniasis (see Chapter 52), amebiasis (see Chapter 53), schistosomiasis (see Chapter 55), and others. An important, although clinically silent, part of the life cycle of malarial parasites also takes place in the liver.

Cholecystitis and Cholangitis

Case

Ms. F., an obese 48-year-old mother of eight with a vague history of intermittent "stomach problems," awoke with moderate midepigastric pain. Approximately 2 hours before going to bed, she had eaten a large meal of fried chicken and mashed potatoes. The pain soon shifted to her right upper quadrant and was occasionally felt in the area of the right scapula. She vomited several times and felt better but had residual pain for several days with numerous similar but less intense attacks. By the sixth day, she felt sick again and developed jaundice and a shaking chill. In the emergency department she was in obvious pain and had a temperature of 40°C. Her skin was slightly yellowish. The right upper quadrant of her abdomen was markedly tender to palpation. An 8-cm tubular mass was felt under the margin of the right ribs. Her white blood cell count was elevated (14,000/mm^3), suggesting a bacterial infection. Her serum bilirubin and alkaline phosphatase levels were elevated, suggesting biliary obstruction.

Blood was cultured and antibiotic therapy begun. An ultrasound examination showed that her gallbladder was markedly distended and contained several stones. The diagnosis of acute cholecystitis was made. Within 36 hours of

admission, the pain improved and the fever resolved. The blood cultures grew enterococci and *E. coli*. Ms. F. was scheduled for surgery to remove the affected gallbladder and stones.

This case raises several questions:

1. What risk factors contributed to the development of cholecystitis in Ms. F.?
2. What are the possible complications of this disease?

PATHOBIOLOGY

Infections of the gallbladder (**cholecystitis**) and the bile duct (**cholangitis**) are secondary consequences of obstruction. The process begins with obstruction and distention, resulting in inflammation of the gallbladder wall. The disease may not progress, but the process increases the risk of infection caused by the small number of bacteria normally present in bile. Patients with cholecystitis commonly have a history of recurrent attacks of biliary colic resulting from obstruction of the biliary outlet. It is possible that Ms. F.'s vague "stomach problems" of the past were episodes of mild biliary colic caused by transient or partial obstructions of the duct by gallstones. In the most recent episode, infection developed, and the character of her illness changed.

Once bacterial infection becomes established, tissue damage may be accelerated by the resulting inflammatory response. Healing is unlikely to occur without surgical or spontaneous relief of the obstruction and specific antimicrobial therapy.

A particularly rapid and severe form of gallbladder infection can occur in patients with compromised arterial blood supply to the gallbladder wall, such as diabetics or the elderly. If the infecting organisms invade the gallbladder wall, they may produce a condition called **emphysematous cholecystitis**. The condition is distinguished by rapid clinical onset, extensive gangrene, presence of gas in the gallbladder wall (when gas-forming species, such as clostridia or *E. coli* are present), and a high mortality rate. Surgical removal of the gallbladder (cholecystectomy) is required because of the frequent occurrence of gangrene, perforation, and extensive peritonitis.

The usual clinical presentation of cholangitis is similar to cholecystitis, as in Ms. F.'s case, but it is often accompanied by high spiking fever, chills, jaundice, and constant pain. The most common obstructing causes are gallstones and neoplasms, but occasionally a helminthic infection, such as *Ascaris lumbricoides*, is responsible. Considerable pressure within the duct seems to be a prerequisite for infection. Experiments in dogs have shown that the normal common duct pressure of 70 mm H_2O must be raised to 250 mm H_2O before *E. coli* injected into the bloodstream produces infection in the gallbladder. It is not known why the resulting distention facilitates bacterial invasion of the duct wall, but microscopic tears or ischemic damage are obvious possibilities.

Organisms that infect the gallbladder and bile duct are usually derived from the GI tract, *E. coli* being the most frequent agent. Approximately 40% of infections in the gallbladder and bile duct are caused by a mixed facultative and strictly anaerobic flora that ascends from the duodenum.

Typhoid bacilli have an unusual predilection for the gallbladder (see Chapter 17). The organisms may persist for a prolonged period within gallstones, where they are protected from the effects of antibiotics. They produce little or no inflammation, and the person may not be aware he or she is a carrier. All carriers, cognizant or not, shed the typhoid bacteria into the environment and can infect other people.

DIAGNOSIS

When the clinical presentation of cholecystitis is typical, as in Ms. F.'s case, a tentative diagnosis can be made on clinical grounds. Unfortunately, the disease is prone to misdiagnosis because it often presents in an atypical form. Abdominal ultrasound is a useful test to establish the diagnosis of cholecystitis; the imaging technique can reliably visualize obstruction or distention in the biliary system. Direct culture of the infected bile is rarely performed because it is difficult to obtain a specimen; antibiotics are chosen on the basis of expected flora. The diagnosis is confirmed when blood cultures grow the causative organisms, but cultures are often negative.

PREVENTION AND TREATMENT

Patients with cholangitis should receive antibiotics appropriate for the expected mixed bacterial species typically present, before the diagnosis is confirmed and bacteria are identified in the blood but not before blood cultures are obtained. Correct antibiotics are not sufficient, however. To effect a definitive cure, the underlying obstruction must be relieved. Relief of the obstruction may occur spontaneously or with surgery. The timing and need for surgery to remove stones and an inflamed gallbladder is controversial, and the surgeon's decision depends on many factors specific to each patient.

Infections of the Small and Large Intestine

The diseases discussed here illustrate the diversity of infectious problems of the gut, based on host factors and

virulence attributes of the causative organisms. Examples of other classic infections of the intestines caused by bacteria are discussed in Chapters 16 and 17, and Chapters 53 and 54 describe intestinal infections caused by animal parasites.

The anatomy and physiology of our alimentary tract ensure that our bodies have first crack at the food we eat (Fig. 60-3). Thanks to the sterilizing power of the stomach and the defenses of the small intestine, we absorb most of our nutrients without microbial competition. The upper intestinal contents, rich in unabsorbed sugars, fats, and other nutrients, do not normally come in contact with large numbers of bacteria (see Table 60-1).

The presence of a large microbial biomass in the absorptive small intestine leads to competition for certain vitamins and malabsorption of fats and produces a disease known as **bacterial overgrowth syndrome.** The study of bacterial overgrowth in the small intestine has helped us understand the normal relationship of the gut flora to gut function.

FIGURE 60-3 ▪ **Schematic representation of host barriers faced by intestinal pathogens.**

Bacterial Overgrowth Syndrome

Case

At the age of 63 years Mr. O. had an operation to remove a tumor that obstructed his stomach outlet. The surgeon excised part of the stomach and duodenum and connected the remainder of the stomach with the jejunum (gastrojejunostomy), bypassing the unresected duodenum. Two years later Mr. O. developed chronic diarrhea, and his weight dropped from 139 lb to 97 lb. Because his food intake was adequate, anorexia could not account for his weight loss. The diarrhea had recently become bulky, smelly, and greasy. Mr. O. felt fatigued, was short of breath on exertion, and had numbness and tingling in his hands and feet. On examination he was extremely thin and appeared ill with a pale complexion.

Laboratory tests showed a severe anemia with large red blood cells (i.e., megaloblastic anemia) and leukopenia with many neutrophils with extra nuclear lobes. Serum levels of vitamin A and its precursor, carotene, were depressed, and vitamin B_{12} was undetectable, although intrinsic factor was present in his gastric juice. Specific tests of intestinal function revealed malabsorption. The diagnosis of bacterial overgrowth syndrome was made. (Although not done in this case, intubation of the small bowel might have revealed approximately 10^9 *Bacteroides fragilis* and 10^6 *E. coli* per milliliter of small bowel content). Fat-soluble vitamins and vitamin B_{12} were replaced, and Mr. O. was treated with a course of ciprofloxacin. The diarrhea resolved, and the tests of absorptive function improved. He continued on antibiotic therapy, and after several months he returned to his normal weight and felt entirely well.

This case raises several questions:

1. What is the underlying cause of the numbness and tingling experienced by Mr. O.?
2. What is the mechanism of the diarrhea that Mr. O is experiencing?

PATHOBIOLOGY

Prior surgery left Mr. O. with a loop of small bowel diverted from the main flow of intestinal contents. The result of this "blind loop" was **stasis of the intestinal contents** caused by the absence of the continuous flushing action of the intestinal secretions. Bacterial proliferation occurred, leading to impaired absorption of fats and fat-soluble vitamins.

Bacterial overgrowth in the small intestine can arise from other causes, such as motor abnormalities that depress peristalsis (e.g., diabetic neuropathy, scleroderma, or gastric atony) or gastric achlorhydria, which permits large bacterial inocula to reach the proximal small bowel. Under those conditions bacterial overgrowth begins. As stagnation progresses, the small number of bacteria normally present increases dramatically. Careful anaerobic sampling of the small intestines of patients with depressed peristalsis has revealed bacteria counts as high as 10^{10}/mL, levels comparable to those in the colon. By far the most numerous bacteria and those most likely to be responsible for the physiological derangement are strict anaerobes, mainly *Bacteroides* species.

DAMAGE

Bacterial overgrowth in the small intestine may have the following effects:

- **Increased fecal fat, or steatorrhea:** Malabsorption of fat resulting from depletion of the bile acid pool is the primary cause of steatorrhea. Why is the pool depleted? Bile acids such as cholic acid are normally conjugated with glycine or taurine in the liver, secreted in the bile, and reabsorbed in the terminal ileum in the conjugated form. The bacterial overgrowth flora can deconjugate those compounds, making them unavailable for reabsorption and ultimately depleting the bile salts needed to form fat micelles necessary for fat absorption in the proximal gut.

- **Deficiency of vitamin B_{12}:** Normally vitamin B_{12} (or cobalamin) is bound to intrinsic factor from the stomach, and this complex is absorbed from the terminal ileum. With bacterial overgrowth, dietary B_{12} is used by bacteria, making it unavailable for uptake by the host. With prolonged B_{12} malabsorption (longer than 1 year), endogenous stores are depleted. Cellular systems with a high rate of turnover and DNA synthesis (e.g., bone marrow, central nervous system, and gut epithelium) are severely impaired, possibly leading to megaloblastic anemia or structural gut abnormalities. The epithelial villi are shortened when the turnover and atrophy of enterocytes decrease, reducing the absorptive area. Thus, bacterial overgrowth sets off a cascade of malabsorptive events. Vitamin B_{12} also is required for myelin synthesis, and its deficiency results in degeneration of the spinal cord, producing the classic neurological syndrome of pernicious anemia.

- **Diarrhea:** Defined as an increase in fecal water and electrolyte excretion above normal amounts, diarrhea occurs in all patients with bacterial overgrowth. It usually results from the degradation by the normal flora of malabsorbed oligosaccharides reaching the colon. When the concentration of osmotically active solutes increases and water moves across the mucosa to maintain isosmolarity, the result is **osmotic diarrhea**. Deconjugated bile salts in the colon also can cause osmotic diarrhea.

- **Malabsorption of vitamins A and D:** Poor absorption of fat-soluble vitamins (A, D, E, and K, but particularly A and D) causes severe visual disturbance (night blindness) and softening of the bones (osteomalacia). Interestingly, vitamin K deficiency is rare. The reduced absorption of that fat-soluble vitamin is offset by the markedly increased vitamin production by the plentiful bacteria, ordinarily our main source of vitamin K.

DIAGNOSIS AND TREATMENT

Bacterial overgrowth syndrome is usually diagnosed when malabsorption and nutritional deficiencies are present together with predisposing anatomic or physiological conditions, such as intestinal blind loops. Noninvasive breath tests are available to document the presence of the overgrowth flora in the proximal small bowel. Treatment requires correction of the surgical or medical predisposing condition in conjunction with careful nutritional repletion and, most importantly, broad-spectrum antibiotic therapy. Relapse can occur, and repeated courses of therapy may be necessary.

Diarrhea and Dysentery

Diarrhea is the final common pathway of intestinal responses to many inciting agents, both infectious and noninfectious (see Chapter 16). **Dysentery**, in contrast, is a distinctive syndrome involving the colon, in which a brisk inflammatory response results in abdominal pain and **small-volume stools consisting of blood, pus, and mucus** (see Chapter 17). Dysentery is a more severe problem than bloody diarrhea. Not only is its pathophysiology distinctive but so too are the organisms involved, usually *Shigella* species. Therapy is directed toward elimination of the pathogen using antibiotics, an issue now complicated by multiple antibiotic resistance.

In contrast, foodborne outbreaks of bloody diarrhea have occurred in recent years, primarily in young children and the elderly, associated with clinical signs resulting from the formation of platelet-fibrin thrombi in the glomeruli or the brain. A group of *E. coli* that produce toxins related to shiga toxin (from *Shigella dysenteriae* type 1), most notably *E. coli* O157:H7, are responsible. This is truly a new and emerging infectious disease.

The cases presented here illustrate distinctive ecological features of the pathogens and their interactions with the host.

Case

Cholera

Approximately 2 days after returning from Mardi Gras in New Orleans, Mr. V., a 24-year-old student who was the runner-up in the raw oyster–eating contest, abruptly started to vomit. Within hours he was restricted to the bathroom with voluminous and nearly continuous but painless watery diarrhea. Soon thereafter, he became lightheaded, with a rapid pulse and a feeling of marked lethargy and weakness. Later that evening his roommate brought him to the emergency department, where Mr. V. was found to be afebrile but profoundly dehydrated, with severely altered levels of serum electrolytes.

In the hospital his stool was composed of an opaque fluid with small flecks of mucus, giving it a typical "**rice water**" appearance (so called because it resembles the starchy water in which rice has been washed), and without a fecal, bloody, or bilious appearance. Although the diagnosis is often missed in the United States, the emergency department physician had worked in a Rwandan refugee camp and recognized the cholera syndrome. Vigorous intravenous rehydration was administered. When Mr. V.'s fluid losses were reversed and the diarrhea rate slowed, fluid balance was maintained with an oral rehydration solution until the diarrhea ceased. The physician requested that the laboratory culture the stool for *V. cholerae,* and a specimen was inoculated onto a special medium called TCBS agar (thiosulfate–citrate–bile salt sucrose). *V. cholerae* was isolated in 24 hours. No antibiotics were used, and by the end of the fourth hospital day, he was discharged with all symptoms and abnormalities resolved.

This case raises several questions:

1. How did *V. cholerae* cause Mr. V's dramatic clinical presentation?
2. Why didn't the treating physicians think to prescribe antibiotics for Mr. V.?
3. Where in the United States has cholera occurred in the 20th century?

Case

Shigellosis

Ms. T., a 26-year-old former Peace Corps worker in East Africa, returned from a visit to the village she had lived in with a low-grade fever and mild watery diarrhea. The next morning her symptoms were worse, with a fever of 40°C, abdominal pain, mostly in the left lower quadrant, and the presence of blood in the stool. Ms. T. thought the problem might be *Shigella* infection and went to the local hospital. The clinician examined the stool under light microscopy and noted the presence of **sheets of neutrophils,** consistent with shigellosis. Ms. T. was given an oral fluoroquinolone antibiotic and sent home with instructions to return if the symptoms worsened. The next day *S. flexneri* was isolated and was found to be resistant to ampicillin and trimethoprim-sulfamethoxazole. Ms. T. steadily improved over the next 48 hours.

This case raises several questions:

1. What is the significance of sheets of neutrophils in the stool of Ms. T.?
2. Should anti-motility agents have been used to treat Ms. T's illness?

Case

Rotavirus Infection

A., a 9-month-old girl, had been enrolled in a child care facility for the past month. Usually a satisfied and happy child, she suddenly became irritable, began to vomit, and had a low-grade fever. She also developed mild upper respiratory symptoms, with cough, nasal discharge, and pharyngitis. Watery diarrhea, without blood or leukocytes, developed and persisted for 2 days. The infant was brought to the pediatrician, who made the clinical diagnosis of rotavirus gastroenteritis. An enzyme-linked immunosorbent assay (ELISA) to detect **rotavirus** antigen in the stool was positive. The pediatrician prescribed an oral rehydration solution to be given at home, and A. made an uneventful recovery by the sixth day.

This case raises several questions:

1. How did A. become infected with rotavirus?
2. Is there a vaccine to prevent rotavirus disease?

Case

Yersinia Infection

Mr. D. took his family to southern Sweden to visit his parents who were dairy farmers outside Malmö. S., a 5-year-old boy, and I., a 12-year-old girl, enjoyed helping their grandparents care for the many domestic animals on the farm and loved the home-cured meat and fresh raw milk served to them. Between 7 and 10 days after arrival, all members of the D. family became ill. S. developed watery, mucoid diarrhea with occasional flecks of blood, low-grade fever, and diffuse abdominal pain, all of which resolved spontaneously after 4 days. I.'s episode began similarly but worsened after 3 days, when her pain localized to the right lower quadrant and became associated with high fever and leukocytosis. She was brought to the local hospital, and a tentative diagnosis of acute appendicitis was made. During surgery, her appendix was found to be normal; however, the terminal ileum was inflamed, with many **enlarged mesenteric lymph nodes**.

Cultures of stool obtained on admission were incubated at 25°C and after several days grew *Yersinia enterocolitica.* By that time I. had made a nearly complete recovery. Mr. D., like S., developed an acute mucoid diarrhea, abdominal pain, and fever that remitted by the fourth day. Three weeks later Mr. D. developed painful swelling of several joints and a painful raised rash over his shins (**erythema nodosum**). Although he had no gastrointestinal symptoms, his stool tested positive for *Y. enterocolitica,* and he was treated with trimethoprim-sulfamethoxazole. The rash and arthritis slowly resolved, returned several months later, and then spontaneously remitted, not to return again.

This case raises several questions:

1. Why did the clinical manifestations of *Yersinia* infection differ in S. and I.?
2. Describe the pathogenesis of the arthritis and rash that developed in Mr. D.?

Case

Hemolytic–Uremic Syndrome

L., a 3-year-old girl, became ill with cramps, fever, and mild watery diarrhea 24 hours after eating at a fast-food hamburger restaurant. Her pediatrician advised giving fluids but did not prescribe antibiotics. The diarrhea turned bloody on day 3, and the child was hospitalized. Laboratory tests revealed moderate leukocytosis but no other abnormalities.

On day 5, *E. coli* 0157:H7 was isolated from the initial stool culture. Laboratory studies the next day revealed a leukocytosis of 27,000 with 85% neutrophils and 5% bands, anemia (hematocrit of 30%), thrombocytopenia (34,000 platelets/mm^3), and an elevated creatinine of 8.8 mg/dL). Erythrocyte fragments characteristic of red cell damage secondary to endothelial cell injury (**microangiopathic hemolytic anemia**) were seen on the blood smear.

Over the next 2 days, L.'s anemia, thrombocytopenia, and uremia progressed, without evidence of consumptive coagulopathy. Those signs established the diagnosis of **hemolytic–uremic syndrome** (HUS). L. required a week of hemodialysis for oliguria, hypertension, and uremia. She also received transfusions of red cells and platelets. She was discharged after 3 weeks, and by 3 months all laboratory tests had returned to normal. L. remained well after two additional years of follow-up.

This case raises several questions:

1. What was the source of the *E. coli* that led to L.'s disease?
2. What is the basis for the renal manifestations of hemolytic-uremic syndrome?
3. Should antibiotics have been administered to L.?

ENCOUNTER

The list of intestinal pathogens is expanding as well-known organisms appear in unexpected frequency and in new settings, and as new organisms are recognized (Table 60-2). Other chapters have discussed some of the more common agents of intestinal infections (see Chapters 16, 17, 37, 51, 53, 54, and 76). This chapter adds a few more to the list. *Campylobacter jejuni,* formerly thought to be a rare cause of diarrhea in the United States, has now emerged as one of the most common. It is **transmitted by poultry,** which are almost always colonized by the organism. Within the last several years *Aeromonas hydrophila* and *Plesiomonas* species have become established as occasional agents of waterborne or shellfish-associated outbreaks. Other common agents of diarrhea here and abroad include the protozoan *Cryptosporidium* (see Chapter 53), which was responsible for a massive waterborne outbreak in Milwaukee, Wisconsin, in 1993 involving almost one-half million people, and a newly described foodborne coccidian parasite, *Cyclospora*

table **60-2**	Some Etiologic Agents of Diarrhea
ORGANISM	**SOURCE**
Escherichia coli	Food contaminated with human feces
Salmonella species	Contaminated food, especially poultry products
Shigella species	Fecal–oral
Campylobacter species	Farm animals, contaminated food (e.g., raw eggs)
Yersinia enterocolitica	Animal products
Vibrio cholerae	Water and shellfish
Vibrio parahaemolyticus	Seafood (e.g., sardines, shellfish)
Bacillus cereus	Contaminated food (e.g., reheated rice)
Clostridium perfringens	Contaminated food (e.g., reheated meat)
Entamoeba histolytica	Fecal–oral and water
Giardia lamblia	Fecal–oral and water
Cryptosporidium and *Cyclospora* species	Fecal–oral and water

cayetanensis (transmitted in a 1996 U.S. outbreak by contaminated imported raspberries; see Chapter 53). Another protozoal group, **microsporidia** (including *Enterocytozoon bieneusi* and *Septata intestinalis*), can cause chronic diarrhea in persons with AIDS. Viral diarrhea is common in all age groups. Agents of viral diarrhea include enteric adenovirus, astrovirus, norovirus, and rotavirus, among others, in normal young children and adults as well as viruses associated with diarrhea and inflammatory enteritis in immunocompromised persons (e.g., CMV and HSV). As the list of enteric pathogens lengthens and an understanding of how they produce disease emerges, the practical challenge of diagnosis and treatment increases.

The cases described here illustrate the relationship of microbial ecology to the transmission of certain microorganisms. *V. cholerae* serogroup O1, long thought to be a human-adapted pathogen, is actually a marine organism inhabiting coastal waters, where it lives in association with plankton. In the United States, it is endemic in the Gulf of Mexico near New Orleans and in the Chesapeake Bay near the nation's capital. Because shellfish can concentrate bacteria present in the waters in which they live, Mr. V., the cholera patient, was undoubtedly infected by eating a large helping of uncooked contaminated oysters. He may have been at greater risk owing to achlorhydria (which was not evaluated), or his meal may have been contaminated by an unfortunately high concentration of the organism.

In areas endemic to cholera, infected persons can transport the bacteria to other areas and initiate epidemics of cholera where water and food cannot be protected and environmental sanitation is poor. Those

events occurred in Latin America in early 1993, resulting in more than 1 million cases of cholera over the subsequent 2 years and approximately 5,000 to 10,000 deaths. Interestingly, **the segment of DNA that encodes cholera toxin is actually contained on a filamentous bacteriophage** (called CTX) that infects the cholera bacteria. The possibility that a functional set of cholera toxin genes can be acquired by phage transduction raises questions about the safety of cholera vaccines based on deletions of the toxin gene. Attesting to the constant evolution of microbes and emerging diseases, a new epidemic serotype of *V. cholerae*, previously unknown and now designated O139 (Bengal), was first detected in India in 1992 and spread in epidemic fashion beginning in 1993 (see Fig. 16-1). The new strain resulted from deletion of O1 lipopolysaccharide (LPS) synthesis genes and insertion of new LPS synthesis genes into the current pandemic serogroup O1 cholera strain. The O139 strain causes severe clinical cholera, and it continues to spread in Asia.

In contrast, *Shigella* infection is found only in close association with humans. Relatively few organisms are required to cause shigellosis (also known as bacillary dysentery). As a result, the disease readily spreads among persons in close contact. It is most commonly a disease of children and, in the United States the most common species, *S. sonnei*, is a frequent cause of self-limited watery diarrhea in infants and children in child care centers. The species infecting Ms. T., *S. flexneri*, is no longer common in the United States but remains an important cause of infection in developing countries, where *S. sonnei* is rare. *Y. enterocolitica* has yet another ecological characteristic; it is often zoonotic (acquired from infected animals; see Chapter 73) and may be transmitted by drinking raw milk or consuming undercooked meat such as pork.

Diarrhea affecting children who are younger than 2 years of age is most likely of viral etiology, with rotavirus by far the most common cause. In temperate regions rotavirus diarrhea is seasonal and produces "winter vomiting disease"; in tropical zones it occurs year-round. Adults may be infected when a child introduces the virus into the household, but adults often do not experience symptoms, presumably because of preexisting immunity. In areas where malnutrition is prevalent, severe diarrhea is associated with measles, which is highly contagious and kills large numbers of infants. The use of the measles vaccine in those populations could reduce the incidence of the life-threatening complication.

A distinct group of enteric infections is seen in homosexual men. Anal intercourse permits infection of the distal bowel with pathogens typically associated with sexually transmitted diseases. Proctocolitis due to *Chlamydia trachomatis*, HSV, *Neisseria gonorrhoeae*, or *Treponema pallidum* has been recognized as the "gay bowel syndrome." Modifications of sexual practices initiated following the AIDS epidemic have diminished the frequency of these infections among gay men.

PATHOBIOLOGY AND DAMAGE

The diarrheal disease pathogens have distinctive sets of virulence properties and preferentially infect specific areas of the bowel (Table 60-3). Therefore, this chapter considers the small and large intestine separately.

Infections of the Small Intestine

The mechanisms involved in diarrhea arising in the small intestine differ according to the type of pathogenic agent:

- **Viruses that cause death or dysfunction of intestinal epithelial cells:** The main agents are the rotaviruses (the case of A.) and noroviruses. These viruses **cause diarrhea by destroying or altering the function of enterocytes at the villi, but they do not affect those in the crypts.** Villus cells are sodium-absorbing cells, whereas crypt cells secrete chloride ions. One theory of virus-induced diarrhea is that damage of villus cells leads to decreased sodium and water absorption, which results in net accumulation ("secretion") of fluid in the lumen and damage to the disaccharidase-containing microvillus membranes, leading to sugar malabsorption. Instead of being hydrolyzed locally and absorbed, these sugars enter the colon where they are metabolized by the bacterial flora to osmotically more active products. As a result, fluid is drawn into the lumen, which worsens the

diarrhea. It is also partly responsible for a postenteritic syndrome seen in children, in whom mild diarrhea persists for considerable time after the infection is resolved.

- **Bacteria that colonize the upper small intestine** (e.g., enterotoxigenic *E. coli* and *V. cholerae*): In enterotoxigenic *E. coli* infections and cholera, diarrhea is secondary to the production of toxins by the organisms. The **toxins activate the enzymes responsible for synthesis of cyclic nucleotide mediators** (cAMP and cGMP), which in turn **stimulate net chloride secretion and inhibit sodium uptake** resulting in fluid loss. These mechanisms are described in detail in Chapter 9.

- **Protozoa, *Giardia* and *Cryptosporidium*,** which infect the small bowel (see Chapter 53): It is not known if a toxin is involved in these infections, or how the organisms colonize or invade the gut epithelium.

- Bacteria that cause true food poisoning: This form of diarrhea occurs when toxigenic bacteria (e.g., *Bacillus cereus* and *S. aureus*) multiply in food some time before it is eaten. As a result, toxins accumulate and are ingested along with the food. Because the signs and symptoms of food poisoning are not caused by bacterial multiplication in the body, the effects are often felt within a few hours after the tainted meal is eaten. Examples are discussed in Chapter 76.

Clearly not all infections of the small intestine produce a secretory diarrhea. Some organisms such as *C. jejuni* or *Y. enterocolitica* (as illustrated by the D. family) may infect the terminal ileum, producing watery, sometimes bloody stools. The varied presentations of illness in the D. family also illustrate the age-related differences in disease caused by a single organism. *Y. enterocolitica* is unique in that respect, and little is known about the reasons for the diversity. *Y. enterocolitica* infects primarily the terminal ileum and colon in all patients, but in children who are younger than 5 years of age, infection manifests as watery diarrhea. In older children, like S., bacteria from the intestine invade the mesenteric lymph nodes and cause focal inflammatory responses. Interestingly, diarrhea may be minimal or absent, and the mesenteric adenitis can mimic acute appendicitis. Many adults infected with *Y. enterocolitica* develop reactive arthritis within weeks after the onset of diarrhea. The same symptoms occur after *C. jejuni*, *S. flexneri*, and nontyphoidal *Salmonella* gastroenteritis. **Reactive arthritis** is probably an immunological phenomenon because organisms are not found in the joint fluid. Interestingly, individuals affected most severely by arthritis often possess the major histocompatibility antigen HLA-B27.

Infections of the Large Intestine

Bacterial pathogens that infect the large intestine tend to produce epithelial damage, mucosal inflammation, and bloody diarrhea, known as the dysentery syndrome. The major pathogens that invade the large bowel and cause dysentery are *Shigella* species and the ameba *E. histolytica*. Because inflammation in shigellosis is prominent and

table 60-3	Clinical Features of Diarrheal Disease	
FEATURE	**SMALL BOWEL**	**LARGE BOWEL**
Pathogens	*Vibrio cholerae*	*Shigella*
	Escherichia coli (enterotoxigenic, or ETEC)	*E. coli* (enteroinvasive, EIEC)
	Rotavirus	Campylobacter
	Norovirus	Entamoeba histolytica
	Giardia	
	Cryptosporidium	
	Cyclospora	
Location of pain	Midabdomen	Lower abdomen, rectum
Volume of stool	Large	Small
Type of stool	Watery	Mucoid
Blood in stool	Rare	Common
White blood cells in stool	Rare	Common (except in amebiasis)
Proctoscopy	Normal	Mucosal ulcers; hemorrhagic friable mucosa

usually located in the distal large bowel, pain often worsens with bowel movements, a symptom known as tenesmus. The mucosa is easily damaged and looks ulcerated when examined by proctoscopy. The stools may be watery and substantial initially but later decrease in volume and consist of blood, mucus, and pus. White blood cells are typically scarce in amebic dysentery because they are lysed by a toxin produced by the amebic trophozoites present in the lesions. Certain bacteria (e.g., species of *Campylobacter, Salmonella,* and *Yersinia*) produce inflammatory illness in the terminal ileum. The inflammation is associated with bloody diarrhea containing leukocytes and occasionally extends to the colon, resulting in dysentery.

E. coli O157:H7 is a normal inhabitant of the intestine of meat and dairy cattle as well as other ruminants (e.g., sheep, goats, and deer). In about 50% of cases contaminated beef products, most often ground beef, is the source of infection, although other sources such as water and fresh produce (e.g., lettuce) have been associated. *E. coli* O157:H7 and a number of other serotypes of shiga toxin–producing *E. coli* (STEC) infect the large bowel. Collectively, the organisms are known as enterohemorrhagic *E. coli* (EHEC). They adhere to colonic epithelial cells, causing a characteristic lesion in which the brush border is effaced by a dramatic change in cytoskeletal structures beneath the attached organism. This lesion causes diarrhea that appears to be almost pure blood, a syndrome known as **hemorrhagic colitis.** A different disease is caused by *Clostridium difficile* and its toxins. *C. difficile* infection usually arises after administration of antibiotics, which deplete or alter the other resident flora. This infection is characterized by an **adherent pseudomembrane with considerable mucosal inflammation** and damage but without tissue invasion (see Chapter 20).

Serious complications arise occasionally from infection of the colon by invasive organisms. Shigellosis may be associated with severe malnutrition, leading to a protein deficiency syndrome in children known as kwashiorkor. Shigellosis sometimes results in rectal prolapse or in a frequently fatal distention of the colon known as toxic megacolon, with a complete cessation of colonic peristalsis. Systemic complications also can occur, leading to HUS, leukemoid reactions with high white blood cell counts, encephalopathy, and other consequences. Amebiasis may cause intestinal perforation or obstruction, or the organisms may spread to produce abscesses in other organs, especially in the liver.

STEC (or EHEC) infections are associated with the production of one of two related and potent toxins called **Shiga toxin 1 and 2** (STX1 and STX2, also called shigalike toxins or verotoxins). These toxins appear to cross the intestinal mucosa and injure the endothelium of the intestinal lamina propria, the glomeruli, and the brain. The toxins cause HUS in children and a more prominent neurological disease in older adults, usually called thrombotic thrombocytopenic purpura (TTP). HUS is associated with an immediate mortality rate of 5 to 10% and an unknown frequency of renal failure after many years. In the past TTP was usually fatal, but the mortality rate has dropped to 20% with improved therapy and the use of exchange transfusion.

Other Gastrointestinal Infections

Infections of Gut-Associated Lymph Tissue

A different type of enteric infection is exemplified by typhoid fever (see Chapter 17). It is characterized by *Salmonella typhi* invasion of the gut-associated lymph tissue of the small bowel. From there the organisms disseminate to the liver and spleen where they proliferate. When the number of organisms is sufficient, they enter the bloodstream, causing the **persistent bacteremia and fever characteristic of enteric fever.** Diarrhea may be absent or transient; some patients may even complain of constipation. Other characteristic findings are a low white blood cell count in relation to fever and enlargement of the liver and spleen. With sustained bacteremia, the organisms invade the lymphatic tissue of Peyer patches and may cause severe inflammatory lesions, bleeding, and perforation. The mortality rate is high if the disease is untreated. Early use of effective antibiotics curtails the acute illness but predisposes to relapse, presumably by interfering with the protective immune response.

Surgical Complications of Intestinal Infections

Perforation of the wall of either the small or the large intestine may be caused by certain intestinal infections that induce inflammatory responses and tissue damage. Trauma, such as a penetrating knife injury or motor vehicle collision, can also cause perforation of the wall of the gut. Perforation results in spillage of intestinal contents into the normally sterile peritoneal cavity. The severity of the resulting peritonitis is generally related to the volume of the spill, its spread in the abdomen, and the ability of the omentum to wall off (contain) the abscess. A small amount of fecal contents may be handled by the defenses in the peritoneum, but a large inoculum can easily overwhelm them; the presence of blood worsens the response. Typically, peritonitis is severe and, if untreated, is often life threatening. Peritoneal infections are most often caused by a mixture of strict anaerobes, in particular *Bacteroides fragilis* and facultative Gram-negative bacteria of the Enterobacteriaceae family. The pathogenic mechanisms are discussed in Chapter 15.

DIAGNOSIS

Most patients with acute diarrhea have a mild and self-limited course and never seek medical attention. It is not practical or necessary to search for enteric pathogens in all patients with diarrhea. In a large percentage of cases it is sufficient to replenish fluids and electrolytes, usually by oral rehydration, and avoid the use of intravenous fluids unless the patient is in hypovolemic shock. A careful history of symptoms is the most important part of the investigation and often narrows the diagnostic possibilities. The clues that suggest disease requiring specific therapy (e.g., antimicrobial drugs) include fever, tenesmus, and persistent or severe abdominal pain (the triad of dysentery), weight loss, blood in the stool, recent antibiotic use, raw seafood meals, male homosexual practices, foreign travel, especially to developing countries, and prolonged duration of symptoms.

Culturing of stool samples for enteric pathogens is primarily intended to isolate *E. coli* O157:H7 and species of *Campylobacter*, *Salmonella*, and *Shigella*. Isolation or identification of other enteric pathogens requires special culture techniques, evaluation of serotype, or tests for toxin production that are not part of routine laboratory practices (see Chapter 58). Animal parasites, protozoa, or helminths are detected by various methods including enzyme immunoassays or direct microscopy of fresh or appropriately preserved stools, but the specimens may require special concentration or staining procedures. Therefore, it is important to narrow the list of possible organisms that are sought. For example, if cholera is suspected, the laboratory should be instructed to inoculate TCBS agar, which is not used in routine stool cultures. Similarly, if *E. coli* O157:H7 is suspected, the laboratory should inoculate sorbitol-containing MacConkey agar (SMAC) because that serotype of *E. coli* usually does not ferment sorbitol and stands out from the other sorbitol-fermenting *E. coli* of the normal flora. However, the SMAC test does not distinguish the non-O157:H7 shiga toxin–producing *E. coli*, which are an important group of organisms that cause a disease similar to that caused by *E. coli* O157:H7. A commercial enzyme immunoassay is available to detect the STX toxins in stool produced by any shiga toxin–producing *E. coli*.

If nonbloody diarrhea persists or remains unexplained, tests for protozoa, especially *Cyclospora* species and *Giardia lamblia*, are indicated. If the patient is infected with HIV, samples should be examined for *Cryptosporidium parvum*, *Isospora belli*, and microsporidia species. Immunoassays to detect antigens of *Cryptosporidium* and *Giardia* are also available. *Cryptosporidium*, *Cyclospora*, and *Isospora* infections can be readily diagnosed in stool or in biopsy specimens because the organisms are visible when stained by the acid-fast technique used for mycobacteria, an unusual feature among protozoa.

The clinical value of a particular test depends on whether the results will affect the management of the patient. Sometimes the information is used not for treatment of the individual but to determine if special isolation measures are warranted. Thus, the presence of rotavirus in A.'s stool did not materially change the treatment plan. However, the positive ELISA test for rotavirus suggested that if she were hospitalized or near other susceptible infants, she would have to be isolated.

TREATMENT

Most acute infectious diarrheas are mild, self-limited, and best treated with oral fluid replacement and continued feeding. The decision to employ specific antimicrobial or more aggressive intravenous fluid replacement therapy is determined by the severity or duration of diarrhea or the presence of shock or dysenteric symptoms. In general, infections caused by toxigenic and invasive *E. coli*, *Shigella* species, and *V. cholerae* are improved with antibiotics, but those infections often resolve before the diagnosis is made. In contrast, the use of antibiotics in the treatment for STEC (e.g., *E. coli* O157:H7) **can increase the risk for developing HUS.** The disadvantage of treating all infections with antibiotics is that the organisms may develop drug resistance. Furthermore, rather than altering the disease course, antibiotic treatment could increase the risk of inducing a carrier state, with the potential of increased spread of the infection, as with *Salmonella*. Other specific antimicrobials are prescribed for *Cyclospora*, *E. histolytica*, *G. lamblia*, and *Isospora*. To date, *Cryptosporidium* species defy truly effective therapy.

Antidiarrheal agents can reduce the frequency of stools and improve their consistency, but no evidence suggests that the drugs shorten the course of illness or (with the exception of loperamide) reduce the volume of fluid lost. In fact, by decreasing gut transit time, antimotility agents may impair pathogen clearance, thereby prolonging the infection and enhancing its severity. In addition, anticholinergics or opiates can produce the life-threatening condition of intestinal stasis known as toxic megacolon, especially in children and those with inflammatory diarrhea.

An important medical breakthrough has been the development of **oral rehydration therapy** for mild to moderate diarrhea. Following the discovery that sodium and glucose transport are coupled in the small intestine, it was observed that the oral administration of glucose with essential electrolytes dramatically accelerates absorption of sodium, with water following passively (i.e., without the expenditure of energy) to maintain osmolality. Moderate dehydration associated with cholera or other small bowel diarrheas should now be corrected with oral replacement. Even in severe dehydration, which requires rapid intravenous fluids to correct or prevent shock, oral rehydration may later be used alone for maintenance of adequate hydration. The impact of this simple concept on worldwide mortality from dehydration cannot be overstated, especially in the poorest areas of the world where the problem is prevalent and severe. In those areas the use of intravenous therapy is too expensive, and trained personnel are too scarce to provide it to more than a small proportion of affected persons. Technically uneducated people can be trained to mix the proper ingredients (sometimes using bottle caps as measuring devices) or dissolve prepackaged mixtures. The recipe for oral rehydration is remarkably simple.

To 1 L of water add:

½ teaspoon salt (3 g)
¼ teaspoon bicarbonate (1.5 g)
¼ teaspoon KCl (1.5 g)
4 tablespoons sugar (20 g)

Conclusion

With approximately 76 million cases of foodborne disease in the United States each year resulting in more than 300,000 hospitalizations, many of which are due to gastroenteritis, upsets to the digestive system are a major burden on the health care system. These numbers do not include patients with peptic ulcer disease, gallbladder disease, and other disorders of the alimentary tract that may be related to infection. One key point to remember in relation to many of the agents discussed in this chapter is that foodborne disease is generally preventable through careful handling and appropriate cooking of food combined with proper personal hygiene. Thus, many gastrointestinal illnesses can be avoided with appropriate care.

Generally, the intestinal system is well designed to defend against pathogenic microbes, but with the growing number of persons who are either immunocompromised or taking medications that alter gastric acidity, physicians must take care to provide advice about preventative strategies to avoid infections of the GI tract. Because a properly functioning digestive system is important for good nutrition, and good nutrition is critical for the prevention of many other diseases, it is important to understand infectious diseases of the intestine and the measures employed in their diagnosis and treatment.

chapter 61

Infections of the Central Nervous System

Roberta L. DeBiasi and Kenneth L. Tyler

Hundreds of pathogens are capable of infecting the human central nervous system (CNS), including viruses, bacteria, mycobacteria, fungi, protozoa, and parasites. The involvement of specific anatomical structures results in distinct clinical presentations of CNS infection, including meningitis, encephalitis, myelitis, and focal suppurative infections such as brain abscess and empyema. CNS infections are among the most serious diseases affecting humans, causing significant morbidity and mortality even when diagnosed and treated appropriately. Antimicrobial therapies have reduced the overall mortality attributable to many CNS infections to less than 10%, but that rate is still unacceptably high. **Neurologic sequelae** resulting from these diseases may lead to significant impairment in daily functioning and have the potential to greatly alter normal cognitive and motor development when occurring in childhood. Prompt diagnosis of CNS infection is essential to maximize the likelihood of a positive response to therapy.

ANATOMIC DEFINITIONS AND THE BLOOD-BRAIN BARRIER

The brain and spinal cord are suspended in **cerebrospinal fluid (CSF)** and are surrounded by three layers of meninges: the **pia mater** and **arachnoid mater**, which together constitute the leptomeninges, and the **dura mater** or pachymeninges (Fig. 61-1). From a microbiological point of view, the brain and spinal cord have distinct features that simultaneously afford significant protection from infection, but some features put the patient at risk for serious consequences should infection occur. A significant degree of mechanical protection and isolation is provided by the skull and vertebral column, but the intracranial and intravertebral spaces are restrictive, and inflammation and swelling of the brain or spinal cord can lead to dramatic changes in intracranial pressure, resulting in irreparable damage or even death. The **blood-brain barrier**—including of the endothelial cells that line brain capillaries and are cemented together by intercellular tight junctions—provides an important barrier to the passage of microorganisms and toxic substances into the brain and CSF. However, the blood-brain barrier also impedes the passage of protective components of the humoral and cellular immune system into the CSF and reduces the penetration of many antimicrobial drugs, resulting in decreased efficacy of available therapeutic agents.

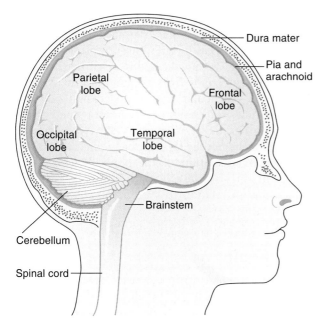

FIGURE 61-1 ▪ **Gross anatomy of the cranium.** The brain is located within a closed space, surrounded by the meninges (pia mater, arachnoid mater, and dura mater in close approximation to mucosal surfaces containing commensal flora (the nasopharynx).

CLINICAL DISEASE DEFINITIONS

Infections of the CNS can be categorized by the anatomic part of the brain affected. Infection of brain parenchyma results in **encephalitis** or **brain abscess,** infection of meninges causes **meningitis,** and infection of spinal cord tissue leads to **myelitis.** That categorization of CNS infections is somewhat artificial, because all areas of the brain are in anatomic communication with each other and can be infected simultaneously. In addition to direct injury from pathogens, CNS disease can result from postinfectious immune-mediated injury. Postinfectious encephalitis (acute disseminated encephalomyelitis) occurs weeks after acute viral infection and is thought to result from immune-mediated cross-reactivity against components of the normal brain, such as myelin, rather than from direct injury of brain tissue by the virus. In addition to acute infections, some organisms produce chronic or persistent infections. "Slow virus disease" (such as subacute sclerosing panencephalitis caused by measles virus) is thought to result from viral persistence within the CNS in conjunction with altered immune mechanisms that facilitate persistent infection, leading to a slowly destructive process occurring over years following infection. Other types of chronic progressive, uniformly fatal CNS infections (such as bovine spongiform encephalopathy and kuru) are caused by **prions,** which are a novel class of infectious agents consisting of abnormally folded proteins (see Chapter 56).

MICROBIOLOGY

CNS infections are caused by viruses, rickettsiae, bacteria, mycobacteria, fungi, amebas, or parasites. The most frequent etiologic agents and the types of disease with which they are most commonly associated fall into distinct categories (Table 61-1). For example, certain bacteria (e.g., *Streptococcus pneumonia, Haemophilus influenzae, Neisseria meningitidis*) classically cause meningitis but rarely cause infections of brain parenchyma, whereas others (e.g., *Staphylococcus aureus,* anaerobic streptococci) commonly cause brain abscesses but seldom cause meningitis. Some viruses are more likely to cause encephalitis

table **61-1**	**Categorization of Central Nervous System Infections and Frequent Etiologic Agents**
Acute meningitis	
Bacteria	
Streptococcus pneumoniae	
Neisseria meningitidis	
Haemophilus influenzae type B	
Group B streptococci	
Escherichia coli	
Viruses	
Arboviruses	
Enteroviruses	
Chronic meningitis	
Bacteria	
Mycobacterium tuberculosis	
Fungi	
Cryptococcus neoformans	
Others	
Acute encephalitis	
Viruses	
Arboviruses	
Enteroviruses	
Herpesviruses	
Acute brain abscess	
Bacteria	
Staphylococci	
Mixed anaerobic and aerobic flora	
Group A or D streptococci	
Chronic Brain Abscess	
Bacteria	
Mycobacterium tuberculosis	
Fungi	
Cryptococcus neoformans	
Parasites	
Taenia solium (cysticercosis)	
Toxoplasma	

(e.g., herpes simplex virus, or HSV), whereas others more commonly cause meningitis (e.g., enteroviruses).

Not all pathogens that infect humans can invade the CNS; organisms that do so possess special characteristics enabling them to infect cells of the nervous system, a property called **neurotropism.** Certain viruses show marked **tropism** for certain neural cell types (e.g., poliovirus for motor neurons of the spinal cord and medulla and mumps viruses for ependymal cells lining the ventricles in the fetal brain). The basis for such tropism is probably the distribution of viral receptors on specific neural cells. An example of a microbiologic attribute conferring the capacity of bacteria to infect the CNS is encapsulation. Over half the strains of *Escherichia coli* that infect the CNS have a capsule composed of **K1 antigen,** suggesting that neuropathogenic strains have been selected from the many antigenically distinct strains of *E. coli.* In contrast to other *E. coli* capsular antigens, K1 is a **polysaccharide rich in sialic acid,** as are capsular polysaccharides of group B streptococci. Polysaccharides containing sialic acid assist in bacterial adherence to the meninges and resultant bacterial growth. K1 antigen also possesses antiphagocytic properties and inhibits the alternative pathway of complement activation, resulting in impeded clearance of the organism. Additional factors that can influence tropism include the site of entry of a pathogen into the host and its mechanism of spread. For example, viruses that spread through neural routes have a different pattern of tropism than those that spread predominantly through the bloodstream.

ENTRY, REPLICATION, AND SPREAD

An infectious agent can invade the CNS using one of three routes: (1) hematogenously, through the systemic circulation; (2) through neural pathways; or less commonly (3) through direct inoculation (usually associated with trauma or congenital anatomical defects; Fig. 61-2).

Hematogenous Route

Most cases of CNS infection are caused by entry of the microorganisms from the **circulation** (see Fig. 61-2). Pathogens can gain access to the bloodstream by various routes, such as following colonization and penetration of the respiratory epithelium (e.g., meningococci), the bite of an arthropod (e.g., West Nile virus), the bite of a mammal (e.g., rabies virus), or transplacentally (e.g., rubella virus). Once an organism is in the bloodstream, the precise mechanism by which it penetrates the blood-brain barrier is not well understood. Some organisms enter the CNS at sites where the blood-brain

barrier is less restrictive because of the lack of tight junctions between endothelial cells, such as the choroid plexus. Choroid plexus infection in turn provides direct access to the CSF within the ventricular system. Infection spreads sequentially from the blood to the choroid plexus to the ventricular CSF to ependymal cells lining the ventricles to periventricular brain tissues. Other viruses, including many arboviruses, have the capacity to directly infect endothelial cells, including those of the microvascular circulation of the brain. Regardless of the route of entry to the CNS, the likelihood of infection increases in relation to the microbial load in the bloodstream.

Neural Route

Although many neurotropic viruses reach the CNS through the bloodstream, a few use special neural pathways (see Fig. 61-2). For example, following inoculation by the bite of a rabid animal, rabies virus enters the axons of peripheral nerves and travels inside nerve axons via axoplasmic transport to reach nerve cell bodies in sensory ganglia and the spinal cord. HSV spreads through nerves from sites of primary infection in the oropharynx (HSV-1) or genital area (HSV-2) to infect trigeminal (HSV-1) or sacral (HSV-2) ganglia, where the virus becomes latent in sensory neurons (see Chapter 41). Reactivation results in spread of virus along sensory nerves to mucosal surfaces, producing recurrent herpes labialis (cold sores) or herpes genitalis. Following chicken pox, which results from primary infection with varicella-zoster virus (VZV), virus spreads from the skin through sensory nerves to become latent in neurons in sensory ganglia. Reactivation results in spread of virus through sensory nerves to produce zoster, or shingles.

Some viruses and other infectious agents can penetrate the body through olfactory nerve endings, which are the only elements of the nervous system in direct contact with the external environment. Experimental studies suggest that herpesviruses reach the brain by this route, and nasal infections have been shown to occur with rabies virus and some arboviruses under conditions with high airborne concentrations of virus, as in caves filled with infected bats. The freshwater ameba *Naegleria fowleri,* which causes a rare but lethal meningoencephalitis, is thought to penetrate the CNS through traumatic gaps in the cribriform plate, allowing access to the olfactory bulbs, perhaps induced when a person dives into water containing the organisms.

LOCAL IMMUNE RESPONSES

The CNS is a sequestered compartment with more restricted immunological defense mechanisms than most other regions of the body. For example, complement

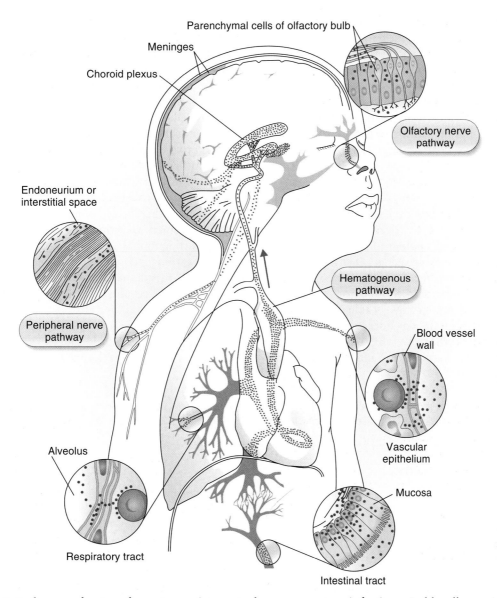

FIGURE 61-2 ▪ **Pathways of entry of agents causing central nervous system infections.** In bloodborne infections, agents from the respiratory tract, gut, or vascular epithelium enter via the choroid plexus. Inside the CNS, microorganisms can spread either by contiguous dissemination from cell to cell or through extracellular spaces. Some neurotropic viruses reach the brain through peripheral nerves or olfactory nerve endings.

levels are low in the CSF, apparently owing to both poor penetration from the blood and the presence of substances that can inactivate complement. Therefore, complement-dependent lysis or phagocytosis of bacteria does not readily occur in the brain, the meninges, and the CSF. However, the CNS is not as immunologically restricted as was once thought. The CNS possesses an intrinsic immunological surveillance mechanism in the **microglia.** Microglial cells have many cell type–specific markers identical to those of peripheral blood monocytes, suggesting that microglia are derived from blood monocytes that enter the CNS and differentiate. In addition, the CNS has a lymphlike system consisting of the Virchow-Robin spaces (the perivascular sheaths

surrounding the blood vessels as they enter the brain). These spaces contain macrophages and lymphocytes and are thought to be sites where those cells enter the CSF. In certain CNS infections, the host immune response maintains the infecting microorganisms in a latent state; active disease results only when immune mechanisms are compromised by drugs, HIV infection, or other forms of immunosuppression. Examples of such infections include tuberculosis and toxoplasmosis.

Immunodeficient persons are at risk for more severe or unusual presentations of CNS disease not seen in immunocompetent individuals. For example, patients with acquired immunodeficiency (e.g., Hodgkin disease and other lymphomas, AIDS, patients receiving immunosuppressive drug regimens) can develop **progressive multifocal leukoencephalopathy (PML)**. PML is caused by reactivation of a polyomavirus called JC virus, which is usually acquired in early childhood. Acute infection with JC virus is either asymptomatic or results in self-limited mild illness before becoming latent within the CNS. However, immunosuppression allows reactivation and replication of latent virus, leading to progressive CNS destruction.

EPIDEMIOLOGY

The most important epidemiological determinants of CNS infection are the age and geographic location of the affected individual and the time of year. For example, certain bacteria are more likely to cause meningitis in persons of defined age groups (Table 61-2). That information is important to consider when choosing empiric antimicrobial therapy while awaiting CSF culture results. Thus, in newborn infants, bacterial

meningitis is most commonly caused by *E. coli* and group B streptococci (*Streptococcus agalactiae*). Likewise, *Listeria monocytogenes* is a more frequent cause of bacterial meningitis in neonates and the elderly than in other age groups. The season in which clinical illness develops also can suggest which specific pathogens are the most likely etiology (Table 61-3). For example, spread of arboviruses by mosquito and tick vectors occurs more commonly in summer months, when mosquito breeding and likelihood of exposure is greatest, and wanes in winter months (see Chapter 33). Enteroviral infections usually peak in the late summer and fall. On the other hand, some pathogens do not have specific seasonal variation and occur with equal frequency throughout the year; among these pathogens is HSV, the most common cause of sporadic viral encephalitis in adults. The geographic distribution of several arboviruses is suggested by their names (e.g., California encephalitis virus, St. Louis encephalitis virus, and West Nile virus), although they often misrepresent the modern host ranges of the viruses. For example, although St. Louis encephalitis virus was

table 61-2 Etiology and Empiric Therapy of Bacterial Meningitis by Patient Category

		BACTERIAL PATHOGEN		
AGE	UNDERLYING DISEASE	MOST COMMON	OTHER	INITIAL EMPIRIC THERAPY
Birth to 3 months	None	*Streptococcus agalactiae* (group B)	*Escherichia coli*	Ampicillin and cefotaxime (or gentamicin)
			Listeria monocytogenes	
			Other Gram-negative organisms	
3–60 months	None	*Streptococcus pneumoniae*	*Neisseria meningitidis*[a]	Vancomycin and cefotaxime (or ceftriaxone)
			(*Haemophilus influenzae* type B)[b]	
> 60 months	None	*Streptococcus pneumoniae*	*N. meningitidis*[a]	Vancomycin and cefotaxime (or ceftriaxone)
			L. monocytogenes	
			Other Gram-negative organisms	
Any age	Cranial surgery	*Staphylococcus aureus*	*Staphylococcus epidermidis*	Vancomycin and cefepime
			Gram-negative organisms including *Pseudomonas aeruginosa*	
Any age	Immunosuppression (malignancy, drug induced, AIDS)		*L. monocytogenes*	Ampicillin (or vancomycin) and cefepime
			Gram-negative organisms, including *P. aeruginosa*	

[a] Occurs in epidemics.
[b] Only in unimmunized populations.

table **61-3**	**Viruses Causing Encephalitis**			
VIRUS	**GEOGRAPHIC LOCATION**	**MAJOR AGE GROUP**	**PREDOMINANT SEASON**	**NOTABLE FEATURES**
Herpes simplex viruses 1 and 2	All	All	None	Focal symptoms
West Nile virus	All	Older adults	Summer through fall	Weakness, movement disorders, poliomyelitis syndrome
St. Louis encephalitis	All	Older adults	Summer through fall	Most cases mild
Eastern equine encephalitis	Atlantic and Gulf coasts, Great Lakes	Children	Summer through fall	High mortality (50–80%) and morbidity (80% with neurologic sequelae)
Western equine encephalitis	Western United States and Canada	Infants and older adults	Summer through fall	Higher mortality (10–20%) and morbidity in infants (50%)
California (La Crosse) encephalitis	Midwest and northeast United States, southern Canada	Older children	Summer through fall	Less than 1% mortality and rare morbidity
Enteroviruses	All	Infants and children more than adults	Summer	Severity inverse to age
Rabies	All	All	All	Animal bite (bats)
Varicella-zoster virus	All	Children and immunocompromised adults	Winter	Rare
HIV	All	Adults more than children	All	Dementia in AIDS patients

named for the city in which it was first isolated from patients with encephalitis, it occurs throughout the United States. Similarly, although West Nile virus was first isolated from the West Nile Valley in Uganda, it is now widely distributed throughout the United States and many other regions of the world. West Nile virus also provides a dramatic example of how the host range of an infectious agent can change dramatically over a relatively short period: the range of the virus expanded across the entire 48 contiguous United States from 1999 to 2004.

DAMAGE

Tissue dysfunction resulting from CNS infection occurs by several mechanisms. Death of CNS cells can result from the action of bacterial toxins, lytic cycles of viral replication, or intracellular growth of bacteria and fungi. In most infections, however, some component of cellular death and tissue destruction results from the immune response of the host. Multiplication and spread of microorganisms within the CNS elicits an inflammatory response similar to but generally less intense than that produced in other areas of the body. Infiltration of microglia and proliferation of **astrocytes** are characteristic of the inflammatory response within the CNS. As in other parts of the body, the CNS inflammatory response has both humoral and cellular components. Inflammation can lead to vasogenic edema caused by increased capillary permeability. Neutrophils and macrophages then infiltrate the area and phagocytize microorganisms and dead cells. Lysis of infiltrating neutrophils releases enzymes, leading to further tissue destruction.

Swelling of the brain resulting from inflammation within the closed cranial vault (cerebral edema) can produce neurologic symptoms as a consequence of decreased capillary perfusion of brain tissue. More severe forms of cerebral edema can cause herniation of the temporal lobe through the falx or the brainstem into the foramen magnum, producing severe brain damage or death. Thus, neurological symptoms that arise during infection of the CNS can be caused by focal tissue destruction that produces specific functional deficits or by cerebral edema that leads to global loss of cortical function.

The localization of specific functions in different areas of the brain, combined with differences in the capacity of microorganisms to infect those areas, provides clues to the diagnosis of specific infections. For example, psychosis, impairment of memory, and seizures suggest HSV encephalitis (because of the preferred involvement of the frontal and temporal lobes); stiffness of the neck without severe impairment of cerebral function is characteristic of enteroviral meningitis; and flaccid paralysis of the lower extremities suggests injury to the motor neurons of the spinal cord from poliovirus or

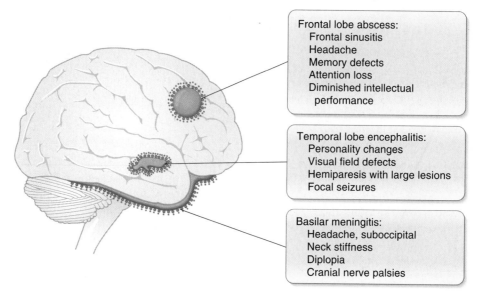

FIGURE 61-3 ▪ **Anatomic basis of localization of symptoms in CNS infections.** Focal involvement of the cerebral cortex produces specific signs and symptoms depending on the primary function of that part of the brain. In contrast, pyogenic meningitis produces global cerebral cortical dysfunction as a result of diffuse cerebral edema.

West Nile virus. Focal symptoms likely to result from specific CNS infections are shown in Figure 61-3.

The following case histories and discussion describe characteristic infections of the CNS and their diagnoses. They include cases of acute bacterial meningitis, acute viral (aseptic) meningitis, chronic tuberculous meningitis, acute viral encephalitis, and brain abscess.

Meningitis

Most cases of meningitis can be classified in the following manner:

- By clinical presentation: acute, subacute, or chronic
- By etiology: bacterial, viral, or fungal
- By epidemiology: sporadic or epidemic

Acute meningitis is usually characterized by the rapid onset of symptoms, occurring within hours of contact with the infectious agent and possibly days before presentation for medical evaluation. Acute meningitis is usually bacterial or viral in etiology. In all cases of suspected bacterial meningitis, antimicrobial therapy must be administered immediately. The predominant etiology of acute bacterial meningitis varies with the age of the patient. In infants younger than 3 months of age, acute bacterial meningitis is caused chiefly by *E. coli*, group B streptococci, or *L. monocytogenes*. The most common etiologic organisms in children more than 3 months of age, adolescents, and adults are *N. meningitides* (meningococci), and *S. pneumonia* (pneumococci). Until recently, *H. influenzae* type B was the most common

cause of bacterial meningitis in children. However, with the introduction of effective *H. influenzae* conjugated vaccines in the mid-1980s, in which *H. influenzae* type B capsular carbohydrate is covalently linked to a protein carrier (tetanus or diphtheria toxoids), that type of bacterial meningitis has been nearly eradicated in immunized populations. Children who are not immunized or only partially immunized remain susceptible to infection with *H influenzae* type B. Meningitis can also be caused by nontypeable *Haemophilus* species, but those agents are seen less often than are other causes of bacterial meningitis. Acute viral meningitis (the most common etiology of the clinical entity referred to as aseptic meningitis) is usually caused by enteroviruses and occurs most frequently in the late summer and fall in annual epidemics.

Subacute or chronic meningitis is most commonly caused by fungi (such as *C. neoformans*) or mycobacteria (such as *Mycobacterium tuberculosis*), organisms that cause chronic, inflammatory, granulomatous tissue reactions. Persons with subacute or chronic meningitis often present with weeks to months of less fulminant clinical symptoms than those associated with acute meningitis, but an acute worsening could prompt the decision to seek medical evaluation.

Acute Bacterial Meningitis

ENCOUNTER AND ENTRY

The two most common agents of acute bacterial meningitis, pneumococci and meningococci, are acquired by

Case

Bacterial Meningitis

One week after arriving at the Army recruit camp at Fort Ord, California, Pvt. W. became the first of three cases of meningitis. He had a precipitous onset of fever and headache and felt a pain in his neck when he moved his head. When he arrived at the infirmary he had a petechial rash on his lower extremities. On lumbar puncture his opening pressure was slightly elevated at 220 mm H_2O (normal range is less than 180 mm H_2O). CSF cell count revealed white blood cells (WBCs) at 500/mm³ (80% polymorphonuclear cells), the CSF glucose was 30 mg/dL (decreased), and protein was 100 mg/dL (increased). A smear of the CSF revealed small Gram-negative coccobacilli and numerous leukocytes (Fig. 61-4).

Antimicrobial therapy was instituted immediately with intravenous vancomycin and ceftriaxone, pending culture results. Twenty-four hours later, the CSF culture grew *N. meningitides.* Vancomycin was discontinued and, following 10 days of intravenous ceftriaxone therapy, Pvt. W. recovered completely. Pvt. H. had developed the same symptoms 24 hours after Pvt. W. When Pvt. B. was diagnosed the next morning with the same illness, the other soldiers in the camp became alarmed. Their fears calmed when the medical corps personnel explained that further spread of infection could be halted by the prophylactic administration of antibiotics to all close contacts of the infected cases.

FIGURE 61-4 ▪ **Gram stain of CSF from a patient with meningococcal meningitis.** Gram-negative coccobacilli and neutrophils are evident.

Case

Viral Meningitis

While Privates W., H., and B. were being treated for their infections, Pvt. E. left the Fort Ord camp for his assignment at Fort Leonard Wood, Missouri. When he arrived he had a fever, severe headache, and some nausea. The next day, when putting on his boots, he noticed that his neck was stiff. He also became very sensitive to bright sunlight. When he was evaluated at the infirmary, a lumbar puncture was performed. The CSF opening pressure was 90 mm H_2O (in the normal range). The CSF contained 76 WBCs/mm³ (90% lymphocytes), 70 mg/dL of protein (mildly increased), and 66 mg/dL of glucose (normal). He was observed in the hospital for 2 days, without institution of antibiotics, pending results of CSF bacterial and viral cultures and CSF enterovirus polymerase chain reaction (PCR). The CSF cultures were negative, but the enteroviral PCR returned positive 36 hours after admission. His symptoms resolved without antimicrobial therapy, and he was discharged from the hospital with a diagnosis of aseptic meningitis caused by enterovirus.

These two cases raise two questions:

1. Why did meningococcal meningitis, the etiology of Pvt. W.'s illness, produce alarm and warrant aggressive treatment and measures to prevent spread of infection, whereas viral aseptic meningitis, the etiology of Pvt. E.'s illness, did not require specific therapy?
2. How do the CSF findings in Pvt. W.'s case (bacterial meningitis) compare with those in Pvt. E.'s case (viral meningitis)?

does not, however, always correlate directly with outbreaks, because individual strains of meningococci vary considerably in virulence. The reason so many people become colonized but only a few get sick is not well understood. The best clue comes from the observation that susceptible individuals lack antibodies against the meningococcal capsular antigen, whereas carriers have protective antibodies. Moreover, a striking association has been made between congenital deficiency in the late components of the complement cascade and neisserial infection, particularly with meningococci. Those findings suggest that the immunological status of an individual plays a role in determining whether disease develops.

SPREAD, MULTIPLICATION, AND DAMAGE

Acute bacterial meningitis can be an isolated clinical event or part of overwhelming bacterial septicemia. In

the respiratory route through inhalation of aerosol droplets from asymptomatic human carriers. It is likely that in the meningococcal outbreak at Ford Ord (see Case: Bacterial Meningitis), most of the recruits were exposed to the organism from another individual, because meningococci are found in the oropharynx of about 10% of healthy people. The frequency of colonization the latter case the symptoms of meningitis only add to an already grave clinical picture; the presence of large numbers of organisms in the blood causes severe nonneural manifestations, such as shock and disseminated intravascular coagulation. In the case of meningococcal disease those signs reflect the high blood content of Gram-negative endotoxin.

The clinical manifestations of acute meningitis, caused by meningococci or other bacteria, include fever, stiff neck (nuchal rigidity), headache, and occasionally global or focal CNS dysfunction. Those symptoms are caused by the inflammatory response to meningeal invasion. The extent of inflammation caused by pathogens varies and is influenced by the intrinsic virulence of the organism and the immune response of the patient. Pus in the subarachnoid spaces can spread over the brain, the cerebellum, and the spinal cord. Pneumococcal infections and those caused by members of the Enterobacteriaceae family are marked by particularly thick accumulations of pus that block CSF flow and readsorption, leading to elevated intracranial pressure. In meningococcal meningitis the CSF pressure is usually only mildly elevated. Increased intracranial pressure from cerebral edema invariably leads to nausea and vomiting, severe headache, and progressive depression in the level of consciousness.

In general, the incidence of neurologic sequelae is lower when bacterial meningitis is caused by meningococci than it is when the cause is some other bacteria. *H. influenzae* meningitis often results in deafness, mental retardation, or both in affected patients. Neurologic sequelae from pneumococcal meningitis also tend to be severe and frequent.

DIAGNOSIS

Acute bacterial infection of the CNS is a medical emergency. Appropriate antibiotic therapy must be urgently initiated after a patient arrives in an emergency department or physician's office. Fortunately, examination of a Gram stain of the CSF obtained by lumbar puncture can rapidly yield a presumptive diagnosis. Examination of the CSF is absolutely necessary when acute meningitis is suspected. The characteristic patterns of inflammation in the CSF in the setting of various CNS infections are summarized in Table 61-4.

The elements of inflammatory response in the CSF also can help in determining whether the infection is likely to be bacterial or viral and may even point to a specific infectious agent as the etiology. A large number of neutrophils suggests bacterial infection, whereas a predominance of lymphocytes or mononuclear cells suggests a nonbacterial (most commonly, but not always, viral) etiology. Gram stain examination of the CSF should be a routine procedure because it reveals infecting bacteria in about 60–90% of the cases of bacterial meningitis.

Culture of CSF can definitively establish the etiology of bacterial meningitis and guide the choice of antibiotic therapy. Rapid tests based on identification of bacterial antigens are unreliable, with unacceptably low sensitivity and specificity to be useful in diagnosis. Polymerase chain reaction (PCR) testing for enterovirus has excellent sensitivity and specificity (greater than 95% each), with results often available in less than 24 hours. PCR tests for bacteria are not yet clinically available.

TREATMENT

To treat bacterial meningitis effectively, antibiotics to which the bacteria are susceptible must penetrate the CSF in an active form. β-**Lactam antibiotics** are frequently used to treat bacterial meningitis. The drugs are highly polar and have relatively low penetration through blood-brain and blood-CSF barriers. The average drug concentration normally achieved in CSF is about 15% of that in serum. However, β-lactam drugs also enter the CSF

table **61-4**	Usual Composition of Cerebrospinal Fluid in Various Central Nervous System Infections					
FACTOR	**NORMAL**	**ACUTE BACTERIAL MENINGITIS**	**CHRONIC MYCOBACTERIAL AND FUNGAL MENINGITIS**	**ACUTE VIRAL MENINGITIS**	**VIRAL ENCEPHALITIS**	**BRAIN ABSCESS**
Leukocytes (/mm³)	0–6	> 1,000	100–500	10–1,000, usually < 300	10–500	10–100
% Neutrophils	0	> 50	< 10	May predominate in first 24 hours, then < 50	May predominate in first 24 hours, then < 50	< 50
Red blood cells (/mm³)	0–2	0–10	0–2	0–2	10–500 (HSV)	0–2
Glucose (mg/dL)[a]	40–80	< 30	≤ 40	40–80	40–80	40–80
Protein (mg/dL)	20–50	> 100	50–100 (fungal), > 100 (mycobacterial)	50–100	50–100	50–100

[a] Diagnostic values are best interpreted as the ratio of glucose levels in CSF compared with serum. Ratios less than 0.4 are considered diminished.

through capillary leaks enhanced by inflammation, enabling the drugs to reach therapeutic levels in patients with meningitis. Newer β-lactam antibiotics, such as **cefotaxime** and **ceftriaxone,** are very potent and produce CSF concentrations that exceed those required to kill bacteria by 20 times or more. Yet the emergence of β-lactam resistance among pneumococcal isolates in the United States (up to 50% of isolates are partially or completely resistant in several parts of the country) makes it imperative to use combination therapy with vancomycin (a glycopeptide antibiotic with a mechanism of action different from that of β-lactam drugs) for empiric therapy of bacterial meningitis, until resistance to cephalosporins has been definitively excluded by culture and susceptibility testing.

An important aspect of the treatment of meningitis is the control of increased intracranial pressure. Cerebral edema can further decrease the already diminished cerebral blood flow and depress oxidative glucose metabolism. Death from compression of the brainstem into the foramen magnum (i.e., herniation) is possible. Supportive measures must ensure that the patient is adequately oxygenated and that blood glucose is in the normal range. Dexamethasone, a glucocorticoid with potent anti-inflammatory activities, has been shown to decrease the incidence of deafness as a consequence of *H. influenzae* meningitis in children more than 3 months of age. Dexamethasone has the same beneficial effect on meningitis caused by pneumococci and perhaps other bacteria in adults.

PREVENTION

Vaccines are currently available for *N. meningitides, S. pneumoniae,* and *H. influenzae* type B, the most common causes of bacterial meningitis. Routine vaccination against meningococci is limited to high-risk groups, such as military recruits. However, many colleges currently recommend or require vaccination of incoming students because outbreaks frequently occur in that population. The meningococcal vaccine contains capsular polysaccharides of type A and C meningococci, the most common types implicated in recent meningococcal epidemics, and two other rare types. An effective vaccine against type B meningococci is not currently available. Chemoprophylaxis with rifampin, quinolone antibiotics, or ceftriaxone effectively eradicates nasopharyngeal carriage of meningococci in the majority of recipients and is indicated for all close contacts of index cases. A multivalent polysaccharide pneumococcal vaccine is available for persons older than 2 years of age who are at risk for acquiring invasive pneumococcal disease (asplenic persons and those with certain forms of primary immunodeficiency). Conjugated pneumococcal vaccine is now recommended as part of the routine immunization schedule for all children in the United States beginning at 2 months

of age. Widespread pneumococcal immunization could lead to a much lower incidence of pneumococcal meningitis in the next decade, as observed following widespread use of the *H. influenzae* type B vaccine among children.

Viral Meningitis
PATHOBIOLOGY

Viruses are the most common cause of the syndrome known as aseptic meningitis. In its traditional sense, the term "aseptic" is a misnomer because it refers only to the fact that the CSF of patients with the syndrome is sterile on routine bacteriological culture. However, aseptic meningitis also results from infections caused by various agents that do not grow on standard bacteriological media (e.g., fungi, leptospira, and *Treponema pallidum*). In addition, aseptic meningitis can result from noninfectious etiologies, such as cancer or autoimmune disease.

DIAGNOSIS AND TREATMENT

Compared with bacterial meningitis, viral meningitis produces a milder disease with low to moderate inflammatory reaction in the CSF consisting primarily of lymphocytes. Pvt. E. had the clinical disease and CSF findings typical of viral meningitis (chiefly, a mildly increased number of CSF leukocytes and normal glucose level; see Table 61-4). Therefore, he did not receive antibiotics and was observed in the hospital. His improvement without antibacterial treatment further supported a viral etiology. The positive CSF PCR for enterovirus confirmed the diagnosis of the most common etiology of viral meningitis. However, many other viruses can cause the disease, including arboviruses and the herpesviruses (HSV-1, HSV-2, and VZV). Although viral meningitis can be confirmed by isolating a virus by culture from the CSF, that process is time consuming and many viruses cannot be cultivated. Isolating a virus known to cause aseptic meningitis from the throat or stool of a patient with appropriate symptoms suggests, but does not prove, that the suspect virus is the cause of aseptic meningitis. If the enterovirus PCR had been negative and Pvt. E. had not improved, other causes for his symptoms and the presence of leukocytes in the CSF would have been pursued.

In infants less than 1 year of age, it is often difficult to distinguish bacterial from aseptic meningitis. The newborn has a limited set of immune responses when the CNS is infected, and the relative immaturity of the reticuloendothelial system at that age may not permit an adult-type inflammatory response. As a result, most infants with symptoms of acute meningitis and leukocytes in the CSF are treated empirically with intravenous antibiotics, even if a viral etiology is suspected.

Case

Tuberculous Meningitis

Ms. G., a 32-year-old native of South America, immigrated to the United States 1 year ago with her husband and three children. Four weeks later her oldest child returned from child care with chickenpox. In another 2 weeks Ms. G. and the rest of her family developed the disease. All recovered uneventfully. However, as Ms. G.'s rash faded, she developed a headache and again had fever. Over the next week she lost her appetite and vomited a few times. Those symptoms persisted for another week, and she became apathetic. When she developed stupor 4 days later, she was taken to a local hospital.

On physical examination Ms. G. was noted to have impaired eye movements. A chest radiograph showed right upper lobe pneumonia. A cranial computerized tomography (CT) scan showed enlarged ventricles suggestive of acute hydrocephalus. A lumbar puncture revealed an opening pressure of 310 mm H_2O (highly elevated), and the CSF showed 350 WBCs/mm^3, of which 87% were lymphocytes. The CSF protein was 168 mg/dL (increased) and the glucose was 20 mg/dL (decreased) with coincident serum glucose of 120 mg/dL. Gram stain and acid-fast stain did not show organisms.

Additional studies of the CSF included detection of tuberculostearic acid and a positive mycobacterial PCR, which led the physician to diagnose tuberculous meningitis (see Chapter 23). Subsequently, *M. tuberculosis* grew from her CSF and was found to be susceptible to isoniazid, rifampin, pyrazinamide, and streptomycin. Ms. G. was treated with urgent ventricular drainage, the four antituberculosis drugs tested, and steroids for 2 months. With resolution of her symptoms, ventricular drainage was discontinued, and she was discharged to receive 10 additional months of therapy with isoniazid and rifampin.

This case raises several questions:

1. What is the explanation for Ms. G.'s eye movement abnormalities?
2. How do the CSF findings in tuberculous meningitis compare with those in viral and bacterial meningitis?
3. Why are multiple drugs required for the treatment of tuberculous meningitis?

Chronic Meningitis

PATHOBIOLOGY

Ms. G. came from a geographic region in which pulmonary tuberculosis is endemic. During primary pulmonary infection, tubercle bacilli may be deposited in multiple organs (including the brain), where they are contained within granulomas and remain quiescent (termed latent tuberculosis). Ms. G.'s chickenpox suppressed her cell-mediated immunity, enabling the tubercle bacilli to multiply and cause inflammation. In the brain, granulomas located near the ventricles may spill tubercle bacilli into the CSF. The organisms then spread throughout the subarachnoid space and characteristically become most prevalent in the basilar cisterns. As cell-mediated immunity returns, it elicits an intense delayed-type hypersensitivity reaction to the organisms. Granulomas and inflammation around cranial nerves cause them to malfunction. In Ms. G.'s case the nerves affected were cranial nerves III and VI, as indicated by the impaired eye movements. Inflammation of the base of the brain compromises CSF circulation from the fourth ventricle into the cisterna magna, which causes acute hydrocephalus and increased intracranial pressure, leading to stupor and the possibility of coma.

DIAGNOSIS

Ms. G.'s CSF findings (lymphocytic pleocytosis, decreased glucose, and increased protein) and indolent course are consistent with chronic meningitis. Both fungi and *M. tuberculosis* are potential etiologies that should be considered in such cases. Acid-fast stain of CSF has poor sensitivity for the diagnosis of tuberculous meningitis, being positive in only 5 to 25% of cases. Thus, the test cannot be used to exclude disease. Mycobacterial culture may require up to 6 weeks for growth and identification of the organism. The presence of a **tubercular lipid** (tuberculostearic acid) in the CSF made the diagnosis of tuberculous meningitis likely in the case of Ms. G. The diagnosis was later confirmed by PCR amplification of mycobacterial DNA and isolation of *M. tuberculosis* from the CSF.

Because the diagnosis of tuberculous meningitis is so important, many research groups are working to develop sensitive and specific DNA-based methods to detect mycobacteria in the CSF, employing PCR primers specific for certain genes of *M. tuberculosis*. Although PCR of CSF has not yet achieved adequate sensitivity or specificity to replace more standard methods, it may be useful as an adjunctive diagnostic method. An intradermal skin test using purified protein derivative may or may not be positive in fulminant tuberculosis, but it should be positive when repeated after weeks to months of effective antituberculous therapy.

TREATMENT

The emergence of drug-resistant strains of *M. tuberculosis* in most parts of the world makes combination therapy with at least three and preferably four drugs with different mechanisms of action the standard of care for the treatment of active tuberculosis, particularly with involvement of the CNS. If the organism is isolated from the CSF (which may take up to 6 weeks) susceptibility testing should be performed to verify selection of the proper drug regimen for long-term therapy (usually 12 months). Steroids are used for treatment of CNS disease because the intense inflammatory response to the organism is a major component of neural dysfunction and damage to the brain and meninges. With successful treatment CSF cultures should become sterile within one month, and CSF glucose should become normal by 1 to 2 months. CSF cell counts and protein may take 1 year to normalize.

Acute Viral Encephalitis

Case

HSV Encephalitis

Sixty-year-old Mr. R. was brought to the hospital with confusion, right-sided weakness, and fever. His daughter, who was visiting him, reported that when she arrived he thought "there were devils in the room." On the way to the hospital he hallucinated intermittently, telling her that he smelled roses. Three days previously he had complained of mild nausea and vomited once. When he arrived at the emergency department, Mr. R. had a generalized seizure.

A CT scan of the head was normal, but a magnetic resonance imaging (MRI) scan documented T1-hypointense and T2-hyperintense signal in the cortex and gray–white matter junction in the left temporal lobe. CSF obtained by lumbar puncture contained 50 WBCs/mm³ (90% mononuclear cells) and 300 RBCs/mm³, glucose in the normal range (70 mg/dL), and elevated protein (100 mg/dL). CSF was sent for bacterial and viral culture and enterovirus and HSV PCR. An electroencephalogram (EEG) revealed periodic high-voltage spike wave activity from the left temporal region.

Intravenous acyclovir was started immediately. By the next day, the CSF enterovirus PCR was negative and the HSV PCR was positive. Mr. R. was continued on intravenous acyclovir for 3 weeks, which halted the progression of his neurological symptoms. However, he had many residual signs of neurological impairment and required extensive rehabilitation therapy.

This case raises two questions:

1. What is the best single diagnostic method to establish a diagnosis of HSV encephalitis?
2. What is the prognosis for patients who survive HSV encephalitis?

■ ■ ■ ■

PATHOBIOLOGY

Approximately 20,000 cases of encephalitis occur in the United States each year, almost all of which are caused by viruses. The hallmark of encephalitis is the acute onset of a febrile illness accompanied by headache and **altered mental status.** The presence of altered mental status (e.g., disorientation, hallucination, or behavioral disturbances) and focal or diffuse neurologic signs (e.g., hemiparesis or seizures) help distinguish encephalitis from meningitis. HSV is the most frequent etiology of sporadic encephalitis in the United States, accounting for approximately 10% of cases in the United States annually. Arboviruses, including West Nile virus, are the most important cause of epidemic encephalitis (see Table 61-3 and Chapters 33 and 41).

HSV-1 (and rarely HSV-2) is usually associated with severe focal encephalitis in adolescents and adults. Untreated, the disease carries a 70% mortality rate, and 97% of untreated survivors are left with permanent neurologic deficits. Fibers emerging from the trigeminal ganglia, in which HSV-1 resides in the latent state following primary infection, innervate the dura of the middle and anterior fossae and the meningeal arteries of the area. HSV may use this route to spread to the meninges and meningeal arteries and, from there, to the contiguous cortex. That postulated pattern might explain the frequent localization of HSV in the temporal and frontal lobes.

Fifty percent of newborns who acquire HSV (usually HSV-2), either transplacentally or at the time of delivery from the maternal genital tract, develop CNS infection. CNS disease occurs predominantly in two forms: (1) nondisseminated neuronal transmission, with disease limited to the CNS, and (2) hematogenous dissemination with multiorgan involvement, including the CNS. Many of the manifestations of HSV encephalitis result from destruction of neurons, especially within the temporal and frontal lobes, accompanied by inflammation with infiltration of mononuclear cells from the perivascular sheaths (Virchow-Robin spaces). Portions of the temporal lobe responsible for the sense of smell may be affected, resulting in olfactory hallucinations (e.g., smelling roses in the case of Mr. R.).

DIAGNOSIS

The diagnosis of herpes encephalitis is suspected if patients have fever and focal cerebral cortical lesions, particularly in the frontal and temporal lobes. CSF abnormalities are generally similar to those found in viral meningitis. Modest pleocytosis (predominantly mononuclear) occurs in 95% of cases, along with the presence of red blood cells in 75% of cases. Increased CSF protein occurs in 90% of cases but rarely exceeds 200 mg/dL; CSF glucose is almost always normal. EEG abnormalities can also provide diagnostic clues because 90% of patients have focal or generalized slowing. The presence of periodic sharp wave complexes in the temporal leads superimposed on a slow amplitude background is highly suggestive of HSV encephalitis. MRI scans show abnormal areas involving the temporal lobes and orbitofrontal cortex in more than 90% of cases of herpes encephalitis. MRI scans are much more sensitive than CT scans early in the illness, but eventually more than 60% of patients will show some abnormality on CT scans.

In the past, cerebral biopsy with virus isolation was employed as the standard for diagnosis of HSV encephalitis. However, biopsy has been replaced by detection of herpes simplex virus DNA in the CSF by polymerase chain reaction. If performed with optimal techniques in an experienced laboratory, specificity is 100% and sensitivity is 95%. However, recent reports indicate that PCR performed on HSV-infected CSF within the first 48 hours of illness may have decreased sensitivity. The frequency of positive PCR tests also declines with treatment and duration of illness. The CSF PCR becomes negative for HSV in the majority of treated patients within 14 days. Therefore, negative PCR results should be interpreted based on the timing during illness and the clinical setting. HSV is rarely cultured from CSF in patients with encephalitis.

TREATMENT

Early recognition of HSV encephalitis is essential because effective antiviral therapy (acyclovir) is available, and prompt treatment can significantly decrease the morbidity and mortality of the disease. Acyclovir acts by inhibiting the viral DNA polymerase, thus interfering with viral replication. In adults with HSV encephalitis, acyclovir has reduced mortality from 70 to 19%. However, even in treated patients, neurologic impairment can occur in 40 to 60% of survivors. Outcome is related to the severity of disease at the time antiviral therapy is begun, hence the urgency to begin treatment as soon as the diagnosis is considered. Intravenous therapy should be continued for 14 to 21 days. As with bacterial meningitis, supportive care must be instituted, including close attention to seizure control, monitoring for hyponatremia secondary to the syndrome of inappropriate antidiuretic hormone secretion, and treatment of increased intracranial pressure. Neurologic sequelae can include seizures, paralysis, and cognitive impairment (e.g., memory loss and difficulty with speech, concentration, and attention).

Brain Abscess

Case

Acute Abscess Caused by a Bacterial Infection

Twenty-nine-year old Ms. M. complained of earache. She had had many such episodes in the past, especially involving the left ear, but the most recent episode was associated with a headache that made her nauseated. She vomited once. After 4 days of those symptoms she was driven to the hospital because she had developed a large blind spot in her right field of vision. At the hospital Ms. M. had a low-grade fever of 38.1°C. A CT scan of her head revealed a 4×3-cm mass in her left occipital lobe, consistent with an abscess (Fig. 61-5).

A neurosurgeon performed a needle aspiration of the abscess under CT guidance. A smear of the aspirate revealed Gram-positive cocci and Gram-negative rods. The abscess fluid was sent for culture under both aerobic and anaerobic conditions. She was empirically treated with broad-spectrum antibiotics, including nafcillin, ceftriaxone, and metronidazole, while awaiting the results of the culture. The aspirate grew only *S. aureus*. She was treated with intravenous nafcillin (to cover *S. aureus*) and metronidazole (to cover anaerobic bacteria) for 6 weeks. During that period, serial CT examinations showed the abscess to be shrinking. She recovered completely, but a small blind spot remained in her right visual field.

This case raises two questions:

1. Why was antimicrobial therapy with both nafcillin and metronidazole continued even though no anaerobic bacteria grew from culture?
2. What was the relationship between Ms. M.'s earache and the location of her brain abscess?

PATHOBIOLOGY

A **brain abscess** is a focal infection of the brain parenchyma, which may be caused by bacteria, fungi, or parasites. Microorganisms that cause brain abscess reach the brain by direct extension from a contiguous focus of infection (such as the paranasal sinuses, middle ear, or mastoids), hematogenous dissemination (as in acute bacterial endocarditis or cyanotic congenital heart disease), or direct penetration (following skull fractures or surgical procedures involving the brain or spinal column). In the case of infections of the middle ear, mastoid, or sinuses, veins that bridge the surrounding bony structures and the cerebral cortex can become infected (septic thrombophlebitis), leading to a decrease in local blood supply and providing a reservoir of bacteria.

Abscesses can appear at many locations within the brain parenchyma and the subdural or epidural meningeal spaces. Infarction of the superficial cerebral cortex during meningitis can produce a subdural abscess that is poorly localized, a condition called **subdural empyema.** If an empyema is not completely drained, it slowly resolves, as do abscesses in other parts of the body. In contrast with intracerebral abscesses, **epidural abscesses,** located external to the dura mater, are invariably related to contiguous infection of bone, sometimes

FIGURE 61-5 ▪ Contrasted computerized tomography scan of a patient with left occipital brain abscess. The necrotic material in the abscess center appears dark (hypodense). The white rim surrounding the abscess is its wall, which is visualized because of its vascularization and contiguous vasodilation. There is surrounding hypodensity, representing edema.

secondary to infection of the paranasal sinuses or mastoids. A spinal epidural abscess can be a complication of epidural anesthesia.

The symptoms caused by brain abscesses are the result of increased intracranial pressure and tissue destruction at specific locations. When the frontal lobe is involved, diminished intellectual performance, memory deficits, drowsiness, and perhaps some memory loss can occur (see Fig. 61-3). Temporal lobe involvement can result in visual field defects and occasionally in difficulty speaking. In some patients, mastoiditis predisposes to cerebellar abscess, resulting in coordination problems and ataxia.

Acute abscesses in the CNS are frequently caused by a mixed bacterial flora consisting of strict and facultative anaerobes. That mixture is similar to the combination of bacteria found in the mouth or a parameningeal focus such as an infected middle ear, mastoid, or sinus. Because anaerobic bacteria are particularly difficult to culture, most patients should receive empiric therapy for anaerobes, regardless of culture results. Staphylococci are more likely to be isolated from brain abscesses in the setting of septic emboli from infected heart valves, trauma, or

surgical procedures. Nosocomial Gram-negative organisms also can cause postsurgical brain abscesses.

Chronic abscesses are located in either the meninges or brain tissue. The most common causative agents are mycobacteria, *Cryptococcus* species, and other fungi. Although chronic abscesses are invariably the result of metastatic spread from foci elsewhere, the CNS manifestations sometimes are the first indication of the presence of infection. Usually running a course of remission and relapse, chronic abscesses are often associated with loss of cell-mediated immunity, when the causative agents are no longer kept in check at the primary focus.

DIAGNOSIS

Diagnosis of a brain abscess is aided by imaging techniques. Cranial CT scans classically demonstrate a mass with a central hypointense nonenhancing center, surrounded by a faint ring that becomes hyperintense with contrast, surrounded by nonenhancing hypointense edema. T-1 weighted MRI scans often demonstrate similar findings, whereas T-2 weighted scans show the inverse. Lumbar puncture is inadvisable in a person suspected of having a brain abscess because the increased intracranial pressure could cause brainstem herniation with lumbar decompression. Furthermore, a lumbar puncture is rarely diagnostic, unless the abscess has ruptured into the ventricular space to produce acute ventriculitis and meningitis.

Aspiration of the abscess cavity yields material for cytological analysis, Gram stain, and culture. Anaerobes are common in brain abscess, and the aspirate should be cultured using both aerobic and anaerobic conditions. Often a smear will show the presence of many Gram-positive cocci, Gram-positive rods, and perhaps a few Gram-negative rods, yet only S. *aureus* will grow in culture. The bacteria that failed to grow can be assumed to be oxygen-sensitive anaerobes.

TREATMENT

Like abscesses elsewhere in the body, brain abscesses usually must be drained to effect resolution. In addition, aspiration of the contents of an abscess helps lower the intracranial pressure and improves CNS function. Focal symptoms due to tissue destruction will not improve, but the lesion can be contained from further increase in size by the administration of antibiotics. Antibiotic therapy is not always effective in the treatment of brain abscesses. Inflammation of the meninges is usually too slight to enhance penetration of antibiotics into the CSF. In addition, most antibiotics function poorly in an abscess. Ideally, an antibiotic should be chosen based on the susceptibility of organisms isolated from the abscess cavity, but aspiration of material for culture and susceptibility testing is not always practical. Usually, β-lactam antibiotics with activity against staphylococci (e.g., nafcillin) and oral flora and Gram-negative enteric organisms (e.g., ceftriaxone or cefotaxime) are administered in combination with a lipophilic antibiotic active against anaerobes (e.g., metronidazole). Antimicrobial therapy can be tailored based on the organisms recovered, except anaerobic coverage is usually maintained regardless of whether anaerobes are successfully cultured. Mortality from brain abscess remains high at 10 to 20%, with the majority of deaths occurring in patients who present in coma or have a major complicating illness that is the source of the brain abscess organism (e.g., endocarditis).

Conclusion

Anatomic and physiological protective mechanisms effectively limit access of microorganisms into the CNS. However, once a microbe gains access to the CNS, various serious consequences may result, including meningitis, encephalitis, and brain abscess. The most frequent infections of the CNS are caused by relatively few agents. Encephalitis is almost exclusively caused by viruses, acute meningitis by viruses and bacteria, and chronic meningitis by tubercle bacilli and fungi. Brain abscesses, in contrast, are frequently caused by a mixture of bacteria derived from the normal flora of the mouth and oropharynx.

Infections of the CNS are often severe and life threatening. Many require immediate action based on rapid and accurate clinical assessment in conjunction with appropriate application of radiographic and microbiologic testing. The single most helpful diagnostic procedure in many cases of CNS infection is evaluation of the CSF for cell counts, chemistries, and the presence of microorganisms. Rapid and sensitive diagnostic tests, such as PCR, have improved the speed and reliability of specific diagnoses, as is the case for enteroviral meningitis and herpes encephalitis. Improved diagnostic methods have allowed more effective application of antimicrobial therapies with proven efficacy in reducing the high mortality and morbidity associated with these diseases.

Respiratory System Infections

MeiLan King Han and Fernando Martinez

The respiratory tract is the most common site for infection by pathogenic microorganisms. Perhaps because respiratory infections are so common and typically mild, their impact is often underestimated. In fact, however, they represent an immense disease burden on our society. Upper respiratory infections (URIs) account for more visits to physicians than any other diagnosis. It has been estimated in the United States that pharyngitis alone accounts for 40 million physician visits annually. Furthermore, some respiratory infections can have severe consequences, especially in immunocompromised individuals. Pneumonia, the most severe form of respiratory infection, is the sixth leading cause of death in the United States and the number one cause of death from infectious diseases.

It is not surprising that the respiratory tract becomes infected frequently. It is in direct contact with the environment and is continuously exposed to microorganisms suspended in the air we breathe. The lungs also have the greatest epithelial surface area in continuous contact with the external environment of any organ. Nevertheless, most microorganisms do not cause infection unless other factors interfere with host defenses. One of the questions that this chapter addresses is why these frequent infections are not even more frequent.

The clinical syndromes associated with infection at various locations within the respiratory tract are shown in Figure 62-1. Infections of the middle ear and the paranasal sinuses are included because these areas are contiguous to the respiratory tract and are lined by respiratory epithelium. Several important diseases of the respiratory system are discussed in other chapters (see Chapters 13, 19, 23, 27, 29, 32, 34, 36, and 68).

The clinical manifestations of respiratory tract infections depend on the causative agent. Thus, viruses are important pathogens in the upper respiratory tract and account for most cases of pharyngitis. Bacteria are the most important causes of otitis media, sinusitis, pharyngitis, epiglottitis, bronchitis, and pneumonia. Fungi and protozoa rarely cause serious respiratory tract infections in healthy individuals but are important causes of pneumonia in immunocompromised hosts. Some of the common pathogens that produce infection at various locations in this system are listed in Table 62-1.

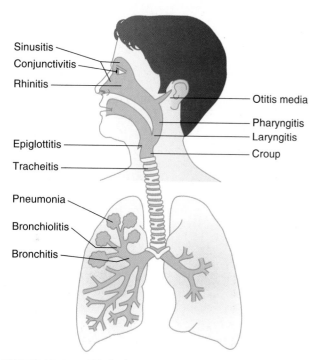

FIGURE 62-1 ▪ Clinical syndromes associated with infection at different locations within the respiratory tract.

table **62-1**	Pathogens Producing Disease at Various Levels of the Respiratory Tract	
LOCATION	**COMMON PATHOGENS**
Nasopharynx	Rhinovirus, coronavirus, other respiratory viruses, *Staphylococcus aureus*
Oropharynx	Group A streptococcus (*Streptococcus pyogenes*), *Corynebacterium diphtheriae*, Epstein-Barr virus, adenovirus, enterovirus
Middle ear and paranasal sinuses	*Streptococcus pneumoniae, Haemophilus influenzae, Moraxella* (*Branhamella*) *catarrhalis*, group A streptococcus (*Streptococcus pyogenes*)
Epiglottitis	*Haemophilus influenzae*
Larynx–trachea	Parainfluenza viruses, *S. aureus*
Bronchi	*S. pneumoniae, H. influenzae, Mycoplasma pneumoniae*, influenza viruses, measles virus
Bronchioles	Respiratory syncytial virus
Lungs	See Table 62-3

Infections of the Nose and Throat

Group A streptococcal pharyngitis is most frequently seen in school-aged children during the winter. Although no clinical features are diagnostic for a specific cause of pharyngitis, fever, tonsillar exudates, and tender cervical

Case

Group A Streptococcal Pharyngitis

F., a 5-year-old boy who had been in good general health, was brought to the pediatrician because of fever and sore throat that began 2 days earlier. On examination F. had a temperature of 38.3°C. His oropharynx was erythematous. His tonsils were enlarged and coated with patchy white exudates. His anterior cervical lymph nodes were also enlarged and tender. The remainder of the examination was unremarkable. A throat culture was positive for group A streptococcus. F. was treated with intramuscular penicillin, and his symptoms resolved over the next week.

This case raises two questions:

1. What common organisms cause pharyngitis?
2. Why is it important to distinguish streptococcal pharyngitis from other forms of the disease?

adenopathy increase the likelihood of group A streptococcal infection; conjunctivitis, cough, coryza, and diarrhea decrease the likelihood. It can be difficult to differentiate between viral and bacterial pharyngitis on the basis of clinical findings. Therefore, a throat culture or a rapid diagnostic test should be performed to detect group A streptococci. It is important to recognize streptococcal infection because it is associated with several complications, including peritonsillar and retropharyngeal abscesses, otitis media, sinusitis, pneumonia, acute glomerulonephritis, and rheumatic fever.

The next most common causes of pharyngitis are respiratory viruses, including rhinoviruses, adenoviruses, coronaviruses, influenza viruses, and parainfluenza viruses (Table 62-2). The adenovirus group may be suspected if conjunctivitis is also present. In adolescents and young adults, Epstein-Barr virus is a common cause of pharyngitis, which is one of the manifestations of infectious mononucleosis. The enteroviruses, especially the group A coxsackieviruses, sometimes produce small vesicles on the mucous membrane of the throat, a clinical picture known as **herpangina.**

Despite extensive evaluation, in approximately one third of patients with pharyngitis, a pathogen cannot be identified. Recent studies suggest that *Chlamydophila pneumoniae* (formerly *Chlamydia pneumonia*) may be a common cause of pharyngitis. Non–group A β-hemolytic streptococci account for a small proportion of cases, as do gonococci in sexually active individuals. Another organism, *Arcanobacterium haemolyticum*, has been found to cause some cases of pharyngitis in older children and young adults but is easily overlooked in a routine

table **62-2**	Common Causes of Pharyngitis	
AGENT	**RELATIVE IMPORTANCE**	
Streptococcus pyogenes (group A β-hemolytic)	+ + + +	
Rhinovirus	+ +	
Adenovirus	+ +	
Coronavirus	+ +	
Epstein-Barr virus	+ +	
Herpes simplex virus	+	
Parainfluenza virus	+	
Influenza virus	+	
Coxsackie virus	+	
Chlamydia pneumonia	+	
Mixed anaerobic bacteria	+	
Neisseria gonorrhoeae	+	
Corynebacterium diphtheriae	+	
Corynebacterium hemolyticum	+	
Mycoplasma pneumoniae	+	
Unknown	+ + + +	

throat culture. *Mycoplasma pneumoniae,* although more commonly an agent of bronchitis and pneumonia, can cause pharyngitis as well.

Infections of the nasopharynx are generally caused by viruses and give rise to the signs and symptoms known collectively as the common cold. **Approximately 40 to 50% of colds are caused by the rhinovirus group** (see Chapter 32). **Coronaviruses** are the next most common group of agents, accounting for approximately 10% of colds. The agents of the remaining percentage of colds are various respiratory viruses, including parainfluenza viruses, respiratory syncytial virus (RSV), influenza viruses, and adenoviruses. Although the patient with a cold may experience a "scratchy" throat, nasal symptoms are usually more prominent. Bacterial infection of the nose occurs occasionally, but is not common.

Infections of the Epiglottis

Acute epiglottitis, also called supraglottitis, is probably the most serious form of URI. This distinct clinical syndrome can be rapidly fatal because the airway can become completely obstructed from swelling of the epiglottis and surrounding structures. Acute epiglottitis

Case

Acute Epiglottitis

P., an unvaccinated 3-year-old girl, was put to bed by her parents with a low-grade temperature. In the middle of the night she awoke crying, and her parents found that her fever was higher and that she was having trouble breathing. The family pediatrician told the parents to take P. immediately to the local hospital. On examination in the emergency department P. had a temperature of 38.9°C. She appeared anxious, was sitting upright, and drooling. Nasal flaring was noted. A presumptive diagnosis of epiglottitis was made, and the child was taken to the operating room, where an endotracheal tube was inserted. A radiograph of the lateral neck that had been taken on the way to the operating room revealed swelling of the epiglottis (Fig. 62-2). When her throat was examined as she was being intubated, her epiglottis was seen to be very red and swollen. She was treated with nafcillin, which is effective against influenza B. The next day, the laboratory reported that blood and epiglottis cultures grew *Haemophilus influenzae.* She responded promptly to treatment and recovered completely.

This case raises one question:

Why was P. started on therapy for influenza B before culture results had returned?

FIGURE 62-2 ▪ Radiograph of the neck taken in a lateral projection reveals marked swelling of the epiglottis (arrow).

occurs most often in children 2 to 7 years of age, with the most common cause being influenza B. Fortunately, since immunization of infants against influenza B has become universal, this feared clinical entity has become less common. In adults influenza B is still occasionally pathogenic, but other common etiologic agents, such as *Streptococcus pneumoniae* and group A streptococci, are more frequent than they are in children. Despite the current rarity of this condition, the practitioner must remain vigilant because early recognition of acute epiglottitis can make the difference between life and death. Why influenza B displays a marked tropism for the epiglottis is not well understood.

If a child presents with the characteristic manifestations of epiglottitis as described in the case of P., ensuring maintenance of the airway should be the physician's first priority. If a patient presents early in the course of diagnosis, radiographs of the lateral neck may help show an enlarged epiglottis protruding from the anterior wall of the hypopharynx (see Fig. 62-2). In adults, nasopharyngolaryngoscopy can aid the diagnosis. The first step in treatment is securing the airway with endotracheal intubation if necessary; then epiglottitis responds readily to treatment with antibiotics, and the outcome is generally good.

Infections of the Larynx and Trachea

Laryngotracheitis in small children, referred to as **croup**, is characterized by the sudden onset, and often sudden resolution, of a barking cough and difficult respiration.

Case

Laryngotracheitis

H., a 19-month-old boy, developed a runny nose, hoarseness, cough, and a low-grade temperature. His pediatrician diagnosed a viral URI and prescribed no specific treatment. That night, H. had a barking cough. His breathing was forced and noisy, especially with inspiration. Alarmed, the parents called the pediatrician, who told them that the child probably had croup. He advised them to take H. into the bathroom and to fill the room with steam by running the hot water in the shower. He also advised them to call back 15 minutes later if the respiratory difficulty worsened. In fact, it subsided and H. fell back to sleep. A similar but milder episode occurred the next night. Over the next few days, all the symptoms gradually resolved.

This case raises one question:

Why did the pediatrician suspect a viral pathogen?

Because children's airways are smaller and their tracheal walls have nonexpendable rings of cartilage, mucous membrane edema is more likely to result in narrowing of the tracheal lumen. This narrowing is worse during inspiration and results in inspiratory stridor. Almost all cases are caused by viruses, especially the parainfluenza viruses. Infection with parainfluenza virus types 1 through 3 is common in young children, and repeated infections can occur. In rare cases bacteria, particularly *Staphylococcus aureus*, cause clinical findings similar to those of viral croup. Typically, mild upper respiratory symptoms such as nasal discharge and dry cough are present days before the signs of airway obstruction become evident. In most cases the illness is self-limited and resolves after 5 to 7 days. No specific drug treatment for parainfluenza virus infection is currently available. Management of croup consists of providing oxygen, administering epinephrine by aerosol in some cases, and supporting the airway if needed.

In adults, the major clinical manifestation of infection of the larynx is **hoarseness**. As in children, most acute laryngeal infections in adults are self-limited conditions caused by respiratory viruses. *Moraxella catarrhalis* and *H. influenzae* have also been reported to cause acute laryngitis in adults. Although antibiotic therapy can shorten the duration of illness, the hoarseness generally resolves over the course of a week, regardless of therapy.

Infections of the Large Bronchi

Acute tracheobronchitis is one of the most common causes of office visits to family practitioners. Infection is the major cause, but inhalation of irritants can also lead to this clinical syndrome. Viruses that have been implicated include rhinoviruses, coronaviruses, RSV, influenza viruses, and adenoviruses. Bacterial infections that can cause bronchitis include *M. pneumoniae*, *Chlamydophila pneumoniae*, and *Bordetella pertussis*. *B. pertussis* causes **whooping cough**, which is a highly contagious disease characterized by paroxysmal, productive coughs occurring primarily in infants and young children (see Chapter 19). In the United States the disease occurs infrequently because of vaccination, although its incidence may be increasing.

In general, acute tracheobronchitis tends to run a short, self-limited course requiring only symptomatic treatment. The role of antibiotics in patients with no underlying lung disease has been controversial because most cases result from viral infections. Studies have shown little to no benefit from antibiotics, yet antibiotic prescriptions for acute bronchitis account for a significant percentage of all prescriptions written in adult

Case

Acute Tracheobronchitis

Dr. V., a 28-year-old physician, developed symptoms of cough, myalgias (aches and pains in the muscles), headache made worse by coughing, substernal chest pain, and high fever. She suspected influenza because an outbreak was in progress and she had recently cared for several patients with similar symptoms. During the next 3 days she was bedridden because of weakness and a persistent temperature of 38.9°C. The symptoms gradually resolved over the next few days without specific treatment. After 10 days, Dr. V. was able to resume her usual activities. A viral throat culture she took on the first day of illness confirmed the diagnosis of influenza.

This case raises one question:

Do most cases of tracheobronchitis resolve on their own, or are antibiotics usually required?

Infections of the Lungs

Many pathogens cause pneumonia, or infection of the lung parenchyma, sometimes with distinctive clinical manifestations. Thus, pneumonia represents a variety of diseases that share a common anatomic location. Although pneumonias can be categorized in various ways, this chapter uses clinical and epidemiological classification (Table 62-3). Because its perspective is that of the clinician, this classification can form the basis for managing the patient's illness even before a specific cause has been proven.

The first important distinction that the classification makes is between **acute pneumonia** (fairly sudden onset with progression of symptoms over a very few days), and **subacute or chronic pneumonia**. Among the acute pneumonias, a second important distinction is made between community- and hospital-acquired (nosocomial) pneumonias. Hospital-acquired pneumonias are classified

practice. Patient education is an important first step in decreasing the use of unnecessary antibiotics.

An important distinction should be made between bronchitis in otherwise healthy patients and those with underlying structural lung disease. Patients with chronic obstructive pulmonary disease (a disease usually related to smoking) may have excessive sputum production, also known as chronic bronchitis. Chronic bronchitis can lead to **acute exacerbation of chronic bronchitis (AECB)**, a clinical diagnosis based on the patient's history of increased cough and sputum production, increased sputum purulence, and increased shortness of breath. The presence of at least two if not all three of those symptoms increases the likelihood of a bacterial infection as the etiology, particularly in the presence of sputum purulence. The role of bacterial infection as the causative agent of AECB has been controversial. However, when viewed collectively, studies show a modest but significant improvement in clinical recovery for patients treated with antibiotics. Thus, treatment for AECB usually includes supportive care and antibiotics effective against *H. influenzae*, *M. catarrhalis*, and *S. pneumoniae*. In selected patients coverage of Gram-negative enteric pathogens may be important.

Infections of the Bronchioles

Bronchiolitis is a common clinical syndrome in the first two years of life and is usually associated with **respiratory syncytial virus** (see Chapter 34).

table **62-3**	**Classification of Pneumonia Syndromes**

Acute

Community acquired

Person-to-person transmission
  Streptococcus pneumoniae, Mycoplasma pneumoniae, Haemophilus influenzae, Chlamydia pneumoniae, Staphylococcus aureus, Klebsiella pneumonias and other enteric Gram-negative rods, *Moraxella catarrhalis, Neisseria meningitides, Streptococcus pyogenes,* influenza viruses

Animal or environmental exposure
  See Table 62-4

Pneumonia in infants and young children
  Chlamydia trachomatis, respiratory syncytial virus and other respiratory viruses, *S. aureus,* group B streptococci, cytomegalovirus, *Ureaplasma urealyticum* (?), *Pneumocystis carinii* (?), *S. pneumoniae, H. influenzae* type B

Hospital acquired (nosocomial)
  S. aureus, Enterobacteriaceae species, *K. pneumonia, Escherichia coli, Serratia marcescens, H. influenzae, S. pneumoniae, Pseudomonas aeruginosa, Acinetobacter* species, influenza A, *Legionella* species, *Aspergillus*

Subacute or chronic

Pulmonary tuberculosis
  Mycobacterium tuberculosis and nontuberculous mycobacteria

Fungal pneumonia
  Histoplasma capsulatum, Blastomyces dermatitidis, Coccidioides immitis, Cryptococcus neoformans

Aspiration pneumonia and lung abscesses
  Mixed anaerobic and aerobic bacterial organisms

Pneumonia in immunocompromised patients

  P. carinii, cytomegalovirus, atypical mycobacteria, *Nocardia, Aspergillus, Phycomycetes, Candida* separately because the responsible pathogens are frequently different from those that produce pneumonia in nonhospitalized individuals.

Most of the common forms of **acute community-acquired pneumonia** are caused by pathogens transmitted from person to person. Transmission is typically airborne over short distances or by contaminated secretions or fomites. On encountering some pathogens—*S. pneumoniae, H. influenzae,* and *S. aureus,* for example—most individuals become colonized, but only a few develop disease directly or after a variable period of colonization. A second group of pneumonia pathogens, encountered less frequently, have animal or environmental reservoirs. In many cases of pneumonia caused by these agents, diagnosis is difficult unless the physician seeks out the circumstances of exposure (e.g., exposure to a parrot leading to psittacosis). The mode of transmission of most of these organisms is the airborne route, although some have insect vectors. Community-acquired pneumonias in infants and young children are placed in a third group because they have a distinctive etiological spectrum.

In contrast to patients with acute pneumonia are those with infections that have been present for weeks or months. Several forms of subacute and chronic pneumonias can be distinguished. These forms include tuberculosis, fungal pneumonia, and anaerobic lung abscesses. It is important to realize that although this classification is based on the common clinical patterns of disease, exceptions do occur. For example, patients with tuberculosis,

histoplasmosis, or lung abscesses sometimes experience acute, rapidly progressing disease. Physicians must also be aware that patients infected with HIV and presenting with acute community-acquired pneumonia may be severely immunocompromised and thus at risk for pneumonias caused by opportunistic pathogens. These pathogens, like *Pneumocystis carinii,* usually cause infections only in immunocompromised individuals.

ENTRY AND SPREAD

Pathogens can reach the lungs by one of five routes: (1) direct inhalation, (2) aspiration of upper airway contents, (3) spread along the mucous membrane surface, (4) hematogenous spread, and rarely, (5) direct penetration. Of these, inhalation and aspiration are the most common.

DEFENSE MECHANISMS OF THE LUNGS

The defense of the lungs begins in the nose, where specialized hairs, known as vibrissae, filter large particles suspended in inhaled air (Fig. 62-3). Large particles (more than 10 μm in diameter) tend to settle at points

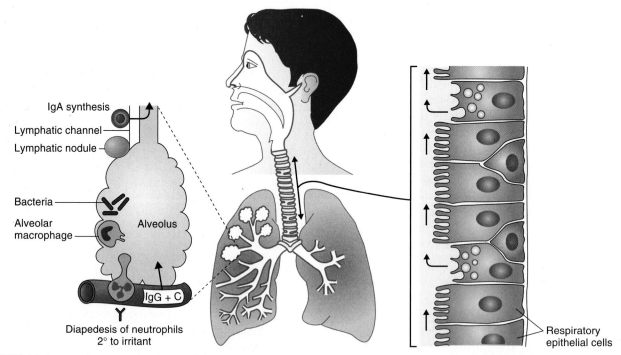

FIGURE 62-3 ▪ **Defense mechanisms of the respiratory tract.** Aerodynamic factors include the presence of vibrissae in the nasal passage and abrupt changes in the direction of flow of the air column. The epiglottis and cough reflex prevent introduction of particulate matter into the lower airway. The ciliated respiratory epithelium propels the overlying mucus layer (red) upward toward the mouth. In the alveoli, macrophages, humoral factors (including immunoglobulins and complement), and neutrophils (when inflammation is present) assist in preventing or clearing infection.

where abrupt changes in the direction of airflow occur, such as the posterior nasopharynx. Smaller particles (less than 3 μm in diameter) are likely to elude those barriers and reach the terminal bronchioles and alveoli. The importance of the upper airway structures in defending the lungs is illustrated in patients in whom these structures are bypassed. **Endotracheal tubes** used during mechanical ventilation provide a conduit from the outside environment to the lower airway; thus, intubated patients are markedly predisposed to pneumonia.

The respiratory epithelium itself has specialized defenses against infection. Epithelial cells from the nose to the terminal bronchioles are covered with **cilia** that beat coordinately. Overlying these cilia is a covering of mucus containing antimicrobial compounds such as **lysozyme, lactoferrin,** and **secretory IgA** antibodies. The cilia move the overlying mucus layer upward toward the larynx; together they are called the mucociliary escalator. Many patients with impaired ciliary function have frequent respiratory infections that ultimately lead to **bronchiectasis** (permanent abnormal dilation of the small airways). Recent evidence suggests that in patients with cystic fibrosis, abnormal sodium and chloride transport in the respiratory epithelial cells decreases the volume of the mucous layer and impairs ciliary function. Impaired clearance of mucous predisposes these patients to chronic infection and inflammation, making them particularly susceptible to infections with *S. aureus* and *Pseudomonas aeruginosa*.

The final lung defenses are found in the alveoli. The alveoli contain IgA antibodies, complement components, and most importantly, alveolar macrophages. These phagocytic cells function as active scavengers, ingesting and killing invading pathogens. When they cannot contain infection by themselves, they are helped by other phagocytic cells that do not normally reside in the lungs, especially neutrophils. Macrophages and neutrophils are especially important in fighting bacterial infections. In viral infection, histopathological studies of the lungs (or other affected tissues) show infiltration by large numbers of lymphocytes and plasma cells, suggesting that viral infection stimulates the recruitment of lymphoid cells rather than neutrophils. Lymphocytes contribute to host defense by producing antibodies and attacking infected cells through cytotoxic T lymphocytes, natural killer cells, and antibody-dependent cell-mediated cytotoxicity.

Acute Pneumonias

Community-Acquired Pneumonia

Community-acquired pneumonia (CAP) afflicts between 4 million and 6 million people in the United States each year, nearly 1 million of whom require hospitalization. In elderly and chronically ill patients, CAP can be associated with prolonged hospitalizations and high mortality. Presenting symptoms frequently include fever and cough. Sometimes the patient complains of chest pain,

Case

Thirty-six-year-old Ms. T., who has a history of smoking 20 packs of cigarettes a year, presented to the emergency department of her local hospital after 3 days of fevers to 39.2°C, chills, cough, and pain on her left side, which was worse with breathing. On examination her respiratory rate was elevated at 22 breaths per minute, but her pulse oximetry was normal at 96%. Auscultation of her lungs revealed rales in her left lower lung fields. A chest radiograph showed an infiltrate in her left lower lobe consistent with pneumonia. Her blood work revealed an elevated white blood cell count of 16,000/mm³. Ms. T. was diagnosed with a community-acquired pneumonia, prescribed a course of antibiotics, and discharged. Over the next several days her fevers resolved, and within two weeks her symptoms had disappeared. A chest radiograph performed at her physician's office 3 months later was normal.

This case raises two questions:

1. How did the physician differentiate bronchitis from pneumonia?
2. What organisms should a physician be concerned about when treating community-acquired pneumonia?

frequently pleuritic (exacerbated by respiratory motion). Patients with extensive involvement of the lungs may have shortness of breath, rapid respiration, and **cyanosis** (bluish tinge to the skin indicative of hypoxemia). Auscultation may reveal **crackles** (also called **rales**), which are usually indicative of alveolar disease.

Both bacteria and viruses cause CAPs, as outlined in Tables 62-3 and 62-4, although in approximately one half of patients an organism is never identified. Traditionally, organisms have been divided into two groups, typical and atypical, based on the belief that the clinical and radiographic features of presentation suggest certain etiologic agents. A typical presentation (as demonstrated by Ms. T.) is characterized by high fever, shaking chills, chest pain, and lobar consolidation. An atypical presentation is characterized by less severe illness, dry cough, headache, and other systemic complaints. Although studies have shown that it is very difficult to predict an etiologic agent based on presentation, the classification of organisms as typical and atypical persists. *S. pneumoniae* is the most common cause of CAP and, along with *H. influenzae, S. aureus,* and other Gram-negative bacteria, is classified as a typical organism. *M. pneumoniae, C. pneumoniae,* and legionellae are among the atypical organisms.

Although considerable overlap exists in the clinical manifestations of pneumonia, certain pathogens tend to be associated with characteristic presentations or tend to affect certain patient populations. For instance, *M. pneumoniae* and *C. pneumoniae* are seen with high frequency in patients with less severe presentations of pneumonia. Pneumococcal pneumonia can occur at any age, but it has a predilection for the very young and the elderly, particularly those with **chronic obstructive pulmonary disease (COPD)**. It usually has a rapid onset and an acute course. Patients with a history of COPD are also at increased risk for infection with *H. influenzae* and *M. catarrhalis*. Alcoholics are at increased risk for contracting *S. pneumoniae*, *Klebsiella pneumonia*, *S. aureus*, and anaerobic pathogens (by aspiration). Nursing home residents, immunocompromised patients, and people with underlying structural lung disease are at increased risk for contracting *Pseudomonas aeruginosa*, Gram-negative enteric bacteria (derived from the gut), and *S. aureus*.

Several pneumonias result from agents found in animals or in the environment (Table 62-4). These infections occur when peoples' activities bring them into contact with the organisms. For example, *Chlamydia psittaci* is a common cause of disease in birds, and psittacosis (parrot fever) may be acquired by inhalation (see Chapter 27). This illness is unlikely to be diagnosed correctly unless the physician obtains the history of contact with birds. Another example is Q fever, caused by the rickettsia *Coxiella burnetii* and usually acquired from sheep, goats, or cattle. The organism is stable in the environment, and infection can occur after exposure to contaminated material from infected animals. As with psittacosis, diagnosis of Q fever is difficult unless the physician elicits the history of exposure to animals or their environment. Another agent of CAPs, *Legionella pneumophila*, is often associated with contaminated environmental water sources such as air conditioners and water-cooling towers.

In children under 2 years of age, the agents of acute pneumonias are more often viruses than bacteria. Illnesses caused by RSV, influenza or parainfluenza viruses, or adenoviruses tend to be milder, and spontaneous recovery is the rule unless the child's immunity is compromised. In other age groups viruses are infrequent causes of community-acquired pneumonia. Although influenza viruses can lead to pneumonia in adults, the pneumonia usually is caused by bacterial superinfection.

Diagnosis of CAP is generally based on appropriate clinical history and chest radiographs. The most important diagnostic finding is a chest radiograph that reveals a shadow, or **infiltrate.** The radiographic pattern may be a clue to the identity of the pathogen. Focal lobar consolidation is more commonly seen with *S. pneumoniae*, *K. pneumoniae* (a Gram-negative rod), and infections caused by aspiration (with a predilection for the lower lobes because of lung anatomy). Diffuse interstitial infiltrates can be seen with infections of *M. pneumoniae*, *C. pneumoniae*, and *P. carinii*. Organisms that tend to cavitate include *S. aureus*, aerobic Gram-negative bacteria, and *Mycobacterium tuberculosis*. Skilled interpretation is important, because other processes, tumors, pulmonary edema, or pulmonary hemorrhage can produce radiographic changes very similar to those of pneumonia.

The decision to admit a patient to the hospital for CAP treatment rather than administering outpatient therapy can be a difficult one, but factors like severity of illness and medical comorbidities are used as general guidelines. Several prediction rules have been proposed to identify patients at increased risk of a complicated course. These are generally based on identifying host factors associated with more virulent organisms or an impaired response to infection. A patient with relatively mild illness managed outside the hospital usually does not undergo sputum Gram stain and culture tests, whereas those tests are performed for patients admitted to hospitals if possible. In most cases the choice of antibiotic therapy is empiric based on the patient's risk factors for certain organisms and the severity of illness.

Opinion-based recommendations by multispecialty experts have been published to provide guidance for empiric antimicrobial therapy based on clinical scenarios and host factors (Table 62-5). Increasing antimicrobial nonsusceptibility among respiratory pathogens, especially *S. pneumoniae*, have altered initial antimicrobial therapy recommendations. Risk factors for drug-resistant *S. pneumoniae* (DRSP) include recent respiratory infection; recent antimicrobial use; advanced age; medical comorbidities, including being immunocompromised or living in a high-risk area (e.g., a residential institution, a day care center). Individuals with at least one of these risk factors or who live in areas with endemic DRSP may be better managed with antimicrobial agents with greater activity against *S. pneumoniae*.

table **62-4**	**Community-Acquired Pneumonias Transmitted by Animals or Environmentally**	
DISEASE	**CAUSATIVE ORGANISM**	**SOURCE**
Psittacosis	*Chlamydia psittaci*	Infected birds
Q fever	*Coxiella burnetii*	Infected animals
Histoplasmosis	*Histoplasma capsulatum*	Infected soil, bats
Coccidioidomycosis	*Coccidioides immitis*	Soil
Cryptococcosis	*Cryptococcus neoformans*	Soil, pigeons
Plague	*Yersinia pestis*	Infected animals, insect vectors
Melioidosis	*Pseudomonas pseudomallei*	Soil
Tularemia	*Francisella tularensis*	Infected animals, ticks
Legionnaire disease	*Legionella pneumophila*	Contaminated water

table **62-5**	**Initial Empiric Antimicrobial Therapy for Community-Acquired Pneumonia in Immunocompetent Adults**
CLINICAL SCENARIO	**PREFERRED THERAPY**
Outpatient	
Previously healthy	
No recent antimicrobial therapy	Macrolide or doxycycline
Recent antimicrobial therapy	Respiratory fluoroquinolone
	Advanced macrolide plus high-dose amoxicillin
Comorbidity	
No recent antimicrobial therapy	Advanced macrolides plus high-dose amoxicillin-clavulanate
Recent antimicrobial therapy	Advanced macrolides or respiratory fluoroquinolone
Suspected aspiration with infection	Respiratory fluoroquinolone
Influenza with bacterial superinfection	Advanced macrolides plus β-lactam
	Amoxicillin-clavulanate or clindamycin
	β-lactam or respiratory fluoroquinolone
Inpatient	
Medical ward	
No recent antimicrobial therapy	Respiratory fluoroquinolone or advanced macrolides plus β-lactam
Recent antimicrobial therapy	Advanced macrolides plus β-lactam or respiratory fluoroquinolone alone
Intensive care unit	
Pseudomonas infection unlikely	β-lactam plus either advanced macrolides or respiratory fluoroquinolone
Pseudomonas infection unlikely and patient has β-lactam allergy	Respiratory fluoroquinolone, with or without clindamycin
Pseudomonas infection possible	Antipseudomonal agent plus ciprofloxacin or antipseudomonal agent plus aminoglycoside plus respiratory fluoroquinolone or macrolides
Pseudomonas infection possible and patient has β-lactam allergy	Aztreonam plus levofloxacin or aztreonam plus moxifloxacin or gatifloxacin, with or without an aminoglycoside

Adapted from Mandell LA, Bartlett JG, Dowell SF, File TM Jr., Musher DM, Whitney C. Update of practice guidelines for the management of community-acquired pneumonia in immunocompetent adults. Clin Inf Dis. 2003;37:1405–1433.

Hospital-Acquired Pneumonia

Hospital-acquired pneumonia (HAP) is defined as a new parenchymal lung infection appearing 48 or more hours after admission to the hospital. It is the leading cause of death from hospital-acquired infections, with an estimated mortality of 20 to 50%. Symptoms suggesting a diagnosis of HAP include fever, cough, purulent sputum production, shortness of breath, and pleuritic chest pain. Physical exam may reveal fever, **tachycardia** (elevated heart rate), and **tachypnea** (elevated respiratory rate). Signs of consolidation on physical exam include course crepitations and bronchial breath sounds. Tactile fremitus and dullness to percussion may also be present.

Microaspiration of bacteria from the oropharynx is considered the most common route of infection. Intubated patients may be directly inoculated with bacteria through the endotracheal tube, resulting in **ventilator-associated pneumonia (VAP)**. Factors influencing the risk of pneu-

monia are the types of bacteria colonizing the pharynx and prior exposure to antibiotics. The oropharynx of hospitalized patients can become colonized with Gram-negative bacteria within several days of admission. Furthermore, illness and medications can disrupt the gastric pH, leading to colonization of the stomach with bacteria. Aspiration of bacteria-contaminated gastric contents can increase oropharyngeal colonization and heighten the risk of HAP. Patients with advanced age; poor nutrition; history of smoking, alcoholism, or intravenous drug use; or other underlying chronic illnesses are also at increased risk for developing nosocomial pneumonia.

The bacteria most commonly causing HAP are enteric Gram-negative rods and *S. aureus*. Common Gram-negative rods include members of the Enterobacteriaceae family, *K. pneumonia*, *Proteus* species, and *Escherichia coli*. Mechanically ventilated patients frequently are infected with multiple organisms. Other organisms reported include *H. influenzae*, *Serratia marcescens*, and *S.*

Case

At 52 years of age Mr. L., who had a history of chronic alcoholism, was admitted to the hospital for an emergent appendectomy. The procedure went well, but on postoperative day 3 he was noted to have a fever of 38.5°C, an elevated heart rate of 115 beats per minute, pulse oximetry of 89%, a cough productive of green sputum, and increased shortness of breath. Examination revealed an ill-appearing patient in moderate respiratory distress. In his left lung base he had bronchial breath sounds on auscultation. Chest radiograph revealed a large left-sided infiltrate (Fig. 62-4). The patient was started on oxygen therapy by nasal cannula. Gram stain and sputum culture were performed. Broad-spectrum antibiotics were started. The sputum culture was reported to have a heavy growth of *K. pneumoniae*, one of the Enterobacteriaceae. Mr. L.'s 3-week hospital course was stormy, and he required mechanical ventilation for 4 days. He was discharged to a chronic care hospital and eventually recovered.

This case raises two questions:

1. How do most patients in the hospital contract pneumonia?
2. Which patients are at increased risk for developing hospital-acquired pneumonia?

FIGURE 62-4 ▪ Pneumonia caused by *Klebsiella pneumoniae*. Chest radiograph shows extensive consolidation of the left lower lobe. Cavity formation is apparent within the involved area (arrow).

pneumoniae. In patients who have more severe infections, have been exposed to broad-spectrum antimicrobial agents, or have had more prolonged hospitalizations, *P. aeruginosa* and *Acinetobacter* species are more common. Rare etiologic agents include influenza A, RSV, *Legionella* species, and *Aspergillus* species.

Diagnosis of HAP in clinical practice can be difficult. Fever, elevated white blood cell count, and purulent sputum are suggestive but not definitive. Chest radiograph showing a new infiltrate is sensitive but not specific because other conditions (e.g., congestive heart failure and pulmonary embolus) can cause similar radiograph abnormalities. Sputum Gram stain and culture are frequently obtained. Unfortunately, the microscopic examination of sputum has limitations. Some patients cannot produce sputum. The presence of squamous epithelial cells in large numbers indicates contamination by oropharyngeal contents, and a culture of such a specimen can yield misleading information. Finding a predominant organism in the Gram stain may point toward the etiological agent. If an organism is cultured, it can be difficult to differentiate a colonizing organism from one causing active disease. Bronchoscopic sampling of the lower airways by bronchoalveolar lavage may be more helpful in establishing an etiologic agent but is generally reserved for immunocompromised patients, individuals with severe disease, and those with illness not resolving with standard therapy.

As with CAP, the choices in initial antibiotic therapy for HAP are generally empiric, based on severity of illness and patient risk factors. Antibiotic therapy is based on the likelihood of infection with **multidrug-resistant (MDR) pathogens**. Risk factors for infection with MDR pathogens include antimicrobial therapy in the preceding 90 days, current hospitalization of 5 days or more, high frequency of MDR organisms in the community or hospital unit, immunosuppressive disease and/or therapy, presence of risk factors for Heath Care Associated Pneumonia (HCAP) such as chronic dialysis, home infusion therapy, or a family member with an MDR pathogen. If risk factors for infection by MDR pathogens are present, broad-spectrum agents are generally used; if not, limited-spectrum therapy is generally recommended. With appropriate therapy many patients display improvement 48 to 72 hours after treatment is initiated. However, many patients with severe infections may develop complications and require prolonged mechanical ventilation. Patients with pleural effusions associated with pneumonia (parapneumonic effusion) should have the fluid evaluated for evidence of infection of the pleural space. Pus in the pleural space is called an empyema and requires surgical drainage.

Subacute Pneumonias

Lung abscesses such as those of Mr. A. are usually a consequence of gross aspiration of oropharyngeal or gastric

Case

Mr. A., who is 46 years old with a poorly controlled seizure disorder, was brought to a physician after 2 weeks of coughing, fever, and weight loss. Physical examination revealed an ill-appearing man with a temperature of 38.3°C and foul-smelling breath. He had amphoric breath sounds (resembling those produced by blowing across the mouth of a bottle), suggestive of a lung cavity. A chest radiograph showed a large cavity in the left midlung with extensive surrounding inflammation (Fig. 62-5). Mr. A. was admitted to the hospital and treated with high-dose intravenous penicillin. He began to feel better almost immediately, his fever disappeared over the course of a week and he was then discharged. After 3 months on oral penicillin, he was judged to be cured.

This case raises one question:

Which organisms can cause cavitary lung lesions?

FIGURE 62-5 ■ **Lung abscess.** Chest radiograph showing a cavitary lesion (arrow) with surrounding infiltrate.

contents. The typical lung abscess represents a polymicrobial infection with multiple species of bacteria. The bacteria most commonly involved are anaerobes and microaerophilic organisms from the normal flora of the mouth. Lung abscesses can also result from infection with other organisms that can also destroy lung tissue, including *S. aureus, K. pneumoniae,* mycobacteria, and others. The resulting infection has a number of distinguishing features. The clinical course tends to be less acute than that of most other forms of bacterial pneumonia. Mr. A. may have been ill for several weeks or even months before seeking medical attention. Definitive diagnosis is usually made on the basis of a chest radio-

graph. Prolonged antibiotic therapy is generally required. If not treated promptly, lung abscess can spread to involve the pleural space, resulting in empyema that might require surgical intervention.

Other frequent causes of infectious subacute pulmonary diseases are fungi and mycobacteria. Fungi that affect the lungs include *Histoplasma capsulatum, Blastomyces dermatitidis, Coccidioides immitis,* and *Cryptococcus neoformans* (see Chapters 47 and 48). *H. capsulatum* and *B. dermatitidis* are dimorphic fungi found in the soil and are endemic to the midwestern and south-central United States, although *B. dermatitidis* extends farther north. *C. immitis* is found in the deserts of the southwestern United States and *C. neoformans* in areas frequented by pigeons. The latter is frequently but not exclusively found in individuals who are immunocompromised. Other causes of subacute pneumonias include infections with *M. tuberculosis* (see Chapter 23) and nonmycobacterial tuberculi, such as *M. avium intracellulare* infection, actinomycosis, and nocardiosis.

Pneumonia in the Immunocompromised Patient

Pneumonia is a common occurrence in immunocompromised individuals, including individuals who undergo cancer chemotherapy, have HIV infection, are taking immunosuppressive medications, or have congenital immunodeficiencies (see Chapters 69 and 70). In addition to being at risk for contracting the same kinds of infections to which individuals with normal immune systems are susceptible, immunocompromised patients often become infected with opportunistic pathogens that rarely cause infections in normal individuals. Examples include *P. carinii*, which is typically seen in patients with HIV whose CD4 lymphocyte count is less than 200 cells/mm^3.

Case

Mrs. S., who is 53 years old and has HIV infection, presented to her internist with a 1-month history of low-grade fevers, cough, and fatigue. On examination her temperature was 37.7°C, and she was not in respiratory distress. Her pulse oximetry was 94% on room air but dropped with exertion. Auscultation and percussion of the chest was normal. Chest radiograph revealed a diffuse, bilateral interstitial infiltrate. Sputum was induced by having her breathe nebulized hypertonic saline. PCR of the sputum confirmed the diagnosis of *P. carinii*. Mrs. S. underwent a 3-week course of trimethoprim and sulfamethoxazole. Repeat chest radiograph 2 months later showed no infiltrate, and Mrs. S.'s energy level returned to normal.

This case raises one question:

Which patients are at increased risk for developing *P. carinii* pneumonia?

Other opportunistic infections include the fungus *Aspergillus fumigatus* and the cytomegalovirus, which can be seen in patients receiving immunosuppressive therapy for organ transplants. The etiologic agent in patients who develop pneumonia in the setting of an immunosuppressed status depends, in part, on the basis of the defect in the host immune system. Many of these infections can be diagnosed only by carrying out invasive procedures such as bronchoscopy or lung biopsy.

Conclusion

The lungs are in continuous exposure with the external environment, yet most microorganisms do not cause infection unless other factors impair host defenses. Lung infections can become very serious if they affect the patency of a patient's airway or the ability of the lungs to exchange oxygen and carbon dioxide. Familiarity with which pathogens affect which parts of the respiratory tree and knowledge of pathogenic predilections for certain patient populations can help physicians obtain rapid diagnoses of diseases affecting the lungs. Awareness of the natural course of infections and potential complications of infections helps the physician identify patients needing immediate attention and treatment.

Urinary Tract Infections

Lindsay E. Nicolle

Urinary tract infections are the most common bacterial infections in humans. They affect a substantial proportion of otherwise healthy women, are common in both men and women with structural or functional abnormalities of the genitourinary tract, and frequently are the cause of both community- and hospital-acquired infections. At least 20% of women experience urinary tract infections by the age of 30 years, and more than 50% have at least one urinary tract infection in their lives (Fig. 63-1). One in 10 women experience frequent recurrent infections for at least some period. An estimated 3 million office visits for the complaint take place each year in the United States. Nosocomial (hospital-acquired) urinary tract infections account for about 40% of all infections acquired in acute care facilities. From 25 to 50% of nursing home patients have bacteriuria at any time.

DEFINITIONS

Urinary tract infection (UTI) can occur at any site in the urinary tract but usually involves the bladder, kidneys, or prostate. Urethritis is infection of the urethra and is characteristic of some sexually transmitted diseases, including those caused by *Neisseria gonorrhea* and *Chlamydia pneumoniae* (see Chapters 14 and 27). **Acute uncomplicated urinary tract infection** presents as acute cystitis (bladder or lower-tract infection) in otherwise healthy women. **Acute nonobstructive pyelonephritis,** also called acute uncomplicated pyelonephritis, is kidney infection (renal or upper-tract infection) that occurs in the same group of otherwise healthy women. **Complicated urinary tract infection** is seen in individuals with underlying structural or functional abnormalities of the genitourinary tract; it may be infection limited to the bladder, or it may affect both the bladder and kidneys. **Asymptomatic bacteriuria** is bacteria present in the urine without symptoms or signs attributable to urinary tract infection. **Bacterial prostatitis** is bacterial infection of the prostate gland. **Acute bacterial prostatitis** is a severe infection of acute onset. **Chronic bacterial prostatitis** is the persistence of bacteria in the prostate. The contribution of chronic bacterial prostatitis to chronic pelvic and urinary symptoms in men is uncertain. **Renal abscess** is uncommon but can occur with severe pyelonephritis or following bacteremic spread of infection from other body sites.

An individual who experiences one episode of UTI is usually at risk for recurrent episodes. Recurrent infection is considered **reinfection** when a new organism is isolated, or if a previously isolated organism is reintroduced into the urinary tract from

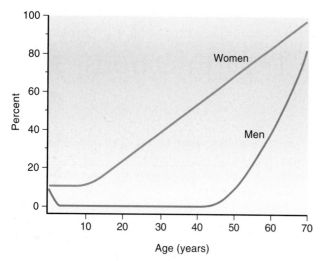

FIGURE 63-1 ▪ **Prevalence of any urinary infection according to age and gender.**

the colonizing gut or genital flora. **Relapse** is recurrent infection with bacteria that remained within the urinary tract, usually the kidney or prostate, despite apparently effective antimicrobial therapy. Chronic bacterial prostatitis is a frequent source for relapsing UTI in older men.

PATHOGENESIS

Urinary tract infection usually results when colonizing flora of the periurethral area and, in women, the vagina ascend the urethra and enter the bladder. Factors promoting ascension and subsequent persistence of bacteria in the bladder include host and organism variables (Fig. 63-2).

Source of Infecting Organisms

Bacteria causing UTIs usually originate from the normal gut flora. The greater frequency of infection in women is thought to be attributable to the shorter female urethra, allowing easier access of bacteria to the bladder. Most bacteria that ascend to the bladder will be flushed out with the next normal voiding. For infection to take place, bacteria must be able to persist and reproduce in the bladder. Pyelonephritis occurs when organisms travel from the bladder to the kidneys, transported either in a column of urine in the ureter or with reflux of urine from the bladder up the ureter in individuals with incompetent ureteral sphincters. Bacterial infection of the prostate gland also happens primarily through ascension

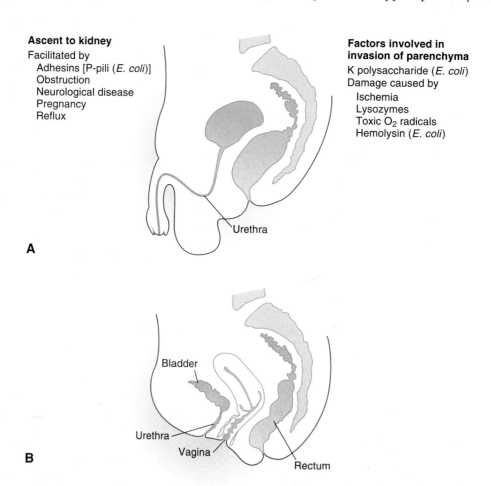

FIGURE 63-2 ▪ **Pathogenesis of urinary tract infections. A.** Male urinary tract. **B.** Female urinary tract.

of organisms from the urethra into the prostate ducts. This process is facilitated by turbulent urine flow, which is common in men with prostate hypertrophy.

Occasionally, UTI follows bacteremic dissemination of organisms through the bloodstream from another infected site. The characteristic pathologic feature of hematogenous dissemination is multiple small renal cortical abscesses. Ascending infection is primarily associated with the renal medulla. Some microorganisms, including *Staphylococcus aureus* and *Candida* species, are more common with hematogenous spread.

Microbiology

The most important uropathogen is *Escherichia coli*. However, a wide spectrum of other organisms may be isolated, depending on the clinical syndrome.

Acute Uncomplicated Urinary Tract Infection

E. coli is isolated from 80 to 85% of episodes of acute cystitis. The *E. coli* virulence characteristic necessary for acute cystitis is expression of the **mannose-sensitive fimbria**, or **FimH**. This protein receptor facilitates adherence of *E. coli* to bladder uroepithelial cells through attachment to mannosylated glycoproteins that line the bladder mucosa. FimH is widespread in *E. coli* strains, and found in more than 80% of cystitis isolates. It is also present in the majority of fecal strains, so additional factors must also contribute to infection. *Staphylococcus saprophyticus*, a Gram-positive organism, is isolated from 5 to 15% of the remaining episodes of acute cystitis. This organism shows a temporal variation, being isolated more frequently in the fall than in other times of year. Organisms such as *Klebsiella* species, *Proteus* species, and group B streptococcus are isolated from the few remaining episodes.

E. coli is also isolated from 85 to 90% of episodes of acute nonobstructive pyelonephritis. The organism virulence factor most often associated with this clinical presentation is another adhesin, **P fimbriae**. The receptor for this adhesin is the **glycosphingolipid Gal(α1–4) Galβ disaccharide**. Attachment of *E. coli* to renal cells mediated by P fimbriae enhances bacterial persistence and inflammation in the urinary tract. Additional *E. coli* virulence factors associated with pyelonephritis include **aerobactin** (which scavenges for iron that the bacteria need to grow) and **hemolysin** (which may lyse host cells). These virulence factors can come together on "**pathogenicity islands**" on the *E. coli* chromosome. Other factors are also likely to be involved because certain *E. coli* serotypes are known to be more frequently associated with pyelonephritis.

Complicated Urinary Tract Infection

E. coli is also the most common pathogen isolated from patients with complicated UTI. However, the organism appears in patients with the complicated syndrome less frequently than in those with uncomplicated UTI. *E. coli* strains isolated from complicated renal infection are characterized by a lower frequency of virulence factors than present in acute uncomplicated pyelonephritis. This is consistent with the concept that host rather than organism factors are the principal determinants of infection.

A wide variety of organisms other than *E. coli* are associated with complicated UTI. These include members of the Enterobacteriaceae family such as species of the genera *Klebsiella, Enterobacter,* and *Citrobacter,* and nonfermenting Gram-negative organisms, particularly *Pseudomonas aeruginosa*. Urease-producing organisms like *Proteus mirabilis, Morganella morganii,* and *Providencia* species are common. These organisms have additional pathogenic potential because they metabolize urea to ammonia, which damages the kidney, and they form struvite (infection) stones, which cause obstruction and further damage. *Enterococcus* species and coagulase negative staphylococci are the most common Gram-positive organisms. Yeast species are occasionally isolated. *Candida albicans* is the most common, but other species include *C. tropicalis, C. glabrata,* and *C. parapsilosis*.

Bacteria isolated from patients with complicated UTI are also characterized by an increased prevalence of antimicrobial resistance, largely attributable to repeated antimicrobial exposure with frequent recurrent infection. Many patients also undergo invasive genitourinary interventions to assess or manage underlying abnormalities. These procedures may be associated with nosocomial acquisition of organisms that have increased resistance.

Individuals with complicated urinary tract infection often have indwelling urologic devices, such as an indwelling urethral catheter, ureteric stent, or nephrostomy tube. The devices are continually bathed in the urinary stream and become coated with a biofilm. The biofilm consists of microorganisms, extracellular substances produced by the organisms, and urinary components such as proteins, calcium, and magnesium. From three to five organisms are usually present in the biofilm and exist in an environment that protects them from both antibiotics and host immune defenses. They are difficult to eradicate without removing the device and are a frequent source of relapsing infection.

Asymptomatic Bacteriuria

The spectrum of organisms isolated from persons with asymptomatic bacteriuria generally mirrors the anticipated spectrum of isolates for symptomatic UTI in the same patient group. Thus, *E. coli* is most common in otherwise healthy women. *E. coli* strains isolated from individuals with asymptomatic bacteriuria are characterized by a low prevalence of potential virulence factors. Gram-positive organisms of low virulence such as *Enterococcus* species and coagulase-negative staphylococci are also isolated more frequently in patients with asymptomatic bacteriuria.

Bacterial Prostatitis

Acute bacterial prostatitis is an uncommon infection primarily caused by *S. aureus* or *E. coli*. The prevalence of virulence factors of *E. coli* in prostate isolates is intermediate between strains isolated from acute cystitis and from pyelonephritis. Chronic bacterial prostatitis is associated with many organisms. Prostate stones that form in men as they age are a nidus for organisms persisting in the prostate and sources of bacteria for relapsing cystitis.

Host Factors

The most important host defense against urinary tract infection is periodic, complete, normal voiding. Urination removes bacteria in the bladder as well as desquamated uroepithelial cells to which bacteria adhere.

Uncomplicated Urinary Tract Infection

Women who experience acute uncomplicated UTI have normal voiding. The ability of organisms to access the bladder and persist is facilitated by genetic and behavioral factors. Women with recurrent acute uncomplicated UTI are more likely to have first-degree female relatives (mother, sisters, daughters) who also experience recurrent infection. Genetic predisposition is partly mediated through being a **nonsecretor of the ABH blood group antigens.** These antigens are secreted at mucosal surfaces and bind to receptors on bacterial cells to prevent attachment to the uroepithelium. Persons who are nonsecretors, about 20% of the population, have bacterial cell surface receptors that remain free for attachment of bacteria to host uroepithelial cells.

The most important behavioral risks for acute cystitis in premenopausal women are **sexual intercourse** and **spermicide use for birth control.** Sexual intercourse mechanically facilitates the ascension of organisms from the periurethral area into the bladder. Bacteria enter the bladder following about 30% of episodes of intercourse. Usually, the next voiding clears the bacteria, but symptomatic or asymptomatic infection can occur. An increased frequency of intercourse is associated with an increased frequency of symptomatic episodes. The normal **lactobacillus** flora of the vagina maintains an acidic pH and prevents colonization by potential uropathogens such as *E. coli*. **Spermicide kills the normal flora,** allowing uropathogens such as *E. coli* to colonize the vagina and cause infection.

Other behavioral risk factors of less importance include having a new sexual partner, using a diaphragm (even without spermicide), and receiving antimicrobial therapy. A new sexual partner increases exposure to new strains of *E. coli*, some of which are uropathogens. Using a diaphragm without spermicide can obstruct the urethra and impair complete bladder emptying. However, spermicide use is typical among women who use diaphragms

and thus remains the major determinant of infection in this group of women. Condom use without spermicide or use of birth control pills does not increase the risk of infection. Recent antimicrobial therapy may also suppress normal colonizing flora, leading to overgrowth of potential uropathogens. Behavioral factors not associated with an increased risk for UTI include voiding practices before and after intercourse, wiping practices after toileting, use of douches or tampons, types of underwear, or bathing in a tub rather than showering.

The genetic propensity to acute uncomplicated UTI persists throughout a woman's lifetime, from childhood through the postmenopausal years. Older women have additional risk factors, including increased postvoid residual urine and abnormalities such as cystoceles or diverticula, which are consistent with complicated urinary tract infection. Estrogen deficiency can also increase the likelihood of infection for some women, but further study of the association is needed. Uncomplicated UTI is rarely seen in healthy young men. Risk factors for men include having a new sexual partner and anal sex. This syndrome is so uncommon in men, however, that any infection occurring in a man is generally considered complicated UTI.

Complicated Urinary Tract Infection

Patients with complicated UTI have structural or functional abnormalities of the genitourinary tract that compromise voiding. Age and gender are not factors in complicated UTI. The specific defects include obstruction to urinary flow, decreased clearance of organisms in protected environments such as stones or biofilm, and/or increased access of organisms through reflux or catheters. Urinary tract infections in pregnant women may be considered complicated because urinary stasis from hormonal effects on autonomic muscles and ureteric obstruction from pressure of the fetal head at the pelvic brim are likely to promote pyelonephritis.

Host Response

Women with acute cystitis have an inflammatory response in the urinary tract characterized by recruitment of leukocytes with **local cytokine production** such as **interleukin 6 (IL-6), IL-8,** and **IL-10.** A local IgA and IgG antibody response specific to the infecting organism also develops. The natural history of untreated acute uncomplicated cystitis is resolution for about 50% of episodes by 2 to 4 weeks, but the contribution of the immune response to resolution is not known. The **local immunity** that develops with an episode of acute cystitis **does not protect from subsequent episodes.**

For acute uncomplicated pyelonephritis, the initial local response is again inflammatory, manifested by **pyuria,** or leukocytes in the urine, and cytokine production. A systemic inflammatory response includes fever, leukocytosis, and elevated C-reactive protein. Systemic antibodies develop, with IgM antibodies predominating for the first infection and IgG antibodies in subsequent infections. IgG antibodies to lipid A correlate with severity of renal infection. The inflammatory response in the kidney likely contributes to tissue damage and renal scarring. The degree of protection for subsequent renal infection provided by this host response is unclear. The role of cell-mediated immunity is also unclear.

The host immune response is not well studied in individuals with complicated UTI. The inflammatory and immune response are likely similar to uncomplicated infection, depending on whether the site of infection is the bladder or kidney. Spontaneous resolution of bacteriuria is less frequent in individuals with complicated UTI, although replacement by another organism is common.

Patients with asymptomatic bacteriuria also usually have pyuria. When pyuria is not present, spontaneous resolution is more likely to occur. Gram-positive organisms such as *Enterococcus* species and coagulase-negative staphylococci are also less often accompanied by pyuria. Some individuals with asymptomatic bacteriuria also manifest a local immune response, with elevated urinary IgG and IgA antibodies and local cytokine production, but the significance of this response is not clear.

DIAGNOSIS

The definitive diagnosis of urinary tract infection requires isolation of bacteria from the urine. However, the clinical presentation characterizes the site of infection, identifies underlying host factors, and determines the management approach.

Clinical Presentation

Uncomplicated Cystitis or Pyelonephritis

Acute cystitis in women presents with lower-tract irritative symptoms such as dysuria (pain on voiding), frequency (frequent urination), urgency (need to void immediately once the urge is felt), and suprapubic or low-back discomfort. Some women also experience gross hematuria. These symptoms vary in intensity from mild to severe in different patients and for different episodes in the same patient. The physical examination is normal in women presenting with acute cystitis. If vaginal symptoms such as discharge or irritation are present, a diagnosis of vaginitis or a sexually transmitted disease must be considered.

Women with acute uncomplicated pyelonephritis present with costovertebral angle pain and tenderness due to renal inflammation. This is usually unilateral, but bilateral renal involvement can occur. The systemic inflammatory response accompanying pyelonephritis manifests with fevers and, in severe cases, nausea, vomiting, and hemodynamic instability consistent with sepsis syndrome. Pyelonephritis may also be accompanied by lower-tract irritative symptoms. Some patients with only lower-tract symptoms also have bacteria present in the kidney. This is referred to as subclinical pyelonephritis and is of uncertain clinical significance.

Complicated Urinary Tract Infection

Individuals with complicated UTI present with symptoms consistent with either acute cystitis or pyelonephritis, depending on the level of urinary tract involvement. If an indwelling catheter is present, urinary tract infection may present with fever alone. Some patients with neurologic impairment have altered clinical presentations. Patients with spinal cord injuries may complain of increased spasticity of the lower limbs or, if the injury is high in the cervical area and affects the brainstem, autonomic dysreflexia. Some multiple sclerosis patients complain of increased fatigue and a deterioration of neurologic symptoms.

Bacterial Prostatitis

Acute bacterial prostatitis presents with severe local and systemic systems. These include **high fever, pelvic pain, and urinary retention.** Physical examination reveals a swollen and tender prostate, but is not recommended as digital rectal examination may precipitate bacteremia. Chronic bacterial prostatitis is characterized by recurrent episodes of acute cystitis from relapses of bacteria persisting in the prostate. Complaints of chronic pelvic discomfort and voiding symptoms previously attributed to chronic bacterial prostatitis are no longer considered infectious in etiology.

Urine Culture

The microbiologic diagnosis of urinary tract infection requires isolation of bacteria from the urine in appropriate quantitative counts (Table 63-1). When voided urine specimens are obtained for culture, external secretions

table **63-1**	Quantitative Criteria for Identification of Significant Bacteriuria in Selected Groups
POPULATION	**BACTERIA COUNTS (CFU/ML)**
Asymptomatic bacteriuria	
In women	$\geq 10^5$, usually in two consecutive specimens
In men	$\geq 10^5$
Acute uncomplicated pyelonephritis	$\geq 10^5$
Acute dysuria in women	$\geq 10^2$, with pyuria
Specimens collected by catheter	$\geq 10^2$

from the periurethral area or the vagina cause contamination, leading to false-positive results. Urine collection methods must limit such contamination. For men, a clean-voided or clean-catch specimen collected during the middle of voiding is also adequate. Contamination is more common for women, but a clean-catch midstream urine specimen is usually adequate. If a woman is unable to cooperate, in and out catheterization may be necessary for specimen collection.

Infecting and contaminating bacteria are distinguished by quantifying the number of organisms growing from the urine specimen. **Colony counts of contaminants in voided specimens are low, while infecting organisms achieve high concentrations** (Figure 63-3). However, small numbers of bacteria in urine grow well at room temperature, so specimens must be promptly forwarded to the laboratory following collection. A single organism is isolated from most patients with urinary tract infection. Some patients with complicated UTI have more than one organism isolated, particularly when chronic urethral catheters or other chronic devices are present.

Urine specimens collected through biofilm-coated devices will reflect the microbiology of the biofilm as well as the urine. The biofilm usually has both a greater number and higher quantitative count of organisms. A patient with a chronic indwelling catheter should have the catheter replaced and a urine specimen collected through the new biofilm-free catheter before starting antimicrobial therapy. This specimen samples bladder urine and is representative of the infecting organisms.

Any quantitative count of a potential uropathogen is consistent with urinary tract infection for women with acute uncomplicated UTI (see Table 63-1). From 50 to 70% of these women will have counts of at least 10^5 colony-forming units (CFU)/mL, and 30 to 50% have lower counts. For acute uncomplicated pyelonephritis or complicated urinary tract infection, at least 10^5 CFU/mL is the appropriate quantitative count. Asymptomatic bacteriuria in women is usually identified by two consecutive urine specimens with counts of at least 10^5 CFU/mL. If an initial specimen is positive at that quantitative count, a second consecutive voided specimen is positive in only 80% of women. Any quantitative count of organisms isolated from a urine specimen obtained by catheterization is consistent with infection.

Some patients, such as those experiencing diuresis from diuretics, renal failure, or frequent voiding, may have lower quantitative counts isolated because organisms do not have sufficient time to grow to high concentrations in bladder urine. In these patients quantitative urine culture results must be interpreted in the context of the clinical presentation. Rarely, the urine culture from an infected patient is negative. This occurs with complete ureteric obstruction and infection proximal to the obstruction. Fastidious organisms, such as *Haemophilus influenzae* and *Ureaplasma urealyticum,* infrequently cause infection and are not isolated with routine laboratory methods. The most common reason for a negative urine culture, however, is that the specimen was obtained after initiation of antimicrobial therapy.

Other Laboratory Tests

Pyuria is measured by microscopic examination of the urine or a dipstick leukocyte esterase test. Although pyuria is a consistent finding in patients with symptomatic UTI, the majority of persons with persistent asymptomatic bacteriuria also have pyuria. In addition, pyuria is not specific for urinary tract infection. It occurs with noninfectious conditions, such as interstitial nephritis and diabetic nephropathy, and with contamination from vagi-

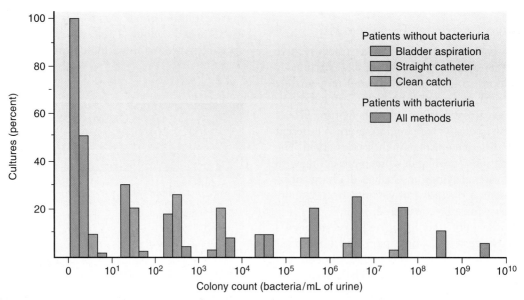

FIGURE 63-3 ▪ **Quantitative colony counts for microbiologic diagnosis of urinary tract infection with various clinical presentations.**

nal secretions. Thus, pyuria does not diagnose UTI or differentiate symptomatic from asymptomatic infection. The absence of pyuria in a urine specimen, however, is good evidence for the absence of UTI.

Patients presenting with severe systemic manifestations or with urinary obstruction may have bacteremia, and blood cultures should be obtained. The peripheral leukocyte count gives information about the severity of illness and may be used to monitor response to therapy. Those patients should also have renal function assessed, initially with a blood urea nitrogen and creatinine measurement.

TREATMENT

The treatment of UTI requires specific antimicrobial therapy directed at the presumed or known infecting organism. Antimicrobials excreted in the urine are preferred because those agents achieve very high urinary levels. For cystitis, which is considered a superficial mucosal infection, only urinary antibacterial activity is needed. For pyelonephritis, treatment requires adequate antimicrobial levels in both urine and tissue. Other variables considered in selecting therapy include patient tolerance, renal and hepatic function, potential adverse effects, drug interactions, and cost (Table 63-2).

Acute Uncomplicated Cystitis

Acute uncomplicated cystitis is usually treated empirically. Antimicrobial therapy is initiated on the basis of consistent symptoms, and a pretherapy urine culture is not routinely obtained. Women who experience re-

Case

A 23-year-old woman presented with a 48-hour history of dysuria, frequency, and gross hematuria. She had had a similar episode about 8 months ago. At the time she had a single sexual partner and used a condom with spermicide for birth control.

This case raises several questions:

1. What is the most likely diagnosis in this woman?
2. What factors have contributed to this episode of infection?
3. Should a urine specimen for culture be obtained?
4. What is optimal antimicrobial treatment of this episode?
5. What might prevent further episodes of infection?

current acute cystitis are 95% accurate in self-diagnosis based on their symptoms. In addition, the microbiology of acute cystitis is highly predictable, and urine culture results are not generally available for 48 to 72 hours. Because short-course therapy lasting 3 days is preferred for acute cystitis, antimicrobial therapy is complete by the time the culture result is available. A pretherapy urine specimen for culture should be obtained, however, in women with inconsistent symptoms if empiric therapy is not effective and for any woman who is pregnant. Obtaining pretherapy urine cultures may also be desirable for women with this syndrome to monitor local *E. coli* susceptibilities.

Considerations in selecting empiric therapy include efficacy for UTI, patient tolerance, and local prevalence of resistance in community *E. coli*. Trimethoprim-

table 63-2	Approaches to Treatment of Urinary Tract Infections for Different Clinical Presentations	
TYPE OF INFECTION	**TREATMENT**	**RATIONALE**
Cystitis	Short course (3 days) preferred	Effective for bacterial cystitis; not effective in patients with early pyelonephritis or resistant bacteria, which are detected by follow-up culture or by relapse of symptoms
Pyelonephritis	10–14 days, full doses; antimicrobial prescription based on susceptibility tests; drug with urinary excretion preferred	Requires antimicrobials that achieve high concentrations in renal tissue as well as urine
Asymptomatic bacteriuria	Indicated only for pregnant women or patients about to undergo traumatic urologic procedures	24–40% of pregnant women with asymptomatic bacteriuria develop pyelonephritis if not treated; bacteremia and sepsis likely following procedures with potential mucosal trauma and bleeding
Recurrent or multiple reinfections	Prophylaxis: long term (6–12 months) low dose or postintercourse	Eradicates colonizing flora; repeatedly sterilizes urine
Relapse	Long-term treatment (e.g., 4–8 weeks or longer)	Suggests tissue invasion or structural abnormality and merits investigation

sulfamethoxazole (TMP/SMX) or trimethoprim (TMP) are the drugs of first choice for 3-day therapy. If those drugs are not appropriate, second-line choices include a fluoroquinolone given for 3 days or nitrofurantoin for 7 days. Amoxicillin is not used for empiric therapy because resistance rates of *E. coli* approach 30 to 50%. Cephalosporins are not generally recommended because they share with other β-lactam antibiotics a somewhat lower efficacy, especially with short-course therapy. However, cephalosporins are useful for treating pregnant women, for whom fetal safety is a concern. Fosfomycin trometamol as a single dose is also available for acute cystitis but is somewhat less effective than other agents.

Acute Uncomplicated Pyelonephritis

A urine specimen for culture should be obtained before the start of antimicrobial therapy whenever pyelonephritis is a diagnostic consideration. The potential seriousness of this infection means the infecting organism and susceptibilities must be identified to facilitate appropriate antimicrobial therapy. A peripheral leukocyte count and blood and urine cultures should be obtained. The severity of illness is assessed clinically by the presence of fever, hemodynamic status, and other systemic symptoms. Important information also includes whether the patient can tolerate oral therapy, has conditions that require close monitoring (e.g., diabetes, pregnancy), or is likely to have structural abnormalities requiring investigation or intervention.

Based on the clinical assessment, the decision is made to manage the patient as an outpatient with oral therapy, with hospitalization for initial parenteral therapy, or for short-term observation and initial parenteral therapy in the emergency department. Empiric therapy is initiated and reviewed when culture results are available, usually after 48 to 72 hours. For oral therapy, TMP/SMX, TMP,

or a fluoroquinolone may be used depending on anticipated susceptibilities. For parenteral therapy, an aminoglycoside, extended spectrum cephalosporin, or fluoroquinolone is appropriate. Generally, 10 to 14 days of therapy are recommended. If clinical improvement has not occurred within 48 to 72 hours, urinary obstruction or other abnormality should be excluded by appropriate diagnostic imaging studies.

Complicated Urinary Tract Infection

The wide variety of potential infecting organisms and greater likelihood of antimicrobial resistance means a urine specimen for culture should be obtained prior to antimicrobial therapy for every episode of complicated infection. When symptoms are mild, antimicrobial therapy should be withheld until the culture results are available so specific therapy can be prescribed. If symptoms are severe, empiric therapy selected on the basis of anticipated organism susceptibilities is initiated and then reassessed when urine culture results are available. Patients who are significantly ill with high fever, nausea, and vomiting or hemodynamic stability, or patients infected with highly resistant organisms, may require hospitalization and initial parenteral therapy. The genitourinary abnormality must be characterized for all patients and may require additional or repeated urologic and diagnostic imaging investigations.

Case

A 39-year-old man with a history of T6 paraplegia for 8 years and bladder emptying managed by condom drainage presented with complaints of increased bladder and lower-leg spasms. He attributed the symptoms to urinary tract infection, having had two similar episodes in the past year. A urine specimen for culture grew more than 10^5 CFU/mL of *Klebsiella pneumoniae* resistant to fluoroquinolones and aminoglycosides.

This case raises several questions:

1. Why is this man experiencing urinary tract infections?
2. Why is the isolate resistant to some antimicrobials?
3. How should antimicrobial therapy to treat the infection be selected?
4. What additional management should be considered for this patient with complicated UTI and a recent increase in infection frequency?

Case

A 32-year-old nonpregnant woman presented with fever, rigors, back pain, nausea, vomiting, and mild dysuria. Her symptoms had increased in severity over 48 hours. The patient described two or three previous episodes consistent with cystitis. Her temperature was 39.2°C, and right costovertebral angle tenderness was present.

This case raises several questions:

1. What is the most likely infecting organism, and what virulence factor is characteristic?
2. What initial investigations should be obtained to confirm the diagnosis and assess the clinical status of this woman?
3. What antimicrobial regimen should be initiated?

Asymptomatic Bacteriuria

Asymptomatic bacteriuria is common in many populations, including nursing home residents. In most patients it should not be treated. An important exception is pregnant women, for whom treatment is always indicated. A

Case

An 87-year-old woman with chronic incontinence appeared somewhat lethargic to the staff at the nursing home where she lived. The nurses also noticed that her urine was cloudy and had a urine specimen sent for culture. The culture result returned 5 days later and was reported as more than 10^5 CFU/mL of *E. coli*. By that time she was no longer lethargic, but the urinalysis also showed pyuria, with white cells too numerous to count.

This case raises two questions:

1. What is the diagnosis in this woman?
2. What antimicrobial treatment should be given for the *E. coli* grown in culture?

woman with asymptomatic bacteriuria identified in early pregnancy has a 20 to 30% risk of pyelonephritis later in pregnancy if the bacteriuria is not treated. Pyelonephritis occurs most frequently at the end of the second trimester or early in the third trimester, when hormonal effects are greatest. Any febrile illness at that point in gestation may be associated with premature labor and delivery and is a risk for the fetus. Identifying and treating asymptomatic bacteriuria in early pregnancy can prevent the complication. A second group of patients for whom identification and treatment of asymptomatic bacteriuria is recommended comprises those who require urological procedures with potential mucosal trauma and bleeding. Bacteriuric patients are at high risk for bacteremia and sepsis following mucosal injury, but those risks can be minimized by treating the bacteriuria before performing urological procedures.

For all other patient groups, treatment of asymptomatic bacteriuria does not benefit patients. Treatment does not prevent symptomatic UTI or improve potential long-term complications such as hypertension or renal failure. Treatment of bacteriuria is, however, associated with increased adverse effects of drug therapy, resistant organisms in reinfections, and high treatment costs. It follows that screening for asymptomatic bacteriuria is not indicated except in pregnant women or patients undergoing traumatic urologic procedures.

Recurrent Urinary Tract Infection

The more difficult clinical problem in the management of urinary tract infection is not treatment of a single episode but management of patients who have recurrent

infection, including some with very frequent recurrences. Occasionally, a patient requires prolonged antimicrobial therapy, either as prophylactic therapy to prevent reinfections or as suppressive therapy to prevent symptomatic relapse when a cure is not possible.

Acute Uncomplicated Urinary Tract Infection

For women with frequent symptomatic reinfections, generally defined as two episodes every 6 months or 3 every year, prophylactic antimicrobial therapy can prevent 90 to 95% of acute symptomatic episodes. This type of treatment is given as long-term low-dose therapy daily or every other day, or following intercourse. For pregnant women prophylaxis is indicated following two documented infections, either symptomatic or asymptomatic. Prophylactic antimicrobials appear to be effective through at least two mechanisms. Antimicrobials such as TMP-SMX, TMP, and fluoroquinolones reduce Gram-negative flora colonizing the gut, vagina, and periurethral area, preventing reinfection with those organisms. Nitrofurantoin is as effective as those antimicrobials but has no impact on colonizing flora. It is likely effective through intermittent sterilization of the urine with high urinary antimicrobial levels.

Complicated Urinary Tract Infection

Prophylactic antimicrobial therapy is not effective for patients with complicated urinary tract infection. Suppressive therapy may be indicated, infrequently, for patients with recurrent symptomatic infection and urologic abnormalities that cannot be corrected or when bacteria cannot be effectively eradicated. Because prolonged antimicrobial therapy can cause resistant organisms to emerge, suppressive therapy is used only in highly selected patients who do not respond to other approaches.

Conclusion

Urinary tract infections are important bacterial infections affecting all ages and both sexes. To understand the epidemiology, pathogenesis, and management of UTIs, it is necessary to appreciate the differences between normal and abnormal genitourinary tracts. Effective management of a UTI requires appropriately collecting specimens and interpreting urine cultures, as well as addressing host factors that contribute to the occurrence of infection.

chapter 64

Infections of the Skin and Soft Tissue

Dennis L. Stevens

Inflamed hangnails, infected cuts, and athlete's foot occur so frequently that we scarcely notice. Those mild and usually inconsequential conditions represent one extreme of the infections of the skin. The other extreme comprises less frequent but more serious diseases like herpes zoster, candidiasis, and certain bacterial infections, such as cellulitis, necrotizing fasciitis, and gas gangrene. Infections of the skin may be caused by viruses, fungi, or bacteria. In addition, many diseases that affect other organs have cutaneous manifestations. Visible skin lesions may indicate systemic infections by viruses (e.g., smallpox, measles, chickenpox), fungi (e.g., cryptococcosis, blastomycosis), or bacteria (e.g., syphilis, tuberculosis, scarlet fever, meningococcemia, endocarditis).

Primary infections of the skin and systemic infections with cutaneous manifestations are discussed throughout this book in the context of specific agents: staphylococci (see Chapter 11), streptococci (see Chapter 12), *Pseudomonas aeruginosa* (see Chapter 18), paramyxoviruses (see Chapter 34), warts (see Chapter 40), and fungal infections (see Chapter 49). This chapter is limited to bacterial skin infections and emphasizes those with important pathobiological implications. The chapter also recognizes that these infections frequently involve the soft tissues underlying the skin, subcutaneous fat, and superficial fascia.

ANATOMY AND PHYSIOLOGY

An understanding of the pathogenesis of skin and soft tissue infections requires knowledge of skin anatomy and physiology. The skin is divided into three distinct layers: the epidermis, dermis, and fat layer. The **epidermis** is a thin, self-renewing epidermal sheet that covers the body. It is about the thickness of two sheets of this book (0.1 mm) over most of the body and is devoid of vessels and nerves. The basal cells of the epidermis, the **keratinocytes**, divide, differentiate, mature, and are eventually sloughed from the skin surface. As they rise from the basal layer to the skin surface, they become more stratified and produce a cornified layer of dead cells, the **stratum corneum.** This outermost epidermal layer consists of dead keratinocytes rich in the tough fibrous protein **keratin** and is held together by intercellular neutral lipids. The stratum corneum is the major physical barrier preventing environmental chemicals and microorganisms from entering the body. In addition to the keratinocytes, the epidermis contains the **Langerhans cells** and the pigment-containing **melanocytes.** Langerhans cells are fixed tissue macrophages. They represent a distant outpost of the immune system and process antigens that breach the stratum corneum.

Skin appendages, including hairs, sebaceous (oil) glands, and sweat glands, originate from the basal layer of the epidermis. They invaginate into the dermis and exit at the surface through the epidermis. Bacteria may bypass the stratum corneum by traversing these conduits.

The **dermis** is several millimeters thick and is separated from the epidermis by a basement membrane. The fibrous proteins **collagen** and **elastin** are embedded in a glycoprotein matrix and constitute the strong supportive dermal structure. A rich plexus of blood vessels and lymphatics courses through the dermis. Interruption of dermal blood flow predisposes to infection by restricting access of humoral and cellular defenses against invaders and by compromising oxygen delivery and nutrition of the epidermal barrier.

Subcutaneous fat, the third layer of the skin, consists predominantly of lipid cells. Those cells serve as heat insulators, shock absorbers, and depots of caloric reserves. The final layer is **superficial fascia** that separates skin from muscles. Any or all of these layers of soft tissue may be involved in a given infectious process.

ENCOUNTER

The skin is sterile in utero and during birth, but it is soon colonized by both anaerobic and aerobic bacteria ranging from 10^2 to 10^4 colony-forming units (CFU) per square centimeter of surface. Many factors affect the distribution, composition, and density of this flora. These factors include not only the environmental climate, which differs throughout the world, but also the microclimates of the body. The intertriginous areas of the axilla and groin are markedly different from the drier areas of the back, forearms, and calves of the leg.

The two properties that make the skin hostile to bacterial growth are **exfoliation** and **dryness.** The constant sloughing of the stratum corneum dislodges many of the bacteria that adhere to its surface. The importance of dryness can be seen when occlusive dressings are applied: within 2 or 3 days bacteria counts may increase from 10^2 to more than 10^7 CFU/cm^2. Accordingly, bacteria counts are much higher in the moister areas of the skin than in the drier regions. Other factors that help limit bacterial growth are low pH, low temperature, and chemical composition. The skin has a pH of approximately 5.5, the result of hydrolysis of sebum lipids by the skin bacteria themselves. Growth of some microorganisms is further hindered by the skin's low temperature, which averages about 33°C. The saltiness of some parts of the skin, the result of the evaporation of sweat, may encourage the growth of salt-resistant species, such as *Staphylococcus epidermidis.* In addition, some organisms are inhibited by the lipid content of the skin surface.

The bacterial flora of skin, like that of mucous membranes, also helps protect the host from invasion by pathogens; skin infections are more likely to occur when the flora is wiped out. The precise mechanisms involved in the skin-protecting ability of the normal flora are not known but may include saturation of binding sites, competition for nutrients, and production of bacteriocins and other inhibitory chemicals by endogenous microbes.

Members of the resident flora of the skin are of low virulence and rarely cause significant infections. Included in the flora are **resident bacteria,** which multiply on the skin and are regularly present, and **transient bacteria,** which survive on the skin for only a short period. Members of the transient flora are deposited on the skin either from mucous membrane "fallout" or from the environment. Evidence suggests that specific adhesins are required for some bacteria to adhere to the skin before they are able to colonize it.

The dry and exposed areas of the skin are normally colonized with Gram-positive bacteria (including *S. epidermidis,* micrococci, anaerobic Gram-positive cocci, and both anaerobic and aerobic diphtheroids). *Propionibacterium acnes,* a Gram-positive rod, thrives in the sebaceous areas. Facultative and anaerobic Gram-negative rods more often colonize the axilla and groin regions and other moist areas, such as the webs of the toes. For unknown reasons, the skin of bedridden patients with serious medical illnesses often has increased colonization of Gram-negative bacilli.

The most important organisms of the transient flora are the common pathogens of cutaneous infections, *Staphylococcus aureus* and *Streptococcus pyogenes.* Those organisms are found more often on exposed skin than on areas normally protected by clothing. *S. aureus* is found commonly in the nose and on the face and upper body rather than on the trunk and legs, probably because the upper respiratory tract is the reservoir for the organism. The box titled "Members of the Skin Flora and the Infections They Cause" lists some of the important pathogens that transiently colonize the skin and cause infections.

ENTRY, SPREAD, AND MULTIPLICATION

Infectious agents enter the skin and its underlying soft tissues by two routes:

- **From the outside:** through cuts, wounds, insect bites, skin disease, or other breaks in the integrity of the stratum corneum
- **From within:** through underlying tissue or carried by blood or lymph

Members of the Skin Flora and the Infections They Cause

RESIDENT FLORA

- *Propionibacterium acnes*
- *Staphylococcus epidermidis:* infection around foreign bodies (prosthetic devices, etc.)
- Micrococci
- Anaerobic Gram-positive cocci
- Aerobic Gram-negative bacilli (low numbers)
- *Pityrosporum ovale* (a yeast)

TRANSIENT FLORA

- Bacteria
  - Frequent:
    - *Staphylococcus aureus:* folliculitis, furuncles, carbuncles, toxic shock syndrome, and bacteremia
    - *Streptococcus pyogenes:* cellulitis, lymphangitis, impetigo, erysipelas, necrotizing fasciitis, toxic shock syndrome
  - Infrequent:
    - *Haemophilus influenzae:* cellulitis
    - *Clostridium* species: gas gangrene
    - *Francisella tularensis:* tularemia
    - *Bacillus anthracis:* anthrax
    - *Pseudomonas aeruginosa:* infections resulting from hot-tub use
    - *Burkholderia cepacia:* foot infection ("foot rot")
    - *Mycobacterium marinum:* "fish tank cellulitis"
- Fungi
  - *Candida albicans:* diaper rash, chronic paronychia
  - Dermatophytes: tinea infections (ringworm)
- Viruses
  - Frequent:
    - Herpes simplex virus 1 and 2: perioral ("cold sore") and genital infection
    - Papillomaviruses: warts
  - Infrequent:
    - *Molluscum contagiosum:* wartlike lesions

Once microorganisms have penetrated the skin, they can spread locally and invade the lymphatics or the bloodstream. As a result, infections originally confined to the skin and soft tissues may ultimately cause complications in other areas of the body.

The spread of some bacteria is associated with specific virulence factors; an example is **hyaluronidase** (also called **spreading factor**), an extracellular enzyme made by both *S. aureus* and *S. pyogenes*. Other enzymes, such as hemolysins, lipases, collagenase, and elastases, are elaborated by cutaneous pathogens and probably play a role in pathogenesis (see Chapter 9). In general, **S. aureus infections tend to localize**, forming abscesses, for example, whereas *S. pyogenes* **infections spread more extensively through tissues**, causing cellulitis.

What is the role of cellular and humoral immunity in the skin? Neutrophils are attracted to the infected area by chemoattractants elaborated by bacteria, tissue macrophages, and activation of complement through the alternative pathway. A local antimicrobial effort is mounted by the epidermal macrophages, the Langerhans cells, through the elaboration of cytokines. Persons with acquired and congenital immunodeficiencies have an increased frequency of certain skin infections (e.g., candidiasis), suggesting that cellular immunity is important in skin defenses. When microorganisms breach the stratum corneum and begin to multiply, the host's defenses are mobilized to the skin. When the defenses are defective, infections of the skin become frequent events, and more extensive infection may be manifest.

DAMAGE

Cellular damage to the skin and soft tissues can be mediated by toxins, degradative enzymes, and the induction of host defense mechanisms that destroy tissues. The manifestations of infection caused by the invasion of microorganisms in the skin depend on the level of penetration, the virulence factors of the microbe, and the host response. Infections of skin and soft tissue are divided into three groups:

- **Exogenous infections** resulting from direct invasion from the external environment
- **Endogenous infections** caused by invasion from an internal source, such as the blood or an infected organ
- **Toxin-induced infections** produced by toxins formed at a distant site

Exogenous Infections

Controversy exists about whether potent pathogens are capable of directly penetrating the normal skin when present in high concentrations or whether they enter through imperceptible microscopic lesions. Without a noticeable break in the skin, high numbers of potent pathogens are required to produce exogenous skin and soft tissue infection. Experimental studies show that colonization of the skin by *S. aureus* at a density of more than 10^6 CFU/cm^2 is required to cause skin infections. Normally, bacteria grow to densities that high only under special circumstances, such as when the skin is very dirty or kept moist for prolonged periods. Once the skin barrier is broken from trauma, surgery, or a foreign body such as suture material, a sliver, or an intravenous catheter, *S. aureus* infection can be caused by as few as 10 to 100 CFU/cm^2. Thus, a number of conditions predispose to skin invasion, including excessive moisture, trauma, introduction of a foreign body, pressure, and compromised blood supply.

Excessive moisture can result from the use of occlusive dressings or from wet diapers on babies. Obese people accumulate moisture in their intertriginous folds. **Immersion infection** is seen in people who spend long periods in wet or swampy areas and cannot allow their footwear to dry out, such as troops during training or combat. Moisture induces skin **maceration** and breakdown of the stratum corneum. It is estimated that among U.S. foot soldiers in Vietnam, disability was more often associated with skin infections than with combat-associated wounds. Staphylococci and streptococci are frequently responsible for immersion infections, but waterborne Gram-negative bacteria also can be involved. Bathing in hot tubs containing high numbers of *Pseudomonas aeruginosa* is another mechanism of immersion infection (see Chapter 18).

Trauma is the most common factor leading to skin and soft tissue infection. Trauma may be mild, as in a torn hangnail or cracks in the skin caused by athlete's foot. Major forms of trauma that place the patient at risk include surgery (considered "organized trauma"), gunshot wounds, crush injuries (e.g., automobile accidents), or burns, in which large areas of skin are denuded and left open. Infections in surgical wounds are a major cause of morbidity in postoperative patients. Infection also is the primary cause of mortality in burn victims.

Many procedures used in the hospital breach the skin. The most common procedure is the use of **percutaneous** ("through the skin") **catheters.** The list of such devices is enormous and includes central venous lines, peritoneal dialysis catheters, tubes to drain body cavities, temporary pacemaker lines, chemotherapy infusion lines, and parenteral nutrition lines. Indeed, the most common reason for premature removal of percutaneous catheters is bacterial infection. Another type of skin infection in hospitalized patients is the **decubitus ulcer,** the cutaneous lesion that develops secondary to pressure injury and is informally referred to as a bed sore. Constant pressure against the skin of a paralyzed or immobile patient leads to skin necrosis and frequently to secondary infection.

table 64-1	Frequent Exogenous Infections of the Skin and Soft Tissues
DISEASE	**ORGANISMS**
Folliculitis	Staphylococci, *Pseudomonas* species
Carbuncles, furuncles	Staphylococci
Impetigo	Streptococci, staphylococci
Erysipelas	Streptococci
Lymphangitis	Streptococci
Cellulitis	Streptococci, staphylococci, *Haemophilus influenzae* (in unimmunized children)
Synergistic cellulitis	Streptococci, enteric bacteria, anaerobes
Gas gangrene	Clostridia
Necrotizing fasciitis	Streptococci, enteric bacteria, anaerobes

Any condition that compromises the blood supply predisposes the skin to invasion by causing barrier breakdown and limiting host defenses. Blood supply compromise can occur acutely following trauma or chronically as a result of peripheral vascular disease, as in patients with diabetes or vasculitis or in elderly people. In the diabetic patient, compromise of the vascular supply is often accompanied by peripheral sensory neuropathy, which limits the patient's awareness of traumatic damage to the skin. Secondary infections can also follow certain noninfectious skin diseases such as atopic dermatitis or pemphigus vulgaris.

The skin responds to invading microorganisms in a limited number of ways that fall into three general categories:

- **Spreading infections:** called **impetigo** when confined to the epidermis, **erysipelas** when involving the dermal lymphatics, and **cellulitis** when the major focus is the subcutaneous fat layer
- **Abscess formation:** known as folliculitis, boils (furuncles), and carbuncles
- **Necrotizing infections,** including fasciitis and gas gangrene (myonecrosis)

The organisms commonly implicated in exogenous infections are listed in Table 64-1. Cellulitis is illustrated in the following case.

Streptococcal Cellulitis, Impetigo, Erysipelas, and Lymphangitis

Case

Ms. W., a 27-year-old emergency medical technician, was evaluated by a physician for a slight infection around the nail of her left index finger (called a **paronychia**). The physician drained the lesion, and a culture of the pus grew a group A β-hemolytic streptococcus (*S. pyogenes*). Ms. W. was not given antimicrobial therapy because the physician thought that drainage was sufficient. Five days later, Ms. W. complained of fever and severe pain in the forearm, which had become swollen and red (erythematous). Her temperature was 40.2°C, and she was sweaty and hot. A patchy rash extended from her left upper arm to her shoulder. Lymph nodes in the axilla were enlarged and tender. Ms. W. was admitted to the hospital with a diagnosis of **streptococcal cellulitis.** She was treated successfully with high doses of penicillin. Blood cultures obtained before starting antimicrobial therapy also yielded *S. pyogenes.*

This case raises several questions:

1. What risk factors predisposed Ms. W. to the development of cellulitis?
2. What virulence determinants are expressed by *S. pyogenes*?
3. What antibiotic should have been administered at the time of the incision and drainage?

Cellulitis is an acute inflammatory process that involves subcutaneous tissue, characterized by areas of redness, induration, heat, and tenderness (Fig. 64-1). The borders of these areas are usually indistinct. Cellulitis can spread rapidly and is often accompanied by lymphangitis and inflammation of the draining lymph nodes. More than 90% of cases are caused by *S. aureus* and group A streptococci, while the rest are attributed to a variety of bacteria. In unimmunized children, infection with *Haemophilus influenzae* type B is an important cause of cellulitis, and it may be characterized by a blue tint of the

FIGURE 64-1 ▪ **Cellulitis of the toe.** The infection began adjacent to the nail as a paronychia but spread proximally to involve the shaft of the toe as cellulitis.

FIGURE 64-2 ▪ **Streptococcal impetigo.** Weeping and crusting lesions are typical of impetigo.

overlying erythema. Cellulitis associated with bites or scratches from cats or dogs is often the result of *Pasteurella multocida* (see Chapter 73). A normal inhabitant of the oral flora of many domestic and wild animals, *P. multocida* spreads rapidly and causes painful cellulitis when injected into human skin through a bite or scratch.

The pathological processes in cellulitis develop rapidly and may progress within 24 to 48 hours from a minor injury to severe septicemia. Characteristically, the tissues contain few organisms but undergo a marked inflammatory response, probably caused by toxins elaborated by the invading bacteria and products of inflammation such as cytokines and prostaglandins. The ability of group A streptococci to spread through the tissues is aided by hyaluronidase and other spreading factors previously mentioned.

Impetigo is a characteristic infection of the epidermis, manifested by intraepidermal vesicles that are filled with exudate and eventually become weeping and crusting lesions (Fig. 64-2). Caused by either group A streptococci or staphylococci, impetigo is a common disease of children and is seen mainly in exposed areas of the body during warm, moist weather. Although not usually associated with systemic signs or symptoms, impetigo caused by nephrogenic group A streptococci can lead to post-streptococcal glomerulonephritis.

Erysipelas is a more serious disease characterized by tender, superficial erythematous and edematous lesions. The infection spreads primarily in the superficial lymphatics of the dermis (Fig. 64-3). The rash is usually confluent, salmon red in color, and sharply demarcated from the surrounding, normal skin. It is seen most frequently in adults with edema of the extremities and often occurs on the face. The most common organisms that cause erysipelas are group A streptococci. Infection of the deep lymphatics, or **lymphangitis,** also is caused by group A streptococci. Erysipelas used to be one of the most serious complications of surgery (see Chapter 12), and it carried a high mortality rate. Its severity and incidence have markedly decreased over the last few decades. The decline can be explained only partially by the widespread use of penicillin to treat streptococcal infections.

FIGURE 64-3 ▪ **Erysipelas.** The rash on the right side of the face is confluent and salmon red in color.

FIGURE 64-4 ▪ **Staphylococcal carbuncle.** The posterior shows multiple follicular abscesses discharging purulent material.

Folliculitis, Furuncles, and Carbuncles Caused by *Staphylococcus aureus*

Case

Mr. C., a 37-year-old roofer, came to the emergency department with fever and a painful swelling on the left side of his neck. He had previously been healthy except for occasional boils. Three days before he had noted a minor irritation around some whiskers. The lesion progressed to the size of a walnut, which prevented him from buttoning his shirt. Physical examination revealed a febrile (temperature 38.8°C) healthy man in mild distress. A 2-to-3–cm mass with a soft center was noted on his left anterior neck at the beard line, surrounded by a rash. Needle aspiration of the mass yielded about 1 mL of pus that, under the microscope, showed large Gram-positive cocci in clusters and many neutrophils. A culture grew *S. aureus*. The abscess was incised and drained, and he was successfully treated with antibiotics.

This case raises several questions:

1. What was the source of the *S. aureus* in the case of Mr. C.?
2. Should the physician suspect any underlying immune deficiency.
3. What should be suspected if the infection fails to respond to β-lactam antibiotics?

▪ ▪ ▪ ▪

Cutaneous abscesses usually begin as superficial infections in and around hair follicles, called **folliculitis.** Folliculitis is a pustular eruption usually associated with *S. aureus*. In the follicle, bacteria are somewhat sequestered from defense mechanisms and are capable of forming microabscesses. If not controlled, the abscesses enlarge to become **furuncles,** better known as **common boils.** If a

number of boils cluster together to form a large multifocal infection, the lesion is called a **carbuncle** (Fig. 64-4). Furuncles may be a recurring and frustrating problem in some individuals, especially young people who are chronic nasal carriers of virulent *S. aureus*. Although the lesions are confined to the skin, they can be a source of bacteremia and complications.

The pathological processes leading to abscess formation include a massive influx of neutrophils and walling-off of the infected site. That process is caused by deposition of fibrin (fostered by staphylococcal coagulase) and stimulation of fibroblasts to produce a fibrous capsule. The result is a well-organized infection containing necrotic white blood cells and huge numbers of bacteria (i.e., pus). Steps that lead to abscess formation include tissue destruction by the invading organisms and massive release of lysosomal enzymes from lysing neutrophils, as well as the deposition of fibrin (see Chapter 11). The unique physicochemical characteristics of abscesses are discussed in Chapter 30. Therapy of an abscess is usually two-pronged: removal of pus by incision and drainage and, when patients have systemic evidence of infection, treatment with antimicrobial agents.

Necrotizing Soft Tissue Infections

Case

A 57-year-old woman with type II diabetes mellitus, Mrs. S. came to the emergency department slightly feverish after 2 days of pain in her right forefoot. When the pain started, she had noted tenderness and serous (watery) discharge between her third and fourth toes. She had been bothered before by an ulcer on the sole of her foot, apparently caused by constant scraping against her shoe. On physical examination she appeared ill and had a temperature of 39.8°C. Her right foot was swollen with patchy erythema, cyanosis, and signs of necrosis. Crusting and oozing was evident around her third and fourth toes.

Cultures of the exudate and blood were obtained, and Mrs. S. was treated with antibiotics. After 24 hours she showed no clinical improvement, and the infection continued to ascend proximally. She was taken to the operating room, and multiple incisions revealed necrotic fasciitis extending to the upper thigh. As much of the necrotic tissue was removed as possible. Cultures from the wound grew the anaerobic Gram-negative rod *Bacteroides fragilis* and an enteric bacterium, *Enterobacter*. Her blood cultures were negative. Mrs. S. slowly recovered and underwent a second operation for closure of her wound.

This case raises several questions:

1. How does diabetes mellitus predispose to the development of skin infections?
2. Would antibiotics alone have been effective in eradicating this infection?

The case of Mrs. S. illustrates **necrotizing fasciitis,** probably started by the entry of bacteria through the ulcer on the sole of the patient's foot. Persons with diabetes frequently suffer from poor skin circulation and lack of local sensation, which may have been the reason for the development of the ulcer. The infection spread rapidly along the superficial fascia that separates subcutaneous fat and muscle. The vessels and nerves that supply the skin course that fascia, and their destruction leads to the patchy necrosis and cutaneous anesthesia that characterize such a rapidly spreading and dangerous infection.

Although tissue necrosis occurs to some extent in most infections, the term **necrotizing (or gangrenous) infection** is reserved for one in which extensive necrosis is the outstanding characteristic. Mrs. S.'s case illustrates a necrotizing fasciitis caused by multiple bacteria (i.e., polymicrobial). In addition to diabetes, loss of integrity of mucous membranes of the gastrointestinal or genitourinary tract can lead to necrotizing fasciitis of the perineum (Fournier gangrene), which is also caused by mixed aerobic and anaerobic bacteria colonizing those sites. Gas from bacterial metabolism is sometimes found in lesions from Fournier gangrene.

Necrotizing fasciitis can be caused by monomicrobial etiologies, such as group A streptococci, *Vibrio vulnificus,* or *Aeromonas hydrophila.* Necrotizing infection of muscle is called myonecrosis, and when caused by gas-producing *Clostridium* bacteria, *C. perfringens, C. septicum, C. histolyticum,* or *C. sordellii,* the illness is called gas gangrene (see Chapter 20). **Myonecrosis** is also found in about 50% of patients with necrotizing fasciitis caused by group A streptococci. If a necrotizing infection is suspected, the diagnosis should be confirmed by inspection of the fascia and muscle by surgical exploration. Interestingly, Gram stains of wound drainage or debrided tissue show few if any white blood cells but large numbers of bacteria in deep infections caused by clostridia (large Gram-positive rods) and group A streptococci (Gram-positive cocci in chains).

The major factors that predispose to clostridial infection are interruption of the blood supply from penetrating trauma such as crush injury, gunshot wound or stabbing, and contamination of a wound with soil or dirty clothing. Injection of black tar heroin into the skin also has been associated with a variety of skin infections, including necrotizing fasciitis and myonecrosis. Thus, traumatic wounds, particularly those grossly contaminated with dirt, should be meticulously cleansed, debrided, irrigated copiously with normal saline, and left open to heal by secondary intention. Infection can be caused by vegetative bacilli or by endospores that germi-

Sources of Endogenous Skin Infections

DIRECT EXTENSION

- Osteomyelitis: draining sinus
- Septic arthritis: draining sinus
- Lymphadenitis
  - Tuberculosis
  - Atypical mycobacteriosis
  - Streptococcal or staphylococcal infection
- Oral infection: dental sepsis (Ludwig angina)
  - Actinomycosis (lumpy jaw)
  - Mixed cellulitis
- Intra-abdominal: necrotizing infection
- Herpes simplex virus
- Varicella-zoster virus

HEMATOGENOUS SPREAD

- Bacteremia
  - Meningococci
  - Staphylococci
  - *Pseudomonas aeruginosa*
- Endocarditis
- Fungemia: candidiasis
- Viremia
  - Varicella-zoster virus
  - Measles virus
- Rickettsioses
  - Rocky Mountain spotted fever
  - Epidemic or endemic typhus

nate only under anaerobic conditions. Antibiotics are ineffective against spores. Antibiotic treatment alone is rarely successful, probably because of the compromised blood supply; extensive surgical debridement is mandatory. Clostridia produce potent toxins such as hemolysins and phospholipases that cause rapid tissue destruction. Experimental studies suggest that suppression of toxin production by antibiotics that inhibit protein synthesis (e.g., clindamycin and tetracycline) in combination with β-lactam antibiotics is more efficacious treatment than with β-lactam antibiotics alone (see the section on toxic shock syndromes later in this chapter).

Endogenous Infections

The skin can become infected by microorganisms that spread from another infected site, either by direct extension from an underlying focus or through the bloodstream. Such secondary infections occur in both immunocompetent and immunosuppressed hosts but with different degrees of incidence and severity. Some of the types of skin infections that occur from within are listed in the box titled "Sources of Endogenous Skin Infections." Systemic infections are manifested in various ways. **Abscesses** can result from intravascular infections such as endocarditis, particularly when caused by *S. aureus*. **Necrosis** seen in chronic meningococcemia or overwhelming meningococcal septicemia can involve large areas of of the skin. Called **purpura fulminans,** the confluent necrosis is the skin manifestation of disseminated intravascular coagulation (Fig. 64-5). Milder forms of necrosis are also seen, for example, in disseminated gonorrhea.

Immunocompromised hosts like Mr. A. are susceptible to a unique skin lesion called **ecthyma gangrenosum,** usually seen with *P. aeruginosa* septicemia. One of the characteristics of endogenous infection with this organism is arteritis resulting in infarction of the skin from vascular insufficiency. *P. aeruginosa* grows in the infarcted area and causes necrosis by the production of

FIGURE 64-5 ▪ **Purpura caused by disseminated intravascular coagulation.**

Case

Fifty-two-year-old Mr. A. underwent chemotherapy with cytotoxic agents for an aggressive lymphoma. As a result of chemotherapy his white blood cell count fell to fewer than 100/mm³. Suddenly, Mr. A. developed shaking chills and fever and complained of pain over his left shoulder. Examination of the area showed an erythematous round area with a central vesicle (Fig. 64-6). Because of the suspicion of Gram-negative bacteremia, Mr. A. was treated with broad-spectrum antibiotics. Within a few hours the area on the left shoulder developed a necrotic center with surrounding erythema, a lesion known as **ecthyma gangrenosum.** A biopsy of the lesion showed an infarcted blood vessel teeming with bacteria. Cultures of the biopsy material and the blood grew *P. aeruginosa.* Mr. A responded to the antimicrobial therapy with resolution of fever and clearing of the skin lesions.

This case raises several questions:

1. What alteration in host defense most directly contributed to the development of *p. aeruginosa* bacteremia in Mr. A.?
2. What is the pathogenesis of the skin lesions?
3. Why was antibiotic therapy initiated prior to obtaining culture results?

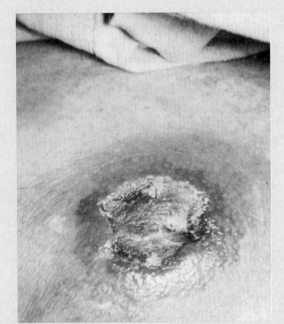

FIGURE 64-6 ▪ Ecthyma gangrenosum, a necrotic skin lesion caused by *Pseudomonas aeruginosa.*

exotoxin A and other toxins (see Chapter 18). In Mr. A.'s case, biopsy of the necrotic area revealed no neutrophil infiltrate because of the patient's granulocytopenia. Instead, infarction of blood vessels by bacterial emboli occurred, with destruction of the arterial wall and bacterial invasion of the surrounding tissues. Besides *P. aeruginosa,* other Gram-negative rods such as *Klebsiella* and *Serratia* species also may be involved, and occasionally *S.*

table **64-2**	**Some Viral Diseases With Cutaneous Manifestations**	
DISEASE	**ETIOLOGICAL AGENT**	**PRINCIPAL CUTANEOUS MANIFESTATION**
Herpes labialis	Herpes simplex virus (most often HSV-1)	Vesicles on the lip ("cold sores")
Herpes genitalis	Herpes simplex virus (most often HSV-2)	Vesicles in the genital area
Herpes zoster	Varicella-zoster virus	Vesicles over specific dermatomes ("shingles")
Chickenpox (varicella)	Varicella-zoster virus	Vesicles, becoming purulent, then dry, crusted lesions
Measles	Measles virus	Maculopapular rash
German measles	Rubella virus	Maculopapular rash
Smallpox (eradicated)	Smallpox virus	Uniform pustular vesicles

aureus can cause these manifestations. Disseminated fungal infections, including those due to *Aspergillus* and *Cryptococcus*, can produce the same characteristic lesions. It is imperative that the physician treat an ecthyma gangrenosum early, before bacteriological confirmation, because the mortality rate in untreated granulocytopenic patients with Gram-negative bacteremia is 50% within 24 hours.

Exanthems, or rashes, are seen in a large variety of infections caused by rickettsiae, other bacteria, and viruses. They are subdivided into hemorrhagic rashes, often accompanied by necrosis (as in meningococcemia; see the box titled "Sources of Endogenous Skin Infections"), and macular (spotted) rashes (as in typhoid fever or Rocky Mountain spotted fever). Rashes prominent in several viral infections, such as measles and rubella, are known as the **viral exanthems** (see Chapter 34 and Table 64-2).

Many cutaneous lesions are themselves **noninfectious** but are secondary to septicemia or other systemic infections. They include hemorrhages, petechiae, and special manifestations of subacute bacterial endocarditis called Osler nodes and Janeway lesions and are caused by vasculitis, probably as a result of deposition of immune complexes (see Chapter 67).

Cutaneous Responses to Bacterial Toxins (Toxic Shock Syndromes and Scarlet Fever)

Case

At the age of 24 years Mr. N. had an operation to repair an inguinal hernia. Five days later he developed shaking chills extremities. He became progressively more ill over the next and a rash on his trunk that rapidly spread to his head and

48 hours, developing a sore throat, headache, myalgias (muscle pains), vomiting, diarrhea, and postural dizziness (dizzy when upright, suggesting low blood pressure). On physical examination Mr. N. had a diffuse rash with some blanching on pressure. His eyes were inflamed with conjunctivitis, and he had an erythematous pharynx and a "strawberry" tongue. His inguinal wound was draining a brown, odorless material.

Laboratory examination revealed a high white blood cell count and elevated serum creatinine value (5.7 mg/dL), indicating acute renal failure. A Gram stain of the material from the wound showed Gram-positive cocci in clusters and grew *S. aureus.* The organism tested positive for the toxic shock syndrome toxin. The patient ultimately showed desquamation of his hands and trunk (Fig. 64-7). He was placed on antibiotics and eventually recovered.

This case raises several questions:

1. What conditions place persons at risk for the development of toxic shock syndrome?
2. What other organisms can produce this disease?
3. How does toxic shock syndrome toxin-1 (TSST-1) cause shock and organ failure?

FIGURE 64-7 ▪ Desquamation of the skin of the palm in a patient with staphylococcal toxic shock syndrome.

The skin responds to toxins elaborated during infections that take place at a distant site. An example is scarlet fever, a pharyngitis caused by certain strains of group A streptococci that elaborate an exotoxin called **erythrogenic factor** or **pyrogenic exotoxin**. The toxin spreads through the bloodstream and is responsible for the red rash familiarly known as strawberry tongue and for desquamation of the skin on the extremities. Scarlet fever used to be a serious disease of childhood; the marked decrease in its severity over the last century has defied explanation.

Staphylococci cause two specific toxin-induced skin diseases: **scalded skin syndrome** and **toxic shock syndrome** (TSS; see Chapter 11). Staphylococcal scalded skin syndrome, a disease of infants, results from the action of a toxin, **exfoliatin,** that separates the epidermis by destroying the intercellular connections (desmosomes). The result resembles skin scalded with hot water.

The case of Mr. N. is a typical clinical presentation of TSS, which is caused by exotoxins produced by certain strains of *S. aureus*. TSS was first described in children in the early 1970s but became widely known in the early 1980s when young menstruating women using "superabsorbent tampons" developed the syndrome. Characteristically, patients develop hypotension, tachycardia, multiorgan dysfunction, and a diffuse red rash resembling sunburn. Patients require aggressive fluid resuscitation to maintain adequate blood pressure. Toxic shock syndrome toxin 1 (TSST-1) has been implicated in menstrual cases. Today tampon-associated TSS is rare, and most cases of TSS are related to the production of enterotoxins, particularly type B, and follow a soft tissue infection, as illustrated in the case of Mr. N.

A similar syndrome also can occur in patients with severe and disseminated *S. pyogenes* infection and is referred to as streptococcal toxic shock syndrome (streptococcal TSS). In contrast to staphylococcal TSS, streptococcal TSS has been associated with necrotizing fasciitis and bacteremia. Interestingly, group A streptococcus produces a myriad of pyrogenic exotoxins which, like staphylococcal TSST-1 and enterotoxins, are superantigens that induce massive cytokine production by both lymphocytes and antigen-presenting cells such as monocytes and macrophages. Antibiotics that inhibit protein synthesis (e.g., clindamycin and tetracycline) shut off toxin production and enhance the efficacy of antibiotics that inhibit bacterial cell wall synthesis in animal models of TSS and in some retrospective clinical reviews.

Methicillin-Resistant *Staphylococcus aureus* Infections

Methicillin-resistant *S. aureus* (MRSA) strains have emerged over the last 30 years in hospitals throughout the world. Since 2000, community-acquired MRSA infections also have dramatically increased in most parts of the world and have been associated with a variety of skin and soft tissue infections, including impetigo, cellulitis, furunculosis, necrotizing soft tissue infections, and TSS. In addition to the general increase in the prevalence of these strains, epidemics of MRSA soft tissue infections have occurred among wrestlers, football players, and prison inmates. Genetic evidence suggests that a higher percentage of MRSA strains possess potent toxins such as TSST-1, enterotoxins, and the Panton-Valentine leukocidin compared with methicillin-susceptible strains. Clearly, empiric treatment of presumed staphylococcal infections of any type may fail if nafcillin, dicloxacillin, or any of the cephalosporins are used. Thus, in patients who have systemic manifestations, or very aggressive soft tissue infections, empiric treatment should include an agent that is reliably active against MRSA, such as vancomycin, linezolid, or daptomycin.

Conclusion

The skin and its underlying soft tissues protect the body from hostile influences in the environment. Traumatic breaks, animal bites, or other skin diseases often facilitate the penetration of these barriers by infectious agents. Microorganisms also may lodge in the skin and soft tissues as the result of hematogenous or lymphatic dissemination. The resulting diseases are extraordinarily varied and are caused by a wide variety of mechanisms. Because of the diverse causes of soft tissue infection, a careful history and physical examination are crucial. Obtaining appropriate samples from aspirates, biopsies, surgical debridement, or blood cultures is essential not only to establish a diagnosis but also to determine the specific susceptibility of the microbes to various antibiotics.

Infections of the Bones, Joints, and Muscles

Jeffrey Parsonnet and Joseph J. Nania

Infections of the bones, joints, and muscles are a diverse collection of diseases that have a number of common features. Organisms with a predilection for these sites vary by the age of the affected individual and share certain virulence determinants. Bone, joint, and muscle infections may develop as a consequence of either hematogenous dissemination or extension from a contiguous site. Complications of these infections can lead to local anatomic compromise and systemic spread. The emergence of antibiotic-resistant bacteria poses new challenges for the treatment of bone, joint, and muscle infections. The pathogenesis of each entity is discussed in this chapter, with an emphasis on microbial etiologies and comorbidities that lead to an increased risk of these infections by certain pathogens.

Bone Infections

Infections of the bones, or **osteomyelitis,** can result from bloodborne infections (hematogenous) or from the direct introduction of microorganisms from external (environmental) or contiguous sources (soft tissues or joints). A special type of infection from contiguous sources occurs in the foot bones of individuals with diabetes. The pathophysiologies of the diseases, the types of infecting agents, and the treatments and prognoses vary among the infections. This chapter discusses both hematogenous and contiguous infections as well as the special cases of bone infection in diabetic patients and chronic osteomyelitis.

Hematogenous Osteomyelitis

PATHOPHYSIOLOGY

Bone has a high rate of synthesis and resorption, two processes that depend on a rich vascular supply. Hematogenous osteomyelitis thus occurs primarily in childhood and adolescence, times in life when long bones are growing rapidly. The most frequent sites of infection are the growing ends, or metaphysis, of long bones, where growth and rapid bone turnover occur. Osteomyelitis is most likely to develop when the bone

Case

O., a 15-year-old boy, received an injury to the lower part of his right thigh in a high school football game. The pain was so intense that he had to leave the game. Although it subsided later that night, the pain returned the next evening, accompanied by chills and a fever to 39.5°C. The following morning O.'s parents took him to the family physician, who noted that O.'s lower right thigh was tender just above the knee. Minimal swelling and erythema were evident in the area of tenderness, and the knee joint was normal with a full range of motion. The physician noted several small boils on O.'s neck and chest. Some were scarred and crusted, and O. admitted to having squeezed them in the past 2 days. Chest radiograph of the right femur showed soft tissue swelling without any abnormalities of the bone.

This case raises several questions:

1. What is the most likely cause of O's infection?
2. How did the bacterium spread to the bone?
3. What are the complications of untreated osteomyelitis?

O. was diagnosed with acute hematogenous osteomyelitis. That diagnosis becomes even more plausible when the pathophysiology of the infection is understood.

Several features of the history and physical examination of the patient point to the diagnosis:

- The trauma to the leg suffered in the football game damaged the distal femur and probably resulted in the rupture of small blood vessels and formation of hematoma or blood clot in the bone. Disruption of the normal anatomical barriers made the bone more susceptible to infection.
- Manipulation of the boils by the patient probably resulted in bacteremia, with *Staphylococcus aureus* being the most likely infecting organism. Bloodborne *S. aureus* could have then seeded the traumatized bone and caused the infection.
- The history of chills and fever, as well as worsening pain and inflammation over the area of trauma, suggests that the patient developed an infection. The normal plain film of the leg did not exclude osteomyelitis because it usually takes several weeks for characteristic radiographic changes in bone to appear (periosteal proliferation or elevation, loss of bone cortex, and bone lysis). A radionuclide bone scan is more likely to be positive early in the disease because the technique measures inflammation, although not infallibly (Fig. 65-1A). Magnetic resonance imaging (MRI), which detects bone marrow edema early in the course of infection, is another useful method as an early diagnostic tool (Fig. 65-1B).

FIGURE 65-1 ■ **Vertebral osteomyelitis in an adult. A.** Radionuclide bone scan shows retention of the tracer in a thoracic vertebra (arrow). Notice also the uptake in the pelvis and hip (also a result of osteomyelitis), the maxilla (caused by a dental abscess), and slight uptake in both shoulders (a result of inflammatory arthritis). The liver and spleen are routinely visualized with this technique. **B.** Magnetic resonance imaging scan of the thoracic spine of the same patient. In the T1 image (left), loss of bony structure in a vertebra is seen (arrow). In the T2 image (right), the high signal intensity owing to water molecules shows edema and infiltrate in the same vertebra.

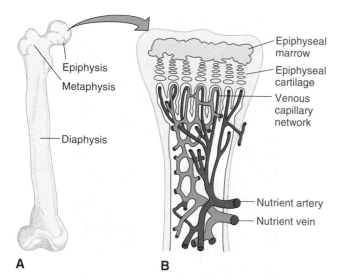

FIGURE 65-2 ▪ **Structure of the femur. A.** Femur showing epiphysis, metaphysis, and diaphysis. **B.** Schematic representation of the vascular supply of a long bone.

has suffered trauma, with resultant disruption of blood vessels and hematoma formation.

The anatomy of the vascular supply of the metaphysis predisposes the area to infection. The capillaries from the nutrient arteries of bone make sharp loops close to the growth plate. They then expand to large sinusoidal vessels that connect with the venous network of the medullary cavity. The sudden increase in the diameter of those vessels slows blood flow and results in sludging of red blood cells (Fig. 65-2). Areas where sludging of blood cells occurs are ideal for the growth of bacteria because microclots form spontaneously in areas of slow blood flow. Clots retain bacteria and shield them from neutrophils, thus allowing the bacteria to proliferate. The result is inflammation, small areas of bone necrosis, and an acidic pH, all of which cause more tissue destruction and more bacterial growth. Endothelial cells in the capillary loops and sinusoids in the bone lack phagocytic properties, which also predisposes those areas to infection. In adults, hematogenous osteomyelitis often starts at the intervertebral disc, which has a rich blood supply, and spreads to adjacent vertebral bodies (see Fig. 65-1); trauma also often precedes this type of infection.

DIAGNOSIS AND TREATMENT

In the case of O., local pain and the presence of systemic signs of infection suggested a serious disease, acute osteomyelitis, which usually calls for admission to the hospital for administration of parenteral antibiotics and often demands surgical drainage. Blood cultures, which are positive in about one third of patients, should be obtained. When possible, a bone aspirate of the site of suspected infection should be attempted. The

procedure has the potential to both make a microbiologic diagnosis and evaluate the need for immediate surgery to drain a bony abscess, as would be indicated by yield of frank pus from needle aspiration. With culture of both blood and material obtained from direct tissue sampling, the infecting organism is isolated in as many as 90% of cases.

Treatment should be initiated with antibiotics after obtaining cultures but before the return of results. Because about 90% of patients with this clinical presentation are infected with *S. aureus* (including children previously vaccinated against *Haemophilus influenzae*), a β-lactamase–resistant penicillin (such as nafcillin or oxacillin) or a first-generation cephalosporin (such as cefazolin) has historically been the treatment of choice. However, in places where methicillin-resistant *S. aureus* has become a common community-acquired pathogen, it is advisable to use vancomycin instead of, or in addition to, a β-lactam antibiotic until culture and sensitivity results are available.

In some circumstances hematogenous osteomyelitis is more likely to be caused by an organism other than *S. aureus* (Table 65-1). For example, *Salmonella* species often cause infection in children with sickle cell disease; *Pseudomonas aeruginosa*, *Candida albicans*, and oral flora in injection drug users; and *Escherichia coli* and enterococci in adults with urinary tract obstruction. In such cases, or when blood cultures are negative and the patient does not respond appropriately to initial therapy, aspiration or biopsy of bone for culture is important to guide definitive antibiotic therapy.

Treatment of acute hematogenous osteomyelitis requires high doses of antibiotics, usually administered parenterally, and long courses of therapy, traditionally in the range of 4 to 6 weeks. High serum levels of antibiotic are necessary to penetrate bone tissue, including areas of infection-induced necrotic bone that shield bacteria from host defenses. Outpatient administration of

table **65-1**	**Some Predisposing Causes and Etiologic Organisms Leading to Osteomyelitis**
PREDISPOSING CAUSES	**ETIOLOGIC ORGANISMS**
Infancy	Group B streptococci
Unvaccinated child	*Haemophilus influenzae*
Sickle cell disease	*Salmonella* spp.
Immunosuppression	Opportunistic fungi, *Nocardia* spp., *Pseudomonas* spp.
Residing in an endemic area	*Coccidioides immitis*, *Histoplasma capsulatum*
Trauma to the jaw	*Actinomyces israelii*
Animal exposure	*Bartonella henselae*, *Brucella* spp.
Pulmonary tuberculosis	*Mycobacterium tuberculosis*

parenteral therapy has become a common practice that has been facilitated by the use of antibiotics with long serum half-lives (such as ceftriaxone), employment of peripherally inserted central catheters (PICC lines), and increasing experience with and financial incentives for the therapeutic approach. In addition, studies have demonstrated that many children with hematogenous osteomyelitis can be successfully treated with an abbreviated course of parenteral therapy followed by high doses of an oral agent, presumably because of the excellent blood supply to the area of infection. However, such patients must be selected carefully and followed closely, preferably by someone with expertise in the practice.

If appropriate treatment is initiated early in the course of infection, before significant bone necrosis occurs, patients usually respond quickly, and cure can be achieved in more than 90% of cases. If fever and pain continue for longer than 48 hours after initiation of treatment, surgical drainage of a subperiosteal collection or soft tissue abscess may be required. Computerized tomography (CT) scans are useful in demonstrating focal collections and in guiding the surgeon's hand should drainage be necessary. Persistent fever also may suggest a metastatic focus of infection, such as endocarditis or a visceral abscess.

Hematogenous Osteomyelitis at Various Ages

Infants

The clinical presentation of hematogenous osteomyelitis depends a great deal on the age of the patient. Osteomyelitis in an infant most commonly begins at the metaphysis of a long bone. The bones of an infant are soft, and the periosteum is loosely attached to the cortex. Therefore, infection originating in medullary bone can easily spread and rupture through the thin cortex into the subperiosteal space. Subperiosteal abscesses are common in this age group and lead to a stimulation of periosteal bone formation at an inappropriate site, as periosteal cells transform into osteoblasts. The new bone formation is disorganized and produces a weakened bone called an **involucrum** (Fig. 65-3).

Osteomyelitis in an infant can be a devastating disease because early in life the capillaries of the metaphysis extend into the epiphyseal growth plate. Infection can spread by that route into the epiphysis and adversely affect growth of the bone. Consequently, osteomyelitis in an infant can be a destructive process resulting in permanent deformity of bone and abnormalities of growth (Fig. 65-4).

Children

In children between the age of 1 year and puberty, bone infection also occurs most frequently in long bones but is generally contained within the metaphysis because

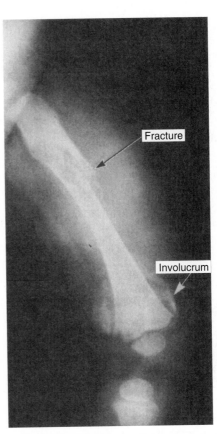

FIGURE 65-3 ▪ Involucrum secondary to extensive periosteal reaction and fracture caused by weakened infected bone.

the cortex is thicker than that of infants and no vessels connect the metaphysis and the epiphysis. Also, the periosteum adheres more tightly to the cortex in this age group; thus, rupture of infection into the subperiosteal space and formation of involucrum is less likely. However, within the bone itself, pressure can increase and cause occlusion of arterioles and clot formation in the capillaries. The end result is often necrosis of bone, and

FIGURE 65-4 ▪ Deformity resulting from pathological fracture secondary to osteomyelitis.

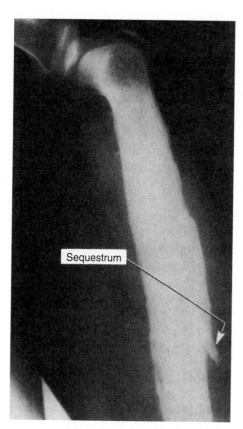

FIGURE 65-5 ■ Radiograph showing changes in more advanced osteomyelitis with extensive bone lesions. A sequestrum is indicated.

in advanced cases a sequestrum can form (Fig. 65-5). Tissue in a sequestrum is no longer in contact with the vasculature and acts essentially as a foreign body in which organisms can proliferate out of reach of both host defenses and antibiotics. Ultimately, the sequestrum must be resorbed (by the body) or removed surgically if the infection is to be cured. As children age, this complication is even more likely because the bone is more calcified and the periosteum even more tightly attached to bone.

Adults

Hematogenous osteomyelitis seen in adults most frequently involves the vertebral bodies. The reason for that predilection is uncertain but may stem from degenerative bony changes and vascular proliferation in the disc space between the vertebrae, which normally occur with age. The infection usually begins in the disc space and then spreads to the contiguous vertebrae; the radiographic finding of an abnormal disc space with erosion of the adjacent vertebral plates is highly suggestive of infection rather than malignancy (see Fig. 11-2). Frequent complications of vertebral osteomyelitis are spinal epidural abscess, which, if not treated appropriately, can cause irreversible loss of neurologic function, and psoas abscess, which often requires surgical drainage for cure.

S. aureus is the most common cause of vertebral osteomyelitis (presumably resulting from bacteremia from a cutaneous source), but enteric Gram-negative bacteria, viridans streptococci, *Mycobacterium tuberculosis,* and enterococci are also common etiologic agents. These organisms may seed the disc space and adjacent vertebrae by hematogenous spread from primary infection in the bowel, gallbladder, or urinary tract, especially among persons over the age of 60 years with diverticular disease, obstructive uropathy, or other predisposing processes. Infection of vertebrae can also result from drainage of infected pelvic organs through pelvic veins into the complex, interconnected venous networks surrounding the spinal column known as Batson plexus.

Because the possible causes of vertebral osteomyelitis are numerous, it is imperative to obtain material from the infected area for culture (unless blood cultures already have yielded causal organisms). This usually can be accomplished by closed aspiration or needle biopsy of the disc space under the guidance of fluoroscopy or a CT scan. Vertebral osteomyelitis usually responds to medical therapy alone, but the neurologic status of the patient must be monitored closely because infection can spread from the vertebral body into the subdural or subarachnoid space through the rich venous and arterial plexus of the paravertebral circulation. The development of sensory or motor changes requires urgent surgical drainage to prevent irreversible neurologic damage.

Osteomyelitis Secondary to Contiguous Foci of Infection

Bone infection can result from the direct introduction of microorganisms from an external source or spread from a contiguous source. Penetrating trauma is an obvious cause of this type of infection. An additional common setting for contiguous bone infection is following insertion of orthopedic hardware, such as a joint prosthesis or bone fixation device (Fig. 65-6). These infections are difficult to eradicate because the bone has been traumatized (reducing the effectiveness of host defenses), and the foreign body acts as an avascular sanctuary for the persistence of bacteria. Bacteria, especially staphylococci, can grow and reside in biofilms on the surface of foreign bodies and are thus sheltered from antibiotics.

In the face of active infection, deciding whether to remove a fixation device or joint prosthesis to facilitate cure is often difficult and emotionally traumatic. On one hand, such a device may be necessary to achieve bony union or to allow ambulation or proper joint function; on the other hand, its presence may prevent cure of the infection. In some infections involving orthopedic prostheses, the devices can be salvaged, especially if the infection is caught early, the organism is exquisitely susceptible to antibiotics (as are streptococci), and there has not been loosening of the prosthesis. However, infections caused by *S. aureus,* Gram-negative bacilli, or fungi

FIGURE 65-6 ▪ Osteomyelitis in bone with a prosthetic fixation device.

are infrequently cured without removal of the devices. Treatment decisions require close interactions between surgeons and internists (or pediatricians) to determine if and when removal is necessary and in the best overall interest of the patient.

S. aureus is the organism that most commonly causes contiguous osteomyelitis, but the presence of a foreign body and the disruption of host defenses predispose to infection with other bacteria that are normally less pathogenic. The identity of the pathogen often reflects the circumstances of the trauma and the part of the body involved. Contamination of a wound by dirt or water often leads to infection with Gram-negative bacteria, including *P. aeruginosa*, whereas postoperative infections are frequently caused by *S. aureus*, the prototypical nosocomial pathogen. A wound may become contaminated with bacteria that are constituents of fecal flora, particularly in an incontinent patient with a hip fracture. Coagulase-negative staphylococci are more likely to cause infections in the presence of a prosthesis.

Osteomyelitis in Persons with Diabetes

A special category of osteomyelitis occurs in persons with diabetes as a consequence of the large vessel and microvascular disease and neuropathy that frequently complicate the condition. Skin and soft tissue ulcerations on the feet may go unnoticed because of sensory neuropathy, persist because of impaired host defenses, and ultimately penetrate into bone. The bone infections

are more likely than others to be polymicrobial in nature. *S. aureus*, streptococci, enterococci, and Gram-negative bacteria are common pathogens, and anaerobic bacteria may be involved as well because of poorly oxygenated and necrotic tissue.

Bone infections in diabetic patients are especially difficult to treat owing to the poor vascular supply to necrotic bone. The most important determinant of successful therapy is adequate debridement of necrotic bone and soft tissue, with antibiotics serving an adjunctive role. It is especially important to determine the bacterial etiology of the infections because of the frequent involvement of inherently resistant organisms such as enterococci and *P. aeruginosa*. Results of surface cultures correlate poorly with those taken from bone and deep tissue and should not be relied on. In the absence of definitive culture results from bone or deep tissues, antibiotics must target a wide range of Gram-positive and Gram-negative bacteria, including anaerobic bacteria. Unfortunately, amputation is frequently the result of what may have started out as a trivial soft tissue infection of the foot, in spite of appropriate surgical and medical management. Good foot care is essential in preventing foot infections in diabetic patients.

Chronic Osteomyelitis

An important complication of untreated acute osteomyelitis is chronic osteomyelitis. Chronic osteomyelitis can remain dormant, and affected patients can be asymptomatic for years or even decades. Exacerbations are often associated with purulent drainage from a fistulous tract to the skin and may be accompanied by worsening pain, fever, and elevations in C-reactive protein and erythrocyte sedimentation rate. Antibiotic therapy often results in resolution of such episodes, and patients generally feel entirely well between them. Over time, however, chronic osteomyelitis can cause progressive bone destruction. Thorough debridement of infected and necrotic bone along with adjunctive, often lifelong therapy may result in cure or prolonged suppression of the infection.

Joint Infections
PATHOPHYSIOLOGY

A swollen, red, warm, painful joint in a patient with fever raises the question of septic arthritis. In evaluating a patient presenting with a joint in that condition, the physician must make three determinations. The first question is whether the joint inflammation is the result of infection. Noninfectious inflammatory joint disease can be caused by gout, pseudogout, rheumatoid arthritis or other connective tissue diseases, or viral infection, and these entities may be difficult to distinguish clinically from a bacterial process. Second, the physician must determine the pathophysiology of the infections process. As with osteomyelitis, a joint can be seeded during the course of bacteremia from another primary focus, bacteria can be introduced directly into the joint by trauma or a surgical procedure, or bacteria can extend into the joint space from adjacent bone. Third, the physician must identify the infecting organism. Usually, a physician can make all three determinations by obtaining a complete history, performing a careful physical examination, and analyzing fluid obtained by aspiration of the joint. The diagnosis of infection is supported by the finding of numerous white blood cells, predominantly neutrophils, in joint fluid, a positive Gram stain or culture of the fluid, and an absence of other potential causes for inflammation, such as crystals.

Synovial fluid consists of water, electrolytes, and other low molecular weight substances filtered from plasma, as well as components synthesized and secreted by synovial cells. Serum proteins are present in normal synovial fluid but in lower concentrations than in plasma. Because fibrinogen is absent, normal synovial fluid does not clot. The inflammatory reaction in synovial fluid is caused by the interaction of serum proteins, phagocytic host cells, and microorganisms.

It is important to recognize that the diagnosis of one type of joint disease does not preclude the presence of a second. Therefore, a joint deformed by arthritis can become infected with bacteria, particularly if that joint has recently been operated on or if steroids have been injected into it. The key to understanding the disease process is to obtain joint fluid for analysis and culture.

Infections of the joints can be caused by viruses, bacteria, and fungi. These possibilities can be differentiated by the clinical presentation of the patient and by the results of laboratory tests of the joint fluid. In general, bacterial infections are more common than the other types of infections and produce a higher number of white blood cells in the joint fluid, with a predominance of neutrophils. The frequency with which specific bacterial agents cause septic arthritis varies with age. Again, *S. aureus* is the most common overall cause and affects all age groups. *H. influenzae* type B, formerly the most frequent cause in children between the ages of 6 months and 3 years, has become uncommon since the introduction in 1988 of an effective vaccine for the bacterium. In children less than 2 years of age, *Kingella kingae,* an oral commensal, is a frequent cause of septic arthritis. However, it is much more common in some areas of the world than in others. The gonococcus is the leading cause of septic arthritis in sexually active adults and accounts for 30 to 50% of hospital admissions for this diagnosis in adults less than 30 years of age.

The etiologic organism causing septic arthritis can be identified by Gram stain and culture of joint fluid. Even if the Gram stain is negative, antibiotic treatment should be started immediately after joint fluid and blood are obtained for culture to prevent continued infection and destruction of the structures in the joint. The relative frequencies in which organisms infect certain age groups are listed in Table 65-2.

Some organisms, like *Neisseria gonorrhea, S. aureus,* streptococci, and several spirochetes have an unusual tropism for the joints. The reason for that predilection is unknown.

table 65-2 Most Frequent Causes of Bacterial Arthritis by Age

ORGANISM	NEONATES	CHILDREN 2 MONTHS TO 2 YEARS	CHILDREN 3–10 YEARS	ADULTS
Staphylococcus aureus	10–25%	25–50%	25–50%	25–75%
Streptococcus spp. (group A, viridans, microaerophilic, anaerobic, S. pneumoniae)	1–10%	10–25%	10–25%	10–25%
Group B streptococci	10–25%	Rare	Rare	1–10%
Kingella kingae	Rare	1–40%	Rare	Rare
Haemophilus influenzae type B[a]	Rare	Rare	Rare	Rare
Neisseria spp.	Rare	1–10%	10–25%	10–25%[b]
Gram-negative bacilli	5–15%	1–10%	1–10%	1–10%
Anaerobes	Rare	Rare	Rare	Rare
Other	1–10%	Rare	1–10%	Rare

[a] Occurs only in unvaccinated or undervaccinated children.
[b] Generally, adults less than 30 years of age.

TREATMENT

In addition to appropriate high-dose antibiotic therapy given parenterally, the infected synovial fluid should be drained. Drainage can be performed by repeated aspirations or by open surgical drainage. Usually, aspiration is attempted first, and surgery is used only when aspiration fails. Open drainage is always performed in septic arthritis of the hip joint and is required to prevent necrosis of the head of the femur, which can result because the blood supply to that part of the bone is tenuous. Unlike osteomyelitis treatment, in which antibiotic levels achieved in infected bone are low, treatment of septic arthritis is facilitated by the ability of most antibiotics to penetrate synovial fluid well and efflux slowly back into serum, resulting in synovial fluid concentrations of drug that exceed serum levels. Therefore, after patients with septic arthritis respond clinically to drainage and parenteral antibiotics, it is common practice to complete therapy with an equivalent oral agent. Total length of treatment for septic arthritis is generally 3 to 4 weeks.

Muscle Infections
PATHOPHYSIOLOGY

All of us have experienced the muscle aches and stiffness (myalgia) that commonly occur when we have a viral illness ("the flu"). In fact, myalgias are prominent features of a variety of infections, including viral illnesses, rickettsial infections, and even osteomyelitis and bacterial endocarditis. Fever is often accompanied by muscle pains or myalgias. Infecting organisms are rarely directly involved in myalgias. More often, muscle involvement is indirect, probably because of the accelerated catabolism of skeletal muscle, part of the so-called acute phase response that accompanies sepsis and trauma. Catabolism is probably mediated by several products of macrophages (monokines), including interleukin 1 and tumor necrosis factor. The systemic symptoms resulting from macrophage products are mediated by the increased synthesis of prostaglandin E2, which in turn activates muscle proteases. Interleukin-1 and tumor necrosis factor also act on the hypothalamus, resulting in the production of fever. These events explain why inhibitors of prostaglandin synthesis, like aspirin, help resolve both fever and muscle aches.

SPECIFIC MUSCLE INFECTIONS

Several of the more common causes of infectious myositis and their specific clinical presentations are listed in Table 65-3. Specific infections of skeletal muscle are unusual. When myositis does occur it may be the result of one of a wide variety of organisms that includes viruses, bacteria, fungi, and parasitic agents. Muscles may be invaded either from contiguous sites of infection or by hematogenous spread from a distant focus. The kinds of infection and their frequency depend on the host, geographic area, and dietary history.

Clinical presentations of some types of muscle infections are so distinctive that they readily suggest the etiologic agent. For example, crepitus, the physical sign that indicates the presence of gas in muscle, suggests gas gangrene secondary to *Clostridium perfringens*. Generalized muscle pain and peripheral eosinophilia in a patient who has eaten undercooked pork should raise the possibility of trichinosis.

table **65-3**	**Pathogenesis of Muscle Infections**	
PATHOGENESIS	**CLINICAL PRESENTATION**	**PRINCIPAL ETIOLOGIES**
Localized and spread from a contiguous site	Gas gangrene	*Clostridium perfringens*, occasionally other clostridial species
	Synergistic myositis or gangrene	Mixed infections with anaerobic bacteria and enteric bacteria
	Muscle abscesses	*Staphylococcus aureus*, group A streptococci
	Gram-negative bacteria	
	Miscellaneous	*Actinomyces* spp., *Nocardia* spp., *Mycobacterium* spp., fungi
Hematogenous spread	Bacterial	Groups A and B streptococci, *S. aureus*, Gram-negative bacteria
	Fungal	*Aspergillus* spp., *Candida* spp., *Coccidioides immitis*, *Histoplasma capsulatum*
	Mycobacterial	*Mycobacterium tuberculosis*, nontuberculous mycobacteria
	Parasitic	*Dracunculus medinensis*, *Trichinella spiralis*
	Viral	Coxsackievirus, echovirus

TREATMENT

Therapy of nonspecific myalgia is usually symptomatic. When a specific etiologic agent is identified, therapy should be directed toward eradication of the organism. Prompt drainage of abscesses and extensive surgical debridement may be necessary if necrotic tissue is present.

Conclusion

Infections of the musculoskeletal system occur at all ages as a result of invasion of microorganisms from contiguous tissues, the bloodstream, or external sources. Although pain and constitutional symptoms are relatively nonspecific complaints of many ill patients, the presence of focal pain in a febrile patient should raise suspicion of an infection involving a bone, joint, or muscle. Careful physical examination in such patients will often reveal swelling, warmth, erythema, or reproducible pain of the musculoskeletal tissues. Radiologic studies are often helpful in supporting the diagnosis, and aspiration of affected sites is generally indicated to make a specific microbiologic diagnosis. Given the need for urgent treatment before culture results are available, knowledge of the organisms commonly found at specific sites of infection and in various patient age groups is essential to guide the initiation of therapy.

Sepsis

Suzanne F. Bradley

Despite improvements in antibiotic therapy, sepsis remains the leading cause of death among critically ill patients. Of the 750,000 cases of sepsis diagnosed in the United States annually, almost one third die. The following cases illustrate the different responses of two hosts to a disseminated infection.

DEFINITION

Sepsis is an ancient Greek word meaning, roughly, "putrefaction." Today sepsis is a general clinical term that describes signs and symptoms of a generalized and often uncontrolled inflammatory response. An infection can remain localized or begin to disseminate with signs of generalized infection such as fever, abnormal white blood cell count, and abnormal clinical symptoms and signs. A classification scheme has been developed to characterize the various progressive stages of this generalized inflammatory response from **systemic inflammatory response syndrome (SIRS)** to **sepsis, severe sepsis, septic shock,** and **multiorgan dysfunction syndrome (MODS)**. This classification reflects a progressive worsening of symptoms, inflammatory signs, and organ failure that frequently result in death (see the box titled "Clinical Syndromes Associated With Disseminated Infection").

A generalized and abnormal inflammatory state can also occur in response to massive tissue injury and necrosis (burns) or owing to drugs or chemical reactions. SIRS is generally referred to as sepsis when infection is the presumed or identified as the cause.

ETIOLOGY

The presence of bacteria in the bloodstream (**bacteremia**) is the most common cause of sepsis, but **fungemia, viremia, parasitemia,** and microbial toxins also can lead to the inflammatory response. Localized infections of the skin and the urinary, respiratory, and gastrointestinal tracts are the most frequent sources of bloodstream infection (**secondary bloodstream infection**). Occasionally, patients have bacteremia without an obvious source (**primary bloodstream infection**).

All bloodstream infections do not lead to a generalized inflammatory response or sepsis. Asymptomatic and transient low-grade bacteremia occurs in all of us on a daily basis following minor mucosal damage caused by toothbrushing or defecation, but those organisms are rapidly removed from the circulation and rarely ever cause

Case

Infection from a Wound

Mr. D., a 48-year-old farmer, cut his thumb while working. The next morning the thumb was sore and the skin surrounding the cut was red. Nevertheless, Mr. D. worked around the farm as usual and did not return home until well after dark. By that time his thumb was swollen and throbbing, and some yellow–white pus was oozing out. Mr. D. noticed two red streaks going up the inside of his forearm, and he suddenly had a shaking chill and felt queasy. His wife drove him 17 miles to the county hospital. When they arrived at the emergency department Mr. D.'s temperature was 39.7°C. He was flushed and ill appearing, his pulse was 125 beats per minute, and his blood pressure was 100/60 mm Hg, much lower than his usual of 145/85 mm Hg. Blood cultures were drawn, and Mr. D. was started on intravenous fluids and an antibiotic active against staphylococci and streptococci. By morning he was somewhat better, and by the following day his symptoms had disappeared. His subsequent recovery and wound healing were uneventful. The blood cultures were found to be positive for *Staphylococcus aureus* on the second day of his illness.

Case

Postsurgery Infection

At 59 years of age Mrs. J. underwent extensive pelvic surgery to remove a cervical carcinoma, including removal of all pelvic organs, removal of a segment of ileum to construct a new bladder, and a colostomy. At first she seemed to be recovering well. During the evening of the third postoperative day, the nurse on the evening shift noticed that Mrs. J.'s respiratory rate, which had been 16 to 18 breaths per minute, was 26. Mrs. J. said she did feel sick. She was not short of breath or in much pain, and her temperature was actually subnormal at 36.2°C.

The next morning Mrs. J. had some fever, 38.3°C, but she continued to feel fairly well. Her wound showed no sign of infection, and her abdomen was no more tender than expected. That afternoon, however, Mrs. J. was clearly in trouble. She was flushed, anxious, and restless; her blood pressure was down from 135/75 to 105/58 mm Hg and her temperature was 39.2°. Blood cultures were drawn, antibiotics were started, and intravenous fluids were infused rapidly, which brought her blood pressure up. Nevertheless, Mrs. J.'s condition worsened. The following morning, she was short of breath and had excess fluid throughout her lungs. Intravenous fluids were cut back, and a vasopressor was required to maintain her blood pressure. She was moved to the intensive care unit for monitoring. To better assess her hemodynamic status, the superior vena cava and one pulmonary artery were catheterized (the latter through the

jugular vein, right atrium, and right ventricle). Mrs. J. was found to have a cardiac output nearly double the normal for a resting adult of her size. However, her systemic vascular resistance was extremely low, which accounted for her low blood pressure despite the high cardiac output.

Over the next 24 hours Mrs. J. continued to do poorly; her urine output dropped to nearly zero, and she required mechanical ventilation to maintain oxygenation. The surgeon decided that reexploration was warranted because of persistent sepsis in the presence of broad-spectrum antimicrobial therapy. At surgery, the suture line attaching the ileum to the colon was found to be partially disrupted, with leakage of bowel contents, intense inflammation of the mesentery, and early abscess formation. Appropriate repairs were made and drains inserted. Thereafter, Mrs. J. recovered slowly but completely. The blood cultures remained sterile.

These cases raise two questions:

1. How did Mr. D.'s clinical course differ from that of Mrs. J., and why was his response to infection less severe?
2. Why was an infecting organism not isolated from Mrs. J.?

us any harm. Why then does sepsis occur in some settings but not in others? The answer is that the risk of sepsis is complex and involves both microbial virulence factors and patient risk factors. Any microbe can lead to a systemic inflammatory response if it is present in the bloodstream in high enough numbers (**inoculum effect**). Some pathogens can cause sepsis more readily at low inoculum because they have virulence factors that facilitate host invasion and dissemination of infection (*Streptococcus pyogenes*), provoke an intense inflammatory response (pneumococci), or produce microbial toxins. The following defects in host defenses are also major risk factors for disseminated infection and sepsis:

- **Disruption or penetration of intact skin and mucosa:** Penetration by trauma or devices, necrosis resulting from impairment of the blood supply, and medications can disrupt mucocutaneous barriers. Drugs (chemotherapy) that damage rapidly dividing mucosal cells lining the mouth and gastrointestinal tract can lead to ulcerations that form a portal of entry for pathogens. Necrotic tissue has no blood supply and serves as a rich culture medium. Lack of blood supply to tissues also impedes the ability of phagocytes, antibody, and complement to defend against invasion.

- **Granulocytopenia and defective granulocyte function:** Neutrophils are the first line of defense against many bacteria as well as many fungi. Granulocytopenia that occurs following chemotherapy predisposes patients to many infections from their own normal flora (**endogenous infections**) or, less often, from

Clinical Syndromes Associated With Disseminated Infection

Systemic inflammatory response syndrome (SIRS)	Defined as having two or more of the following: Fever Elevated or low white blood cell count (leukocytosis or leukopenia) Elevated heart rate (tachycardia) Elevated respiratory rate (tachypnea)
Sepsis Severe sepsis	SIRS, as defined above, plus confirmed infection SIRS, as defined above, plus low blood pressure (hypotension) Corrected by administration of fluids
Septic shock	SIRS, as defined above, plus persistent hypotension Aggressive fluid resuscitation not effective Drugs to increase vascular tone required
Multiorgan dysfunction syndrome (MODS)	SIRS, as defined above, plus persistent hypotension leading to the following: Evidence of clotting disorders or failure of renal, hepatic, cardiac, or cognitive function Accumulation of products of metabolism that cannot be cleared (e.g., lactic acidosis)

the environment (**exogenous infection**). In poorly controlled diabetes the number of granulocytes is normal, but adherence, chemotaxis, ingestion, oxidative burst, and killing are all impaired.

- **Complement defects:** Homozygous deficiencies in classical pathway components and in C3 are associated with bacteremia and sepsis in some affected patients. A rare defect in the alternative pathway, properdin deficiency, predisposes to fulminant sepsis with Neisseria meningitidis. Deficiencies in late components (C5 through C9) also create a susceptibility to neisserial infections, but those infections are apt to be less severe. Cirrhosis and severe burn injury are complement-deficient states because of decreased syntheses and increased complement; the result is impaired neutrophil chemotaxis. Premature infants comprise another complement-deficient group of patients with an increased incidence of sepsis.
- **Immune defects:** Loss of opsonic and bactericidal antibodies (humoral defects) and loss of the ability to activate macrophages in response to specific antigenic stimuli (cellular defects) predispose to sepsis. Humoral immune defects, as seen in B-cell malignancies; protein-losing states, as in burns; and the late stages of AIDS are particularly associated with bacterial infections, including sepsis.
- **Splenic malfunction or absence:** Loss of the spleen creates a humoral immunodeficiency, particularly in primary antibody responses. Additionally, without the

spleen the body's ability to clear encapsulated bacteria from the blood is impaired. A person lacking a functioning spleen is susceptible to fulminant sepsis caused by bacteria such as *Streptococcus pneumoniae, Haemophilus influenzae,* and N. meningitidis. That person would have to be immunized and warned to seek emergent medical attention at the first sign of illness. Some people without a functioning spleen take antibiotics on a long-term basis in the hope of preventing an episode of severe infection.

- **Genetic predisposition:** Studies in mice and humans suggest that minor changes in some genes (genetic polymorphisms) may explain why some hosts are more susceptible to sepsis than others.

SPREAD AND MULTIPLICATION

Host Response: A Delicate Balance

Following the introduction of infection, high levels of **proinflammatory cytokines**—typically, **tumor necrosis factor-α (TNF-α)** and **interleukin 1 (IL-1)**, IL-6, and IL-8, among others—are rapidly released, often within minutes. The proinflammatory cytokines are produced primarily by the **cellular innate immune system.** Secondary stimulation and release of other inflammatory mediators, like cytokines, **prostaglandins, leukotrienes, toxic oxygen products, adhesion proteins,** and **proteases,** occurs so rapidly that it is often difficult to discern what factor is contributing to damage of tissues. Rapid activation of **plasma protein systems,** including the complement and coagulation cascades and the **kallikrein-kinin system,** also ensues.

In the absence of an inflammatory response, the patient dies of overwhelming infection. However, an unopposed inflammatory process can also be detrimental. Fortunately, a **compensatory anti-inflammatory response syndrome (CARS)** typically occurs, leading to increased levels of **anti-inflammatory cytokines** (e.g., IL-4, IL-10, IL-11, **transforming growth factor-β**). The levels of other anti-inflammatory factors, such as soluble TNF-receptors and IL-1 receptor antagonists, and stress hormones also rise in response to the inflammatory response.

In severe sepsis, septic shock, and MODS, the delicate balance of proinflammatory and anti-inflammatory responses is dysregulated. Until recently, it was thought that excessive proinflammatory cytokine was the sole cause of severe symptoms and signs, multiorgan system failure, and death. Now it appears that an unopposed anti-inflammatory response may also play a detrimental role late in sepsis. Leukocytes of septic patients are hyporesponsive to infectious stimuli and in a state of excessive immunosuppression. Thus, patients with sepsis are at risk of acquiring secondary nosocomial infection.

Stimulation of Inflammatory Mediators

All infectious agents do not have the same ability to cause sepsis. Components of the cell walls of various microbes have varying abilities to stimulate the production of proinflammatory cytokine production. The cell wall components of Gram-negative bacilli, **lipopolysaccharide (LPS)** or **lipid A,** are among the most potent stimulators of cytokines. It is therefore not surprising that those organisms are closely associated with septic shock. Less potent stimulators of cytokines have been found in the cell walls of Gram-positive bacteria (**lipoteichoic acid, peptidoglycan**), mycobacteria (**lipoarabinomannan**), and fungi (**mannan**).

To understand how microbes and their components interact with the innate immune system, initial interest was focused on LPS. It was discovered that LPS shed from Gram-negative bacteria into the circulation binds to an **LPS-binding protein** that isolates individual LPS molecules from complexes, permitting them to be presented to a cellular receptor. The identification of the LPS receptor **CD14** on macrophages, dendritic cells, and neutrophils was initially thought to explain how those cells might generate proinflammatory cytokines in response to infection with Gram-negative bacilli. However, it is now known that CD14 forms a receptor complex with one of a class of signal transduction molecules known as **pattern recognition receptors.**

Pattern recognition receptors were first identified in fruit flies and called **toll receptors.** When similar molecules were identified in mammals, they were termed **toll-like receptors (TLRs).** The receptor for LPS is now thought to consist of a complex of CD14, TLR4, and at least one other cellular protein.

The characterization of numerous other TLRs have begun to explain how various microbes and even drugs and tissue necrosis can lead to stimulation of cytokines and sepsis by different components of the innate immune system (Table 66-1). Generalizations are difficult because considerable overlap exists among TLRs, their ligands, and various pathogens. However, LPS and Gram-negative bacteria are primarily recognized by TLR4, and Gram-positive bacterial components and yeast by TLR2. After binding of microbial ligands to TLRs, intracellular signaling occurs through pathways similar to those used by cytokine receptors, eventually leading to an activation of **nuclear factor κB,** cytokine production, and release. Another possible reaction is cytokine release by T cells following the nonspecific binding of superantigens—for example, toxic shock syndrome toxin 1, streptococcal pyrogenic exotoxins, and staphylococcal enterotoxins—with cells presenting the positive-sense major histocompatibility complex class II. Recent discovery of TLR mutations and genetic polymorphisms for TNF-α and other cytokines may explain why some patients develop sepsis following infection and others do not.

DAMAGE

Elucidating the secondary effects of the proinflammatory mediators is complex. It is not always clear whether a given mediator produces its toxic effects directly or through additional mediators. Some of the mediators of sepsis and their effects are shown in Table 66-2. The two most common physiologic effects are **capillary leak** and **hypotension,** which account for many of the clinical findings seen in the septic patient (Fig. 66-1). Hypotension, which is caused by vascular and cardiac factors, leads to dysfunction, necrosis, and failure of other vital organs (brain, lungs, kidney, liver, and gastrointestinal tract) and accumulation of toxic metabolites (**lactic acidosis**).

The impact that sepsis has on the body is summarized in this list:

- **Vasculature:** Early dilation of blood vessels in response to the infection (decreased **systemic vascular resistance**) and leakage of fluids from blood vessels into extravascular tissues contribute to decline in blood pressure and increased cardiac work.
- **Heart:** Infection can directly affect the ability of the heart to function as a pump by depressing **myocardial contractility.** Eventually, **stroke volume** is decreased to

table 66-1 Toll-Like Receptors and Their Ligands

RECEPTOR	CELL TYPE EXPRESSING TOLL-LIKE RECEPTORS	ORIGIN/RECEPTOR LIGAND
TLR1	All cells	Works in concert with TLR2, bacteria, lipoproteins, lipopeptides, *Neisseria* species, soluble factor
TLR2	Monocytes, dendritic and NK cells	See TLR1, TLR6, TLR10
TLR3	Dendritic and NK cells	Viral RNA (double stranded)
TLR4	Macrophages, dendritic cells, endothelial cells	Works in concert with CD14, Gram-negative bacteria, lipopolysaccharide, capsules, mycobacteria, heat labile factor, cytomegalovirus/retroviruses, F protein, envelope protein
TLR5	Monocytes, young dendritic cells, epithelial cells, NK and T cells	Bacterial flagella (flagellin)
TLR6	Primarily B cells, monocytes and NK cells to a lesser degree	Works in concert with TLR2, mycoplasma, lipopeptides, yeast, Gram-positive bacteria, peptidoglycan, staphylococci, modulin
TLR7	B cells and some dendritic cells	Antiviral/antitumor drugs
TLR8	Primarily monocytes, NK and T cells	Unknown
TLR9	B cells, macrophages, neutrophils, NK cells, microglia, some dendritic cells	Bacterial CpG DNA
TLR10	B cells, some dendritic cells	Works in concert with TLR2, Gram-positive bacteria, lipoteichoic acid, Gram-negative bacteria, capsules, mycobacteria, lipoarabinomannan, glycolipids, measles, hemagglutinin, spirochetes, glycolipids, protozoa

NK cells, natural killer cells; TRL, toll-like receptor.

table 66-2 Putative Proinflammatory Mediators of Sepsis

MEDIATOR	PHYSIOLOGIC EFFECTS
Tumor necrosis factor-α (TNF-α)	Mimics sepsis syndrome; margination of neutrophils is particularly striking after TNF-α administration
Interleukin 1	Fever, increased adhesiveness of endothelial cells and leukocytes, endothelial procoagulant activity
Interleukins 2, 6, 8	Hypotension, capillary leak, decreased myocardial contractility, synthesis of "acute phase" proteins (e.g., fibrinogen) by the liver, leukocyte chemotaxis
Hageman factor (factor XII), tissue factor, factor X	Coagulation, fibrinolysis
Complement cascade	Neutrophil chemotaxis, neutrophil aggregation, capillary leak
Endorphins	Hypotension
Leukotrienes and thromboxane	Platelet aggregation, neutrophil adhesion, capillary leak, decreased myocardial contractility
Prostaglandins (especially E_2 and I_2)	Hypotension, neutrophil adhesion to endothelium, fever, muscle aches, muscle proteolysis
Bradykinin (via factor XII and kallikrein)	Hypotension, capillary leak
Serotonin	Pulmonary hypertension, capillary leak
Histamine	Hypotension, capillary leak
Platelet-activating factor (PAF)	Hypotension, capillary leak, platelet aggregation, leukocyte activation, decreased myocardial contractility
Phagocyte products–lysosomal proteins, oxygen free radicals	Endothelial cell damage, capillary leak
Myocardial depressant factor	Decreased myocardial contractility
Endothelin 1	Vasoconstriction, especially in the kidney
Endothelial relaxing factor	Hypotension

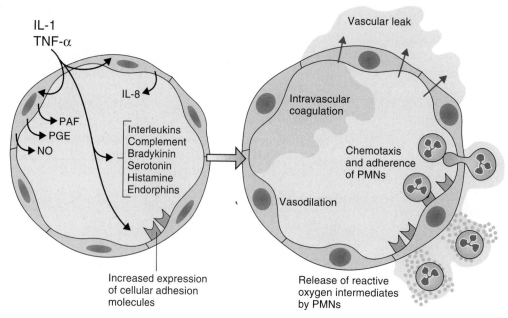

FIGURE 66-1 ▪ **Vasculature effects in sepsis.** The release of interleukin 1 (IL-1) and tumor necrosis factor-α (TNF-α) causes the outpouring of a number of cytokines and other effectors. In turn, that outpouring leads to intravascular coagulation, vasodilation, increased neutrophil adherence to vessel walls, and vascular leakage. NO, nitric oxide; PAF, platelet-activating factor; PGE, prostaglandin E; PMN, polymorphonuclear leukocyte.

the point where a compensatory increase in heart rate (**tachycardia**) can no longer maintain the increase in **cardiac output** needed to maintain blood pressure. Early in the course of sepsis, the combination of very low blood pressure (in adults, defined as less than 90 mm Hg systolic or more than 40 mm Hg below baseline) and low high cardiac output has been termed **warm shock** because the patient is vasodilated with warm or even flushed skin. In some cases of late sepsis, cardiac output falls and peripheral vasodilation is replaced by vasoconstriction in an attempt to shunt blood to vital organs. The skin becomes pale and cold, the hands and feet are blue–purple in color, and the patient expires in **cold shock.**

- **Brain:** Hypotension, decreased perfusion of the brain, and direct effects of the infection itself can render patients confused, delirious, stuporous, or comatose.
- **Lung:** Capillary endothelial damage and leak may be enhanced by activated neutrophils that adhere to the pulmonary endothelium in large numbers, spewing oxygen radicals. Fluid exudes into the interstitium and alveolar spaces, the lung becomes soggy and stiff, and adequate gas exchange is impossible. This condition is called the **adult respiratory distress syndrome (ARDS).** Oxygen must be pumped into the patient's lungs under pressure using a ventilator.
- **Kidney:** Hypotension and infection lead to **acute tubular necrosis** and renal failure. Dialysis is frequently required in septic patients to remove dangerous metabolites that accumulate.
- **Liver:** Necrosis of the liver and impaired gallbladder

function frequently lead to jaundice and impairment of hepatic functions such as drug metabolism, production of albumin, and clotting factors. Lack of albumin contributes to leakage of fluid out of blood vessels into tissues (**edema**) and can contribute to further decline in intravascular blood pressure.

- **Gastrointestinal tract:** Hypotension can cause ischemia and necrosis of the bowel mucosa and wall leading to hemorrhage.
- **Clotting system:** Endothelial damage following hypotension can lead to extensive microvascular thrombosis, or **disseminated intravascular coagulation (DIC).** DIC consumes platelets and clotting factors, which increases the tendency of bleeding. As a result, thrombosis and bleeding may be present at the same time. Activation of the fibrinolytic system counteracts the thrombosis but adds to the coagulopathy because some fibrin degradation products inhibit clotting.
- **Endocrine and metabolic effects:** Sepsis is a **catabolic state,** with massive proteolysis, lipolysis, and glycogenolysis. Stress hormones (**cortisol, cate-cholamines, glucagon**) circulate in high levels. Oxygen metabolism is abnormal, with a high fraction of oxygen sent to the tissues returning to the heart unused. Impaired oxygen use results from some organs not being perfused or their cells being too metabolically impaired to use the oxygen delivered to them. Either way, in a low oxygen state, glycolysis by cells leads to the formation of pyruvic acid and the accumulation of lactic acid, resulting in **lactic acidosis.**

TREATMENT

The mainstays of therapy of sepsis are to control the infection and to preserve and maintain the function of the patient's vital organs. As characterized in the preceding section, sepsis is a state of relative oxygen deprivation. Measures to promote oxygen delivery include supplying the patient with air that has a high oxygen content, using a ventilator to keep the airways under pressure throughout the respiratory cycle, providing intravenous fluids to maintain blood volume, and transfusing to maintain adequate hemoglobin concentrations. Hypotension may be treated with intravenous fluids and drugs that stimulate **adrenergic receptors.** These **vasopressor** drugs cause vasoconstriction and increase myocardial contractility, thus maintaining tissue perfusion pressure. Bactericidal antibiotics are generally given in high doses intravenously and are directed against the most likely pathogens if unknown. In addition, surgical removal or debridement of devitalized tissue and drainage of pus are essential, as illustrated by Mrs. J., who did not get better, despite antibiotics, until her abscess was drained.

Newer treatments based on an understanding of cytokine biology have been disappointing. **Hyperimmune globulin** and **monoclonal antibodies** have been tried unsuccessfully as a strategy to inactivate LPS or prevent its binding to CD14. It is thought that the cytokine cascade and its damage occur so quickly that therapeutic interventions cannot be given soon enough to impact the course of sepsis. Consequently, antibodies directed against TNF-α, IL-1, or their receptors have not been effective, nor have anti-inflammatory agents that antagonize the production of cytokine and prostaglandins, such as glucocorticoids and cyclooxygenase inhibitors. Similarly, strategies to inhibit **oxygen free radicals, bradykinin, complement, platelet-activating factor,** and **free radical production** have also been tried, and colony-stimulating factors have been proposed as a means of reversing the state of immunodepression in late sepsis. Reversal of coagulopathy by **activated protein C** replacement has been shown to be of some benefit and is now available for clinical use.

Conclusion

Major strides in understanding the pathophysiology of sepsis have been made in just the past few years. Advances in technology and antimicrobial agents have greatly increased the options available to physicians who treat critically ill patients. Unfortunately, little impact has been made on the outcome of this most serious of infectious syndromes.

chapter 67

Intravascular Infection

Adolf W. Karchmer

Many microorganisms gain entry to the intravascular space and are passively carried throughout the circulatory system, either suspended in the plasma or within various cellular components of blood. Usually, entry of microorganisms into the circulation represents a brief phase of an infection centered primarily in another organ system. However, for some bacteria and protozoa, the primary site of infection is within the vascular system—that is, the cellular components of blood or the structural elements of the circulatory system. For example, *Plasmodium* species (the cause of malaria), *Babesia microti* (the cause of babesiosis), and *Bartonella bacilliformis* (the agent of Oroya fever) produce disease by invading or adhering to erythrocytes. Occasionally, microorganisms infect the endothelial surface of a specific component of the cardiovascular system. Intravascular infection of an artery is called **endarteritis;** of an endothelial site in the heart, **endocarditis;** and of the lumen of a vein, **phlebitis.**

Infective phlebitis occurs mainly by direct spread from an adjacent focus of infection or when intravascular foreign bodies (such as catheters) implanted in veins become infected. **Infective endarteritis** arises in an analogous manner and, on rare occasions, when congenital arterial anomalies (e.g., patent ductus arteriosus, coarctation of the aorta) or diseased arterial endothelium (e.g., atherosclerotic plaques) become infected during transient bacteremia. **Infective endocarditis**, with the exception of episodes that arise as a consequence of cardiac surgery or intracardiac instrumentation, results from seeding of endothelial sites by microorganisms that are transiently present in the circulatory tree. Most vascular endothelial infections are caused by bacteria and, rarely, by fungi. Infective endocarditis is the prototype of spontaneously occurring intravascular endothelial infection and is the focus of this chapter. The term *endocarditis* will refer here to infective endocarditis.

Endocarditis

Case

Mrs. Q., who at 75 years of age had a history of a systolic ejection heart murmur and mild aortic stenosis, hypertension, and diabetes, was admitted to the hospital because of 6 weeks of intermittent fevers, malaise, weakness, and loss of appetite. The day before admission she noted her temperature was 41.2°C and discovered that she was 14 lb below her usual weight.

On examination Mrs. Q. was pale, her temperature was 38.1°C, heart rate 100 beats per minute, and blood pressure 150/90 mm Hg. Three small hemorrhages were noted on the right palpebral conjunctiva. The fundi were normal. She was edentulous. On cardiac examination a grade III/VI systolic ejection heart murmur was heard at the base of the heart, suggesting aortic stenosis; and a grade I/VI brief, high-pitched decrescendo diastolic murmur was heard at the left sternal border, indicating aortic insufficiency. The spleen could not be palpated.

Laboratory tests revealed hematocrit of 27% (normal is greater than 36%), normal leukocyte count, sedimentation rate of 92 mm/hr (normal is less than 15 mm/hr), and creatinine level of 1.9 mg/dL (normal is less than 1.3 mg/dL). Urine analysis showed 25 to 30 red blood cells per high-power field but no white blood cells or casts. Six blood cultures obtained over 48 hours were all positive for *Streptococcus bovis.*

Treatment for subacute bacterial endocarditis was started with 3 million units of penicillin intravenously every 4 hours. On the sixth hospital day, Mrs. Q. was found unresponsive with a dilated left pupil. An emergency cranial CAT scan revealed a large left parietal hematoma. Mrs. Q died on the eighth hospital day.

Autopsy confirmed vegetations on the aortic valve at the closure line. The valve was bicuspid and thickened. A Gram stain of the vegetation confirmed the presence of Gram-positive cocci. Small embolic infarcts were noted in the myocardium and in the spleen. Changes of focal glomerulonephritis and several small infarcts were found in both kidneys. Also noted was a massive subarachnoid and left parietal intracerebral hemorrhage from an apparent leaking aneurysm (a mycotic aneurysm or saclike dilatation, which results from growth of bacteria in the vessel wall).

This case raises several questions:

1. What underlying medical condition placed Mrs. Q. at risk for developing endocarditis?
2. What virulence factors elaborated by *S. bovis* contributed to endocarditis?
3. What is the significance of the urinalysis showing 25 to 30 red blood cells per high-power field?

DEFINITIONS AND CLASSIFICATIONS

Infective endocarditis is usually localized on one of the cardiac valves, but it can also occur on one of the cordae tendineae or on areas of the atrial or ventricular wall. Endocarditis can be classified according to the tempo of the clinical illness, the microbiological cause, or the clinical setting or site of infection. Patients presenting with markedly febrile, toxic courses lasting only days to several weeks have **acute endocarditis.** In contrast, patients with **subacute endocarditis** have lower fevers and illnesses marked by anorexia, weakness, and weight loss, and are symptomatic for longer than several weeks. Subacute endocarditis, which is usually caused by less virulent nonpyogenic bacteria, attacks structurally abnormal valves. Acute endocarditis, which is caused by more-invasive pyogenic bacteria, can involve structurally abnormal or normal valves.

Current practice is to avoid classifications in favor of brief descriptions that include the microbiological cause, the type and site of the infected valve, and predisposing events. For example, the diagnoses "α-hemolytic streptococcal native valve endocarditis," "*Staphylococcus aureus* tricuspid valve endocarditis in an injection drug user," or "*Staphylococcus epidermidis* prosthetic aortic valve endocarditis" are more precise and give specific indications regarding therapy and prognosis.

EPIDEMIOLOGY

Over the past two decades the incidence of endocarditis in developed countries has ranged from 1.7 to 4.2 cases per 100,000 population each year. Endocarditis accounts for approximately 1 in 1,000 admissions to large general hospitals. The median age of patients with endocarditis has increased steadily since the preantibiotic era; in the 1920s the median age was less than 30 years, whereas currently more than 50% of cases involve people older than 50 years of age.

The type of structural heart disease that serves as the predisposing factor for endocarditis also has changed. **Acute rheumatic fever** and subsequent rheumatic heart disease has declined in developed countries as a predisposing factor for endocarditis. The common predisposing factors for endocarditis are now **congenital cardiac defects** (especially bicuspid aortic valves, ventricular septal defects, tetralogy of Fallot, and patent ductus arteriosus), **degenerative valvular disease** (calcific valvular disease), and **mitral valve prolapse** with mitral regurgitation. In recent reports about 20% of patients with endocarditis were found to have infection on a prolapsing regurgitant mitral valve. **Prosthetic heart**

valves also have become an important site for the establishment of endocarditis. Between 15 and 30% of patients with endocarditis are not known to have had a prior valvular abnormality.

Endocarditis can affect older people for the following reasons:

- People with congenital heart disease now live longer.
- Prosthetic valves to correct valve dysfunction are implanted more frequently in this age group.
- The age of the general population and therefore that of persons with degenerative valve disease has increased.
- The prevalence of rheumatic heart disease (a disease with onset at a younger age) has decreased.
- The precipitating circumstances for transient bacteremia resulting in endocarditis, such as genitourinary tract infections and manipulations, colonic pathology (benign polyps and malignancy), and health care–associated bacteremias (occurring both during hospitalization and among outpatients) are more common in the elderly.

However, the current epidemic of injection drug use has raised the incidence of endocarditis among younger persons. Different structures are affected by infections in patients of different age groups. Typically, endocarditis in persons who do not abuse drugs involves a previously abnormal **aortic** or **mitral valve.** In injection drug users, not only does it affect previously abnormal left heart valves, but also in half the cases it involves a normal **tricuspid valve.**

ENCOUNTER

Endocarditis is caused by a large variety of microorganisms but the most prevalent are staphylococci, streptococci, and enterococci (Table 67-1). In studies reporting cases occurring from 2000 to 2005, *Staphylococcus aureus* was found to be the most common causative organism, reflecting the interaction of its pathogenicity and the frequency of events leading to *S. aureus* bacteremia, health care–associated infections, and drug abuse. Specific organisms show preferences for the type of valve infected (native or prosthetic) and the event or site causing the endocarditis-inciting bacteremia (e.g., dental source, injection drug use, or nosocomial infection).

The organisms that cause native valve endocarditis present as either acute or subacute infections. In acute endocarditis, *S. aureus* accounts for 60% of cases, with the rest caused by pneumococci, streptococci, or aerobic Gram-negative bacilli. In contrast, in subacute endocarditis, α-hemolytic and nonhemolytic streptococci cause 60% of infection, with enterococci, coagulase-negative staphylococci, and fastidious Gram-negative rods causing the remainder. Among the streptococci causing subacute illness, *Streptococcus mitior, S. bovis, S. sanguis,* and *S. mutans* predominate and account for 70% of the isolates.

The organisms that cause infection among injection drug users vary depending on whether infection involves the tricuspid valve (or occasionally the pulmonic valve)

table **67-1**	**Microbiology of Infective Endocarditis in Specific Populations at Risk**[a]					
	NATIVE VALVE IE			**PROSTHETIC VALVE IE**		
ORGANISM	**COMMUNITY ACQUIRED** **(N = 683)**	**NOSOCOMIAL** **(N = 82)**	**IE IN INJECTION DRUG USERS**[b] **(N = 550)**	**≤ 2 MONTHS** **(N=161)**	**2–12 MONTHS** **(N = 31)**	**>12 MONTHS** **(N = 194)**
Staphylococci	269 (39)	53 (65)	313 (57)	87 (55)	15 (48)	56 (29)
S. aureus	240 (35)	45 (55)	313 (57)	36 (22)	4 (12)	34 (18)
Coagulase-negative	29 (4)	8 (10)		51 (32)	11 (32)	22 (11)
Streptococci	228 (33)	6 (7)	50 (9)	5 (3)	3 (9)	61 (31)
Viridans	151 (22)					
Other	77 (11)					
Enterococci	57 (8)	13 (16)	55 (10)	13 (8)	4 (12)	22 (11)
HACEK	22 (3)					11 (6)
Fungi	5 (1)	3 (4)	25 (5)	12 (7)	4 (12)	3 (1)
Other bacteria	63 (9)	5 (6)	91 (16)	32 (20)	3 (9)	25 (14)
Culture negative	38 (6)	2 (2)	16 (3)	7 (7)	2 (6)	16 (8)

HACEK, *Haemophilus, Actinobacillus, Cardiobacterium, Eikenella,* and *Kingella* species of bacteria; IE, infective endocarditis.
[a] Data derived from large series reported from 1990 to 2004.
[b] Of 550 cases, 346 involved right-sided valves, largely tricuspid, and 77% of total cases were caused by *S. aureus.*

or the valves of the left heart. Among injection drug users *S. aureus* causes 75% of right-sided endocarditis, whereas a broader range of organisms cause left-sided infection (*S. aureus,* 25%; streptococci, 15%; enterococci, 25%; fungi, 10%; and Gram-negative bacilli, 8%). *S. aureus* isolated from injection drug users with endocarditis are often resistant to methicillin. Advances in blood culture technology, molecular analysis of surgically removed vegetations, and serologic testing have led to the identification of a rickettsia, *Coxiella burnetii* (especially in western Europe), and *Bartonella* species as infrequent but important causes of subacute endocarditis. Previously, endocarditis caused by those organisms was often classified as culture negative (unknown cause).

The microbiology of prosthetic valve endocarditis depends on the time after surgery when infection becomes symptomatic. In the first year after valve placement, many infections are nosocomial and often the result of perioperative wound contamination. As with other nosocomial infections, staphylococci cause 55% of endocarditis cases occurring in that first year, with Gram-negative rods, corynebacteria, and fungi each accounting for 5%. Prosthetic valve endocarditis with symptoms beginning more than 1 year after valve surgery is community acquired and a consequence of

transient bacteremias similar to those that give rise to native valve endocarditis. Accordingly, streptococci, *S. aureus*, enterococci, and fastidious Gram-negative coccobacilli are the causes of later-onset endocarditis. Coagulase-negative staphylococci remain an important cause of prosthetic valve infections. In persons who have acquired endocarditis in the first year after valve replacement, 80% of coagulase-negative staphylococci are β-lactam antibiotic–resistant *S. epidermidis*, whereas in patients who become infected later, other staphylococcal species, often those that are β-lactam sensitive, are more common. That pattern suggests that late-onset staphylococcal prosthetic endocarditis is probably acquired as a consequence of transient bacteremia.

ENTRY, SPREAD, AND MULTIPLICATION

Transient bacteremia is a common event (see Chapter 66). It occurs when heavily colonized mucosal surfaces are traumatized and spontaneously when mucosal surfaces are diseased (Table 67-2). For example, spontaneous

table 67-2 Frequency of Transient Bacteremia in Selected Settings

EVENT	PERCENTAGE OF PATIENTS WITH BACTEREMIA	COMMON ORGANISMS RECOVERED
Oral cavity		
Dental extraction	30–80	Streptococci, diphtheroids, *Staphylococcus epidermidis*
Tooth rocking	85	
Chewing paraffin	50	
Gingival surgery	30–85	
Airway		
Tonsillectomy	38	Streptococci, *Haemophilus* spp., diphtheroids
Bronchoscopy (rigid scope)	15	Streptococci, *S. epidermidis*, aerobic Gram-negative rods
Gastrointestinal tract		
Upper gastrointestinal endoscopy	8–12	Streptococci, *S. epidermidis*, diphtheroids, *Neisseria* spp.
Colonoscopy	2–10	Aerobic Gram-negative rods, streptococci, *Bacteroides* spp.
Urinary tract		
Urethral dilation	20–36	Aerobic Gram-negative rods, diphtheroids, streptococci
Cystoscopy	17	
Transurethral prostatic resection	10–45	
Genital tract		
Parturition	0–5	Aerobic Gram-negative rods, streptococci
Intrauterine device insertion/removal		

Adapted from Everett ED, Hirschmann JV. Transient bacteremia and endocarditis prophylaxis. A review. Medicine. 1977;56:61–77.

bacteremia was documented in 10% of patients with severe gingival disease who were studied before undergoing a dental procedure. Despite the frequency of bacteremia and the broad spectrum of organisms that gain entry into the circulatory system, endocarditis remains a relatively rare occurrence. A small group of bacteria, most of which are not notably virulent, cause the majority of cases. Also puzzling is that these infections are confined primarily to the aortic and mitral valves and do not usually involve the vast expanse of the remaining vascular endothelial surface. What factors operate to produce this uniform pattern?

Role of Nonbacterial Thrombotic Vegetations

Normal vascular endothelium is resistant to bacterial infection, as can be inferred from the relative infrequency of endocarditis involving normal heart valves as well as from the difficulty of inducing endocarditis in laboratory animals. Microscopic examination of the traumatized valve in experimental animal models of endocarditis reveals that intravenously injected bacteria initially adhere to aggregates of platelets and fibrin, the so-called **nonbacterial thrombotic vegetations.**

Several lines of evidence suggest that nonbacterial thrombotic vegetations play a prominent permissive role in the development of endocarditis in humans. First, this type of vegetation occurring in persons with chronic disease and malignancy (marantic endocarditis) is seen at the exact valve sites most commonly involved in infective endocarditis. Second, the cardiac abnormalities associated with endocarditis promote the formation of platelet–fibrin aggregates at these sites. Cardiac abnormalities that allow blood to flow from an area of very high pressure through a narrowing into a low-pressure reservoir (e.g., ventricular septal defects and mitral and aortic valve regurgitation) are commonly associated with endocarditis. That flow pattern results in a **Venturi effect,** in which a low-pressure area is formed immediately downstream and to the sides of the narrowed orifice. When combined with turbulent flow, the Venturi effect allows platelet–fibrin aggregates to form on the endothelium at the low-pressure side of regurgitant aortic or mitral valves and ventricular septal defects. Additionally, high-velocity jet streams of blood flowing through the regurgitant valves and septal defects injure the endothelium on the wall of the left atrium, the right ventricle, or the chordae tendineae–anterior mitral valve leaflet. In turn, platelet–fibrin thrombi form at the sites of endothelial injury and serve as a niche for infective endocarditis (Fig. 67-1). Interestingly, cardiac lesions that result in low-pressure gradients (ostium secundum atrial septal defect) or low flow and reduced turbulence (chronic congestive heart failure) are rarely associated with infective endocarditis.

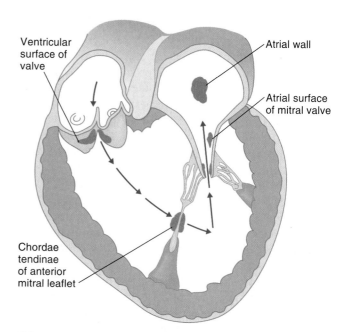

FIGURE 67-1 ▪ The location of endocarditic vegetations resulting from high-velocity regurgitant blood flow. The arrows indicate the high-velocity stream of blood. Regurgitant flow through the orifice of an incompetent aortic valve results in vegetations on the ventricular surface of the valve or on the chordae tendineae of the anterior mitral leaflet. Regurgitant flow across the incompetent mitral valve into the low-pressure left atrium allows vegetations to form on the atrial surface of the mitral valve (or at the site of jet stream impact on the atrial wall).

Microbial Virulence Factors

Although a broad array of bacteria gain entry into the circulation, only a limited number are common causes of endocarditis. To cause endocarditis, organisms must not only enter the circulation but also survive host defenses, adhere to the thrombotic vegetation or valve endothelium, replicate on the valve surface, and promote further vegetation formation. For that sequence to culminate in endocarditis requires a complex interaction between infective agent, host defenses, endothelium, plasma components of the coagulation system, platelets, and host proteins. The precise molecular and quantitative interactions vary among specific agents and are not completely understood. However, some elements of those interactions have been inferred by studies of organisms causing endocarditis and their capacity to do so in animal models.

To cause endocarditis, organisms that reach the cardiac valves must be resistant to the complement-mediated bactericidal activity of serum, as well as escape phagocytosis and killing by neutrophils. Moreover, the organisms must be able to adhere to the thrombotic vegetation or the valve endothelium. Structures in the bacterial cell wall or extracellular polysaccharides have been implicated in interactions with host tissue receptors that result in the adherence of selected organisms. The common bacteria causing endocarditis, *S. mutans, S. sanguis, S. mitior,* and *S. bovis,* produce extracellular dextran, which mediates vigorous adherence of the organisms to platelet–fibrin aggregates on the aortic valve. In addition, the ability to produce dextran by streptococci isolated from blood cultures is strongly associated with endocarditis. Adherence of streptococci to fibrin also is facilitated by a bacterial protein, FimA, previously identified as an oral cavity adhesin; that protein has been associated with the virulence of streptococcal strains in an animal model of endocarditis. Cell wall lipoteichoic acid and a protein with major homology to the streptococcal oral adhesins may promote adherence of enterococci to platelet–fibrin aggregates.

Endocarditis-producing organisms, including *S. aureus, Enterococcus faecalis, S. mutans,* and *S. sanguis,* bind more vigorously to fibronectin than do organisms rarely implicated in the disease, suggesting a role for that host protein in mediating microbial adherence to cardiac valves. Binding of *S. aureus* and coagulase-negative staphylococci to fibronectin-coated foreign devices correlates with device infection and has been suggested as a possible important step in initiating prosthetic valve infection as a consequence of bacteremia. Fibronectin is present on the surface of nonbacterial thrombotic vegetations and is exposed as subendothelial matrix when the endothelium is injured. However, the protein is not present on intact normal endothelium.

On the other hand, fibrinogen is both present in nonbacterial thrombotic vegetations and binds to normal endothelial cells and is a key target for the adherence of *S. aureus* to thrombotic vegetations and to normal valve endothelium in the absence of platelet–fibrin thrombi. The initial adherence is mediated through a fibrinogen-binding protein of the *S. aureus* cell surface (clumping factor) and may account for acute endocarditis without prior valvular disease. Interestingly, coagulase, which is used to identify *S. aureus* (versus coagulase-negative species), does not promote adherence to thrombotic vegetations and is not a virulence factor associated with endocarditis. The reason may be that coagulase is secreted into the medium rather than being bound to the bacterial surface. Some streptococci and *S. aureus* possess microbial surface components recognizing adhesive matrix molecules that bind to extracellular matrix molecules acting as specific ligands, causing adherence of organisms to thrombotic vegetations and injured endothelium.

After adherence to the valve, bacteria must survive and replicate if endocarditis is to occur. The virulence factors that initially favor bacterial survival are not well known. Fibronectin-binding proteins of *S. aureus* facilitate the invasion of endothelial cells by that organism and the subsequent production by the cells of tissue factor, a glycoprotein that acts as a procoagulant for thrombin formation. Streptococci and *S. epidermidis*

induce tissue factor activity as well but by interactions with locally recruited monocytes. Growth and maturation of the vegetation and the resulting envelopment of the microorganisms aid in organism survival and replication, which ultimately lead to overt endocarditis.

Platelets activated by thrombin release low molecular weight, cationic, microbicidal proteins that kill some *S. aureus* and α-hemolytic streptococci. Resistance of adherent organisms to the platelet microbicidal proteins, termed thrombocidins, may be an important factor in progression from valvular adherence to endocarditis. A capsular polysaccharide expressed by coagulase-negative staphylococci may enhance their resistance to clearance by host defenses and thus facilitate development of prosthetic valve endocarditis by strains that contaminate the valve intraoperatively.

Vegetation formation and bacterial growth feed on each other. When a vegetation is colonized by bacteria, it tends to grow by continued deposition of platelets and fibrin. α-hemolytic streptococci and *S. aureus* promote platelet adhesion and aggregation and vegetation growth by complex unique and independent mechanisms unrelated to the elaboration of tissue factor and its procoagulant activity. Protected within the vegetation, bacterial proliferation proceeds unimpeded, leading to dense populations of organisms (10^8 to 10^9 bacteria per gram of tissue). The relative absence of phagocytic cells in vegetations is likely a factor that permits bacterial growth to continue without interruption. On the other hand, experimental data suggest that phagocytic cells limit infection at extracardiac intravascular sites and on the tricuspid valve (perhaps a reason why bacteremic infection of these sites is infrequent). When animals with experimental endocarditis are treated with anticoagulation or fibrinolytic therapy, the size of the vegetation is reduced. However, that strategy has not been translated to effective adjunctive therapy for endocarditis in humans.

DAMAGE

A vegetation is the cardinal pathologic feature of infective endocarditis (Fig. 67-2). Classically, vegetations occur along the line of valve closure on the low-pressure surface of the regurgitant valve or septal defect, or at the site of a jet stream lesion. Vegetations vary in size from a few millimeters to a centimeter or larger and may be single or multiple. Microscopically, vegetations are a mass of fibrin, platelets, and clumps of bacteria; neutrophils are rare. Microorganisms deep in vegetations are often metabolically inactive, whereas the more superficial ones are actively proliferating. A broad array of symptoms and signs are associated with endocarditis (Table 67-3). The following events are the causes of those symptoms and signs:

FIGURE 67-2 ▪ **Vegetation on a heart valve from a patient with bacterial endocarditis.**

- Persistent bacteremia
- Release of cytokines, resulting in constitutional symptoms
- Tissue destruction by infecting organisms
- Fragmentation of vegetations into the circulation, causing peripheral emboli with resultant organ injury
- Induction of antibodies, which combine with bacterial antigens to form circulating immune complexes

Organisms proliferating near the surface of the vegetation are continuously shed into the blood. Although the number of organisms in the blood varies over time, infective endocarditis is characterized by continuous bacteremia. Bacteremia mediates the release of cytokines, resulting in the constitutional symptoms

table **67-3**

Symptoms and Signs Associated With Infective Endocarditis

SYMPTOM	FREQUENCY (%)	SIGN	FREQUENCY (%)
Fever	90	Fever	90
Weakness	50	Murmur	85
Sweats	30	Embolic event	35
Anorexia	50		
Weight loss	60	Osler nodes	10
Malaise	60	Petechiae	25
Myalgia, arthralgia	15	Janeway lesions	5–10
		Retinal lesion	<5
Back pain	10	Stroke	20
Confusion	10	Splenomegaly	25–50
		Septic complications	20

associated with endocarditis: fever, sweats, fatigue, anorexia, and weight loss.

Damage of tissues in endocarditis may occur at the intracardiac site of infection or at a remote site that has been infected during bacteremia. **Intracardiac damage** most commonly involves distortion and destruction of valve leaflets, rupture of a chordae tendineae, or in the case of infected prosthetic valves, destruction of a valve leaflet, impaired mobility of the valve mechanism, and paravalvular flow caused by dehiscence from the annulus. The resulting valvular dysfunction may precipitate congestive heart failure. Infection can extend beyond the valve leaflet into the annulus to cause a perivalvular abscess.

Clinical clues to invasive infection, especially following aortic valve endocarditis, include fever that persists despite appropriate antimicrobial therapy, new electrocardiographic conduction changes (a consequence of the anatomic proximity of the atrioventricular conduction system, the bundle of His, and the bundle branches to the mitral and aortic annuli), and pericarditis (a consequence of the infection extending into the pericardial space). Vegetations, valve function, hemodynamic status, and perivalvular–myocardial abscess are now demonstrable by transthoracic or transesophageal echocardiography. Although intracardiac complications can occur with all microbial causes of endocarditis, they are more common when virulent pyogenic bacteria are responsible or when infection involves prosthetic valves (particularly within the initial year after valve surgery). Those complications, if not repaired surgically, are the major causes of death from endocarditis.

Infection of remote sites often complicates endocarditis caused by pyogenic bacteria. Included among such infections are septic arthritis, osteomyelitis, splenic or kidney abscesses, and meningeal or parenchymal brain abscesses. Infection in the vasa vasorum of larger arteries and arteritis beginning at the site of arterial occlusion from septic emboli in patients with *S. aureus* endocarditis give rise to **mycotic aneurysms.** Those lesions, which can occur in any artery, are usually asymptomatic until they rupture (as in the case of Mrs. Q.).

Emboli are recognized clinically in 25 to 35% of patients with endocarditis and are found in 45 to 65% of those who die from the disease. Arterial occlusion, infarction, and other secondary complications in virtually any organ can result from emboli. Clinically, they are most notable as the cause of embolic stroke; acute myocardial infarction; and abdominal, flank, and back pain resulting from intestinal, splenic, and renal infarction, respectively. In tricuspid valve endocarditis caused by *S. aureus*, septic pulmonary artery emboli with secondary pneumonia, lung abscess, or pyopneumothorax are prominent components of the clinical picture.

Circulating **immune complexes** that contain antigen from the causative organisms are detectable in most patients; the concentration of those complexes has been correlated with prolonged duration of the disease, occurrence of extracardiac manifestations, and reduced serum complement concentrations. Tissue injury mediated by deposition of circulating immune complexes has been described in the skin, choroid plexus, spleen, and synovium. Clinical findings such as Osler nodes, petechiae, vasculitic purpura, and arthralgia have been attributed to the deposition of immune complexes in the skin, arterial wall, and synovium.

Glomerulonephritis is the best-documented immune-mediated complication of endocarditis (see Chapter 12). Endocarditis is associated with a continuum of immune renal injury, from focal embolic glomerulonephritis (a lesion with few clinical consequences) to diffuse proliferative glomerulonephritis that results in an active urine sediment (i.e., containing erythrocytes and erythrocyte casts) and is commonly associated with decreased creatinine clearance. In patients with prolonged episodes of subacute streptococcal endocarditis, circulating immune complexes, which form intravascularly under conditions of antibody excess, deposit in a subepithelial location along the glomerular basement membrane. Immunofluorescence studies reveal IgG and early complement components on the glomerular basement membrane in a lumpy distribution (Fig. 67-3). Among patients with subacute endocarditis, glomerulonephritis is frequent, generally mild (primarily focal), and remits with effective therapy of the infection. Acute staphylococcal endocarditis causes an immune-mediated glomerulonephritis as a consequence of antigen deposition at the glomerular basement membrane and activation of the alternative complement pathway. That type of lesion is found in more than 25% of patients with *S. aureus* endocarditis of less than 2 weeks' duration.

DIAGNOSIS

The diagnosis of endocarditis is suggested by the clinical presentation and is confirmed by documenting persistent bacteremia through multiple positive blood cultures for the same organisms over 24 to 48 hours. Likewise, blood cultures positive for organisms that commonly cause endocarditis should raise suspicion of the diagnosis, even in the absence of other clinical findings. Without prior antibiotic therapy, at least 95% of patients with endocarditis have positive blood cultures. In almost all those cases, one of the initial two cultures is positive. Depending on the susceptibility of the organism, administration of antibiotics during the preceding 2 weeks may significantly reduce the frequency of positive blood cultures. Therefore, to avoid false-negative results, blood cultures should be obtained before antibiotics are given. Transthoracic echocardiography, followed by transesophageal echocardiography if necessary, is a highly sensitive and specific approach to the identification of vegetations on valves and intracardiac complications. Although that approach is

FIGURE 67-3 ▪ Immune complex glomerulonephritis. A. Immunofluorescence staining of the glomerulus stained with antibodies directed against C3 showing deposits in the capillary walls and the mesangium. **B.** Electron micrograph of a glomerular tuft revealing electron-dense immune complex deposits in the mesangium (single arrow) and subendothelial capillary space (double arrow). The basement membrane splits to surround the subendothelial deposits, giving rise to the double-contoured appearance noted in part A. These deposits will be stained by fluorescent-tagged antihuman IgG in a lumpy distribution. CL, capillary lumen; Ep, epithelial cell; Mes, mesangium; US, urinary (Bowman) space.

not suitable for screening patients with little clinical evidence of endocarditis, it can aid in identifying typical vegetations in patients in whom the disease is highly suspected and thus confirm the diagnosis. Other laboratory tests that are frequently abnormal in patients with endocarditis—including hematocrit, sedimentation rate, urine analysis, circulating immune complex concentration, and rheumatoid factor—are not helpful in making a specific diagnosis.

TREATMENT

Effective treatment for endocarditis requires identifying the causative agent and determining its antimicrobial susceptibility. That information enables the design of an effective antimicrobial regimen. Because host defenses are not very effective at inhibiting bacteria within vegetations, bactericidal antibiotics or combinations of antibiotics are required for optimal therapy. Antibiotics are administered parenterally to achieve high serum concentrations, which are necessary to penetrate the depths of relatively avascular vegetations. The reduced metabolic state of organisms deep in vegetations may render the bacteria difficult to eradicate and supports the use of prolonged antibiotic courses for most patients with infective endocarditis.

The increasing prevalence of enterococci that are resistant to penicillins, vancomycin, and the aminoglycosides (high-level resistance to streptomycin and gentamicin)—as well as staphylococci resistant to methicillin (also resistant to all semisynthetic penicillinase-resistant penicillins, cephalosporins, and carbapenems)—may result in endocarditis that is difficult to treat with antibiotics. Fungi and antibiotic-resistant Gram-negative rods also may cause endocarditis that is difficult to treat with antibiotics. Surgery to excise valves infected by antibiotic-resistant organisms might help eradicate those infections. Additionally, the survival of patients with intracardiac complications, such as valve dysfunction that leads to congestive heart failure or perivalvular abscess, has been greatly enhanced by surgery to debride sites of infection, restore anatomic defects, and replace a dysfunctional valve with a prosthesis.

PREVENTION

The value of prophylactic antibiotics to prevent endocarditis in patients at risk is uncertain because carefully controlled studies have not been performed. Nonetheless, animal studies support the use of antibiotic prophylaxis. Persons at risk usually include those with heart valve lesions who undergo procedures that can lead to bacteremia with organisms that are the most common causes of endocarditis. Therefore, it is recommended that persons with known endocarditis-prone rheumatic heart disease, prosthetic valves, or heart valve malformations from other causes be given amoxicillin just before and for a short time after procedures like tooth cleaning and extraction. To provide prophylaxis against enterococci, an aminoglycoside should be added to the penicillin prior to invasive maneuvers in the gastrointestinal or genitourinary tracts. Prophylactic use of antibiotics is particularly important for people with prosthetic heart valves, in whom bacterial endocarditis has such a poor prognosis that attempts to prevent it are mandatory.

Conclusion

In spite of improvements in health care, endocarditis remains an important life-threatening infection with a stable incidence of 1.7 to 4.2 cases per 100,000 population every year. The evolving epidemiology of the infection in the developed world reflects new predispositions in an aging, health care–supported population and new behavioral practices with attendant risks. *S. aureus* has become the predominant causative organism. An understanding of the complex interaction of bacteria and host resulting in endocarditis is better but still incomplete. Echocardiography has facilitated diagnosis and patient assessment. Potent antibiotics for therapy and surgical intervention have improved survival rates, but challenges still exist. Prevention of morbidity, especially from emboli and ruptured mycotic aneurysms, remains an important objective. Endocarditis prophylaxis is a cherished yet elusive goal of endocarditis research.

Head and Neck Infections

Preeti N. Malani and Mark A. Zacharek

Infections of the head and neck occur most commonly when organisms spread from contiguous mucosal surfaces into soft tissue and interstitial spaces. Less often, infection results from hematogenous seeding of organisms from the bloodstream. Regardless of the route, clinical manifestations of head and neck infections primarily involve **inflammation**. The resultant swelling is often readily recognized, as when it causes facial cellulitis or it acutely affects a physiological function like swallowing or breathing.

The **air-filled cavities** of the head (sinuses, mastoids, middle ear) are lined by respiratory epithelium (Fig. 68-1). Infections of those spaces result when **normal drainage routes become obstructed**. The ciliated respiratory epithelium normally removes bacteria by trapping them in mucus and propelling the mucus out. When drainage is blocked, the epithelium cannot function normally. As aerobic bacteria reach their maximum growth, oxygen in the affected cavity becomes depleted, permitting anaerobes to grow. Bacteria release fragments of cell wall (such as lipopolysaccharide or murein subunits) that elicit a cytokine response, leading to more inflammation and obstruction.

ENCOUNTER AND ENTRY

The common cold (**rhinitis**) and sore throats (**pharyngitis**) account for most head and neck infections (see Chapters 32 and 12, respectively, for more detail on those topics). Frequently, a more invasive infection follows a viral or streptococcal infection that disrupts the mucosal epithelium. Histological examination of respiratory mucosa during acute infection demonstrates loss of ciliated epithelial cells and thinning of the mucosal layer. The resulting loss of continuity allows bacteria to enter the underlying soft tissue (**cellulitis**) or overwhelm the defenses in the lymph nodes (**lymphadenitis**).

In **sinusitis**, the ostia can become blocked because of a viral upper respiratory infection or allergies, both of which produce **edema**. In the **middle ear,** eustachian tube dysfunction can occur congenitally (e.g., in infants with cleft palates), as a result of an upper respiratory tract infection, or secondary to allergies. Because the cavity of the middle ear is contiguous with the mastoid air cells, individuals with **acute otitis media** also have **mastoiditis,** an acute inflammatory reaction in the mastoid air cells.

The most common infections of the head and neck are listed in Table 68-1. The bacteria associated with the infections are mostly those isolated from the upper

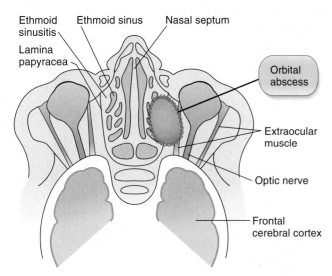

FIGURE 68-1 ▪ **Superior axial view of the face through the level of the ethmoid sinus.**

table **68-1**	**Infections of the Head and Neck**

Infections of air-filled cavities

Otitis media (acute and chronic)

Sinusitis

Mastoiditis

Infections of structures contiguous to air-filled cavities

Orbital cellulitis or abscess

Cavernous sinus thrombosis or thrombophlebitis

Lateral sinus thrombosis or thrombophlebitis

Cervical adenitis

Infections of soft tissues

Rhinitis

Pharyngitis, exudative and non-exudative

Conjunctivitis

Facial cellulitis

Abscess of canine fossa

Lymphadenitis

Oropharyngeal abscess

Paratonsillar infection

Pterygomaxillary infection

Lateral neck infection

Thyroiditis

Infections of embryonic remnants

Branchial cleft cellulitis or abscess

Thyroglossal duct cellulitis or abscess

respiratory tract, including *Streptococcus pneumoniae, Haemophilus influenzae, Staphylococcus aureus, Streptococcus pyogenes,* and anaerobic bacteria. The six clinical cases presented in this chapter illustrate common manifestations of head and neck infections.

Otitis Media

Otitis media is among the most common infections seen by primary care providers. The majority of cases occur in children between 6 and 36 months of age, with an average child having two episodes per year during the first 3 years of life. Children are especially susceptible to otitis media for several reasons. One predisposing factor is that the medial orifice of the eustachian tube is more open in infancy than later in life. Supine feeding (giving a bottle at bedtime) permits reflux of pharyngeal contents into the lumen of the eustachian tubes, producing irritation that results in inflammation and occlusion. Additionally, the eustachian tube is shorter and more horizontal in young children, which allows reflux of nasopharyngeal organisms into the middle ear. Eustachian tube dysfunction is also facilitated by viral infections of the lymphoid tissue around the medial orifice (the adenoidal pad), such as those caused by respiratory syncytial virus, influenza A or B, or adenovirus. With inflammation and occlusion, normal upper respiratory flora can proliferate in the middle ear. The most common bacteria associated with otitis media are *S. pneumoniae, H. influenzae,* and *Moraxella catarrhalis.* Viral infections can promote bacterial replication in the middle ear by direct damage to the respiratory epithelium lining.

Case

E., a 14-month-old girl, came down with the same "cold" that her older sister had had for the past 3 days. She became irritable, stopped taking her bottle, and developed a temperature of 39.8°C, prompting her mother to take her to the family's physician. In the office the nurse used a tympanometer to measure the mobility of E.'s eardrum and told the mother that E. had an ear infection. On further otoscopic examination, the physician agreed and prescribed oral amoxicillin.

This case raises several questions:

1. Should E.'s sister be brought in and checked for an ear infection?
2. Should a culture be obtained before antibiotics are prescribed?
3. How can the physician be sure that amoxicillin is the right antibiotic for E.?
4. Could E. have complications of her ear infection?

DIAGNOSIS AND TREATMENT

The signs and symptoms of middle ear inflammation reflect the anatomy of the region. Early in the course, submucosal edema and hemorrhage lead to the outpouring of exudate into the middle ear space. As the cavity fills with fluid, the tympanic membrane becomes less mobile, resulting in a **conductive hearing loss.** Mobility can be measured by pneumatic otoscopy (changing the air pressure on the eardrum while looking at it), or by **tympanometry** (a technique that measures the compliance of the tympanic membrane). In a healthy ventilated ear, tension on the tympanic membrane varies with the pressure exerted on it. When fluid is present in the middle ear, the tympanic membrane cannot stretch with changes in pressure (poor compliance).

In **chronic otitis media** the epithelium of the middle ear undergoes marked histological changes. Bacterial cell wall components and secreted toxins cause mucus-secreting cells to increase in number. Mucin is secreted into the middle ear, possibly in an effort to entrap and remove bacteria and inflammatory debris. The usual exit route for fluids, the eustachian tube, remains occluded. Accordingly, an essential part of treatment is fluid drainage. That can be accomplished indirectly by administering medications that restore eustachian tube function or directly by incising and placing a tube through the tympanic membrane (**myringotomy** and placement of **pressure equalization tubes**).

The middle ear can become infected with any of the bacteria present in the upper respiratory tract. In acute disease the primary pathogens are pneumococci and nontypeable *H. influenzae* (together accounting for about 80% of infections overall). Antimicrobial drugs active against those two species have proven effective in the treatment of otitis media, alone or in combination with other measures. Thus, empirical treatment directed against the most common pathogens is justifiable in acute otitis media. However, several studies suggest that acute otitis media can resolve without antimicrobial medication. Some authorities advocate observation with limited antimicrobial use in older children. On the other hand, infants are almost always treated with antimicrobials because of an increased incidence of complications. Aspiration of the middle ear fluid (**tympanocentesis**) is not routinely performed for culture and susceptibility testing. Besides being a painful and risky procedure, the results do not significantly impact management because the microbiology is predictable in acute disease.

COMPLICATIONS

Although most ear infections treated with antimicrobial medications resolve without complications, chronic and recurrent episodes of otitis media can lead to infectious and noninfectious sequelae such as facial nerve paralysis, brain abscess, and epidural or subdural abscess. Some patients develop perforated tympanic membranes. In those cases the associated pathogens occasionally include not only the upper respiratory flora but also Gram-negative bacilli, particularly *Pseudomonas aeruginosa* and *Proteus* species.

Another complication of otitis media is persistent middle ear fluid leading to conductive hearing loss. Uncorrected, the hearing loss can impact speech and language development. Children experiencing recurrent bouts of otitis media should be referred to an otolaryngologist for further evaluation. Some patients benefit from myringotomy and the surgical placement of pressure equalization tubes. In general, that procedure is considered when a patient has had recurrent episodes of acute otitis media (usually five to seven infections in a year), a persistent effusion lasting more than 12 weeks, and an associated conductive hearing loss. Prospective clinical studies demonstrate that children treated with tubes experience improved hearing and fewer recurrences of otitis media. Additionally, a child's nutritional status can improve along with quality of life parameters for parents and children. Like any surgical procedure, tube placement carries risk. Risks of tube placement include the development of chronic **otorrhea** (persistent drainage through the puncture site), tympanic membrane perforation, and very rarely, ossicular chain injury and sensorineural hearing loss.

PREVENTION

Increasing antimicrobial resistance has encouraged novel approaches to the prevention of otitis media. In 2000 a capsule-protein conjugate vaccine against pneumococcal disease became available. The vaccine offers protection against the seven serotypes of *S. pneumoniae* responsible for a large portion of invasive and/or drug-resistant infections. Initial results suggest that pneumococcal conjugate vaccine has excellent efficacy against invasive pneumococcal disease. Although the vaccine may not directly prevent otitis media, reduction of upper respiratory tract colonization appears to decrease transmission of resistant strains within families. More recently, annual influenza vaccination has been expanded to young children, particularly those less than 2 years of age. Theoretically, that will have a beneficial effect on otitis media.

Orbital Cellulitis

Orbital cellulitis involves acute inflammation of the connective tissue of the eye socket and is a serious complication of acute sinusitis. The lateral borders of the ethmoid sinuses form the medial wall of the orbit, also

Case

B., a 14-year-old girl, has had ongoing problems with allergic rhinitis generally manifesting as a runny nose, watery eyes, and episodes of fullness in the front of her face. One morning she awoke with headache, cough, and a foul taste in her mouth. Interpreting that as another episode of her allergies, B. took an antihistamine and some acetaminophen. The next morning her headache had become severe and she was unable to open her left eye. Feeling terribly ill, she went to see her pediatrician, who noted marked erythema and swelling around B.'s eye and a slight exudate from the eyelids. B. had a temperature of 38.3°C and a heart rate of 120 beats per minute. When the doctor retracted B.'s eyelids, she found that the left eye was slightly deviated inferiorly and laterally and noted limitation in extraocular eye movements. She immediately referred B. to an otolaryngologist as she likely had a serious illness, orbital cellulitis.

This case raises several questions:.

1. Why should B. see an otolaryngologist if the problem is with her eye?
2. How are B.'s allergies related to the development of orbital cellulitis?
3. Are antimicrobials necessary?

known as the **lamina papyracea** (Latin for "paper thin"). Infection in the ethmoid sinus can erode through the lamina papyracea and enter the orbit. If the cellulitis becomes localized, an intraorbital but extraocular abscess, known as a **subperiosteal abscess,** can develop (see Fig. 68-1). By convention, orbital cellulitis is graded clinically based on the severity and extent of disease, ranging from preseptal cellulitis to cavernous sinus thrombosis. The approach to treatment varies with the extent of disease.

DIAGNOSIS

Clinical findings helped B.'s physician quickly recognize the disease. Because the superior and medial region of the orbit was affected, the eye was displaced inferiorly and laterally. Had she measured it, the physician would have found that the eyeball was proptotic (protruding out of the orbit). **Proptosis** is caused by the edema and inflammatory exudate in the orbit, literally making the cavity smaller and forcing the eye outward. Other signs of orbital cellulitis include limitation of extraocular eye muscles caused by the structures becoming edematous. In addition, stretching of the optic nerve can decrease visual acuity and can result in blindness.

TREATMENT AND PREVENTION

Because the source of orbital cellulitis is the sinus, treatment may require surgical drainage of the involved ethmoid. An external drainage procedure or an endoscopic transnasal decompression of the abscess can be performed to allow the globe to return to its normal position. Antimicrobials are also vital to treatment. As with other infections of the head and neck, bacteria associated with orbital cellulitis are from the oral and pharyngeal flora. More virulent infections, such as that experienced by B., are likely caused by *S. aureus*. Accordingly, clinicians should select antimicrobials active against *S. aureus* as well as members of the upper respiratory tract flora. Orbital cellulitis identified at an early stage (**preseptal cellulitis**) is usually treated with antimicrobials, steroids, and close observation. Surgical drainage is imperative with advanced disease.

Facial Cellulitis

EPIDEMIOLOGY

Facial cellulitis in infants is almost exclusively caused by *H. influenzae* type B. Had R. been immunized with the conjugate *H. influenzae* vaccine, the disease could have been prevented. The pathogenesis is not entirely clear, but it is likely that minor facial trauma allows blood to seep into the soft tissues. When transient *H. influenzae* bacteremia occurs, the organisms seed and grow in the traumatized subcutaneous tissue using the

Case

R., a 14-month-old unvaccinated boy, awoke from his nap fussy, with a low-grade temperature and slight swelling of his right cheek. His mother thought R. might have bumped it with a bottle while feeding himself in the crib. That evening when she put R. to bed, he seemed improved but remained irritable. His right cheek was more swollen and had developed a slight purplish hue. Aside from a fever, he appeared well. The next morning his temperature was 41.6°C, prompting his mother to take R. to the family doctor. The physician told her that R. would need hospitalization for parenteral antibiotics to treat **facial cellulitis**.

This cases raises two questions:

1. How did the bacteria get into R.'s cheek?
2. Why did R. need to receive intravenous antibiotics for cellulitis?

extravasated red blood cells as a source of nutrition (*haemophilus* is Latin for "blood loving"). Because the soft tissue was seeded through the bloodstream, R. was at risk for other more serious complications of *H. influenzae* bacteremia, including meningitis, septic arthritis, and osteomyelitis.

DIAGNOSIS AND TREATMENT

Because *H. influenzae* does not make cell-damaging exotoxins, tissue inflammation is often minimal. At times the distinction between a slight bruise on the face and cellulitis is difficult to make. The important clinical findings are fever and swelling out of proportion to the magnitude of facial trauma. R.'s physician suspected *H. influenzae* because of the typical purplish (not reddish) hue of the inflamed region and his knowledge that the family refused *H. influenzae* type B vaccine for religious reasons.

 H. influenzae cellulitis resolves with the administration of appropriate antimicrobials. Because secondary diseases owing to *H. influenzae* are very serious, the usual treatment is to administer antibiotic therapy intravenously until the cellulitis has completely resolved.

Oropharyngeal Abscess
DIAGNOSIS

Ms. J. had the typical symptoms of an oropharyngeal abscess. In her case the most likely diagnosis was that of a **peritonsillar abscess**, as evidenced by examination of

Case

Before going to bed one evening, Ms. J., a 19-year-old college student, noticed "a scratchy throat" with slight pain. Over the next 4 days she had an increasingly sore throat and her right ear began to ache. She thought she had a fever and took some aspirin. On the sixth day of her illness Ms. J. could barely open her mouth to eat breakfast. When she did get food into her mouth, it was difficult to swallow. Her roommate noted that her voice was of lower pitch and volume, as though she had something hot in her mouth. At the campus health clinic, the physician looked in Ms. J.'s mouth and then recommended hospitalization for additional tests and possibly surgery.

 This case raises several questions:

1. Why did Ms. J.'s sore throat not go away by itself?
2. Why might she need surgery?
3. Does Ms. J.'s roommate have to worry about catching the illness?

the oral cavity. The tonsils lie between the anterior and posterior pillars (mucosa that covers the palatoglossus and palatopharyngeus muscles, respectively; Fig. 68-2). The superior tonsillar poles overlie part of the superior pharyngeal constrictor muscle and the medial pterygoid muscle. Inflammation behind the tonsil adjacent to those structures causes their dysfunction. **Trismus,** the inability to open one's mouth, is caused by dysfunction of the medial pterygoid, and the inability to initiate swallowing results from dysfunction of the superior pharyngeal constrictor. Failure to elevate the palate results from edema, leading to a muffled, "hot potato" voice, even though the tongue is unaffected. Ms. J. could swallow because

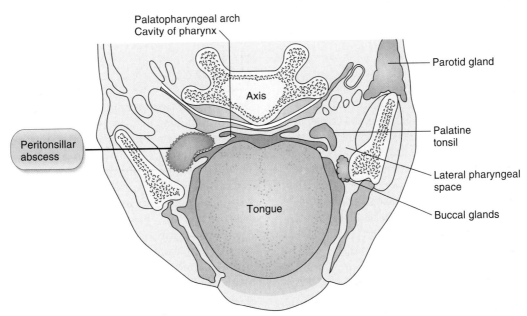

FIGURE 68-2 ▪ **Axial view of the oropharynx through the level of the palatine tonsil.**

there was no mechanical obstruction to food entering her esophagus, but inflammation of the superior constrictor made it difficult to initiate the process. With peritonsillar abscess, the tonsil appears displaced, medially and downward. The uvula is deviated away from the involved tonsil. On palpation, the tonsil may feel fluctuant because of pus in the underlying fascial plane.

Group A streptococci are responsible for about half the cases of peritonsillar abscess. However, commensals are also frequently involved. The process begins as a cellulitis of the peritonsillar tissues, followed by local necrosis. The aerobic and anaerobic oral flora then gain access to the necrotic tissue.

TREATMENT

The primary therapy is surgical drainage. Antimicrobial drugs are also necessary and should include an agent active against common oropharyngeal flora as well as *S. aureus*. In most cases the drug of choice is a semisynthetic penicillin resistant to staphylococcal β-lactamase. Patients allergic to penicillin can be treated with clindamycin.

Conjunctivitis

DIAGNOSIS

Conjunctivitis is a very common infection that physicians see primarily in children and young adults and must distinguish from more serious ocular conditions such as **keratitis** and **iritis**. Distinguishing features of keratitis include eye pain, photophobia, and impaired vision in addition to diffuse inflammation of the eye, a gritty irritation, and excessive lacrimation. When bacterial conjunctivitis occurs alone, the most common causative agents include nontypeable *H. influenzae*, adenovirus, pneumococcus, *M. catarrhalis*, and staphylococci.

Adenoviral and bacterial conjunctivitis can usually be distinguished clinically. Adenoviral disease is generally accompanied by upper respiratory symptoms. Also notable are hyperplasia of lymphoid follicles beneath the conjunctiva, hyperemia of the palpebral conjunctiva, and conjunctival hemorrhages on the globe. In many patients adenoviral conjunctivitis is characterized by a diffuse superficial keratitis that can result in transient blurring of the vision. Adenoviral keratoconjunctivitis is more commonly associated with preauricular lymphadenopathy. In C.'s case, a thorough history and physical examination enabled the physician to make the correct diagnosis.

Generally, organisms are introduced into the eye by direct contact with a carrier's hands. Rarely, the infecting agent is spread by respiratory droplets. Serious infections of the anterior portion of the eye are associated with herpes simplex virus, *Pseudomonas aeruginosa* (contact lens wearers), and, *Chlamydia trachomatis* (people in developing nations). In addition to the usual symptoms of conjunctivitis, herpes simplex virus (and varicella-zoster virus) cause vesicular lesions on the eyelid. Herpes simplex conjunctivitis progresses to keratitis in 50% of cases and is among the most common causes of severe corneal ulceration and acquired blindness in the United States. Because of the serious nature of herpes keratoconjunctivitis and the high risk of recurrence, patients must be referred to an ophthalmologist. Varicella-zoster conjunctivitis occurs in approximately 4% of children with chickenpox. Because the virus is delivered to the skin through the vascular compartment, vesicles present on the lateral aspect of the tip of the nose predict involvement of the eye and reflect involvement of the nasociliary branch of the first division of the trigeminal nerve. Thus, subsequent involvement of the anterior structures of the eye is inevitable.

Case

C. was an active 9-year-old boy who returned from summer camp in good health. The next day he awoke with the sensation that he had "something stuck" in his eye and conjunctival irritation. Later C. developed blurred vision in the right eye, but his left eye felt fine. His mother took him to a physician when she noted that the inside of eyelids looked "bloody" and tears from that eye were blood-tinged. The physician noted a tender, preauricular lymph node and a runny nose. After placing a patch over C.'s eye, the physician told the mother that C. had a "virus" and should improve in a few days.

This case raises two questions:

1. Could C.'s mother and father develop the eye infection?
2. Why did the physician not prescribe antibiotics for the infection?

TREATMENT

Symptomatic treatment of adenoviral conjunctivitis consists of removing exudates with saline-moistened cotton and patching to relieve pain. Antivirals active against adenovirus are not available. In patients with presumed bacterial conjunctivitis, application of an antimicrobial ointment four times a day improves the rate of resolution. Such ointments most often contain polymyxin and bacitracin.

Viral keratitis is treated with antivirals, either topically or systemically. Agents include idoxuridine, trifluorothymidine, vidarabine, acyclovir, and valacyclovir. Available data suggest that most herpetic corneal ulcers treated with trifluorothymidine applied every 1 to 2 hours resolve within 2 weeks. Close follow-up with an ophthalmologist is imperative.

Within 3 days, C.'s signs and symptoms were gone. The physician removed his eye patch, and no further treatment was needed. Had C. failed to improve, a reasonable approach would have been to reexamine the eye, looking for evidence of herpetic infection. If no herpes simplex virus was seen but exudate was still present, a trial of antibiotic ointment could have been administered.

Cervical Lymphadenitis
ENCOUNTER AND ENTRY

Cervical adenitis, inflammation of the lymph nodes in the neck, can be caused by numerous infectious agents. Depending on the nature of the infecting agent in the lymph node, the influx of cells causing the swelling consists of neutrophils or histiocytes and lymphocytes. In general, bacterial infections result in necrosis of the center of the lymph node (**suppuration**). In contrast, viral infections of the cervical lymph nodes are rarely localized to one region, such as the neck; **lymphadenopathy** can be readily detected in other parts of the body.

DIAGNOSIS

Given the number of agents of this cervical adenitis, a physician's approach to a patient with the disease relies heavily on epidemiology. Infections by certain agents occur in certain parts of the world (i.e., trypanosomiasis in tropical countries and *Pseudomonas pseudomallei* infection in southeast Asia). Other important historical

Case

Ms. M., an 18-year-old Caucasian college student, had lived in Minneapolis all her life. Six weeks after arriving at the University of Wisconsin she experienced a mild sore throat and a low-grade temperature (37.8°C). While going to bed, she noted a small, slightly tender lump beneath the angle of her jaw. The next morning the lump was the size of a walnut and more tender. She felt feverish, although her temperature was the same as the night before.

At the student health clinic, a physician told Ms. M. that she had cervical adenitis and that a throat culture and blood tests were needed to ascertain the bacterial agent of the infection (he suspected group A streptococcus) and determine the appropriate treatment. The blood tests were a complete blood count with differential and a screen for heterophile antibody.

This case raises several questions:

1. Is this a life-threatening illness?
2. Why did she need blood tests?
3. Should the physician prescribe antimicrobial drugs?

data include contact with animals (tularemia, plague, or cat scratch disease), immunization status (measles, rubella, or mumps), and exposure to tuberculosis.

Tuberculosis of the cervical lymph glands occurs in patients with pulmonary tuberculosis who inoculate the mouth through coughing. Rarely, it is acquired through the ingestion of milk contaminated with *Mycobacterium tuberculosis*. In the United States most of *M. tuberculosis* infections (other than those in HIV-infected patients) occur in immigrants, Native Americans, and homeless individuals. In Ms. M.'s case *M. tuberculosis* is unlikely on epidemiological grounds, and clinically the rapid onset of swelling is evidence against tuberculosis.

The major etiological agents that needed to be considered in Ms. M.'s case are group A streptococcus, *S. aureus*, and Epstein-Barr virus (EBV) infection. Clinically apparent primary infection with EBV usually causes sore throat, fever, and swelling in the neck. In addition, many patients experience headache, loss of appetite, malaise, and muscle aches. Extensive exudate in the posterior oral pharynx can be seen with Epstein-Barr virus or with group A streptococcal infection. Because EBV infection does not localize to one side of the pharynx, clinical findings are generally bilateral. The test ordered by Ms. M.'s physician was a titer for **heterophile antibody**, which is present in about 90% of Epstein-Barr virus cases. Another common, but nonspecific, finding is the demonstration of atypical lymphocytes on a complete blood count.

Most cases of bacterial cervical adenitis present with unilateral swelling of a single lymph node and minimal upper respiratory or constitutional complaints. The most common bacterial etiology for cervical adenitis is group A streptococcus or *S. aureus*. Demonstration of group A streptococcus in the pharynx would impact the treatment plan because at least 10 days of antimicrobials are needed to prevent immune-mediated sequelae. Needle aspiration of the lymph node is a more definitive means of establishing the diagnosis.

Conclusion

Head and neck infections are among the most common diseases seen by primary care providers. Clinical history, physical exam, and an awareness of head and neck anatomy are essential for accurate diagnosis and management. Bacteria associated with infections in the head and neck regions are often commensals. Treatments for acute otitis media and sinusitis are major sources of antimicrobial use. Increasing antimicrobial resistance, especially pneumococcal, can make treatment of such infections a challenge. The long-term clinical impact of widespread application of the conjugate pneumococcal vaccine remains to be seen. However, early results are promising and suggest that the vaccine may impact invasive infection in a manner similar to the conjugate *H. influenzae* vaccine.

chapter **69**

Sexually Transmitted Diseases

John Richard Ebright and Jack D. Sobel

exually transmitted diseases (**STDs**) are a broad but relatively well-defined group of infectious diseases, generally with acute manifestations that often progress to a chronic clinical picture. STDs rank among the most important of all infectious diseases because of the physical, psychological, and economic damage they cause.

As shown in Table 69-1, the agents of STDs are representatives of widely varying groups that include the pyogenic cocci (*Neisseria gonorrhoeae*), spirochetes (*Treponema pallidum* of syphilis), fastidious Gram-negative rods (*Haemophilus ducreyi* of chancroid), strict intracellular bacteria (*Chlamydia trachomatis*), viruses (herpes simplex viruses 1 and 2, human papillomaviruses, and HIV), protozoa (*Trichomonas vaginalis*), and arthropods (scabies, pubic lice). Other agents of STDs exist but are encountered less frequently in developed countries.

EPIDEMIOLOGY

Magnitude of the Problem

In the last half of the twentieth century the incidence of STDs increased dramatically worldwide. Currently, more than 25 diseases are known to spread primarily through sexual activity. In the United States more than 65 million people are living with an incurable STD and an additional 15 million people will become infected with one or more STDs each year (Table 69-2). Approximately one fourth of new STD infections are in teenagers, underscoring the sobering reality that adolescents and minority populations in the United States are disproportionately affected.

In 2002 more than 350,000 new cases of gonorrhea were reported in the United States, 25 percent of which were in teenagers. The disease imposes enormous physical, emotional, and social costs. In the United States an estimated $1 billion is spent each year to diagnose and treat gonorrhea. In addition, gonococcal antibiotic resistance has been increasing for two decades. Chlamydial infections have an even higher incidence than gonorrhea, with 3 million new cases estimated to occur annually in the United States.

Chancroid, an STD that causes genital ulcer disease, has declined since 1987 but with syphilis remains an important problem in certain areas of the United States, such as the rural south and in inner cities, particularly among African Americans. In those settings the cycle of infection reflects failure to diagnose and treat the disease, a pattern that is driven by poverty and lack of access to health care. Genital herpes

table 69-1	Sexually Transmitted Diseases and Their Agents
DISEASE	**AGENT**
Chlamydial infection	*Chlamydia trachomatis* (all biovars but L)
Gonorrhea	*Neisseria gonorrhoeae*
Genital herpes	Herpes simplex virus type II and type I
Warts, anogenital cancer	Human papillomavirus
Trichomoniasis	*Trichomonas vaginalis*
AIDS	HIV
Chancroid	*Haemophilus ducreyi*
Syphilis	*Treponema pallidum*
Lymphogranuloma venereum (LGV)	*Chlamydia trachomatis* (L biovars)
Granuloma inguinale	*Donovania granulomatis*
Candidiasis	*Candida albicans*
Bacterial vaginosis	*Gardnerella vaginalis*
Pubic lice (crab lice)	*Pthirus pubis*
Scabies	*Sarcoptes scabiei*

(HSV), on the other hand, does not appear to be decreasing in any segment of the population or region. Of the estimated 47 million North Americans afflicted with HSV, 80% are unaware of being infected.

Certain types of human papillomavirus (HPV) infection have been recognized as the cause of cervical cancer. An estimated 28 million North Americans are infected with genital HPV. Although most of those infections are low-risk types associated with genital warts, some involve cervical dysplasias and cervical cancer. For reasons that are not understood but are likely to be linked to a functional immune system, only a small number of infected women (15,000 per year) progress to cervical cancer, and one in three die of the surgically treatable condition. Recently, an HPV type-specific vaccine has been tested using HPV type 16, the most prevalent cancer-associated type. Early studies have shown protection against acquiring HPV infection and developing precancerous changes, indicating the potential for using a vaccine to prevent cervical cancer.

Population Dynamics

Efforts at prevention and control of STDs require an understanding of the factors that contribute to their spread and progression. Although STDs share a common mode of transmission, each disease presents unique challenges to diagnosis, therapy, and prevention. Additionally, many biological and social forces are involved in the dynamics of STD transmission. To make sense of

the multitude of variables related to STDs, it is convenient to separate them according to a model proposed by May and Anderson. According to the model, the rate of movement of an STD throughout the population depends on three variables: (1) the **transmissibility** (or infectivity rate) of the infectious agent, (2) the **rate of new partner acquisition** as well as the partners' sexual history, and (3) the **duration of infectiousness**. Each variable in the model is affected by biological, behavioral, and social risk factors.

Transmissibility of the Agent

The transmissibility, or infectivity rate, of an agent is defined as the risk of acquiring infection during a single contact with an infected partner. For each STD, the rate varies not only with the type of sexual activity but also the biological properties of the infecting organism and possibly the immune status of the host. Behavioral factors, including drug and alcohol use, contraceptive practices, circumcision, and douching, also affect the infectivity rate. Consider HIV, which possesses specific surface molecules for attachment to host cell receptors found primarily on rectal epithelial cells as well as lymphocytes. Sexual behavior is an especially important factor in HIV transmission because anal intercourse facilitates the spread of the virus. Several behavioral studies have shown that risk-taking may be characteristic of a subset of the teenage population. Thus, smoking, alcohol and other substance abuse, excessive automobile speeding, and a high number of sexual partners are interrelated high-risk behaviors of certain teens.

table 69-2	Dimensions of the Problem of Sexually Transmitted Diseases in the United States	
DISEASE	**REPORTED NEW CASES, 2002[a]**	**ESTIMATED NEW CASES PER YEAR[b]**
Chlamydial infection	834,555	3 Million
Gonorrhea	351,852	650,000
Genital herpes	—	1 Million
Papillomavirus infection	—	5.5 Million
Trichomoniasis	—	5 Million
AIDS	42,745	886,575[c]
Chancroid	67	—
Syphilis	6,662[d]	70,000
PID	5,722	1 Million

[a] Of all the STDs, only syphilis, gonorrhea, chlamydia, and AIDS are reportable in every state.
[b] 1999 estimates.
[c] Total cumulative cases from start of epidemic through 2002.
[d] Primary or secondary syphilis.

STD Complications Experienced Only by Women

Pelvic inflammatory disease
Infertility
Chronic pelvic pain
Ectopic pregnancy

Cervical cancer
Spontaneous abortion
Premature delivery
Congenital and neonatal infections of newborns

Rate of New Partner Acquisition

The rate of new partner acquisition is defined as the number of new partners an individual has over a specified period. The parameter depends on the probability that any given partner may be infected. The greater the number of partners, the greater the chance that one of them is infected. Surveys indicate that most people have only a few sexual partners over their lifetimes and that propagation of STD epidemics is actually attributable to a small number of individuals with a large number of sexual partners, referred to as the **core**. Thus, the number of sexual partners an individual has determines membership in the core. Common characteristics of STD core members include living in an urban environment, low socioeconomic status, age within the range of 15 to 30 years, minority ethnicity, and illicit drug use and prostitution. Sexual activity among core members sustains the disease, and sexual activity outside the core spreads the disease.

Duration of Infectivity

The duration of infectivity is the length of time an individual is capable of transmitting infection. Included in this factor are biological characteristics of both the pathogen and the host. Some pathogens (e.g., chlamydiae) commonly cause asymptomatic disease; carriers of chlamydiae do not know they are infected and do not seek treatment. Thus, they remain able to transmit the disease. Antimicrobial sensitivity is also an important factor in duration of infectivity; if an agent is drug-resistant, treatment will fail and the infective period will be increased.

The duration of infectivity can also depend on patients' access to and use of health care as well as attitudes and behaviors of health care providers. Access to health care is affected by the location of the clinic, the speed with which care can be obtained, and the cost of services. The likelihood that an individual will seek care is influenced by such factors as the stigma associated with using an STD facility, knowledge of the existence of the facility, and the perception of the quality of services provided. The availability of effective screening programs, **partner notification** systems, effective treatment protocols, and the patient's willingness to change high-risk behavior also contribute to duration of infectivity.

Groups at Risk

The multiple, long-term, devastating consequences of STDs disproportionately affect women and infants (see the box titled "STD Complications Experienced Only by Women"). STDs are especially prevalent among the young. In the United States 63% of STD cases occur in persons less than 25 years old. Sexually experienced teenagers are three times more likely to be diagnosed with pelvic inflammatory disease (PID) than are 25- to 29-year old women. Biological factors compound behavioral risk factors. Thus, features of the cervical anatomy of adolescents (primarily cervical ectopy) increase the likelihood of chlamydial or gonococcal infection and thereby heighten the risk of PID.

The current STD epidemic in the United States also disproportionately affects minority groups. Both the incidence of STDs and long-term sequelae are consistently higher among non-Caucasian men and women. In the second half of the 1980s syphilis increased enormously among low-income, inner-city heterosexuals and their children. In the 1980s the incidence of gonorrhea decreased in Caucasians of both sexes but increased in African Americans. A survey conducted from 1988 to 1994 showed that African American males were at least two times more likely than Caucasians to be seropositive to herpes simplex virus type 2 (HSV-2). The difference among females was even greater.

ENCOUNTER AND ENTRY

Most of the STD-causing agents enter the body at local sites, through the mucosal or squamous epithelial layers of the cervix, urethra, rectum, oral pharynx or, to a lesser extent, the vagina. An exception is HIV. Although HIV is transmitted primarily by sexual contact, contaminated blood products or hypodermic needles also are sources of infection.

Nearly all the agents of STDs are relatively sensitive to chemical and physical factors and are practically never found free in the environment. Animal reservoirs also are unknown for most of STD agents, making the asymptomatic human carrier the most frequent reservoir. The limited distribution of STD agents makes the diseases theoretical candidates for eradication, but formidable medical, social, and behavioral obstacles lie in the way of achieving it.

SPREAD AND MULTIPLICATION

All the agents that cause STDs are able to resist the host's nonspecific defense mechanisms and are infectious—that is, able to attach to and enter tissue with relative ease. The fact that chronic manifestations of STDs are relatively frequent indicates that the agents often cause asymptomatic disease and are not easily eliminated by specific immune responses. The strategies employed to withstand antimicrobial defenses are varied and should be reviewed by reading the chapters on specific agents.

DAMAGE

The acute manifestations of the most frequent STDs fall into two groups: (1) **mucopurulent cervicitis and urethritis,** as in gonorrhea and chlamydial infection; and (2) **genital ulcer disease,** as in syphilis, chancroid, and genital herpes. With the exception of HIV, the agents of STDs tend to cause primary lesions at or near the sites of entry. It is not uncommon for the lesions to be so indolent as to go unnoticed or to be located at anatomical sites that render them invisible. Consequently, diagnosis and treatment are often delayed, enabling the transmission and progression of the disease to continue.

The most serious effects of STDs relate to their progression to chronic infections such as the following:

- **Pelvic inflammatory disease (PID),** an ascending infection of the uterus and fallopian tubes most commonly caused by gonococci and chlamydiae
- **Anogenital cancer, including cervical cancer,** caused by some human papillomavirus types
- **Secondary and tertiary syphilis**
- **Recurrent herpes infection**

Many of these chronic infections cause additional adverse sequelae, including the following:

- **Fallopian tube scarring and adhesions** of surrounding tissues, resulting in **ectopic pregnancy, infertility,** and **chronic pelvic pain**
- **Congenital diseases,** as in syphilis, herpes, papillomatosis, and chlamydial infection
- **Increased risk of acquiring HIV** owing to genital ulcers (found in syphilis, chancroid, and herpes) or altered genital mucosa (found in gonorrhea and chlamydial infection)

- **Adverse outcomes of pregnancy,** including premature termination, fetal wastage, low birth weight, and premature rupture of membranes

Pelvic Inflammatory Disease

Pelvic inflammatory disease, or **female upper reproductive tract infection,** is an ascending infection of the uterus, fallopian tubes, ovaries, and adjacent peritoneal linings. PID frequently results in severe, irreversible sequelae such as infertility, ectopic pregnancy, and chronic pelvic pain. A case of postchlamydial PID is described in Chapter 14.

Accurate data on the incidence and prevalence of PID is difficult to obtain because the clinical diagnosis of acute symptomatic disease is imprecise. In addition, approximately 60% of cases are subclinical, with women experiencing no or only mild symptoms and not seeking medical care until late sequelae such as infertility or ectopic pregnancy occurs. It is estimated that approximately 1 million women experience an episode of acute PID each year in the United States and more than 100,000 become infertile each year as a result of the infection. The incidence of PID is particularly high among young, nonwhite, single or divorced women from urban areas.

Pathobiology

The events that lead to PID are not well understood. It is likely that almost all cases involve the ascending spread of infection from the lower to the upper genital tract. Some cases progress to develop chronic sequelae.

Most cases of PID are caused by the sexually transmitted organisms N. gonorrhoeae or C. trachomatis and follow cervicitis or urethritis. Other organisms implicated in the etiology of PID include *Mycoplasma hominis, Mycoplasma genitalium, Ureaplasma urealyticum,* and numerous aerobic and anaerobic bacteria such as *Escherichia coli* and *Prevotella* species. These bacteria are referred to as **endogenous** because they are often isolated from the lower genital tract in the absence of any disease. Little is known about the pathogenesis of the infections. Usually, a primary episode of gonococcal and chlamydial PID is followed by subsequent episodes of PID caused by the endogenous organisms. The pathogenesis of gonococcal and chlamydial PID probably includes nonspecific inflammatory responses to bacterial invasion that result in tissue damage, as well as the specific immune responses to gonococci and chlamydiae. In addition, several anatomical factors appear to be important in the pathogenesis of gonococcal and chlamydial PID. For instance, gonococcal and chlamydial cervical infections can damage the endocervical canal, break down the mucus plug in the endocervix, and allow the pathogens, as well as endogenous vaginal organisms, to ascend to the upper genital tract. Another contributing factor in adolescent females is a larger **zone of ectopy** (extension of columnar epithelium from the endocervical canal to the ectocervix) than in older women. Unprotected by cervical mucus, the zone of ectopy is highly susceptible to gonococcal and chlamydial infections because columnar cells are preferential sites of microbial attachment and invasion.

Other host defenses are probably useful in preventing centripetal spread of organisms. The most relevant host defenses are tubal ciliary movement (unidirectional towards the uterus), flow of mucus in the tubal lumen (towards the uterus), and myometrial contractions during menses (resulting in sloughing of the endometrium).

Several additional risk factors appear to be important in the pathogenesis of PID. **Oral contraceptives** may decrease the risk of chlamydial (but perhaps not gonococcal) PID, whereas intrauterine devices appear to increase the risk of PID within the first few months of placement. Vaginal douching also is associated with increased risk. Most cases of gonococcal (and possibly chlamydial) PID occur during or near the end of menses; hormonal changes during the menstrual cycle can lead to changes in the cervical mucus plug, permitting passage of organisms, particularly when estrogen levels are high and progesterone levels are relatively low. The reflux of infected blood during menstrual uterine contractions can also provide a route of entry into the fallopian tubes.

Types of PID

Gonococcal PID

Investigators studying the pathogenesis and epidemiology of gonococcal infections have found strain typing of *N. gonorrhoeae* to be very useful. Strain typing is based on two methodologies: (1) defining the specific amino acid and nucleoside nutritional requirements of the isolate (auxotype); and (2) serotyping based on another membrane protein known as porin, which can be divided into two classes, PorA and PorB, each of which is composed of many serovars. Interestingly, strains of *N. gonorrhoeae* that have been found to cause PID are not the same as those that have been found to cause disseminated disease.

The pathophysiological changes that occur have been studied in fallopian tube explants exposed to gonococci (see Chapter 14). In the presence of the organisms, the motility of ciliated epithelial cells slows and ultimately ceases. Ciliated cells are selectively sloughed from the epithelial surface, apparently because of the toxic action of lipopolysaccharide (LPS) or murein fragments. Gonococci attach to nonciliated epithelial cells by pili

and an outer membrane protein known as **Opa** (so named because of the opacity of colonies on plates when this protein is expressed). After attachment, the gonococci-expressing Opa induce phagocytosis. The organisms replicate within phagosomal vesicles, move to the basal portion of the cells, and exit into the subepithelium to cause inflammation.

Progressive mucosal cell damage and submucosal invasion are accompanied by a vigorous polymorphonuclear leukocyte response, contributing to local inflammation, microabscess formation, and purulent exudate. Tissue damage appears to result especially from two components of the gonococcal cell surface: lipo-oligosaccharide (LOS) and peptidoglycan. The toxic portion of LOS almost certainly is the lipid A portion. Experimental evidence suggests gonococci paradoxically may be protected by a coating of antibodies directed to an outer membrane protein (reduction modifiable protein, or Rmp). Those "blocking antibodies" inhibit the ability of otherwise bactericidal IgM antibodies in normal human sera to effectively recognize their target on LOS.

Chlamydial PID

The steps in infection of chlamydial PID include attachment of the organisms to cells, probably via certain receptor–ligand interactions, but the specifics of the attachment process have not been confirmed. The major outer membrane protein of the chlamydiae appears to be involved in the interactions. The organisms actively induce uptake by stimulating endocytosis. Phagolysosomal fusion does not occur, probably owing to the function of ill-defined surface components of the **elementary bodies** (the infectious form of the organism). The chlamydiae-containing phagosomes, referred to as **inclusions**, are visible in histologic preparations. Within the phagosomes, elementary bodies differentiate into **reticulate bodies** (the metabolic form of the organism). Ultimately, the reticulate bodies reorganize into new elementary bodies and, in time, are released from the host cell to infect adjacent cells. The life cycle of the organisms is described in detail in Chapter 27.

Chlamydial infections incite a greater mononuclear immune response than those caused by gonococci, but neutrophils are also seen, mainly in the early phases of the inflammatory response. The chronic sequelae of chlamydial disease may result from a cell-mediated immune response. A surface protein of the organisms, known as the 57 kDal heat-shock protein, may be the target antigen of a delayed hypersensitivity reaction. In epidemiological studies, high titers of antibodies against that protein have been shown to be prognosticators of tubal scarring, a long-term sequelae of PID.

Coinfections by Gonococci and Chlamydiae

The high prevalence of gonococcal and chlamydial coinfection has prompted recommendations that patients with either infection be treated for both. Experimentally, simultaneous gonococcal infection facilitates chlamydial replication in cervical epithelia by about a hundredfold. It has been proposed that stimulation of endocytosis in nonciliated epithelial cells by the first parasite leads to alterations in the surface structure of the cells, allowing ready uptake of the second parasite. Thus, one pathogen may facilitate the engulfment of the second.

Bacterial Vaginosis and PID

Bacterial vaginosis is an asymptomatic or symptomatic disruption of the normal vaginal flora characterized clinically by a malodorous vaginal discharge. The normally dominant colonizing lactobacilli (especially species that produce hydrogen peroxide) are markedly reduced, while a variety of species including *Gardnerella vaginalis,* anaerobic streptococci, *Prevotella* species, and genital mycoplasmas, increase in numbers. Several investigators have demonstrated an association between bacterial vaginosis and PID, independent of chlamydial and gonococcal infections.

HIV and STDs

The AIDS pandemic has focused attention on STDs for several reasons. The relationships between HIV infection and other STDs are complex and intriguing. They explain, in part, the global spread of the HIV epidemic and may provide insights into the pathogenesis of all sexually transmitted infections. Furthermore, the relationships have compelling implications for efforts to control HIV.

Aside from sexual behavior, the two obvious relationships between HIV infection and other STDs are (1) increased transmission of HIV because of other STDs; and (2) alteration in the natural history, diagnosis, or response to therapy of other STDs in the presence of HIV infection.

Bidirectional Interplay Between HIV and STDs

The risk of HIV transmission is increased threefold to fivefold in the presence of genital ulcer diseases like syphilis, nonulcerative diseases like gonorrhea or chlamydial infections, or vaginal diseases like bacterial vaginosis, candida vaginitis, or trichomonal vaginitis. Human papillomavirus infection and anogenital warts do not appear to facilitate HIV transmission, perhaps because they do not usually cause breaks in the skin or mucous membranes.

The compromised immune system of patients with AIDS can result in more severe manifestations of other STDs. Mucocutaneous genital and perirectal herpes infections, for example, can cause extensive and persistent ulcers that can be more difficult to treat in HIV-positive patients than in those who are HIV negative. *Molluscum contagiosum,* a cutaneous poxvirus infection, is seen more often in HIV-infected persons and can cause extensive and disfiguring lesions. Kaposi sarcoma, a malignancy at least partially attributable to a sexually transmitted herpesvirus (human herpesvirus type 8), was one of the first AIDS-defining conditions recognized at the outset of the epidemic in the United States. In HIV-infected patients, genital warts caused by papillomavirus may be extensive and more likely associated with cervical dysplasia, and chancroid may be less responsive to treatment and heal more slowly.

In the past the potential significance of the bidirectional interplay between HIV infection and other STDs was not fully appreciated. Because HIV coinfection prolongs the infectivity and severity of certain STDs, and the same STDs facilitate transmission of HIV, the two infections amplify one another. The increases in HIV and STD incidence may well contribute to the rapid spread of HIV in some heterosexual populations and may represent "epidemiological synergy" between diseases that are linked by a common mode of transmission.

How is the Transmission of HIV Enhanced by Other STDs?

It is likely that the inflammatory changes that accompany STDs facilitate HIV entry by altering the barrier function of the genital mucosal epithelium. In fact, HIV has been isolated directly from genital ulcers in both men and women. It is recognized that intercourse during menses increases the risk of HIV transmission; therefore, it is likely that mucosal irritation, friability, and bleeding may shorten the route to target cells and impair the function of natural defenses. Those defenses normally include an intact mucus layer and tight junctions between epithelial cells. Ulcer-producing STDs provide an easy portal of entry for HIV, and all STDs with enhanced superficial inflammation provide inflammatory cells as targets for viral invasion and dissemination. Local inflammation, even in the absence of ulcer formation, also results in proinflammatory cytokine production, which can enhance local HIV replication.

Molecular interactions may also contribute to the pathogenesis of HIV infection and other STDs. For example, herpes simplex virus may potentiate HIV infection by stimulating the expression of the surface receptors needed for HIV attachment. Conversely, HIV gene products have been shown to be potent intracellular transactivating factors. Those factors may enhance the growth of herpesvirus and human papillomavirus.

PREVENTION AND CONTROL

Prevention and control of sexually transmitted diseases comprise a multifaceted problem. Depending on the circumstances, the objective may be prevention and control of infection, transmission, disease, or disease progression. Those objectives can be achieved through several approaches: effective vaccines, interruption of transmission and progression through behavioral interventions, and curative medical interventions. The tools necessary to achieve those objectives include information about the prevalence of known high-risk behaviors and corresponding effective behavioral interventions; safe, efficacious vaccines; diagnostic tests; effective therapeutics; an efficient network of health care facilities; and well-trained, highly skilled health care professionals.

In reality, almost all those tools are still far from being fully developed and available. We have no vaccines for STDs except for hepatitis B, and that vaccine is underused. Recent success with HPV vaccine and some encouraging results with the use of a herpes simplex vaccine in women suggest potential breakthroughs. For some STDs medical therapy is either unavailable (e.g., viral diseases) or problematic (e.g., antimicrobial resistance). Given the need to facilitate practical goals, how should technological advances be prioritized?

Development and use of inexpensive, simple, rapid diagnostic tests that are appropriate for resource-limited settings, such as inner cities (where the majority of STDs occur), is a fundamental component of STD prevention and control. Such tests are particularly important for diagnosis of STDs in women. In resource-limited settings, clinical algorithms based on recognition of symptoms and signs of STDs have been useful for diagnosis and treatment of urethritis and genital ulcer disease in men but are far less useful for diagnosis of STDs in women. The special requirements of resource-limited settings lead to the conclusion that useful diagnostic tests should be (1) inexpensive, with the cost to the provider less than $1.00 per patient; (2) simple, with no equipment and minimal training required; (3) rapid, with results available before the patient leaves the clinic; (4) performed on convenient specimens that are simple to collect, socioculturally acceptable, and require no separation or preparation; (5) designed to use stable reagents, with long shelf life and no refrigeration required; (6) packaged simply, based on functionality and low cost; and (7) appropriately sensitive and specific, dependent in part on the potential morbidity and cost for undetected infection and the cost of the resulting treatment.

Examples of diagnostic tests with the appropriate format are the occult fecal blood card and the urine glucose dipstick. Recently, progress has been made in developing methods to screen for sexually transmitted chlamydial infections using a ligase chain reaction (LCR) on samples of urine. In addition, relatively easily performed and rapid assays are available for detecting HIV infection. Obviously much more progress is needed in expanding the number of such tests and in reducing their cost.

Treatment of STDs would be greatly enhanced if safe, effective antimicrobial agents could be administered as single oral doses. Noncompliance is a formidable problem when treatment regimens involve multiple-dose therapy for prolonged periods, especially when treatment exceeds the duration of symptoms. Again, therapies should be inexpensive, have a long shelf life, have minimal side effects, and be safe for use during pregnancy. Theoretically, that approach would decrease the likelihood of antibiotic resistance. An example of such an advance is the recent development of azithromycin (an erythromycin-like macrolide antibiotic), a single-dose (although relatively expensive) treatment for chlamydial infection.

There is general consensus that prevention of sexually transmitted STDs, including HIV infection, will be facilitated by the development of safe and effective female-controlled **chemical barriers** called topical **microbicides.** A microbicide effective not only against the most common agents of STDs but also those of genital ulcers would have a substantial impact on HIV transmission. The male condom, which is very effective if used consistently and correctly, requires male partner cooperation and is too often not accepted or used. Just as hormonal contraceptives and intrauterine devices have dramatically enhanced women's ability to avoid unwanted pregnancy, effective female-controlled microbicides are urgently needed to enhance a woman's ability to avoid STDs. In addition, effective chemical barriers may reduce female-to-male as well as male-to-female transmission.

The ideal microbicide would be colorless, odorless, tasteless, stable, easy to store, fast acting, effective pre- and postcoitus, inexpensive, available without prescription, and safe for repeated use. A microbicide like that could ideally be formulated with or without spermicidal activity. Noncontraceptive microbicides would be very useful for women who wish to become pregnant.

The role of the health care provider is an integral part of an STD prevention and control program. Currently many medical school curricula lack focused STD training. Ideally, an integrated approach, including basic biomedical, clinical, epidemiological, and behavioral training, would be most effective.

Conclusion

The STD epidemic is a complex, multifaceted problem that mandates multifaceted approaches for prevention and control. Vaccines, diagnostics, therapeutics, health care delivery systems, and behavioral interventions will play important roles in achieving those interrelated goals.

Infections of the Immunocompromised Patient

E. Turner Overton and William G. Powderly

A person is considered to be immunocompromised when suffering either from the disruption of specific defenses of a particular organ or system or from systemic abnormalities of humoral or cellular immunity. Usually, it is possible to predict the general type of infection an immunocompromised patient is likely to acquire based on the component of the defense mechanisms that is disturbed. However, when the immune deficiency is general and profound, the patient could acquire one or several of a number of different infections.

Researchers have learned a great deal about the body's normal defense mechanisms by studying what happens when they become impaired. In fact, our knowledge of the relative importance of humoral and cellular immunity is derived from observing patients with immunodeficiencies. Thus, we note that persons with agammaglobulinemia are especially susceptible to extracellular bacteria that cause acute inflammation, whereas people with defects in cell-mediated immunity fall prey more readily to viruses, fungi, mycobacteria, and other intracellular agents of chronic diseases. Opportunistic infections have assumed immense importance in modern medicine, primarily because many of the major technological advances in therapeutics have been accompanied by iatrogenic disruption of body defense mechanisms. The practical need to understand the risk factors associated with defects in defenses against invading microorganisms cannot be overestimated.

Most infections acquired by immunocompromised patients are caused by commonly known pathogens. However, severe forms of immunocompromise open the door to infections by organisms not typically considered virulent, including many in the normal flora or in the environment. Unexpected extremes have been reached in scattered cases of infections of heart valves and other vital tissues transmitted by mushrooms (in their mycelial form) and colorless algae. This underscores how the definition of virulence must include not only the obvious pathogenic properties of microorganisms but also the range of susceptibility of the patient.

This chapter recapitulates the consequences of risk factors mentioned throughout the book, presenting them according to the type of abnormality or defect in specific defense mechanisms.

Patients who have undergone bone marrow transplantation provide an extreme example of the profound disturbances of normal body defenses that can predispose to infection. For example, disruption of anatomic barriers by radiation and chemotherapy, resulting in skin and mucosal ulcerations, provides entry sites for invasive organisms. Severe neutropenia is characteristic of the period immediately following transplantation, and although granulocyte recovery begins in the third week after the procedure, qualitative defects remain for some time. Cellular immune function, which in the bone marrow recipient depends on donor macrophages and T

Case

At 17 years of age, V. came to the hospital with fever and bruising and was eventually diagnosed with acute myelogenous leukemia (AML). Induction chemotherapy was initiated with cytarabine and daunorubicin to achieve remission of the AML. Seven days after the initiation of chemotherapy, V. developed burning mouth pain and white plaques. The mucosa subsequently sloughed off, leaving painful ulcers throughout her mouth.

With chemotherapy V.'s AML went into remission, and **allogeneic** (nontwin) bone marrow transplantation was attempted in the hope of achieving a cure. Five days after transplantation V. had no detectable circulating white blood cells, and 2 days thereafter she became febrile. She denied any localizing signs or symptoms such as headache, cough, chest pain, abdominal pain, dysuria, or diarrhea. V. continued to complain of oral pain and difficulty swallowing as well as fatigue and malaise. Blood cultures taken at that time were positive for *Escherichia coli*. She responded well to antibiotics, and her temperature dropped rapidly.

Eight days later V. again became febrile, and blood cultures were positive for *Candida albicans*. Although she was placed on antifungal therapy, she remained febrile for 4 days. However, her temperature rapidly dropped to normal after removal of a venous catheter that had been implanted in her subclavian vein for intravenous drug administration. Nineteen days posttransplantation, white blood cells started to appear in her circulation, indicating that the transplanted marrow had successfully engrafted and was beginning to function.

Thirty-one days after transplantation, V. complained of shortness of breath, and a chest radiograph showed a diffuse pneumonia. A lung biopsy revealed the presence of *Pneumocystis carinii*. Treatment with trimethoprim-sulfamethoxazole was started, and she slowly responded to therapy. She was discharged from the hospital 2 months after her transplantation, but 10 days later she developed a painful cutaneous herpes zoster infection. Following treatment V. regained her health and remained well for the next 3 months, although she had developed mild chronic graft-versus-host disease. She returned again to the hospital 5 months after her transplantation, complaining of fever and shortness of breath. Physical examination and chest radiograph revealed a lobar pneumonia, and both blood and sputum cultures grew *Streptococcus pneumoniae*. She responded well to penicillin therapy and remained healthy thereafter.

This case raises several questions:

1. What risk factors predispose V. to the bacteremia with *E. coli*?
2. What risk factors predisposed V. to the fungemia with *C. albicans*?
3. What risk factors predisposed V. to the pneumonia with *P. carinii*?
4. What risk factors predisposed V to the pneumonia and bacteremia with *S. pneumoniae*?

cells, remains abnormal for several months. It is also compromised by the use of immunosuppressive therapy to treat graft-versus-host disease. Although IgG and IgM levels may return to normal after 45 months, B-cell function remains disturbed, and antibody levels to specific organisms, such as pneumococci, can remain depressed for years.

In the following sections, we review the disturbances in various body defense mechanisms and their consequences in affected individuals.

Abnormalities of Host Defense Barriers

The body is protected from microbial invasion by the barrier provided by skin and mucous membranes and by the presence of a normal commensal flora. Those tissues not only serve as structural barriers preventing invasion by possible pathogens but also have other key antimicrobial factors preventing infection, including pH, temperature, local protective bacterial flora, and proteins with antimicrobial activity such as lysozyme. Disruption of local mechanical barriers can result from instrumentation (e.g., intravenous or urinary catheterization), surgery, drugs (including chemotherapeutic agents), or burns. Chemotherapeutic agents pose a specific problem because their antiproliferative properties have deleterious effects on tissues with a high turnover rate, such as the mucosal surfaces. That tissue damage gives infecting organisms a portal of entry into the body. Furthermore, the commensal flora resident at the entry site can also invade and cause infection. For example, breaching the skin with intravenous catheters can introduce *Staphylococcus epidermidis* into the bloodstream, with subsequent septicemia.

The consequences of immunological or biochemical impairment at the level of the integuments are less well understood. For example, it is not known with certainty if secreted IgA immunoglobulins or lysozyme contributes to resistance to infection. The suspicion is, however, that people with IgA deficiency are more prone to sinusitis, pneumonia, and gastrointestinal infections (e.g., giardiasis). Individuals with genetic defects in lysozyme have not been found.

Burns are an extreme example of the critical role of intact integument on resistance to infection. Necrotic skin tissue is an excellent culture medium for bacteria, thus increasing the size of the inoculum. In addition, the thermal injury itself leads to a poorly understood suppression of white blood cell function. It is not surprising that skin and subcutaneous tissue infections and septicemias with *Staphylococcus aureus* or *Pseudomonas aeruginosa* are major challenges in the management of patients with severe burns.

The normal bacterial flora can be disrupted by antibiotic treatment, which may in turn lead to superinfection by organisms resistant to the antibiotic being administered. This happens particularly often in the intestine, sometimes as a result of antibiotic "prepping" of patients for abdominal surgery in which the normal flora of the gastrointestinal tract is killed, allowing the overgrowth of resistant pathogens such as *Clostridium difficile*, which causes pseudomembranous colitis, a complication of such therapy.

Some tissues possess additional local defense mechanisms. In the lungs, for example, the combination of mucous production by goblet cells and the ciliary activity of the respiratory epithelial cells traps microbes and carries them out of the lungs. Disruption of that disposal system predisposes to pneumonia. An extreme example is cystic fibrosis, a chronic hereditary condition characterized by the production of abnormally thick mucus. Cystic fibrosis patients experience recurrent pneumonia, and their lungs are often colonized by the opportunistic bacterium *P. aeruginosa*. Most patients are unable to clear the organism from the respiratory tract and may die from respiratory failure after repeated episodes of pneumonia.

Innate Immunity

Once the first line of defense is breached, the innate immune defense assumes the critical role in checking the spread of invasive disease. This arm of the immune system is nonspecific and reacts rapidly (in the first 96 hours of infection) to the presence of foreign antigens. Complement activation occurs immediately and leads to the generation of soluble molecules that direct the innate immune response. Soluble mediators such as opsonins and chemoattractants recruit neutrophils, macrophages, and natural killer (NK) cells to the site of inflammation and infection.

The **neutrophil** is the key player of the innate immune response and kills pathogens either directly by phagocytosis or indirectly by recruitment of other cells through the release of cytokines. Defects in neutrophil activity, either qualitative or quantitative, predispose patients to infection with certain bacteria and fungi (Table 70-1). Examples of defects include a decreased number of phagocytic cells, impairment of their chemotactic response, and lowering of their ability to engulf and kill microorganisms.

Granulocytopenia, which is a decrease in the number of circulating neutrophils, clearly predisposes to infection. **Myelosuppressive cancer chemotherapy** is the most common cause of granulocytopenia in hospitals. Neutropenia also occurs in bone marrow failure caused by aplasia, autoimmune disease, hematological malignancy, or invasion of the bone marrow by a tumor. Serious infections, usually accompanied by bacteremia, are a frequent and often life-threatening problem in neutropenic hosts. The most important correlation is between the number of circulating neutrophils and the risk of infection. The rate of infection clearly increases as the number

table 70-1	Common Causes of Compromised Immunity and Their Consequences		
IMPAIRED FUNCTION	**DEFECT**	**COMMON INFECTING ORGANISMS**	**SITES COMMONLY AFFECTED**
Barrier			
	Damaged integument	Pyogenic cocci, enteric bacteria	Skin, subcutaneous connective tissue
	Loss of normal microbial flora	Pyogenic cocci, enteric bacteria, *Clostridium difficile*, *Candida albicans*	Skin, intestine
Phagocyte functions			
	Chemotactic dysfunction	*Staphylococcus aureus*, enteric bacteria	Skin, respiratory tract
	Neutropenia	*S. aureus*, enteric bacteria	Skin, respiratory tract
	Abnormal microbial killing	*S. aureus*, *Aspergillus* species	Skin, visceral abscesses
Humoral functions			
	Hypogammaglobulinemia	Pyogenic bacteria	Any site
	IgA deficiency	Pyogenic bacteria	Respiratory tract
	Lack of spleen	Pneumococcus, *Haemophilus influenzae*	Septicemia
	Complement deficiencies (early components)	Pyogenic bacteria	Bacteremia, meningitis
	Complement deficiencies (late components)	*Neisseria* species	Meningitis, arthritis
Cell-mediated immunity			
	Abnormal number or function of macrophages or T cells	Viruses, fungi, protozoa, intracellular bacteria	Any site

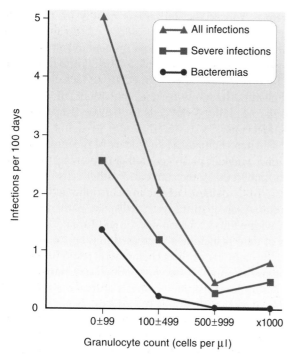

FIGURE 70-1 ▪ **Relationship between the incidence of infection and the absolute neutrophil count in patients with acute leukemia.** The incidence of infection rises as the neutrophil count decreases.

of neutrophils decreases (Fig. 70-1). Additionally, **the duration of neutropenia increases a person's risk to develop a severe infection not only from bacterial pathogens but also fungi and viruses.** Disruptions in the integrity of the skin and gastrointestinal tract, which are often the result of chemotherapy or radiation therapy, are also important in the pathogenesis of these infections. The organisms responsible are usually derived from the patient's own flora, particularly that of the bowel. Gram-negative enteric bacilli and staphylococci are the most common bacterial pathogens. Prolonged antibacterial therapy also predisposes to colonization by fungi. *Candida* and *Aspergillus* infections are the most important causes of fungal sepsis and mortality among patients taking antibacterial drugs for extended periods.

Chemotactic dysfunction of phagocytes is uncommon and usually congenital in origin. Defective neutrophil chemotaxis may result from inadequate signaling of the neutrophil, abnormalities of neutrophil receptors for chemoattractants, or disorders in cell locomotion. *S. aureus* is the most important pathogen in patients with chemotactic dysfunction, who are usually seen with recurrent cutaneous or deep abscesses.

Abnormalities in microbial killing power are usually inherited. Of the many disorders that have been described, the most common is **chronic granulomatous disease (CGD)**, a condition in which neutrophils fail to mount a respiratory burst during phagocytosis. The cause of CGD is a defect in the enzyme **NADPH oxidase,**

and **hydrogen peroxide** is not formed. Patients with the disorder are at **risk of infection with catalase-positive organisms,** especially *S. aureus,* fungi, and granuloma formation. Infections in these patients are usually localized to the respiratory tract, the skin, the liver, and the lymph nodes. The following organisms are the most commonly encountered pathogens in patients with CGD: *S. aureus, Burkholderia cepacia, Serratia marcescens, Nocardia* species, and *Aspergillus* species. Those organisms are relatively resistant to the **nonoxidative killing mechanisms** of neutrophils, which include antibacterial proteins and peptides stored in the **neutrophil-specific granules.** On the other hand, bacteria like pneumococci and streptococci, which generate their own hydrogen peroxide but have no catalase, are likely to be killed by the defective neutrophils. CGD neutrophils still contain the enzyme **myeloperoxidase,** which uses the hydrogen peroxide made by the bacteria's metabolism to produce lethal radicals. In effect, the bacteria commit suicide. Patients with CGD are given antibiotic prophylaxis with trimethoprim-sulfamethoxazole to prevent infections of bacterial pathogens, particularly *S. aureus.*

Adaptive Immunity

The **adaptive immune system** requires time to develop a functional response to invasive pathogens. That response is highly specific to the antigen of the invasive pathogen and is directed by antigen-specific lymphocytes. Adaptive immunity has both cellular and humoral components. **CD4+ T cells** are critical to antigen recognition; the subsequent development of cellular immunity, which is key to the destruction of intracellular pathogens such as viruses, fungi, and mycobacteria; and the development of humoral immunity, which protects us from extracellular pathogens.

T cells play a critical role in the development of both the cellular and humoral components of the adaptive immune response. Once stimulated by antigen recognition, CD4+ T cells differentiate into Th1 or Th2 cells, which play an immunomodulator role. **Th1 cells produce interferon-γ and interleukin 2 (IL-2),** which activate CD8+ T cells, macrophages, and NK cells to clear intracellular infections through lysis of infected cells. **Th2 cells produce IL-4, IL-5, and IL-10,** which cause differentiation of B cells and a highly specific antibody response against extracellular pathogens. Additionally, specialized populations of memory T and B cells develop as a result of the adaptive immune response. Those long-lived lymphocytes provide immunologic memory to respond rapidly to the re-presentation of the antigen that initially stimulated their development. The progressive depletion of CD4+ T cells in HIV infection and the development of opportunistic infections in AIDS exemplify the critical role of T cells in the maintenance of the adaptive immune response.

Abnormalities in Humoral Defense

The **humoral immune response** protects the host from extracellular bacteria that have evaded the cellular component of the innate immune system. The immediate response is carried out by the **complement** cascade, a nonspecific response leading to the production of nonspecific molecules that serve as opsonins and chemoattractants and effect bacteria lysis. The subsequent expansion of the B-cell population produces highly specific immunoglobulins that coat the extracellular microorganisms and lead to their clearance by the spleen. As stated previously, a subset of the B cells develops into memory cells to provide the host with long-term protection against subsequent infections.

Immunoglobulin deficiency can be congenital (e.g., **Bruton X-linked agammaglobulinemia**) or acquired (e.g., **common variable immunodeficiency**). Acquired hypogammaglobulinemia also arises as a result of conditions that lead to protein loss (e.g., nephrotic syndrome, intestinal lymphangiectasia), cancers of cells that make immunoglobulins (e.g., multiple myeloma, chronic lymphocytic leukemia), or burns. Defective B-lymphocyte function also occurs following bone marrow transplantation, as in V.'s case. The predominant infectious diseases seen in persons with immunoglobulin deficiencies are recurrent infections of the upper and lower respiratory tract caused by encapsulated bacteria, reflecting **the important role of antibodies in opsonization of encapsulated bacteria** such as *Streptococcus pneumoniae* and *Haemophilus influenzae*.

The rare cases of **complement deficiencies** are characterized by predisposition to infection with encapsulated bacteria. *Neisseria* **species are a special problem for patients with deficiencies of any of the late complement components** (C6, C7, C8, or C9) because complement-mediated lysis is required to kill those organisms. Many bacteria infect patients with defects earlier in the complement cascade. Most clinically significant complement deficiencies are congenitally acquired.

The **spleen** plays an important role in humoral immunity, both as a source of complement- and antibody-producing B cells and as the organ **primarily responsible for the removal of opsonized microbes from the bloodstream.** Defects in spleen function can result from splenectomy or diseases such as sickle cell anemia and put patients at risk of infection with encapsulated bacteria (e.g., pneumococci and *Haemophilus*). Bacterial infections can be fulminant in patients with splenic deficiency. Bacteremia and septic shock often result, and mortality is high unless patients receive appropriate therapy rapidly.

Disorders of Cell-Mediated Immunity

Defects in the function or number of macrophages and T lymphocytes lead to an increased risk of infection with bacteria that survive intracellularly, as well as with viruses, fungi, and protozoa (see Table 70-1). Patients with defective cell-mediated immunity are divided into two groups, depending on whether the defect is congenital or acquired. Primary disorders of cell-mediated immunity are usually diagnosed in childhood, and patients usually die from opportunistic infections before adulthood. An example of this immunodeficiency is **severe combined immunodeficiency (SCID)**, an inherited disease in which persons are born with no T cells but normal B-cell populations. The disease manifests early in life with failure to thrive, intestinal infections, and interstitial pneumonias caused by pathogens such as *Pneumocystis carinii*, *Candida* species, *Aspergillus* species, and viruses. Vaccination with live, attenuated viruses or bacille Calmette-Guérin (BCG) vaccine could lead to possibly fatal disseminated infections. SCID patients should be given prophylactic therapy with trimethoprim-sulfamethoxazole for *P. carinii* and acyclovir to prevent herpetic infections.

Acquired defects in cell-mediated immunity are seen in an increasingly large population of patients treated in hospitals. The enormous success of transplant surgery is a consequence of the development of drugs (such as **cyclosporin**) that suppress the graft-versus-host response and prevent rejection of the transplant. However, those **immunosuppressive drugs** also interfere with normal cell-mediated immunity, and all transplantation patients are at increased risk of opportunistic infection. Some immunosuppressive drugs, especially **corticosteroids**, are used to treat various inflammatory diseases. Cell-mediated immunity is also disturbed in patients with lymphoma.

The most profound example of defective cell-mediated immunity occurs in AIDS patients. HIV infection depletes CD4$^+$ helper T cells, leading almost inevitably to death from uncontrolled opportunistic infection or malignancy. AIDS patients have profound disturbances of cell-mediated immunity, especially that mediated by cytotoxic lymphocytes and macrophages, and **develop infections with eukaryotic agents** (e.g., *Pneumocystis carinii*), **viruses** (e.g., cytomegalovirus), and **intracellular bacteria** (e.g., mycobacteria).

Management of Infection in Immunocompromised Hosts: General Considerations

The presentation of infection in the immunocompromised patient can be subtle. Fever may be the only indication that the patient has an active infection, and the maximal temperature may be blunted by the level of immunosuppression. A thorough history and physical examination are crucial to effective management. History of previous infections and procedures and recent antibiotic and chemotherapeutic therapy should be assessed. In neutropenic patients the physical examination may be unrevealing because inflammation may not be evident without the presence of neutrophils. The physician should do a complete examination, paying particular attention to the oropharynx, sites of indwelling catheters, the perineum, scalp, and skin.

As with all patients, treatment of infections in the immunocompromised person should be directed against the specific infecting organism. However, defective host response heightens the risk of severe infection, and the need may be urgent to begin treatment presumptively, based on the most likely etiological possibilities. Knowing the type of immune defect, the likely resident microbial flora, the site and clinical features of the infection, and some epidemiological features often makes it possible to predict the likely infecting organism. For example, in granulocytopenic patients, broad-spectrum antibiotics with activity against both Gram-positive bacteria and Gram-negative bacteria (including those in the Enterobacteriaceae family) should be given at the first sign of infection, such as fever. Patients with decreased spleen function should be treated with drugs active against pneumococci and *H. influenzae*. A diffuse pneumonia involving most of the lung in a patient with AIDS is likely caused by *P. carinii*. However, that is not always the case, and in some patients specifically identifying the causative organism is necessary to start appropriate treatment or avoid toxic therapy.

Therefore, whenever possible, specimens should be obtained before starting therapy for infections in immunocompromised patients. The clinician and the microbiology laboratory should coordinate to ensure the recovery and identification of opportunistic pathogens. Unless warned, the microbiological laboratory may consider *S. epidermidis* a contaminant from the skin and not report it.

It is particularly important to attempt to reverse the immune defect; whenever practical, iatrogenic causes should be eliminated. Catheters should be removed, or at least changed, and immunosuppressive drugs should be discontinued whenever possible. In some transplant recipients it may even be necessary to allow the transplant to be rejected by suspending immunosuppressive therapy to permit an adequate host response to infection. In other cases replacement therapy is beneficial. Passive administration of immunoglobulins decreases the incidence of infection in patients with hypogammaglobulinemia. Granulocyte transfusions may benefit some granulocytopenic patients with refractory Gram-negative bacterial infections.

Preventive measures are also important in the care of immunocompromised patients. Simple procedures such as care with use and insertion of catheters, careful hand washing, and appropriate isolation techniques may reduce the incidence of opportunistic infection acquired in hospitals. Some vaccines (e.g., against influenza virus or pneumococci) may be beneficial. It is essential to remember that live vaccines should be given with caution to immunocompromised patients, who can acquire severe disease even from attenuated viruses. Prophylactic antibiotics are rarely beneficial; major exceptions are the use of penicillin to prevent pneumococcal infections in children with sickle cell disease and the use of trimethoprim-sulfamethoxazole to prevent pneumocystic pneumonia in patients with severe defects in cell-mediated immunity.

Conclusion

The immune system is a complex system that protects us from many pathogens. The congenital absence or acquired loss of any component of the immune system can lead to immunodeficiency and the development of life-threatening infections. With improvements in chemotherapeutic agents for malignancies, greater success in transplantation, and prolonged survival of patients with congenital immune defects, the number of patients with compromised immune systems continues to expand. Immunocompromised patients are susceptible not only to pathogens encountered in normal hosts but also to opportunistic infections with less virulent organisms that are easily cleared by a functioning immune system. The key to successful management of these patients lies in the ability to recognize their immune deficits and the risks that those defects create. Once the defects are identified, immunocompromised patients can be treated appropriately by minimizing their level of immune deficiency when possible, giving prophylactic antimicrobial therapy when indicated, aggressively seeking diagnosis early with appropriate tests and procedures, and recognizing the importance of pathogens associated with specific defects.

Acquired Immunodeficiency Syndrome

Richard K. Groger and William G. Powderly

As of 2003 the World Health Organization estimated that approximately 40 million people were infected with human immunodeficiency virus (HIV), the causative agent of acquired immunodeficiency syndrome (AIDS). Of those approximately 790,000 to 1.2 million lived in North America. Worldwide the number of new infections has averaged 5 million per year, and the number of deaths was approximately 3 million in 2003 alone. In many parts of sub-Saharan Africa, AIDS is the leading cause of death among young adults.

The impact of AIDS cannot be overemphasized. In 1995 the syndrome was the leading cause of death in the United States among men 20 to 45 years of age and was rapidly rising among women. By 2002 more than 500,000 people had died of AIDS in the United States. In some parts of Africa AIDS is the leading cause of death among young adults. Thanks to advances in treatment, deaths from AIDS declined sharply in the United States, from a peak of about 50,000 per year in 1995 to about 15,000 per year in 2002, even though the number of people living with HIV continued to rise. Unfortunately, only 10 percent of the people living with HIV worldwide have access to antiretroviral medications. Unless curative therapy is developed, most infected individuals will develop AIDS and eventually die from its consequences. In the interim, infected individuals may infect others.

AIDS is a constellation of clinical illnesses, primarily opportunistic infections and malignancies that can occur when HIV destroys the immune system. The syndrome is the final manifestation of an HIV infection that occurred many years previously (10 years on average). The continuous and relentless progression of HIV infection has been well characterized, and several methods are used to classify its stages. Chapter 38 describes the basic virology of HIV and the course of a typical HIV infection in terms of its progressive stages. This chapter focuses on one clinical case to describe the progression from HIV infection to AIDS, the manifestations of the syndrome, patient management, and preventive measures.

Early Acute HIV Infection

Mr. F.'s complaints and manifestations are nonspecific and common. His presentation is typical of many viral infections, including those caused by HIV and the Epstein-Barr virus. A clinician should consider the possibility of HIV infection if a patient presenting with the signs and symptoms of a viral infection is a gay or bisexual man or an intravenous drug user. Mr. F. has three risk factors for HIV infection: he is a bisexual man, he has had multiple sex partners who may have been infected, and he is a hospital phlebotomist.

Case

Mr. F., a 26-year-old married bisexual man who worked as a hospital phlebotomist, was seen in his physician's office complaining of a 1-week history of fever, swollen lymph nodes, and headache. He stated that he had unprotected sexual contact with a new male partner 3 weeks previously. On examination he had a red and inflamed pharynx, enlarged cervical lymph nodes, and a splotchy rash all over his body.

At this point the case raises two questions:

1. Could Mr. F. have been infected with HIV?
2. Can HIV be diagnosed at the initial stage?

Acute illness occurs in 50 to 90% of persons 24 weeks after infection by HIV. In most cases the only symptoms are mild fever and sore throat. A small subgroup may have fever, myalgias, lethargy, pharyngitis, arthralgias, lymphadenopathy, and a maculopapular rash of the trunk. Some patients have aseptic meningitis, and the headache that Mr. F. complained of may have been caused by mild meningeal irritation. The illness typically lasts 3 to 14 days, and complete recovery is the rule, even in patients with neurologic complications.

Antibodies against HIV are usually not detectable initially. However, various methods of detecting viral RNA in the blood have been developed. Although patients with acute HIV infection usually have high levels of viral RNA, follow-up serological testing is needed to confirm a diagnosis. No specific therapy is available for acute HIV disease. Although at the initial stage of infection a patient is likely to have a negative HIV antibody test, the result can be used to establish a baseline for future testing.

Case

After counseling about the implications and possible outcome of HIV testing, Mr. F. had an HIV test, which was negative. He returned for a follow-up 6 weeks later. His symptoms had resolved completely and he felt well. Serological testing at the time revealed a positive **enzyme-linked immunosorbent assay (ELISA)** for HIV signifying antibodies specific to HIV. A **Western blot** confirmed that result.

At this point the case raises two questions:

1. How accurate are the tests for HIV?
2. Can Mr. F. be sure he is infected?

Diagnostic Tests

Measurement of viral RNA by polymerase chain reaction (PCR) methodologies can detect HIV early in infection. However, because of its cost, a PCR test is not used to screen for infection unless the clinician suspects acute infection. Instead, HIV infection is typically diagnosed by detecting circulating antibodies to the virus. Unlike most antibody tests, in which the presence of specific antibodies signifies past infection with the agent in question, a positive HIV antibody test signifies current infection. Any individual who has HIV antibodies must be assumed to have active infection that can be transmitted to others. It is important, therefore, that individuals with positive HIV antibody tests receive counseling about the issues involved in transmission so that spread can be minimized.

Specific anti-HIV antibodies generally appear 6 to 12 weeks after infection. However, studies using PCR to test for specific HIV RNA have shown that in rare cases infected individuals do not develop antibodies for several months or years after exposure. Those unusual individuals have false-negative serological tests for HIV. In addition, some patients in the terminal phases of AIDS have negative serological tests (presumably because of **severe B-cell dysfunction**). Fortunately, patients with advanced disease can usually be identified by other than serological means; however, B-cell dysfunction also complicates the serologic diagnosis of several of the opportunistic infections that occur in AIDS.

The most common method for testing for HIV antibodies is the ELISA. This test is performed by adding a sample of the patient's serum to small wells to which HIV antigens are bound. If antibodies are present, they will complex with the antigen. An anti-immunoglobulin antibody linked to an identifier enzyme is then added to bind to the complex. Although the ELISA is a highly sensitive test (more than 99%), it is not completely specific, and false-positive results occur. When screening a large population (such as all adults in the United States), **even a false-positive rate of less than 0.01% would mean that many uninfected individuals would be misidentified.** Persons with false-positive test results could face discrimination in insurance, employment, and housing. The incidence of false-positives, no matter how low, is a strong argument against indiscriminate testing without obtaining the permission of the patient.

Consequently, positive ELISA results should be verified with a more specific test. In most laboratories that test is a **Western blot,** which detects antibodies to specific viral polypeptides. The Western blot is a sensitive and specific way to test for HIV antibodies; however, it is too time consuming and expensive to be used for primary screening purposes.

Rarely, some people exhibit nonspecific cross-reactivity in serological HIV tests and may be difficult to distinguish from patients with early HIV infection. The true pattern can usually be determined by repeating the Western blot after 3 or 4 months. By then a person with true infection will usually have developed new antibodies to different epitopes (which show up in the Western blot), whereas those with nonspecific reactivity will have the same pattern as before. Waiting for repeat HIV tests can be a difficult time for patients, who will need counseling and support to help them understand the limitations of technology.

Other assays to determine the presence of HIV infection are available but are not always useful. The **p24 antigen** is the viral core protein produced by the *gag* gene, and its presence denotes active viral replication. However, the antigen is not detectable in the serum of all patients and thus not useful diagnostically. HIV can be cultured from lymphocytes of most infected individuals, but that test is technically difficult and is rarely used outside research settings. HIV DNA PCR, which amplifies chromosomally integrated HIV provirus, is a highly sensitive and specific method of detecting early infection. It is most commonly used to identify HIV-infected infants born to HIV positive mothers, for whom maternal antibodies could complicate serologic diagnostic tests. Although the DNA test becomes positive only slightly later than the HIV RNA PCR, the RNA test can occasionally become undetectable in established infection, even in the absence of antiretroviral therapy, and the DNA test does not. Both DNA and RNA PCR tests can give false-positive results in cases of laboratory cross-contamination. Therefore follow-up serologic confirmation of a positive test is necessary. Additionally, genetic drift causes mismatch with the primers used in PCR assays and can give false-negative results, particularly in some HIV **clades,** or clonally related groups. HIV RNA PCR is most commonly used to assess the need for and effectiveness of antiretroviral therapy.

HIV Transmission

Mr. F. has clearly seroconverted (from negative to positive) and is infected with HIV. How did he get his infection? HIV is transmitted primarily by direct inoculation of infected blood or body fluids into the host. Thus, the epidemiology of HIV mirrors that of viruses spread by that means (e.g., hepatitis B and C). **Most cases of HIV infection are acquired sexually,** and sexual practices associated with trauma, such as receptive anal intercourse, facilitate the spread of the virus. Other sexually transmitted diseases, especially chancroid, are associated with an increased risk of HIV transmission, possibly because the epithelial barrier is breached by the genital ulcers. In the United States and other western countries, HIV initially infected mainly homosexual men and was wrongly perceived as an exclusive disease of that community. However, in other parts of the world, sexual transmission of HIV is predominantly heterosexual. In the United States the number of cases of HIV infection acquired by heterosexual contact has risen steadily. Some studies suggest that women are more easily infected than men, but transmission clearly occurs in both directions.

Contact with infected blood or blood products is another important form of transmission of HIV. Transmission through infected blood and blood products has considerably diminished since blood donor testing and treatment of plasma to inactivate the virus was instituted. However, that mode of transmission has not been eliminated completely. Because of the "window period" in early infection, blood donors with early HIV infection may not have developed HIV antibodies.

Bloodborne spread of HIV remains a considerable problem among intravenous drug users who share needles and syringes. Individuals who exchange sex for drugs may then infect their sexual partners. Infected women can infect their children in utero or intra partum (**vertical transmission**). Additional risk of transmission occurs with breast-feeding. Without antiretroviral therapy for HIV infected mothers, between 13 and 40% of their infants will be infected with the virus. Antiretroviral therapy for HIV-infected pregnant women may substantially lower the risk of transmission to their babies—to less than 1%, under optimal circumstances. The reason all children with HIV-infected mothers are not infected is unknown, although it may be related, in part, to maternal immune responses to HIV and to the level of HIV circulating in the mother's blood.

HIV is also an occupational problem for health care workers. Exposure to HIV-infected blood, predominantly through needlestick injuries, is now a significant hazard for health care workers. The risk of infection after such exposure is low; it is estimated that 1 in 300 exposures leads to infection. Cases of AIDS resulting from needlestick injuries have been documented. Transmission in the opposite direction (i.e., from an infected health care worker to a patient) has also been documented. **Universal precautions** (assuming all blood or other fluids are potentially infected) are important to prevent transmission of HIV infection in health care settings.

Thus, Mr. F. could have been infected in a number of ways. He is a bisexual man with a recent new sexual partner, and he is a phlebotomist who may have had exposure to infected blood. Statistically, it is most likely that he acquired HIV from sexual contact.

When should people be tested for HIV infection? Persons with HIV disease seek medical attention at various stages of the disease. Many patients with early HIV infection do not seek medical attention and do not know they are infected until they develop AIDS. However, most patients are seen by a physician before they develop AIDS. Many want to be tested for HIV because they perceive that some aspect of their lifestyle puts them at risk. Others consult a physician with complaints that are not obviously caused by HIV disease, and the diagnosis is made when their physician counsels them to be tested for HIV.

Case

Mr. F. returned to his physician's office 2 weeks later to get the results of his antibody tests. When told he was HIV positive, he became anxious and asked, "Does that mean I have AIDS?" In addition to informing his male and female sexual partners that he is HIV-positive and taking precautions not to infect them, Mr. F. needs to consider his occupation. If his hospital duties include the performance of invasive procedures, he should think about transferring to another position.

At this point the case raises two questions:

1. Will Mr. F. get AIDS?
2. What kind of lifestyle changes should Mr. F. consider making to minimize the risk of spreading the infection to others and to maintain his health as much as possible?

Consequences of Being HIV Positive

The period following a definitive diagnosis of HIV infection is a difficult time for a patient. Anxiety about the possibility of AIDS and concern about transmission of the virus to close family members are common reactions. Counseling patients is, therefore, important at that point. Patients should be taught how the virus is spread and educated fully about their duty to protect other people, especially their sexual contacts. Infected persons should be informed that abstinence from sexual intercourse is the only sure way of avoiding transmission. **Sexual practices that do not involve contact with semen or vaginal secretions are considered safe.** Condom use is essential if patients are going to continue to have sexual intercourse. Patients should be reassured that casual contact with others does not pose a risk of transmission.

The probability of progression to AIDS can be estimated by determining the degree of immunodeficiency. The most helpful measurement is the level of **T-lymphocytes** subsets. Because the **CD4$^+$ (T4** or **helper-inducer) T cells** are a specific target of HIV, measurement of the number and percentage of those cells in the circulation indicates the degree of immune impairment and thus the risk of developing AIDS. The normal CD4$^+$ T-cell count in adults ranges from 800 to 2,000 cells/mm^3. Progressive loss of the cells over time is the usual pattern of progressive HIV infection (Fig. 71–1). The probability of AIDS-related opportunistic infections rises sharply when a patient's CD4$^+$ T-cell count falls below 200 cells/mm^3, and the types of infections to which the individual is susceptible varies according to the degree of immunosuppression. The rate of decline of CD4$^+$ T cells over time can also give important prognostic clues. In addition, the **viral load,** as reflected by measurements of the HIV plasma RNA, also provides important prognostic information, perhaps even more important than the CD4$^+$ T-cell count. The higher the viral load in the plasma, the more rapid the progression of a patient to clinical AIDS or death.

Once HIV enters the body, it rapidly disseminates to many organs, especially the lymphoreticular system and the brain. Initial infection may, in fact, be associated with a profound, albeit temporary, loss of CD4$^+$ T cells (and even opportunistic infections in occasional patients). With the appearance of a cellular immune response, the levels of viral RNA in the plasma decrease dramatically. However, active viral replication continues at a high rate within lymph nodes. Recent information

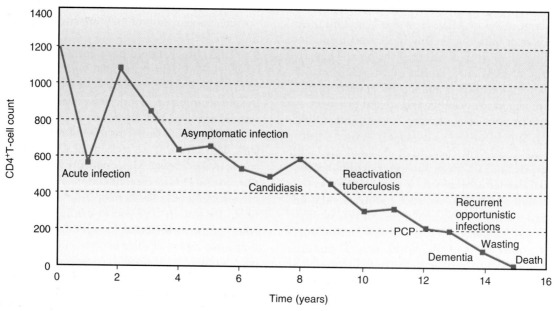

FIGURE 71-1 ▪ **The natural history of HIV disease.**

suggests that a high turnover of virus and of CD4$^+$ T cells occurs on a daily basis until the body's reserve of lymphocytes is depleted. Pathologically, the lymph nodes are progressively destroyed at the same time, and ultimately the virus escapes the partial surveillance, and high plasma levels of virus are seen again as the disease progresses.

Symptoms or clinical illnesses that suggest immunodeficiency also help identify patients who are likely to progress more rapidly to AIDS. Consequently, a careful history should be taken regarding fever, night sweats, unintentional weight loss, or unexplained diarrhea. The presence of *Candida* infection in the mouth (thrush) also indicates a poor prognosis. Despite those prognostic markers, precisely how quickly a particular patient will progress to AIDS cannot be foretold. The mechanisms controlling the rate of progression are not well understood, and factors such as genetic variability (i.e., the host), viral phenotype, and viral load are potentially important.

Because most HIV-infected individuals develop progressive immunodeficiency, they should be assessed for occult infections that may become problematic later. Tuberculin skin testing and a chest radiograph should be performed when a patient has a history of a positive tuberculin skin test because the risk of reactivation tuberculosis is dramatically increased in HIV-infected persons. Patients who test positive to the skin test and thus do not have active tuberculosis should be treated prophylactically with isoniazid. Patients with positive serology for syphilis require antitreponemal therapy, particularly if neurosyphilis is suspected. Baseline **cytomegalovirus (CMV)** and *Toxoplasma gondii* antibody testing identifies persons at risk for reactivation disease by those agents. HIV-positive individuals are also candidates for vaccination against pneumococcal disease and annual immunization against influenza. Because patients are also at risk for hepatitis B, they should be tested for antibodies against that virus, and those who are negative should be offered vaccination against it.

Case

Mr. F.'s CD4$^+$ T-cell count was measured and found to be 750 cells/mm^3. He was otherwise completely well. His physician advised him that he had no evidence of significant immune impairment and should return for a checkup every 6 months for CD4$^+$ T-cell measurement and evaluation.

Unfortunately, Mr. F. did not keep his scheduled appointments. Four years passed before he returned to his physician's office complaining of a blistering rash on his left shoulder and upper torso. He also complained of sore throat and white spots in his mouth. Examination showed oral thrush; enlarged, nontender cervical, axillary, and inguinal lymph nodes; and a vesicular (blistering) rash in a dermatomal distribution consistent with shingles. Mr. F.'s CD4$^+$ T-cell count was 280 cells/mm^3.

At this point the case raises two questions:

1. By ignoring his physician's advice and not having regular checkups, has Mr. F. caused himself irreparable harm?
2. What kind of treatment and management should Mr. F. receive?

■ ■ ■ ■

Progression to AIDS

Acute HIV infection is followed by a latent period during which infected individuals are asymptomatic and appear healthy. The duration of that period is variable, ranging from **several months to more than 15 years;** the median time is about 10 years. Although the period is referred to as asymptomatic, many patients in fact have complaints that are not obviously linked to HIV infection or to the associated immunodeficiency. For example, HIV-infected persons are particularly prone to skin complaints. The reason is unknown, but infection of the epidermal Langerhans cells may be a contributory factor. Many patients complain of excessively dry skin or pruritus, **seborrheic dermatitis with eczema folliculitis,** or **psoriasis.** Onset of severe psoriasis, eczema, or folliculitis in a previously healthy adult should raise the possibility of HIV infection. Furthermore, reactivation of **herpes zoster (shingles),** as occurred with Mr. F., can also be a sentinel of HIV infection. Patients are also prone to recurrent **herpes simplex** infection, **molluscum contagiosum,** and drug eruptions. In addition, a type of skin cancer, cutaneous **Kaposi sarcoma,** may be the first manifestation of AIDS. It is characterized by blue–violet palpable, nonpruritic, painless lesions.

Patients in the latent stage of infection may also present with localized or generalized lymphatic enlargement, as Mr. F. did. **Painless generalized lymphadenopathy** is a common manifestation of HIV disease, but **has no prognostic significance.** On the other hand, localized adenopathy or changes in already enlarged nodes can be early signs of infection or malignancy and should be investigated.

Recurrent mucocutaneous candidiasis (vaginal or oral in women, oral in men) and extensive oral aphthous ulcerations (canker sores) are common early manifestations of HIV infection and identify patients at greater risk of soon developing AIDS. **Hairy leukoplakia** (plaques of thickened mucosa on the tongue and elsewhere in the mouth) is caused by Epstein-Barr virus and also occurs early in HIV disease. Another feature of early HIV disease is the appearance of abnormal laboratory findings. For instance, many infected individuals have isolated hematologic cytopenias, usually anemia, lymphopenia, or thrombocytopenia. Abnormalities in liver function tests, which are also common, are usually a result of previous or concurrent viral hepatitis.

The progressive loss of CD4[1] T cells and the oral *Candida* infection suggest that Mr. F.'s cell-mediated immunity has significantly diminished since his physician last saw him. Mr. F. does not yet have AIDS. However, the drop in CD4[1] T cells and the oral candidiasis are poor prognostic signs and an indication for starting specific antiretroviral treatment. Mr. F. should also start prophylactic therapy to prevent *Pneumocystis jiroveci (Pneumocystis carinii)* infection.

The status of patients in the natural progression of HIV infection is routinely assessed in three ways:

- Ongoing clinical evaluation for HIV- and AIDS-related conditions
- CD4$^+$ T-cell count
- Quantification of HIV viral burden

HIV viral burden is typically measured in blood using a nucleic acid–based test, such as a DNA probe or PCR assay. Those tests have been shown effective in predicting progression to AIDS and long-term survival. The decision to initiate antiretroviral therapy is usually based on one or more of the three standard assessments. Although when antiretroviral therapy should begin in early HIV infection is still a controversial question, the presence of an AIDS-defining illness, a CD4$^+$ T-cell count less than 350 cells/mm^3, or a viral burden of 55,000 viral genomes/mm^3 of blood have been used as criteria for initiating therapy.

Treatment with **zidovudine (AZT)** as a single agent showed that the progression to AIDS could be modestly delayed, but certain indicators of HIV progression, such as CD4$^+$ T-cell counts and viral burden, progress in spite of therapy after a few months. The progression of disease in spite of antiretroviral treatment results from the emergence of resistant HIV viruses during therapy. Resistant mutants arise promptly because the viral reverse transcriptase is prone to errors. In the case of AZT and other reverse transcriptase inhibitors, the mutations occur in the viral gene encoding the enzyme. Similarly, mutations within the protease gene are associated with resistance to protease inhibitors. The emergence of resistance can be prevented by combining several different antiretroviral agents that act at different steps of viral replication or that require distinct mutations to confer resistance (Fig. 71-2). Most patients are treated initially with three or more active drugs (e.g., two reverse transcriptase inhibitors and a protease inhibitor). Combination antiretroviral regimens typically induce long-lasting reductions in viral burden and increases in CD4$^+$ T-cell counts, and the regimens have contributed to a recent and significant reduction in AIDS-related deaths in the United States.

Pneumocystic pneumonia is a preventable disease. Prospective studies of HIV-positive patients have shown that at least one third of patients with CD4$^+$ T-cell counts less than 200 cells/mm^3 develop pneumocystic pneumonia within 3 years in the absence of prophylactic therapy. The risk is considerably greater if the patients are also symptomatic (i.e., have fever, night sweats, weight loss, or oral candidiasis). The risk of infection can be substantially reduced with prophylactic therapy such as trimethoprim-sulfamethoxazole. Pneumocystic pneumonia is less clearly correlated with CD4$^+$ T-cell counts in children. HIV-infected infants with CD4$^+$ T-cell counts less than 1,500 cells/mm^3 should be considered candidates for prophylaxis.

Case

Mr. F.'s physician prescribed combination antiretroviral therapy and trimethoprim-sulfamethoxazole tablets. When he broke out in an itchy rash 10 days later, Mr. F. stopped taking all his medications but did not inform his doctor. Six months later he arrived at a local emergency department complaining

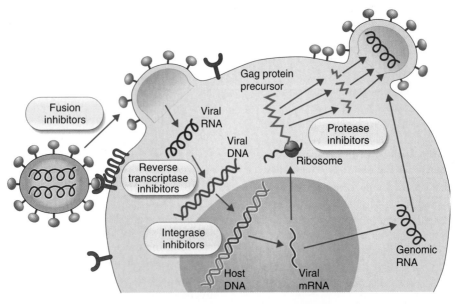

FIGURE 71-2 ▪ **Possible sites of intervention in the inhibition of HIV replication.**

of a 6-day history of gradually worsening dry cough and shortness of breath. His temperature was 40°C and a chest radiograph showed a diffuse bilateral interstitial pneumonia. Examination of fluid from bronchoalveolar lavage revealed *P. jiroveci.* Mr. F.'s infection had advanced to AIDS.

At this point the case raises two questions:

1. What other infections might Mr. F. acquire?
2. Can any treatment help him avoid those infections at this stage?

Clinical Manifestations of AIDS

The signs and symptoms of pneumocystic pneumonia place Mr. F. in the category of AIDS patients, but any of a number of other opportunistic infections, singly or in groups, would lead to the same diagnosis. The box titled "AIDS-Defining Illnesses" (see below) indicates the major infections associated with AIDS, most of which are caused by intracellular agents usually controlled by cell-mediated immunity. These infections are often the result of endogenous reactivation of previously acquired organisms, rather than newly acquired infection.

Most AIDS-related infections do not occur until the CD4$^+$ T-cell count falls below 200 cells/mm^3. Kaposi sarcoma is the major exception to that rule because its occurrence seems to be independent of the underlying T-cell depletion, although it is more frequent at lower CD4$^+$ T-cell counts. Reactivation tuberculosis, which is the most frequent presenting opportunistic infection worldwide, can also occur with CD4$^+$ T-cell counts above 200 cells/mm^3, but the risk of reactivation increases with progressive immunodeficiency. Infections in AIDS patients are characterized by a high density of organisms and disseminated disease, as well as infections with multiple organisms. The infections are rarely cured. Control of disease consequently requires prolonged acute therapy as well as long-term use of antimicrobial agents to prevent relapses.

Lung Infections

Pneumonia caused by *P. jiroveci* is the most frequent opportunistic infection associated with AIDS and occurs in 25 to 60% of patients. The typical symptoms are **fever, cough,** and **shortness of breath.** Although the infection typically affects the lung, it can involve other sites, especially the liver, lymph nodes, and choroid. Pneumocystic pneumonia is treatable yet is associated with a mortality rate of 10 to 20% from irreversible respiratory failure.

An opportunistic infection such as pneumocystic pneumonia does not mean that patients will automatically develop multiple medical problems and soon die. The use of specific antiretroviral therapy and anti–*P. jiroveci* drugs has led to an improvement in the quality and length of life for AIDS patients. Many people are able to live and work normally for long periods. In

AIDS-Defining Illnesses^a

1. Multiple or recurrent bacterial infections (two in a 2-year period) affecting a child less than 13 years of age: septicemia, pneumonia, meningitis, bone or joint infection, or internal abscess caused by *Haemophilus influenzae,* streptococci, or other pyogenic bacteria
2. Candidiasis of the esophagus, trachea, bronchi, or lungs
3. Disseminated coccidioidomycosis
4. Extrapulmonary cryptococcosis
5. Chronic cryptosporidiosis, with diarrhea for more than 1 month
6. Cytomegalovirus infection
7. Mucocutaneous herpes simplex virus infection persisting for more than 1 month
8. HIV encephalopathy
9. Disseminated histoplasmosis
10. Isosporiasis, with diarrhea for more than 1 month
11. Kaposi sarcoma
12. Primary lymphoma of the brain
13. Non-Hodgkin lymphoma of B-cell or unknown phenotype, including Burkitt lymphoma
14. Lymphoid interstitial pneumonia affecting a child less than 13 years of age
15. Disseminated mycobacterial infection (not *Mycoplasma tuberculosis*)
16. Extrapulmonary tuberculosis
17. *Pneumocystis jiroveci (Pneumocystis carinii)* infection
18. Progressive multifocal leukoencephalopathy
19. Recurrent *Salmonella* infection
20. Toxoplasmosis of the brain

^{a}Any of these diseases indicates a diagnosis of AIDS in the presence of laboratory evidence of HIV infection.

patients who achieve optimal responses to antiretroviral medications, there is usually significant reconstitution of cellular immune responses, with concomitant reduction in the risk of opportunistic infections for as long as the retroviral replication can be suppressed. Nevertheless, no curative therapy is available, and the emergence of resistant virus or the inability of patients to tolerate side effects or pill burden can limit the success of antiretroviral regimens. Progressive deterioration with repeated episodes of infection is the normal pattern for patients with advanced HIV disease, for whom suppression of viral replication cannot be achieved.

Case

After the episode of pneumonia, Mr. F. made a complete recovery and was able to return to work. He took zidovudine, **lamivudine,** and **efavirenz** for his HIV and **trimethoprim-sulfamethoxazole** as prophylaxis for pneumocystic pneumonia. Mr. F. had no problems for about a year until he went to his physician complaining of difficulty swallowing and diarrhea. He also admitted that he had not been taking his medications regularly. His diarrhea was intermittent but could be as severe as 20 bouts of loose watery stools per day. On examining his mouth, the physician noticed multiple white plaques on his palate and tongue.

At this point the case raises two questions:

1. Why did Mr. F. have difficulty swallowing?
2. What caused his diarrhea?

Gastrointestinal Infections

Gastrointestinal problems are common in patients with AIDS. Candidiasis of the mouth and pharynx is almost universal in patients with profound immunodeficiency but is usually manageable. A substantial number of patients go on to develop esophageal candidiasis, which can cause pain and difficulty on swallowing, leading to considerable weight loss. Esophageal infection can also be caused by the herpes viruses, herpes simplex and CMV, although they more typically involve other sites. Herpes simplex causes recurrent skin infections, especially perirectally, that can become resistant to therapy. CMV typically causes disseminated disease with viremia. Involvement of the colon can lead to severe abdominal pain and diarrhea. CMV infection of the eye presents as blurred vision and may lead to blindness. Diarrhea is a common problem in patients with advanced AIDS and may be severe and difficult to diagnose and treat. It can be caused by a large number of agents:

- CMV and other viruses
- Enteric Gram-negative bacteria such as *Salmonella* and *Shigella* species (with accompanying bacteremia)
- Mycobacterial infection (especially the *Mycobacterium avium* complex) that affects the small bowel and colon and causes malabsorption and diarrhea

- Intestinal parasites such as *Giardia, Isospora,* and *Cryptosporidium* species and microsporidia

Malignancies such as Kaposi sarcoma or lymphoma involving the stomach or colon may also cause gastrointestinal symptoms. Furthermore, HIV itself may infect the cells of the gastrointestinal tract and cause an enteropathy leading to diarrhea.

Investigating intestinal distress in AIDS patients requires culturing stool for bacteria and examining it microscopically for parasites. If the examination does not give an answer, it may be necessary to perform invasive tests.

Case

Mr. F., was found to have esophageal candidiasis and *Salmonella* infection. Following treatment his symptoms resolved. His virus had now developed multiple mutations in the reverse transcriptase gene, and he was started on a new regimen. Unfortunately, he was not able to take his medications regularly. Two months later he was admitted to the hospital with a high fever, cough, and shortness of breath. A chest radiograph showed a lobar pneumonia, and sputum cultures grew *Streptococcus pneumoniae.* He responded rapidly to penicillin treatment.

At this point the case raises two questions:

1. What other agents of pneumonia is Mr. F. susceptible to?
2. Is he at risk for tuberculosis, and is it treatable?

Mycobacterial and Fungal Infections

Although *P. jiroveci* is a frequent cause of pneumonia in AIDS patients, other causes must be considered, such as pneumococci, *Haemophilus influenzae,* and enteric Gram-negative rods. Tuberculosis is another important cause of pneumonia in AIDS, and it can disseminate widely to cause lymphadenitis, hepatitis, or meningitis.

Although most opportunistic infections occur during severe immunodeficiency, tuberculosis is an exception and can occur earlier, when the immune function of AIDS patients is only mildly impaired (i.e., in the "asymptomatic" phase). Consequently, **HIV infection should be considered in the event of pulmonary tuberculosis in previously healthy young adults or adolescents.** Infected patients can easily spread tuberculosis to household members and other close contacts. Indeed, the rise in incidence of tuberculosis in the United States that began in the late 1980s can be attributed largely to the spread of tuberculosis among HIV-infected persons and their close contacts. Fortunately, tuberculosis is treatable in patients with HIV infection and remains one of the few AIDS-associated opportunistic infections that does not require lifelong suppressive treatment after a prolonged course of curative therapy.

Disseminated infection with the *Mycobacterium avium* complex is also common in AIDS. Although the MAC organism can cause pneumonia, it more typically causes disseminated disease, particularly in the lymphoreticular organs and the gastrointestinal tract. Typically, patients develop fever, night sweats, weight loss, and enlarged livers and spleens; some also develop diarrhea. Similar symptoms are seen in patients with disseminated fungal infection, such as **histoplasmosis**, which is common in patients from the Midwest and Latin America. Disseminated **coccidioidomycosis** is found in patients from the southwestern United States.

Case

On recovering from pneumonia, Mr. F. returned to work. He went back to see his physician 4 months later when he developed high fever and headache. Although his examination was normal the physician obtained a rapid test for cryptococcal antigen on the patient's serum. This test was positive, and the physician then recommended a spinal tap. The cell count and glucose and protein levels on the cerebrospinal fluid were normal, but an India ink smear of cerebrospinal fluid showed it to be packed with encapsulated yeast. Mr. F. responded well to antifungal treatment.

At this point the case raises one question:

1. Why did the physician perform a serum cryptococcal antigen test despite Mr. F.'s normal examination?

Infections of the Nervous System

Opportunistic infections can also cause neurological problems in AIDS patients. Fever and headache are the most common presentations of infection with the fungus *Cryptococcus neoformans*, which typically causes meningitis. Mr. F.'s case illustrates one of the major problems of treating such infections in a patient with AIDS. His spinal fluid was teeming with fungi, yet because of his immune defect, he was unable to mount an effective inflammatory response (which explains his normal cell count and glucose and protein levels).

Other opportunistic infections can affect the brain. Reactivation of infection with the parasite *Toxoplasma gondii* typically causes a **multifocal infection in the brain.** Patients may present with headache, confusion, or seizures. Infection with another virus, the **JC virus,** causes a progressive and fatal encephalopathy (**progressive multifocal leukoencephalopathy,** or **PML**). CMV causes retinitis and occasionally encephalitis.

Case

Mr. F. became increasingly concerned about his weight loss. In fact, on reviewing Mr. F.'s records the physician found that his weight loss over the previous year was 90 lb, although Mr. F. reported he was eating fairly well. He continued to have difficulty adhering to antiretroviral therapy, and multiple muta-

tions were detected in both the reverse transcriptase and protease genes. He also noted fevers, night sweats, and intermittent bouts of severe diarrhea. Mr. F. has progressive AIDS.

At this point the case raises one question:

1. What caused Mr. F.'s significant weight loss?

Direct Manifestations of HIV Itself

HIV itself can directly affect many organs of the body, such as the intestine and the kidney. **HIV nephropathy** is manifested by proteinuria, the nephrotic syndrome, and kidney failure and may respond to antiretroviral therapy. **Myopathy** and **myositis** both occur and may be related to HIV infection or the effects of drug therapy. **Cardiomyopathy** also occurs. One of the most distressing features of late AIDS is a **wasting syndrome** that is characterized by profound weight loss with concomitant loss of muscle mass. The pathogenesis of wasting syndrome in AIDS is unclear; however, it carries a grave prognosis and usually portends death.

Case

A few days later Mr. F. returned to his physician with several purple–red skin lesions on his legs and trunk. The lesions were biopsied, and Kaposi sarcoma was diagnosed.

At this point the case raises one question:

1. What is Kaposi sarcoma?

Oncological Manifestations in Advanced AIDS

It is important to realize that the illnesses we associate with AIDS are changing in frequency and importance. As physicians become more adept in treating and preventing infections like pneumocystic pneumonia, other infections (e.g., those caused by mycobacteria and CMV) assume greater importance. Neurological manifestations of HIV in its later stages (discussed in the next section) and malignancies have also assumed more importance. As patients live longer with profound immunodeficiency, malignancies are seen more frequently. The two most common malignancies are Kaposi sarcoma and lymphoma.

Kaposi sarcoma is associated with **human herpes virus 8.** It is most commonly seen in male homosexuals with HIV disease. Its occurrence is independent of underlying immunocompromise, although it behaves more aggressively and is more difficult to treat as the $CD4^+$ T-cell count falls. In its mildest form, it may merely cause localized skin disease without significant morbidity. Severe cases of Kaposi sarcoma present with widely disseminated lesions; involve the lymph nodes, gastrointestinal tract, and lungs; and can be fatal.

Both Hodgkin disease and non-Hodgkin lymphoma occur more frequently in HIV-infected patients. The latter is an increasingly important problem. Involvement of the central nervous system is common and usually associated with poor prognosis. Epstein-Barr virus has been associated with most cases of central nervous system lymphoma, suggesting a probable role for this virus in the pathogenesis of this tumor.

Case

Mr. F. missed his next two appointments with his physician, and the next time he came to the office he was accompanied by his parents, who reported that he had become more forgetful and withdrawn. They informed the physician that Mr. F. had been fired from his job because he was constantly late and could not concentrate on tasks. When his physician examined him, Mr. F. appeared inattentive and, although he knew who and where he was, he had problems remembering simple commands. The physician ordered a computerized tomography (CT) scan of his head, which showed profound brain atrophy.

At this point the case raises one question:

1. What is Mr. F.'s prognosis?

Neurological Manifestations in Advanced AIDS

Although opportunistic infections and lymphomas can involve the nervous system in AIDS, by far the most common neurological problems are caused by HIV itself. HIV is a lentivirus and, like many others in that group, is neurotropic. Infection of the nervous system occurs early in the disease, probably soon after exposure. The presence of HIV in the nervous system has been documented by viral culture of brain tissue, in situ hybridization demonstrating viral DNA sequences, and electron micrographic identification of retroviral particles. Within the central nervous system, the virus resides predominantly in macrophages and cells derived from macrophages, although the pathogenesis of HIV-associated neuronal damage is unclear.

Manifestations of nervous system involvement can occur at any stage of HIV disease. Acute primary infection may be complicated by aseptic meningitis, encephalitis, myelitis, or inflammatory neuropathies such as Guillain-Barré syndrome. Later in HIV disease patients may have peripheral neuropathies, both motor and sensory, or spinal cord syndromes, resembling subacute combined degeneration of the cord. The most common form of neurological disease, however, is HIV-associated

encephalopathy, which leads to progressive dementia, as in the case of Mr. F.

In its earliest form, HIV dementia may consist of generalized mental slowing, difficulty concentrating, and forgetfulness, all of which must be differentiated from the depression that often accompanies HIV infection. In the later stages of HIV dementia, patients have profound deficits in cognitive, motor, and sensory functions and may be totally unable to care for themselves. CT scans of the brain often show considerable atrophy (Fig. 71-3). Severe dementia is almost inevitably fatal.

Outcome

Mr. F.'s outcome is typical of the usual course of untreated HIV infection. Although HIV disease is, as yet, incurable and fatal, its progression varies. With improved antiretroviral therapy and use of prophylactic

FIGURE 71-3 ▪ **Computerized tomography scan of the brain of a patient with AIDS. A. Normal CT scan. B.** Scan from the same patient 4 months later when he presented with mental slowing and confusion. Note the profound loss of brain substance and consequent enlargement of the fluid-filled ventricles.

Case

Two weeks later, Mr. F.'s parents called the physician to tell him that Mr. F. had died at home that day.

■ ■ ■ ■

antimicrobial therapy, HIV infection is increasingly a chronic disease in many patients.

Genetic and Developmental Predisposition to AIDS

Would the course of Mr. F.'s illness have been different if he had been a female? Probably not, although some of the indicator diseases may have been different. As mentioned earlier, recurrent **vaginal candidiasis** may be a common and troublesome complaint in HIV-infected women. In addition, increasing evidence shows that human papillomavirus infection may behave more aggressively in persons with HIV infection. Consequently, **cancer of the uterine cervix** emerged as an important complication.

Host-specific genetic determinants that likely affect the rate of progression of disease in HIV infection are only beginning to be elucidated. In addition, slight differences may exist among patients regarding the toxicity of antiretroviral agents, depending on patients' genetic backgrounds. It should be noted that there are no indications that drug treatment is ineffective or harmful; thus, no person should go untreated because he or she belongs to a particular racial group or gender.

HIV infection in children follows a similar course, with progressive immunodeficiency, recurrent opportunistic infections, and neurological involvement. However, the pace of the disease is much more rapid in infants. Transmission is usually vertical (i.e., acquired from the mother), and 13 to 40% of babies born to HIV-infected mothers acquire the infection. Combination antiretroviral therapy of HIV-infected mothers during the last two trimesters and during labor may reduce the transmission rate to less than 2%.

Most children with vertically acquired HIV infection have an indolent course with slow progression (8 or more years) to clinical disease; however, 15 to 20% of those children rapidly progress to symptomatic disease and death within 2 to 4 years after birth without medical intervention. In addition to their opportunistic infections, the infants fail to thrive (i.e., have abnormal growth rates), and many have developmental delays secondary to HIV brain infection. Recurrent bacterial infections (e.g., otitis, pneumonia) are common and are related to B-cell dysfunction. However, as with adults,

antiretroviral treatment and prophylactic therapy for infection improve the quality and extent of life.

Management of HIV-Infected Patients

Management of the HIV-infected patient involves a long-term commitment from physicians and other members of the health care team not only to provide medical treatment and management but also to support and educate the patient and the family. Patients need to be alerted about symptoms that require prompt medical attention, such as changes in fever patterns or new onsets of cough or headache. Physicians must be prepared to deal with the many complaints that develop and distinguish those that herald important complications. Patients must be educated about the modes of transmission so that new cases can be prevented. In addition, the members of the health care team need to help the patient cope with the changing social dimensions of the disease. Confidentiality and maintenance of employment and insurance benefits are prime concerns. Most patients with AIDS wish to be treated as much as possible at home. Family and friends also need support and education.

Starting antiretroviral therapy early in the disease has been shown to delay the progression of HIV infection. Later in the disease those therapies can prolong survival. Nucleoside analogs such as zidovudine, **didanosine**, and nonnucleoside reverse transcriptase inhibitors such as efavirenz and **nevirapine** target the retroviral-specific DNA polymerase (see Chapter 38). Several inhibitors of HIV protease have been developed and have been shown to prevent viral replication and to prolong survival (given alone or in combination with nucleoside analogs) in patients with advanced infection. One fusion inhibitor, **enfuvirtide**, is available. Other agents in that class, which block viral adherence to target cells, are in development. Additionally, inhibitors of **HIV integrase**, an enzyme essential for integration of provirus into host chromosomal DNA, are in earlier stages of development. In a manner analogous to the therapy of tuberculosis, chemotherapy for HIV involves combinations of agents acting at different sites to achieve synergism and delay the emergence of resistant viruses. As with tuberculosis, failure to adhere to correct schedule of therapy often leads to drug resistance, as occurred in Mr. F's case.

Prevention

By far the best approach to AIDS is prevention. Development of an effective vaccine would eliminate the future threat of the disease. However, development of an HIV vaccine has been hampered by many problems. One is an incomplete understanding of the host immune response to the virus; although many individuals develop neutralizing antibodies to HIV, their role in vivo is unclear. Thus, circulating antibodies effectively clear the bloodstream of infectious virus yet fail to prevent the progression of HIV infection. In addition, HIV shows great variability in its major antigens (Chapter 38). Finally, the testing of HIV vaccines for protective efficacy requires putting people at risk for infection and thus raises ethical concerns. Even after vaccines are developed and applied, it may be decades before AIDS ceases to be a major problem.

Until vaccines are developed, education to reduce transmission of HIV remains the only effective way of stemming its spread. Controversial though they may be, the most effective approach to AIDS prevention is education and the use of measures to reduce sexual spread (such as condoms) and intravenous drug use.

Conclusion

AIDS is a devastating disease that will continue to have a profound effect on society. Scientifically, it has enhanced our understanding of the human immune system. The practice of medicine has been irrevocably changed with the recognition of this new incurable disease. In Western society the crisis has forced people to face issues such as the economics and inequity of health care delivery and discrimination in employment and insurance. Despite greater recognition of those problems, the sobering truth is that mortality from AIDS will continue to increase and the devastation caused by HIV will continue for the foreseeable future. AIDS will decimate communities in the developing world that lack the resources to treat infected individuals or to prevent further transmission. Little relief is in sight.

Congenital and Perinatal Infections

Charles G. Prober

Fetuses and neonates are susceptible to a variety of unique infections. Congenital (also called intrauterine or prenatal) infections occur during fetal life and result from transplacental transmission from mother to fetus. Perinatal infections occur during the first 4 weeks after birth and are contracted from the mother at birth or during the neonatal period, from either maternal or nonmaternal sources. Infectious agents most commonly associated with congenital infection include cytomegalovirus (CMV), *Toxoplasma gondii, Treponema pallidum,* and rubella virus. Less common causes of congenital infection include herpes simplex virus (HSV), varicella-zoster virus (VZV), parvovirus, and HIV. Infectious agents most commonly responsible for perinatal infections include group B streptococci (GBS), Gram-negative enteric pathogens (especially *Escherichia coli*), *Listeria monocytogenes,* HSV, hepatitis B virus (HBV), and HIV.

Special Immunological Problems of the Fetus and Neonate

Fetuses and neonates are immunocompromised hosts. All the components of their immune systems—the phagocytic system, natural killer cells, complement, B lymphocytes, and T lymphocytes—are deficient compared with those in the immune systems of older children and adults. The degree of deficiency is inversely related to gestational age and birth weight, although even term infants are immunologically naive.

Fortunately, the fetus is partially sheltered from infection by the fetal membranes and the placenta, which serve as barriers against many maternal microorganisms. Further protection is afforded by the transfer of considerable quantities of maternal immunoglobulins, largely of the IgG class. At term, the fetal concentration of IgG antibodies may be greater than that of the mother, because the placenta actively transports the molecules into the fetal circulation. Conversely, a baby born prematurely may not have received a full complement of maternal antibodies, further contributing to the preterm infant's already heightened risk of infection. Some degree of protection is afforded by breast milk, which contains secretory IgA antibodies that reduce the likelihood of nursing infants contracting severe infections caused by certain pathogens.

Congenital Infection

Case

Baby L. was born at 37 weeks' gestation, following an uneventful pregnancy to a 28-year-old healthy mother. On physical examination about 30 minutes after delivery, the baby was found to weigh 2 kg and to have a head circumference of 28 cm (both measurements falling below the third percentile). He was pale and had numerous nonblanching purple spots on his trunk, back, face, and extremities. His vital signs were stable and his cardiopulmonary examination was unremarkable. He had an enlarged liver and spleen. Urine obtained on Baby L.'s second day of life was positive for CMV on viral culture, establishing the diagnosis of congenital CMV infection.

This case raises several questions:

1. How did Baby L. become infected inside the womb?
2. What are the signs and symptoms of intrauterine CMV infection?
3. What is the prognosis for Baby L.?
4. Could Baby L.'s mother have done anything to prevent her son's infection?

The physician reassured Baby L.'s parents that they had not done anything to contribute to the child's disease. The answer to the question of how a baby can get an infection before birth requires an understanding of the pathogenesis of intrauterine infections.

Baby L. presents clinical signs and symptoms typical of congenital infections, including poor intrauterine growth and evidence of multisystem disease (including microcephaly, a rash compatible with hematologic problems, and hepatosplenomegaly). Notably, the symptoms of infection were present at birth. Also characteristic of many intrauterine infections is the mother being asymptomatic during her pregnancy.

DETERMINANTS OF FETAL INFECTION

The most important determinant of the likelihood and consequences of congenital infection is the timing of gestational infection. For most pathogens, including CMV, rubella virus, parvovirus, and *T. gondii*, maternal infection during the first trimester results in the most severe fetal consequences. Infection with these organisms late in pregnancy usually has no adverse effects on the fetus. In contrast, although the placenta can be breached by *T. pallidum* early in pregnancy, induction of pathologic changes in fetal tissue usually does not result before the fifth month of gestation. The

table **72-1**	Approximate Annual Incidence of Congenital Infections in the United States	
AGENT	**INCIDENCE PER 100,000 BIRTHS**	**APPROXIMATE NUMBER OF CASES**
Cytomegalovirus	1,000	40,000
Toxoplasmosis	100	4,000
Syphilis	80	3,200
Rubella	50	2,000

approximate incidence of congenital infection caused by the four agents most common in the United States is summarized in Table 72-1.

DAMAGE

Three types of effects on the growing and developing fetus can result from intrauterine infection. One is interference with the normal development of tissues and organs, leading to structural abnormalities. For example, congenital rubella can cause cataracts and defects of the retina, patent ductus arteriosus, pulmonary artery stenosis, pulmonary valvular stenosis, or sensorineural deafness. The second effect on the developing fetus results from the inflammatory reaction in response to infection. For example, congenital CMV or toxoplasmosis infections can result in cerebritis, which can lead to cerebral atrophy and intracranial calcifications. The third effect results from direct placental infection, which leads to placental insufficiency. Inflammation, edema, and fibrosis associated with placental infection may compromise normal growth and development of the fetus, leading to low birth weight, premature birth, or fetal death.

Although the damage to fetal cells and organs occurs prenatally, the effects of the damage may not become clinically apparent until several months after birth. For example, deafness or mental retardation as a result of congenital rubella or CMV infection may not become evident until infected children have reached an age at which language and other cognitive skills can be reliably evaluated. In addition, certain tissue damage continues after birth in some congenital infections (e.g., rubella, CMV, untreated syphilis) as the microbes continue to replicate after delivery.

Some of the most common clinical manifestations associated with congenital infection are listed in the box titled "Common Manifestations of Congenital Infection." Although certain malformations may suggest a specific pathogen as the cause of congenital infection, the patterns of abnormalities induced by the infectious agents overlap too much to allow a definitive diagnosis to be made without laboratory confirmation.

Common Manifestations of Congenital Infection

Prematurity
Intrauterine growth retardation
Congenital defects

- Abnormal head size
  - Microcephaly
  - Hydrocephaly
- Intracranial calcifications
  - Periventricular
  - Diffuse

- Eye abnormalities
  - Chorioretinitis
  - Cataracts
  - Microphthalmia
- Hearing loss
- Hepatosplenomegaly
- Hematologic abnormalities
  - Thrombocytopenia
  - Anemia
- Bone lesions
- Inflammation of cerebral spinal fluid

DIAGNOSIS

Recognizing exposure of a pregnant woman to an infectious agent that may result in fetal or neonatal injury is important if documentation of infection might result in specific therapy or a recommendation to consider pregnancy termination. Detection of either IgM antibodies specific for the microbial agent or a rising titer of specific IgG antibodies in the mother's serum may be helpful in assessing the risk of congenital toxoplasmosis, CMV, HIV, rubella, or syphilis. Other specific tests, such as darkfield microscopy, antigen detection, or polymerase chain reaction (PCR), may be warranted under certain clinical circumstances. If maternal infection is strongly suspected, antenatal-specific testing of amniotic fluid or fetal blood may be useful to determine if fetal infection has occurred. Unfortunately, most agents that cause congenital infection produce minimal or no symptoms in the mother and consequently arouse no suspicion until after the infant is born.

Attempts should be made to identify the presence of an infecting agent in an ill infant, such as the one presented in Baby L.'s case. Serologic tests are of limited value in diagnosing congenitally infected neonates because IgG antibodies readily pass from mother to infant through the placenta. Therefore, the mere presence of such antibodies in the baby is not sufficient to diagnose intrauterine infection. Although not of immediate diagnostic utility, the serial performance of serologic tests on an infant may support the diagnosis of congenital infection. Because the half-life of maternal IgG is approximately 28 days, most of the mother's IgG is lost several months after she gives birth, and any IgG detectable in the baby is most likely to be of infant origin. Thus, in the congenitally infected baby, the level of IgG antibody remains the same or increases over time, whereas in an uninfected baby, specific antibodies of maternal origin eventually disappear.

Maternal IgM antibodies, on the other hand, do not readily cross the placenta. Therefore, the presence of CMV, rubella virus, or *T. gondii*–specific IgM antibodies in a baby suggests that the baby has been infected. Unfortunately, IgM antibody assays are not well standardized, resulting in high rates of false-positive and false-negative results.

In contrast to the limitations of serologic testing, isolation of a specific pathogen provides definitive evidence of congenital infection. In evaluating infants for possible congenital infection, urine, saliva, leukocytes (buffy coat), and cerebrospinal fluid (CSF) specimens should be cultured for CMV; nasopharyngeal specimens, urine, buffy coat, and CSF should be cultured for rubella virus. Techniques for culturing *T. gondii* and *T. pallidum* are not available in routine diagnostic laboratories. However, darkfield microscopy of material from the base of an oral or skin lesion can reveal the presence of *T. pallidum,* and an immunoassay can identify *T. pallidum* antigens in tissue specimens. Also, inspection for placental trophozoites by a skilled pathologist may facilitate prompt detection of congenital infection with *T. gondii.* PCR techniques that amplify organism-specific DNA in appropriate specimens can enhance the ability to detect even small numbers of pathogens.

TREATMENT

Penicillin G is effective in treating neonates congenitally infected with syphilis. Infants with congenital toxoplasmosis have been successfully treated with a combination of pyrimethamine and sulfadiazine. Infants congenitally infected with CMV have been treated with ganciclovir, although the therapeutic benefit appears to be limited to a modest reduction in hearing impairment. There is no antiviral therapy for congenital rubella syndrome. Management of many types of congenital infection requires multidisciplinary supportive care.

PREVENTION

Appropriate immunization against rubella during childhood effectively prevents congenital rubella syndrome. Routine prenatal serologic testing detects syphilis in infected mothers, and treatment of the mother with penicillin more than one month prior to delivery prevents most cases of congenital syphilis. Avoiding contact with cat litter boxes and not eating undercooked meat protects most susceptible pregnant mothers from contracting *T. gondii* infection. Preventing congenital *T. gondii* infection by treating acutely infected pregnant women with spiramycin followed by pyrimethamine and sulfonamide has been reported to decrease fetal mortality and improve long-term outcome. Meticulous hand washing reduces the likelihood of contracting CMV infection from exposure to the secretions and body fluids of young children (frequently older siblings) who may be excreting CMV.

Perinatally Acquired Infection

Case

Fourteen days after her birth Baby C. was brought to the emergency department with a 24-hour history of fever (38.9°C), poor feeding, lethargy, and irritability. Born at term to a 22-year-old mother following an uneventful pregnancy, Baby C. was discharged with her mother 24 hours after delivery. The mother reported that Baby C. had been doing well until the day before admission, when the mother had to wake her for feeding. The baby then nursed only weakly and for a short period.

Evaluation in the emergency department revealed that Baby C. had a high peripheral white blood cell count (24,000/mm³ with 68% segmented neutrophils, 20% bands, and 12% lymphocytes). Examination of the CSF revealed 230 white blood cells, 90% of which were neutrophils; a protein concentration of 830 mg/dL; and glucose concentration of 20 mg/dL. Gram-positive cocci in short chains were present on Gram stain of the CSF, and the culture grew group B streptococci. Baby C. was treated with ampicillin and gentamicin. After a difficult 21-day course of antibiotic therapy in the hospital, characterized by apneic spells, seizures, and poor feeding, she was sent home. At age 8 months she was delayed in achieving appropriate developmental milestones.

Baby C. was apparently healthy and normal at birth and developed acute symptoms suggestive of infection at 2 weeks of age. Thus, the infection was likely contracted during or after birth rather than before it. The presence of an inflammatory reaction and the recovery of pathogenic bacteria from CSF confirm the diagnosis of bacterial meningitis.

This case raises several questions:

1. To which infectious agents are newborns susceptible?
2. How do group B streptococci cause meningitis in newborn infants?
3. Could Baby C.'s mother have done anything to prevent her daughter's infection?

DETERMINANTS OF NEONATAL INFECTION

Although neonates receive transplacental maternal antibodies, they are not protected against organisms to which their mothers have not generated an immune response. In addition, newborns are unable to generate antibodies against certain types of antigens, particularly polysaccharides. Terminal components of the complement cascade, especially important for defense against Gram-negative enteric bacteria, are present at a concentration less than 20% of that found in older children and adults. Also, the neonatal cellular immune system is suppressed, as evidenced by low natural killer cytotoxicity and antibody-dependent cell-mediated cytotoxicity. Phagocytic defenses are compromised by a small neutrophil storage pool, limited ability to adhere to endothelium and migrate to infectious foci, and variable deficiencies in the ingestion and killing of microbes. Secretory IgA and other elements of mucosal immunity are not adequately developed until several weeks or more after birth. Thus, even normal, healthy neonates should be considered immunocompromised hosts.

The immune system of a premature infant is even more compromised than that of a term infant. In addition, the mucoepithelial surfaces of chronically hospitalized premature neonates are colonized by multiresistant bacterial flora, often selected by their exposure to repeated courses of broad-spectrum antibiotics. Therefore, the risk of severe, life-threatening infection is substantially greater in premature babies than in term infants.

MICROBIAL AGENTS

The most common types of bacteria that cause perinatally acquired infections are present in the maternal vaginal tract and include group B streptococci, *E. coli* and other members of the Enterobacteriaceae family, and *L. monocytogenes*. Other bacteria present in the baby's postnatal environment also can cause neonatal infection, including antibiotic-resistant Gram-negative enteric bacilli and, less frequently, *Staphylococcus aureus* and coagulase-negative staphylococci. *Chlamydia trachomatis* and *Neisseria gonorrhoeae* can infect the ocular and respiratory mucous membranes during birth and cause neonatal conjunctivitis.

Several viruses are unique in their predilection for neonates. HSV and the enteroviruses can cause serious multiorgan systemic infection that clinically resembles acute bacterial sepsis. Perinatal transmission of VZV also can result in overwhelming infection with multiorgan failure, when maternal varicella infection occurs within 5 days of delivery. This results from the virus readily crossing the placenta before protective maternal antibodies have been formed. HBV and HIV can be transmitted perinatally, usually through exposure to infected maternal blood; infected babies usually are asymptomatic during the neonatal period. Respiratory syncytial virus and other respiratory viruses can cause nonspecific symptoms in neonates, including apnea. They also can cause mild-to-severe lower respiratory tract infection. Species of *Candida,* including *C. albicans,* are increasingly important causes of perinatal infection, especially among infants born prematurely.

ENCOUNTER AND ENTRY

Babies are exposed to the agents causing perinatal infections in a variety of ways. Most bacteria responsible for infection during the first week of life colonize (or infect) the maternal vaginal tract and are acquired by neonates as they pass through the birth canal. Within the first hours of life, babies become colonized with the organisms, particularly on their nasopharynx, skin, and around the umbilical stump; colonization of the neonatal gastrointestinal tract occurs more slowly. Babies also can be exposed at the time of delivery to bloodborne agents that do not readily cross the placenta. That is the most common mechanism of perinatal acquisition of HBV and HIV.

Many types of environmental factors serve to promote neonatal infection following exposure to viruses, bacteria, and fungi. During labor, many infants are evaluated for evidence of fetal distress by the application of monitoring devices to the fetal scalp. This procedure can facilitate the translocation of organisms from the skin to the bloodstream. In addition, after the umbilical cord is severed the healing stump provides a potential route for bacterial invasion. Many prematurely born newborns require intensive medical support such as endotracheal intubation with artificial ventilation, hyperalimentation, antibiotic therapy through intravenous catheters, and several other therapeutic or diagnostic procedures that are invasive or potentially injurious to the otherwise protective barriers of the skin and mucous membranes.

DAMAGE

The effect of perinatally acquired infections on the neonate is variable and depends on the specific pathogen, organs infected, and the degree of compromised immunity. Early clinical manifestations of infection are often nonspecific and can include poor feeding, lethargy, or irritability. Bacterial sepsis or meningitis can progress rapidly to severe neonatal illness or death within 12 to 24 hours. Even with timely, appropriate antibiotic therapy the mortality of neonatal sepsis is between 10 and 40%, and significant neurological sequelae occur in 20 to 50% of survivors of neonatal meningitis.

The extent of involvement and the morbidity associated with perinatally acquired viral infections vary markedly. For example, HSV infection may involve a single organ such as the skin, with cutaneous vesicles being the only sign of infection, or it may cause multiorgan systemic infection involving the liver, central nervous system, and lungs and result in death or severe brain injury. In contrast, HBV is generally asymptomatic in neonates, but neonates infected with HBV are at very high risk (more than 90%) of becoming chronic carriers of HBV. Chronic HBV infection is associated with high susceptibility to hepatic cirrhosis or hepatocellular carcinoma in adulthood.

DIAGNOSIS

The diagnosis of a perinatally acquired infection depends on the recognition of suggestive symptoms and signs. Temperature instability, poor feeding, lethargy, or irritability may be the only presenting symptoms and signs of neonatal septicemia or meningitis and may be very subtle. Thus, the possibility of perinatal infection should be considered in neonates exhibiting even nonspecific symptoms. More specific signs, such as conjunctivitis or skin rash, may suggest a more focal infectious process.

Definitive diagnosis relies on the detection of an etiological agent in infected body sites. However, the causative agents may not always be recovered by culture, sometimes because of antimicrobial therapy given before the collection of specimens or because specimens likely to reveal the organism cannot be easily obtained (e.g. lung, liver, or brain tissue). Detection of viral or bacterial antigens or nucleic acids in serum, urine, or CSF may reveal the causative agent. Antigen detection is available for group B streptococci, *E. coli* K1, HBV, and HIV. PCR has become a valuable diagnostic tool for enterovirus and HSV infections involving the central nervous system.

TREATMENT

The outcome of perinatal infections in babies is influenced by the type of pathogen, availability of specific antimicrobial therapy, severity of infection, and the presence of comorbidities. Several effective antimicrobial agents are available for the treatment of neonatal infections caused by most bacteria. In addition, antifungal agents can be effective in treating *Candida* infections. The antiviral agent acyclovir is useful in the therapy of neonates infected with HSV.

In general, antimicrobial treatment is most effective if initiated early after the onset of infection. Because identification of the specific pathogen is not immediate, selection of antimicrobial therapy usually is made empirically. The dosages and dosing intervals of drugs differ in neonates from those in older children or adults because neonates have decreased renal and hepatic elimination of most drugs and increased volumes of distribution of many drugs. Careful surveillance during therapy is necessary to ensure successful eradication of the infection, minimize potential antimicrobial toxicity, and institute appropriate supportive therapy as needed.

PREVENTION

Because prematurely born infants are at greater risk of perinatal infection than are full-term neonates, prevention of premature delivery substantially reduces the frequency of perinatal infections. Prematurely born babies often require prolonged hospital care and invasive medical interventions. Therefore, strict attention to infection control practices in the care of vulnerable neonates (e.g., hand washing and equipment decontamination) also decreases the risk of infection.

Other potential preventive strategies are focused on the mother. Maternal immunization against tetanus, for example, provides protective transplacental antibodies to infants greater than 28 weeks' gestation, greatly reducing the potential for neonatal tetanus. Gestational screening for maternal HBV infection permits effective immunoprophylaxis for the infant at birth. Detecting HIV infection in the mother prompts institution of antiretroviral therapy and Casarian delivery, both of which serve to reduce mother-to-child transmission of HIV. Intrapartum maternal administration of penicillin significantly reduces the risk of early onset group B streptococcal disease in newborn infants.

Conclusion

Congenital and perinatal infections are an important cause of neonatal mortality and long-term morbidity. A variety of pathogens, including viruses, bacteria, and protozoa, can cause these infections. Immaturity of host defenses plays an important role in the pathogenesis of infections in newborn infants. Attention to their prevention through adherence to current recommendations for immunization, antibiotic prophylaxis, and infection control practices is incumbent upon health care providers. Recognition of these infections and the provision of appropriate therapy, when available, may ameliorate some of their important consequences.

Zoonoses

Daniel S. Shapiro

Zoonoses are infections normally found in nonhuman vertebrates that are transmitted to humans. The diversity of zoonoses is extraordinary; they include viral (e.g., rabies), bacterial (e.g., anthrax), mycobacterial (e.g., bovine tuberculosis), fungal (e.g., some skin infections caused by dermatophytes), and parasitic (e.g., trichinellosis) infections, and even prion disease (the agent of bovine spongiform encephalopathy, or "mad cow disease," in cattle and variant Creutzfeldt-Jakob disease in humans). Some controversy surrounds what constitutes a zoonotic infection. For example, the numerous arthropod-borne viral infections in which humans are bitten by an infected mosquito are not considered zoonoses by some experts but are by others.

In recent years recognition of the importance of zoonotic infections has increased, partly because of the significant overlap of zoonoses within two areas of public health: emerging infectious diseases and potential agents of bioterrorism (Fig. 73-1). Thus, the potential for significant illness and death from zoonotic infections is of major concern. Not only is conventional public health of importance in the recognition and control of zoonoses, but also high-quality veterinary public health, which is not readily available in countries with limited resources, is essential. Both types of public health strategies help to ensure a safe food supply for humans, which is important to human health and the economic vitality of countries that export food products or animals.

Contact Between Humans and Animals

The means of contact between humans and animals and humans and animal products are numerous (Table 73-1). Humans are in contact with animals as a result of occupational exposures, as in farming and veterinary medicine, and as a result of having pets. Less obvious, but of no less importance, is that our omnivorous diet puts us in contact with animal products during food preparation and ingestion.

Domestic Animals

The effect of a growing human population is of great importance in numerous threats to public health, including zoonotic infections. The tremendous number of

FIGURE 73-1 ■ **A schematic diagram of the interplay between zoonoses, emerging diseases, and potential agents of bioterrorism.**

animals with which humans have daily contact includes more than 100 million dogs and cats in the United States and huge numbers of cattle, pigs, goats, sheep, horses, chickens, and other domestic animals raised for food or their products (e.g., hides, fur). As the human population increases, so do the domestic animal population and the number of potential human–animal interactions. In addition, the need to dispose of the excrement of domestic animals poses substantial challenges. Large-scale factory farming includes hog farms that house many thousands of animals in a relatively small space and results in wastewater "lagoons" that have been implicated in the contamination of the environment with resistant bacteria. Broiler chickens in the United States are often raised in confinement pens that house between 10,000 and 20,000 birds.

Antibiotics in Feed

The practice of including antibiotics in animal feed, which results in selection of antibiotic-resistant bacteria that can be transmitted to humans, continues to be widely practiced in the United States. One recent estimate is that 27.5 million pounds of antibiotics are used for purposes that include growth promotion and disease prophylaxis in animals in the United States, whereas 2 million pounds are used for therapeutic purposes in ani-

mals. This awesome selection pressure has significant implications for disease risk in humans.

Population Increase

The increase in human population has resulted in people moving into areas where only wildlife had existed. The potential for exposure to zoonoses in those settings is significant, including not only diseases caused by direct contact with animals or their excreta but also diseases transmitted by arthropod vectors, such as Lyme disease. As humans enter new areas, the potential emerges for exposure to pathogens that previously have not infected our species.

Transmission of Zoonotic Infections to Humans

Some zoonotic infections can be acquired by humans through many routes, as illustrated for tularemia in Figure 73-2. In most cases, however, a zoonosis can only be passed from an animal to a human through one of the six routes described in the following sections.

table **73-1**	Contact Between Humans and Animals Documented to Result in the Transmission of Zoonoses
TYPE OF CONTACT	**EXAMPLES**
Occupational	Animal groomer Butcher Cook Farmer Fisherman Furrier Hunter Laboratory animal caretaker Leather worker Sewer worker (contact with water contaminated by rat urine) Slaughterhouse worker Trapper Veterinarian Veterinary assistant Wildlife scientist (e.g., mammalogist) Wool sorter Pet store worker Zoo worker
Common activities	Camping Drinking milk Eating Preparing food Owning a pet Swimming Visiting a petting zoo or farm
Injuries	Animal bites Animal scratches Bites by ectoparasites (e.g., fleas, ticks) Fish fin injuries

Direct Contact

Through **direct contact** with an animal or an animal product, a person can acquire various diseases, ranging from dermatophyte infections, which are common among veterinary assistants through contact with cat fur, to cutaneous anthrax, which is seen among workers handling contaminated animal hides (Table 73-2). Through **contact with urine,** sewer workers can acquire leptospirosis as a result of exposure to water that contains the urine of infected rats. Leptospirosis can also spread as a result of flooding.

Animal Bites or Scratching

Acquisition of infection through **animal bites or scratches** is a common mechanism of zoonotic infection (Table 73-3). For example, the bite of an infected dog, bat, wolf, fox, or other mammal can lead to rabies in-

fection in humans. Bacterial infections also can be acquired by this mechanism, such as infection by *Pasteurella multocida* following the bite or scratch of a cat (typically) or a dog (less frequently).

Inhalation

Zoonotic infections can be acquired by **inhalation** of an infectious agent from the excreta of an animal, as occurs in the hantavirus pulmonary syndrome (Table 73-4). Inhalation anthrax, which also is known as wool sorter's disease, is caused by inhaling spores of *Bacillus anthracis* present in the wool of sheep. The organism was used when spores were sent in envelopes through the United States mail. That act of bioterrorism resulted in a number of infections, both cutaneous and inhalation anthrax, and several deaths among individuals who were exposed to the spores, including postal workers in facilities that used mail-sorting machines.

Inhalation also is a means of acquiring the pneumonic form of plague. That infection can result from exposure to a person with pneumonic plague who generates an infectious aerosol of *Yersinia pestis* by coughing or sneezing. *Y. pestis* can also spread through contact with infected cats or inhalation of an aerosol that has been engineered to serve as a weapon. Pulmonary tularemia has not been transmitted from person to person, but the disease can be acquired by individuals who work outside and mow over an infected animal or animal excreta, resulting in an infectious aerosol (see Fig. 73-2). In addition to pulmonary involvement, the aerosol can inoculate the conjunctiva.

Ingestion

Infections acquired through **ingestion** of undercooked meat or fish include trichinellosis, which results from eating undercooked pork contaminated by *Trichinella spiralis* (Table 73-5). Drinking milk that has not been pasteurized, a process involving rapid heating and cooling, can cause bovine tuberculosis if the cows were infected with *Mycobacterium bovis*. Other common foodborne bacteria include *Salmonella* species and *Yersinia enterocolitica*.

Contamination of a food at any step of the production process, from animal slaughter or milking to food preparation or storage, can result in human infection. Examples include outbreaks of *Escherichia coli* O157:H7 infection from contaminated ground beef used in hamburgers served at fast-food restaurants and large-scale outbreaks of salmonellosis among Inuit communities where people ate meat from a dead, rotting whale that had birds feeding on the

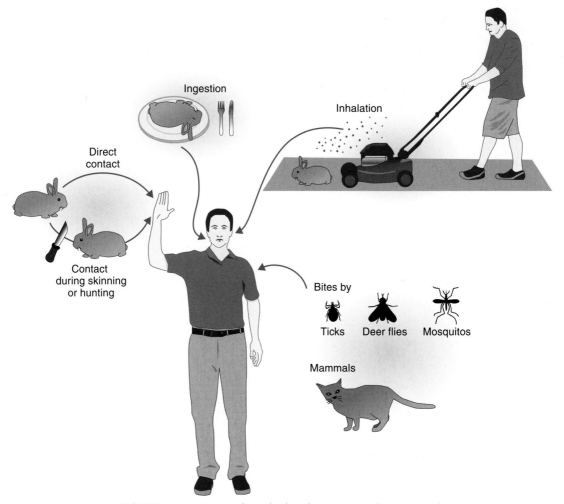

FIGURE 73-2 ▪ **Means by which tularemia can be acquired.**

carcass. An important concern for the consumption of beef is the transmission of variant Creutzfeldt-Jakob disease, a prion disease that epidemiologic and laboratory evidence has linked to cattle infected with bovine spongiform encephalopathy (BSE). In addition to the United Kingdom, where more than 100 people have been infected with variant Creutzfeldt-Jakob disease, France has had a large number of cases of BSE, and isolated cases have been detected in cattle in other European countries, Canada, and the United States.

Fecal–Oral Transmission

Acquisition of zoonotic infection by the **fecal–oral route** is quite common. All vertebrates potentially can be infected by *Salmonella* species and excrete the organism in their feces. Thus, contact with animal feces can result in human cases of salmonellosis. The risk of *Salmonella* infection is of particular importance to individuals who have pet reptiles, which commonly serve as carriers of salmonellosis and may excrete the organism intermittently in their feces, especially when stressed. Other possibilities include the many para-

sitic diseases for which an infective form appears in animal feces, such as the oocysts of *Toxoplasma gondii* in cat feces. Because *T. gondii* is an organism that may cause an infection that crosses the placenta and affects the fetus, pregnant women should avoid contact with cat feces and wear gloves if they must dispose of cat litter.

Another documented route of fecal–oral transmission is contaminated public water supplies. This mode of transmission includes not only the lack of a clean source of potable water in resource-poor countries but also problems with the treatment of water in countries with good public health infrastructures. In 1993 in Milwaukee, Wisconsin, approximately 400,000 people became infected with *Cryptosporidium* protozoa as a result of incomplete removal of the organisms by filtration of contaminated water from Lake Michigan.

Arthropod Bites

Many pathogens are transmitted to humans through the **bites of arthropods** (Table 73-6). Infection can occur as a result of mechanical transmission of the

table 73-2 Direct Skin Penetration

DISEASE	ORGANISM NAME	GROUP	ANIMAL
Bacterial			
Anthrax[a,b]	Bacillus anthracis	Gram-positive aerobic spore former	Domestic mammals (herbivores)
Brucellosis[a,b]	Brucella melitensis	Gram-negative rods	Goats, sheep
	B. abortus		Cattle
	B. suis		Swine
	B. canis		Dogs
Erysipeloid	Erysipelothrix rhusiopathiae	Gram-positive rods	Swine, poultry, fish
Leptospirosis	Leptospira interrogans	Spirochete	Rodents, dogs, domestic animals
Glanders[a]	Pseudomonas mallei	Gram-negative rods	Equines
Tularemia[a,b,c,d]	Francisella tularensis	Gram-negative rods	Rabbits, rodents, cats
Viral			
Orf (contagious ecthyma)	Parapoxvirus	Poxvirus family	Sheep, goats
Vesicular stomatitis	Vesicular stomatitis virus	Rhabdovirus family	Cattle, horses
Parasitic			
Cutaneous larva migrans (creeping eruption)	Ancylostoma caninum (dog hookworm)	Nematode	Dogs, cats, carnivores
	Ancylostoma braziliense (dog and cat hookworm)	Nematode	
Fungal			
Dermatophytes	Zoophilic trichophyton, microsporum	Fungi	Dogs, cats, cattle, other mammals

Alternative portals:
[a]Inhalation
[b]Ingestion
[c]Arthropod vector
[d]Animal bite

table 73-3 Animal Bite or Scratch

DISEASE	ORGANISM NAME	GROUP	ANIMAL
Bacterial			
Pasteurellosis[a,b]	Pasteurella multocida	Gram-negative rods	Cats, dogs, and wild mammals
Rat bite fever[a,c]	Spirillum minor	Spirochete	Rats and other rodents
	Streptobacillus moniliformis	Gram-negative rods	Rats, rodents, turkeys
Capnocytophaga canimorsus	Capnocytophaga canimorsus	Gram-negative rods	Dogs
Cat scratch disease[d]	Bartonella henselae	Gram-negative rods	Cats, dogs suspected
Viral			
Rabies	Rabies virus	Rhabdovirus	Bats, skunks, foxes, opossums, domestic mammals
Herpes B encephalomyelitis[d]	Cercopithecine herpesvirus 1	Herpesvirus	Rhesus macaques
Fungal			
Blastomycosis	Blastomyces dermatitidis		Dogs (very rare)

Alternative portal:
[a]Skin penetration
[b]Inhalation
[c]Ingestion
[d]Conjunctival inoculation

table 73-4	Inhalation			
DISEASE	**ORGANISM NAME**	**GROUP**	**ANIMAL RESERVOIR**	**INHALANT**
Bacterial				
Anthrax[a,b] (wool sorter's disease)	*Bacillus anthracis*	Gram-positive aerobic spore-forming rod	Goats, sheep, cattle	Spores from wool, animal hides
Ornithosis (psittacosis)	*Chlamydophila psittaci*	Chlamydia	Parrots, turkeys, birds	Dried excreta from infected birds
Plague[c]	*Yersinia pestis*	Gram-negative rods	Rats, rodents, cats (contact with infected cats especially likely to result in pneumonic form of plague)	Respiratory contact with humans with pneumonic plague and infected cats
Q fever	*Coxiella burnetii*	Rickettsia	Domestic animals	Soil and fomites contaminated with animal excretions, especially placental products
Tuberculosis[d]	*Mycobacterium bovis*	Acid-fast bacillus	Domestic mammals	Contaminated respiratory secretions
Tularemia[a,b,e,f]	*Francisella tularensis*	Gram-negative rods	Wild rabbits, rodents, wild mammals, cats that hunt outdoors	Excreta or aerosolized small animals
Fungal				
Histoplasmosis	*Histoplasma capsulatum*	Fungi	Birds, bats	Microconidia from contaminated soil
Viral				
Lymphocytic choriomeningitis	Lymphocytic choriomeningitis virus	Arenavirus family	Mice, hamsters, other rodents	Infected aerosols
Hantavirus pulmonary syndrome	Sin Nombre virus and other viruses	Bunyavirus family	Mice, other rodents	Infected aerosols

Alternative portals:
[a] Skin penetration   [d] Ingestion of milk
[b] Animal bite   [e] Ingestion of infected animal
[c] Flea bite   [f] arthropod bite

pathogen, as when an arthropod vector bites an infected animal and subsequently bites a human. With that form of transmission, no intervening stages of development in the life cycle of the pathogen take place within the arthropod. For example, transmission of *Francisella tularensis*, the etiologic agent of tularemia, can occur following the bite of a tick, deer fly, or (in parts of northern Europe) mosquito that has bitten an infected animal. In contrast, the life cycle of the parasite *Babesia microti* involves both a rodent host and a tick. After the introduction of sporozoites into the rodent host, the parasite differentiates into male and female gametes. After the gametes are ingested by the deer tick host as part of a blood meal from an infected rodent, the gametes unite, ultimately resulting in sporozoites. If a tick that contains sporozoites bites a human rather than a rodent, the sporozoites can be introduced into the human, who will become infected.

Global Concerns About Zoonoses

The range of species a given pathogen can infect is known as the **host range** of the pathogen. For most viruses the host range is narrow; one exception is rabies virus, which can infect many species. A broad host range also is seen with the bacterial cause of tularemia, *F. tularensis*, which is able to infect more than 100 mammal species. The capacity of a pathogen to make the "species jump" to humans is of great concern because the new (to humans) pathogen must be detected, identified, and rapidly contained, although the pathogenesis and epidemiology of the pathogen in its nonhuman host may be unknown (see the box titled "Newly Recognized Zoonosis Caused by a Change in the Environment").

| table **73-5** | **Ingestion** | | | |

DISEASE	ORGANISM NAME	GROUP	ANIMAL RESERVOIR	INGESTANT (CONTAMINATED FOODSTUFF)
Bacterial				
Brucellosis[a,b]	*Brucella melitensis* *B. abortus, B. snis, B. canis*	Gram-negative rods	Goats, cattle	Dairy products
Campylobacter	*Campylobacter jejuni*	Gram-negative rods	Domestic mammals, fowl	Milk, water, meat, poultry
Listeriosis[a]	*Listeria monocytogenes*	Gram-positive rods	Domestic mammals, rodents, birds	Meat, cheese, vegetables
Salmonellosis	*Salmonella* species (not *S. typhi*)	Gram-negative rods	Fowl, domestic mammals, turtles	Milk, eggs, meat, poultry, shellfish
Tuberculosis[b]	*Mycobacterium bovis*	Acid-fast bacillus	Cattle	Milk
Yersiniosis	*Yersinia enterocolitica*	Gram-negative rods	Pigs, cattle	Milk (particularly unpasteurized milk), pig intestines
Helminthic				
Anisakiasis	*Anisakis simplex*	Nematode	Marine fish	Larvae in undercooked fish
Tapeworm infection	*Taenia saginata*	Cestode	Cattle	Larvae (cysticercus) in undercooked beef
	Taenia solium	Cestode	Pigs	Larvae (cysticercus) in undercooked pork
	Diphyllobothrium latum	Cestode	Fish	Larvae in raw fish
	Echinococcus	Cestode	Dogs, sheep, reindeer, caribou, wolves	Ova from infected dogs via the fecal–oral route
Trichinellosis	*Trichinella spiralis*	Nematode	Pigs, domestic mammals, wild mammals, rodents	Larval cysts
Visceral larva migrans	*Toxocara canis* (roundworm of dogs)	Nematode	Dogs	Ova in soil from infected dogs via the fecal–oral route
Protozoal				
Cryptosporidiosis	*Cryptosporidium*		Cattle	Oocysts in fecally contaminated water
Toxoplasmosis[c,d]	*Toxoplasma gondii*		Cats	Oocysts from cat feces, tissue cyst from uncooked meat
Other				
Variant Creutzfeldt-Jakob disease		Prion	Cattle	Beef

Alternative portals:
[a]Skin penetration   [c]Transplacental
[b]Inhalation   [d]Organ transplantation

Another major concern that must be quickly addressed is whether a new pathogen can spread efficiently from person to person. This capability varies dramatically among pathogens. For example, rabies virus, which has a broad host range and can be transmitted to humans from many animals, has rarely been transmitted from human to human and only by extraordinary means (e.g., corneal transplant or organ transplant). In contrast, HIV-1, which has spread globally, appears to have been introduced into the human population from a single species, chimpanzees (*Pan troglodytes troglodytes*). A current major public health concern is the introduction of avian strains of influenza A (e.g., H5N1) into the human population in Asia. The new influenza virus strains

table 73-6 Arthropod Vectors

DISEASE	VECTOR	ORGANISM NAME	MICROBIAL GROUP	ANIMAL RESERVOIR
Bacterial				
Lyme disease	Tick	*Borrelia burgdorferi*	Spirochete	Rodents, deer
Plague, bubonic[a]	Flea	*Yersinia pestis*	Gram-negative rods	Urban rats, rodents
Relapsing fever	Tick	*Borrelia species*	Spirochete	Rodent, wild mammals
Tularemia[a,b,c]	Tick, biting flies, mosquitoes (northern Europe)	*Francisella tularensis*	Gram-negative rods	Wild rabbits, rodents, wild mammals, cats that hunt outdoors
Rocky Mountain spotted fever	Tick	*Rickettsia rickettsii*	Rickettsia	Wild rodents, dogs
Scrub typhus	Mite (chigger)	*Rickettsia tsutsugamushi*	Rickettsia	Wild rodents, rats
Murine typhus	Flea	*Rickettsia typhi*	Rickettsia	Rats, opossums
		Rickettsia felis		
Rickettsialpox	Mite	*Rickettsia akari*	Rickettsia	Mice
Ehrlichiosis	Ticks	*Ehrlichia species*	Ehrlichia	Deer, elk, rodents, dogs
Viral				
Yellow Fever	Mosquito	Flavivirus	Flavivirus family	Primates (sylvatic cycle)
Encephalitis Eastern equine Venezuelan equine Western equine	Mosquito	Alphavirus	Togavirus family	Birds
West Nile	Mosquito	Flavivirus	Flavivirus family	Birds
St. Louis	Mosquito	Flavivirus	Flavivirus family	Birds
California	Mosquito	Bunyavirus	Bunyavirus family	Mammals, wild rodents
Rift Valley fever[a]	Mosquito	Bunyavirus	Bunyavirus family	Sheep, goats, cattle
Crimean-Congo hemorrhagic fever[a]	Tick	Bunyavirus	Bunyavirus family	Domestic mammals, rodents
Colorado tick fever	Tick	Orbivirus	Reovirus family	Rodents
Protozoal				
Babesiosis	Tick	*Babesia species*		Domestic and wild animals
Leishmaniasis (kala-azar, cutaneous leishmaniasis)	Sandfly	*Leishmania species*		Dogs, foxes, rodents, wild mammals
American trypanosomiasis	Reduviid bug (kissing bug)	Trypanosoma cruzi		Dogs, cats, opossums, armadillos, wild mammals
African sleeping sickness	Tsetse fly	*Trypanosoma species*		Cattle, wild animals

Alternative portals:
[a]Skin penetration
[b]Ingestion
[c]Inhalation

could eventually develop into a strain that is efficiently spread from person to person, resulting in a pandemic in which millions of people perish.

The host range and efficiency of spread of viral pathogens depend on the molecular biology of the virus and the human host. A virus (really a viral population) with a high frequency of mutation or recombination prompts concern that strains will be selected that are able to both make the species jump to humans and spread efficiently from person to person. For some

Newly Recognized Zoonosis Caused by a Change in the Environment

In May 1993 an outbreak of unexplained respiratory illness occurred in the Four Corners region of the United States, an area of the southwest shared by New Mexico, Arizona, Colorado, and Utah. The outbreak was notable for a severe illness in previously healthy young adults. They suddenly developed acute respiratory distress, and approximately one half of the infected persons died. Usual and unusual (e.g., pneumonia, plague) causes were excluded by appropriate testing.

An active investigation to determine the cause and epidemiology of the outbreak was successful. Tissues from infected individuals were sent to the Centers for Disease Control and Prevention (CDC), where molecular virology studies demonstrated an association between the pulmonary syndrome and a previously unknown hantavirus. This association led to the designation hantavirus pulmonary syndrome (HPS) for the disease. Active collection of rodents, the hosts of hantaviruses, was performed, and in November 1993 the virus that caused the outbreak, a previously unknown hantavirus, was isolated by the Special Pathogens Branch at CDC from tissue of a deer mouse (*Peromyscus maniculatus*) that had been trapped near the New Mexico home of a patient. Approximately 1,700 rodents representing various species had been trapped and studied during the investigation, and approximately 30% of the deer mice tested showed evidence of the infection.

Because the convention for naming hantaviruses is to use the name of the location where the virus was first isolated, the HPS hantavirus was initially named Muerto Canyon virus. However, that area is sacred to the Navajo, and the name was subsequently changed to Sin Nombre virus. The virus is a member of the genus *Hantavirus*, family Bunyaviridae. Studies of archived tissue from patients who were ill with respiratory infections demonstrated that there had been cases of HPS before 1993.

Why this outbreak occurred at the time and location it did was investigated by public health authorities. In 1993 the mouse population in the Four Corners area was unusually large. Following a drought that had plagued the area for several years, a marked increase in precipitation in early 1993 resulted in burgeoning plant growth. The availability of food for the deer mice increased dramatically, leading to an increase in their reproductive rate. At the time of the first cases of the outbreak, May 1993, 10 times as many mice inhabited the area as had been there a year earlier. The explosion in the mouse population led to a greater probability of mice interacting with humans, including the potential for human inhalation of virus from mouse excreta. According to the CDC, from May 1993 to July 2005, Sin Nombre virus caused 396 cases of severe respiratory disease with a mortality rate of 36%. The virus has been recognized in 32 states (Fig. 73-3).

The discovery of Sin Nombre virus as the cause of HPS spurred a great deal of research on it and related hantaviruses. Many hantaviruses have caused HPS in persons from Canada to South America. Fortunately, there is no evidence of person-to-person transmission of HPS, with the exception of HPS caused by Andes virus, a newly described hantavirus isolated in Argentina.

---

pathogens, the reservoir in nature may be unaffected by chronic infection. In contrast, the biology of the infection in a host of a different species cannot be easily predicted.

Evaluation for Possible Zoonoses

When a patient presents to the physician with an illness, consideration should be given to obtaining an animal exposure history. The specific animal or exposure can provide clues to the patient's diagnosis. Of equal importance is the public health impact of establishing a diagnosis of a zoonotic infection, because many infections occur in clusters as a result of common exposure (e.g., a large foodborne outbreak). The need to consider bioterrorism, or the need to take appropriate action to safeguard the population from a mosquito-borne illness is especially significant. Being able to establish a broad differential diagnosis on the basis of the type of animal to which an individual is exposed and to generate a list of the possible types of exposure once a zoonotic infection is diagnosed are essential tools for the health of the patient and the community.

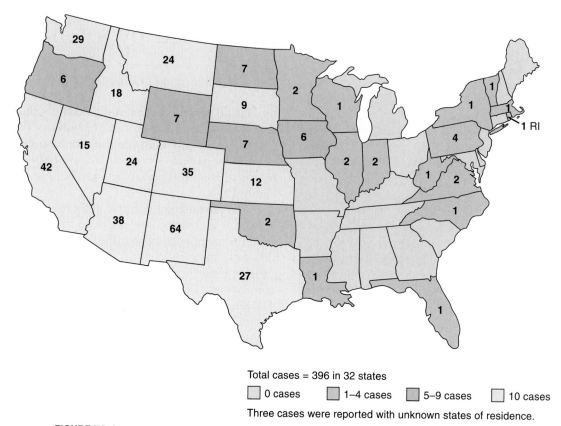

Total cases = 396 in 32 states

☐ 0 cases   ▨ 1–4 cases   ▧ 5–9 cases   ☐ 10 cases

Three cases were reported with unknown states of residence.

FIGURE 73-3 ▪ Hantavirus pulmonary syndrome cases by state of residence, United States, May 1993 to July 2005.

Conclusion

An awareness of zoonoses and their tremendous impact on human health—and the devastating potential of the introduction of new zoonotic agents into the human population—has led to increases in both surveillance for these agents and research in areas ranging from wildlife biology to molecular biology. These efforts require the coordinated work of veterinarians, physicians, basic researchers, entomologists, and public health experts. Because many of the potential pathogens are found in developing countries that lack a public health infrastructure, the recognition of an outbreak of an established or novel pathogen may be delayed, with potentially disastrous consequences not only for the country of origin but also worldwide. Similarly, war often results in a breakdown in public health and an unwillingness to provide information by the government (or group) that is in power. These types of barriers are difficult, if not impossible, to overcome in the absence of the political will of the international community to recognize emerging zoonotic infections as a threat that knows no boundaries.

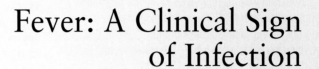

Fever: A Clinical Sign of Infection

Suzanne F. Bradley

Not all elevations in body temperature are fever, nor are they necessarily caused by infection. An elevation of temperature that is a normal variant or reflects increased generation of body heat or an inability to dissipate it is called **hyperthermia**. An elevation of temperature caused by the release of inflammatory mediators in response to various foreign or exogenous stimuli is called **fever**. Although many people fear the complications of fever, it is a normal reaction to invasion by certain microorganisms and may actually play a beneficial role in the host response to infection. However, infection is only one of many causes of fever. Occasionally, the causes of prolonged temperature elevations may be difficult to diagnose. **Fever of unknown origin (FUO)** can be one of the greatest challenges for the infectious diseases consultant to solve.

What Is Normal Body Temperature?

Rigors (shivering), sweats, chills, flushing, tachycardia, lethargy, and increased warmth of skin have been recognized as signs and symptoms of disease since ancient times. Although crude mercury thermometers had been available for more than a century, the significance of increased body temperature and its association with the signs and symptoms of disease (fever) were not fully appreciated until 1871, when Carl Wunderlich reported his detailed studies of body temperature.

Generally, **normal body temperature** ranges from 36.3° to 37.5°C (97.3° to 99.5°F) in healthy humans. Body temperature normally fluctuates 1° to 1.3°C (1.8° to 2.4°F), with the lowest measurements noted between 2 and 8 AM and the highest between 4 and 9 PM. The daily, cyclic variation in temperature is called **diurnal variation**. Temperature measurements vary when measured at different body sites. Rectal temperature measurements are generally 0.8°C (1°F) higher than oral temperature measurements. Normal temperatures may be higher in females and lower in newborns and in the debilitated elderly. Therefore, the accepted "normal temperature" of 37°C (98.6°F), an average value, may have little clinical meaning for a given individual. Within these limitations temperatures above 37.5°C (99.4°F) orally and 38.0°C (100.4°F) rectally are generally accepted as abnormal in immunocompetent adults. Abnormal temperatures in newborns and the elderly may be lower. Mr. J's temperature at 38.9°C is definitely abnormal.

Case

At 82 years of age Mr. J. had been feeling well until he noted a significant decline in his vision, intermittent jaw pain, and headaches associated with night sweats. Over the following year his symptoms extended to include anorexia, weight loss of 20 lb, and occasional temperatures greater than 38.6°C. Examination revealed a decline in vision, mild anemia, and an erythrocyte sedimentation rate (ESR) of 129 mm/hr (normal is 0 to 20 mm/hr).

Mr. J. had no allergies and took no medications. A retired insurance salesman, he had traveled throughout the United States. He lived with his wife, a dog, and a cat. His medical and family histories were unremarkable. He looked relatively well, but his clothes fit loosely. Physical examination was unremarkable except for a temperature of 38.9°C, a resting pulse of 105 beats per minute, and tenderness over the right temple. No sinus tenderness was elicited by palpation and the chest examination was normal.

The change in vision, anemia, anorexia, and elevated ESR were ascribed to "old age" and the jaw pain to poor dentition. He was treated with multiple antibiotics for sinusitis and bronchitis, although he denied productive cough or pain over his sinuses.

This case raises several questions:

1. Does Mr. J. have a fever?
2. Is his temperature elevation a danger to him?
3. Is his illness caused by infection?
4. How might Mr. J.'s physician begin to evaluate the potential causes of his symptoms?

Every elevated temperature does not necessarily require evaluation for underlying disease. Normal elevations of body temperatures of 0.6° to 0.8°C (1° to 1.5°F) may be observed transiently in healthy persons after vigorous exercise or eating. A brief local increase in oral temperature measurements can occur after smoking, gum chewing, or drinking warm liquids. Following a self-limited febrile infection, some patients continue to take their temperatures even though their illnesses have resolved. A diary that details early morning and evening temperatures, measurements when the patient feels warm, and associated activities may be a helpful tool to determine whether a temperature is abnormal or merely reflects daily activities or normal diurnal variation.

Hyperthermia: Abnormal Thermoregulation

Humans regulate their body temperature by voluntary and involuntary means. A person who feels too cool will move to a warmer environment or put on warmer clothing. To minimize loss of body heat, **peripheral vasoconstriction** occurs through α-adrenergic receptors of the sympathetic nervous system. Heat may be generated through the involuntary contraction of skeletal muscle (shivering) and increased catabolism. Conversely, cooling is accomplished through movement to a cooler environment, removal of excess clothing, vasodilatation mediated by β-adrenergic receptors, and sweating (mediated by cholinergic receptors). Dysregulation of normal thermoregulatory mechanisms leading to increased body temperature is termed **hyperthermia**.

Patients with mild hyperthermia (**heat exhaustion**) may feel lethargic and thirsty and present with clammy skin and signs of mild dehydration. In patients with severe hyperthermia (**heat stroke**), high temperatures, delirium, coma, warm dry skin, signs of severe dehydration, organ failure, cardiac arrhythmias, and death may ensue. Treatment includes rehydration and immersion in cooling baths.

Persons with impairment of any aspect of thermoregulation may be at increased risk of hyperthermia. Elderly or demented individuals or patients with cerebrovascular accidents or other neuropsychiatric disorders may have impaired thermal perception. Conditions that impair mobility can prevent an individual from leaving a warm environment. Drugs with α-adrenergic activity can prevent vasodilatation, and drugs that increase fluid loss (diuretics) or have anticholinergic side effects (antipsychotics, antiemetics) can impede sweating. Patients with skin disorders that prevent them from sweating normally may be at risk for hyperthermia, as are those with cervical spinal cord injuries that have damaged the sympathetic nervous system, leading to dysregulated thermoregulatory responses. Endocrine disorders such as hyperthyroidism and pheochromocytoma or increased skeletal muscle activity as seen in generalized seizures can also lead to hyperthermia. None of those conditions was evident in the case of Mr. J., suggesting that the cause of his temperature elevation was fever, not hyperthermia.

Pathophysiology of Fever

Fever is a normal physiologic phenomenon regulated by the central nervous system. Thus, fever differs in its pathophysiology from the dysregulated phenomenon of hyperthermia. Fever is caused by the release of **inflammatory mediators** (**endogenous pyrogens**) often stimulated by invading pathogens like bacteria, viruses, fungi, and parasites (see Chapter 6). The microbial products that elicit this response are generally microbial surface components (e.g., endotoxin, lipoteichoic acids, muramyl dipeptide, mannan) or exotoxins (staphylococcal toxic shock syndrome toxin 1). Antigen–antibody complexes can also stimulate endogenous pyrogen production.

Endogenous pyrogen activity has been attributed to several pyrogenic **cytokines:** interleukin 1 (IL-1), tumor necrosis factor (TNF), IL-6, and interferon-γ. In addition, factors such as granulocyte-macrophage colony-stimulating factor, IL-2, and others may indirectly cause fever by stimulating the production of those cytokines. The relative contributions of each cytokine to the febrile response are not clear. Many different cells contribute to the production of the mediators, but most are probably produced by monocytes and macrophages. Endogenous pyrogens presumably travel to the brain through the circulation, although TNF and IL-1 are usually not detected by assays of the blood in patients with overwhelming infection.

Circulating endogenous pyrogens probably act at areas of the brain with fenestrated capillaries and thus lack a complete blood-brain barrier. Those areas, called the **circumventricular organs,** are close to the preoptic (anterior) hypothalamus and brainstem, which are important regulatory centers for autonomic and endocrine functions. One circumventricular organ, the **organum vasculosum of the lamina terminalis (OVLT),** appears to be important in the development of fever and recognition of cytokines in certain animals. It is not known which specific cells within the circumventricular organ respond to endogenous pyrogens.

The result of the action of endogenous pyrogens is an increase in local levels of **prostaglandin E_2 (PGE_2).** Local PGE_2 production in the OVLT may stimulate neuronal pathways to the hypothalamus and brainstem, which in turn results in the development of fever. Areas within the preoptic hypothalamus are important in thermoregulation (preoptic area), the secretion of hormones such as vasopressin and corticotropin-releasing hormone, regulation of blood flow (paraventricular nucleus), and the control of appetite (lateral hypothalamus). Those areas, in addition to the sleep-wake centers located in the hypothalamus and brainstem, account not only for the generation of fever but also for its associated symptoms of chilling, rigors, cool and clammy skin, anorexia, and lethargy.

Fever does not increase unimpeded while an infection persists. The preoptic hypothalamus contains multiple cell populations whose firing rate is temperature dependent. It has been suggested that such **warmth-sensitive neurons** have an inhibitory effect on other neurons responsible for the generation of heat. Endogenous pyrogens may work by inhibiting those "warm" neurons, leading to an increase in the normal **thermoregulatory set point in the hypothalamus.** Essentially, the body's thermostat is turned up.

The newly elevated thermoregulatory set point is maintained by a complex negative feedback loop. Endogenous pyrogen production leads to increased corticotropin-releasing, factor-mediated stimulation of the hypopituitary-adrenal axis. The **adrenal glucocorticoids** produced by this stimulation inhibit cytokine production and attenuate fever. Other factors with antiendogenous pyrogen activity, such as melanocyte-stimulating hormone and arginine vasopressin, may also be produced by the central nervous system. In addition, increased levels of the endogenous pyrogens themselves may downregulate their own production. When stimulated by cytokines, cells of target end organs may decrease their responsiveness to a specific mediator by downregulating the expression of the surface receptors, or in some instances by shedding them. As a result, a patient who has reached the hypothetical thermoregulatory set point begins to sweat, and vessels dilate to dissipate excess heat. If the patient's temperature falls below the thermoregulatory set point, the cycle begins again with rigors, chills, and vasoconstriction to raise the body temperature. External means of cooling a patient with fever, such as using ice packs and cooling blankets, only further stimulate the body to reach its higher thermoregulatory set point. Frequent bouts of rigors and chills may be more uncomfortable to the patient than the fever itself.

To prevent recurrence of fever, the disease that causes the fever must be treated and the thermoregulatory set point lowered through the use of **antipyretic agents** (aspirin, nonsteroidal anti-inflammatory drugs, and acetaminophen) that inhibit endogenous pyrogen and PGE_2 production. In contrast to fever, hyperthermia is not mediated by endogenous pyrogens. Therefore, antipyretics are not effective in lowering the body temperature of patients with hyperthermia.

Fever as a Beneficial Host Response

In the last two centuries, fever has been perceived as a dangerous affliction to be eliminated by physician and layperson alike. However, until the 1800s and the advent of antipyretics, fever was seen as a potent ally, purging patients of the bad humors that caused disease. In fact, scientific evidence supports the concept that fever in the face of infection confers a survival advantage to the host. For example, numerous unrelated species of animals have evolved this mechanism as a common response to infection, and they each produce multiple cytokines with redundant endogenous pyrogen activity. Inhibiting fever in infected reptiles and fish results in increased mortality with infection. Similarly, humans with bacteremia or peritonitis who are unable to mount a febrile response are more likely to die than those who develop fever. Inhibition of the febrile response with antipyretics has been associated with prolonged shedding of rhinoviruses and delayed healing of varicella lesions.

Endogenous pyrogens not only cause fever but also influence the recruitment and function of many types of cells. Not unexpectedly, some of those cells function optimally at higher body temperatures. Thus, phagocytosis and **killing by neutrophils and macrophages is enhanced** at elevated temperatures. Antigen presentation by macrophages, helper T cell–dependent antibody production, lymphocyte proliferation, cytotoxic T-cell function, and production of IFN-γ, IL-1, and IL-2 all increase at higher temperatures. Endogenous pyrogens also decrease the levels of trace metals (iron and zinc) that many bacteria require for growth. In addition, temperatures of 39° to 41°C directly inhibit the growth of some bacteria (pneumococci, gonococci, *Treponema pallidum, Mycobacterium leprae*), fungi (*Sporothrix schenckii*), and some parasites in vitro. Motility, capsule formation, and cell wall formation may be inhibited and antimicrobial susceptibility may increase at higher temperatures. Because many microorganisms prefer to grow at cooler temperatures, they may preferentially infect distal appendages. Local heating has been reported to be effective as a treatment of infection caused by chromomycosis, sporotrichosis, chancroid, and leishmaniasis.

In the past physicians used artificial **fever therapy,** probably induced by infection with malaria, to treat leprosy, tumors, and other diseases. Recently, the artificial induction of fever in mammals has been shown to increase resistance to bacterial, fungal, and viral infections. In 1927 malarial therapy for neurosyphilis was sufficiently successful to earn its discoverer the Nobel Prize. In animal studies injection of recombinant endogenous pyrogens before or within a few hours of infection has been shown to reduce mortality, and sometimes the microbial load. Conversely, increased mortality has been seen when antibodies to endogenous pyrogens were given before some infections. Thus, evidence exists that fever may have a beneficial role in the host response to infection.

Fever as an Adverse Host Response

Unfortunately, the story of fever versus microbes is not as simple as hero versus villain. Excessive production of endogenous pyrogens may provoke the **sepsis syndrome** and result in necrosis of tissues, end-organ failure, shock, and even death. Monoclonal antibodies against TNF and its receptors, an antagonist of the IL-1 receptor, and other cytokine inhibitors appear to confer protection in animals, but subsequent studies in humans have shown less promise for their therapeutic use. Future therapies must aim to control excessive endogenous pyrogen production without loss of the beneficial effects of these cytokines.

Moderate fever alone is not dangerous and generally does not require medical intervention except for patient comfort. Although one could argue that inhibiting fever

may be detrimental, it should be recognized that an increase in temperature of 1°C or more over 37°C leads to a 13% rise in oxygen consumption. Very high fevers (41°C, or 106°F) considerably increase host metabolic demands and place substantial stress on the cardiovascular system, resulting in congestive heart failure and ischemia. Thus, decreasing body temperature is essential in some patients. In the setting of very high fever, external cooling to rapidly reduce body temperature is appropriate when used in conjunction with antipyretics. Organ damage and death can theoretically occur when temperatures exceed 41.7°C (107°F). In the absence of serious underlying disease, such as in the case of Mr. J., low-grade fevers can be tolerated without adverse consequences.

Temperatures higher than 40°C (103°F) have been associated with generalized **seizures in children.** Children who have experienced seizures previously are likely to experience them again with high fevers, and there is little evidence that the early use of antipyretics and anticonvulsants is helpful in preventing further seizures. Fortunately, neurologic sequelae and resulting learning disabilities are very rare. Congenital malformations in the newborns of women who had high fevers while pregnant have also been reported.

Evaluation of Elevated Temperature

Elevated body temperature is a sign of possible disease. The temperature amplitude itself does not predict whether a patient has serious disease. Classic fever patterns, when present, may suggest specific diseases: Hodgkin disease (recurrent episodes, or Pel-Ebstein fever), malaria (fever every other day or every third day), yellow fever or dengue (saddle back or biphasic fever), or penicillin treatment of spirochetal diseases (Jarisch-Herxheimer reaction).

A careful clinical history, including present illness, past medical history, prescription and nonprescription medications, travel history, pets, family history, and review of systems is essential to narrowing the diagnostic possibilities. A thorough physical examination looking for signs involving specific organ systems may further confirm or exclude clinical suspicions. How quickly the evaluation is performed and treatment initiated depends on the clinical status of the patient. A patient who appears clinically well can be evaluated and treated at a more leisurely pace than the patient who appears severely ill.

Infections are the most common causes of fever. Fortunately, the majority of infections encountered in routine practice get better with time, regardless of whether treatment is initiated. Malignancies, granulomatous diseases, vasculitis, autoimmune diseases, drug reactions, and other conditions may also present as febrile illnesses. Sometimes the etiology of fever defies easy diagnosis. This uncommon clinical syndrome, termed **fever of unknown (or undetermined) origin (FUO)** as demonstrated in the case of Mr J., remains one of the greatest clinical challenges in medicine.

Fevers of Unknown Origin

Mr J. had an FUO of longstanding duration. He looked relatively well, so it was not likely that he had an occult abscess, tuberculosis, or malignancy. His workup did not necessarily require hospitalization. Dismissing patient symptoms as normal consequences of aging is unwise. Declining vision, jaw pain, and ESR greater than 100 mm/hr in an elderly man strongly suggests the diagnosis of **temporal arteritis,** a noninfectious inflammatory disease. An outpatient temporal artery biopsy revealed granulomas consistent with this diagnosis. With corticosteroid therapy, Mr. J.'s fever and jaw pain resolved, he regained weight, and his vision and anemia rapidly improved.

DEFINITION

A fever of unknown origin is usually defined as the presence of temperatures higher than 38.3°C (101°F) noted on multiple occasions over a 3-week period. A possible etiology of that fever must not be evident following reasonable intensive diagnostic evaluation over a period of approximately 1 week. That definition excludes most self-limited causes of fever that usually resolve spontaneously or prolonged fevers that are diagnosed promptly.

The diseases that cause FUO usually are not rare or unusual but often are the **atypical presentation of common diseases.** Diagnosis is frequently delayed not because too few tests were ordered but because the physician overlooked significant clues to the diagnosis or misinterpreted their significance. Diagnosis may be particularly difficult in a patient who is either very young or very old and is unable to adequately perceive, interpret, and communicate symptoms. Repeated clarification of the history and reexamination of the patient can be extremely valuable. Each symptom, physical finding, and laboratory abnormality should be thoroughly evaluated and used to guide the judicious ordering of invasive or expensive diagnostic tests.

The spectrum of diseases responsible for FUOs changes with time as technological advances lead to

table 74-1	Differential Diagnosis of Fevers of Unknown Origin (FUO)	
CATEGORY		**CASES (%)**
Infections		30–40
Abscesses (intra-abdominal) Hepatic, biliary Tuberculosis Endocarditis Cytomegalovirus infection HIV infection		
Malignancies		20–30
Hematologic Leukemias (monocyte derived) Lymphomas (Hodgkin disease, non-Hodgkin lymphoma) Solid tumors Hypernephroma (renal) Hepatoma (liver)		
Collagen vascular diseases		9–29
Rheumatoid arthritis (Still disease) Systemic lupus erythematosus Rheumatic fever Arteritis (temporal arteritis, polyarteritis nodosa)		
Granulomatous diseases		5–10
Sarcoidosis Inflammatory bowel disease (Crohn disease) Granulomatous hepatitis		
Miscellaneous		10–20
Pulmonary embolus Drug fever Hematoma Occupational (metal fume fever) Periodic (familial Mediterranean fever) Thermoregulatory disorders[a] Cervical spinal cord injuries Endocrine diseases (hyperthyroidism, Addison disease) Congenital skin disorders Factitious or fraudulent fever[b]		
No diagnosis		10–15

[a] Elevated body temperature in a thermoregulatory disorder is not fever but hyperthermia.
[b] Both types of fever are illusory; patients with factitious fever manipulate temperature-measuring devices, and patients with fraudulent fever inject themselves with pyrogenic substances.

improvements in diagnosis. The advent of computerized tomography, magnetic resonance imaging, and radionucleotide imaging has removed from the FUO category many patients with **abscesses, bacterial endocarditis,** and **collagen vascular diseases** (autoimmune or immune complex–mediated diseases) because those diseases are more easily diagnosed now than in the past.

Although physicians have become more successful in determining many causes of FUO, changes in the population result in new challenges. The spectrum of diseases causing FUO can vary in patients who are immunocompromised, including HIV-infected patients, transplant recipients, elderly persons, and those who develop FUO in the hospital. In general, infection remains the most common cause of FUO, followed by neoplasms, collagen vascular diseases, and granulomatous diseases (Table 74-1). Very rarely, patients will cause fever by injecting themselves with pyrogenic substances (fraudulent fever) or manipulate the temperature-measuring device to give the appearance of having fever (factitious fever).

TREATMENT

Even with improvements in diagnostic technology, 10% of FUO patients still defy diagnosis. Fortunately, most patients with undiagnosed FUO do well. More than 95% of patients under the age of 35 years spontaneously recover without therapy. In persons more than 65 years old, spontaneous resolution is rare, and usually a serious disease is ultimately discovered. Empiric trials of antitubercular therapy, corticosteroids, and anti-inflammatory agents may be tried in patients with persistent FUO, but only if the patient's clinical condition is deteriorating rapidly and only after exhaustive attempts to make a diagnosis have failed.

Conclusion

It is important to interpret elevated body temperature measurements only after careful assessment of the patient. Not all elevated body temperatures are fever. The treatment of hyperthermia is different from that of fever. Some elevations of body temperature require treatment, others only careful observation. Fever may be a beneficial host response. The general rule is to treat the underlying cause, not just the elevated body temperature. Some etiologies of fever may be difficult to discern. A careful approach is essential for diagnosis, and empirical therapy should be used only as a last resort.

Health Care–Associated Infections

David R. Snydman

Approximately 5% of patients develop infections while they are in hospitals. An infection acquired during a hospital stay is called a **nosocomial infection.** An infection resulting from intervention by a physician, in or out of a hospital, is known as an **iatrogenic infection.** Because of the complexity of home care and nursing care and the need to distinguish clearly between infections associated with medical care from those that are not, a new term, **health care–associated infections,** has recently been adopted as the standard terminology. A nosocomial infection can result in a prolonged hospital stay and be extraordinarily costly in terms of morbidity and even mortality. It is estimated that about $5 billion is spent each year for the management of hospital-acquired infections in the United States.

Several factors related to hospitalization predispose patients to the risk of hospital-acquired infections. The most important factors are those that violate the host's own defenses. Invasive procedures produce **new portals of entry** for microorganisms from the patient's own flora or from the environment. Examples of invasion are the use of devices like endotracheal tubes, mechanical ventilators, and intravenous or intra-arterial catheters as well as surgical procedures in general.

Broadly speaking, the incidence of a nosocomial infection is related to the severity of the underlying disease; that is, patients who have a high likelihood of dying during their hospitalizations also are most at risk of developing nosocomial infections. In contrast, patients admitted with less severe disease are less likely to acquire infections in the hospital. This underscores the need for improved management of the severely compromised patients. Unfortunately, it is estimated that only about one third to one half of nosocomial infections are preventable, even under the most favorable conditions.

Agents of Health Care–Associated Infections

Generally, the organisms that cause health care–associated infections are similar to those found elsewhere in the community. The most common causative agents may not be especially pathogenic; in fact, sometimes they are even less pathogenic than those that cause disease outside the hospital.

A salient example is the emergence of *Serratia marcescens* as a hospital-acquired pathogen. The bacterium was thought to be so benign that it was used in the 1950s

table **75-1**	Common Hospital-Acquired Infections and Frequently Associated Organisms
TYPE OF INFECTION	**MOST COMMON ORGANISM**
Surgical wounds	*Staphylococcus aureus* *Escherichia coli* *Enterococcus* spp.
Pneumonia	*Klebsiella pneumoniae* *Pseudomonas aeruginosa* *Staphylococcus aureus* *Enterobacter* spp. *Escherichia coli*
Intravenous catheter	*Staphylococcus epidermidis* *Staphylococcus aureus* *Enterococcus* spp. *Candida* spp.
Urinary catheter	*Escherichia coli* *Enterococcus* spp. *Pseudomonas aeruginosa* *Klebsiella* spp.

to trace the movement of air in a subway system and to determine the movement of bacteria into the urethra through the catheter–meatal interface. This "nonpathogen" has become the source of significant nosocomial infections, although it rarely causes disease outside the hospital.

Like many pathogens associated with nosocomial infections, *S. marcescens* has acquired significant antibiotic resistance. Gram-negative bacterial strains that possess plasmid-mediated, multiple antibiotic resistance are commonly encountered in nosocomial infections. Plasmid transfer occurs among various strains of the same species and even among various genera. **Transfer of antibiotic resistance** has been demonstrated in the urine of patients with Foley catheters and on patients' skin. Presumably, transfer of antibiotic resistance takes place in the gastrointestinal tract as well. Antibiotic-resistant pathogens have become so common that methicillin-resistant *Staphylococcus aureus* and aminoglycoside-resistant Gram-negative bacteria are regularly encountered in nosocomial infections. Examples of nosocomial pathogens are listed in Table 75-1. The list of pathogens that can cause health care–associated infections encompasses the agents of practically all infections. However, health care–associated infections generally have a greater degree of antibiotic resistance among both Gram-negative and Gram-positive organisms.

ENCOUNTER

A hospital is a microenvironment in which organisms can be transferred in many ways from one individual to another, or from the hospital staff to patients (Fig. 75-1).

Transmission between individuals can be direct by hand contact or indirect by inhalation, ingestion, or puncture through the integument. For example, methicillin-resistant staphylococci spread directly among patients or through hospital personnel. Tubercle bacilli are transmitted through aerosolization and inhalation. Viral agents, such as those of varicella-zoster or influenza, can be spread through the air to susceptible immunocompromised individuals. Blood used for transfusions may be contaminated with hepatitis A, B, or C virus or HIV. Food handlers may contaminate food eaten by patients, and physicians and nurses can introduce microorganisms into deeper tissues during operations or while dressing surgical or other wounds. Unusual epidemics can sometimes be traced to **specific carriers** among members of the hospital staff. For example, well-documented epidemics caused by group A streptococci have been attributed to carriers who had contact with patients in the operating room. In one epidemic the organisms were located in the carrier's vagina and presumably were aerosolized through normal body movements.

Microorganisms that spread to patients may be **endemic** to the hospital environment. Notable examples include the fungi that cause aspergillosis, which may be present as more or less visible mildew on moist room walls or construction panels. Infections by exogenous organisms can also be acquired from improperly sterilized surgical instruments and even contaminated disin-

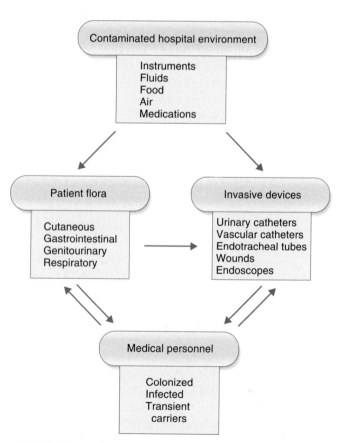

FIGURE 75-1 ▪ **Sources of hospital-acquired infections.**

fectant solutions. Fortunately, those events are rare in most hospitals.

Patients acquire nosocomial infections as the result of breaks in their own defenses and from their inability to combat infection. Host defense breaks usually occur as the result of **invasive diagnostic or therapeutic interventions** that physicians perform on patients. Thus, the most common nosocomial infections affect the urinary tract, because catheterization of the bladder is frequently used with bedridden patients. The commonly used Foley catheter bypasses the normal mucosal barriers and facilitates the entry of organisms that colonize the skin or the urinary introitus. The next most frequent types of nosocomial infections are surgical wound infections and respiratory tract infections, both of which result from invasive procedures.

ENTRY

Skin Penetration

The skin barrier is breached by intravenous catheters or devices used to measure intravascular pressure. **The longer devices stay in place, the higher the risk of both local infection and bacteremia.** That underscores the need for vigilance in the care of patients with indwelling devices. National surveys conducted in the United States indicate that in the 1980s the rate of nosocomial bacteremia almost doubled and the rate of *Staphylococcus epidermidis* infection tripled. In the author's institution, 1 in 100 patients develops hospital-acquired bacteremia; half those cases result from the implantation of intravascular devices.

The role of the normal skin in protecting from microbial invasion is also evident in burn victims. Frequently, patients who have extensive second- or third-degree burns will become colonized with bacteria, especially *Pseudomonas aeruginosa*. Necrotizing lesions at the site of skin damage are accompanied by sepsis, the major cause of death in burn victims.

Inhalation

The most common cause of nosocomial pneumonia is the use of an **endotracheal tube,** a device that bypasses the normal epithelial defenses and allows the entry of organisms through aerosols. In the early 1960s, when mechanical ventilation of the lungs was being developed, epidemics of Gram-negative pneumonia occurred because nebulized mists contained bacteria-laden aerosols. An understanding of the problem prompted changes in ventilator design that have virtually eliminated the ventilator as a source of hospital-acquired pneumonia. Patients with endotracheal tubes still develop pneumonia, but now the offending organisms tend to come from the patient's stomach or intestine to colonize the nasophar-

ynx. From there the bacteria can be aspirated into the lungs. Other examples of nosocomial infections acquired by inhalation can be seen in hospital epidemics of influenza, respiratory syncytial virus, and varicella-zoster, which are particularly dangerous for immunocompromised patients.

Ingestion

Epidemics of nosocomial infection sometimes result from the ingestion of pathogenic bacteria. The organisms are often those associated with community-acquired infections, including those caused by *Salmonella* species, hepatitis A virus, and rotavirus, the latter being most frequent among neonates or infants. Epidemics of salmonellosis in hospitals usually result from eating foods contaminated during preparation. Another source of salmonellosis outbreaks is the use of contaminated carmine dye or other animal products for diagnostic purposes. The **gastrointestinal tract of hospitalized patients is a reservoir for antibiotic-resistant microorganisms** to which patients may be exposed in the environment. For example, vancomycin-resistant enterococci may be ingested from a contaminated environment, colonize patients, and then lead to a health care–associated infection, such as a bloodstream or urinary tract infection (see the cases presented later in the chapter).

Inanimate Environment

The complexity of a hospital environment provides innumerable opportunities for the encounter of patients with microorganisms. Some encounters are specific to the hospital environment and do not usually occur elsewhere. An example is the use of **contaminated intravenous solutions,** which have caused many epidemics. Contamination rarely takes place at the point of manufacture but more commonly occurs during the **handling of bottles and infusion lines.**

Instruments and dressings improperly sterilized before surgery also provide a possible source of infection. A separate technology has developed to solve the problem of determining if autoclaves and sterilizing ovens perform their expected tasks. Thus, it is customary to insert a vial containing bacterial spores with the material to be autoclaved and to determine spore viability afterward. Deviance from established procedures can result in improper sterilization and in contamination of surgical or other wounds.

Environmental contamination can occur quite easily with organisms carried in the stool of patients, such as vancomycin-resistant enterococci or *Klebsiella pneumoniae* that harbor plasmids conferring resistance to late-generation cephalosporins, so-called extended-spectrum β-lactamase–producing organisms (ESBL), and even methicillin-resistant *S. aureus,* as well as other

Gram-negatives such as *Enterobacter* species. Once the environment is contaminated, if hospital personnel do not pay attention to cleanliness and hand washing when making patient contacts, those organisms can be transmitted from the environment to the patient.

Model Infections

Nosocomial Urinary Tract Infection

The case of Mr. H. is a classic example of a nosocomial infection of the urinary tract. The use of Foley catheters for more than 1 or 2 days often results in contamination of the bladder, especially by fecal coliforms. Most catheters include an expandable collection bag for urine, thus making a closed system. Nonetheless, the risk of bacteriuria is cumulative and still occurs at a rate of 5 to 8% of patients with catheters per day. The risk of bacteriuria is related to the skill of the person inserting the catheter, the sex and age of the patient, and the duration of catheterization.

Nosocomial Wound Infection

This case illustrates the problem of surgical wound infections and the serious impact they can have on patient recovery. Wound infections of the mediastinum complicate from 1 to 5% of open-heart surgeries. If the infection reaches deep portions of the chest, its effect can be extremely serious. Patients frequently require multiple surgical interventions with removal of devitalized bone, cartilage, and other tissue.

Case

At 67 years of age Mr. H. underwent a transurethral prostatectomy for cancer of the prostate. Because of concern about postoperative bleeding from straining during urination, he had a Foley catheter placed into the bladder. Three days later Mr. H. developed a urinary tract infection with low-grade fever, some pain, and pyuria. Quantitative urine counts yielded 3×10^5 colonies of *Escherichia coli* per milliliter of urine. The organisms were resistant to all tested antibiotics except for the aminoglycosides. Within 2 days Mr. H. developed bacteremia with hypotension and shock. Physicians were eventually able to control the bacteremia with gentamicin therapy. Fortunately, Mr. H. recovered completely and was discharged.

This case raises several questions:

1. How did Mr. H. acquire this infection?
2. What are the most likely organisms?
3. How can this scenario be prevented?

Case

Ms. Z., an 82-year-old patient with rheumatic heart disease, underwent a mitral valve replacement and coronary artery bypass graft. Her postoperative course was complicated by bleeding in the mediastinum, which required more surgery. Subsequently, she recovered well and was discharged after 12 days. Three weeks later Ms. Z. noticed some purulent drainage along the wound site on her chest. She continued to have pain but did not tell her family, assuming that the pain was related to her healing process. When she returned to see the surgeon 1 month later, she reported her pain and low-grade fever. The surgeon noted considerable drainage at the wound site. Probing the wound, he noticed a lot of pus.

Ms. Z. was hospitalized again for radical debridement (cleaning) of her chest wound. Cultures of the pus yielded *S. epidermidis*. Her wound was debrided, the wires in her sternum were removed, and she was treated intravenously with vancomycin for 6 weeks. At the end of that period she required a plastic surgical device and a muscle flap to close the wound. After 2 more months of hospitalization, she was discharged and continued her convalescence at home.

This case raises several questions:

1. How did Ms. Z develop her infection?
2. What are the most common organisms?
3. What is cost of such infections in morbidity?

Surgical wound infections are the most costly of all nosocomial infections. Some are clearly preventable. Many are caused by *S. aureus*, but *S. epidermidis*, a normal skin commensal, is another significant pathogen. In the case of Ms. Z. the source of the infection was probably the **normal flora on her skin**. As with other infections, establishment of a surgical wound infection depends on the size of the inoculum, the pathogenic potential of the invading organisms, and the state of host defenses. All those factors should be taken into account before planning surgical treatment. When infection would be devastating to the patient's outcome—for instance, in an artificial hip implant—surgeons go to great lengths to prevent wound infections, such as using laminar airflow systems and prophylactic antibiotics.

Nosocomial Bacteremia

This case is an example of primary bacteremia, which is defined as bacteremia that cannot be ascribed to another focus of infection. Primary bacteremia is frequently either the result of a contaminated intravenous line or associated with granulocytopenia in the immunosuppressed leukemic patient.

From the bottle to the intravenous catheter, intravenous therapy provides many potential sources of contamination. The risk of intravenous catheter-related in-

Case

Fifty-nine-year-old Mr. S. was hospitalized with acute myocardial infarction. His disease was so severe that he required a catheter to measure his cardiac pressure and output. Unfortunately, the catheter was left in place for several more days than was probably necessary. Six days after his infarction Mr. S. developed fever, leukocytosis, and inflammation at the site of insertion of the catheter. Four blood cultures all revealed the presence of *S. aureus*. He was treated with intravenous antibiotics; however, a new cardiac murmur was noted 7 days into therapy. An echocardiogram revealed the development of a tricuspid valve vegetation. Mr. S. required 4 weeks of antibiotic therapy for his hospital-acquired, catheter-related endocarditis.

This case raises several questions:

1. Where did the organisms arise in Mr. S infection?
2. How do the organisms enter the patient?
3. What is the best prevention?

fection is generally influenced by the type of catheter and the duration of catheterization. Patients who have large-bore catheters that require surgical insertion have the highest risk. If the catheter is left in place for 48 hours or longer, the patient has a 23% risk of bacteremia. In the example cited, the patient developed endocarditis, a rare but recognized complication. The usual pathogen of endocarditis is *S. aureus*, *S. epidermidis*, a variety of Gram-negative rods, or *Candida* species (see Table 75-1).

Another example of primary bacteremia is seen in leukemia and lymphoma patients who are granulocytopenic as a result of cancer chemotherapy. Typically, the source of the bacteremia is an intestinal pathogen, most often Gram-negative rods originating endogenously from the patient's normal flora or exogenously from the hospital.

Case

Ms. I. was hospitalized for a coronary artery bypass procedure. Because the 76-year-old woman had difficulty breathing when off the ventilator, physicians attempted extubation. However, Ms. I. aspirated, and over the next 24 to 48 hours she developed a cough, was suctioned for purulent sputum, and had a pulmonary infiltrate. The culture grew *P. aeruginosa*. Treatment was initiated, and Ms. I. eventually recovered, but not without a prolonged hospitalization.

This case raises several questions:

1. Where did the organisms arise?
2. What are the most common?
3. What preventive methods are there?

Case

Dr. M. developed a needlestick injury while recapping a needle used on a patient who abused intravenous drugs. About 2 months later Dr. M. developed arthralgias, fatigue, malaise, and jaundice. Diagnosed as having hepatitis B, he lost 3 months of work but slowly recovered.

This case raises several questions:

1. What is likelihood of transmission of HIV, HBV or HCV following needlestick?
2. What steps can be taken to prevent transmission?

Nosocomial Pneumonia

Nosocomial pneumonia can be a devastating illness. Risk factors for development usually are the need for **mechanical ventilation, intubation, thoracoabdominal surgery, failure to be able to wean from a ventilator,** and **older age.** The case of Ms. I. illustrates the role that intubation and aspiration play in the acquisition of organisms that cause nosocomial pneumonia. Often patients aspirate stomach or nasopharyngeal contents as a result of their debilitation. Infections acquired resulting from aspiration are frequently caused by organisms colonizing the back of the nasopharynx. Unfortunately, nosocomial pneumonia is difficult to prevent and is associated with the highest mortality rate among all hospital-acquired infections.

Nosocomial Bloodborne Disease

For decades hepatitis B has been recognized as a nosocomial hazard for both health care workers and patients. Needlestick transmission is a recognized hazard, with rates of transmission approaching 25%. Blood transfusions constituted a major threat to patients before the early 1970s. Fortunately, the risk of transmission of hepatitis B virus has been recognized, and using hepatitis B surface antigen (HBsAg) screening has significantly reduced the bloodborne transmission of the virus.

The incidence of needlestick injuries has been significantly reduced by the practice of not recapping needles and the use of safety devices, which are now prevalent. For health care workers needlestick transmission of hepatitis B is now infrequent because a vaccine is available to prevent transmission. Prior to the availability of vaccination, the rate of needlestick transmission of hepatitis B was from 3 to 20%. However, needlestick transmission of hepatitis C and HIV still occurs at a rate of about 3%. For hepatitis C no vaccination exists; thus, avoidance of needlestick is of the utmost importance. Current protocols try to treat early-onset HCV infection to "revert" the infection. For HIV, needlestick transmission occurs in approximately 0.3% of needlestick injuries. There is evidence that use of antiretroviral agents within 8 hours of the needlestick can reduce the risk by about 60%.

CONTROL AND PREVENTION

Control of nosocomial infections requires awareness by all health care professionals. **Using hand hygiene techniques** between patient contacts is a simple but much-neglected procedure. It has been estimated that only one third of patient contacts are accompanied by appropriate hand hygiene. **Alcohol-based hand-rubbing solutions** are available to make it much easier for medical personnel to disinfect their hands before coming into contact with patients. Appropriate hand hygiene has become a focus for all hospitals and even licensing agencies because of its importance in decreasing transmission of microorganisms between hospital staff and patients. The use of **aseptic techniques** during surgical and other invasive procedures, as stressed in surgical training, is also a significant step in preventing infections.

Another control measure instituted by hospitals is the **infection control committee,** which is responsible for overseeing all aspects of infection control within the institution. The committee's oversight duties include su-pervising surveillance of hospital-acquired infections, establishing policies and procedures to prevent infections, and intervening when necessary in investigations of epidemics or other problems. Most hospitals have specific personnel, called **infection control practitioners,** who are assigned these tasks and function as the "eyes and ears" of the committee. The practitioners are responsible for tracing epidemics, monitoring infection rates, and determining the level of isolation of patients. However, hospitals still have much to learn. Intense efforts are directed at preventing infections in the increasing number of immunocompromised patients and in devising effective means to prevent nosocomial pneumonias.

Conclusion

Every physician encounters health care–associated infections. It is incumbent on the medical profession to minimize the occurrence of such infections by paying attention to isolation precautions, practicing scrupulous hand hygiene, and using safety devices when appropriate.

Foodborne Diseases

David R. Snydman

Foodborne infections are a significant public health problem. In the United States these infections are a major cause of morbidity, although an infrequent cause of mortality. Between 1983 and 1987, 909 outbreaks were reported to the Centers for Disease Control and Prevention from nearly all 50 states. The number of ill people reported to the health authorities as a result of the outbreaks totaled more than 50,000, with 134 deaths. Studies suggest that the true incidence of infection related to food probably is 10 to 100 times higher.

A foodborne disease outbreak is defined by two criteria: (1) two or more persons must experience a similar illness, usually gastrointestinal, after ingestion of the same food; and (2) epidemiological analysis must implicate the food as the source of the illness. However, exceptions to that definition exist. For example, one case of botulism constitutes an outbreak for the purposes of epidemiological investigation and control because of the high probability that other cases may be involved.

The most common diseases acquired by **ingestion of contaminated food** in the United States are those usually called **food poisoning**. A case of food poisoning results from the consumption of food contaminated with bacteria, bacterial toxins, parasites, viruses, or chemicals. Bacteria cause approximately two thirds of the foodborne disease outbreaks in the United States for which an etiology can be determined (Table 76-1). However, it should be noted that in only 44% of foodborne disease outbreaks is the etiology confirmed. This chapter discusses major food-poisoning illnesses that occur in the United States. The chapter is organized according to the three main types of foodborne illnesses:

- **Intoxications caused by a toxin preformed in the food:** In these cases the organism does not have to be alive to cause disease. Examples of causative bacteria are *Staphylococcus aureus*, *Clostridium botulinum*, and *Bacillus cereus*.
- **Intoxications caused by toxins manufactured in the body:** These cases emerge after live organisms such as *Vibrio cholerae* or *Clostridium perfringens* are ingested.
- **Intestinal invasive diseases:** The most common of these diseases is gastroenteritis caused by invasive organisms like *Salmonella* and *Campylobacter* species.

The distinction between foodborne illnesses caused by toxin-producing organisms and those caused by invasive pathogens is important clinically and epidemiologically. In general, **diseases caused by toxin-forming organisms** like *S. aureus* have a short incubation period and are characterized by upper gastrointestinal complaints, such as nausea and vomiting. Diarrhea is less frequent, and constitutional symptoms, including fever and chills, are uncommon. In contrast, **food poisonings caused by invasive organisms**—*Salmonella* species, for example—usually have a longer incubation period and are characterized by fever, chills, and lower gastrointestinal

table **76-1**	**Recent Major Outbreaks of Foodborne Disease in the United States**[a]	
YEAR	**ETIOLOGIC AGENT**	**CIRCUMSTANCES**
2002–03	Norovirus	Multiple cruise ship outbreaks with very high attack rates disrupted operations for several cruise lines for weeks to months
1997	Hepatitis A	153 cases associated with eating frozen strawberries imported from Mexico and served in Michigan public schools
1996	*Cyclospora cayetanensis*	More than 40 individual outbreaks and more than 850 persons ill owing to contaminated raspberries imported from Guatemala and distributed nationwide
1996	Enterohemorrhagic *Escherichia coli*	Juice and cider made with "dropped" apples harvested from the ground. Sixty-six illnesses and one death in western United States and Canada
1994	*Salmonella enteritidis*	Multistate outbreak caused by a national brand of ice cream contaminated at the factory; an estimated 224,000 persons became ill
1993	Enterohemorrhagic *E. coli*	More than 500 cases of hemorrhagic colitis associated with undercooked hamburgers served at 93 fast food restaurants in several states (four children died)
1991	*Vibrio cholerae*	Four cases in nontravelers associated with tainted coconut milk imported from Thailand
1990	*Clostridium perfringens*	700 cases of food poisoning associated with beef and chicken tacos served in a Missouri prison
1988	*Campylobacter jejuni*	120 cases traced to raw milk served at a vacation Bible school in Kansas
1988	*Shigella sonnei*	3,175 illnesses among people who ate raw tofu salad at an outdoor music festival in Michigan (117 hospitalized)

[a]Selected from among approximately 500 outbreaks each year reported to the Centers for Disease Control and Prevention.

complaints. Diarrhea, often bloody or containing pus or mucus, is more prominent in invasive diseases than are nausea or vomiting. Therefore, ascertaining the type of food poisoning is generally a matter of determining whether the symptoms are more indicative of intoxication or invasion. Some overlap exists in this classification scheme, because organisms such as species of *Shigella* and *Salmonella* may have invasive properties as well as the ability to produce toxin.

In the United States the most frequently recognized agents of bacterial food poisoning are generally limited to a dozen organisms (see Table 76-1). *Salmonella* infections dominate the confirmed outbreaks and constitute more than half the reported cases of foodborne illness. That dominance is partly the result of the ease with which the infections are recognized as well as the awareness of physicians and the public. Shigellae are the next most frequent cause of foodborne disease outbreaks and are associated with 20% of reported cases. *S. aureus* and *C. perfringens* are the next most frequent and together are associated with 56% of reported cases. *Campylobacter* species, hepatitis A and norovirus, and other pathogens cause illness less frequently. Parasites and chemical agents acquired from food are the least frequent causes of foodborne disease. Features of the principal foodborne diseases are shown in Table 76-2.

table **76-2**	**Some Characteristics of Bacterial Food Poisoning**			
ORGANISM	**MECHANISM**	**INCUBATION PERIOD (HR)**	**VEHICLES**	**FEATURES**
Staphylococcus aureus	Heat-stable toxin	1–6	Ham, pastry, baked goods	Vomiting
Bacillus cereus	Heat-stable toxin	1–6	Fried rice	Vomiting
	Heat-labile toxin	8–24	Cream sauce	Diarrhea
Salmonella species	Invasion	16–48	Chicken, beef, eggs, milk	Fever, diarrhea
Campylobacter species	Invasion	16–48	Chicken, beef, milk	Fever, diarrhea
Vibrio parahaemolyticus	Invasion (toxin?)	16–72	Shellfish	Fever, diarrhea
Yersinia enterocolitica	Invasion (toxin?)	16–72	Milk, tofu	Diarrhea
Escherichia coli	Toxin	16–72	Salads	Diarrhea
	0157:H7 (vero toxin)	16–48	Beef	Fever, diarrhea
Clostridium perfringens	Toxin	8–12	Beef, poultry, gravy	Diarrhea

It is important to note that **etiological patterns vary throughout the world.** Etiology depends on many factors, such as food preferences, awareness by physicians and the public, and laboratory capabilities. For example, in the United States food poisoning by *Salmonella* and *Shigella* species represents about 70% of the outbreaks. In contrast, *C. perfringens* is implicated in more than 90% of the recognized foodborne illness in England and Wales. Japan has yet another etiological pattern, with *Vibrio parahaemolyticus* gastroenteritis representing more than 50% of reported outbreaks. For U.S. citizens traveling to countries like Mexico, the most common cause of traveler's diarrhea ("turista") is an enterotoxigenic strain of *Escherichia coli*.

Intoxications

Staphylococcus aureus

ENCOUNTER

Outbreaks of staphylococcal foodborne disease are characterized by explosive onset 1 to 6 hours after consuming contaminated food. Attack rates are usually quite high because very small quantities of staphylococcal enterotoxin can cause illness. In outbreaks involving single families and uniform doses of enterotoxin, virtually 100% of individuals are affected. The **staphylococcal enterotoxin**

Case

As the aircraft cruised at 35,000 feet, the cabin attendants passed out a lunch meal that included ham sandwiches. Two hours later two thirds of the passengers aboard the Boeing 747 jet developed nausea and vomiting. Diarrhea occurred in about one third of those affected. The waiting lines for the toilets trailed down the aisle. As a result of this and similar epidemics, rules for serving the cockpit crew different meals went into effect.

This case raises two questions:

1. What was the cause of the outbreak?
2. How could one kind of meal have affected such a large number of individuals?

It was later discovered that two thirds of the passengers on the flight were served ham sliced by a chef who had a pustular lesion on his hand. *S. aureus* was isolated from the lesion, and an identical strain was isolated from the ham. The passengers had ingested food contaminated with one of the many *S. aureus* toxins (see Chapter 11).

is resistant to heat and can remain in food after cooking, even though the causative organism has been killed.

Outbreaks from staphylococci can occur at any time of the year, but most are reported during the warm weather months. Staphylococci are carried by so many people that food preparation in almost any setting can act as a means of transmission. Most outbreaks are reported from places where many people gather—for instance, in school cafeterias, group picnics, club dining halls, and restaurants. Many different foods have been implicated, including ham, canned beef, pork, or any salted meat and cream-filled cakes or pastries like cream puffs. Potato and macaroni salads are occasionally involved. Foods that have a high content of salt (ham) or sugar (custard) selectively favor the growth of staphylococci.

Foods that are involved in outbreaks have usually been cut, sliced, grated, mixed, or ground by workers who are carriers of enterotoxin-producing strains of staphylococci. Although animal carcasses may be contaminated before processing, competitive growth from other members of the normal flora usually limits the staphylococci. Therefore, transmission is from the food handler to the food product. Most commonly, the contaminated food has been allowed to sit at room temperature for some time before preparation or cooking, thus allowing the toxin to be produced in significant quantities.

DIAGNOSIS

The signs and symptoms of staphylococcal food poisoning are primarily profuse vomiting, nausea, and abdominal cramps, often followed by diarrhea. Notably, fever and other signs of inflammation are absent. In severe cases blood may be observed in the vomitus or stool. Rarely, hypotension and marked prostration occur, but recovery is usually complete within 24 to 48 hours.

Staphylococcal food poisoning should be considered in anyone with severe vomiting, nausea, cramps, and some diarrhea. A history of ingesting meats of high salt or sugar content may be helpful. The best epidemiological clue, especially if many individuals are ill, is the short incubation period (1 to 6 hours). Of the bacterial foodborne diseases, only *B. cereus* has similar symptoms, with a short incubation period and a marked vomiting syndrome. However, because the *B. cereus* vomiting syndrome is closely associated with rice consumption, the epidemiological distinction can usually be made easily.

Diagnosis can be confirmed by culturing the suspected food, the skin or nose of the food handler, or occasionally, the vomitus or stools of affected individuals. The recovered *S. aureus* may be typed either by phage or pulsed field gel electrophoresis to prove that the isolated strains are identical (see Chapter 11). Detection of staphylococcal enterotoxin is the ultimate means of making the diagnosis when an appropriate test becomes generally available.

Clostridium perfringens

ENCOUNTER

The lengthy time between ingestion of suspected food and onset of symptoms, the clinical manifestations, and the fact that most of the persons present at the meal got sick point to *C. perfringens* as the likely cause of the outbreak. *C. perfringens* food poisoning is the fourth most common cause of foodborne disease in the United States. Because the diagnosis is often difficult to establish, reported cases probably represent a small fraction of the actual cases that occur.

Epidemics of *C. perfringens* are usually characterized by high attack rates. The incubation period in most outbreaks varies between 8 and 14 hours (median of 12 hours), but can be as long as 74 hours. For reasons that are not clear, more cases of *C. perfringens* food poisoning are reported in the fall and winter months. The nadir of reported cases occurs in the summer, in marked contrast to outbreaks of *Salmonella* and staphylococcal food poisoning. It may be that the kinds of food usually implicated in *C. perfringens* outbreaks, such as stews, are eaten less frequently in the summer.

Outbreaks caused by this organism are often reported from institutions and large gatherings. The latter is probably a reporting artifact, because only large groups recognize the illness as food poisoning. In the late 1940s it was discovered that *C. perfringens* caused outbreaks of a severe and often lethal intestinal disease labeled **enteritis necroticans** that affected people in Germany and New Guinea (where it is termed pig-bel, as discussed in the next section).

PATHOPHYSIOLOGY

Food poisoning from *C. perfringens* often occurs when dishes prepared with poultry, meat, or fish are cooked

Case

A group of college dormitory residents sat down for a turkey feast at a nearby restaurant at 6 PM. They consumed turkey, giblets, gravy, and "all the fixin's." At approximately 2 AM, the first of many of the group awoke with severe intestinal cramps and watery diarrhea. Most of the other students in the group became ill with similar symptoms at approximately 6 AM. Several students had to spend the night in the college infirmary. Fortunately, the wave of diarrhea resolved within 24 hours.

This case raises several questions:

1. What is the likely agent of this disease?
2. What is the pathophysiology of this type of diarrhea?
3. How could such an outbreak be prevented?

and then allowed to cool slowly without proper refrigeration for extended periods. Spores of the organisms present in the meat or fish resist the first heating and then germinate and grow in the unrefrigerated food. When the food is reheated, the already-multiplied bacteria form spores again. Illness occurs either when a large number of vegetative bacteria that survive reheating or a large number of spores are ingested with the food. Most commonly, ingested spores germinate in the intestine and release clostridial toxin in vivo.

The heat-labile protein enterotoxin has a molecular weight of approximately 34,000 daltons. The clostridial toxin differs from cholera toxin in several respects. Its activity is maximal in the ileum and minimal in the duodenum, which is opposite to that of cholera toxin. Clostridial enterotoxin inhibits glucose transport, damages the intestinal epithelium, and causes protein loss into the intestinal lumen; no such effects are observed with cholera toxin. Recently, *C. perfringens* enterotoxin has been detected in the stools of affected individuals. Enterotoxin activity disappears quickly from the stool but can be measured in serum.

Immunity in *C. perfringens* intoxication is not well understood. One study has found that 65% of Americans and 84% of Brazilians have antienterotoxin activity in serum. The significance of that finding is unknown at present; in none of the outbreaks studied to date has blood drawn before an outbreak been available. Such samples would permit the study of a possible correlation between antienterotoxin immunity and the disease. In animal studies, enterotoxin antiserum blocks the action of the toxin on ligated rabbit loops. It is not known, however, if the presence of antibody in serum has any effect on toxin activity in the intestine.

Another disease rarely seen in the United States but caused by *C. perfringens* is enteritis necroticans (pig-bel), which is characterized by high attack rates in children in New Guinea, coupled with a high mortality. Although enteritis necroticans and *C. perfringens* food poisoning are caused by the same organism, the two diseases are quite different. Outbreaks of pig-bel have been clearly associated with the consumption of pork at large native feasts. At the feasts, improperly cooked pork was consumed in large quantities over 3 or 4 days.

As its name suggests, enteritis necroticans is a severe necrotizing disease of the small intestine. After a 24-hour incubation period, illness ensues with intense abdominal pain, bloody diarrhea, vomiting, and shock. The mortality rate is about 40%, usually as a result of intestinal perforation. The disease is caused by a toxin known as α-toxin, a 35-kilodalton protein unusually sensitive to proteases and thus rapidly inactivated by the intestinal enzyme trypsin. The disease usually affects people who eat large, high-protein meals that overwhelm the ability of the intestinal trypsin to neutralize the toxin.

CLINICAL FEATURES

C. perfringens food poisoning is generally characterized by watery diarrhea and severe cramping abdominal pain, usually without vomiting, beginning 8 to 24 hours after the suspected meal. Fever, chills, headache, or other signs of infection are usually not present. The illness lasts 24 hours or less. Rare fatalities have been recorded in debilitated or hospitalized patients who are victims of clostridial food poisoning.

DIAGNOSIS

The diagnosis of *C. perfringens* food poisoning should be considered in any diarrheal illness characterized by abdominal pain and moderate to severe diarrhea, unaccompanied by fever and chills. Many individuals usually are involved in the outbreak; the suspected food is beef or chicken that has been stewed, roasted, or boiled and then allowed to stand without proper refrigeration. The incubation period is 8 to 14 hours; occasional outbreaks have incubation periods as short as 5 to 6 hours or as long as 22 hours.

A form of food poisoning caused by *B. cereus* may have similar symptoms and can only be ruled out by bacteriological study. Enterotoxigenic *E. coli* can also produce the symptoms associated with *C. perfringens* food poisoning, although low-grade fever is often present. *V. cholerae* produces more profuse diarrhea, which helps differentiate it from clostridial intoxication. *Salmonella* or *Campylobacter* infections are usually accompanied by fever, a longer incubation period, and more marked systemic signs.

Because *C. perfringens* can be isolated from normal stools, it is helpful to use an established serotyping schema to distinguish between the approximately 20 different serotypes. In an outbreak the same serotype of *C. perfringens* should be recovered from all affected individuals and from the food they ate. If food specimens are not available, the diagnosis can be made by isolating organisms of the same serotype from the stool of most ill individuals but not from that of suitable controls. In the absence of either of those findings, culturing 10^5 or more organisms per gram of the suspected food is highly suggestive of the diagnosis.

Bacillus cereus

ENCOUNTER

B. cereus has been recognized as an increasingly significant cause of food poisoning since about 1970. One percent or less of all food-poisoning outbreaks in the United States are caused by the organism. Data from other countries are still generally sparse.

Case

Six medical students returned to class after a lunch break in Chinatown. The meal consisted of hot and sour soup, spring rolls, fried rice, and three other Chinese entrées. Two hours later, while listening to Professor S. expound on the hazards of mushroom poisoning, four of the six students felt the urge to vomit and had to excuse themselves from class.

This case raises two questions:

1. Which food is most likely to have contributed to this early-onset form of food poisoning?
2. How could the food have become contaminated?

The incubation period for the outbreaks of emetic illness is usually 2 or 3 hours, whereas that for the diarrheal outbreaks is 6 to 14 hours. The clear-cut association between the vomiting syndrome and fried rice deserves emphasis. Most outbreaks of *B. cereus* vomiting syndrome in the United States and Great Britain implicate that dish as the vehicle. The diarrheal illness, however, has been caused by a variety of foods, including boiled beef, sausage, chicken soup, vanilla sauce, and puddings.

B. cereus is found in about 25% of foodstuffs sampled, including cream, pudding, meat, spices, dry potatoes, dry milk, spaghetti sauces, and rice. Contamination of food products generally occurs before they are cooked. The organisms grow if the food is maintained at 30° to 50°C during preparation. Spores survive extreme temperatures and, when allowed to cool relatively slowly, germinate and multiply. No evidence exists that human carriage of the organism or other means of contamination play a role in transmission.

Contamination of rice by *B. cereus* is attributed to the practice common in Oriental restaurants of allowing large portions of boiled rice to drain unrefrigerated to avoid clumping. The flash frying in the final preparation of certain rice dishes (e.g., fried rice) does not raise the temperature sufficiently to destroy the preformed heat-stable toxin.

PATHOPHYSIOLOGY

Several **extracellular toxins** produced by strains of *B. cereus* may contribute to their virulence, including an enterotoxin that causes fluid accumulation in the rabbit intestine and stimulates the adenylate cyclase–cyclic adenosine monophosphate (cAMP) system in intestinal epithelial cells (see Chapter 9).

A second presumptive toxin has been isolated from a strain of *B. cereus* implicated in an outbreak of vomiting-type illness. Cell-free culture filtrates from that strain do not produce fluid accumulation in rabbit intestine, do not stimulate the adenyl cyclase–cAMP system, and only produce vomiting when fed to rhesus monkeys. This "vomiting toxin" is heat stable.

CLINICAL FEATURES

Food poisoning caused by *B. cereus* has two main clinical manifestations, diarrheal and emetic. The diarrheal form of the illness is characterized by a long incubation period, diarrhea (96%), abdominal cramps (75%), and vomiting (23%); fever is uncommon. The duration of disease ranges from 20 to 36 hours, with a median of 24 hours.

The predominant symptoms of the emetic form of the illness are vomiting (100%) and abdominal cramps (100%). Diarrhea is only present in one third of affected individuals. The duration of the illness ranges from 8 to 10 hours with a median of 9 hours. In both types of illness the disease is usually mild and self-limited. The vomiting syndrome must be differentiated from *S. aureus* food poisoning. As stated earlier, the association with fried rice is epidemiologically useful in differentiating the two organisms.

Food Poisoning Caused by Invasive Organisms

Salmonella Gastroenteritis

This case underscores the invasive potential of several bacteria associated with food poisoning. Although many organisms are invasive, the most common agents are species of *Salmonella* and *Campylobacter*. Relatively uncommon invasive bacteria are *Vibrio parahaemolyticus*, *Yersinia enterocolitica*, and a specific strain of *E.*

Case

Forty-eight hours after eating poorly cooked chicken, Mr. T. developed fever, shaking chills, abdominal cramps, and blood-tinged diarrhea. The illness lasted several days, and fever and diarrhea gradually abated. Sixty-five years old, Mr. T. had a silent abdominal arterial aneurysm. Unbeknownst to him or his physician, the organisms causing his febrile diarrheic episode seeded the bloodstream and invaded the aneurysm. Ten days after the initial episode Mr. T. developed more fever and chills, and his aneurysm expanded. Blood cultures were positive for *Salmonella typhimurium*. Surgery and antibiotics were required. Fortunately, Mr. T. survived.

■ ■ ■ ■

coli. Invasiveness is generally associated with the presence of neutrophils in the stool and systemic signs such as fever, chills, myalgias, and headache. These organisms are discussed in more detail in Chapters 16 and 17.

Vibrio parahaemolyticus

Like *V. cholera*, *V. parahaemolyticus* is often associated with contaminated shellfish. The organism tends to behave as one of the invasive pathogens, rather than as a toxin-producing pathogen such as *V. cholera*.

Yersinia enterocolitica

Y. enterocolitica is a Gram-negative rod that has recently been implicated as a cause of food poisoning. Contaminated milk has been one well-documented source. The type of infection caused by the organism is generally invasive, although a heat-stable enterotoxin has been described. Tissue invasion, frequently mimicking acute appendicitis, is common in *Y. enterocolitica* infection. At surgery the appendix of an infected patient may be normal, but the mesenteric lymph nodes surrounding the appendix will be markedly inflamed.

Escherichia coli

Although *E. coli* is part of the host's normal flora, some toxigenic and enteropathogenic strains are associated with food poisoning. Toxigenic *E. coli* occurs in about 50% of traveler's diarrhea (see Chapter 16). Travelers ingest the organisms in contaminated salads, raw fruits, and vegetables. This syndrome is usually associated with watery diarrhea; fever is less common. The organisms make both a heat-labile and heat-stable enterotoxin.

Another toxigenic strain of *E. coli* causes a syndrome of bloody diarrhea, generally without fever. The causative agent is a shiga toxin–producing strain of *E. coli* (serotype O157:H7). The mechanism of action of this toxin appears to be identical to that of *Shigella*, the agent of bacillary dysentery. A rare consequence of this illness in children is hemolytic–uremic syndrome, which can lead to severe kidney damage and hemolytic anemia and potentially death (see Chapter 17). The agent has been epidemiologically connected to poorly cooked hamburger or other poorly cooked beef products.

Listeria monocytogenes

Increasingly recognized as a foodborne pathogen, *Listeria monocytogenes* is a Gram-positive, motile rod that is relatively heat resistant; it withstands pasteurization of milk. The bacteria is widely distributed in nature and is found in the intestinal tracts of various animals and humans, as well as in sewage, soil, and water.

The syndromes usually associated with listeriosis include meningitis, bacteremia, or focal metastatic disease. Frequently, gastrointestinal symptoms such as diarrhea precede the bacteremic disease. The organism has a propensity to affect adults who are either immunosuppressed or pregnant. The evidence that listeriosis is foodborne is accumulating from investigations of several recent epidemics. Contaminated cole slaw and raw and pasteurized milk have been implicated as vehicles for epidemic listeriosis. The source of sporadic *Listeria* infection is less well understood.

Nonbacterial Forms of Food Poisoning

Several agents have gained attention as prominent causes of food poisoning in the past decade. Waterborne outbreaks of *Cryptosporidium parvum* have affected whole cities. In Milwaukee, Wisconsin, an estimated 350,000 cases of diarrhea resulted from contamination of the drinking water and other sources of potable water. Outbreaks of viral gastroenteritis have become very common, especially in crowded populations or those sharing common environmental conditions, such as cruise ships. Outbreaks of norovirus infections have had attack rates of more than 50% on some cruise ships, effectively requiring that the cruises be aborted, people brought to shore, and the ships decontaminated. However, the difficulty in eliminating the virus by cleaning and the very high attack rates in susceptible patients have made the norovirus a problematic organism. It is thought that food handlers excrete the virus and contaminate food during preparation. The incubation period is short and the attack rate quite high. Fortunately, patients recover after being ill with nausea, vomiting, and diarrhea for 24 to 72 hours.

TREATMENT

Because foodborne diseases are generally self-limited and, for the most part, toxin-mediated, **antibiotics play no major role** either in therapy or prophylaxis. Occasionally, individuals with diseases caused by the more invasive pathogens like *Salmonella*, *Shigella*, *Listeria*, or *Campylobacter* require antibiotic therapy. **Fluid replacement** is a major consideration in all foodborne illnesses.

CONTROL AND PREVENTION

The common theme that characterizes all foodborne illnesses is the improper handling of food before its consumption. A study of factors responsible for foodborne disease outbreaks in the United States over a 15-year period showed that inadequate refrigeration was the single most frequent factor (Table 76-3). Usually, other factors are also associated with a specific outbreak, such as advance preparation of food without adequate storage or improper reheating. To a lesser degree, contaminated equipment, cross-contamination, and poor personal hygiene of food preparation personnel contribute to outbreaks.

The ubiquity of *Salmonella* and *Campylobacter* species, *B. cereus*, and *C. perfringens* makes it mandatory that food be cooked properly and stored at low temperatures. Control of foodborne illnesses is based on the inhibition of bacterial growth, prevention of contamination after preparation, and destruction of potential pathogens with cooking. In general, foods should be heated to internal temperatures of 74°C, but lower temperatures for longer periods of time are also effective. (People should probably think twice before ordering steak tartare, sushi, or other uncooked or undercooked meat or fish.) Once cooked or processed, foods must be held at temperatures of 4.4°C or below.

Although those control measures are standard, many places where food preparation takes place do not abide by them. It is through diligent efforts of public health officials that reported outbreaks are investigated and food preparation techniques corrected. Therefore, recognition and reporting of foodborne illness becomes essential in the control of the problem. Education of the public, nurses, physicians, and eating establishment personnel is crucial to the control of foodborne illness. Carriage of most of the organisms considered in this chapter

table **76-3**	Factors That Contributed to Foodborne Disease Outbreaks in the United States

FACTOR	PERCENTAGE IMPLICATED[a]
Inadequate refrigeration	47
Food prepared too far in advance of service	21
Infected person with poor personal hygiene	21
Inadequate cooking	16
Inadequate holding temperature	16
Inadequate reheating	12
Contaminated raw ingredient	1
Cross-contamination	7
Dirty equipment	7

[a] Percentage values total more than 100% because more than one factor may contribute to one foodborne disease outbreak.

is not a problem, with the exception of staphylococci. Because staphylococcal carriage is necessary for the development of foodborne illness, food handlers must be educated to watch for boils and pustules.

Conclusion

Food poisoning caused by enterotoxins may occur after ingestion of preformed toxin in food or by production of toxin by organisms in the intestinal tract. Most cases of intoxication cause nausea, vomiting, or diarrhea; they do not typically cause fever. Some foodborne disease is associated with invasive intestinal pathogens such as *Salmonella* and *Listeria* species. These illnesses may present with gastrointestinal symptoms as well as inflammatory features, such as fever, and they may require treatment with antibiotics. Most foodborne illnesses occur because food is improperly handled and are preventable if food handlers are appropriately educated and observant of public health guidelines.

Index

Note: Page numbers followed by f indicate figures; those followed by t indicate tables.